PHARMACOEPIDEMIOLOGY
Fourth Edition

Edited by

BRIAN L. STRC

University of Pennsylvania, Philad

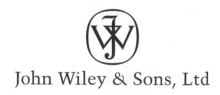

John Wiley & Sons, Ltd

Other Wiley Editorial Offices

John Wiley & Sons Inc., 111 River Street, Hoboken, NJ 07030, USA

Jossey-Bass, 989 Market Street, San Francisco, CA 94103-1741, USA

Wiley-VCH Verlag GmbH, Boschstr. 12, D-69469 Weinheim, Germany

John Wiley & Sons Australia Ltd, 33 Park Road, Milton, Queensland 4064, Australia

John Wiley & Sons (Asia) Pte Ltd, 2 Clementi Loop #02-01, Jin Xing Distripark, Singapore 129809

John Wiley & Sons Canada Ltd, 22 Worcester Road, Etobicoke, Ontario, Canada M9W 1L1

Wiley also publishes its books in a variety of electronic formats. Some content that appears in print
may not be available in electronic books.

Library of Congress Cataloging in Publication Data

Pharmacoepidemiology / edited by Brian L. Strom.—4th ed.
    p. ; cm.
  Includes bibliographical references and index.
  ISBN 0-470-86681-0 (alk. paper)
  1. Pharmacoepidemiology. 2. Pharmacology. I. Strom, Brian L.
  [DNLM: 1. Pharmacoepidemiology—methods. QZ 42 P536 2005]
  RM302.5.P53 2005
  615'.7042—dc22

                       2005047360

British Library Cataloguing in Publication Data

A catalogue record for this book is available from the British Library

ISBN-13 978-0-470-86681-8 (H/B)
ISBN-10 0-470-86681-0 (H/B)

Typeset in 9/11pt Times by Integra Software Services Pvt. Ltd, Pondicherry, India
Printed and bound in Great Britain by Antony Rowe Ltd, Chippenham, Wiltshire
This book is printed on acid-free paper responsibly manufactured from sustainable forestry
in which at least two trees are planted for each one used for paper production.

PHARMACOEPIDEMIOLOGY

Fourth Edition

Contents

Contributors

SYED RIZWANUDDIN AHMAD, MD, MPH Medical Epidemiologist, Division of Drug Risk Evaluation, Office of Drug Safety, FDA, CDER, 10903 New Hampshire Avenue, Silver Spring, MD 20993, USA, ahmads@cder.fda.gov

ELIZABETH B. ANDREWS, PhD, MPH RTI Health Solutions, 3040 Cornwallis Road, PO Box 12194, Research Triangle Park, NC 27709-2194, USA, eandrews@rti.org

PETER ARLETT, BSc, MBBS, MRCP, MFPM Principal Administrator, Pharmaceuticals Unit, European Commission, Honorary Senior Lecturer, Department of Medicine, University College London, 36 Fairbridge Road London, N19 3HZ, UK, peter.arlett@cec.eu.int

MARK I. AVIGAN, MD, CM Office of Drug Safety, Center for Drug Evaluation and Research, US Food and Drug Administration, 10903 New Hampshire Avenue, Silver Spring, MD 20993, USA, aviganm@cder.fda.gov

DAVID W. BATES, MD, MSc Chief, General Medicine Division, Professor of Medicine, Brigham and Women's Hospital, 1620 Tremont St., 3rd Fl, BC3-2M, Boston, MA 02120-1613, USA, and Medical Director, Clinical and Quality Analysis, Partners HealthCare System, Inc., dbates@partners.org

PATRICIA BECK, BSP, MSc Research Consultant, Research Services, Saskatchewan Health, 3475 Albert Street, Regina, Saskatchewan S4S 6X6, Canada, pbeck@health.gov.sk.ca

ULF BERGMAN, MD, PhD Professor, Division of Clinical Pharmacology, Karolinska Institutet, Karolinska University Hospital—Huddinge, SE-141 86 Stockholm, Sweden, Ulf.Bergman@karolinska.se

JESSE A. BERLIN, ScD Senior Director, Statistical Science, Johnson & Johnson Pharmaceutical Research and Development, LLC, 1125 Trenton-Harbourton Road, PO Box 200 (mail stop 67), Titusville, NJ 08560, USA, jberlin@prdus. jnj.com

JEAN-FRANÇOIS BOIVIN, MD, ScD Professor, Department of Epidemiology and Biostatistics, McGill University, 1020 Pine Avenue West, Montreal, Quebec H3A 1A2, Canada, jean-f.boivin@mcgill.ca

ROSELIE A. BRIGHT, ScD Epidemiologist, Center for Devices and Radiological Health, United States Food and Drug Administration, 1350 Piccard Drive, HFZ-541, Rockville, MD 20850, USA, rxb@cdrh.fda.gov

ROBERT M. CALIFF, MD Associate Vice Chancellor for Clinical Research, Director, Duke Clinical Research Institute, Professor of Medicine, Duke University Medical Center, 2400 Pratt Street, room 0311 Terrace Level, Durham, NC 27705, USA, califf001@mc.duke.edu

ARTHUR CAPLAN, PhD Robert and Emanuel Hart Professor of Bioethics, Director, Center for Bioethics, University of Pennsylvania, 3401 Market Street, Suite 320, Philadelphia, PA 19104-3308, USA, caplan@mail.med.upenn.edu

JEFFREY L. CARSON, MD Richard C. Reynolds Professor of Medicine, Chief, Division of General Internal Medicine, UMDNJ-Robert Wood Johnson Medical School, 125 Paterson Street, New Brunswick, New Jersey 08903, USA, carson@umdnj.edu

DAVID CASARETT, MD, MA Center for Health Equity Research and Promotion at the Philadelphia VAMC, Assistant Professor, Division of Geriatrics, University of Pennsylvania, 3615 Chestnut Street, Philadelphia, PA 19104, USA, casarett@mail.med.upenn.edu

K. ARNOLD CHAN, MD, ScD Associate Professor of Medicine, Harvard School of Public Health, 677 Huntington Avenue, Boston, MA 02115, USA, kachan@hsph.harvard.edu

ROBERT T. CHEN, MD, MA Immunization Safety Branch, National Immunization Program, Centers for Disease Control and Prevention, 1600 Clifton Road, NE, Atlanta, GA 30333, USA, bchen@cdc.gov

JEAN-PAUL COLLET, MD, PhD, MSc Professor, Department of Epidemiology and Biostatistics, McGill University, Director, Randomized Clinical Trial Unit, Jewish General Hospital, 3755 Cote-Ste-Catherine Road, Montreal, Quebec, H3T IE2, Canada, jean-paul.collet@gereq.net

PATRICIA F. COOGAN, ScD Associate Professor of Epidemiology, Slone Epidemiology Center, Boston University, 1010 Commonwealth Ave, 4th floor, Boston, MA 02215, USA, pcoogan@slone.bu.edu

ILONA CSIZMADI, PhD, MSc Postdoctoral Fellow, Division of Population Health and Information, Alberta Cancer Board, 1331-29 Street NW, Calgary, Alberta, T2N 4N2, Canada, ilona.csizmadi@cancerboard.ab.ca

HASSY DATTANI BSc, MRPharmS, MBA EPIC, Regeneration House, York Way, London N1 0UZ, UK, Hassy.Dattani@epic-uk.org

ROBERT L. DAVIS, MD, MPH Professor, Epidemiology and Pediatrics, University of Washington, Seattle, WA 98195, USA, rdavis@u.washington.edu

GRETCHEN S. DIECK, PhD Vice President, Risk Management Strategy, Pfizer, Inc., 235 East 42nd Street, New York, New York 10017, USA, gretchen.dieck@pfizer.com

WINANNE DOWNEY, BSP Manager, Research Services, Saskatchewan Health, 3475 Albert Street, Regina, Saskatchewan S4S 6H6, Canada, wdowney@health.gov.sk.ca

I. RALPH EDWARDS, MB, ChB Professor and Director, WHO Collaborating Centre for International Drug Monitoring, Uppsala Monitoring Centre, Stora Torget 3, S-753 20 Uppsala, Sweden, ralph.edwards@who-umc.org

GARY D. FRIEDMAN, MD, MS Adjunct Investigator (Former Director), Division of Research, Kaiser Permanente Medical Care Program of Northern California, 2000 Broadway, 3rd Floor, 031R16, Oakland, CA 94612-2304, and Consulting Professor, Stanford University School of Medicine, Department of Health Research and Policy, Redwood Building, Room T210, Stanford, CA 94305-5405, USA, Gary.Friedman@kp.org

JOEL M. GELFAND, MD, MSCE Medical Director, Clinical Studies Unit, Assistant Professor of Dermatology, Associate Scholar, Center for Clinical Epidemiology and Biostatistics, University of Pennsylvania, 3600 Spruce Street, 2 Maloney Building, Philadelphia, PA 19104, USA, joel.gelfand@uphs.upenn.edu

KATE GELPERIN, MD, MPH Office of Drug Safety, Center for Drug Evaluation and Research, US Food and Drug Administration, 10903 New Hampshire Avenue, Silver Spring, MD 20993, USA, GelperinK@cder.fda.gov

DALE B. GLASSER, PhD Medical Director, Sexual Health, Pfizer, Inc., 235 East 42nd Street, New York, New York 10017, USA, dale.glasser@pfizer.com

HENRY A. GLICK, PhD Assistant Professor of Medicine, Division of General Internal Medicine, University of Pennsylvania School of Medicine, 1211 Blockley Hall, 423 Guardian Drive, Philadelphia, PA 19104, USA, hlthsvrs@mail.med.upenn.edu

ROGER A. GOETSCH, RPh, PharmD Special Assistant for Regulatory Affairs, Electronic Submission Coordinator, Office of Drug Safety (HFD-430), 12300 Twinbrook Parkway, Suite 240, Rockville, Maryland 20851, USA, goetsch@cder.fda.gov

DAVID J. GRAHAM, MD, MPH Associate Director for Science and Medicine, Office of Drug Safety, Center for Drug Evaluation and Research, US Food and Drug Administration, 10903 New Hampshire Avenue, Silver Spring, MD 20993, USA, grahamd@cder.fda.gov

HARRY A. GUESS, MD, PhD Professor, Department of Epidemiology, School of Public Health CB#7435, The University of North Carolina at Chapel Hill, Chapel Hill, NC 27599-7435, USA, harry_guess@unc.edu

MARGARET J. GUNTER, PhD Vice President and Executive Director, Lovelace Clinic Foundation, Lovelace Health Systems, 2309 Renard Place SE, Suite 103-B, Albuquerque, New Mexico 87106, USA, maggie@lcfresearch.org

JERRY H. GURWITZ, MD Executive Director, Meyers Primary Care Institute, Fallon Foundation and University of Massachusetts Medical School, The Dr John Meyers Professor of Primary Care Medicine, University of Massachusetts Medical School, 630 Plantation Street, Worcester, MA 01605, USA, jgurwitz@meyersprimary.org

GORDON H. GUYATT, MD Professor, Clinical Epidemiology and Biostatistics/Department of Medicine, McMaster University, Hamilton, ON L8N 3Z5, Canada, guyatt@mcmaster.ca

SEAN HENNESSY, PharmD, MSCE, PhD Assistant Professor of Epidemiology and Pharmacology, Department of Biostatistics and Epidemiology, Center for Clinical

Epidemiology and Biostatistics, University of Pennsylvania School of Medicine, 803 Blockley Hall/423 Guardian Drive, Philadelphia, PA 19104-6021 USA, shenness@cceb.med.upenn.edu

DAVID A. HENRY, MB, ChB Professor, Discipline of Clinical Pharmacology, Faculty of Health, University of Newcastle, Newcastle Mater Hospital, Waratah, NSW 2298, Australia, david.henry@newcastle.edu.au

LISA J. HERRINTON, PhD Investigator, Division of Research, Kaiser Permanente Northern California, 2000 Broadway, Oakland, CA 94612, USA, Lisa.Herrinton@kp.org

SUZANNE HILL, BMed, PhD Associate Professor, Discipline of Clinical Pharmacology, Faculty of Health, University of Newcastle, Newcastle Mater Hospital, Waratah NSW 2298, Australia, Suzanne.Hill@newcastle.edu.au

BRUCE HUGMAN, BA, MA, Diploma in Education Communications Consultant to the Uppsala Monitoring Centre, Senior Academic Adviser, Naresuan University, Phayao Campus, Thailand, PO Box 246, Amphur Muang, Chiang Rai 57000, Thailand, mail@brucehugman.net

ROMAN JAESCHKE, MD, MSc Clinical Professor of Medicine, Department of Medicine, St Joseph's Hospital, 301 James Street S, Hamilton, Ontario L8N 3A6, Canada, jaeschke@mcmaster.ca

ERIC S. JOHNSON, PhD Senior Research Associate, Center for Health Research, Kaiser Permanente Northwest, 3800 N Interstate Ave, Portland, OR 97227-1110, USA, eric.johnson@kpchr.org

JUDITH K. JONES, MD, PhD President, The Degge Group, Ltd, Suite 1430, 1616 N Ft Myer Drive, Arlington, VA 22209-3109, USA, jkjones@deggegroup.com

JASON KARLAWISH, MD Assistant Professor of Medicine, Institute on Aging, Division of Geriatrics and Center for Bioethics, University of Pennsylvania School of Medicine, 3615 Chestnut Street, Philadelphia, PA 19104, USA, jasonkar@mail.med.upenn.edu

RAINU KAUSHAL, MD MPH Instructor in Medicine, Harvard Medical School, Division of General Internal Medicine, Brigham and Women's Hospital, 1620 Tremont St, Boston MA 02120, USA, rkaushal@partners.org

CARIN J. KIM, MS Graduate Student, Division of Biostatistics, Department of Biostatistics and Epidemiology, University of Pennsylvania School of Medicine, 501 Blockley Hall, 423 Guardian Drive, Philadelphia, PA 19104-6021, USA, cakim@cceb.upenn.edu

STEPHEN E. KIMMEL, MD, MSCE Associate Professor of Medicine and Epidemiology, Department of Medicine, Cardiovascular Division, Center for Clinical Epidemiology and Biostatistics, University of Pennsylvania School of Medicine, 717 Blockley Hall, 423 Guardian Drive, Philadelphia, PA 19104, USA, skimmel@cceb.med.upenn.edu

DAVID LEE, MD Deputy Director, Technical Strategy and Quality, Center for Pharmaceutical Management, Management Sciences for Health, Inc. 4301 N Fairfax Drive Suite 400, Arlington, VA 22203-1627, USA, dlee@msh.org

SAMUEL M. LESKO, MD, MPH Director of Research and Medical Director, Northeast Regional Cancer Institute, University of Scranton Campus, 334 Jefferson Avenue, Scranton, PA 18510, USA, leskos2@scranton.edu

HUBERT G. LEUFKENS, PhD Chair, Department of Pharmacoepidemiology and Pharmacotherapy, Utrecht Institute for Pharmaceutical Sciences (UIPS), PO Box 80082, 3508 TB, Utrecht, The Netherlands, H.G.M.Leufkens@pharm.uu.nl

MARIE LINDQUIST, MSc, PhD Head, Data Management and Research, General Manager, Uppsala Monitoring Centre, WHO Collaborating Centre for International Drug Monitoring, Uppsala Monitoring Centre, Stora Torget 3, S 753 20 Uppsala, Sweden, marie.lindquist@who-umc.org

HELENE LEVENS LIPTON, PhD Professor of Pharmacy and Health Policy, Department of Clinical Pharmacy, School of Pharmacy, Institute for Health Policy Studies, School of Medicine, University of California at San Francisco, 3333 California Street Suite 265, St Laurel Heights, San Francisco, CA 94143-0936, USA, lipton@itsa.ucsf.edu

THOMAS M. MacDONALD MD, MPH, PhD Professor of Clinical Pharmacology and Pharmacoepidemiology, Department of Clinical Pharmacology and Therapeutics, Division of Medicine and Therapeutics, University of Dundee, Ninewells Hospital and Medical School, Dundee, Scotland, UK DD2 5NN, t.m.macdonald@dundee.ac.uk

LEANNE K. MADRE, JD, MHA Program Director, CERTs Coordinating Center, Duke University Medical Center, PO Box 17969, Durham, NC 27715, USA, madre005@mc.duke.edu

SUMIT R. MAJUMDAR, MD, MPH Associate Professor, Division of General Internal Medicine, Department of Medicine, University of Alberta, Edmonton, Alberta T6G 2B7, Canada, me2.majumdar@ualberta.ca

DAVID J. MARGOLIS, MD, MSCE, PhD Associate Professor of Dermatology and Epidemiology, Center for

Clinical Epidemiology and Biostatistics, Room 815 Blockley Hall, 423 Guardian Drive, Philadelphia, PA 19104, USA, dmargoli@cceb.med.upenn.edu

NORMAN S. MARKS, MD, MHA Medical Director, MedWatch Program, US Food and Drug Administration, CDER/Office of Drug Safety/Division of Surveillance, Research and Communication Support, 10903 New Hampshire Avenue, Silver Spring, MD 20993, USA, marksn@cder.fda.gov

BENTSON H. McFARLAND, MD PhD Professor of Psychiatry, Public Health and Preventive Medicine, Oregon Health and Science University, Adjunct Investigator, Kaiser Permanente Center for Health Research, 3181 S.W. Sam Jackson Park Road, mail code CR-139, Portland, Oregon 97239, USA, mcfarlab@ohsu.edu

PATRICIA McGETTIGAN, MB, B Pharm, MD Senior Lecturer in Clinical Pharmacology, Discipline of Clinical Pharmacology, Faculty of Health, University of Newcastle, Newcastle Mater Hospital, Waratah, NSW 2298, Australia, Patricia.McGettigan@newcastle.edu.au

KENNETH L. MELMON (the late), MD Professor of Medicine and Molecular Pharmacology, Associate Dean of Post Graduate Medical Education, 341 Medical School Office Building, Stanford University School of Medicine, Stanford, CA 94305, USA

ALLEN A. MITCHELL, MD Director, Slone Epidemiology Center, Professor of Epidemiology and Pediatrics, Boston University Schools of Public Health & Medicine, 1010 Commonwealth Avenue, Boston, Massachusetts 02215, USA, amitchell@slone.bu.edu

JANE MOSELEY, MSc MFPM Team Leader, Pharmacoepidemiology Research Team, Medicines and Healthcare products Regulatory Agency (MHRA), Room 15-206, Market Towers, 1 Nine Elms Lane, London SW8 5NQ, UK, jane.moseley@mhra.gsi.gov.uk

ANDREW D. MOSHOLDER, MD, MPH Office of Drug Safety, Center for Drug Evaluation and Research, US Food and Drug Administration, 10903 New Hampshire Avenue, Silver Spring, MD 20993, USA, mosholdera@cder.fda.gov

WINNIE W. NELSON, PharmD, MS Research Associate, HealthPartners Research Foundation, 8100 34th Avenue S, PO Box 1524, Minneapolis, MN 55440, USA, Winnie.W.Nelson@healthpartners.com

JAMES L. NICHOL, B Admin Research Consultant, Research Services, Saskatchewan Health, 3475 Albert Street, Regina, Saskatchewan S4S 6X6, Canada, jnichol@health.gov.sk.ca

STEN OLSSON, MSc, Pharm Head of External Affairs, Uppsala Monitoring Centre, WHO Collaborating Centre for International Drug Monitoring, Uppsala Monitoring Centre, Stora Torget 3, S-753 20 Uppsala, Sweden, sten.olsson@who-umc.org

WILLIAM OSEI, MD, MPH Provincial Epidemiologist, Saskatchewan Health, 3475 Albert Street, Regina, Saskatchewan S4S 6X6, Canada, wosei@health.gov.sk.ca

JULIE R. PALMER, ScD Professor of Epidemiology, Boston University School of Public Health, Senior Epidemiologist, Slone Epidemiology Center at Boston University, 1010 Commonwealth Avenue, Boston, MA 02215, USA, jpalmer@slone.bu.edu

JOHN PARKINSON, PhD Client Services Director, Medicines Monitoring Unit, Division of Medicine and Therapeutics, University of Dundee, Ninewells Hospital & Medical School, Dundee, DD2 5NN, UK, jp@memo.dundee.ac.uk

RICHARD PLATT, MD, MSc Professor of Ambulatory Care and Prevention, Harvard Medical School and Harvard Pilgrim Health Care, 126 Brookline Ave, Suite 200, Boston, MA 02215, Richard_Platt@harvard.edu

DANIEL POLSKY, PhD Research Associate Professor of Medicine, Division of General Internal Medicine, University of Pennsylvania School of Medicine, 1212 Blockley Hall, 423 Guardian Drive, Philadelphia, PA 19104-6021, USA, polsky@mail.med.upenn.edu

CHARLES POOLE, MPH, ScD Associate Professor, Department of Epidemiology (CB 7435), University of North Carolina School of Public Health, Pittsboro Road, Chapel Hill, NC 27599-7435, USA, poolec@email.unc.edu

MARSHA A. RAEBEL, PharmD Research and Education Manager, Kaiser Permanente of Colorado, 2550 S Parker Road, Suite 300, Aurora, CO 80014, USA, Marsha.A.Raebel@kp.org

NIGEL S.B. RAWSON, MSc, PhD Pharmacoepidemiologist, GlaxoSmithKline, 2030 Bristol Circle, Oakville, ON, L6H 5V2, Canada, nigel.s.rawson@gsk.com

WAYNE A. RAY, PhD Professor and Director, Division of Pharmacoepidemiology, Vanderbilt University School of Medicine, A-1106 MCN, Nashville, TN 37232, USA, wayne.ray@vanderbilt.edu

TIMOTHY R. REBBECK, PhD Professor of Epidemiology, Center for Clinical Epidemiology and Biostatistics, University of Pennsylvania School of Medicine, 904 Blockley Hall, 423 Guardian Dr., Philadelphia, PA 19104, USA, trebbeck@cceb. med.upenn.edu

ROBERT F. REYNOLDS, ScD Director, Global Epidemiology, Pfizer, Inc., 235 East 42nd Street, New York, New York 10017, USA, robert.reynolds@pfizer.com

PHILIP H. RHODES PhD Immunization Safety Branch, National Immunization Program, Centers for Disease Control and Prevention, Atlanta, GA 30333, USA, prhodes@cdc.gov

ROBIN ROBERTS, MSc Professor Emeritus, Department of Clinical Epidemiology and Biostatistics, Faculty of Health Sciences, McMaster University, Hamilton, Ontario, Canada, robertsr@mcmaster.ca

DOUGLAS W. ROBLIN, PhD Investigator, Research Department, Kaiser Permanente Georgia, 3495 Piedmont Road, NE Bldg 9, Atlanta, Georgia 30305, USA, douglas.roblin@kp.org

LYNN ROSENBERG, ScD Associate Director, Slone Epidemiology Center, Boston University, 1010 Commonwealth Ave, 4th floor, Boston, MA 02215, USA, rosenberg@slone.bu.edu

KATHLEEN W. SAUNDERS, JD Analyst/Programmer, Center for Health Studies, Group Health Cooperative, 1730 Minor Ave, Suite 1600, Seattle, WA 98101, USA, saunders.k@ghc.org

RITA SCHINNAR, MPA Senior Research Analyst and Project Manager, Center for Clinical Epidemiology and Biostatistics, University of Pennsylvania School of Medicine, 807 Blockley Hall/423 Guardian Drive, Philadelphia, PA 19104-6021, USA, rschinna@cceb.med.upenn.edu

KEVIN A. SCHULMAN, MD Professor of Medicine, Director, Center for Clinical and Genetic Economics, Duke Clinical Research Institute, Duke University Medical Center, PO Box 17969, Durham, NC 27715 USA, schul012@onyx.dcri.duke.edu

HOLGER SCHÜNEMANN, MD, PhD Associate Professor of Medicine, Preventive Medicine, Clinical Epidemiology and Biostatistics, University at Buffalo, McMaster University (PT), Department of Medicine, ECMC-CC142, 462 Grider St, Buffalo, NY 14215, USA, hjs@buffalo.edu or schuneh@mcmaster.ca

JOE V. SELBY MD, MPH Director, Division of Research, Kaiser Permanente Northern California, 2000 Broadway, Oakland, CA 94612, USA, Joe.Selby@kp.org

PAUL J. SELIGMAN, MD, MPH Director, Office of Pharmacoepidemiology and Statistical Science, United States Food and Drug Administration, HFD-030, Room 15B-03, 5600 Fishers Lane, Rockville, MD 20857, USA, seligmanp@cder.fda.gov

SAAD A.W. SHAKIR, MB, ChB, LRCP & S, FRCP, FFPM, MRCGP Drug Safety Research Unit, Bursledon Hall, Blundell Lane, Southampton, SO31 1AA, UK, saad.shakir@dsru.org

DEBORAH SHATIN, PhD Senior Researcher, Center for Health Care Policy and Evaluation, UnitedHealthGroup, 12125 Technology Drive, Minneapolis, MN 55440-1459, USA, deborah_shatin@uhc.com

DAVID H. SMITH, RPh, PhD Investigator, Center for Health Research, Kaiser Permanente Northwest, 3800 N Interstate Ave, Portland, OR 97227, USA, david.h.smith@kpchr.org

STEPHEN B. SOUMERAI, ScD Professor of Ambulatory Care and Prevention, Harvard Medical School and Harvard Pilgrim Health Care, 133 Brookline Avenue, 6th floor, Boston, MA 02215, USA, ssoumerai@hms.harvard.edu

MARYROSE STANG, PhD Research Consultant, Research Services, Saskatchewan Health, 3475 Albert Street, Regina, Saskatchewan, S4S 6X6, Canada, mstang@health.gov.sk.ca

ANDY STERGACHIS, PhD, RPh Professor of Epidemiology and Adjunct Professor of Pharmacy, Interim Chair, Pathobiology, Northwest Center for Public Health Practice, School of Public Health & Community Medicine, University of Washington, 1107 NE 45th St, Ste 400, Box 354809, Seattle, WA 98105, USA stergach@u.washington.edu

BRIAN L. STROM, MD, MPH George S. Pepper Professor of Public Health and Preventive Medicine, Professor of Biostatistics and Epidemiology, Medicine, and Pharmacology, Chair, Department of Biostatistics and Epidemiology, Director, Center for Clinical Epidemiology and Biostatistics, Associate Vice Dean, University of Pennsylvania School of Medicine, Associate Vice President for Strategic Integration, University of Pennsylvania Health System, 824 Blockley Hall, 423 Guardian Drive, Philadelphia, PA 19104-6021, USA, bstrom@cceb.med.upenn.edu

SAMY SUISSA, PhD James McGill Professor of Epidemiology and Biostatistics, McGill University, Director, Division of Clinical Epidemiology, Royal Victoria Hospital, 687 Pine

Avenue West, R4 29, Montreal, Quebec H3A 1A1, Canada, samy.suissa@clinepi.mcgill.ca

ANNE TONKIN, BSc, BM, BS, PhD Associate Professor, Department of Clinical and Experimental Pharmacology, University of Adelaide, South Australia, Medical School North, Room N522, Adelaide SA 5005, Australia, anne.tonkin@adelaide.edu.au

JOHN URQUHART, MD 975 Hamilton Ave, Palo Alto, CA 94301, USA, urquhart@ix.netcom.com

LI WEI, MBChB MSc PhD Research Fellow, University of Dundee, Medicines Monitoring Unit, Health Information Centre, University of Dundee, MacKenzie Building, Kirsty Semple Way, Dundee, DD2 4BF, UK, l.wei@chs.dundee.ac.uk

SUZANNE L. WEST, MPH, PhD Associate Professor, Department of Epidemiology (CB 7435), University of North Carolina, School of Public Health, Pittsboro Road, Chapel Hill, NC 27599-7435, USA, Sue_West@med.unc.edu

Preface

The history of drug regulation in the United States is a history of political responses to epidemics of adverse drug reactions, each adverse reaction of sufficient public health importance to lead to political pressure for regulatory change.

The initial law, the Pure Food and Drug Act, was passed in 1906. It was a response to the excessive adulteration and misbranding of the foods and drugs available then. The 1938 Food, Drug, and Cosmetic Act was a reaction to an epidemic of renal failure resulting from a brand of elixir of sulfanilimide being dissolved in diethylene glycol. The 1962 Kefauver–Harris Amendments were a response to the infamous thalidomide disaster, in which children exposed to thalidomide *in utero* were born with phocomelia, that is with flippers instead of limbs. The resulting regulatory changes led, in part, to the accelerated development of the field of clinical pharmacology, the study of the effects of drugs in humans.

The 1970s, 1980s, and 1990s continued to see a series of accusations about major adverse events possibly associated with drugs. Those discussed in the first edition of this book included liver disease caused by benoxaprofen, subacute myelo-optic-neuropathy (SMON) caused by clioquinol, the oculomucocutaneous syndrome caused by practolol, acute flank pain and renal failure caused by suprofen, liver disease caused by ticrynafen, and anaphylactoid reactions caused by zomepirac. Added in the second edition were arrhythmias from astemizole, hypertension, seizures, and strokes from postpartum use of bromocriptine, deaths from fenoterol, suicidal ideation from fluoxetine, hypoglycemia from human insulin, birth defects from isotretinoin, cancer from depot-medroxyprogesterone, multiple illnesses from silicone breast implants, memory and other central nervous system disturbances from triazolam, arrhythmias from terfenadine, and hemolytic anemia and other adverse reactions from temafloxacin. Further added in the third edition were liver toxicity from amoxicillin-clavulanic acid, liver toxicity from bromfenac, cancer and myocardial infarction from calcium channel blockers, arrhythmias with cisapride interactions, primary pulmonary hypertension and cardiac valvular disease from dexfenfluramine and fenfluramine, gastrointestinal bleeding, postoperative bleeding, deaths, and many other adverse reactions associated with ketorolac, multiple drug interactions with mibefradil, thrombosis from newer oral contraceptives, myocardial infarction from sildenafil, seizures with tramadol, eosinophilia myalgia from tryptophan, anaphylactic reactions from vitamin K, and liver toxicity from troglitazone. New in this edition are ischemic colitis from alosetron, cardiac arrhythmias from astemizole, myocardial infarction from celecoxib, rhabdomyolysis from cerivastatin, cardiac arrhythmias from grepafloxin, myocardial infarction from naproxen, stroke from phenylpropanolamine, bronchospasm from rapacuronium, myocardial infarction and stroke from rofecoxib, and many others. Most of these resulted in drug withdrawals. Recently published data also suggest that adverse drug reactions could be as much as the fourth leading cause of death. These and other serious but uncommon drug effects have led to the development of new methods to study drug effects in large numbers of patients. Academic investigators, the pharmaceutical industry, regulatory agencies, and the legal community have turned for these methods to the field of epidemiology, the study of the distribution and determinants of disease in populations.

As this edition goes to press, in response to a series of accusations about myocardial infarctions and strokes caused by analgesics, each detected in long-term prevention trials rather than in normal use of the drugs, questions are being asked in the US about the roles of industry and the FDA in these events. New changes are expected in organization, regulation, and possibly legislation. Further, a new study by the Institute of Medicine of the US National Academy of Sciences is just being commissioned, to make recommendations about how our drug safety system should be designed, a study that will undoubtedly lead to additional modifications.

The joining of the fields of clinical pharmacology and epidemiology has resulted in the development of a new field: pharmacoepidemiology, the study of the use of and the effects of drugs in large numbers of people. Pharmacoepidemiology applies the methods of epidemiology to the content area of clinical pharmacology. This new field has become the science underlying postmarketing drug surveillance, studies of drug effects that are performed after a drug has been released to the market. In recent years, pharmacoepidemiology has expanded to include many other types of studies as well.

The field of pharmacoepidemiology has grown enormously since the publication of the first edition of this book. The International Society of Pharmacoepidemiology, an early idea when the first edition of this book was written, has grown into a major international scientific force, with over 800 members from 37 countries, an extremely successful and well-attended annual meeting, a large number of very active committees, and its own journal. At least four other journals have been founded as well (most of which have already disappeared), all competing to publish the work of this field, and a number of established journals have targeted pharmacoepidemiology manuscripts as desirable. As new scientific developments occur within mainstream epidemiology, they are rapidly adopted, applied, and advanced within our field as well. We have also become institutionalized as a subfield within the field of clinical pharmacology, with a vigorous Pharmacoepidemiology Section within the American Society for Clinical Pharmacology and Therapeutics, and with pharmacoepidemiology a required part of the Clinical Pharmacology board examination.

Most of the major international pharmaceutical companies have founded special units to organize and lead their efforts in pharmacoepidemiology, pharmacoeconomics, and quality-of-life studies. The continuing parade of drug safety crises continues to emphasize the need for the field, and some foresighted manufacturers have begun to perform "prophylactic" pharmacoepidemiology studies, in order to have data in hand and available when questions arise, rather than waiting to begin to collect data after a crisis has developed. Pharmacoepidemiologic data are now routinely used for regulatory decisions, and many governmental agencies have been developing and expanding their own pharmacoepidemiology programs. Risk management programs are now required by regulatory bodies with the marketing of new drugs, as a means of improving drugs' benefit/risk balance, and manufacturers are scrambling to respond. Requirements that a drug be proven to be cost-effective have been added to national, local, and insurance health care systems, either to justify reimbursement or even to justify drug availability. A number of schools of medicine, pharmacy, and public health have established research programs in pharmacoepidemiology, and a few of them have also established pharmacoepidemiology training programs in response to a desperate need for more pharmacoepidemiology manpower. Pharmacoepidemiologic research funding is now more plentiful, and even limited support for training is now available. An international foundation was formed, with one of its missions to support pharmacoepidemiology work, and then disbanded.

In the United States, drug utilization review programs are required, by law, of each of the 50 state Medicaid programs, and have been implemented as well in many managed care organizations. Now, years later, however, the utility of drug utilization review programs is being questioned. In addition, the Joint Commission on Accreditation of Health Care Organizations now requires that every hospital in the country have an adverse drug reaction monitoring program and a drug use evaluation program, turning every hospital into a mini-pharmacoepidemiology laboratory. As this book goes to press, the United States is planning the implementation of a new drug benefit as part of Medicare, that is, paying for drugs for those over age 65. This should generate an enormous new interest in this field, and potentially new data and new funding, as a major branch of the Federal Government becomes concerned about the costs of and effects of prescription drugs. Stimulated in part by the interests of the World Health Organization and the Rockefeller Foundation, there is even substantial interest in pharmacoepidemiology in the developing world. Yet, throughout the world, the increased concern by the public about privacy has made pharmacoepidemiologic research much more difficult.

In the first edition, my goal was to help introduce this new field to the scientific world. The explosion in interest in the field, the rapid scientific progress that has been made, and the unexpected sales of the first edition led to the second edition. The continued maturation of what used to be a new field, the marked increase in sales of the second edition over the first, and the many requests I had from people all over the world led me to organize the third edition. Since then, much in the field has changed, and so a new edition is in order. Most chapters in the new edition have been thoroughly revised. A number of new chapters have been added, along with many new authors. Overall, the book has continued to expand in size, although with some careful pruning of old chapters, the net growth has been kept to only four new chapters.

As in earlier editions, Part I of this book provides background information on what is included in the field of pharmacoepidemiology, a description of the study designs it uses, a description of its unique problem—the requirement for very large sample sizes—and a discussion about when one would want to perform a pharmacoepidemiology study. Also included is a chapter providing analogous basic principles of clinical pharmacology. Part II presents a series of discussions on the need for the field, the contributions it can make, and some of its problems, from the perspectives of academia, industry, and regulatory agencies. Part III describes the systems that have been developed to perform pharmacoepidemiology studies, and how each approaches the problem of gathering large sample sizes of study subjects in a cost-effective manner. This Part is now subdivided into two sections, one on *ad hoc* data sources, and one on automated data systems. A number of new data resources have been developed, others were discontinued, and some were discontinued and then revived. Part IV is new, and describes selected special opportunities for the application of pharmacoepidemiology to address major issues of importance. These are of particular interest as the field continues to turn its attention to questions beyond just those of adverse drug reactions. Part V presents state-of-the-art discussions of some particular methodologic issues that have arisen in the field. Finally, Part VI provides my personal speculations about the future of the field. My expectation is that Parts I, II, III, and VI of this book will be of greatest interest to the neophyte. In contrast, Parts III, IV, V, and VI should be of greatest interest to those with some background, who want a more in-depth view of the field.

This book is not intended as a textbook of adverse drug reactions, i.e. a compilation of drug-induced problems organized either by drug or by problem. Rather, it is intended to elucidate the methods of investigating adverse drug reactions, as well as other questions of drug effects. It is also not intended as a textbook of clinical pharmacology, organized by disease or by drug, or a textbook of epidemiology, but rather a text describing the overlap between the two fields.

It is my hope that this book can serve as both a useful introduction to pharmacoepidemiology and a reference source for the growing number of people interested in this field, in academia, in regulatory agencies, in industry, and in the law. It will also hopefully be useful as a text for the numerous courses now under way in this field. I have been excited by the rapid progress and growth that our field has seen, and delighted that this book has played a small role in assisting this. With this new edition, it will document the major changes the field has seen. In the process, my hope is that it can continue to serve to assist the field in its development.

Brian L. Strom, MD, MPH, 2005

Acknowledgments

There are many individuals and institutions to whom I owe thanks for their contributions to my efforts in preparing this book. Over the years, my pharmacoepidemiology work has been supported by cooperative agreement FD-U-000079 from the US Food and Drug Administration; NIH grants and contracts R01-HL 27433, R01-AM/HD 31865, 1-R01-AM32869, R01-HD24316, R01-HD21726, R01-HD20531, R01-HL39000, R01-HD 29201, R01-AG14601, NICHD CRE-91–3, PO1-CA77596, R01-CA45762, K08-DK02589, K08-MH01584, MO1-RR00040, K23-DK02897, K23-HL04243, K23-AG01056, and R01-CA45762; grants from the Agency for Healthcare Research and Quality for a Center for Education and Research on Therapeutics (U18-HS10399), a Center for Excellence in Patient Safety Research and Practice (P01-HS11530), and the CERTs Prescribing Safety Program (U18-HS11843); grants from the Joint Commission on Prescription Drug Use, the Asia Foundation, the Charles A. Dana Foundation, the Rockefeller Foundation, the Andrew W. Mellon Foundation, and the International Clinical Epidemiology Network, Inc.; and grants from Alza Corporation, Bayer Corporation, Berlex Laboratories, the Burroughs Wellcome Company, Ciba-Geigy Corporation, Health Information Designs, Inc., Hoechst-Roussel Pharmaceuticals, Hoffman-La Roche, Inc., Integrated Therapeutics, Inc., a subsidiary of Schering-Plough Corporation, International Formula Council, Marion Merrell Dow, Inc., McNeil Consumer Products, McNeil Pharmaceuticals, Mead Johnson Pharmaceuticals, Merck and Company, Novartis Pharmaceuticals Corp., Pfizer Pharmaceuticals, A.H. Robins Company, Rowell Laboratories, Sandoz Pharmaceuticals, Schering Corporation, Smith Kline and French Laboratories, Sterling Winthrop Inc., Syntex, Inc., the Upjohn Company, and Wyeth-Ayerst Research. In addition, generous support to our pharmacoepidemiology training program has been provided by Alza Corporation, Aventis Pharmaceuticals, Inc., Berlex Laboratories, Inc., Ciba-Geigy Corporation, Genentech, Inc., Hoechst-Marion-Roussel, Inc., Integrated Therapeutics Group, Inc., Johnson and Johnson, Merck and Company, Inc., McNeil Consumer Product Company, McNeil Consumer Healthcare, Novartis Pharmaceuticals Corporation, Pfizer, Inc., SmithKline Beecham Pharmaceuticals, Whitehall-Robins Healthcare, and Wyeth-Ayerst Research. While none of this support was specifically intended to support the development of this book, without this assistance, I would not have been able to support my career in pharmacoepidemiology. Finally, I would like to thank my publisher, John Wiley & Sons, Ltd, for their assistance and insights, both in support of this book, and in support of the field's journal, *Pharmacoepidemiology and Drug Safety*.

Jane Sinopoli-Sosa was her usual dedicated and hardworking self, assisting me in the myriad arrangements that the book required. Rita Schinnar reviewed virtually all of the chapters, editing them in detail and posing additional questions and issues for the authors to address. Finally, Anne Saint John provided superb help in preparing both the manuscripts for my chapters and the formatted versions of all of the other chapters.

I would like to thank my parents for the support and education that were critical to my being able to begin my career. I would also like to thank Paul D. Stolley, MD, MPH and the late Kenneth L. Melmon, MD, who unfortunately passed away since the third edition, for their direction, guidance, and inspiration in the formative years of my career. I would like to thank my trainees, from whom I learn at least as much as I teach. Last, but certainly not least, I would like to thank my family—Lani, Shayna, and Jordi—for accepting the time demands of the book, for tolerating my endless hours working at home on it, and for their ever present love and support.

Part I

INTRODUCTION

1

What is Pharmacoepidemiology?

BRIAN L. STROM

University of Pennsylvania School of Medicine, Philadelphia, Pennsylvania, USA.

A desire to take medicine is, perhaps, the great feature which distinguishes man from other animals.
Sir William Osler, 1891

In recent decades, modern medicine has been blessed with a pharmaceutical armamentarium that is much more powerful than what it had before. Although this has given health care providers the ability to provide better medical care for their patients, it has also resulted in the ability to do much greater harm. It has also generated an enormous number of product liability suits against pharmaceutical manufacturers, some appropriate and others inappropriate. In fact, the history of drug regulation parallels the history of major adverse drug reaction "disasters." Each change in pharmaceutical law was a political reaction to an epidemic of adverse drug reactions. Recent data indicate that 100 000 Americans die each year from adverse drug reactions (ADRs), and 1.5 million US hospitalizations each year result from ADRs; yet, 20–70% of ADRs may be preventable.[1] The harm that drugs can cause has also led to the development of the field of pharmacoepidemiology, which is the focus of this book. More recently, the field has expanded its focus to include many issues other than adverse reactions, as well.

To clarify what is, and what is not, included within the discipline of pharmacoepidemiology, this chapter will begin by defining pharmacoepidemiology, differentiating it from other related fields. The history of drug regulation will then be briefly and selectively reviewed, focusing on the US experience as an example, demonstrating how it has led to the development of this new field. Next, the current regulatory process for the approval of new drugs will be reviewed, in order to place the use of pharmacoepidemiology and postmarketing drug surveillance into proper perspective. Finally, the potential scientific and clinical contributions of pharmacoepidemiology will be discussed.

DEFINITION OF PHARMACOEPIDEMIOLOGY

Pharmacoepidemiology is the study of the use of and the effects of drugs in large numbers of people. The term pharmacoepidemiology obviously contains two components: "pharmaco" and "epidemiology." In order to better appreciate and understand what is and what is not included in this new field, it is useful to compare its scope to that of other related fields. The scope of pharmacoepidemiology will first be

compared to that of clinical pharmacology, and then to that
of epidemiology.

PHARMACOEPIDEMIOLOGY VERSUS CLINICAL PHARMACOLOGY

Pharmacology is the study of the effects of drugs. *Clinical pharmacology* is the study of the effects of drugs in humans (see also Chapter 4). Pharmacoepidemiology obviously can be considered, therefore, to fall within clinical pharmacology. In attempting to optimize the use of drugs, one central principle of clinical pharmacology is that therapy should be individualized, or tailored to the needs of the specific patient at hand. This individualization of therapy requires the determination of a risk/benefit ratio specific to the patient at hand. Doing so requires a prescriber to be aware of the potential beneficial and harmful effects of the drug in question and to know how elements of the patient's clinical status might modify the probability of a good therapeutic outcome. For example, consider a patient with a serious infection, serious liver impairment, and mild impairment of his or her renal function. In considering whether to use gentamicin to treat the infection, it is not sufficient to know that gentamicin has a small probability of causing renal disease. A good clinician should realize that a patient who has impaired liver function is at a greater risk of suffering from this adverse effect than one with normal liver function.[2] Pharmacoepidemiology can be useful in providing information about the beneficial and harmful effects of any drug, thus permitting a better assessment of the risk/benefit balance for the use of any particular drug in any particular patient.

Clinical pharmacology is traditionally divided into two basic areas: pharmacokinetics and pharmacodynamics. *Pharmacokinetics* is the study of the relationship between the dose administered of a drug and the serum or blood level achieved. It deals with drug absorption, distribution, metabolism, and excretion. *Pharmacodynamics* is the study of the relationship between drug level and drug effect. Together, these two fields allow one to predict the effect one might observe in a patient from administering a certain drug regimen. Pharmacoepidemiology encompasses elements of both of these fields, exploring the effects achieved by administering a drug regimen. It does not normally involve or require the measurement of drug levels. However, pharmacoepidemiology can be used to shed light on the pharmacokinetics of a drug, such as exploring whether aminophylline is more likely to cause nausea when administered to a patient simultaneously taking cimetidine. However, to date this is a relatively unusual application of the field.

Specifically, the field of pharmacoepidemiology has primarily concerned itself with the study of adverse drug effects. Adverse reactions have traditionally been separated into those which are the result of an exaggerated but otherwise usual pharmacological effect of the drug, sometimes called *Type A reactions*, versus those which are aberrant effects, so called *Type B reactions*.[3] Type A reactions tend to be common, dose-related, predictable, and less serious. They can usually be treated by simply reducing the dose of the drug. They tend to occur in individuals who have one of three characteristics. First, the individuals may have received more of a drug than is customarily required. Second, they may have received a conventional amount of the drug, but they may metabolize or excrete the drug unusually slowly, leading to drug levels that are too high. Third, they may have normal drug levels, but for some reason are overly sensitive to them.

In contrast, Type B reactions tend to be uncommon, not related to dose, unpredictable, and potentially more serious. They usually require cessation of the drug. They may be due to what are known as hypersensitivity reactions or immunologic reactions. Alternatively, Type B reactions may be some other idiosyncratic reaction to the drug, either due to some inherited susceptibility (e.g., glucose-6-phosphate dehydrogenase deficiency) or due to some other mechanism. Regardless, Type B reactions are the more difficult to predict or even detect, and represent the major focus of many pharmacoepidemiology studies of adverse drug reactions.

The usual approach to studying adverse drug reactions has been the collection of spontaneous reports of drug-related morbidity or mortality (see Chapters 9 and 10). However, determining causation in case reports of adverse reactions can be problematic (see Chapter 36), as can attempts to compare the effects of drugs in the same class. This has led academic investigators, industry, the FDA, and the legal community to turn to the field of epidemiology. Specifically, *studies of adverse effects* have been supplemented with *studies of adverse events*. In the former, investigators examine case reports of purported adverse drug reactions and attempt to make a subjective clinical judgment on an *individual* basis about whether the adverse outcome was actually caused by the antecedent drug exposure. In the latter, controlled studies are performed examining whether the adverse outcome under study occurs more often in an exposed *population* than in an unexposed population. This marriage of the fields of clinical pharmacology and epidemiology has resulted in the development of a new field: pharmacoepidemiology.

PHARMACOEPIDEMIOLOGY VERSUS EPIDEMIOLOGY

Epidemiology is the study of the distribution and determinants of diseases in populations (see Chapter 2). Since pharmacoepidemiology is the study of the use of and effects of drugs in large numbers of people, it obviously falls within epidemiology as well. Epidemiology is also traditionally subdivided into two basic areas. The field began as the study of infectious diseases in large populations, i.e., epidemics. More recently, it has also been concerned with the study of chronic diseases. The field of pharmacoepidemiology uses the techniques of chronic disease epidemiology to study the use of and the effects of drugs. Although application of the methods of pharmacoepidemiology can be useful in performing the clinical trials of drugs that are performed before marketing[4] (see Chapter 26), the major application of these principles is after drug marketing. This has primarily been in the context of postmarketing drug surveillance, although in recent years the interests of pharmacoepidemiologists have broadened considerably.

Thus, pharmacoepidemiology is a relatively new applied field, bridging between clinical pharmacology and epidemiology. From clinical pharmacology, pharmacoepidemiology borrows its focus of inquiry. From epidemiology, pharmacoepidemiology borrows its methods of inquiry. In other words, it applies the methods of epidemiology to the content area of clinical pharmacology. In the process, multiple special logistical approaches have been developed and multiple special methodologic issues have arisen. These are the primary foci of this book.

HISTORICAL BACKGROUND

The history of drug regulation in the US is similar to that in most developed countries, and reflects the growing involvement of governments in attempting to assure that only safe and effective drug products were available and that appropriate manufacturing and marketing practices were used. The initial US law, the Pure Food and Drug Act, was passed in 1906, in response to excessive adulteration and misbranding of the food and drugs available at that time. There were no restrictions on sales or requirements for proof of the efficacy or safety of marketed drugs. Rather, the law simply gave the Federal Government the power to remove from the market any product that was adulterated or misbranded. The burden of proof was on the Federal Government.

In 1937, over 100 people died from renal failure as a result of the marketing by the Massengill Company of elixir of sulfanilimide dissolved in diethylene glycol.[5] In response, the Food, Drug, and Cosmetic Act was passed in 1938. Preclinical toxicity testing was required for the first time. In addition, manufacturers were required to gather clinical data about drug safety and to submit these data to the FDA before drug marketing. The FDA had 60 days to object to marketing or else it would proceed. No proof of efficacy was required.

Little attention was paid to adverse drug reactions until the early 1950s, when it was discovered that chloramphenicol could cause aplastic anemia.[6] In 1952, the first textbook of adverse drug reactions was published.[7] In the same year, the AMA Council on Pharmacy and Chemistry established the first official registry of adverse drug effects, to collect cases of drug-induced blood dyscrasias.[8] In 1960, the FDA began to collect reports of adverse drug reactions and sponsored new hospital-based drug monitoring programs. The Johns Hopkins Hospital and the Boston Collaborative Drug Surveillance Program developed the use of in-hospital monitors to perform cohort studies to explore the short-term effects of drugs used in hospitals[9,10] (see Chapter 35). This approach was later to be transported to the University of Florida–Shands Teaching Hospital as well.[11]

In the winter of 1961, the world experienced the infamous "thalidomide disaster." Thalidomide was marketed as a mild hypnotic, and had no obvious advantage over other drugs in its class. Shortly after its marketing, a dramatic increase was seen in the frequency of a previously rare birth defect, phocomelia—the absence of limbs or parts of limbs, sometimes with the presence instead of flippers.[12] Epidemiologic studies established its cause to be *in utero* exposure to thalidomide. In the United Kingdom, this resulted in the establishment in 1968 of the Committee on Safety of Medicines. Later, the World Health Organization established a bureau to collect and collate information from this and other similar national drug monitoring organizations (see Chapter 10).

The US had never permitted the marketing of thalidomide and, so, was fortunately spared this epidemic. However, the thalidomide disaster was so dramatic that it resulted in regulatory change in the US as well. Specifically, in 1962 the Kefauver–Harris Amendments were passed. These amendments strengthened the requirements for proof of drug safety, requiring extensive preclinical pharmacological and toxicological testing before a drug could be tested in humans. The data from these studies were required to be submitted to the FDA in an Investigational New Drug Application (IND) before clinical studies could begin. Three explicit phases of clinical testing were defined, which are described in more detail below. In addition, a new requirement was added to the clinical testing, for "substantial evidence that the drug will have the effect it purports or is represented to have." "Substantial evidence" was defined as "adequate and well-controlled investigations, including clinical investigations." Functionally, this has generally been interpreted as requiring randomized clinical trials to document drug efficacy before marketing. This new procedure also delayed drug marketing until the FDA explicitly gave approval. With some modifications, these are the requirements still in place in the US today. In addition, the amendments required the review of all drugs approved between 1938 and 1962, to determine if they too were efficacious. The resulting Drug Efficacy Study Implementation (DESI) process, conducted by the National Academy of Sciences' National Research Council with support from a contract from the FDA, was not completed until relatively recently, and resulted in the removal from the US market of many ineffective drugs and drug combinations. The result of all these changes was a great prolongation of the approval process, with attendant increases in the cost of drug development, the so-called drug lag.[13] However, the drugs that are marketed are presumably much safer and more effective.

The mid-1960s also saw the publication of a series of drug utilization studies.[14-18] These studies provided the first descriptive information on how physicians use drugs, and began a series of investigations of the frequency and determinants of poor prescribing (see also Chapters 27–29).

With all of these developments, the 1960s can be thought to have marked the beginning of the field of pharmacoepidemiology.

Despite the more stringent process for drug regulation, the late 1960s, 1970s, 1980s, and especially the 1990s and 2000s have seen a series of major adverse drug reactions. Subacute myelo-optic-neuropathy (SMON) was found to be caused by clioquinol, a drug marketed in the early 1930s but not discovered to cause this severe neurological reaction until 1970.[19] In the 1970s, clear cell adenocarcinoma of the cervix and vagina and other genital malformations were found to be due to *in utero* exposure to diethylstilbestrol two decades earlier.[20] The mid-1970s saw the discovery of the oculomucocutaneous syndrome caused by practolol, five years after drug marketing.[21] In part in response to concerns about adverse drug effects, the early 1970s saw the development of the Drug Epidemiology Unit, now the Slone Epidemiology Center, which extended the hospital-based approach of the Boston Collaborative Drug Surveillance Program (Chapter 35) by collecting lifetime drug exposure histories from hospitalized patients and using these to perform hospital-based case–control studies[22] (see Chapter 11). The year 1976 saw the formation of the Joint Commission on Prescription Drug Use, an interdisciplinary committee of experts charged with reviewing the state of the art of pharmacoepidemiology at that time, as well as providing recommendations for the future.[23] The Computerized Online Medicaid Analysis and Surveillance System was first developed in 1977, using Medicaid billing data to perform pharmacoepidemiology studies[24] (see Chapter 18). The Drug Surveillance Research Unit, now called the Drug Safety Research Trust, was developed in the United Kingdom in 1980, with its innovative system of Prescription Event Monitoring[25] (see Chapter 12). Each of these represented major contributions to the field of pharmacoepidemiology. These and newer approaches are reviewed in Part III of this book.

In 1980, the drug ticrynafen was noted to cause deaths from liver disease.[26] In 1982, benoxaprofen was noted to do the same.[27] Subsequently the use of zomepirac, another nonsteroidal anti-inflammatory drug, was noted to be associated with an increased risk of anaphylactoid reactions.[28] Serious blood dyscrasias were linked to phenylbutazone.[29] Small intestinal perforations were noted to be caused by a particular slow release formulation of indomethacin.[30] Bendectin®, a combination product indicated to treat nausea and vomiting in pregnancy, was removed from the market because of litigation claiming it was a teratogen, despite the absence of valid scientific evidence to justify this claim[31] (see Chapter 32). Acute flank pain and reversible acute renal failure were noted to be caused by suprofen.[32] Isotretinoin was almost removed from the US market because of the birth defects it causes.[33,34] The eosinophilia–myalgia syndrome was linked to a particular brand of L-tryptophan.[35] Triazolam, thought by the Netherlands in 1979 to be subject to a disproportionate number of central nervous system side effects,[36] was discovered by the rest of the world to be problematic in the early 1990s.[37-39] Silicone breast implants, inserted by the millions in the US for cosmetic purposes, were accused of causing cancer, rheumatologic disease, and many other problems, and restricted from use except for breast reconstruction after mastectomy.[40] Human insulin was marketed as one of the first of the new biotechnology drugs, but soon thereafter was accused of causing a disproportionate amount of hypoglycemia.[41-45] Fluoxetine was marketed as a major new important and commercially successful psychiatric product, but then lost a large part of its market due to accusations about its association with suicidal ideation.[46,47] An epidemic of deaths from asthma in New Zealand was traced to fenoterol,[48-50] and later data suggested that similar, although smaller, risks might be present with other beta-agonist inhalers.[51] The possibility was raised of cancer from depot-medroxyprogesterone, resulting in initial refusal to allow its marketing for contraception in the US,[52] multiple studies,[53,54] and ultimate approval. Arrhythmias were linked to the use of the antihistamines terfenadine and astemizole.[55,56] Hypertension, seizures, and strokes were noted from postpartum use of bromocriptine.[57,58] Multiple different adverse reactions were linked to temafloxacin.[59] Other examples include liver toxicity from amoxicillin-clavulanic acid;[60] liver toxicity from bromfenac;[61,62] cancer, myocardial infarction, and gastrointestinal bleeding from calcium channel blockers;[63–71] arrhythmias with cisapride interactions;[72–75] primary pulmonary hypertension and cardiac valvular disease from dexfenfluramine and fenfluramine;[76–78] gastrointestinal bleeding, postoperative bleeding, deaths, and many other adverse reactions associated with ketorolac;[79–82] multiple drug interactions with mibefradil;[83] thrombosis from newer oral contraceptives;[84–87] myocardial infarction from sildenafil;[88] seizures with tramadol;[89,90] anaphylactic reactions from vitamin K;[91] liver toxicity from troglitazone;[92–95] and intussusception from rotavirus vaccine.[96]

Since the previous edition of this book, drug crises have occurred due to allegations of ischemic colitis from alosetron;[97] rhabdomyolysis from cerivastatin;[98] bronchospasm from rapacuronium;[99] torsade de pointes from ziprasidone;[100] hemorrhagic stroke from phenylpropanolamine;[101] arthralgia, myalgia, and neurologic conditions from Lyme vaccine;[102] multiple joint and other symptoms from anthrax vaccine;[103] myocarditis and myocardial infarction from smallpox vaccine;[104] and heart attack and stroke from rofecoxib.[105] Twenty-two different prescription drug products have been removed from the US market since 1980 alone—alosetron (2000), astemizole (1999), benoxaprofen (1982), bromfenac (1998), cerivastatin (2001), cisapride (2000), dexfenfluramine (1997), encainide (1991), fenfluramine (1998), flosequinan (1993), grepafloxin (1999), mibefradil (1998), nomifensine (1986), phenylpropanolamine (2000), rapacuronium (2001), rofecoxib (2004), suprofen (1987), terfenadine (1998), temafloxacin (1992), ticrynafen (1980), troglitazone (2000), and zomepirac (1983) (see Chapter 8).

The licensed vaccines against rotavirus[96] and Lyme[102] were also recently withdrawn because of safety concerns (see Chapter 30). Between 1990 and 2004, at least 13 non-cardiac drugs were subject to significant regulatory actions because of cardiac concerns,[106] including astemizole, cisapride, droperidol, grepafloxacin, halofantrine, pimozide, rofecoxib, sertindole, terfenadine, terodiline, thioridazine, vevacetylmethadol, and ziprasidone.

In some of these examples, the drug was never convincingly linked to the adverse reaction. However, many of these discoveries led to the removal of the drug involved from the market. Interestingly, however, this withdrawal was not necessarily performed in all of the different countries in which each drug was marketed. Most of these discoveries

have led to litigation, as well, and a few have even led to criminal charges against the pharmaceutical manufacturer and/or some of its employees.

Each of these was a serious but uncommon drug effect, and these and other serious but uncommon drug effects have led to an accelerated search for new methods to study drug effects in large numbers of patients. This led to a shift from adverse effect studies to adverse event studies.

The 1990s and especially the 2000s have seen another shift in the field, away from its exclusive emphasis on drug utilization and adverse reactions, to the inclusion of other interests as well, such as the use of pharmacoepidemiology to study beneficial drug effects, the application of health economics to the study of drug effects, quality-of-life studies, meta-analysis, etc. These new foci are discussed in more detail in Parts IV and V of this book.

Recent years have seen increasing use of these data resources and new methodologies, with continued and even growing concern about adverse reactions. The American Society for Clinical Pharmacology and Therapeutics issued, in 1990, a position paper on the use of purported postmarketing drug surveillance studies for promotional purposes,[107] and the International Society for Pharmacoepidemiology issued, in 1996, Guidelines for Good Epidemiology Practices for Drug, Device, and Vaccine Research in the United States, which was very recently updated.[108] In the late 1990s, pharmacoepidemiologic research has been increasingly hampered by concerns about patient confidentiality[109–113] (see also Chapter 38).

Organizationally, in the US, the Prescription Drug User Fee Act (PDUFA) of 1992 allowed the US FDA to charge manufacturers a fee for reviewing New Drug Applications. This provided additional resources to the FDA, and greatly accelerated the drug approval process. New rules in the US, and in multiple other countries, now permit direct-to-consumer advertising of prescription drugs. The result is a system where more than 330 new medications were approved by FDA in the 1990s. Each drug costs $300–500 million to develop; drug development cost the pharmaceutical industry a total of $24 billion in 1999 and $32 billion in 2002.[114]

Yet, funds from the PDUFA of 1992 were initially prohibited from being used for drug safety regulation. In 1998, whereas 1400 FDA employees worked with the drug approval process, only 52 monitored safety; the FDA spent only $2.4 million in extramural safety research. This has coincided with the growing numbers of drug crises cited above. With the passage of PDUFA III, however, this is markedly changing (see Chapter 8). As another measure of drug safety problems, the FDA's new MedWatch program of collecting spontaneous reports of adverse reactions (see Chapter 9) now issues monthly notifications of label changes, and as of mid-1999, 20–25 safety-related label changes are being made every month. According to a study by the US Government Accounting Office, 51% of approved drugs have serious adverse effects not detected before approval.[115] Further, there is recognition that the initial dose recommended for a newly marketed drug is often incorrect, and needs monitoring and modification after marketing.[116,117]

Recently, with the publication of the results from the Women's Health Initiative indicating that combination hormone replacement therapy causes an increased risk of myocardial infarction rather than a decreased risk,[118,119] there has been increased concern about reliance solely on nonexperimental methods to study drug safety after marketing,[120–123] and we are beginning to see the use of massive randomized clinical trials as part of postmarketing surveillance (see Chapter 39).

There is also increasing recognition that most of the risk from most drugs to most patients occurs from known reactions to old drugs. Yet, nearly all of the efforts by the FDA and other regulatory bodies are devoted to discovering rare unknown risks from new drugs. In response, there is growing concern, in Congress and among the US public at least, that perhaps the FDA is now approving drugs too *fast*.[124] There are also calls for the development of an independent drug safety board, analogous to the National Transportation Safety Board,[125,126] with a mission much wider than the FDA's regulatory mission, to complement the latter. For example, such a board could investigate drug safety crises such as those cited above, looking for ways to prevent them, and could deal with issues such as improper physician use of drugs, the need for training, and the development of new approaches to the field of pharmacoepidemiology.

As an attempt to address the kinds of questions which until now have not been addressed, the US Agency for Healthcare Research and Quality (AHRQ) has funded seven Centers for Education and Research on Therapeutics (CERTs).[127] Discussed more in Chapter 6, the CERTs program seeks to improve health care and patient safety. It has identified specific roles that include: (a) development and nurturing of public–private partnerships to facilitate research on therapeutics; (b) support and encouragement of research on therapeutics likely to get translated into policy or clinical practice; (c) development of educational modules and dissemination strategies to increase awareness of the benefits and risks of pharmaceuticals; and (d) creation of a national information resource on the safe and effective use of therapeutics. Activities include the conduct of research on therapeutics, specifically exploring new uses of drugs,

ways to improve the effective uses of drugs, and risks associated with new uses or combinations of drugs. The CERTs also develop educational modules and materials for disseminating the findings from their research, consistent with their overarching mission to become a national resource for people seeking information about medical products. The CERTs strive to seek public and private sector cooperation to facilitate these efforts.

Another new initiative closely related to pharmacoepidemiology is the Patient Safety movement. In the Institute of Medicine's report, *To Err is Human: Building a Safer Health System*, the authors note that: (a) "even apparently single events or errors are due most often to the convergence of multiple contributing factors," (b) "preventing errors and improving safety for patients requires a systems approach in order to modify the conditions that contribute to errors," and (c) "the problem is not bad people; the problem is that the system needs to be made safer."[128] In this framework, the concern is not about substandard or negligent care, but rather, is about errors made by even the best trained, brightest, and most competent professional health caregivers and/or patients. From this perspective, the important research questions ask about the conditions under which people make errors, the types of errors being made, and the types of systems that can be put into place to prevent errors altogether when possible. Errors that are not prevented must be identified and corrected efficiently and quickly, before they inflict harm. Turning specifically to medications, from 2.4% to 6.5% of hospitalized patients suffer adverse drug events (ADEs), prolonging hospital stays by 2 days, and increasing costs by $2000–2600 per patient.[129–132] Over 7000 US deaths were attributed to medication errors in 1993.[133] Indeed, a recent CERT paper called for a systematic review of the entire drug risk assessment process, perhaps as a study by the US Institute of Medicine.[134] As of the time this chapter goes to press, it appears that study will be initiated, at least in part in response to the circumstances surrounding the withdrawal of rofecoxib. Although these estimates have been disputed,[135–140] the overall importance of reducing these errors has not been questioned. In recognition of this problem, the AHRQ has launched a major new grant program of over 100 projects, with over $50 million/ year of funding. While only a portion of this is dedicated to medication errors, they are clearly a focus of interest and relevance to many. More information is provided in Chapter 34.

Finally, another major new initiative of close relevance to pharmacoepidemiology is risk management. There is increasing recognition that the risk/benefit balance of some drugs can only be considered acceptable with active management of their use, to maximize their efficacy and/or minimize their risk.

In response, there are many initiatives under way, ranging from new FDA requirements for risk management plans, to a new FDA Drug Safety and Risk Management Advisory Committee. More information is provided is Chapters 8 and 33.

THE CURRENT DRUG APPROVAL PROCESS

The current drug approval process in the US and most other developed countries includes preclinical animal testing followed by three phases of clinical testing. Phase I testing is usually conducted in just a few normal volunteers, and represents the initial trials of the drug in humans. Phase I trials are generally conducted by clinical pharmacologists, to determine the metabolism of the drug and a safe dosage range in humans, and to exclude any extremely common toxic reactions which are unique to humans.

Phase II testing is also generally conducted by clinical pharmacologists, on a small number of patients who have the target disease. Phase II testing is usually the first time patients are exposed to the drug. Exceptions are drugs that are so toxic that it would not normally be considered ethical to expose healthy individuals to them, like cytotoxic drugs. For these, patients are used for Phase I testing as well. The goals of Phase II testing are to obtain more information on the pharmacokinetics of the drug and on any relatively common adverse reactions, and to obtain initial information on the possible efficacy of the drug. Specifically, Phase II is used to determine the daily dosage and regimen to be tested more rigorously in Phase III.

Phase III testing is performed by clinician–investigators in a much larger number of patients, in order to rigorously evaluate a drug's efficacy and to provide more information on its toxicity. At least one of the Phase III studies needs to be a randomized clinical trial (see Chapter 2). To meet FDA standards, at least one of the randomized clinical trials usually needs to be conducted in the US. Generally between 500 and 3000 patients are exposed to a drug during Phase III, even if drug efficacy can be demonstrated with much smaller numbers, in order to be able to detect less common adverse reactions. For example, a study including 3000 patients would allow one to be 95% certain of detecting any adverse reactions that occur in at least one exposed patient out of 1000. At the other extreme, a total of 500 patients would allow one to be 95% certain of detecting any adverse reactions which occur in 6 or more patients out of every 1000 exposed. Adverse reactions which occur less commonly than these are less likely to be detected in these premarketing studies. The sample sizes needed to detect drug effects are discussed in more detail in Chapter 3.

POTENTIAL CONTRIBUTIONS OF PHARMACOEPIDEMIOLOGY

The potential contributions of pharmacoepidemiology are only beginning to be realized, as the field is new. However, some contributions are already apparent (see Table 1.1). In fact, since the early 1970s the FDA has required postmarketing research at the time of approval for about one third of drugs.[141] In this section we will first review the potential for pharmacoepidemiology studies to supplement the information available prior to marketing, and then review the new types of information obtainable from postmarketing pharmacoepidemiology studies but not obtainable prior to drug marketing. Finally, we will review the general, and probably most important, potential contributions such studies can make. In each case, the relevant information available from premarketing studies will be briefly examined first, to clarify how postmarketing studies can supplement this information.

SUPPLEMENTARY INFORMATION

Premarketing studies of drug effects are necessarily limited in size. After marketing, nonexperimental epidemiologic studies can be performed, evaluating the effects of drugs administered as part of ongoing medical care. These allow

Table 1.1. Potential contributions of pharmacoepidemiology

(A) Information which supplements the information available from premarketing studies—better quantitation of the incidence of known adverse and beneficial effects

    (a) Higher precision
    (b) In patients not studied prior to marketing, e.g., the elderly, children, in pregnant women
    (c) As modified by other drugs and other illnesses
    (d) Relative to other drugs used for the same indication

(B) New types of information not available from premarketing studies

    (1) Discovery of previously undetected adverse and beneficial effects

        (a) Uncommon effects
        (b) Delayed effects

    (2) Patterns of drug utilization
    (3) The effects of drug overdoses
    (4) The economic implications of drug use

(C) General contributions of pharmacoepidemiology

    (1) Reassurances about drug safety
    (2) Fulfillment of ethical and legal obligations

the cost-effective accumulation of much larger numbers of patients than those studied prior to marketing, resulting in a more precise measurement of the incidence of adverse and beneficial drug effects (see Chapter 3). For example, at the time of drug marketing, prazosin was known to cause a dose-dependent first dose syncope,[142,143] but the FDA requested the manufacturer to conduct a postmarketing surveillance study in the US to quantitate its incidence more precisely.[23] In recent years, there has even been an attempt, in selected special cases, to release selected critically important drugs more quickly, by taking advantage of the work that can be performed after marketing. Probably the best-known example was zidovudine.[144,145] As noted above, the increased sample size available after marketing also permits a more precise determination of the correct dose to be used.[116,117,146,147]

Premarketing studies also tend to be very artificial. Important subgroups of patients are not typically included in studies conducted before drug marketing, usually for ethical reasons. Examples include the elderly, children, and pregnant women. Studies of the effects of drugs in these populations generally must await studies conducted after drug marketing.[148]

Additionally, for reasons of statistical efficiency, premarketing clinical trials generally seek subjects who are as homogeneous as possible, in order to reduce unexplained variability in the outcome variables measured and increase the probability of detecting a difference between the study groups, if one truly exists. For these reasons, certain patients are often excluded, including those with other illnesses or those who are receiving other drugs. Postmarketing studies can explore how factors such as other illnesses and other drugs might modify the effects of the drugs, as well as looking at the effects of differences in drug regimen, compliance, etc.[149] For example, after marketing, the ophthalmic preparation of timolol was noted to cause many serious episodes of heart block and asthma, resulting in over ten deaths. These effects were not detected prior to marketing, as patients with underlying cardiovascular or respiratory disease were excluded from the premarketing studies.[150]

Finally, to obtain approval to market a drug, a manufacturer needs to evaluate its overall safety and efficacy, but does not need to evaluate its safety and efficacy relative to any other drugs available for the same indication. To the contrary, with the exception of illnesses that could not ethically be treated with placebos, such as serious infections and malignancies, it is generally considered preferable, or even mandatory, to have studies with placebo controls. There are a number of reasons for this preference. First, it is easier to show that a new drug is more effective than a placebo than

to show it is more effective than another effective drug. Second, one cannot actually prove that a new drug is as effective as a standard drug. A study showing a new drug is no worse than another effective drug does not provide assurance that it is better than a placebo; one simply could have failed to detect that it was in fact worse than the standard drug. One could require a demonstration that a new drug is more effective than another effective drug, but this is a standard that does not and should not have to be met. Yet, optimal medical care requires information on the effects of a drug relative to the alternatives available for the same indication. This information must often await studies conducted after drug marketing.

NEW TYPES OF INFORMATION NOT AVAILABLE FROM PREMARKETING STUDIES

As mentioned above, premarketing studies are necessarily limited in size. The additional sample size available in postmarketing studies permits the study of drug effects that may be uncommon, but important, such as drug-induced agranulocytosis.[151]

Premarketing studies are also necessarily limited in time; they must come to an end, or the drug could never be marketed! In contrast, postmarketing studies permit the study of delayed drug effects, such as the unusual clear cell adenocarcinoma of the vagina and cervix, which occurred two decades later in women exposed *in utero* to diethylstilbestrol.[20]

The patterns of physician prescribing and patient drug utilization often cannot be predicted prior to marketing, despite pharmaceutical manufacturers' best attempts to predict in planning for drug marketing. Studies of how a drug is actually being used, and determinants of changes in these usage patterns, can only be performed after drug marketing (see Chapters 27 and 28).

In most cases, premarketing studies are performed using selected patients who are closely observed. Rarely are there any significant overdoses in this population. Thus, the study of the effects of a drug when ingested in extremely high doses is rarely possible before drug marketing. Again, this must await postmarketing pharmacoepidemiology studies.[152]

Finally, it is only in the past decade or two that our society has become more sensitive to the costs of medical care, and the techniques of health economics have been applied to evaluate the cost implications of drug use.[153] It is clear that the exploration of the costs of drug use requires consideration of more than just the costs of the drugs themselves. The costs of a drug's adverse effects may be substantially higher than the cost of the drug itself, if these adverse effects result in additional medical care and possibly even hospitalizations.[154] Conversely, a drug's beneficial effects could reduce the need for medical care, resulting in savings that can be much larger than the cost of the drug itself. As with studies of drug utilization, the economic implications of drug use can be predicted prior to marketing, but can only be rigorously studied after marketing (see Chapter 41).

GENERAL CONTRIBUTIONS OF PHARMACOEPIDEMIOLOGY

Lastly, it is important to review the general contributions that can be made by pharmacoepidemiology. As an academic or a clinician, one is most interested in the new information about drug effects and drug costs that can be gained from pharmacoepidemiology. Certainly, these are the findings that receive the greatest public and political attention. However, often no new information is obtained, particularly about new adverse drug effects. This is not a disappointing outcome, but in fact, a very reassuring one, and this reassurance about drug safety is one of the most important contributions that can be made by pharmacoepidemiology studies. Related to this is the reassurance that the sponsor of the study, whether manufacturer or regulator, is fulfilling its organizational duty ethically and responsibly by looking for any undiscovered problems which may be there. In an era of product liability litigation, this is an important assurance. One cannot change whether a drug causes an adverse reaction, and the fact that it does will hopefully eventually become evident. What can be changed is the perception about whether a manufacturer did everything possible to detect it and, so, whether it was negligent in its behavior.

REFERENCES

1. Lazarou J, Pomeranz BH, Corey PN. Incidence of adverse drug reactions in hospitalized patients: a meta-analysis of prospective studies. *JAMA* 1998; **279**: 1200–5.
2. Moore RD, Smith CR, Lietman PS. Increased risk of renal dysfunction due to interaction of liver disease and aminoglycosides. *Am J Med* 1986; **80**: 1093–7.
3. Rawlins MD, Thompson JW. Pathogenesis of adverse drug reactions. In: Davies DM, ed., *Textbook of Adverse Drug Reactions*. Oxford: Oxford University Press, 1977; p 44.
4. Strom BL. Integrating pharmacoepidemiology into the design and conduct of clinical trials. *J Clin Res Drug Dev* 1988; **2**: 161–8.
5. Geiling EMK, Cannon PR. Pathogenic effects of elixir of sulfanilimide (diethylene glycol) poisoning. *JAMA* 1938; **111**: 919–26.
6. Wallerstein RO, Condit PK, Kasper CK, Brown JW, Morrison FR. Statewide study of chloramphenicol therapy and fatal aplastic anemia. *JAMA* 1969; **208**: 2045–50.
7. Meyler L. *Side Effects of Drugs*. Amsterdam: Elsevier, 1952.
8. Erslev AJ, Wintrobe MM. Detection and prevention of drug induced blood dyscrasias. *JAMA* 1962; **181**: 114–9.
9. Cluff LE, Thornton GF, Seidl LG. Studies on the epidemiology of adverse drug reactions. I. Methods of surveillance. *JAMA* 1964; **188**: 976–83.
10. Miller RR, Greenblatt DJ. *Drug Effects in Hospitalized Patients*. New York: John Wiley & Sons, 1976.
11. Caranasos GJ, Stewart RB, Cluff LE. Drug-induced illness leading to hospitalization. *JAMA* 1974; **228**: 713–7.
12. Lenz W. Malformations caused by drugs in pregnancy. *Am J Dis Child* 1966; **112**: 99–106.
13. Wardell WM. Therapeutic implications of the drug lag. *Clin Pharmacol Ther* 1974; **15**: 73–96.
14. Lee JAH, Draper PA, Weatherall M. Prescribing in three English towns. *Milbank Mem Fund Q* 1965; **43**: 285–90.
15. Muller C. Medical review of prescribing. *J Chronic Dis* 1965; **18**: 689–96.
16. Meade TW. Prescribing of chloramphenicol in general practice. *BMJ* 1967; **1**: 671–4.
17. Joyce CRB, Last JM, Weatherall M. Personal factors as a cause of differences in prescribing by general practitioners. *Br J Prev Soc Med* 1968; **22**: 170–7.
18. Muller C. Outpatient drug prescribing related to clinic utilization in four New York City hospitals. *Health Serv Res* 1968; **3**: 142–54.
19. Kono R. Trends and lessons of SMON research. In: Soda T, ed., *Drug-Induced Sufferings*. Princeton, NJ: Excerpta Medica, 1980; p. 11.
20. Herbst AL, Ulfelder H, Poskanzer DC. Adenocarcinoma of the vagina: association of maternal stilbestrol therapy with tumor appearance in young women. *N Engl J Med* 1971; **284**: 878–81.
21. Wright P. Untoward effects associated with practolol administration. Oculomucocutaneous syndrome. *BMJ* 1975; **1**: 595–8.
22. Slone D, Shapiro S, Miettinen OS. Case–control surveillance of serious illnesses attributable to ambulatory drug use. In: Colombo F, Shapiro S, Slone D, Tognoni G, eds, *Epidemiological Evaluation of Drugs*. Littleton, MA: PSG, 1977; pp. 59–82.
23. Joint Commission on Prescription Drug Use. *Final Report*. Washington, DC, 1980.
24. Strom BL, Carson JL, Morse ML, Leroy AA. The Computerized Online Medicaid Analysis and Surveillance System: a new resource for post-marketing drug surveillance. *Clin Pharmacol Ther* 1985; **38**: 359–64.
25. Inman WHW. Prescription Event Monitoring. *Acta Med Scand Suppl* 1984; **683**: 119–26.
26. Ticrynafen recalled. *FDA Drug Bull* 1980; **10**: 3–4.
27. Suspension of benoxaprofen (Opren). *BMJ* 1982; **285**: 519–20.
28. Strom BL, Carson JL, Morse ML, West SL, Soper KA. The effect of indication on hypersensitivity reactions associated with zomepirac sodium and other nonsteroidal antiinflammatory drugs. *Arthritis Rheum* 1987; **30**: 1142–8.

29. Inman WHW. Study of fatal bone marrow depression with special reference to phenylbutazone and oxyphenbutazone. *BMJ* 1977; **1**: 1500–5.

30. Committee on Safety of Medicines. *Osmosin (Controlled Release Indomethacin) Current Problems, no. 11*. London, 1983.

31. Barash CI, Lasagna L. The Bendectin saga: "Voluntary" discontinuation. *J Clin Res Drug Devel* 1987; **1**: 277–92.

32. Strom BL, West SL, Sim E, Carson JL. The epidemiology of the acute flank pain syndrome from suprofen. *Clin Pharmacol Ther* 1989; **46**: 693–9.

33. FDA ponders approaches to curbing adverse effects of drug used against cystic acne. *JAMA* 1988; **259**: 3225–30.

34. Stern RS. When a uniquely effective drug is teratogenic: the case of isotretinoin. *N Engl J Med* 1989; **320**: 1007–9.

35. Hertzman PA, Falk H, Kilbourne EM, Page S, Shulman LE. The eosinophilia–myalgia syndrome: the Los Alamos conference. *J Rheumatol* 1991; **18**: 867–73.

36. Meyboom RHB. The triazolam experience in 1979 in The Netherlands, a problem of signal generation and verification. In: Strom BL, Velo GP, eds, *Drug Epidemiology and Postmarketing Drug Surveillance*. New York: Plenum Press, 1992; pp. 159–67.

37. Triazolam's status in European Community. *Lancet* 1991; **338**: 1586–7.

38. Brahams D. Triazolam suspended. *Lancet* 1991; **338**: 938.

39. Triazolam hearing. *Lancet* 1992; **339**: 1291.

40. Randall T. Penile, testicular, other silicone implants soon will undergo FDA review (news). *JAMA* 1992; **267**: 2578–9.

41. Egger M, Smith GD, Imhoof H, Teuscher A. Risk of severe hypoglycaemia in insulin treated diabetic patients transferred to human insulin: a case control study. *BMJ* 1991; **303**: 617–21.

42. Egger M, Smith GD, Teuscher AU, Teuscher A. Influence of human insulin on symptoms and awareness of hypoglycaemia: a randomised double blind crossover trial. *BMJ* 1991; **303**: 622–6.

43. Colagiuri S, Miller JJ, Petocz P. Double-blind crossover comparison of human and porcine insulins in patients reporting lack of hypoglycaemia awareness. *Lancet* 1992; **339**: 1432–5.

44. Jick H, Hall GC, Dean AD, Jick SS, Derby LE. A comparison of the risk of hypoglycemia between users of human and animal insulins. 1. Experience in the United Kingdom. *Pharmacotherapy* 1990; **10**: 395–7.

45. Jick SS, Derby LE, Gross KM, Jick H. Hospitalizations because of hypoglycemia in users of animal and human insulins. 2. Experience in the United States. *Pharmacotherapy* 1990; **10**: 398–9.

46. Teicher MH, Glod C, Cole JO. Emergence of intense suicidal preoccupation during fluoxetine treatment. *Am J Psychiatry* 1990; **147**: 207–10.

47. Beasley CM, Dornseif BE, Bosomworth JC, Sayler ME, Rampey AH, Heiligenstein JH, *et al*. Fluoxetine and suicide: a meta-analysis of controlled trials of treatment for depression. *BMJ* 1991; **303**: 685–92.

48. Crane J, Pearce N, Flatt A, Burgess C, Jackson R, Kwong T, *et al*. Prescribed fenoterol and death from asthma in New Zealand, 1981–83: case–control study. *Lancet* 1989; **1**: 917–22.

49. Pearce N, Grainger J, Atkinson M, Crane J, Burgess C, Culling C, *et al*. Case–control study of prescribed fenoterol and death from asthma in New Zealand, 1977–81. *Thorax* 1990; **45**: 170–5.

50. Grainger J, Woodman K, Pearce N, Crane J, Burgess C, Keane A, *et al*. Prescribed fenoterol and death from asthma in New Zealand, 1981–7: a further case–control study. *Thorax* 1991; **46**: 105–11.

51. Spitzer WO, Suissa S, Ernst P, Horwitz RI, Habbick B, Cockcroft D, *et al*. The use of beta-agonists and the risk of death and near death from asthma. *N Engl J Med* 1992; **326**: 501–6.

52. Rosenfield A, Maine D, Rochat R, Shelton J, Hatcher RA. The Food and Drug Administration and medroxyprogesterone acetate. What are the issues? *JAMA* 1983; **249**: 2922–8.

53. WHO Collaborative Study of Neoplasia and Steroid Contraceptives. Breast cancer and depot-medroxyprogesterone acetate: a multinational study. *Lancet* 1991; **338**: 833–8.

54. WHO Collaborative Study of Neoplasia and Steroid Contraceptives. Depot-medroxyprogesterone acetate (DMPA) and risk of invasive squamous cell cervical cancer. *Contraception* 1992; **45**: 299–312.

55. Nightingale SL. From the Food and Drug Administration: warnings issued on nonsedating antihistamines terfenadine and astemizole. *JAMA* 1992; **268**: 705.

56. Ahmad SR. Antihistamines alert. *Lancet* 1992; **340**: 542.

57. Rothman KJ, Funch DP, Dreyer NA. Bromocriptine and puerperal seizures. *Epidemiology* 1990; **1**: 232–8.

58. Gross TP. Bromocriptine and puerperal seizures. *Epidemiology* 1991; **2**: 234–5.

59. Finch RG. The withdrawal of temafloxacin: are there implications for other quinolones? *Drug Saf* 1993; **8**: 9–11.

60. Nathani MG, Mutchnick MG, Tynes DJ, Ehrinpreis MN. An unusual case of amoxicillin/clavulanic acid-related hepatotoxicity. *Am J Gastroenterol* 1998; **93**: 1363–5.

61. Hunter EB, Johnston PE, Tanner G, Pinson CW, Awad JA. Bromfenac (Duract)-associated hepatic failure requiring liver transplantation. *Am J Gastroenterol* 1999; **94**: 2299–301.

62. Moses PL, Schroeder B, Alkhatib O, Ferrentino N, Suppan T, Lidofsky SD. Severe hepatotoxicity associated with bromfenac sodium. *Am J Gastroenterol* 1999; **94**: 1393–6.

63. Furberg CD, Psaty BM, Meyer JV. Nifedipine. Dose-related increase in mortality in patients with coronary heart disease. *Circulation* 1995; **92**: 1326–31.

64. Pahor M, Guralnik JM, Furberg CD, Carbonin P, Havlik R. Risk of gastrointestinal haemorrhage with calcium antagonists in hypertensive persons over 67 years old. *Lancet* 1996; **347**: 1061–5.

65. Pahor M, Guralnik JM, Ferrucci L, Corti MC, Salive ME, Cerhan JR, *et al*. Calcium-channel blockade and incidence of cancer in aged populations. *Lancet* 1996; **348**: 493–7.

66. Braun S, Boyko V, Behar S, Reicher-Reiss H, Shotan A, Schlesinger Z, *et al*. Calcium antagonists and mortality in patients with coronary artery disease: a cohort study of 11,575 patients. *J Am Coll Cardiol* 1996; **28**: 7–11.

67. Kostis JB, Lacy CR, Cosgrove NM, Wilson AC. Association of calcium channel blocker use with increased rate of acute

myocardial infarction in patients with left ventricular dysfunction. *Am Heart J* 1997; **133**: 550–7.

68. Jick H, Jick S, Derby LE, Vasilakis C, Myers MW, Meier CR. Calcium-channel blockers and risk of cancer. *Lancet* 1997; **349**: 525–8.

69. Fitzpatrick AL, Daling JR, Furberg CD, Kronmal RA, Weissfeld JL. Use of calcium channel blockers and breast carcinoma risk in postmenopausal women. *Cancer* 1997; **80**: 1438–47.

70. Rosenberg L, Rao RS, Palmer JR, Strom BL, Stolley PD, Zauber AG, *et al.* Calcium channel blockers and the risk of cancer. *JAMA* 1998; **279**: 1000–4.

71. Michels KB, Rosner BA, Walker AM, Stampfer MJ, Manson JE, Colditz GA, *et al.* Calcium channel blockers, cancer incidence, and cancer mortality in a cohort of U.S. women: the Nurses' Health Study. *Cancer* 1998; **83**: 2003–7.

72. Wysowski DK, Bacsanyi J. Cisapride and fatal arrhythmia. *N Engl J Med* 1996; **335**: 290–1.

73. Piquette RK. Torsade de pointes induced by cisapride/clarithromycin interaction. *Ann Pharmacother* 1999; **33**: 22–6.

74. Smalley W, Shatin D, Wysowski DK, Gurwitz J, Andrade SE, Goodman M, *et al.* Contraindicated use of cisapride: impact of food and drug administration regulatory action. *JAMA* 2000; **284**: 3036–9.

75. Weatherby LB, Walker AM, Fife D, Vervaet P, Klausner MA. Contraindicated medications dispensed with cisapride: temporal trends in relation to the sending of "Dear Doctor" letters. *Pharmacoepidemiol Drug Safety* 2001; **10**: 211–8.

76. Kramer MS, Lane DA. Aminorex, dexfenfluramine, and primary pulmonary hypertension. *J Clin Epidemiol* 1998; **51**: 361–4.

77. Connolly HM, Crary JL, McGoon MD, Hensrud DD, Edwards BS, Edwards WD, *et al.* Valvular heart disease associated with fenfluramine-phentermine. *N Engl J Med* 1997; **337**: 581–8.

78. Kimmel SE, Keane MG, Crary JL, Jones J, Kinman JL, Beare J, *et al.* Detailed examination of fenfluramine-phentermine users with valve abnormalities identified in Fargo, North Dakota. *Am J Cardiol* 1999; **84**: 304–8.

79. Strom BL, Berlin JA, Kinman JL, Spitz PW, Hennessy S, Feldman H, *et al.* Parenteral ketorolac and risk of gastrointestinal and operative site bleeding: a postmarketing surveillance study. *JAMA* 1996; **275**: 376–82.

80. Feldman HI, Kinman JL, Berlin JA, Hennessy S, Kimmel SE, Farrar J, *et al.* Parenteral ketorolac: the risk for acute renal failure. *Ann Intern Med* 1997; **126**: 193–9.

81. Hennessy S, Kinman JL, Berlin JA, Feldman HI, Carson JL, Kimmel SE, *et al.* Lack of hepatotoxic effects of parenteral ketorolac in the hospital setting. *Arch Intern Med* 1997; **157**: 2510–4.

82. Garcia Rodriguez LA, Cattaruzzi C, Troncon MG, Agostinis L. Risk of hospitalization for upper gastrointestinal tract bleeding associated with ketorolac, other nonsteroidal antiinflammatory drugs, calcium antagonists, and other antihypertensive drugs. *Arch Intern Med* 1998; **158**: 33–9.

83. Mullins ME, Horowitz BZ, Linden DH, Smith GW, Norton RL, Stump J. Life-threatening interaction of mibefradil and beta-blockers with dihydropyridine calcium channel blockers. *JAMA* 1998; **280**: 157–8.

84. Spitzer WO, Lewis MA, Heinemann LA, Thorogood M, MacRae KD. Third generation oral contraceptives and risk of venous thromboembolic disorders: an international case-control study. *BMJ* 1996; **312**: 83–8.

85. Jick H, Jick SS, Gurewich V, Myers MW, Vasilakis C. Risk of idiopathic cardiovascular death and nonfatal venous thromboembolism in women using oral contraceptives with differing progestagen components. *Lancet* 1995; **346**: 1589–93.

86. WHO Technical Report Series. *Cardiovascular Disease and Steroid Hormone Contraception.* Geneva, Switzerland: World Health Organization, 1998.

87. de Bruijn SF, Stam J, Vandenbroucke JP. Increased risk of cerebral venous sinus thrombosis with third-generation oral contraceptives. *Lancet* 1998; **351**: 1404.

88. Feenstra J, van Drie-Pierik RJ, Lacle CF, Stricker BH. Acute myocardial infarction associated with sildenafil. *Lancet* 1998; **352**: 957–8.

89. Kahn LH, Alderfer RJ, Graham DJ. Seizures reported with tramadol. *JAMA* 1997; **278**: 1661.

90. Jick H, Derby LE, Vasilakis C, Fife D. The risk of seizures associated with tramadol. *Pharmacotherapy* 1998; **18**: 607–11.

91. Pereira SP, Williams R. Adverse events associated with vitamin K$_1$: results of a worldwide postmarketing surveillance programme. *Pharmacoepidemiol Drug Saf* 1998; **7**: 173–82.

92. Misbin RI. Troglitazone-associated hepatic failure. *Ann Intern Med* 1999; **130**: 330.

93. Vella A, de Groen PC, Dinneen SF. Fatal hepatotoxicity associated with troglitazone. *Ann Intern Med* 1998; **129**: 1080.

94. Neuschwander-Tetri BA, Isley WL, Oki JC, Ramrakhiani S, Quiason SG, Phillips NJ, Brunt EM. Troglitazone-induced hepatic failure leading to liver transplantation. A case report. *Ann Intern Med* 1998; **129**: 38–41.

95. Gitlin N, Julie NL, Spurr CL, Lim KN, Juarbe HM. Two cases of severe clinical and histologic hepatotoxicity associated with troglitazone. *Ann Intern Med* 1998; **129**: 36–8.

96. Suspension of rotavirus vaccine after reports of intussusception—United States, 1999. *Morb Mortal Wkly Rep* 2004; **53**: 786–9.

97. Moynihan R. Alosetron: a case study in regulatory capture, or a victory for patients' rights? *BMJ* 2002; **325**: 592–5.

98. Thompson PD, Clarkson P, Karas RH. Statin-associated myopathy. *JAMA* 2003; **289**: 1681–90.

99. Schulman SR. Rapacuronium redux. *Anesth Analg* 2002; **94**: 483–4.

100. Kelly DL, Love RC. Ziprasidone and the QTc interval: pharmacokinetic and pharmacodynamic considerations. *Psychopharmacol Bull* 2001; **35**: 66–79.

101. Kernan WN, Viscoli CM, Brass LM, Broderick JP, Brott T, Feldmann E, *et al.* Phenylpropanolamine and the risk of hemorrhagic stroke. *N Engl J Med* 2000; **343**: 1826–32.

102. Lathrop SL, Ball R, Haber P, Mootrey GT, Braun MM, Shadomy SV, *et al.* Adverse event reports following vaccination for Lyme disease: December 1998–July 2000. *Vaccine* 2002; **20**: 1603–8.

103. Committee to Assess the Safety and Efficacy of the Anthrax Vaccine, Joellenbeck LM, Zwanziger LL, Durch JS, Strom BL, eds, *The Anthrax Vaccine: Is it Safe? Does it Work?* Washington, DC: National Academy Press, 2002.

104. Chen RT, Lane JM. Myocarditis: the unexpected return of smallpox vaccine adverse events. Lancet 2003; **362**: 1345–6.

105. Topol EJ. Failing the public health—rofecoxib, Merck, and the FDA. *N Engl J Med* 2004; **351**: 1707–9.

106. Shah RR. The significance of QT interval in drug development. *Br J Clin Pharmacol* 2002; **54**: 188–202.

107. Strom BL, Members of the ASCPT Pharmacoepidemiology Section. Position paper on the use of purported postmarketing drug surveillance studies for promotional purposes. *Clin Pharmacol Ther* 1990; **48**: 598.

108. International Society for Pharmacoepidemiology. Guidelines for good pharmacoepidemiology practices (GPP). http://www.pharmacoepi.org/resources/guidelines_08027.cfm

109. Neutel CI. Privacy issues in research using record linkage. *Pharmacoepidemiol Drug Saf* 1997; **6**: 367–9.

110. Melton LJ III. The threat to medical-records research. *N Engl J Med* 1997; **337**: 1466–70.

111. Mann RD. Data privacy and confidentiality. *Pharmacoepidemiol Drug Saf* 1999; **8**: 245.

112. Andrews EB. Data privacy, medical record confidentiality, and research in the interest of public health. *Pharmacoepidemiol Drug Saf* 1999; **8**: 247–60.

113. Mann RD. The issue of data privacy and confidentiality in Europe—1998. *Pharmacoepidemiol Drug Saf* 1999; **8**: 261–4.

114. Pharmaceutical Research and Manufacturers of America (PhRMA). *Pharmaceutical Industry Profile 2003*. Washington, DC: PhRMA, 2003; p. 75.

115. US General Accounting Office. *FDA Drug Review: Postapproval Risks 1976–85*. GAO/PEMD-90-15, April 1990; p. 24.

116. Cross J, Lee H, Westelinck A, Nelson J, Grudzinskas C, Peck C. Postmarketing drug dosage changes of 499 FDA-approved new molecular entities, 1980–1999. *Pharmacoepidemiol Drug Saf* 2002; **11**: 439–46.

117. Heerdink ER, Urquhart J, Hubert G, Leufkens HG. Changes in prescribed drug doses after market introduction. *Pharmacoepidemiol Drug Saf* 2002; **11**: 447–453.

118. Manson JE, Hsia J, Johnson KC, Rossouw JE, Assaf AR, Lasser NL, et al. Estrogen plus progestin and the risk of coronary heart disease. *N Engl J Med* 2003; **349**: 523–34.

119. Writing Group for the Women's Health Initiative Investigators. Risks and benefits of estrogen plus progestin in healthy postmenopausal women. Principal results from the Women's Health Initiative randomized controlled trial. *JAMA* 2002; **288**: 321–33.

120. Col NF, Pauker SG. The discrepancy between observational studies and randomized trials of menopausal hormone therapy: did expectations shape experience? *Ann Intern Med* 2003; **139**: 923–9.

121. Grimes DA, Lobo RA. Perspectives on the Women's Health Initiative trial of hormone replacement therapy. *Obstet Gynecol* 2002; **100**: 1344–53.

122. Whittemore AS, McGuire V. Observational studies and randomized trials of hormone replacement therapy: what can we learn from them? *Epidemiology* 2003; **14**: 8–9.

123. Piantadosi S. Larger lessons from the Women's Health Initiative. *Epidemiology* 2003; **14**: 6–7.

124. Kleinke JD, Gottlieb S. Is the FDA approving drugs too fast? Probably not—but drug recalls have sparked debate. *BMJ* 1998; **317**: 899.

125. Wood AJ, Stein CM, Woosley R. Making medicines safer—the need for an independent drug safety board. *N Engl J Med* 1998; **339**: 1851–4.

126. Moore TJ, Psaty BM, Furberg CD. Time to act on drug safety. *JAMA* 1998; **279**: 1571–3.

127. Califf RM. The need for a national infrastructure to improve the rational use of therapeutics. *Pharmacoepidemiol Drug Saf* 2002; **11**: 319–27.

128. Kohn LT, Corrigan JM, Donaldson MS, eds. *To Err Is Human. Building a Safer Health System*. Washington, DC: National Academy Press, 2000.

129. Bates DW, Cullen DJ, Laird N, Petersen LA, Small SD, Servi D, et al. Incidence of adverse drug events and potential adverse drug events: implications for prevention. *JAMA* 1995; **274**: 29–34.

130. Brennan TA, Leape LL, Laird NM, Hebert L, Localio AR, Lawthers AG, et al. Incidence of adverse events and negligence in hospitalized patients. Results of the Harvard Medical Practice Study I. *N Engl J Med* 1991; **324**: 370–6.

131. Classen DC, Pestotnik SL, Evans R, Scott R, Lloyd JF, Burke JP. Adverse drug events in hospitalized patients: excess length of stay, extra costs, and attributable mortality. *JAMA* 1997; **277**: 301–6.

132. Bates DW, Spell N, Cullen DJ, Burdick E, Laird N, Petersen LA, et al. The costs of adverse drug events in hospitalized patients. *JAMA* 1997; **277**: 307–11.

133. Phillips DP, Christenfeld N, Glynn LM. Increase in US medication-error deaths between 1983 and 1993. *Lancet* 1998; **351**: 643–4.

134. The Centers for Education and Research on Therapeutics (CERTs) Risk Assessment Workshop Participants. Risk assessment of drugs, biologics and therapeutic devices: present and future issues. Available from: http://www.interscience. wiley.com/.Accessed: April 8, 2002. D01:10, 1002/pds.699.

135. Manasse HR. Increase in US medication-error deaths (letter). *Lancet* 1998; **351**: 1655.

136. Ferner RE, Anton C. Increase in US medication-error deaths (letter). *Lancet* 1998; **351**: 1655–6.

137. Rooney C. Increase in US medication-error deaths (letter). *Lancet* 1998; **351**: 1656–7.

138. Phillips DP, Christenfeld N, Glynn LM. Increase in US medication-error deaths (letter). *Lancet* 1998; **351**: 1657.

139. McDonald CJ, Weiner M, Hui SL. Deaths due to medical errors are exaggerated in the Institute of Medicine report. *JAMA* 2000; **284**: 93–95.

140. Leape LL. Institute of Medicine error figures are not exaggerated. *JAMA* 2000; **284**: 95–7.

141. Mattison N, Richard BW. Postapproval research requested by the FDA at the time of NCE approval, 1970–1984. *Drug Inf J* 1987; **21**: 309–29.

142. Rosendorff C. Prazosin: severe side effects are dose-dependent. *BMJ* 1976; **2**: 508.

143. Graham RM, Thornell IR, Gain JM, Bagnoli C, Oates HF, Stokes GS. Prazosin: the first-dose phenomenon. *BMJ* 1976; **2**: 1293–4.

144. Kaitin KI. Case studies of expedited review: AZT and L-Dopa. *Law Med Health Care* 1991; **19**: 242–6.

145. Wastila LJ, Lasagna L. The history of zidovudine (AZT). *J Clin Res Pharmacoepidemiol* 1990; **4**: 25–37.

146. Peck CC. Postmarketing drug dosage changes. *Pharmacoepidemiol Drug Saf* 2003; **12**: 425–6.

147. Temple RJ. Defining dose decrease. *Pharmacoepidemiol Drug Saf* 2003; **12**: 151–2.

148. McKenzie MW, Marchall GL, Netzloff ML, Cluff LE. Adverse drug reactions leading to hospitalization in children. *J Pediatr* 1976; **89**: 487–90.

149. May FE, Stewart RB, Cluff LE. Drug interactions and multiple drug administration. *Clin Pharmacol Ther* 1977; **22**: 322–8.

150. Nelson WL, Fraunfelder FT, Sills JM, Arrowsmith JB, Kuritsky JN. Adverse respiratory and cardiovascular events attributed to timolol ophthalmic solution, 1978–1985. *Am J Ophthalmol* 1986; **102**: 606–11.

151. The International Agranulocytosis and Aplastic Anemia Study. Risks of agranulocytosis and aplastic anemia: a first report of their relation to drug use with special reference to analgesics. *JAMA* 1986; **256**: 1749–57.

152. Stewart RB, Forgnone M, May FE, Forbes J, Cluff LE. Epidemiology of acute drug intoxications: patient characteristics, drugs, and medical complications. *Clin Toxicol* 1974; **7**: 513–30.

153. Eisenberg JM. New drugs and clinical economics: analysis of cost-effectiveness analysis in the assessment of pharmaceutical innovations. *Rev Infect Dis* 1984; **6** (suppl 4): 905–8.

154. Morse ML, Leroy AA, Gaylord TA, Kellenberger T. Reducing drug therapy-induced hospitalization: impact of drug utilization review. *Drug Inf J* 1982; **16**: 199–202.

2

Study Designs Available for Pharmacoepidemiology Studies

BRIAN L. STROM

University of Pennsylvania School of Medicine, Philadelphia, Pennsylvania, USA.

Pharmacoepidemiology applies the methods of epidemiology to the content area of clinical pharmacology. Therefore, in order to understand the approaches and methodologic issues specific to the field of pharmacoepidemiology, the basic principles of the field of epidemiology must be understood. To this end, this chapter will begin with an overview of the scientific method, in general. This will be followed by a discussion of the different types of errors one can make in designing a study. Next the chapter will review the "Criteria for the causal nature of an association," which is how one can decide whether an association demonstrated in a particular study is, in fact, a causal association. Finally, the specific study designs available for epidemiologic studies, or in fact for any clinical studies, will be reviewed. The next chapter discusses a specific methodologic issue which needs to be addressed in any study, but which is of particular importance for pharmacoepidemiology studies: the issue of sample size. These two chapters are intended to be an introduction to the field of epidemiology for the neophyte. More information on these principles can be obtained from any textbook of epidemiology or clinical epidemiology.[1–23]

Finally, Chapter 4 will review basic principles of clinical pharmacology, the content area of pharmacoepidemiology, in a similar manner.

OVERVIEW OF THE SCIENTIFIC METHOD

The scientific method is a three-stage process (see Figure 2.1). In the first stage, one selects a group of subjects for study. Second, one uses the information obtained in this sample of study subjects to generalize and draw a conclusion about a population in general. This conclusion is referred to as an association. Third, one generalizes again, drawing a conclusion about scientific theory or causation. Each will be discussed in turn.

Any given study is performed on a selection of individuals, who represent the *study subjects*. These study subjects should theoretically represent a random sample of some defined population. For example, one might perform a randomized clinical trial of the efficacy of enalapril in lowering blood pressure, randomly allocating a total of

Pharmacoepidemiology, Fourth Edition   Edited by B.L. Strom
© 2005 John Wiley & Sons, Ltd

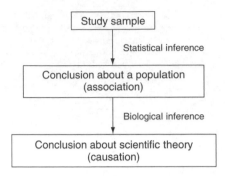

Figure 2.1. Overview of the scientific method.

40 middle-aged hypertensive men to receive either enalapril or placebo and observing their blood pressure six weeks later. One might expect to see the blood pressure of the 20 men treated with the active drug decrease more than the blood pressure of the 20 men treated with a placebo. In this example, the 40 study subjects would represent the study sample, theoretically a random sample of middle-aged hypertensive men. In reality, the study sample is almost never a true random sample of the underlying target population, because it is logistically impossible to identify every individual who belongs in the target population and then randomly choose from among them. However, the study sample is usually treated as if it were a random sample of the target population.

At this point, one would be tempted to make a generalization that enalapril lowers blood pressure in middle-aged hypertensive men. However, one must explore whether this observation could have occurred simply by chance, i.e., due to random variation. If the observed outcome in the study was simply a chance occurrence then the same observation might not have been seen if one had chosen a different sample of 40 study subjects. Perhaps more importantly, it might not exist if one were able to study the entire theoretical population of all middle-aged hypertensive men. In order to evaluate this possibility, one can perform a statistical test, which allows an investigator to quantitate the probability that the observed outcome in this study (i.e., the difference seen between the two study groups) could have happened simply by chance. There are explicit rules and procedures for how one should properly make this determination: the science of statistics. If the results of any study under consideration demonstrate a "statistically significant difference," then one is said to have an *association*. The process of assessing whether random variation could have led to a study's findings is referred to as *statistical inference*, and represents the major role for statistical testing in the scientific method.

If there is no statistically significant difference, then the process in Figure 2.1 stops. If there is an association, then one is tempted to generalize the results of the study even further, to state that enalapril is an antihypertensive drug, in general. This is referred to as *scientific or biological inference*, and the result is a conclusion about *causation*, that the drug really does lower blood pressure in a population of treated patients. To draw this type of conclusion, however, requires one to generalize to populations other than that included in the study, including types of people who were not represented in the study sample, such as women, children, and the elderly. Although it may be obvious in this example that this is in fact appropriate, that may well not always be the case. Unlike statistical inference, there are no precise quantitative rules for biological inference. Rather, one needs to examine the data at hand in light of all other relevant data in the rest of the scientific literature, and make a subjective judgment. To assist in making that judgment, however, one can use the "Criteria for the causal nature of an association," described below. First, however, we will place causal associations into a proper perspective, by describing the different types of errors that can be made in performing a study and the different types of associations that each results in.

TYPES OF ERRORS THAT ONE CAN MAKE IN PERFORMING A STUDY

There are four basic types of associations that can be observed in a study (Table 2.1). The basic purpose of research is to differentiate among them.

First, of course, one could have no association.

Second, one could have an *artifactual association*, i.e., a spurious or false association. This can occur by either of two mechanisms: chance or bias. Chance is unsystematic, or random, variation. The purpose of statistical testing in science is to evaluate this, estimating the probability that the result observed in a study could have happened purely by chance.

Table 2.1. Types of association between factors under study

(1) None (independent)
(2) Artifactual (spurious or false)

    (a) Chance (unsystematic variation)
    (b) Bias (systematic variation)

(3) Indirect (confounded)
(4) Causal (direct or true)

The other possible mechanism for creating an artifactual association is bias. Epidemiologists' use of the term bias is different from that of the lay public. To an epidemiologist, *bias* is systematic variation, a consistent manner in which two study groups are treated or evaluated differently. This consistent difference can create an apparent association where one actually does not exist. Of course, it also can mask a true association.

There are many different types of potential biases.[24] For example, consider an interview study in which the research assistant is aware of the investigator's hypothesis. Attempting to please the boss, the research assistant might probe more carefully during interviews with one study group than during interviews with the other. This difference in how carefully the interviewer probes could create an apparent but false association, which is referred to as interviewer bias. Another example would be a study of drug-induced birth defects that compares children with birth defects to children without birth defects. A mother of a child with a birth defect, when interviewed about any drugs she took during her pregnancy, may be likely to remember drug ingestion during pregnancy with greater accuracy than a mother of a healthy child, because of the unfortunate experience she has undergone. The improved recall in the mothers of the children with birth defects may result in false apparent associations between drug exposure and birth defects. This systematic difference in recall is referred to as recall bias.[25]

Note that biases, once present, cannot be corrected. They represent errors in the study design that can result in incorrect results in the study. It is important to note that *a statistically significant result is no protection against a bias*; one can have a very precise measurement of an incorrect answer! The only protection against biases is proper study design. (See Chapter 47 for more discussion about biases in pharmacoepidemiology studies.)

Third, one can have an indirect, or confounded, association. A *confounding variable*, or *confounder*, is a variable other than the risk factor and outcome under study which is related independently to both the risk factor and the outcome variable and which may create an apparent association or mask a real one. For example, a study of risk factors for lung cancer could find a very strong association between having yellow fingertips and developing lung cancer. This is obviously not a causal association, but an indirect association, confounded by cigarette smoking. Specifically, cigarette smoking causes both yellow fingertips and lung cancer. Although this example is transparent, most examples of confounding are not. In designing a study, one must consider every variable that can be associated with the risk factor under study or the outcome variable under study, in

Table 2.2. Approaches to controlling confounding

(1) Random allocation
(2) Subject selection

    (a) Exclusion
    (b) Matching

(3) Data analysis

    (a) Stratification
    (b) Mathematical modeling

order to plan to deal with it as a potential confounding variable. Preferably, one will be able to specifically control for the variable, using one of the techniques listed in Table 2.2. (See Chapters 40 and 47 for more discussion about confounding in pharmacoepidemiology studies.)

Fourth, and finally, there are true, causal associations.

Thus, there are three possible types of errors that can be produced in a study: random error, bias, and confounding. The probability of random error can be quantitated using statistics. Bias needs to be prevented by designing the study properly. Confounding can be controlled either in the design of the study or in its analysis. If all three types of errors can be excluded, then one is left with a true, causal association.

CRITERIA FOR THE CAUSAL NATURE OF AN ASSOCIATION

The "Criteria for the causal nature of an association" were first put forth by Sir Austin Bradford Hill,[26] but have been described in various forms since, each with some modification. Probably the best known description of them was in the first Surgeon General's Report on Smoking and Health,[27] published in 1964. These criteria are presented in Table 2.3, in no particular order. No one of them is absolutely necessary for an association to be a causal association. Analogously, no

Table 2.3. Criteria for the causal nature of an association

(1) Coherence with existing information (biological plausibility)
(2) Consistency of the association
(3) Time sequence
(4) Specificity of the association
(5) Strength of the association

    (a) Quantitative strength
    (b) Dose–response relationship
    (c) Study design

one of them is sufficient for an association to be considered a causal association. Essentially, the more criteria that are present, the more likely it is that an association is a causal association. The fewer criteria that are met, the less likely it is that an association is a causal association. Each will be discussed in turn.

The first criterion listed in Table 2.3 is *coherence with existing information* or *biological plausibility*. This refers to whether the association makes sense, in light of other types of information available in the literature. These other types of information could include data from other human studies, data from studies of other related questions, data from animal studies, or data from *in vitro* studies, as well as scientific or pathophysiologic theory. To use the example provided above, it clearly was not biologically plausible that yellow fingertips could cause lung cancer, and this provided the clue that confounding was present. Using the example of the association between cigarettes and lung cancer, cigarette smoke is a known carcinogen, based on animal data. In humans, it is known to cause cancers of the head and neck, the pancreas, and the bladder. Cigarette smoke also goes down into the lungs, directly exposing the tissues in question. Thus, it certainly is biologically plausible that cigarettes could *cause* lung cancer.[28] It is much more reassuring if an association found in a particular study makes sense, based on previously available information, and this makes one more comfortable that it might be a causal association. Clearly, however, one could not require that this criterion always be met, or one would never have a major breakthrough in science.

The second criterion listed in Table 2.3 is the *consistency of the association*. A hallmark of science is reproducibility: if a finding is real, one should be able to reproduce it in a different setting. This could include different geographic settings, different study designs, different populations, etc. For example, in the case of cigarettes and lung cancer, the association has now been reproduced in many different studies, in different geographic locations, using different study designs.[29] The need for reproducibility is such that one should never believe a finding reported only once: there may have been an error committed in the study, which is not apparent to either the investigator or the reader.

The third criterion listed is that of *time sequence*— a cause must precede an effect. Although this may seem obvious, there are study designs from which this cannot be determined. For example, if one were to perform a survey in a classroom of 200 medical students, asking each if he or she were currently taking diazepam and also whether he or she were anxious, one would find a strong association between the use of diazepam and anxiety, but this does not mean that diazepam causes anxiety! Although this is obvious, as it is not a biologically plausible interpretation, one cannot differentiate from this type of cross-sectional study which variable came first and which came second. In the example of cigarettes and lung cancer, obviously the cigarette smoking usually precedes the lung cancer, as a patient would not survive long enough to smoke much if the opposite were the case.

The fourth criterion listed in Table 2.3 is *specificity*. This refers to the question of whether the cause ever occurs without the presumed effect and whether the effect ever occurs without the presumed cause. This criterion is almost never met in biology, with the occasional exception of infectious diseases. Measles never occurs without the measles virus, but even in this example, not everyone who becomes infected with the measles virus develops clinical measles. Certainly, not everyone who smokes develops lung cancer, and not everyone who develops lung cancer was a smoker. This is one of the major points the tobacco industry stresses when it attempts to make the claim that cigarette smoking has not been proven to cause lung cancer. Some authors even omit this as a criterion, as it is so rarely met. When it is met, however, it provides extremely strong support for a conclusion that an association is causal.

The fifth criterion listed in Table 2.3 is the *strength of the association*. This includes three concepts: its quantitative strength, dose–response, and the study design. Each will be discussed in turn.

The *quantitative strength* of an association refers to the effect size. To evaluate this, one asks whether the magnitude of the observed difference between the two study groups is large. A quantitatively large association can only be created by a causal association or a large error, which should be apparent in evaluating the methodology of a study. A quantitatively small association may still be causal, but it could be created by a subtle error, which would not be apparent in evaluating the study. Conventionally, epidemiologists consider an association with a relative risk of less than 2.0 a weak association. Certainly, the association between cigarette smoking and lung cancer is a strong association: studies show relative risks ranging between 10.0 and 30.0.[29]

A dose–response relationship is an extremely important and commonly used concept in clinical pharmacology and is used similarly in epidemiology. A *dose–response relationship* exists when an increase in the intensity of an exposure results in an increased risk of the disease under study. Equivalent to this is a *duration–response relationship*, which exists when a longer exposure causes an increased risk of the disease. The presence of either a dose–response relationship or a duration–response relationship strongly implies that

Table 2.4. Advantages and disadvantages of epidemiologic study designs

Study Design	Advantages	Disadvantages
Randomized clinical trial	Most convincing design	Most expensive
(Experimental study)	Only design which controls for unknown or unmeasurable confounders	Artificial. Logistically most difficult. Ethical objections
Cohort study	Can study multiple outcomes Can study uncommon exposures Selection bias less likely Unbiased exposure data Incidence data available	Possibly biased outcome data More expensive If done prospectively, may take years to complete
Case–control study	Can study multiple exposures Can study uncommon diseases Logistically easier and faster Less expensive	Control selection problematic Possibly biased exposure data
Analyses of secular trends	Can provide rapid answers	No control of confounding
Case series	Easy quantitation of incidence	No control group, so cannot be used for hypothesis testing
Case reports	Cheap and easy method for generating hypotheses	Cannot be used for hypothesis testing

an association is, in fact, a causal association. Certainly in the example of cigarette smoking and lung cancer, it has been shown repeatedly that an increase in either the number of cigarettes smoked each day or in the number of years of smoking increases the risk of developing lung cancer.[29]

Finally, *study design* refers to two concepts: whether the study was well designed, and which study design was used in the studies in question. The former refers to whether the study was subject to one of the three errors described earlier in this chapter, namely random error, bias, and confounding. Table 2.4 presents the study designs typically used for epidemiologic studies, or in fact for any clinical studies. They are organized in a hierarchical fashion. As one advances from the designs at the bottom of the table to those at the top, studies get progressively harder to perform, but are progressively more convincing. In other words, associations shown by studies using designs at the top of the list are more likely to be causal associations than associations shown by studies using designs at the bottom of the list. The association between cigarette smoking and lung cancer has been reproduced in multiple well-designed studies, using analyses of secular trends, case–control studies, and cohort studies. However, it has not been shown using a randomized clinical trial, which is the "Cadillac" of study designs, as will be discussed below. This is the other major defense used by the tobacco industry. Of course, it would not be ethical or logistically feasible to randomly allocate individuals to smoke or not to smoke and expect them to follow that for 20 years to observe the outcome in each group.

The issue of causation is discussed more in Chapters 9 and 10 as it relates to the process of spontaneous reporting of adverse drug reactions, and in Chapter 36 as it relates to determining causation in case reports.

EPIDEMIOLOGIC STUDY DESIGNS

In order to clarify the concept of study design further, each of the designs in Table 2.4 will be discussed in turn, starting at the bottom of the list and working upwards.

CASE REPORTS

Case reports are simply reports of events observed in single patients. As used in pharmacoepidemiology, a case report describes a single patient who was exposed to a drug and experiences a particular, usually adverse, outcome. For example, one might see a published case report about a young woman who was taking oral contraceptives and who suffered a pulmonary embolism.

Case reports are useful for raising hypotheses about drug effects, to be tested with more rigorous study designs. However, in a case report one cannot know if the patient reported is either typical of those with the exposure or typical of those with the disease. Certainly, one cannot usually determine whether the adverse outcome was due to the drug exposure or would have happened anyway. As such, it is very rare that a case report can be used to make a statement about causation. One exception to this would be when the outcome is so rare and so characteristic of the exposure that one knows that it was likely to be due to the exposure, even if the history of exposure were unclear. An example of this is clear cell vaginal adenocarcinoma occurring in young women exposed *in utero* to diethylstilbestrol.[30] Another exception would be when the disease course is very predictable and the treatment causes a clearly apparent change in this disease course. An example would be the ability of penicillin to cure streptococcal endocarditis, a disease that is nearly uniformly fatal in the absence of treatment. Case reports can be particularly useful to document causation when the treatment causes a change in disease course which is reversible, such that the patient returns to his or her untreated state when the exposure is withdrawn, can be treated again, and when the change returns upon repeat treatment. Consider a patient who is suffering from an overdose of methadone, a long-acting narcotic, and is comatose. If this patient is then treated with naloxone, a narcotic antagonist, and immediately awakens, this would be very suggestive that the drug indeed is efficacious as a narcotic antagonist. As the naloxone wears off the patient would become comatose again, and then if he or she were given another dose of naloxone the patient would awaken again. This, especially if repeated a few times, would represent strong evidence that the drug is indeed effective as a narcotic antagonist. This type of challenge–rechallenge situation is relatively uncommon, however, as physicians generally will avoid exposing a patient to a drug if the patient experienced an adverse reaction to it in the past. This issue is discussed in more detail in Chapters 9, 10, and 36.

CASE SERIES

Case series are collections of patients, all of whom have a single exposure, whose clinical outcomes are then evaluated and described. Often they are from a single hospital or medical practice. Alternatively, case series can be collections of patients with a single outcome, looking at their antecedent exposures. For example, one might observe 100 consecutive women under the age of 50 who suffer from a pulmonary embolism, and note that 30 of them had been taking oral contraceptives.

After drug marketing, case series are most useful for two related purposes. First, they can be useful for quantifying the incidence of an adverse reaction. Second, they can be useful for being certain that any particular adverse effect of concern does not occur when observed in a population which is larger than that studied prior to drug marketing. The so-called "Phase

IV" postmarketing surveillance study of prazosin was conducted for the former reason, to quantitate the incidence of first-dose syncope from prazosin.[31] The "Phase IV" postmarketing surveillance study of cimetidine[32] was conducted for the latter reason. Metiamide was an H-2 blocker, which was withdrawn after marketing outside the US because it caused agranulocytosis. Since cimetidine is chemically related to metiamide there was a concern that cimetidine might also cause agranulocytosis.[31] In both examples, the manufacturer asked its sales representatives to recruit physicians to participate in the study. Each participating physician then enrolled the next series of patients for whom the drug was prescribed.

In this type of study, one can be more certain that the patients are probably typical of those with the exposure or with the disease, depending on the focus of the study. However, in the absence of a control group, one cannot be certain which features in the description of the patients are unique to the exposure, or outcome. As an example, one might have a case series from a particular hospital of 100 individuals with a certain disease, and note that all were men over the age of 60. This might lead one to conclude that this disease seems to be associated with being a man over the age of 60. However, it would be clear that this would be an incorrect conclusion once one noted that the hospital this case series was drawn from was a Veterans Administration hospital, where most patients are men over the age of 60. In the previous example of pulmonary embolism and oral contraceptives, 30% of the women with pulmonary embolism had been using oral contraceptives. However, this information is not sufficient to determine whether this is higher, the same as, or even lower than would have been expected. For this reason, case series are also not very useful in determining causation, but provide clinical descriptions of a disease or of patients who receive an exposure.

ANALYSES OF SECULAR TRENDS

Analyses of secular trends, also called "ecological studies," examine trends in an exposure that is a presumed cause and trends in a disease that is a presumed effect and test whether the trends coincide. These trends can be examined over time or across geographic boundaries. In other words, one could analyze data from a single region and examine how the trend changes over time, or one could analyze data from a single time period and compare how the data differ from region to region or country to country. Vital statistics are often used for these studies. As an example, one might look at sales data for oral contraceptives and compare them to death rates from venous thromboembolism, using recorded vital statistics. When such a study was actually performed, mortality rates from venous thromboembolism were seen to increase in parallel with increasing oral contraceptive sales, but only in women of reproductive age, not in older women or in men of any age.[33]

Analyses of secular trends are useful for rapidly providing evidence for or against a hypothesis. However, these studies lack data on individuals; they utilize only aggregated group data (e.g., annual sales data in a given geographic region in relation to annual cause-specific mortality in the same region). As such, they are unable to control for confounding variables. Thus, among exposures whose trends coincide with that of the disease, analyses of secular trends are unable to differentiate which factor is likely to be the true cause. For example, lung cancer mortality rates in the US have been increasing in women, such that lung cancer is now the leading cause of cancer mortality in women.[34] This is certainly consistent with the increasing rates of cigarette smoking observed in women until the mid-1960s,[35] and so appears to be supportive of the association between cigarette smoking and lung cancer. However, it would also be consistent with an association between certain occupational exposures and lung cancer, as more women in the US are now working outside the home.

CASE–CONTROL STUDIES

Case–control studies are studies that compare cases with a disease to controls without the disease, looking for differences in antecedent exposures. As an example, one could select cases of young women with venous thromboembolism and compare them to controls without venous thromboembolism, looking for differences in antecedent oral contraceptive use. Several such studies have been performed, generally demonstrating a strong association between the use of oral contraceptives and venous thromboembolism.[36]

Case–control studies can be particularly useful when one wants to study multiple possible causes of a single disease, as one can use the same cases and controls to examine any number of exposures as potential risk factors. This design is also particularly useful when one is studying a relatively rare disease, as it guarantees a sufficient number of cases with the disease. Using case–control studies, one can study rare diseases with markedly smaller sample sizes than those needed for cohort studies (see Chapter 3). For example, the classic study of diethylstilbestrol and clear cell vaginal adenocarcinoma required only 8 cases and 40 controls,[30] rather than the many thousands of exposed subjects that

would have been required for a cohort study of this question.

Case–control studies generally obtain their information on exposures retrospectively, i.e., by recreating events that happened in the past. Information on past exposure to potential risk factors is generally obtained by abstracting medical records or by administering questionnaires or interviews. As such, case–control studies are subject to limitations in the validity of retrospectively collected exposure information. In addition, the proper selection of controls can be a challenging task, and inappropriate control selection can lead to a selection bias, which may lead to incorrect conclusions. Nevertheless, when case–control studies are done well, subsequent well-done cohort studies or randomized clinical trials, if any, will generally confirm their results. As such, the case–control design is a very useful approach for pharmacoepidemiology studies.

COHORT STUDIES

Cohort studies are studies that identify subsets of a defined population and follow them over time, looking for differences in their outcome. Cohort studies generally are used to compare exposed patients to unexposed patients, although they can also be used to compare one exposure to another. For example, one could compare women of reproductive age who use oral contraceptives to users of other contraceptive methods, looking for the differences in the frequency of venous thromboembolism. When such studies were performed, they in fact confirmed the relationship between oral contraceptives and thromboembolism, which had been noted using analyses of secular trends and case–control studies.[37,38] Cohort studies can be performed either prospectively, that is simultaneous with the events under study, or retrospectively, that is after the outcomes under study had already occurred, by recreating those past events using medical records, questionnaires, or interviews.

The major difference between cohort and case–control studies is the basis upon which patients are recruited into the study (see Figure 2.2). Patients are recruited into case–control studies based on the presence or absence of a disease, and their antecedent exposures are then studied. Patients are recruited into cohort studies based on the presence or absence of an exposure, and their subsequent disease course is then studied.

Cohort studies have the major advantage of being free of the big problem that plagues case–control studies: the difficult process of selecting an undiseased control group. In addition, prospective cohort studies are free of the problem

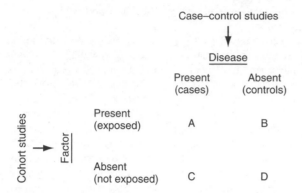

Figure 2.2. Cohort and case–control studies provide similar information, but approach data collection from opposite directions. (Reprinted with permission from Elsevier from Strom BL. Medical databases in post-marketing drug surveillance. *Trends in Pharmacological Sciences* 1986; **7**: 377–80.)

of the questionable validity of retrospectively collected data. For these reasons, an association demonstrated by a cohort study is more likely to be a causal association than one demonstrated by a case–control study. Furthermore, cohort studies are particularly useful when one is studying multiple possible outcomes from a single exposure, especially a relatively uncommon exposure. Thus, they are particularly useful in postmarketing drug surveillance studies, which are looking at any possible effect of a newly marketed drug. However, cohort studies can require extremely large sample sizes to study relatively uncommon outcomes (see Chapter 3). In addition, prospective cohort studies can require a prolonged time period to study delayed drug effects.

ANALYSIS OF CASE–CONTROL AND COHORT STUDIES

As can be seen in Figure 2.2, both case–control and cohort studies are intended to provide the same basic information; the difference is how this information is collected. The key statistic reported from these studies is the relative risk. The *relative risk* is the ratio of the incidence rate of an outcome in the exposed group to the incidence rate of the outcome in the unexposed group. A relative risk of greater than 1.0 means that exposed subjects have a *greater* risk of the disease under study than unexposed subjects, or that the exposure appears to cause the disease. A relative risk less than 1.0 means that exposed subjects have a *lower* risk of the disease than unexposed subjects, or that the exposure seems to protect against the disease. A relative risk of 1.0 means that exposed subjects and unexposed subjects have the same risk

of developing the disease, or that the exposure and the disease appear unrelated.

One can calculate a relative risk directly from the results of a cohort study. However, in a case–control study one cannot determine the size of either the exposed population or the unexposed population that the diseased cases and undiseased controls were drawn from. The results of a case–control study do not provide information on the incidence rates of the disease in exposed and unexposed individuals. Therefore, relative risks cannot be calculated directly from a case–control study. Instead, in reporting the results of a case–control study one generally reports the *odds ratio*, which is a close estimate of the relative risk when the disease under study is relatively rare. Since case–control studies are generally used to study rare diseases, there usually is very close agreement between the odds ratio and the relative risk, and the results from case–control studies are often loosely referred to as relative risks, although they are in fact odds ratios.

Both relative risks and odds ratios can be reported with p-*values*. These p-values allow one to determine if the relative risk is statistically significantly different from 1.0, that is whether the differences between the two study groups are likely to be due to random variation or are likely to represent real associations.

Alternatively, and probably preferably, relative risks and odds ratios can be reported with *confidence intervals*, which are an indication of the range of relative risks within which the true relative risk for the entire theoretical population is most likely to lie. As an approximation, a 95% confidence interval around a relative risk means that we can be 95% confident that the true relative risk lies in the range between the lower and upper limits of this interval. If a 95% confidence interval around a relative risk excludes 1.0, then the finding is statistically significant with a p-value of less than 0.05. A confidence interval provides much more information than a p-value, however. As an example, a study that yields a relative risk (95% confidence interval) of 1.0 (0.9–1.1) is clearly showing that an association is very unlikely. A study that yields a relative risk (95% confidence interval) of 1.0 (0.1–100) provides little evidence for or against an association. Yet, both could be reported as a relative risk of 1.0 and a p-value greater than 0.05. As another example, a study that yields a relative risk (95% confidence interval) of 10.0 (9.8–10.2) precisely quantifies a ten-fold increase in risk that is also statistically significant. A study that yields a relative risk (95% confidence interval) of 10.0 (1.1–100) says little, other than an increased risk is likely. Yet, both could be reported as a relative risk of 10.0 ($p < 0.05$). As a final example, a study yielding a relative risk (95% confidence interval) of 3.0 (0.98–5.0) is strongly suggestive of an association, whereas a study reporting a relative risk (95% confidence interval) of 3.0 (0.1–30) would not be. Yet, both could be reported as a relative risk of 3.0 ($p > 0.05$).

Finally, another statistic that one can calculate from a cohort study is the excess risk, also called the risk difference or, sometimes, the attributable risk. Whereas the relative risk is the ratio of the incidence rates in the exposed group versus the unexposed groups, the excess risk is the arithmetic difference between the incidence rates. The relative risk is more important in considering questions of causation. The excess risk is more important in considering the public health impact of an association, as it represents the increased rate of disease due to the exposure. For example, oral contraceptives are strongly associated with the development of myocardial infarction in young women.[36] However, the risk of myocardial infarction in non-smoking women in their 20s is so low, that even a five-fold increase in that risk would still not be of public health importance. In contrast, women in their 40s are at higher risk, especially if they are cigarette smokers as well. Thus, oral contraceptives should not be as readily used in these women.[36]

As with relative risks, excess risks cannot be calculated from case–control studies, as incidence rates are not available. As with the other statistics, p-values can be calculated to determine whether the differences between the two study groups could have occurred just by chance. Confidence intervals can be calculated around excess risks as well, and would be interpreted analogously.

RANDOMIZED CLINICAL TRIALS

Finally, *experimental studies* are studies in which the investigator controls the therapy that is to be received by each participant. Generally, an investigator uses that control to randomly allocate patients between or among the study groups, performing a *randomized clinical trial*. For example, one could theoretically randomly allocate sexually active women to use either oral contraceptives or no contraceptive, examining whether they differ in their incidence of subsequent venous thromboembolism. The major strength of this approach is random assignment, which is the only way to make it likely that the study groups are comparable in potential confounding variables that are either unknown or unmeasurable. For this reason, associations demonstrated in randomized clinical trials are more likely to be causal associations than those demonstrated using one of the other study designs reviewed above.

However, even randomized clinical trials are not without their problems. The randomized clinical trial outlined above, allocating women to receive contraceptives or no contraceptives, demonstrates the major potential problems inherent in the use of this study design. It would obviously be impossible to perform, ethically and logistically. In addition, randomized clinical trials are expensive and artificial. Inasmuch as they have already been performed prior to marketing to demonstrate each drug's efficacy, they tend to be unnecessary after marketing. They are likely to be used in pharmacoepidemiology studies mainly for supplementary studies of drug efficacy.[37] However, they remain the "gold standard" by which the other designs must be judged. Indeed, with the publication of the results from the Women's Health Initiative indicating that combination hormone replacement therapy causes an increased risk of myocardial infarction rather than a decreased risk,[38–41] there has been increased concern about reliance solely on nonexperimental methods to study drug safety after marketing,[42–44] and we are beginning to see the use of massive randomized clinical trials as part of postmarketing surveillance (see Chapter 39).

DISCUSSION

Thus, a series of different study designs are available (Table 2.4), each with respective advantages and disadvantages. Case reports, case series, analyses of secular trends, case–control studies, and cohort studies have been referred to collectively as *observational study designs* or *nonexperimental study designs*, in order to differentiate them from experimental studies. In nonexperimental study designs the investigator does not control the therapy, but simply observes and evaluates the results of ongoing medical care. Case reports, case series, and analyses of secular trends have also been referred to as *descriptive studies*. Case–control studies, cohort studies, and randomized clinical trials all have control groups, and have been referred to as *analytic studies*. The analytic study designs can be classified in two major ways, by how subjects are selected into the study and by how data are collected for the study (see Table 2.5). From the perspective of how subjects are recruited into the study, case–control studies can be contrasted with cohort studies. Specifically, case–control studies select subjects into the study based on the presence or absence of a disease, while cohort studies select subjects into the study based on the presence or absence of an exposure. From this perspective, randomized clinical trials can be viewed as a subset of cohort studies, a type of cohort study in which the

Table 2.5. Epidemiologic study designs

(A) Classified by how subjects are recruited into the study

    (1) Case–control (case-history, case-referent, retrospective, trohoc) studies

    (2) Cohort (follow-up, prospective) studies

        (a) Experimental studies (clinical trials, intervention studies)

(B) Classified by how data are collected for the study

    (1) Retrospective (historical, non-concurrent, retrolective) studies

    (2) Prospective (prolective) studies

    (3) Cross-sectional studies

---

investigator controls the allocation of treatment, rather than simply observing ongoing medical care. From the perspective of timing, data can be collected *prospectively*, that is simultaneously with the events under study, or *retrospectively*, that is after the events under study had already developed. In the latter situation, one recreates events that happened in the past using medical records, questionnaires, or interviews. Data can also be collected using *cross-sectional studies*, studies that have no time sense, as they examine only one point in time. In principle, either cohort or case–control studies can be performed using any of these time frames, although prospective case–control studies are unusual. Randomized clinical trials must be prospective, as this is the only way an investigator can control the therapy received.

The terms presented in this chapter, which are those that will be used throughout the book, are probably the terms used by a majority of epidemiologists. Unfortunately, however, other terms have been used for most of these study designs as well. Table 2.5 also presents several of the synonyms that have been used in the medical literature. The same term is sometimes used by different authors to describe different concepts. For example, in this book we are reserving the use of the terms "retrospective study" and "prospective study" to refer to a time sense. As is apparent from Table 2.5, however, in the past some authors used the term "retrospective study" to refer to a case–control study and the term "prospective study" to refer to a cohort study, confusing the two concepts inherent in the classification schemes presented in the table. Other authors use the term "retrospective study" to refer to any nonexperimental study, while others appear to use the term to refer to any study they do not like, as a term of derision! Unfortunately, when reading a scientific paper, there is no way of determining which usage the author intended. What is more important than the terminology, however, are the concepts underlying the terms. Understanding these

concepts, the reader can choose to use whatever terminology he or she is comfortable with.

CONCLUSION

From the material presented in this chapter, it is hopefully now apparent that each study design has an appropriate role in scientific progress. In general, science proceeds from the bottom of Table 2.4 upward, from case reports and case series that are useful for suggesting an association, to analyses of trends and case–control studies that are useful for exploring these associations. Finally, if a study question warrants the investment and can tolerate the delay until results become available, then cohort studies and randomized clinical trials can be undertaken to assess these associations more definitively.

For example, regarding the question of whether oral contraceptives cause venous thromboembolism, an association was first suggested by case reports and case series, then was explored in more detail by analyses of trends and a series of case–control studies.[36] Later, because of the importance of oral contraceptives, the number of women using them, and the fact that users were predominantly healthy women, the investment was made in two long-term, large-scale cohort studies.[45,46] This question might even be worth the investment of a randomized clinical trial, except it would not be feasible or ethical. In contrast, when thalidomide was marketed, it was not a major breakthrough; other hypnotics were already available. Case reports of phocomelia in exposed patients were followed by case–control studies[47] and analyses of secular trends.[48] Inasmuch as the adverse effect was so terrible and the drug was not of unique importance, the drug was then withdrawn, without the delay that would have been necessary if cohort studies and/or randomized clinical trials had been awaited. Ultimately, a retrospective cohort study was performed, comparing those exposed during the critical time period to those exposed at other times.[49]

In general, however, clinical, regulatory, commercial, and legal decisions need to be made based on the best evidence available at the time of the decision. To quote Sir Austin Bradford Hill:[26]

> All scientific work is incomplete—whether it be observational or experimental. All scientific work is liable to be upset or modified by advancing knowledge. That does not confer upon us a freedom to ignore the knowledge we already have, or to postpone the action that it appears to demand at a given time.

Who knows, asked Robert Browning, but the world may end tonight? True, but on available evidence most of us make ready to commute on the 8 : 30 next day.

REFERENCES

1. Lilienfeld DE, Stolley P. *Foundations of Epidemiology*, 3rd edn. New York: Oxford University Press, 1994.
2. MacMahon B, Pugh TF. *Epidemiology: Principles and Methods*. Boston, MA: Little, Brown, 1970.
3. Friedman G. *Primer of Epidemiology*, 3rd edn. New York: McGraw Hill, 1994.
4. Mausner JS, Kramer S. *Epidemiology: An Introductory Text*, 2nd edn. Philadelphia, PA: Saunders, 1985.
5. Ahlbom A, Norell S. *Introduction to Modern Epidemiology*, 2nd edn. Chestnut Hill, MA: Epidemiology Resources, 1990.
6. Sackett DL, Haynes RB, Tugwell P. *Clinical Epidemiology: A Basic Science for Clinical Medicine*, 2nd edn. Boston, MA: Little, Brown, 1991.
7. Schuman SH. *Practice-Based Epidemiology*. New York: Gordon and Breach, 1986.
8. Rothman KJ, Greenland S. *Modern Epidemiology*, 2nd edn. Philadelphia, PA: Lippincott-Raven, 1998.
9. Weiss N. *Clinical Epidemiology: The Study of the Outcome of Illness*, 2nd edn. New York: Oxford University Press, 1996.
10. Kelsey JL, Thompson WD, Evans AS. *Methods in Observational Epidemiology*, New York: Oxford University Press, 1986.
11. Hennekens CH, Buring JE. *Epidemiology in Medicine*, Boston, MA: Little, Brown, 1987.
12. Fletcher RH, Fletcher SW, Wagner EH. *Clinical Epidemiology: The Essentials*, 3rd edn. Baltimore, MD: Williams and Wilkins, 1996.
13. Hulley SB, Cummings SR. *Designing Clinical Research: An Epidemiologic Approach*, Baltimore, MD: Williams and Wilkins, 1988.
14. Gordis L. *Epidemiology*, 2nd edn. Philadelphia, PA: Saunders, 2000.
15. Rothman KJ. *Epidemiology: An Introduction*, New York: Oxford University Press, 2002.
16. Nieto FJ, Szklo M. *Epidemiology: Beyond the Basics*, Frederick, MD: Aspen, 1999.
17. Jekel JF, Elmore JG, Katz DL. *Epidemiology, Biostatistics, and Preventive Medicine*, Philadelphia, PA: Saunders, 1996.
18. Aschengrau A, Seage GR. *Essentials of Epidemiology in Public Health*, Sudbury, MA: Jones and Bartlett, 2003.
19. Friis RH, Sellers TA. *Epidemiology for Public Health Practice*, 2nd edn. Frederick, MD: Aspen, 1999.
20. Hulley SB, Cummings SR, Browner WS, Grady D, Hearst N, Newman TB. *Designing Clinical Research: An Epidemiologic Approach*, 2nd edn. Baltimore, MD: Williams and Wilkins, 2001.
21. Greenberg RS, Daniels SR, Flanders WD, Eley JW, Boring JR. *Medical Epidemiology*, 3rd edn. New York: McGraw-Hill, 2001.
22. Wassertheil-Smoller S. *Biostatistics and Epidemiology: A Primer for Health Professionals*, New York: Springer-Verlag, 2003.
23. Katz DL. *Clinical Epidemiology and Evidence-Based Medicine: Fundamental Principles of Clinical Reasoning and Research*, Thousand Oaks, CA: Sage, 2001.
24. Sackett DL. Bias in analytic research. *J Chronic Dis* 1979; **32**: 51–63.
25. Mitchell AA, Cottler LB, Shapiro S. Effect of questionnaire design on recall of drug exposure in pregnancy. *Am J Epidemiol* 1986; **123**: 670–6.
26. Hill AB. The environment and disease: association or causation? *Proc R Soc Med* 1965; **58**: 295–300.
27. US Public Health Service. *Smoking and Health. Report of the Advisory Committee to the Surgeon General of the Public Health Service*. Washington DC: Government Printing Office, 1964; p. 20.
28. Experimental Carcinogenesis with Tobacco Smoke. In: *US Public Health Service: The Health Consequences of Smoking— Cancer. A Report of the Surgeon General*. Washington, DC: Government Printing Office, 1982; p. 181.
29. Biomedical evidence for determining causality. In: *US Public Health Service: The Health Consequences of Smoking— Cancer. A Report of the Surgeon General*. Washington, DC: Government Printing Office, 1982; p. 13.
30. Herbst AL, Ulfelder H, Poskanzer DC. Adenocarcinoma of the vagina: association of maternal stilbestrol therapy with tumor appearance in young women. *N Engl J Med* 1971; **284**: 878–81.
31. Joint Commission on Prescription Drug Use. *Final Report*. Washington, DC, 1980.
32. Humphries TJ, Myerson RM, Gifford LM, Aeugle ME, Josie ME, Wood SL, *et al.* A unique postmarket outpatient surveillance program of cimetidine: report on phase II and final summary. *Am J Gastroenterol* 1984; **79**: 593–6.
33. Markush RE, Seigel DG. Oral contraceptives and mortality trends from thromboembolism in the United States. *Am J Public Health* 1969; **59**: 418–34.
34. National Center for Health Statistics. *Health: United States 1982*. Hyattsville, MD: Department of Health and Human Services, 1982.
35. US Public Health Service. *Smoking and Health. Report of the Advisory Committee to the Surgeon General of the Public Health Service*. Washington, DC: Government Printing Office, 1964; p. A1.
36. Strom BL, Stolley PD. Vascular and cardiac risks of steroidal contraception. In: Sciarra JW ed., *Gynecology and Obstetrics*, vol. 6. Hagerstown, MD: Harper and Row, 1989, pp. 1–17.
37. Bell RL, Smith EO. Clinical trials in post-marketing surveillance of drugs. *Control Clin Trials* 1982; **3**: 61–8.
38. Manson JE, Hsia J, Johnson KC, Rossouw JE, Assaf AR, Lasser NL, *et al.* Estrogen plus progestin and the risk of coronary heart disease. *N Engl J Med* 2003; **349**: 523–34.
39. Herrington DM, Howard TD. From presumed benefit to potential harm—hormone therapy and heart disease. *N Engl J Med* 2003; **349**: 519–21.
40. John B. Hormone-replacement therapy and cardiovascular diseases. *N Engl J Med* 2003; **349**: 521–2.

41. Writing Group for the Women's Health Initiative Investigators. Risks and benefits of estrogen plus progestin in healthy post-menopausal women. Principal results From the Women's Health Initiative randomized controlled trial. *JAMA* 2002; **288**: 321–33.

42. Col NF, Pauker SG. The discrepancy between observational studies and randomized trials of menopausal hormone therapy: did expectations shape experience? *Ann Intern Med* 2003; **139**: 923–9.

43. Grimes DA, Lobo RA. Perspectives on the Women's Health Initiative trial of hormone replacement therapy. *Obstet Gynecol* 2002; **100**: 1344–53.

44. Whittemore AS, McGuire V. Observational studies and randomized trials of hormone replacement therapy: what can we learn from them? *Epidemiology* 2003; **14**: 8–9.

45. Royal College of General Practitioners. *Oral Contraceptives and Health*. London: Pitman, 1974; ch.7.

46. Vessey MP, Doll R, Peto R, Johnson B, Wiggins P. A long-term follow-up study of women using different methods of contraception—an interim report. *J Biosoc Sci* 1976; **8**: 373–427.

47. Mellin GW, Katzenstein M. The saga of thalidomide. *N Engl J Med* 1962; **267**: 1238–44.

48. Taussig HB. A study of the German outbreak of phocomelia. *JAMA* 1962; **180**: 1106–14.

49. Kajii T, Kida M, Takahashi K. The effect of thalidomide intake during 113 human pregnancies. *Teratology* 1973; **8**: 163–6.

3

Sample Size Considerations for Pharmacoepidemiology Studies

BRIAN L. STROM

University of Pennsylvania School of Medicine, Philadelphia, Pennsylvania, USA.

INTRODUCTION

Chapter 1 pointed out that between 500 and 3000 subjects are usually exposed to a drug prior to marketing, in order to be 95% certain of detecting adverse effects that occur in between one and six in a thousand exposed individuals. While this seems like a reasonable goal, it poses some important problems that must be taken into account when planning pharmacoepidemiology studies. Specifically, such studies must generally include a sufficient number of subjects to add significantly to the premarketing experience, and this requirement for large sample sizes raises logistical obstacles to cost-effective studies. This central special need for large sample sizes is what has led to the innovative approaches to collecting pharmacoepidemiologic data that are described in Part III of this book.

The approach to considering the implications of a study's sample size is somewhat different depending on whether a study is already completed or is being planned. After a study is completed, if a real finding was statistically significant, then the study had a sufficient sample size to detect it, by definition. If a finding was not statistically significant, then one can use either of two approaches. First, one can examine the resulting confidence intervals in order to determine the smallest differences between the two study groups that the study had sufficient sample size to exclude.[1] Alternatively, one can approach the question in a manner similar to the way one would approach it if one were planning the study *de novo*. Nomograms can be used to assist a reader in interpreting negative clinical trials in this way.[2]

In contrast, in this chapter we will discuss in more detail how to determine a proper study sample size, from the perspective of one who is designing a study *de novo*. Specifically, we will begin by discussing how one calculates the minimum sample size necessary for a pharmacoepidemiology study, to avoid the problem of a study with a sample size that is too small. We will first present the approach for cohort studies, then for case–control studies, and then for case series. For each design, one or more tables will be presented to assist the reader in carrying out these calculations.

Pharmacoepidemiology, Fourth Edition   Edited by B.L. Strom

SAMPLE SIZE CALCULATIONS FOR COHORT STUDIES

The sample size required for a cohort study depends on what you are expecting from the study. To calculate sample sizes for a cohort study, one needs to specify five variables (see Table 3.1).[3,4]

The first variable to specify is the *alpha* (α) or *type I error* that one is willing to tolerate in the study. Type I error is the probability of concluding there is a difference between the groups being compared when in fact a difference does not exist. Using diagnostic tests as an analogy, a type I error is a false positive study finding. The more tolerant one is willing to be of type I error, the smaller the sample size required. The less tolerant one is willing to be of type I error, the smaller one would set α, and the larger the sample size that would be required. Conventionally the α is set at 0.05, although this certainly does not have to be the case. Note that α needs to be specified as either one-tailed or two-tailed. If only one of the study groups could conceivably be more likely to develop the disease and one is interested in detecting this result only, then one would specify α to be one-tailed. If either of the study groups may be likely to develop the disease, and either result would be of interest, then one would specify α to be two-tailed. To decide whether α should be one-tailed or two-tailed, an investigator should consider what his or her reaction would be to a result that is statistically significant in a direction opposite to the one expected. For example, what if one observed that a drug increased the frequency of dying from coronary artery disease instead of decreasing it, as expected? If the investigator's response to this would be: "Boy, what a surprise, but I believe it," then a two-tailed test should be performed. If the investigator's response would be: "I don't believe it, and I will interpret this simply as a study that does not show the expected decrease in coronary artery disease in the group treated with the study drug," then a one-tailed test should be performed. The more

conservative option is the two-tailed test, assuming that the results could turn out in either direction. This is the option usually, although not always, used.

The second variable that needs to be specified to calculate a sample size for a cohort study is the *beta* (β) or *type II error* that one is willing to tolerate in the study. A type II error is the probability of concluding there is no difference between the groups being compared when in fact a difference does exist. In other words, a type II error is the probability of missing a real difference. Using diagnostic tests as an analogy, a type II error is a false negative study finding. The complement of β is the power of a study, i.e., the probability of detecting a difference if a difference really exists. Power is calculated as $(1 - \beta)$. Again, the more tolerant one is willing to be of type II errors, i.e., the higher the β, the smaller the sample size required. The β is conventionally set at 0.1 (i.e., 90% power) or 0.2 (i.e., 80% power), although again this need not be the case. β is always one-tailed.

The third variable one needs to specify in order to calculate sample sizes for a cohort study is the minimum effect size one wants to be able to detect. For a cohort study, this is expressed as a relative risk. The smaller the relative risk that one wants to detect, the larger the sample size required. Note that the relative risk often used by investigators in this calculation is the relative risk the investigator is expecting from the study. This is *not correct*, as it will lead to inadequate power to detect relative risks which are smaller than expected, but still clinically important to the investigator. In other words, if one chooses a sample size that is designed to detect a relative risk of 2.5, one should be comfortable with the thought that, if the actual relative risk turns out to be 2.2, one may not be able to detect it as a statistically significant finding.

The fourth variable one needs to specify is the expected incidence of the outcome of interest in the unexposed control group. Again, the more you ask of a study, the larger the sample size needed. Specifically, the rarer the outcome of interest, the larger the sample size needed.

Table 3.1. Information needed to calculate a study's sample size

For cohort studies	For case–control studies
(1) α or type I error considered tolerable, and whether it is one-tailed or two-tailed	(1) α or type I error considered tolerable, and whether it is one-tailed or two tailed
(2) β or type II error considered tolerable	(2) β or type II error considered tolerable
(3) Minimum relative risk to be detected	(3) Minimum relative risk to be detected
(4) Incidence of the disease in the unexposed control group	(4) Prevalence of the exposure in the undiseased control group
(5) Ratio of unexposed controls to exposed study subjects	(5) Ratio of undiseased controls to diseased study subjects

The fifth variable one needs to specify is the number of unexposed control subjects to be included in the study for each exposed study subject. A study has the most statistical power for a given number of study subjects if it has the same number of controls as exposed subjects. However, sometimes the number of exposed subjects is limited and, therefore, inadequate to provide sufficient power to detect a relative risk of interest. In that case, additional power can be gained by increasing the number of controls alone. Doubling the number of controls, that is including two controls for each exposed subject, results in a modest increase in the statistical power, but it does not double it. Including three controls for each exposed subject increases the power further. However, the increment in power achieved by increasing the ratio of control subjects to exposed subjects from $2:1$ to $3:1$ is smaller than the increment in power achieved by increasing the ratio from $1:1$ to $2:1$. Each additional increase in the size of the control group increases the power of the study further, but with progressively smaller gains in statistical power. Thus, there is rarely a reason to include greater than three or four controls per study subject. For example, one could design a study with an α of 0.05 to detect a relative risk of 2.0 for an outcome variable that occurs in the control group with an incidence rate of 0.01. A study with 2319 exposed individuals and 2319 controls would yield a power of 0.80, or an 80% chance of detecting a difference of that magnitude. With the same 2319 exposed subjects, ratios of control subjects to exposed subjects of $1:1$, $2:1$, $3:1$, $4:1$, $5:1$, $10:1$, and $50:1$ would result in statistical powers of 0.80, 0.887, 0.913, 0.926, 0.933, 0.947, and 0.956, respectively.

It is important to differentiate between the ratio of the number of controls and the number of control groups. It is not uncommon, especially in case–control studies, where the selection of a proper control group can be difficult, to choose more than one control group. This is done for reasons of validity, not statistical power, and it is important that these multiple control groups not be aggregated in the analysis. In this situation, the goal is to assure that each comparison yields the same answer, not to increase the available sample size. As such, the comparison of each control group to the exposed subjects should be treated as a separate study. The comparison of the exposed group to each control group requires a separate sample size calculation.

Once the five variables above have been specified, the sample size needed for a given study can be calculated. Several different formulas have been used for this calculation, each of which gives slightly different results. The formula that is probably the most often used is modified from Schlesselman:[3]

$$N = \frac{1}{[p(1-R)]^2} \left[Z_{1-\alpha} \sqrt{\left(1 + \frac{1}{K}\right) U(1-U)} \right.$$

$$\left. + Z_{1-\beta} \sqrt{pR(1-Rp) + \frac{p(1-p)}{K}} \right]^2$$

where p is the incidence of the disease in the unexposed, R is the minimum relative risk to be detected, α is the type I error rate which is acceptable, β is the type II error rate which is acceptable, $Z_{1-\alpha}$ and $Z_{1-\beta}$ refer to the unit normal deviates corresponding to α and β, K is the ratio of number of control subjects to the number of exposed subjects, and

$$U = \frac{Kp + pR}{K+1}$$

$Z_{1-\alpha}$ is replaced by $Z_{1-\alpha/2}$ if one is planning to analyze the study using a two-tailed α. Note that K does not need to be an integer.

A series of tables are presented in Appendix A, which were calculated using this formula. In Tables A1–A4 we have assumed an α (two-tailed) of 0.05, a β of 0.1 (90% power), and control to exposed ratios of $1:1$, $2:1$, $3:1$, and $4:1$, respectively. Tables A5–A8 are similar, except they assume a β of 0.2 (80% power). Each table presents the number of exposed subjects needed to detect any of several specified relative risks, for outcome variables that occur at any of several specified incidence rates.

For example, what if one wanted to investigate a new nonsteroidal anti-inflammatory drug that is about to be marketed, but premarketing data raised questions about possible hepatotoxicity? This would presumably be studied using a cohort study design and, depending upon the values chosen for α, β, the incidence of the disease in the unexposed, the relative risk one wants to be able to detect, and the ratio of control to exposed subjects, the sample sizes needed could differ markedly (see Table 3.2). For example, what if your goal was to study hepatitis that occurs, say, in 0.1% of all unexposed individuals? If one wanted to design a study with one control per exposed subject to detect a relative risk of 2.0 for this outcome variable, assuming an α (two-tailed) of 0.05 and a β of 0.1, one could look in Table A1 and see that it would require 31 483 exposed subjects, as well as an equal number of unexposed controls. If one were less concerned with missing a real finding, even if it was there, one could change β to 0.2, and the required sample size would drop to 23 518 (see Table 3.2 and Table A5). If one wanted to minimize the number of exposed subjects needed for the study, one could include up to four controls

Table 3.2. Examples of sample sizes needed for a cohort study

Disease	Incidence rate assumed in unexposed	α	β	Relative risk to be detected	Control: exposed ratio	Sample size needed in exposed group	Sample size needed in control group
Abnormal liver function tests	0.01	0.05 (2-tailed)	0.1	2	1	3 104	3 104
	0.01	0.05 (2-tailed)	0.2	2	1	2 319	2 319
	0.01	0.05 (2-tailed)	0.2	2	4	1 323	5 292
	0.01	0.05 (1-tailed)	0.2	2	4	1 059	4 236
	0.01	0.05 (2-tailed)	0.1	4	1	568	568
	0.01	0.05 (2-tailed)	0.2	4	1	425	425
	0.01	0.05 (2-tailed)	0.2	4	4	221	884
	0.01	0.05 (1-tailed)	0.2	4	4	179	716
Hepatitis	0.001	0.05 (2-tailed)	0.1	2	1	31 483	31 483
	0.001	0.05 (2-tailed)	0.2	2	1	23 518	23 518
	0.001	0.05 (2-tailed)	0.2	2	4	13 402	53 608
	0.001	0.05 (1-tailed)	0.2	2	4	10 728	42 912
	0.001	0.05 (2-tailed)	0.1	4	1	5 823	5 823
	0.001	0.05 (2-tailed)	0.2	4	1	4 350	4 350
	0.001	0.05 (2-tailed)	0.2	4	4	2 253	9 012
	0.001	0.05 (1-tailed)	0.2	4	4	1 829	7 316
Cholestatic jaundice	0.0001	0.05 (2-tailed)	0.1	2	1	315 268	315 268
	0.0001	0.05 (2-tailed)	0.2	2	1	235 500	235 500
	0.0001	0.05 (2-tailed)	0.2	2	4	134 194	536 776
	0.0001	0.05 (1-tailed)	0.2	2	4	107 418	429 672
	0.0001	0.05 (2-tailed)	0.1	4	1	58 376	58 376
	0.0001	0.05 (2-tailed)	0.2	4	1	43 606	43 606
	0.0001	0.05 (2-tailed)	0.2	4	4	22 572	90 288
	0.0001	0.05 (1-tailed)	0.2	4	4	18 331	73 324

for each exposed subject (Table 3.2 and Table A8). This would result in a sample size of 13 402, with four times as many controls, a total of 67 010 subjects. Finally, if one considers it inconceivable that this new drug could *protect* against liver disease and one is not interested in that outcome, then one might use a one-tailed α, resulting in a somewhat lower sample size of 10 728, again with four times as many controls. Much smaller sample sizes are needed to detect relative risks of 4.0 or greater; these are also presented in Table 3.2.

In contrast, what if one's goal was to study elevated liver function tests, which, say, occur in 1% of an unexposed population? If one wants to detect a relative risk of 2 for this more common outcome variable, only 3104 subjects would be needed in each group, assuming a two-tailed α of 0.05, a β of 0.1, and one control per exposed subject. Alternatively, if one wanted to detect the same relative risk for an outcome variable that occurred as infrequently as 0.0001, perhaps cholestatic jaundice, one would need 315 268 subjects in each study group.

Obviously, cohort studies can require very large sample sizes to study uncommon diseases. A study of uncommon diseases is often better performed using a case–control study design, as described in the previous chapter.

SAMPLE SIZE CALCULATIONS FOR CASE–CONTROL STUDIES

The approach to calculating sample sizes for case–control studies is similar to the approach for cohort studies. Again, there are five variables that need to be specified (see Table 3.1). Three of these are α, or the type I error one is willing to tolerate; β, or the type II error one is willing to tolerate; and the minimum odds ratio (an approximation of the relative risk) one wants to be able to detect. These are discussed in the section on cohort studies, above.

In addition, in a case–control study one selects subjects based on the presence or absence of the disease of interest, and then investigates the prevalence of the exposure of interest in each study group. This is in contrast to a cohort study, in which one selects subjects based on the presence or absence of an exposure, and then studies whether or not the disease of interest develops in each group. Therefore, the fourth variable to be specified for a case–control study is the expected prevalence of the exposure in the undiseased control group, rather than the incidence of the disease of interest in the unexposed control group of a cohort study.

Finally, analogous to the consideration in cohort studies of the ratio of the number of unexposed control subjects to the number of exposed study subjects, one needs to consider in a case–control study the ratio of the number of undiseased control subjects to the number of diseased study subjects. The principles in deciding upon the appropriate ratio to use are similar in both study designs. Again, there is rarely a reason to include a ratio greater than 3 : 1 or 4 : 1. For example, if one were to design a study with a two-tailed α of 0.05 to detect a relative risk of 2.0 for an exposure which occurs in 5% of the undiseased control group, a study with 516 diseased individuals and 516 controls would yield a power of 0.80, or an 80% chance of detecting a difference of that size. Studies with the same 516 diseased subjects and ratios of controls to cases of 1 : 1, 2 : 1, 3 : 1, 4 : 1, 5 : 1, 10 : 1, and 50 : 1 would result in statistical powers of 0.80, 0.889, 0.916, 0.929, 0.936, 0.949, and 0.959, respectively.

The formula for calculating sample sizes for a case–control study is similar to that for cohort studies (modified from Schlesselman):[3]

$$N = \frac{1}{(p-V)^2} \left[Z_{1-\alpha} \sqrt{\left(1 + \frac{1}{K}\right) U(1-U)} \right.$$
$$\left. + Z_{(1-\beta)} \sqrt{p(1-p)/K + V(1-V)} \right]^2$$

where R, α, β, $Z_{1-\alpha}$, and $Z_{1-\beta}$ are as above, p is the prevalence of the exposure in the control group, and K is the ratio of undiseased control subjects to diseased cases,

$$U = \frac{p}{K+1} K + \frac{R}{1 + p(R-1)}$$

and

$$V = \frac{pR}{1 + p(R-1)}$$

Again, a series of tables that provide sample sizes for case–control studies is presented in Appendix A. In Tables A9–A12, we have assumed an α (two-tailed) of 0.05, a beta of 0.1 (90% power), and control to case ratios of 1 : 1, 2 : 1, 3 : 1, and 4 : 1, respectively. Tables A13–A16 are similar, except they assume a β of 0.2 (80% power). Each table presents the number of diseased subjects needed to detect any of a number of specified relative risks, for a number of specified exposure rates.

For example, what if again one wanted to investigate a new nonsteroidal anti-inflammatory drug that is about to be marketed but premarketing data raised questions about possible hepatotoxicity? This time, however, one is attempting to use a case–control study design. Again, depending upon the values chosen of α, β, and so on, the sample sizes needed could differ markedly (see Table 3.3). For example, what if one wanted to design a study with one control per diseased subject, assuming an α (two-tailed) of 0.05 and a β of 0.1? The sample size needed to detect a relative risk of 2.0 for any disease would vary, depending on the prevalence of use of the drug being studied. If one optimistically assumed the drug will be used nearly as commonly as ibuprofen, by perhaps 1% of the population, then one could look at Table A9 and see that it would require 3210 diseased subjects and an equal number of undiseased controls. If one were less concerned with missing a real association, even if it existed, one could opt for a β of 0.2, and the required sample size would drop to 2398 (see Table 3.3 and Table A13). If one wanted to minimize the number of diseased subjects needed for the study, one could include up to four controls for each exposed subject (Table 3.3 and Table A16). This would result in a sample size of 1370, with four times as many controls. Finally, if one considers it inconceivable that this new drug could *protect* against liver disease, then one might use a one-tailed α, resulting in a somewhat lower sample size of 1096, again with four times as many controls. Much smaller sample sizes are needed to detect relative risks of 4.0 or greater and are also presented in Table 3.3.

In contrast, what if one's estimates of the new drug's sales were more conservative? If one wanted to detect a relative risk of 2.0 assuming sales to 0.1% of the population, perhaps similar to tolmetin, then 31 588 subjects would be needed in each group, assuming a two-tailed α of 0.05, a β of 0.1, and one control per diseased subject. In contrast, if one estimated the drug would be used in only 0.01% of patients, perhaps like phenylbutazone, one would need 315 373 subjects in each study group.

Obviously, case–control studies can require very large sample sizes to study relatively uncommonly used drugs. In addition, each disease requires a separate case group and, thereby, a separate study. As such, as described in the prior

Table 3.3. Examples of sample sizes needed for a case–control study

Hypothetical drug	Prevalence rate assumed in undiseased	α	β	Odds ratio to be detected	Control: case ratio	Sample size needed in case group	Sample size needed in control group
Ibuprofen	0.01	0.05 (2-tailed)	0.1	2	1	3 210	3 210
	0.01	0.05 (2-tailed)	0.2	2	1	2 398	2 398
	0.01	0.05 (2-tailed)	0.2	2	4	1 370	5 480
	0.01	0.05 (1-tailed)	0.2	2	4	1 096	4 384
	0.01	0.05 (2-tailed)	0.1	4	1	601	601
	0.01	0.05 (2-tailed)	0.2	4	1	449	449
	0.01	0.05 (2-tailed)	0.2	4	4	234	936
	0.01	0.05 (1-tailed)	0.2	4	4	190	760
Tolmetin	0.001	0.05 (2-tailed)	0.1	2	1	31 588	31 588
	0.001	0.05 (2-tailed)	0.2	2	1	23 596	23 596
	0.001	0.05 (2-tailed)	0.2	2	4	13 449	53 796
	0.001	0.05 (1-tailed)	0.2	2	4	10 765	43 060
	0.001	0.05 (2-tailed)	0.1	4	1	5 856	5 856
	0.001	0.05 (2-tailed)	0.2	4	1	4 375	4 375
	0.001	0.05 (2-tailed)	0.2	4	4	2 266	9 064
	0.001	0.05 (1-tailed)	0.2	4	4	1 840	7 360
Phenylbutazone	0.0001	0.05 (2-tailed)	0.1	2	1	315 373	315 373
	0.0001	0.05 (2-tailed)	0.2	2	1	235 579	235 579
	0.0001	0.05 (2-tailed)	0.2	2	4	134 240	536 960
	0.0001	0.05 (1-tailed)	0.2	2	4	107 455	429 820
	0.0001	0.05 (2-tailed)	0.1	4	1	58 409	58 409
	0.0001	0.05 (2-tailed)	0.2	4	1	43 631	43 631
	0.0001	0.05 (2-tailed)	0.2	4	4	22 585	90 340
	0.0001	0.05 (1-tailed)	0.2	4	4	18 342	73 368

chapter, studies of uncommonly used drugs and newly marketed drugs are usually better done using cohort study designs.

SAMPLE SIZE CALCULATIONS FOR CASE SERIES

As described in Chapter 2, the utility of case series in pharmacoepidemiology is limited, as the absence of a control group makes causal inference difficult. Despite this, however, this is a design that has been used repeatedly. There are scientific questions that can be addressed using this design, and the collection of a control group equivalent in size to the case series would add considerable cost to the study. Case series are usually used in pharmacoepidemiology to quantitate better the incidence of a particular disease in patients exposed to a newly marketed drug. For example, in the "Phase IV" postmarketing drug surveillance study conducted for prazosin, the investigators collected a case series of 10 000 newly exposed subjects recruited through the manufacturer's sales force, to quantitate better the incidence of first-dose syncope, which was a well-recognized

adverse effect of this drug.[5,6] Case series are usually used to determine whether a disease occurs more frequently than some predetermined incidence in exposed patients. Most often, the predetermined incidence of interest is zero, and one is looking for any occurrences of an extremely rare illness. As another example, when cimetidine was first marketed, there was a concern over whether it could cause agranulocytosis, since it was closely related chemically to metiamide, another H-2 blocker, which had been removed from the market in Europe because it caused agranulocytosis. This study also collected 10 000 subjects. It found only two cases of neutropenia, one in a patient also receiving chemotherapy. There were no cases of agranulocytosis.[7]

To establish drug safety, a study must include a sufficient number of subjects to detect an elevated incidence of a disease, if it exists. Generally, this is calculated by assuming the frequency of the event in question is vanishingly small, so that the occurrence of the event follows a Poisson distribution, and then one generally calculates 95% confidence intervals around the observed results.

Table A17 in Appendix A presents a table useful for making this calculation.[8] In order to apply this table, one first calculates the incidence rate observed from the study's results, that is the number of subjects who develop the disease of interest during the specified time interval, divided by the total number of individuals in the population at risk. For example, if three cases of liver disease were observed in a population of 1000 patients exposed to a new nonsteroidal anti-inflammatory drug during a specified period of time, the incidence would be 0.003. The number of subjects who develop the disease is the "Observed number on which estimate is based (n)" in Table A17. In this example, it is 3. The lower boundary of the 95% confidence interval for the incidence rate is then the corresponding "Lower limit factor (L)" multiplied by the observed incidence rate. In the example above, it would be $0.206 \times 0.003 = 0.000\ 618$. Analogously, the upper boundary would be the product of the corresponding "Upper limit factor (U)" multiplied by the observed incidence rate. In the above example, this would be $2.92 \times 0.003 = 0.00876$. In other words, the incidence rate (95% confidence interval) would be 0.003 (0.000618–0.00876). Thus, the best estimate of the incidence rate would be 30 per 10 000, but there is a 95% chance that it lies between 6.18 per 10 000 and 87.6 per 10 000.

In addition, a helpful simple guide is the so-called "rule of threes," useful in the common situation where no events of a particular kind are observed.[8] Specifically, if no events of a particular type are observed in a study of X individuals, then one can be 95% certain that the event occurs no more often than $3/X$. For example, if 500 patients are studied prior to marketing a drug, then one can be 95% certain that any event which does not occur in any of those patients may occur with a frequency of 3 or less in 500 exposed subjects, or that it has an incidence rate of less than 0.006. If 3000 subjects are exposed prior to drug marketing, then one can be 95% certain that any event which does not occur in this population may occur no more than 3 in 3000 subjects, or the events have an incidence rate of less than 0.001. Finally, if 10 000 subjects are studied in a postmarketing drug surveillance study, then one can be 95% certain that any events which are not observed may occur no more than 3 in 10 000 exposed individuals, or that they have an incidence rate of less than 0.0003. In other words, events not detected in the study may occur less often than 1 in 3333 subjects.

DISCUSSION

The above discussions about sample size determinations in cohort and case–control studies assume one is able to obtain information on each of the five variables that factor into these sample size calculations. Is this in fact realistic? Four of the variables are, in fact, totally in the control of the investigator, subject to his or her specification: α, β, the ratio of control subjects to study subjects, and the minimum relative risk to be detected. Only one of the variables requires data derived from other sources. For cohort studies, this is the expected incidence of the disease in the unexposed control group. For case–control studies, this is the expected prevalence of the exposure in the undiseased control group. In considering this needed information, it is important to realize that the entire process of sample size calculation is approximate, despite its mathematical sophistication. There is certainly no compelling reason why an α should be 0.05, as opposed to 0.06 or 0.04. The other variables specified by the investigator are similarly arbitrary. As such, only an approximate estimate is needed for this missing variable. Often the needed information is readily available from some existing data source, for example vital statistics or commercial drug utilization data sources. If not, one can search the medical literature for one or more studies that have collected these data for a defined population, either deliberately or as a by-product of their data collecting effort, and assume that the population you will study will be similar. If this is not an appropriate assumption, or if no such data exist in the medical literature, one is left with two alternatives. The first, and better, alternative is to conduct a small pilot study within your population, in order to measure the information you need. The second is simply to guess. In the second case, one should consider what a reasonable higher guess and a reasonable lower guess might be, as well, to see if your sample size should be increased to take into account the imprecision of your estimate.

Finally, what if one is studying multiple outcome variables (in a cohort study) or multiple exposure variables (in a case–control study), each of which differs in the frequency you expect in the control group? In that situation, an investigator might base the study's sample size on the variable that leads to the largest requirement, and note that the study will have even more power for the other outcome (or exposure) variables. It is usually better to have a somewhat larger than expected sample size than the minimum, anyway, to allow some leeway if any of the underlying assumptions were wrong. This also will permit subgroup analyses with adequate power. In fact, if there are important subgroup analyses that represent *a priori* hypotheses that one wants to be able to evaluate, one should perform separate sample size calculations for those subgroups.

Note that sample size calculation is often an iterative process. There is nothing wrong with performing an initial calculation, realizing that it generates an unrealistic sample size, and then modifying the underlying assumptions accordingly. What is important is that the investigator examines his or her final assumptions closely, asking whether, given the compromises made, the study is still worth undertaking.

Note that the discussion above was restricted to sample size calculations for dichotomous variables, i.e., variables with only two options: a study subject either has a disease or does not have a disease. Information was not presented on sample size calculations for continuous outcome variables, i.e., variables that have some measurement, such as height, weight, blood pressure, or serum cholesterol. Overall, the use of a continuous variable as an outcome variable, unless the measurement is extremely imprecise, will result in a marked increase in the power of a study. Details about this are omitted because epidemiologic studies unfortunately do not usually have the luxury of using such variables. Readers who are interested in more information on this can consult a textbook of sample size calculations.[9]

All of the previous discussions have focused on calculating a minimum necessary sample size. This is the usual concern. However, two other issues specific to pharmacoepidemiology are important to consider as well. First, one of the main advantages of postmarketing pharmacoepidemiology studies is the increased sensitivity to rare adverse reactions that can be achieved, by including a sample size larger than that used prior to marketing. Since between 500 and 3000 patients are usually studied before marketing, most pharmacoepidemiology cohort studies are designed to include at least 10 000 exposed subjects. The total population from which these 10 000 exposed subjects would be recruited would need to be very much larger, of course. Case–control studies can be much smaller, but generally need to recruit cases and controls from a source population of equivalent size as for cohort studies. These are not completely arbitrary figures, but are based on the principles described above, applied to the questions which remain of great importance to address in a postmarketing setting. Nevertheless, these figures should not be rigidly accepted but should be reconsidered for each specific study. Some studies will require fewer subjects; many will require more. To accumulate these sample sizes while performing cost-effective studies,

several special techniques have been developed, which are described in Part III of this book.

Second, because of the development of these new techniques, pharmacoepidemiology studies have the potential for the relatively unusual problem of *too large* a sample size. It is even more important than usual, therefore, when interpreting the results of studies that use these data systems to examine their findings, differentiating clearly between statistical significance and clinical significance. With a very large sample size, one can find statistically significant differences that are clinically trivial. In addition, it must be kept in mind that subtle findings, even if statistically and clinically important, could easily have been created by biases or confounders (see Chapter 2). Subtle findings should not be ignored, but should be interpreted with caution.

REFERENCES

1. Makuch RW, Johnson MF. Some issues in the design and interpretation of "negative" clinical trials. *Arch Intern Med* 1986; **146**: 986–9.
2. Young MJ, Bresnitz EA, Strom BL. Sample size nomograms for interpreting negative clinical studies. *Ann Intern Med* 1983; **99**: 248–51.
3. Schlesselman JJ. Sample size requirements in cohort and case–control studies of disease. *Am J Epidemiol* 1974; **99**: 381–4.
4. Stolley PD, Strom BL. Sample size calculations for clinical pharmacology studies. *Clin Pharmacol Ther* 1986; **39**: 489–90.
5. Graham RM, Thornell IR, Gain JM, Bagnoli C, Oates HF, Stokes GS. Prazosin: the first dose phenomenon. *BMJ* 1976; **2**: 1293–4.
6. *Joint Commission on Prescription Drug Use*. Final Report. Washington, DC, 1980.
7. Gifford LM, Aeugle ME, Myerson RM, Tannenbaum PJ. Cimetidine postmarket outpatient surveillance program. *JAMA* 1980; **243**: 1532–5.
8. Haenszel W, Loveland DB, Sirken MG. Lung cancer mortality as related to residence and smoking history. I. White males. *J Natl Cancer Inst* 1962; **28**: 947–1001.
9. Cohen J. *Statistical Power Analysis for the Social Sciences*. New York: Academic Press, 1977.

4

Basic Principles of Clinical Pharmacology Relevant to Pharmacoepidemiology Studies

DAVID A. HENRY[1], PATRICIA McGETTIGAN[2], ANNE TONKIN[3] and SEAN HENNESSY[4]

[1] Faculty of Health, The University of Newcastle, Newcastle, NSW, Australia; [2] Division of Medicine, Newcastle Mater Hospital, Waratah, NSW, Australia; [3] Department of Clinical and Experimental Pharmacology, University of Adelaide, South Australia, Australia; [4] Center for Clinical Epidemiology and Biostatistics, University of Pennsylvania School of Medicine, Philadelphia, Pennsylvania, USA.

INTRODUCTION

Clinical pharmacology comprises all aspects of the scientific study of medicinal drugs in humans.[1] Its overall objective is to provide the knowledge base needed to ensure rational drug therapy. In addition to studying biologic effects of drugs, clinical pharmacology includes the study of non-pharmacologic (e.g., economic and social) determinants and effects of medication use. The development of clinical pharmacology had its roots in the so-called "drug explosion" that occurred between the 1930s and 1960s, which was marked by a pronounced escalation of the rate at which new drugs entered the markets of economically developed nations. With this rapid expansion of the therapeutic armamentarium came the need for much more information regarding the effects and optimal use of these agents, which spurred the growth of clinical pharmacology as a scientific discipline.

Some would define an additional related discipline, *pharmacotherapeutics*, which is the application of the principles of clinical pharmacology to rational prescribing, the conduct of clinical trials, and the assessment of outcomes during real-life clinical practice.

Clinical pharmacology tries to explain the response to drugs in *individuals*, while pharmacoepidemiology is concerned with measuring and explaining variability in outcome of drug treatment in *populations*. However, there is great overlap in the scope of the two disciplines and many clinical pharmacologists are heavily involved in pharmacoepidemiologic research. Pharmacoepidemiology is the application of epidemiologic methods to the subject matter of clinical pharmacology. Of course, neither approach would be justified if responses to drugs were totally predictable. From this perspective, the origins of pharmacoepidemiology can be seen clearly in the disciplines of clinical pharmacology and pharmacotherapeutics.

Pharmacoepidemiology, Fourth Edition   Edited by B.L. Strom
© 2005 John Wiley & Sons, Ltd

In epidemiologic studies of non-drug exposures, it is frequently assumed that the amount and duration of exposure is proportional to the risk of the outcome. For instance, the risk of a stroke or heart attack is often presumed to increase in proportion both to the level of a risk factor, such as elevated blood pressure or blood cholesterol, and to the length of time the risk factor has been present. Likewise, duration of exposure to carcinogens (e.g., cigarette smoke) is sometimes assumed to be linearly related to the level of risk. On occasion, these proportionality assumptions hold true in pharmacoepidemiology. For instance, the risk of endometrial cancer increases in direct proportion to the duration of exposure to estrogens.[2] In other situations, proportionality assumptions are invalid, as is the case with rashes, hepatic reactions, and hematologic reactions to drugs, which often occur in the first few weeks of treatment, the risk declining thereafter. These apparently declining risks may be an artifact of the epidemiologic phenomenon known as "depletion of susceptibles" (where long-term users of a drug class tend to be those who are tolerant of the drug's effects), and/or they may be due to a number of biologic factors that are unique to the ways in which drugs elicit responses, are handled by the body, and are used in clinical practice.

Exposure to a drug is never a completely random event, as individuals who receive a drug almost always differ from those not receiving it. The circumstances leading to a patient receiving a particular drug in a particular dose, at a particular time, are complex and relate to the patient's health care behavior and use of services, the severity and nature of the condition being treated, and the perceived advantages of a drug in a specific setting. For many conditions, physicians alter or titrate the dose of a drug against a response, and will tend to switch medications in the case of non-response. Consequently, the choice of a drug and dose may be determined by factors that are themselves related to the outcome under study. In other words, the association between the drug and the outcome of interest may be confounded by the indication for the drug or other related features (see also Chapter 40). Because of the high probability of confounding beyond that which can be controlled for using measured variables (i.e., residual confounding), pharmacoepidemiologists tend to be cautious about the interpretation of weak associations between drug exposure and outcomes.

When interpreting pharmacoepidemiology studies, it is important to realize that relationships exist between drug response and various biologic and sociologic factors, and to attempt to explore the reasons for them. The discipline of clinical pharmacology has provided us with explanations for some of these variations in response to important drugs,

and knowledge of these is necessary when conducting or interpreting pharmacoepidemiology studies.

This chapter is intended to introduce readers to some of the core concepts of clinical pharmacology. Obviously, a single book chapter cannot convey the entire discipline; many general and topic-specific clinical pharmacology textbooks exist which accomplish this. The emphasis of this chapter will be on concepts that are likely to be important in conducting and understanding pharmacoepidemiologic research. In particular, one of the most important areas of study within clinical pharmacology that is inherently amenable to the use of epidemiologic methods is the variability of drug response that exists across the population. The following sections present some of the central concepts of clinical pharmacology that are important to the pharmacoepidemiologist who is attempting to understand differences in the population with regard to the effects of drugs. Specifically, this chapter will discuss the nature of drugs, the mechanisms of drug action, the concept of drug potency, the role of pharmacodynamics and pharmacokinetics (including genetic factors that influence these functions), and the importance of human behavior in explaining variability in drug effects.

THE NATURE OF DRUGS

A drug may be defined as any exogenously administered substance that exerts a physiologic effect. Taken as a group, drugs vary greatly with regard to their molecular structure. For example, interferon alfa-2a is an intricate glycoprotein, while potassium chloride is a simple salt containing only two elements. Most drugs are intermediate in complexity, and produce their pharmacologic response by exerting a chemical or molecular influence on one or more cell constituents.

Typically, the active drug component of a tablet, capsule, or other pharmaceutical dosage form accounts for only a small percentage of the total mass and volume. The remainder is composed of excipients (such as binders, diluents, lubricants, preservatives, coloring agents, and sometimes flavoring) that are chosen, among other concerns, because they are believed to be pharmacologically inert. This is relevant to the pharmacoepidemiologist because a drug product's ostensibly inactive ingredients can sometimes produce effects of their own. For example, benzyl alcohol, which is commonly used as a preservative in injectable solutions, has been implicated as the cause of a toxic syndrome that has resulted in the deaths of a number of infants.[3]

Also of potential concern to the pharmacoepidemiologist is the fact that, over time, a pharmaceutical product can be reformulated to contain different excipients. Furthermore, because of the marketing value of established proprietary drug product names, non-prescription products are sometimes reformulated to contain different active ingredients, and then continue to be marketed under their original brand name. This is potentially of concern to any pharmacoepidemiologist interested in studying the effects of non-prescription drugs. It also is a potential source of medication errors (see also Chapter 34).

MECHANISMS OF DRUG ACTION

Pharmacology seeks to characterize the actions of drugs at many different levels of study, such as the organism, organ, tissue, cell, cell component, and molecular levels. On the macromolecular level, most drugs elicit a response through interactions with specialized proteins such as enzymes and cell surface receptors. While drug molecules may be present within body fluids either in their free, native state, or bound to proteins or other constituents, it is typically the free or unbound fraction that is available to interact with the target proteins, and is thus important in eliciting a response.

Enzymes are protein catalysts, or molecules that permit certain biochemical reactions to occur more rapidly. By directly inhibiting an enzyme, a drug may block the formation of its product. For instance, inhibition of angiotensin-converting enzyme blocks the conversion of angiotensin I to its active form, angiotensin II, resulting in a fall in arteriolar resistance that is beneficial to individuals with hypertension or congestive heart failure. Other drugs block ion channels, and consequently alter intracellular function. For example, calcium channel blocking drugs reduce the entry of calcium ions into smooth muscle cells, thereby inhibiting smooth muscle contraction, dilating blood vessels, and so reducing arteriolar resistance.[4]

Alternatively, drugs may interact with specialized receptors on the cell surface, which activate a subsequent intracellular signaling system, ultimately resulting in changes in the intracellular milieu. For instance, drugs that bind to and activate β2-adrenoceptors (β2-agonists) in the pulmonary airways increase intracellular cyclic adenosine monophosphate concentrations and activate protein kinases, resulting in smooth muscle relaxation and bronchodilation.[5] Many drugs act through interaction with G-protein-coupled receptors on the surface of cells. These are specialized protein receptors that thread through the double lipid layer in cell membranes and broadcast to the inside of the cell that a drug is on the outside.[5] Other drugs, such as the purine and pyrimidine antagonists that are used in cancer chemotherapy, and the nucleoside analogues that are used in the treatment of HIV and other viral infections, exert their effects by blocking cell replication processes.

DRUG POTENCY

In its pharmacologic usage, the term potency refers to the amount of drug that is required to elicit a given response, and is important when one is comparing two or more drugs that have similar effects. For example, 10 mg morphine has approximately the same analgesic activity as 1.3 mg hydromorphone when both drugs are administered by injection.[6] Thus, we say that 10 mg morphine is approximately "equipotent" to 1.3 mg hydromorphone, and that hydromorphone is approximately 7.7 times as potent as morphine (10/1.3=7.7). As an aside, there is sometimes a tendency to equate potency with "effectiveness," yielding the misconception that because one drug is more potent than its alternative, it is therefore more effective. This view is fallacious. As the active drug component typically accounts for only a small portion of a pharmaceutical dosage form, the amount of drug that can be conveniently delivered to the patient is rarely at issue; if need be, the dose can simply be increased. Milligram potency is rarely an important consideration in therapeutic drug use, while maximal efficacy (which indicates the maximum effect the drug can exert) is much more important.

On the other hand, drug potency may be important in interpreting pharmacoepidemiology studies. For example, if a particular drug is noted to have a higher rate of adverse effects than other drugs of the same class, it is important to investigate whether this is a result of an intrinsic effect of that drug, or if the drug is being used in clinical practice at a higher dose, relative to its potency, than other drugs of the class. For instance, this may explain some of the apparent differences in risks of serious gastrointestinal complications with individual nonsteroidal anti-inflammatory drugs.[7]

PHARMACODYNAMICS AND PHARMACOKINETICS

Clinical pharmacology can be divided broadly into pharmacodynamics and pharmacokinetics. *Pharmacodynamics* quantifies the response of the target tissues in the body to a given concentration of a drug. *Pharmacokinetics* is the study of the processes of drug absorption, distribution, and elimination from the body. Put simply, pharmacodynamics is concerned with the drug's action on the body, while pharmacokinetics is concerned with the body's action on the drug. The combined effects of these processes determine the time course of concentrations of a drug at its target sites and the consequences of the presence of the drug at that concentration. The role of each in contributing to the variability of drug effects among the population will be discussed in turn.

THE ROLE OF PHARMACODYNAMICS IN DETERMINING VARIABILITY OF DRUG RESPONSE

Compared with most non-drug exposures, there is considerable existing knowledge about the effects of a drug by the time it is marketed. This must be incorporated into the design of new studies that seek to gain further information about that drug's actions. This is true whether the design of the new study is experimental or nonexperimental. Further, there is considerable information about determinants of patients' responses to drugs in general. In this section, we present the effects of genetics, adaptive responses, age, disease states, and concomitant drugs in determining variability in drug response.

GENETIC DETERMINANTS OF HUMAN RESPONSES TO DRUGS

This is the most rapidly developing area of research in clinical pharmacology (also see Chapter 37). The science of genomics helps us understand (and possibly predict) who will respond (or not) to a drug and who will develop serious toxicity at doses that are normally therapeutic in effect. Investigations into genetic determinants have concentrated on three main areas: drug actions, drug transporters, and drug metabolism.[8] The latter two topics are discussed later in the sections on pharmacokinetics. Single nucleoside polymorphisms in genes that code for drug receptors can result in variability in responses to certain drugs. Genetic polymorphisms are differences in the sequence of DNA occurring with a frequency of 1% or more, which can lead to the formation of proteins that do not work properly. For example, polymorphism of the β_2 adrenoceptor leads to lack of response to bronchodilators, and genetic variations in the $5HT_{2a}$ receptor lead to resistance to the anti-psychotic agent clozapine.[9] Polymorphisms of different genes affecting platelet and endothelial cell function may be associated with an increased risk of thrombosis, and a relative resistance to the anti-thrombotic effects of low dose aspirin.[10] Polymorphisms in response genes may also predict the risk of adverse reactions. Mutations of multiple genes are associated with the "long QT syndrome" and a propensity to ventricular arrhythmia with drugs such as antihistamines, macrolide antibiotics, and cisapride.[9] The affected genes encode cardiac ion channels (K^+ and Na^+), which have a major role in suppressing arrhythmias initiated by premature beats.[11]

It can be appreciated that gene polymorphisms have potentially important roles in explaining variations in the beneficial and adverse effects to a wide range of drugs.

Pharmacoepidemiology, historically, has estimated the average effects of drugs in populations and the trend has been to pursue efficient designs, particularly through the exploitation of data stored in electronic medical records and administrative databases (see Chapters 13–22), which can be linked in order to study the relationship between exposure and outcome. As the science of pharmacogenomics evolves, there is a growing need to incorporate biologic sampling, either through revisiting more efficient *ad hoc* study designs, or through linkage of medical or administrative records to banks of biosamples. These designs will raise significant ethical issues that have not been features of traditional pharmacoepidemiology studies (see also Chapter 38).

EFFECTS OF ADAPTIVE RESPONSES

It is a general rule of pharmacology that pharmacodynamic responses are often followed by adaptive responses which, crudely put, are the body's attempt to "overcome" or "counteract" the effects of the drug. An example is the increase in the concentration of the membrane-bound enzyme Na^+/K^+ ATPase that occurs during continued treatment with cardiac glycosides such as digoxin. As cardiac glycosides exert their effects by inhibiting Na^+/K^+ ATPase, the localized increase in the concentration, or up-regulation, of this enzyme that occurs during therapy may be responsible for the relatively transient inotropic effects of the drugs that are seen in some individuals.

Cell surface adrenoceptors tend to up-regulate during prolonged administration of β-adrenergic blocking agents such as propranolol, resulting in increased numbers of active β-receptors. If the beta-blocking drug is withdrawn rapidly from a patient, a large number of β-receptors become available to bind to norepinephrine and epinephrine, their natural ligands. This can produce tachycardia, hypertension, and worsening angina—the so-called "beta-blocker withdrawal syndrome."[12]

In some cases, the mechanisms of apparent adaptive responses have not yet been fully explored. For example, among subjects taking nonsteroidal anti-inflammatory drugs (NSAIDs), endoscopic studies have documented gastrointestinal mucosal damage within days of commencing treatment.[13] Endoscopic investigation of patients chronically exposed to aspirin found that the mucosal damage appeared to resolve over time.[14] While this suggests that continued exposure promotes gastric adaptation, the mechanism by which this might occur is unclear. Pharmacoepidemiology studies of gastric ulceration and its complications of bleeding, perforation, and stenosis were in keeping with the observation, suggesting that the risk of gastrointestinal complications was highest in the early weeks of NSAID treatment, and declined thereafter.[15,16] However, more recent evidence has questioned this conclusion. In a record linkage study, MacDonald *et al.* found that the increased risks of admission to hospital with gastrointestinal complications related to NSAID use were constant during continuous exposure and that excess risk appeared to persist for at least a year after the last exposure.[17] So the experimental and observational studies of adaptation are somewhat at odds in their findings, which illustrates that it is not always possible to correlate our biologic understanding with epidemiologic observations; sometimes the latter can inform the former, a reversal of a common view of the discovery process. In the case of NSAIDs, the field of study has tended to be overtaken by the introduction of the controversial COX-2 inhibitor drugs (e.g., rofecoxib), which have a lower risk of causing serious gastrointestinal complications than non-selective NSAIDs, but increase the risk of vascular occlusion.

EFFECTS OF AGE

On the whole, the effects of age on pharmacodynamic responses have been less well studied than its effects on pharmacokinetics. This is particularly so in the very young, who are rarely included in experimental studies to investigate the clinical effects of drugs. Although it may seem counterintuitive, the elderly are often *equally* or even *less* sensitive to the primary pharmacologic effects of some drugs than are the young. But, overall the elderly behave as though they have a "reduced functional reserve" and their secondary homeostatic responses may be impaired. Several examples of the effects of old age on pharmacodynamic responses may be found in the cardiovascular therapeutics:

- It has long been known that elderly subjects are relatively resistant to the effects of both the β-agonist drug isoproterenol and the β-blocking drug, propranolol.[18] The extent to which this is due to elevated levels of plasma catecholamines and alterations in β-receptor numbers is not clear.
- Elegant experimental work has demonstrated that elderly subjects have a blunted primary electrophysiologic response to the calcium channel blocking drug verapamil.[19] The degree of prolongation of the electrocardiographic P-R interval in response to a given concentration of verapamil was *less* pronounced in elderly than in younger subjects.[19] However, in contrast to its effect on the P-R interval, verapamil produces a

greater drop in blood pressure in the elderly than it does in younger subjects. How may the last two observations be reconciled? The likely answer is that both the secondary adaptive physiologic responses and the primary pharmacologic response are impaired in the elderly subjects. Maintenance of blood pressure depends on activation of the sympathetic nervous system, which tends to be less responsive in the elderly.[18] It is likely that impairment of secondary (adaptive) responses, rather than increased sensitivity to the primary pharmacologic actions *per se*, accounts for the increased susceptibility of elderly subjects to the side effects of many drugs.

Homeostatic regulation (the body's control of its internal environment) is often impaired in the elderly and may contribute to the occurrence of adverse events as well as increased sensitivity to drug effects. For example, older individuals have an impaired ability to excrete a free water load, possibly as a result of lower renal prostaglandin production. This may be exacerbated by treatments that further impair either free water excretion, such as diuretics, or renal prostaglandin production, for example, NSAIDs. In either case, there is a risk of dilutional hyponatremia or volume overload.

Postural hypotension (the sudden drop in blood pressure that occurs with standing or sitting up, particularly in patients on antihypertensive drugs) is frequently symptomatic in the elderly; the pathogenesis probably includes decreased baroreceptor response, altered sympathetic activity and responsiveness, impaired arteriolar and venous vasomotor responses, and altered volume regulation. Accordingly, drugs that alter central nervous system function, sympathetic activity, vasomotor response, cardiac function, or volume regulation may exacerbate postural changes in blood pressure. The list of agents is extensive and includes such commonly used drugs as phenothiazines, antihypertensives, diuretics, and levodopa.

EFFECTS OF DISEASE STATES

The effects of disease states on pharmacodynamics have not been widely studied. As most diseases that lead to organ failure are more common in older subjects, the effects of disease can be confounded by age. It is a common clinical observation that individuals with certain diseases can have exaggerated responses to particular drugs. For example, individuals with chronic liver or lung disease sometimes exhibit extreme sensitivity to drugs that depress central nervous system function, such as benzodiazepines and opiates.[20,21] This apparent increase in drug sensitivity may be due to: (i) changes in receptor function, which would increase actual sensitivity to drugs, or (ii) disease-related changes in neuronal function, such as occurs in encephalopathy caused by severe lung or liver disease. A further possibility, in the case of liver failure, is the presence of elevated concentrations of circulating endogenous ligands that bind to the benzodiazepine receptor, the effect of which is additive to that of diazepam.[22]

Another example of the role of disease states in pharmacodynamic variability is the propensity for NSAIDs to impair renal function in certain groups of individuals.[23] Both congestive heart failure and hepatic failure are characterized by high circulating levels of the vasoconstrictor hormones norepinephrine, angiotensin II, and antidiuretic hormone. In response to the presence of these hormones, the kidneys release prostaglandins to modulate their vasoconstrictor effects and thus help preserve renal blood flow in times of physiologic stress. In susceptible individuals, inhibition of prostaglandin synthesis (for example, as a result of NSAID administration) can lead to unopposed vasoconstriction with a marked and rapid reduction in renal blood flow, and a consequent fall in the rate of glomerular filtration.

DRUG–DRUG INTERACTIONS THAT OCCUR THROUGH PHARMACODYNAMIC MECHANISMS

Although many important drug–drug interactions occur through pharmacokinetic mechanisms, a number of important interactions are pharmacodynamic in nature. Pharmacodynamic interactions arise as a consequence of drugs acting on the same receptors, sites of action, or physiological systems and having either synergistic or antagonistic effects. In examining the variability that exists within the population with regard to the effects of drugs, the presence or absence of concomitant medications can play a particularly important role and must be considered as potential causal or confounding variables in pharmacoepidemiology studies.

For example, individuals with any given serum digoxin concentration are more likely to suffer from digoxin toxicity if they are depleted of certain electrolytes, such as magnesium and potassium. Thus, patients on concomitant magnesium-/potassium-wasting diuretics such as furosemide are more likely than those who are not to develop arrhythmias, given the same serum digoxin concentration.

Many drugs have central nervous system depressant effects and these may be potentiated where a number of such agents are used together, such as hypnotics, anxiolytics, antidepressants, opioids, anti-epileptics, antihistamines, and methyldopa. A "serotonergic syndrome" (consisting of mental

changes, muscle rigidity, hypertension, tremor, hyperreflexia, and diarrhea) may be induced in some patients given combinations of proserotonergic drugs such as selective serotonin reuptake inhibitors (SSRIs), tramadol, tricyclic antidepressants, monoamine oxidase inhibitors (MAOIs), carbamazepine, and lithium.

Competition between drugs acting at the same receptor sites usually results in antagonistic effects. These may be desired, as in the case of naloxone or flumazenil given to reverse central nervous system depression or coma resulting from opiate or benzodiazepine overdose, respectively, or unintended, as in the case of the mutual antagonism occurring between β-agonists (bronchodilators) and non-selective β-antagonists (bronchoconstrictors).

Sildenafil selectively inhibits cyclic guanosine monophosphate (cGMP)-specific phosphodiesterase type 5, the predominant enzyme metabolizing cGMP in the smooth muscles of the corpus cavernosum. By doing so, it restores the erectile response to sexual stimulation in men with erectile dysfunction.[24] However, the formation in the first place of cavernosal cGMP is due to the release of nitric oxide in response to sexual stimulation. In men taking concomitant nitrate drugs for heart disease, there is a risk of a precipitous fall in blood pressure due to potentiation by sildenafil of their hypotensive effects, mediated by vascular smooth muscle relaxation. Although concomitant use is contraindicated by the manufacturer, a number of sildenafil-associated deaths are thought to have been due to this drug combination.

Case–control pharmacoepidemiology studies have demonstrated an association between long-term use (>3 months) of certain appetite suppressants (phentermine plus fenfluramine or dexfenfluramine, or dexfenfluramine alone) and cardiac valve abnormalities.[25] The use of amphetamine-like appetite suppressants, mainly fenfluramine and dexfenfluramine, has also been associated with primary pulmonary hypertension.[26] It has been postulated that these unintended effects were due to serotonin accumulation as a consequence of both increased release and reduced removal of serotonin. Serotonin is the predominant mediator of pulmonary vasoconstriction caused by aggregating platelets and has been shown to increase pulmonary vascular smooth muscle proliferation. Prolonged use of fenfluramine and dexfenfluramine may produce an excess of serotonin sufficient to damage blood vessels in the lungs. Serotonin excess is also thought to be responsible for the cardiac damage as the pathological findings in damaged valves resembled those of carcinoid heart disease or heart disease associated with ergotamine toxicity, both of which are serotonin-related syndromes. Both fenfluramine and dexfenfluramine were withdrawn from the worldwide market in 1997.

In conclusion, adaptive responses, age, disease states, and concomitant medications can each have important effects on pharmacodynamic responses, and may result in considerable heterogeneity in the responses to drugs, both between and within individuals. Allowance must be made for this when interpreting pharmacoepidemiologic data.

We will now consider the effects of pharmacokinetic determinants of variability in drug response.

THE ROLE OF PHARMACOKINETICS IN DETERMINING VARIABILITY OF DRUG RESPONSE

As noted earlier, pharmacokinetics is the science that describes the time course of the absorption, distribution, and elimination of drugs within the body, the processes which in turn determine the concentration of drug at its active site. From a research perspective, it is generally easier to measure changing concentrations of drugs in body fluids than it is to characterize the pharmacologic responses to those concentrations. Consequently, the literature on pharmacokinetics is voluminous, and it could be said that clinical pharmacology as a discipline has been overly concerned with its study. However, it must be acknowledged that variation in pharmacokinetic parameters is an important cause of the observed heterogeneity that exists with regard to patients' response to drugs. In this section, we review the processes of absorption, distribution, and elimination of drugs, and then consider the effects of age, genetics, disease, and concomitant medications. First, however, it is useful to define some of the basic mathematical parameters that are used in pharmacokinetics.

BASIC MATHEMATICAL PARAMETERS USED IN PHARMACOKINETICS

Figure 4.1 shows the serum concentration of a hypothetical drug following a single intravenous bolus injection, plotted against time. Because the rate of decline of serum drug concentrations, like many other natural phenomena, frequently appears to be log-linear, the vertical axis is plotted on a logarithmic scale. It was observed that, for some drugs, the initial portion of the log-concentration versus time curve deviates notably from the line that is defined by the terminal portion of the curve. For this reason, the concept of pharmacokinetic compartments was developed. A *pharmacokinetic compartment* is a theoretical space, defined mathematically,

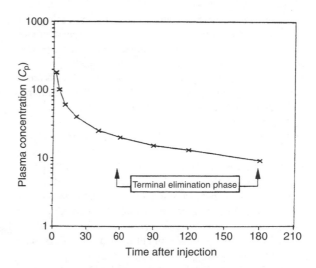

Figure 4.1. Plasma concentration–time curve of a hypothetical drug after intravenous administration. Note the early rapid decline in blood levels which reflects distribution of the drug, a consequence of its lipid solubility and degree of protein binding. The terminal phase of the concentration–time curve is log-linear and reflects elimination of the drug from the central compartment. This may be by renal clearance or hepatic metabolism. In this case, the terminal elimination phase is equivalent to a half-life of about 100 minutes.

into which drug molecules are said to distribute, and is represented by a given linear component of the log-concentration versus time curve. It is not an actual anatomic or physiologic space, but is sometimes thought of as a tissue or group of tissues that have similar blood flow and drug affinity. Because of the rather theoretical basis of mathematical modeling clinical pharmacologists have, more recently, been trying to correlate plasma concentration time curves more closely with physiological parameters such as cardiac output and tissue partition coefficients. The incorporation of these variables sometimes improves the accuracy and predictive ability of kinetic models.

The initial, rapid decline of measured drug concentration (Figure 4.1) is attributed to distribution of drug molecules through plasma and into other well-perfused tissues. This is usually referred to as the *distribution phase*. After the concentration of drug molecules has reached equilibrium across the compartments the more gradual decline in serum concentrations that is seen at the right-hand portion of the curve represents the elimination of drug from the body, and is referred to as the *terminal elimination phase*.

Because the dose of injected drug is known, and the initial plasma concentration immediately following administration (C_p, the peak plasma concentration) can be extrapolated from the points on the curve, a pharmacokinetic parameter known as *apparent volume of distribution*, or V_d, can be calculated by dividing dose by C_p. V_d is expressed in units of volume, such as liters, and is the volume into which the drug *appears* to have been dissolved in order to produce the actual peak concentration. Just as with pharmacokinetic compartments, the apparent volume of distribution is a theoretical, rather than an actual, volume, although it does have some physiologic interpretability. For example, a highly lipid-soluble drug such as a tricyclic antidepressant may have an apparent volume of distribution of hundreds of liters. This is because the drug partitions readily into fatty tissue, leaving little measurable drug in the bloodstream.

The slope of the line that represents the elimination phase is known as the *elimination rate constant*, or K_e, and is expressed in units of reciprocal time, such as hour^{-1}. Because of the linearity of the terminal elimination phase on a semi-log plot, the time that it takes for any given drug concentration to decline to half of this original concentration is constant, and is known as the drug's *half-life*, or $T_{1/2}$. Half-life is expressed in units of time, such as hours. Mathematically, this parameter is calculated from the elimination rate constant using the formula: $T_{1/2} = 0.693/K_e$.

An additional pharmacokinetic parameter, *clearance*, or Cl, can also be defined. Again, this is a theoretical parameter, and refers to the volume whose concentration is being measured that *appears* to be completely cleared of drug, per unit of time, regardless of the clearance mechanism. It is expressed in units of volume per unit time, such as liters per hour. Clearance can be calculated by taking the product of the apparent volume of distribution and the elimination rate constant. It is important to note that both volume of distribution and the rate of clearance together determine the half-life of elimination ($T_{1/2} = (0.693 \times V_d)/Cl$).

When a drug is administered according to a stable dosing regimen, the plasma drug concentration eventually reaches an equilibrium state, in which the amount of drug being administered equals the amount of drug being eliminated from the body (Figure 4.2). This is referred to as *steady state*. The amount of time required for a drug to reach steady state depends on the rate of elimination of the drug from that individual. For the purposes of therapeutic drug monitoring, achieving >95% of the steady state concentration is generally considered sufficient in order to estimate the true steady state concentration. This can be accomplished by obtaining a biologic sample after approximately five

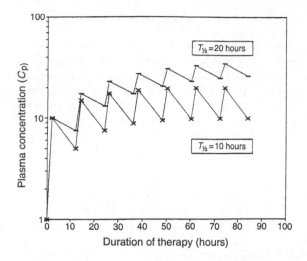

Figure 4.2. Profile of plasma drug concentrations for two hypothetical drugs during repeated 12-hourly dosing schedule. The lower curve relates to a drug with a half-life of 10 hours; steady state concentrations are achieved after 50–60 hours. In contrast, the upper curve relates to a drug with a half-life of 20 hours and the plasma concentrations are still rising at the end of the study.

drug half-lives. The amount of drug that is administered affects the *magnitude* of the steady state drug concentration, but not the *amount of time* that it takes to reach steady state. Under these circumstances a longer half-life results in a longer time to achieve steady state concentrations and a tendency to accumulate. This can lead to toxicity when a long half-life drug is commenced in hospital and suitable arrangements are not made for follow-up and monitoring of either drug concentrations or effects.

EFFECTS OF VARIATIONS IN DRUG ABSORPTION

In clinical practice, most drugs are administered by mouth. Because most drug molecules are small and at least partially lipid soluble, they are absorbed by *passive diffusion* across the large surface area of the mucosa lining the small intestine. The extent of absorption is determined primarily by the physicochemical properties of the drug and the integrity of the small intestine, while the *rate* of absorption depends largely on gastric emptying time and the motility of the small intestine. Both increasing age and the presence of disease states sometimes affect the extent and rate of gastrointestinal absorption of drugs; if they have an effect, both will tend to *decrease* absorption. Reduced absorption can also result from co-ingestion of drugs with chelating agents. For instance, the anion-binding resin cholestyramine (used to bind bile acids and reduce blood cholesterol levels) is capable of binding a variety of drugs, including statins (e.g., fluvastatin, simvastatin), which may be co-ingested by patients with severe hypercholesterolemia.

Rarely, variations in absorption may increase the rate or extent of the systemic availability of a drug and cause adverse effects. This is usually explained by altered bio-availability following a formulation change. An example of this was seen in Australia involving the calcium antagonist nifedipine, which was available both as sustained release tablets and as rapid release capsules. Individuals who were switched inadvertently from the former to the same dose of the latter sometimes experienced hypotension, presumably due to rapid absorption leading to elevated peak concentrations of the drug, with subsequent vasodilatation.[27]

Absorption of drugs is not confined to the gastrointestinal tract. Systemic absorption of drugs may occur following unintended absorption via other routes, such as transdermally, following administration by metered-dose inhaler, or ocular instillation. Each of these may result in adverse drug effects. The ability of lipid-soluble compounds to be absorbed across intact skin has been utilized in the design of transdermal delivery systems for several drugs, including estradiol, nitroglycerin, nicotine, and scopolamine.

Transdermal drug absorption can produce adverse as well as beneficial effects, as illustrated by the hexachlorophene toxicity that occurred in neonates following the mixture of excessive quantities of this antiseptic with talcum powder, and in another instance, following the inadvertent contamination of talcum powder with the anticoagulant warfarin.[28,29] Neonates are particularly susceptible to the effects of transdermal drug exposure because their skin provides a poor barrier to systemic absorption, and because they have a large surface area in proportion to their body weight. In a similar fashion, quantities of corticosteroid sufficient to produce systemic effects can be swallowed following administration from a metered-dose inhaler.[30] Beta-blocking drugs instilled into the eyes can travel down the naso-lachrymal duct to be swallowed and absorbed, inducing bronchospasm or exacerbation of congestive heart failure in susceptible individuals.[31]

In summary, because variability in the absorption of oral dosage forms of drugs from the gastrointestinal tract typically *reduces* absorption it is more important as a cause of lack of efficacy than an increase in adverse effects. However, unintended systemic absorption can occur through a variety of routes, and can have important consequences.

EFFECTS OF VARIATION IN SYSTEMIC DISTRIBUTION OF DRUGS

As drug molecules are absorbed, they are distributed to various tissues at a rate and to an extent that are determined by: (i) the lipid solubility of the drug, (ii) the degree of protein binding of the drug, and (iii) the amount of blood flow received by the different tissues. A high degree of lipid solubility confers an ability to move readily across cell membranes and to accumulate in lipid environments, and therefore results in a higher proportion of drug molecules being distributed to fatty tissues. Extensive binding to plasma proteins will reduce movement of drug molecules out of the central compartment, and thus reduce the drug's apparent volume of distribution. Better perfused tissues will tend to receive a larger amount of drug than tissues which are poorly perfused.

Protein binding is an aspect of drug distribution that receives considerable attention—perhaps more than it deserves. Untoward effects of drugs are often attributed to altered protein binding, which can occur in certain disease states, pregnancy, or when other highly protein-bound drugs are taken concurrently. However, there are relatively few occasions when disease-induced disturbances of protein binding or protein binding drug–drug interactions have been shown to have clinically important effects. The main reason for this is that, while it is the free fraction of drug that interacts with target proteins in order to produce a pharmacologic effect, it is also the free fraction that is available to the clearance mechanisms. Therefore, any increase in the free drug concentration that is caused by either reduced albumin levels or by displacement by other drugs is also accompanied by an increase in clearance, so that the free, active concentration ultimately changes little.[32] The period of time for which there may be an important increase in free concentration is limited to about three half-lives after onset of the interaction. There are occasional situations in which this general rule may not apply, particularly where small changes in concentrations have large effects, or where the drug has a single clearance mechanism that has a limited capacity, and therefore can become saturated.

Research has revealed that not all drug distribution is passive. There is growing interest in the function of drug "transporters." Drug transporters are specialized proteins that mediate the efflux of drugs (i.e., transport out) from cells and tissues.[8] The most studied mediator is P-glycoprotein, which is located in the plasma membrane, and translocates its substrates from the inside of the cells to the outside.[33] Interest in this protein arose from the observation that over-expression of P-glycoprotein in cancer cells leads to low intracellular concentrations of anti-cancer drugs and apparent resistance of the tumors to treatment. Subsequent research has revealed a wider potential for this transporter to explain variations in the actions of a range of compounds, by reducing concentrations in various tissues, including the central nervous system. For instance, recent work has docu-mented polymorphism of the drug transporter gene ABCB1, which codes for P-glycoprotein, and causes resistance to a wide range of anticonvulsant drugs.[34]

In conclusion, changes in drug distribution are often cited as reasons for variability in response to drugs and, therefore, may be implicated when seeking explanations for pharma-coepidemiologic findings. Alterations in the passive phases of drug distribution rarely produce clinically important effects. However, new information on the role of drug trans-porters suggests that variability in these active processes may account for lack of efficacy to various drug classes.

EFFECTS OF VARIATION IN DRUG ELIMINATION

Drugs are excreted from the body either as the unchanged parent compound, or as one or more products of drug metabolism. Although a number of organs, including the biliary system, the lungs, and the skin, participate in drug elimination, the kidneys play the most important role. Most excretory organs remove water-soluble compounds more efficiently than they remove lipid-soluble compounds. Consequently, water-soluble drugs tend to be eliminated unchanged in the urine, while lipid-soluble drugs tend to undergo metabolism to more water-soluble products, usually in the liver, prior to being excreted.

Effects of Variation in Renal Elimination

Virtually all drugs are small enough to be filtered through the glomeruli, the filtering units of the kidney, into the renal tubules. The extent of *glomerular filtration* depends on both the perfusion pressure to the glomeruli, and the protein binding characteristics of the drug. Because only the unbound fraction of a drug in the bloodstream is available to be filtered, a high degree of protein binding and a high affinity of the drug for the binding protein will limit the amount of drug that reaches the renal tubules. Once inside the renal tubules, lipid-soluble drugs are readily reabsorbed into the bloodstream, across the lipid membranes of the cells lining the renal tubules, leaving virtually none of the filtered fraction to be excreted in the urine. Because this process does not involve the consumption of cellular energy, it is known as *passive tubular reabsorption*. Water-soluble drugs, such as aminoglycoside antibiotics and digoxin, do not cross the tubular membrane and therefore remain in the urine and are excreted. *Active tubular secretion* occurs when substances are secreted into the renal tubules by energy-consuming carrier proteins. It is an important clearance mechanism for a number of drugs, including penicillin.

For drugs that are readily ionized at physiologic pH, such as salicylates, pH can be a crucial determinant of renal excretion. Because the non-ionized (uncharged) drug fraction is the most lipid soluble, it is most likely to undergo passive tubular reabsorption. Therefore, the renal excretion of salicylates, which are ionized at high (alkaline) pH, can be enhanced by the pharmacologic alkalinization of the urine. This characteristic is exploited when alkaline diuresis is used to enhance renal clearance in cases of salicylate poisoning.

From a pharmacoepidemiology standpoint, the importance of renal clearance is that it can be estimated and, therefore, individuals can be identified who are at risk of toxicity through accumulation of water-soluble drugs. This is much simpler than estimating hepatic function (see below).

Plasma creatinine concentration is a measure of renal function that is frequently used in clinical practice. The rate at which the kidneys clear creatinine from the blood (creatinine clearance) correlates closely with the glomerular filtration rate. Creatinine concentration at any point in time is a func-tion of production and clearance, both of which tend to decline to a proportionally similar degree with age; the former because of declining muscle mass, the latter because of an age-related decline in numbers of functioning glomeruli. For example, a blood creatinine level of $0.1\,\mathrm{mmol\,l^{-1}}$ in an 80-year-old female reflects a much lower level of renal function than the same creatinine concentration in a 20-year-old male (Figure 4.3).

The importance of considering age when interpreting plasma creatinine concentrations is illustrated in Figure 4.3. If both subjects mentioned in the previous paragraph required treatment with digoxin, the dose used to achieve therapeutic concentrations in the older subject would be less than half that required by the young man. Remember that these individuals have identical blood creatinine concen-trations, illustrating the limitations of relying on this parameter solely as a measure of renal function.

In conclusion, it is important to take account of variation in renal function when conducting pharmacoepidemiology studies of drugs for which this is the principal route of

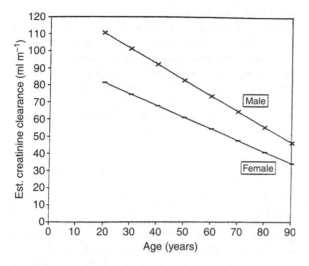

Figure 4.3. Change in estimated creatinine clearance (Cockcroft and Gault formula[35]) with age in a male and a female who maintain a serum creatinine of 0.1 mmol l^{-1} (NR 0.07–0.12 mmol l^{-1}), throughout their lives. In estimating creatinine clearance, it was assumed that the male maintained a weight of 75 kg, and the female a weight of 60 kg. The figure indicates that creatinine clearance declines in a linear fashion with age, and serum creatinine, alone, is an inadequate measure of glomerular filtration. Consequently, the clearance of some drugs is impaired in the elderly. For instance, the female depicted at 80 years (creatinine clearance 45 ml min^{-1}) would require less than half the dose of digoxin taken by the male at 20 years, despite having an identical serum creatinine level.

elimination from the body. Some pharmacoepidemiology studies access clinical laboratory data, enabling estimates of renal function to be made and included in analyses of outcomes. Consequently, it is important to recognize that plasma creatinine concentrations must be adjusted for age and body weight before being used as an estimate of renal function. A number of suitable formulae have been published, with the most widely used being that of Cockcroft and Gault.[35]

Drug–Drug Interactions Involving Renal Elimination

Drugs are capable of interfering with elimination of other substances by the kidney. This can occur through an effect on filtration, tubular reabsorption, or tubular secretion. A thorough discussion of this topic is beyond the scope of this overview, but one or two examples will illustrate the importance of this type of interaction. The deleterious effect of NSAIDs on renal blood flow that occurs in certain clinical states was mentioned earlier. As a result, NSAIDs are capable of inhibiting the clearance of a range of potentially toxic compounds, including lithium and methotrexate. Accumulation of these agents can produce serious adverse effects.

In cases where filtration pressure is maintained by angiotensin II-mediated vasoconstriction of the post-glomerular efferent arteriole, angiotensin converting enzyme inhibitors (ACEIs) or angiotensin receptor antagonists may abruptly decrease the glomerular filtration rate through inhibition of angiotensin II synthesis. This may occur in renal artery stenosis, hypovolemia, and cardiac failure, thereby increasing the effects or the toxicity of concomitantly administered drugs that are renally excreted or that are nephrotoxic. The immunosuppressant cyclosporine induces vasoconstriction of the afferent glomerular arteriole in a dose-related and reversible fashion. An increased risk of acute renal failure exists when cyclosporine is combined with NSAIDs, ACEIs, or other nephrotoxic drugs.

Probenecid, a drug that is used in the treatment of gout, reduces the reabsorption of uric acid by the renal tubules, and inhibits the active tubular secretion of penicillin. These actions explain two therapeutic effects of probenecid—it lowers uric acid concentrations in the blood and enhances the effect of a dose of penicillin. Both mechanisms are exploited in clinical practice.

EFFECTS OF VARIATION IN DRUG METABOLISM

Variability in the metabolism of drugs is an important factor to be considered in the analysis and interpretation of pharmacoepidemiology studies. In this section, we will consider the effects of genetics, age, disease states, and concomitant drugs on the metabolism of drugs. Next, we will discuss some of the implications of active drug metabolites and intrinsic clearance. But first, an overview of drug metabolism is in order.

An Overview of Drug Metabolism

The majority of drugs are too lipid soluble to be effectively eliminated by the kidneys. First, they must be converted into water-soluble metabolites that can then be excreted in the urine, or sometimes in feces, via the bile. The metabolic steps necessary for the conversions occur primarily in the liver. Chemical reactions that result in the metabolism of drugs are classified as either Phase I or II reactions. *Phase I reactions* are usually oxidative (e.g., hydroxylation) and create an active site on the drug molecule that can act as a target for Phase II conjugative (synthetic) reactions. *Phase II reactions* involve the synthesis of a new molecule from the combination of the drug and a water-soluble substrate such as glucuronic or acetic acid (Figure 4.4). The product of this type of reaction, for instance the glucuronide or acetyl derivative of the drug, is highly water soluble, and is excreted in the urine, or occasionally in the feces, if it is of high molecular weight.

Most drugs that undergo Phase I (oxidative) metabolism are transformed by a superfamily of enzymes called the cytochrome P450 (CYP) system. Cytochrome P450 is so named because in a certain form its maximal light absorption occurs at a wavelength of approximately 450 nanometers. Most Phase I drug metabolism involves cytochrome P450 families 1, 2, and 3 (CYP1, CYP2, and CYP3). Specific enzymes exist within CYP families. For example, enzymes CYP2C9, CYP2C10, CYP2C18, and CYP2C19 are responsible for most drug metabolism within the CYP2C group of enzymes. Different drugs may be metabolized by different isoenzymes,[5] or because of incomplete substrate specificity, a given drug may be metabolized by more than one enzyme.

Some drugs are capable of participating in synthetic reactions without prior Phase I metabolism. An example is the benzodiazepine temazepam, which is conjugated directly with glucuronide, and is eliminated in the urine in this form. In contrast, diazepam, another benzodiazepine, must undergo several Phase I oxidative reactions before it can be conjugated and eliminated. Phase I reactions are usually the rate limiting step in this process and are subject to much greater intra- and inter-individual variability than are Phase II reactions. This explains why diazepam metabolism is largely affected by age and disease, while temazepam metabolism is relatively unaffected by these factors.[36,37]

Effect of Genetic Factors on Drug Metabolism

Genetic factors are sometimes important in determining the activity of drug metabolizing enzymes. Studies have shown that half-lives of phenylbutazone and coumarin anticoagulants are much less variable in monozygotic than in heterozygotic twins. The half-lives of these drugs in the overall population display an approximately Gaussian distribution, although the limits are often wide, and may encompass 5- to 10-fold variations.[38]

The metabolism of the anti-tubercular drug isoniazid exhibits a bimodal distribution within the population. The conjugation of isoniazid with acetic acid is an important step in its inactivation and elimination. Variability in the rate of isoniazid acetylation results from a single recessive

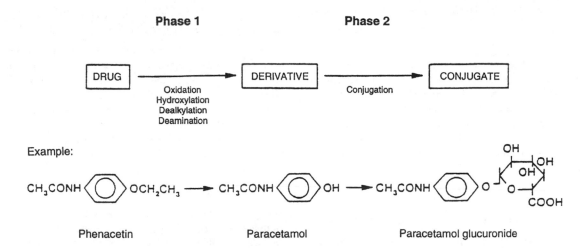

Figure 4.4. Phase I and II reactions often occur sequentially. Phase I reactions usually consist of oxydation, reduction, hydrolysis, and products are often more reactive, and sometimes more toxic, than the parent drug. Phase II reactions involve conjugation and these usually result in inactive compounds. The main effect of this conjugation is to render the substance more water soluble. In the example given, phenacetin is converted to acetaminophen (paracetamol) by dealkylation (Phase I reaction). This introduces a reactive hydroxyl group to which the glucuronyl group can be attached. Both phenacetin and acetaminophen are active, whereas acetaminophen glucuronide is inactive, and water soluble, and is excreted in the urine. (Figure and legend reprinted with permission from Rang *et al. Pharmacology*, 5th edn. Edinburgh: Churchill Livingstone, 2003.)

gene whose distribution shows some racial dependence (acetylation polymorphism). For example, approximately half (50–60%) of most Caucasian communities are slow acetylators, and therefore have a reduced capacity to eliminate the drug.[38] In Japan, the prevalence of the slow acetylator phenotype is only 15%, and slow acetylators have not been identified in Eskimo populations. Although attempts have been made to correlate acetylator phenotype with risk of isoniazid-induced hepatotoxicity, published reports are equivocal, with some showing an association with slow inactivators and others showing an association with rapid inactivators. Recent work has emphasized the possible role of an alternative pathway for isoniazid metabolism. Patients with a particular CYP2E1 genotype had a higher risk of hepatotoxicity with isoniazid after adjustment for acetylator status.[39]

Acetylation polymorphism affects the metabolism of a number of drugs in addition to isoniazid; these include some sulphonamides (including sulphsalazine), hydralazine, procainamide, dapsone, nitrazepam, and caffeine. In general, the clinical implications are that slow acetylators require lower doses both for therapeutic effect and to minimize toxicity and side effects.

Hydroxylation polymorphism was identified in 1977.[40] It has since been established that around 10% of Caucasians and 1% of Asians exhibit hydroxylation deficiency as a result of reduced activity of the enzyme CYP2D6. First described in relation to debrisoquine, the deficiency also affects the metabolism of antidepressants (amitryptyline, clomipramine, desipramine, nortryptyline, mianserin, paroxetine), antiarrhythmics (flecanide, propafenone), antipsychotics (haloperidol, perphenazine, thioridazine), and β-blockers (alprenolol, metoprolol) leading to accumulation of the active parent compound. In the cases of amitryptyline and thioridazine, both parent and active metabolite accumulate. Poor hydroxylators may have markedly increased effects or a prolonged duration of action of the affected drugs.

CYP2C19 polymorphism is described in 2–5% of Caucasians and 12–23% of Asians who have a deficient capacity to hydroxylate S-mephenytoin. CYP2C19 also catalyzes the metabolism of commonly used drugs such as barbiturates, omeprazole, propranolol, diazepam and citalopram.[41]

The clinical consequences of genetic polymorphism have not been fully elucidated, but it is likely that such genetically determined differences may account in some part for the inter-individual and inter-ethnic differences in therapeutic response and side effect profile observed with many drugs.

The CYP2D6 phenotype of a given individual can be determined by testing the metabolic clearance of a test drug, such as debrisoquine or sparteine. This technique can be useful in performing pharmacoepidemiology studies. For instance, Wiholm *et al.* compared debrisoquine hydroxylation in a group of subjects who had developed lactic acidosis while taking phenformin with the expected distribution in the Swedish population.[42] This study illustrates the potential for investigating groups of individuals who display apparently idiosyncratic reactions to certain drugs. Other examples of the use of laboratory techniques to investigate the occurrence of serious adverse reactions include the demonstration of possible familial predispositions to halothane hepatitis and phenytoin-induced hypersensitivity syndromes.[43]

Genetic polymorphism of drug metabolizing enzymes does not just account for adverse effects, it may also lead to lack of efficacy. For instance, individuals who have the extensive metabolism genotype of CYP2C19 need large doses of proton pump inhibitors (e.g., omeprazole) to reduce gastric acid secretion. The slow metabolizer genotype of CYP2D6 will have poor conversion of codeine to morphine and consequently will not experience optimal analgesic effects of the drug.[8]

The large series of well-validated case reports held by many spontaneous reporting systems represent fertile areas for this type of research (see Chapters 9 and 10). However, this requires that the adverse reactions agency maintains a good relationship with those who send in reports. The agency also must have a mechanism for obtaining access to biological or genetic material with the approval of the relevant ethics committees. The use of genetic testing in concert with voluntary adverse drug reaction (ADR) reports and pharmacoepidemiologic methods to predict and explain variability in drug response is a promising new area of research (see also Chapter 37).

Effects of Disease on Drug Metabolism

Hepatic disease can result in reduced elimination of lipid-soluble drugs that are metabolized by this organ. Unfortunately, there are no convenient tests of liver function that are analogous to the measurement of creatinine clearance for estimating renal function. The conventional biochemical tests largely reflect liver damage, rather than liver function. It is quite possible for an individual to have grossly disordered liver function tests, while still metabolizing drugs normally, or alternatively to have apparently normal liver function tests, despite the presence of advanced liver disease with marked impairment of metabolic capacity. To complicate matters further, the liver behaves as though it has a number of "partial functions" that respond differently to disease. For example, bilirubin conjugation may be impaired, while albumin synthesis continues fairly normally. Alternatively, both of these functions may be almost normal, despite the presence of liver disease that has progressed so far that it has resulted in elevated pressure in the portal vein, with subsequent bleeding esophageal varices. It is thus difficult to generalize about the effects of liver disease on hepatic drug metabolism. However, pharmacokinetic studies have shown that liver disease has to be severe, and usually chronic, to result in marked impairment of drug elimination. This is the case, for example, in individuals with cirrhosis or chronic active hepatitis, where Phase I reactions are primarily affected, while conjugative reactions are relatively spared. Other individuals, such as those with biliary obstruction or acute viral hepatitis, may have surprisingly normal drug metabolism.

Drug metabolism may also be affected by disease processes originating in other organs. For example, congestive heart failure can result in severe congestion of the liver, and therefore impair the hepatic clearance of some compounds, while hypoxia has been shown to reduce markedly the metabolism of theophylline.[44] Reduced liver blood flow may also result in reduced extraction and metabolism of high clearance drugs such as morphine and propranolol.

To summarize, liver disease is a relatively uncommon cause of clinically important impaired drug metabolism. Generally, it can be stated that genetic and environmental factors are more important causes of variability in hepatic metabolism of drugs than diseases of the organ itself.

Effects of Active Metabolites

The general rule that drug metabolism produces metabolites that are inactive or markedly less active than the parent drug does not always hold true. This should be considered as a possible explanation for unexpected pharmacoepidemiologic findings. For example, several metabolites of carbamazepine contribute to its pharmacologic activity.[45] The hydroxyl metabolite of propranolol has similar activity to its parent compound.[46] Conjugated metabolites are usually devoid of activity, but morphine-6-glucuronide has been shown to have morphine-like action, and accumulation of this metabolite may explain the prolonged opiate effect of morphine that is found in individuals with advanced renal failure.[47] Likewise, the conjugated acetyl derivative of the antiarrhythmic drug procainamide has been shown to have pharmacologic activity, and may cause toxicity.

Sometimes a metabolite has toxic effects that are not shown by the parent drug. N-acetylbenzo-quinoneimine is the toxic metabolite formed by the oxidative metabolism of acetaminophen. This is normally produced in small quantities but rapidly cleared by reaction with glutathione. In acetaminophen poisoning, the available glutathione reserves are exhausted and the toxic metabolite is free to exert its action on cell membranes, leading to hepatic damage that may on occasions be fatal. More of the metabolite may be formed in the presence of enzyme induction. As a result, chronic heavy drinkers and individuals taking long-term anticonvulsants may be more prone to develop liver damage.[48]

Effects of Presystemic Clearance

Certain orally administered drugs are metabolized substantially in the intestine and/or in the liver before they ever reach the systemic circulation. This phenomenon is known as "first pass" metabolism or "presystemic" clearance. Drugs with high presystemic clearance include morphine, oral contraceptives, prazosin, propranolol, and verapamil. The differences between drugs with high or low presystemic clearances become apparent if hepatic metabolism is impaired by disease or inhibited by another drug or if blood flow to the liver is reduced in shock or in congestive heart failure.

In the case of a drug with low presystemic clearance, a reduction in hepatic metabolism results in a prolongation of the elimination half-life. Generally, it takes approximately five half-lives to reach a new steady state concentration, and accumulation of the drug may cause toxicity. If the drug has a high presystemic clearance, a decline in metabolism will result in increased *bioavailability* of the drug, with elevated, and possibly toxic, concentrations early in the course of treatment, possibly after the first dose, although it will still take five half-lives to reach the new steady state concentration (in a similar fashion as when the dose is increased). Thus, in a study of the adverse effects of drugs in subjects with hepatic impairment or metabolic inhibition by other drugs, the time course of adverse effects can be critically dependent on this factor.

Drug–Drug Interactions Involving Drug Metabolizing Enzymes

Enzyme induction occurs when the chronic administration of a substance results in an increase in the amount of a particular metabolizing enzyme. When such enzymes are induced, the rate of metabolism of a drug can increase several-fold. The subsequent fall in the concentration of the drug in the blood, and, consequently, at its sites of action, may result in a substantial loss of drug activity. For instance, failure of ethinylestradiol-containing oral contraceptives can result from the CYP450 enzyme-inducing effects of some anti-epileptic medications.[49] The rate of metabolism of warfarin is increased by concomitantly administered drugs, including carbamazepine, rifampicin, and barbiturates, leading to reduced steady state plasma concentrations, and therefore a reduced anticoagulant effect.

Enzyme induction proceeds through a mechanism that involves increases in gene transcription, resulting in increased synthesis of new enzyme protein.[5] It can take several weeks to reach its peak (except with alcohol, where the process is quicker), and can persist for some time after the inducing drug is ceased. CYP450 enzymes differ in their ability to be induced in response to a given exposure. For example, theophylline metabolism is readily inducible by cigarette smoking, while phenytoin metabolism is affected to a greater extent by barbiturates and anti-epileptic medications.[44]

Enzyme inhibition occurs when the presence of one substance inhibits the metabolism of another substance. It involves either competition for active sites on the enzyme, or other binding-site interactions that alter the activity of the enzyme. In contrast to induction, enzyme inhibition occurs rapidly, and is rapidly reversed once the inhibiting substance has been withdrawn. As with induction, interacting compounds display considerable specificity, and a number of commonly used drugs have the capacity to inhibit microsomal function. For example, cimetidine is capable of inhibiting the metabolism of many compounds, including warfarin, theophylline, phenytoin, propranolol, and several benzodiazepines.[50] In contrast, omeprazole has been shown to inhibit the metabolism of diazepam and phenytoin, but not of propranolol.[51-53] Erythromycin is a clinically important enzyme inhibitor, well known for its effects on theophylline metabolism. Erythromycin and other macrolide antibiotics have been shown to inhibit the metabolism of the antihistamines terfenadine and astemizole and the prokinetic agent cisapride. These drugs may inhibit the potassium ion channels in the heart with a consequent risk of serious ventricular dysrhythmia, and they have been withdrawn from most markets.[54] Drug–drug interactions are not always harmful. The calcium antagonists diltiazem and verapamil (but not nifedipine) increase cyclosporine plasma concentrations, but with relative sparing of nephrotoxicity, and the interaction has been used in clinical practice to produce an immunosuppressive concentration of cyclosporine at a lower ingested dose.[55] Drug cost savings of 14–48%, attributable to the use of calcium antagonists, have been reported in transplant pharmacotherapy. Similarly, the protease inhibitor ritonavir is used in combination with other drugs in this class (e.g., lopinavir) in low doses as it inhibits their metabolism and "boosts" their blood levels and efficacy.

Recent research has revealed that many inducers and inhibitors of CYP3A4 act similarly on the drug transporter P-glycoprotein. For instance this pumps some drugs (e.g., digoxin) into the intestinal lumen, reducing bioavailability.[8] Macrolide antibiotics may inhibit this transporter and so increase the bioavailability of digoxin, leading to toxicity. Clearly the world of drug–drug interactions is more complex than we could have ever imagined!

Interactions arise not only as a consequence of other drugs; food constituents may affect drug metabolism. For example, the biflavenoids present in grapefruit juice have a strong inhibitory effect on the presystemic metabolism of calcium antagonists, causing a two- to three-fold increase in the systemic absorption of oral nifedipine and felodipine.[56] A similar effect of biflavenoids on cyclosporine concentrations has been observed and has been utilized to reduce the doses, and therefore the side effects and costs, of cyclosporine therapy. Both calcium antagonists and cyclosporine are metabolized by the CYP450 isoenzyme CYP3A4, which is present in the gut wall and in the liver, and the biflavenoids inhibit its activity.

Sometimes dietary constituents can directly antagonize the effects of drugs. For instance, vitamin K-containing foods such as cabbage, brussels sprouts, broccoli, spinach, lettuce, rape seed oil, and soya bean oil, taken in sufficient amounts, may antagonize the effects of warfarin.

CONSEQUENCES OF VARIABILITY IN PHARMACOKINETICS

The foregoing discussion on causes of variability in pharmacokinetics is only of importance if there are clinical consequences that are likely to be detected in pharmacoepidemiology studies. Therefore, it is important to determine the circumstances in which these factors will contribute to variability in drug response.

Several factors are important. The first is the relationship between the concentration of the drug and its effects. Alterations of drug pharmacokinetics tend to be important if they involve drugs that have a low therapeutic ratio. This refers to the ratio of the concentration of drug that produces toxic effects to the concentration that elicits a therapeutic effect. If the ratio is low then small changes in drug concentration will lead to adverse effects. Examples of drugs with this profile are digoxin and lithium, which are primarily excreted unchanged by the kidneys, and theophylline and warfarin, which are primarily inactivated by hepatic metabolism. Cyclosporine also has a narrow therapeutic ratio, but wide variations between individuals in absorption, distribution, and metabolism have made definition of therapeutic, but nontoxic, concentrations difficult. It undergoes both hepatic metabolism and local metabolism in the gut, and the latter may be a major contributor to the variability in absorption.

Regardless of whether we are dealing with a decline in renal function or a reduction or inhibition of hepatic metabolism, the consequences in each case of increases in plasma concentration will be accumulation of the drug, and potential toxicity. In contrast, interactions involving drugs with high therapeutic ratios, for instance penicillin, will rarely produce significant adverse effects.

THE IMPORTANCE OF THE HUMAN FACTOR: PRESCRIBER AND CONSUMER BEHAVIOR

Human behavior may be an even greater source of variability in patterns of drug exposure than any other factor considered so far in this chapter. This is because many of the other factors considered in this chapter did not relate to use but rather to intensity of exposure (e.g., alterations in clearance, or drug–drug interactions). In contrast, non-adherence with therapy will have a more profound effect (see also Chapter 46).

In conducting pharmacoepidemiology studies, it is important to give cognizance to the impact of human behavior upon observed prescribing and consumption patterns. The influences that determine prescribing practices and consumer behavior are complex and have not been studied comprehensively; they are known to include factors related to the illness itself, the doctor, the patient, the doctor–patient interaction, drug costs and availability, perceived and actual benefits and risks of treatment, and pharmaceutical company promotional activities.

TREATMENT OUTCOMES AND INDICATIONS

A primary influence on prescribing may be the natural desire to achieve the best possible treatment outcome for the patient. For example, if the starting dose of the drug of first choice is not effective in a given patient, the prescriber may choose to increase the dose, add another drug, or switch to a different medication. Sometimes, all of these options will be tried in sequence. For many disorders, the intensity of treatment is titrated against a measured response, such as the blood pressure, blood cholesterol measurement, or the distance that the patient can walk before developing anginal pain. As a result, individuals with more severe underlying disease or more resistant symptoms will tend to receive higher doses of drugs, and greater numbers of drugs. In pharmacoepidemiology studies, it may therefore be difficult to determine whether a given disease–drug association is caused by the drug under study, or is confounded by the nature or severity of the underlying disease state (see also Chapters 39, 40, and 47).

The occurrence of adverse events, for example cough with ACE inhibitors or gastrointestinal bleeding with NSAIDs, will clearly cause prescribers to alter drug choices and to avoid the future use of such agents in the affected patients, and perhaps in other patients. Similarly, the existence of contraindications to certain drugs, like β-blockers in asthma, or penicillin allergy, will impact on prescribers' drug choices for certain patients. Underlying pathology frequently directs drug choice—for example, ACE inhibitors are a reasonable first choice for the treatment of hypertension in diabetic patients, but would be regarded by many as an unnecessarily expensive first drug for newly diagnosed simple hypertension in an otherwise well individual. In the absence of information about diagnosis, other pathology, and contraindications, the accurate interpretation of drug use patterns observed in pharmacoepidemiology studies may be difficult.

EXPECTATION AND DEMAND

Patient demand and expectation have been cited as influencing doctors' decisions to prescribe. However, it appears a gap exists between patients' expectations of a prescription and doctors' perceptions of their expectations.[57] After controlling for the presenting condition, patients in general practice who expected a prescription were up to three times more likely to receive one than those who did not. However, patients whom the general practitioner believed expected a prescription were up to ten times more likely to receive one.[58] It is speculated that failure to ascertain patients' expectations is a major reason why doctors prescribe more drugs than patients expect. Other factors that influenced the decision to prescribe in these studies included the doctor's level of academic qualification, practice prescribing rates, patient exemption from prescribing charges, and difficult consultations.[57]

PERCEPTION OF HARMS AND BENEFITS OF TREATMENT

The harms and benefits of treatment may exert influence on prescribing decisions—patients perceived to be at risk of unwanted adverse effects of therapy are less likely than those without such risks to receive treatment.[59] Perception of harm and benefit may vary with the prescriber. For example, it has been found that compared with cardiologists, general physicians overestimate the benefits of certain cardiac treatments.[60]

Information framing, that is, the manner of presentation of risks and benefits, may influence prescribing decisions. Treatment outcomes presented in terms of relative risk reduction are more likely to elicit a decision to treat than those presented in terms of absolute risk reduction or as numbers needed to treat.[61] Promotional materials from pharmaceutical companies frequently present the benefits of treatments in relative as opposed to absolute terms, as do the newspaper articles that quote them.[62] As relative effect measures usually appear more striking than absolute measures, relative effect measures may be judged sufficiently impressive to persuade prescription by prescribers too busy to consider the original data in detail. While the decision to prescribe based on such evidence may be justifiable in cases where the absolute benefit happens to be reasonable, inappropriate prescribing decisions may be made if it is very small or insignificant.

Patients may also be influenced by the manner of presenting data on benefits and harms of treatments.[63] For instance, surgery is more likely to be preferred over medical treatment if results are expressed in a positive frame (survival) than a negative frame (mortality).

All human decisions are subject to cognitive biases. As Greenhalgh *et al.* have pointed out, "these biases include anchoring against what is seen to be 'normal', inability to distinguish between small probabilities, and undue influence from events that are easy to recall. Stories (about the harmful effects of medicines) have a particularly powerful impact, especially when presented in the media as unfolding social dramas."[64]

ECONOMIC INFLUENCES

Economic influences, exerted from various sources, may influence drug use and therefore the interpretation of pharmacoepidemiology studies (see also Chapter 41). As medicines, particularly new ones, become increasingly expensive, budgetary restrictions, or indeed incentives, may impact upon prescribing decisions. For example, in 1993, the German government placed a limit on reimbursable drug costs and announced that a proportion of spending in excess of this limit would be recouped from doctors' remuneration budgets. The changes in prescribing patterns, at least in the early aftermath of the limit, were significant. The numbers of prescriptions fell and there was a move to the use of both generic products and older, less expensive drugs.[65]

In England the Department of Health introduced several schemes intended to contain the costs of National Health Service prescribing. These included setting indicative prescribing budgets for general practices, offering incentives to make prescribing savings, and fundholding schemes whereby practices hold and manage their own budgets for a number of services, including prescribing. The effects on prescribing patterns have been variable. In Australia, pharmaceutical companies are required to provide evidence of the cost-effectiveness of their product, compared with that of an existing alternative, prior to listing on the national list of reimbursable medicines (see also Chapter 25). Generic substitution is encouraged and the costs of "me too" drugs are controlled, in part, by reference pricing. New Zealand also uses pharmacoeconomic analysis and reference pricing, but is unusual among developed countries in also tendering for some of its pharmaceutical needs. This has been highly unpopular among major brand name manufacturing companies.

Other approaches intended to contain prescribing costs have included national formularies and limited lists, patient co-payments, and practice guidelines.

While the approaches outlined above reflect some attempts of governments to contain drug costs by influencing prescribing choices, patients themselves may also exert influence based upon their ability to pay for medicines. Where patients are covered by state or private insurance schemes, medicine expense may not be perceived by the patient or the prescriber to be an issue and drug choice will not be constrained by ability to pay. In fact, more expensive choices than are absolutely necessary may be encouraged. However, for patients required to pay in whole or in part for their medicines, costs may well influence drug choice and, for instance, a diuretic as opposed to an ACE inhibitor or calcium antagonist may be chosen for hypertension treatment, although not necessarily the best choice for the individual concerned. Even in countries with strong social insurance programs patients sometimes have difficulty in affording medications, because of relatively high patient co-payment levels.[66]

Prescribers themselves may have a pecuniary interest in prescribing. Fee for service methods of physician remuneration (as against a capitation fee) have been found to encourage a higher use of services.[67] In Japan, physicians dispense as well as prescribe medicines and the associated financial incentive is considered to contribute to the high numbers of prescriptions per capita and the use of expensive drugs.[68,69] Concerns about the effects on prescribing of incentives offered to doctors by the pharmaceutical industry have led to such practices being discouraged in most countries and manufacturers have voluntarily adopted a code of good promotional practice.

THE PHARMACEUTICAL INDUSTRY

Promotional activities of the pharmaceutical industry can affect prescribing practices in ways that are relevant to pharmacoepidemiology. For example, if a manufacturer promotes a new NSAID as being less prone to cause gastrointestinal toxicity than other NSAIDs, it may be given to individuals who have an intrinsically higher risk of gastrointestinal bleeding, such as those who have developed dyspepsia while receiving other NSAIDs, or who have a past history of gastric ulceration. These individuals would therefore be expected to have an increased risk of subsequent gastrointestinal bleeding in comparison with those receiving other NSAIDs, although such a finding might be wrongly attributed to the new drug. This form of "channeling" has been a particularly strong feature with COX-2 inhibitors and, if not adjusted for in nonrandomized studies, will give a misleadingly pessimistic impression of the gastrointestinal toxicity of this class of drugs.[70]

Pharmaceutical companies may exert influence, direct and indirect, on prescribing choices. This may occur through their representatives who visit doctors to provide information about drug products on a one-to-one basis, the sponsorship of educational meetings, the employment of personnel (for example, nurses at asthma or diabetic clinics), sponsorship to attend international specialty meetings, or invitations to specialists to become "expert advisors" in their particular areas of practice.

PATIENT BEHAVIOR

Consumer behavior must also be considered in pharmacoepidemiology studies. Numerous studies have shown that individuals with some diseases, particularly illnesses that are asymptomatic, such as hypertension and hypercholesterolemia, tend to have poor compliance with prescribed drug therapy regimens. Therefore, if a pharmacoepidemiology study were to be performed in such a situation, and the use of a drug were operationally defined as the dispensing of a prescription, then the number of prescriptions dispensed might overestimate the true exposure to that medication. On the other hand, compliance with some drugs, such as oral contraceptives, tends to be good because consumers are highly motivated to take them. In the case of drugs that are taken for particular symptoms, such as pain or wheezing, individuals may take more medication than is prescribed. If this occurs chronically, it should be reflected in the number of prescriptions that have been dispensed for an individual over a given time period.

The use of non-prescription drugs, which sometimes have the same effects as prescription drugs, also needs to be considered. For example, when examining the effects of NSAIDs using prescription data, it is important to consider the possibility that individuals who appear to be unexposed might actually have been exposed to a non-prescription NSAID. There is a general trend worldwide for a wider variety of drugs, previously only available on prescription, to become available over-the-counter. In many countries, drugs known to have significant potential for causing interactions, such as cimetidine, are included in this non-prescription availability. Of course, the increasing use of dietary supplements, with virtually no quality control or effective regulation, makes this even worse.

Consumers of prescribed medications may differ from nonusers in a number of other ways that may confound pharmacoepidemiology studies, for example, alcohol intake and smoking status. Unfortunately, this information is rarely, if ever, available from some data sources, (e.g., automated databases). Individuals who take certain drugs may use other medical services or have different lifestyles from nonusers. In the case of post-menopausal estrogen therapy, consumers were shown to make greater use of other medical services and to have higher levels of exercise than nonconsumers.[71] This is important, because these factors were potential confounders of the relationship between estrogen use and outcomes such as hip fracture and myocardial infarction (see Chapter 40).

Knowledge of prescriber and consumer behavior is crucial when conducting pharmacoepidemiology studies. Both high doses of drugs and the use of drug combinations are often markers for more severe underlying diseases. Therefore, attempts to link exposure to a drug with a particular outcome must take account of these factors. Disease severity or intolerance to previous medications may be linked in subtle ways to the outcomes of interest, and pharmacoepidemiology studies are subject to these forms of confounding. Economic and promotional influences may affect prescribing patterns in a number of ways, both obvious and subtle, and also require consideration as potential confounders.

CONCLUSIONS

Pharmacoepidemiology is a complex and inexact science. It would be convenient if exposures and outcomes could always be assumed to be dichotomous; the relationships could be assumed to be unconfounded; and if risk could be assumed to increase proportionately with duration of exposure. However, because of the complexity of the use and effects of drugs among the population, these simplifying assumptions are often violated. Users of drugs will often differ in many respects from nonusers, and in ways that are not easily adjusted for. These differences may confound the associations between exposure and outcomes. Responses to drugs are very variable, not only between individuals but also within individuals over time. This variability in inter- and intra-individual responses can result in adverse reactions being manifest early in treatment, and the development of tolerance in long-term users. A study of clinical pharmacology provides us with many insights, and a knowledge of the underlying principles is essential during the conduct, and particularly the interpretation, of pharmacoepidemiology studies.

REFERENCES

1. Royal Australasian College of Physicians. Available from: http://www.racp.edu.au/.

2. Nelson HD, Humphrey LL, Nygren P, Teutsch SM, Allan JD. Postmenopausal hormone replacement therapy: scientific review. *JAMA* 2002; **288**: 872–81.

3. American Academy of Pediatrics Committee on Fetus and Newborn Committee on Drugs. Benzyl alcohol: toxic agent in neonatal units. *Pediatrics* 1983; **72**: 356.

4. Nayler WG. *Calcium Antagonists*. London: Academic Press, 1988.

5. Rang HP, Dale MM, Ritter JM, Moore PK. *Pharmacology*, 5th edn. Edinburgh: Churchill Livingstone, 2003.

6. Jaffe JH, Martin WR. Opioid analgesics and antagonists. In: Gilman AG, Rall TW, Nies AS, Taylor P, eds, *The Pharmacological Basis of Therapeutics*, 8th edn. New York: Pergamon Press, 1990; p. 497.

7. Henry D, Lim LL-Y, Garcia Rodriguez LA, Perez Gutthann S, Carson JL, Griffin M. *et al.* Variability in risk of major upper gastrointestinal complications with individual NSAIDs: results of a collaborative meta-analysis. *BMJ* 1996; **312**: 1563–6.

8. Shenfield G, Le Couter DG, Rivory LP. Updates in medicine: clinical pharmacology. *Med J Aust* 2002; **176**: 9.

9. Ingelman-Sundberg M. Pharmacogenetics: an opportunity for a safer and more efficient pharmacotherapy. *J Intern Med* 2001; **250**: 186–200.

10. Gandhi PJ, Cambria-Kiely JA. Aspirin resistance and genetic polymorphisms. *J Thromb Thrombolysis* 2003; **14**: 51–8.

11. Lu Y, Mahaut-Smith MP, Huang CL-H, Vandenberg JI. Mutant MiRP1 subunits modulate HERG K+ channel gating: a mechanism for pro-arrhythmia in long QT syndrome type 6. *J Physiol* 2003; **551**: 253–62.

12. Kendall MJ, Beeley L. Beta-adrenoceptor blocking drugs: adverse reactions and drug interactions. *Pharmacol Ther* 1983; **21**: 351–69.

13. Lanza FL. Endoscopic studies of gastric and duodenal injury after the use of ibuprofen, aspirin, and other nonsteroidal anti-inflammatory agents. *Am J Med* 1984; **77**: 19–24.

14. Graham DY, Smith JL, Spjut HJ, Torres E. Gastric adaptation. *Gastroenterology* 1988; **95**: 327–33.

15. Garcia-Rodriguez LA, Walker LAM, Perez-Gutthann S. Nonsteroidal anti-inflammatory drugs and gastrointestinal hospitalisations in Saskatchewan: a cohort study. *Epidemiology* 1992; **3**: 337–42.

16. Langman MJS, Weil J, Wainright P. Risk of bleeding peptic ulcer associated with individual nonsteroidal anti-inflammatory drugs. *Lancet* 1994; **343**: 1075–8.

17. MacDonald TM, Morant SV, Robinson GC, Shield MJ, McGilchrist MM, Murray FE, McDevitt DG. Association of gastrointestinal toxicity of nonsteroidal anti-inflammatory drugs with continued exposure: a cohort study. *BMJ* 1997; **315**: 1333–7.

18. Vestal RE, Wood AJ, Shand DG. Reduced beta adrenoceptor sensitivity in the elderly. *Clin Pharmacol Ther* 1979; **26**: 181–6.

19. Abernethy DR, Schwartz JB, Todd EL. Verapamil pharmacodynamics and disposition in young and elderly hypertensive patients. Altered electrocardiographic and hypotensive responses. *Ann Intern Med* 1986; **105**: 329–36.

20. Podoisky DK, Isselbacher KJ. Derangements of hepatic metabolism. In: Wilson JD, Braunwald E, Isselbacher KJ, eds, *Harrison's Principles of Internal Medicine*, 12th edn. New York: McGraw Hill, 1991; pp. 1311–7.

21. Anon. Morphine. In: Dollery C, ed., *Therapeutic Drugs*, vol. 2. Edinburgh: Churchill Livingstone, 1991; pp. M225–33.

22. Grimm G, Ferenci P, Katzenschlager R, Madl C, Schneeweiss B, Laggner AN, Lenz K, Gangl A. Improvement of hepatic encephalopathy treated with flumazenil. *Lancet* 1988; **ii**: 1392–4.

23. Clive DM, Stoff JS. Renal syndromes associated with nonsteroidal anti-inflammatory drugs. *N Engl J Med* 1984; **310**: 563–72.

24. Goldstein I, Lue TF, Padma-Nathan H, Rosen RC, Steers WD, Wicker PA. Oral sildenafil in the treatment of erectile dysfunction. *New Engl J Med* 1998; **338**: 1397–404.

25. Khan MA, Herzog CA, St Peter JV, Hartley GG, Madlon-Kay R, Dick CD. The prevalence of cardiac valvular insufficiency assessed by transthoracic echocardiography in obese patients treated with appetite suppressant drugs. *New Engl J Med* 1998; **339**: 713–8.

26. Abenhaim L, Moride Y, Brenot F, Rich S, Benichou J, Kurz X *et al.* for the International Primary Pulmonary Hypertension Group. Appetite-supressant drugs and the risk of primary pulmonary hypertension. *New Engl J Med* 1996; **335**: 609–16.

27. Anon. Adalat tablets. Approved product information. In: Thomas J, ed., *Prescription Products Guide*. Hawthorne, Victoria: Australian Pharmaceutical Publishing, 1992, pp. 237–8.

28. Larregue M, Bressieux JM, Laidet B, Titi A. Caustic diaper dermatitis and toxic encephalopathy following the application of talc contaminated by hexachlorophene. *Ann Pediatr (Paris)* 1986; **33**: 587–92.

29. Martin-Bouyer G, Khanh NB, Linh PD, Hoa DQ, Tuan LC, Tourneau J, *et al.* Epidemic of haemorrhagic disease in Vietnamese infants caused by warfarin-contaminated talcs. *Lancet* 1983; **i**: 230–2.

30. Law CM, Preece MA, Warner JO. Nocturnal adrenal suppression in children inhaling beclamethasone dipropionate (letter). *Lancet* 1987; **i**: 1321.

31. Anon. Timoptol. Approved product information. In: Thomas J, ed., *Prescription Products Guide*. Hawthorne, Victoria: Australian Pharmaceutical Publishing Company, 1992; p. 17401.

32. Birkett D. Drug protein binding. *Aust Prescr* 1992; **15**: 56–7.

33. Fromm MF. Importance of P-glycoprotein for drug disposition in humans. *Eur J Clin Invest* 2003; **33** (suppl 2): 6–9.

34. Asra S, Reinhold K, Michael EW, Ulrich B. Association of multidrug resistance in epilepsy with a polymorphism in the drug-transporter gene ABCB1. *N Engl J Med* 2003; **348**: 1442–8.

35. Cockcroft DW, Gault MH. Prediction of creatinine clearance from serum creatinine. *Nephron* 1976; **16**: 31–41.

36. Klotz U, Avant GR, Hoyumpa A, Schenker S, Wilkinson GR. The effect of age and liver disease on the disposition and elimination of diazepam in adult man. *J Clin Invest* 1975; **55**: 347–59.

37. Ghabrial H, Desmond PV, Watson KJ, Gijsbers AJ, Harman PJ, Breen KJ, Mashford ML. The effects of age and chronic liver disease on the elimination of temazepam. *Eur J Clin Pharmacol* 1986; **30**: 93–7.

38. Graham-Smith DG, Aronson JK. Pharmacokinetics. In: *Oxford Textbook of Clinical Pharmacology and Drug Therapy*, 2nd edn. Oxford: Oxford University Press, 1992, pp. 94–103.

39. Huang Y-S, Chern H-D, Su W-J, Wu J-C, Chang S-C, Chiang C-H *et al*. Cytochrome P450 2E1 genotype and the susceptibility to antituberculosis drug-induced hepatitis. *Hepatology* 2003; **37**: 924–30.

40. Mahgoub A, Idle JR, Dring LG, Lancaster R, Smith RL. Polymorphic hydroxylation of debrisoquine in man. *Lancet* 1977; **2**: 584.

41. Meyer UA. Molecular mechanisms of genetic polymorphisms of drug metabolism. *Annu Rev Pharmacol Toxicol* 1997; **37**: 269–96.

42. Wiholm BE, Alvan G, Bertilsson L, Sawe J, Sjoqvist F. Hydroxylation of debrisoquine in patients with lactic acidosis after phenformin. *Lancet* 1981; **i**: 1098–9.

43. Ranek L, Dalhoff K, Poulsen HE, Brosen K, Flachs H, Loft S *et al*. Drug metabolism and genetic polymorphism in subjects with previous halothane hepatitis. *Scand J Gastroenterol* 1993; **28**: 677–80.

44. Jusko WJ, Eaten ML. Factors affecting theophylline disposition. In: McLeod SM, Isles A, eds, *Theophylline Therapy Update*. Mississauga, Ontario: Astra Pharmaceuticals Canada, 1982; pp. 19–29.

45. Anon. Carbamazepine. In: Dollery C, ed., *Therapeutic Drugs*, vol. 1. Edinburgh: Churchill Livingstone, 1991; pp. 49–53.

46. Anon. Propranolol. In: Dollery C, ed., *Therapeutic Drugs*, vol. 1. Edinburgh: Churchill Livingstone, 1991; pp. 272–8.

47. Osborne RJ, Joel SP, Slevin ML. Morphine intoxication in renal failure: the role of morphine-6-glucuronide. *BMJ* 1986; **292**: 1548–9.

48. Bray GP, Harrison PM, O'Grady JG, Tredger JM, Williams R. Long-term anticonvulsant therapy worsens outcome in paracetamol-induced fulminant hepatic failure. *Hum Exp Toxicol* 1992; **11**: 265–70.

49. Stockley IH. *Drug Interactions*, 2nd edn. Oxford: Blackwell Scientific, 1991.

50. Anon. Gastrointestinal drugs. In: McEvoy GK, ed., *AHFS Drug Information*. Bethesda: American Society of Hospital Pharmacists, 1990; pp. 1666–70.

51. Gugler R, Jensen JC. Omeprazole inhibits elimination of diazepam (letter). *Lancet* 1984; **i**: 969.

52. Prichard PJ, Walt RP, Kitchingman GK, Somerville KW, Langman MJ, Williams J, Richens A. Oral phenytoin kinetics during omeprazole therapy. *Br J Clin Pharmacol* 1987; **24**: 534–5.

53. Henry D, Brent P, Whyte I, Mihaly G, Devenish-Meares S. Propranolol steady-state pharmacokinetics are unaltered by omeprazole. *Eur J Clin Pharmacol* 1987; **33**: 369–73.

54. Anon. Ventricular arrthythmias due to terfenadine and astemizole. Current problems. *Comm Saf Med* 1992; **35**: 1–2.

55. Kumana CR, Tong MKL, Li C-S, Lauder IJ, Lee JSK, Kou M *et al*. Diltiazem co-treatment in renal transplant patients receiving microemulsion cyclosporin. *Br J Clin Pharmacol* 2003; **56**: 670–8.

56. Bailey DG, Arnold JMO, Spence JD. Grapefruit juice and drugs: how significant is the interaction? *Clin Pharmacokinet* 1994; **26**: 91.

57. Britten N, Ukoumunne O. The influence of patients' hopes of receiving a prescription on doctors' perceptions and the decision to prescribe: a questionnaire survey. *BMJ* 1997; **315**: 1506–10.

58. Cockburn J, Pit S. Prescribing behaviour in clinical practice: patients' expectations and doctors' perceptions of patients' expectations—a questionnaire study. *BMJ* 1997; **315**: 520–3.

59. Nikolajevic-Sarunac J, Henry DA, O'Connell DL, Robertson J. Effects of information framing on general practitioners' intentions to prescribe long term hormone replacement therapy: results of a randomized controlled trial. *J Gen Intern Med* 1999; **14**: 591–8.

60. Freidman PD, Brett AS, Mayo-Smith MF. Differences in generalists' and cardiologists' perceptions of cardiovascular risk and the outcomes of preventive therapy in cardiovascular disease. *Ann Intern Med* 1996; **124**: 414–21.

61. McGettigan P, Sly K, O'Connell D, Hill S, Henry D. The effects of information framing on the practices of physicians. *J Gen Intern Med* 1999; **14**: 633–42.

62. Moynihan R, Bero L, Ross-Degnan D, Henry D, Lee K, Watkins J *et al*. Coverage by the news media of the benefits and risks of medications. *N Engl J Med* 2000; **342**: 1645–50.

63. Moxey A, O'Connell D, McGettigan P, Henry D. Describing treatment effects to patients: how they are expressed makes a difference. *J Gen Intern Med* 2003; **18**: 948–59.

64. Greenhalgh T, Kostopoulou O, Harries C. Making decisions about benefits and harms of medicines. *BMJ* 2004; **329**: 47–50.

65. Bloor K, Freemantle N. Lessons from international experience in controlling pharmaceutical expenditure II: influencing doctors. *BMJ* 1996; **312**: 1525–7.

66. Doran E, Robertson J, Rolfe I, Henry D. Patient co-payments and use of prescription medicines. *Aust N Z J Public Health* 2004; **28**: 62–7.

67. Abel-Smith B, Grandjeat P. *Pharmaceutical Consumption.* Social Policy Series 38. Brussels: Commission of the European Communities, 1978.

68. Rittenhouse BE. Economic incentives and disincentives for efficient prescribing. *Pharmacoeconomics* 1994; **6**: 222–32.

69. Seo T. Prescribing and dispensing of pharmaceuticals in Japan. *Pharmacoeconomics* 1994; **6**: 95–102.

70. Wolfe F, Flowers N, Burke TA, Arguelles LM, Pettitt D. Increase in lifetime adverse drug reactions, service utilization, and disease severity among patients who will start COX-2 specific inhibitors: quantitative assessment of channeling bias and confounding by indication in 6689 patients with rheumatoid arthritis and osteoarthritis. *J Rheumatol* 2002; **29**: 1015–22.

71. Barrett-Connor E. Post-menopausal estrogen and prevention bias. *Ann Intern Med* 1991; **115**: 455–6.

5

When Should One Perform Pharmacoepidemiology Studies?

BRIAN L. STROM

University of Pennsylvania School of Medicine, Philadelphia, Pennsylvania, USA.

As discussed in the previous chapters, pharmacoepidemiology studies apply the techniques of epidemiology to the content area of clinical pharmacology. This chapter will review when pharmacoepidemiology studies should be performed. It will begin with a discussion of the various reasons why one might perform pharmacoepidemiology studies. Central to many of these is one's willingness to tolerate risk. Whether one's perspective is that of a manufacturer, regulator, academician, or clinician, one needs to consider the risk of adverse reactions which one considers tolerable. Thus, this chapter will continue with a discussion of the difference between safety and risk. It will conclude with a discussion of the determinants of one's tolerance of risk.

REASONS TO PERFORM PHARMACOEPIDEMIOLOGY STUDIES

The decision to conduct a pharmacoepidemiology study can be viewed as similar to the regulatory decision about whether to approve a drug for marketing or the clinical decision about whether to prescribe a drug. In each case, decision making involves weighing the costs and risks of a therapy against its benefits.

The main costs of a pharmacoepidemiology study are obviously the costs (monetary, effort, time) of conducting the study itself. These costs clearly will vary, depending on the questions posed and the approach chosen to answer them. Regardless, with the exception of postmarketing randomized clinical trials, the cost per patient is likely to be at least an order of magnitude less than the cost of a premarketing study. Other costs to consider are the opportunity costs of other research that might be left undone if this research is performed.

One risk of conducting a pharmacoepidemiology study is the possibility that it could identify an adverse outcome as associated with the drug under investigation when in fact the drug does not cause this adverse outcome. Another risk is that it could provide false reassurances about a drug's safety. Both these risks can be minimized by appropriate study designs, skilled researchers, and appropriate and responsible interpretation of the results obtained.

Pharmacoepidemiology, Fourth Edition   Edited by B.L. Strom
© 2005 John Wiley & Sons, Ltd

The benefits of pharmacoepidemiology studies could be conceptualized in four different categories: regulatory, marketing, clinical, and legal (see Table 5.1). Each will be of importance to different organizations and individuals involved in deciding whether to initiate a study. Any given study will usually be performed for several of these reasons. Each will be discussed in turn.

Table 5.1. Reasons to perform pharmacoepidemiology studies

(A) Regulatory

    (1) Required
    (2) To obtain earlier approval for marketing
    (3) As a response to question by regulatory agency
    (4) To assist application for approval for marketing elsewhere

(B) Marketing

    (1) To assist market penetration by documenting the safety of the drug
    (2) To increase name recognition
    (3) To assist in repositioning the drug

        (a) Different outcomes, e.g., quality of life and economic
        (b) Different types of patients, e.g., the elderly
        (c) New indications
        (d) Less restrictive labeling

    (4) To protect the drug from accusations about adverse effects

(C) Legal

    (1) In anticipation of future product liability litigation

(D) Clinical

    (1) Hypothesis testing

        (a) Problem hypothesized on the basis of drug structure
        (b) Problem suspected on the basis of preclinical or premarketing human data
        (c) Problem suspected on the basis of spontaneous reports
        (d) Need to better quantitate the frequency of adverse reactions

    (2) Hypothesis generating—need depends on:

        (a) whether it is a new chemical entity
        (b) the safety profile of the class
        (c) the relative safety of the drug within its class
        (d) the formulation
        (e) the disease to be treated, including

           (i) its duration
           (ii) its prevalence
           (iii) its severity
           (iv) whether alternative therapies are available

REGULATORY

Perhaps the most obvious and compelling reason to perform a postmarketing pharmacoepidemiology study is regulatory: a plan for a postmarketing pharmacoepidemiology study is required before the drug will be approved for marketing. Requirements for postmarketing research have become progressively more frequent in recent years. In fact, since the early 1970s the FDA has required postmarketing research at the time of approval for about one third of all newly approved drugs.[1] Many of these required studies have been randomized clinical trials, designed to clarify residual questions about a drug's efficacy. Others focused on questions of drug toxicity. Often it is unclear whether the pharmacoepidemiology study was undertaken in response to a regulatory requirement or in response to merely a "suggestion" by the regulator, but the effect is essentially the same. Early examples of studies conducted to address regulatory questions include the "Phase IV" cohort studies performed of cimetidine[2] and prazosin.[3] These are discussed more in Chapters 1 and 2.

Sometimes a manufacturer may offer to perform a pharmacoepidemiology study with the hope that the regulatory agency might thereby approve the drug's earlier marketing. If the agency believed that any new serious problem would be detected rapidly and reliably after marketing, it could feel more comfortable about releasing the drug sooner. Although it is difficult to assess the impact of volunteered postmarketing studies on regulatory decisions, the very large economic impact of an earlier approval has motivated some manufacturers to initiate such studies. In addition, in recent years regulatory authorities have occasionally released a particularly important drug after essentially only Phase II testing, with the understanding that additional data would be gathered during postmarketing testing. For example, zidovudine was released for marketing after only limited testing, and only later were additional data gathered on both safety and efficacy, data which indicated, among other things, that the doses initially recommended were too large.[4]

Some postmarketing studies of drugs arise in response to case reports of adverse reactions reported to the regulatory agency. One response to such a report might be to suggest a labeling change. Often a more appropriate response, clinically and commercially, would be to propose a pharmacoepidemiology study. This study would explore whether this adverse event in fact occurs more often in those exposed to the drug than would have been expected in the absence of the drug and, if so, how large is the increased risk of the disease. As an example, a Medicaid database was used to study hypersensitivity reactions to tolmetin,[5] following reports about this problem to the FDA's Spontaneous Reporting System.[6]

Finally, drugs are obviously marketed at different times in different countries. A postmarketing pharmacoepidemiology study conducted in a country which marketed a drug relatively early could be useful in demonstrating the safety of the drug to regulatory agencies in countries which have not yet permitted the marketing of the drug. This is becoming increasingly feasible, as both the industry and the field of pharmacoepidemiology are becoming more international, and regulators are collaborating more.

MARKETING

As will be discussed below, pharmacoepidemiology studies are performed primarily to obtain the answers to clinical questions. However, it is clear that a major underlying reason for some pharmacoepidemiology studies is the potential marketing impact of those answers. In fact, some companies make the marketing branch of the company responsible for pharmacoepidemiology, rather than the medical branch.

Because of the known limitations in the information available about the effects of a drug at the time of its initial marketing, many physicians are appropriately hesitant to prescribe a drug until a substantial amount of experience in its use has been gathered. A formal postmarketing surveillance study can speed that process, as well as clarifying any advantages or disadvantages a drug has compared to its competitors.

A pharmacoepidemiology study can also be useful to improve product name recognition. The fact that a study is under way will often be known to prescribers, as will its results once it is publicly presented and published. This increased name recognition will presumably help sales. An increase in a product's name recognition is likely to result particularly from pharmacoepidemiology studies that recruit subjects for the study via prescribers. However, as discussed in Chapter 23, while this technique can be useful in selected situations, it is extremely expensive and less likely to be productive of scientifically useful information than most other alternatives available. In particular, the conduct of a purely marketing exercise under the guise of a postmarketing surveillance study, not designed to collect useful scientific information, is to be condemned.[7] It is misleading and could endanger the performance of future scientifically useful studies, by resulting in prescribers who are disillusioned and, thereby, reluctant to participate in future studies.

Pharmacoepidemiology studies can also be useful to reposition a drug that is already on the market, i.e., to develop new markets for the drug. One could explore different types of outcomes resulting from the use of the drug for the approved indication, for example the impact of the drug on the cost of medical care (see Chapter 41) and on patients' quality-of-life (see Chapter 42). One could also explore the use of the drug for the approved indication in types of patients other than those included in premarketing studies, for example in children or in the elderly. By exploring unintended beneficial effects, or even drug efficacy (see Chapter 40), one could obtain clues to and supporting information for new indications for drug use. Finally, whether because of questions about efficacy or questions about toxicity, drugs are sometimes approved for initial marketing with restrictive labeling. For example, bretylium was initially approved for marketing in the US only for the treatment of life-threatening arrhythmias. Approval for more widespread use requires additional data. These data can often be obtained from pharmacoepidemiology studies.

Finally, and perhaps most importantly, pharmacoepidemiology studies can be useful to protect the major investment made in developing and testing a new drug. When a question arises about a drug's toxicity, it often needs an immediate answer, or else the drug may lose market share or even be removed from the market. Immediate answers are often unavailable, unless the manufacturer had the foresight to perform pharmacoepidemiology studies in anticipation of this problem. Sometimes these problems can be specifically foreseen and addressed. More commonly, they are not. However, the availability of an existing cohort of exposed patients and a control group will often allow a much more rapid answer than would have been possible if the study had to be conducted *de novo*. One example of this is provided by the experience of Pfizer Pharmaceuticals, when the question arose about whether piroxicam (Feldene) was more likely to cause deaths in the elderly from gastrointestinal bleeding than the other nonsteroidal anti-inflammatory drugs. Although Pfizer did not fund studies in anticipation of such a question, it was fortunate that several pharmacoepidemiology research groups had data available on this question because of other studies that they had performed.[8] McNeil was not as fortunate when questions were raised about anaphylactic reactions caused by zomepirac. If the data they eventually were able to have[9] had been available at the time of the crisis, they might not have removed the drug from the market. More recently, Syntex recognized the potential benefit, and the risk, associated with the marketing of parenteral ketorolac, and chose to initiate a postmarketing surveillance cohort study at the time of the drug's launch.[10–12] Indeed, the drug was accused of multiple different adverse outcomes, and it was only the existence of this study, and its subsequently published results, that saved the drug in its major markets.

LEGAL

Postmarketing surveillance studies can theoretically be useful as legal prophylaxis, in anticipation of eventually having to defend against product liability suits. One often hears the phrase "What you don't know, won't hurt you." However, in pharmacoepidemiology this view is shortsighted and, in fact, very wrong. All drugs cause adverse effects; the regulatory decision to approve a drug and the clinical decision to prescribe a drug both depend on a judgment about the relative balance between the benefits of a drug and its risks. From a legal perspective, to win a product liability suit using a legal theory of negligence, a plaintiff must prove causation, damages, and negligence. A pharmaceutical manufacturer that is a defendant in such a suit cannot change whether its drug causes an adverse effect. If the drug does, this will presumably be detected at some point. The manufacturer also cannot change whether the plaintiff suffered legal damages from the adverse effect, that is whether the plaintiff suffered a disability or incurred expenses resulting from a need for medical attention. However, even if the drug did cause the adverse outcome in question, a manufacturer certainly can document that it was performing state-of-the-art studies to attempt to detect whatever toxic effects the drug had. In addition, such studies could make easier the defense of totally groundless suits, in which a drug is blamed for producing adverse reactions it does not cause.

CLINICAL

Hypothesis Testing

The major reason for most pharmacoepidemiology studies is hypothesis testing. The hypotheses to be tested can be based on the structure or the chemical class of a drug. For example, the cimetidine study mentioned above[2] was conducted because cimetidine was chemically related to metiamide, which had been removed from the market in Europe because it caused agranulocytosis. Alternatively, hypotheses can also be based on premarketing or postmarketing animal or clinical findings. For example, the hypotheses can come from spontaneous reports of adverse events experienced by patients taking the drug in question. The tolmetin,[5] piroxicam,[8] zomepirac,[9] and ketorolac[10–12] questions mentioned above are all examples of this. Finally, an adverse effect may clearly be due to a drug, but a study may be needed to quantitate its frequency. An example would be the postmarketing surveillance study of prazosin, performed to quantitate the frequency of first-dose syncope.[3] Of course, the hypotheses to be tested can involve beneficial drug effects as well as harmful drug effects, subject to some important methodologic limitations (see Chapter 40).

Hypothesis Generating

Hypothesis generating studies are intended to screen for previously unknown and unsuspected drug effects. In principle, all drugs could, and perhaps should, be subjected to such studies. However, some drugs may require these studies more than others. This has been the focus of a formal study, which surveyed experts in pharmacoepidemiology.[13]

For example, it is generally agreed that new chemical entities are more in need of study than so-called "me too" drugs. This is because the lack of experience with related drugs makes it more likely that the new drug has possibly important unsuspected effects.

The safety profile of the class of drugs should also be important to the decision about whether to conduct a formal screening postmarketing surveillance study for a new drug. Previous experience with other drugs in the same class can be a useful predictor of what the experience with the new drug in question is likely to be.

The relative safety of the drug within its class can also be helpful. A drug that has been studied in large numbers of patients before marketing and appears safe relative to other drugs within its class is less likely to need supplementary postmarketing surveillance studies.

The formulation of the drug can be considered a determinant of the need for formal screening pharmacoepidemiology studies. A drug that will, because of its formulation, be used mainly in institutions, where there is close supervision, may be less likely to need such a study. When a drug is used under these conditions, any serious adverse effect is likely to be detected, even without any formal study.

The disease to be treated is an important determinant of whether a drug needs additional postmarketing surveillance studies. Drugs used to treat chronic illnesses are likely to be used for a long period of time. As such, it is important to know their long-term effects. This cannot be addressed adequately in the relatively brief time available for each premarketing study. Also, drugs used to treat common diseases are important to study, as many patients are likely to be exposed to these drugs. Drugs used to treat mild or self-limited diseases also need careful study, because serious toxicity is less acceptable. This is especially true for drugs used by healthy individuals, such as contraceptives. On the other hand, when one is using a drug to treat individuals who are very ill, one is more tolerant of toxicity, assuming the drug is efficacious.

Finally, it is also important to know whether alternative therapies are available. If a new drug is not a major therapeutic advance, since it will be used to treat patients who would have been treated with the old drug, one needs to be more certain of its relative advantages and disadvantages. The presence of significant adverse effects, or the absence of beneficial effects, is less likely to be tolerated for a drug that does not represent a major therapeutic advance.

SAFETY VERSUS RISK

Clinical pharmacologists are used to thinking about drug "safety": the statutory standard that must be met before a drug is approved for marketing in the US is that it needs to be proven to be "safe and effective under conditions of intended use." It is important, however, to differentiate safety from risk. Virtually nothing is without some risks. Even staying in bed is associated with a risk of acquiring bed sores! Certainly no drug is completely safe. Yet, the unfortunate misperception by the public persists that drugs mostly are and should be without any risk at all. Use of a "safe" drug, however, still carries some risk. It would be better to think in terms of *degrees of safety*. Specifically, a drug "is safe if its risks are judged to be acceptable."[14] Measuring risk is an objective but probabilistic pursuit. A judgment about safety is a personal and/or social value judgment about the acceptability of that risk. Thus, assessing safety requires two extremely different kinds of activities: measuring risk and judging the acceptability of those risks.[14] The former is the focus of much of pharmacoepidemiology and most of this book. The latter is the focus of the following discussion.

RISK TOLERANCE

Whether or not to conduct a postmarketing surveillance pharmacoepidemiology study also depends on one's willingness to tolerate risk. From a manufacturer's perspective, one can consider this risk in terms of the risk of a potential regulatory or legal problem that may arise. Whether one's perspective is that of a manufacturer, regulator, academician, or clinician, one needs to consider the risk of adverse reactions that one is willing to accept as tolerable. There are several factors that can affect one's willingness to tolerate the risk of adverse effects from drugs (see Table 5.2). Some of these factors are related to the adverse outcome being studied. Others are related to the exposure and the setting in which the adverse outcome occurs.

Table 5.2. Factors affecting the acceptability of risks

(A) Features of the adverse outcome

    (1) Severity
    (2) Reversibility
    (3) Frequency
    (4) "Dread disease"
    (5) Immediate versus delayed
    (6) Occurs in all people versus just in sensitive people
    (7) Known with certainty or not

(B) Characteristics of the exposure

    (1) Essential versus optional
    (2) Present versus absent
    (3) Alternatives available
    (4) Risk assumed voluntarily
    (5) Drug use will be as intended versus misuse is likely

(C) Perceptions of the evaluator

FEATURES OF THE ADVERSE OUTCOME

The severity and reversibility of the adverse reaction in question are of paramount importance to its tolerability. An adverse reaction that is severe is much less tolerable than one that is mild, even at the same incidence. This is especially true for adverse reactions that result in permanent harm, for example birth defects.

Another critical factor that affects the tolerability of an adverse outcome is the frequency of the adverse outcome in those who are exposed. Notably, this is *not* a question of the relative risk of the disease due to the exposure, but a question of the excess risk (see Chapter 2). Use of tampons is extraordinarily strongly linked to toxic shock: the relative risk appears to be between 10 and 20. However, toxic shock is sufficiently uncommon, that even a 10- to 20-fold increase in the risk of the disease still contributes an extraordinarily small risk of the toxic shock syndrome in those who use tampons.[15]

In addition, the particular disease caused by the drug is important to one's tolerance of its risks. Certain diseases are considered by the public to be so-called "dread diseases," diseases which generate more fear and emotion than other diseases. Examples are AIDS and cancer. It is less likely that the risk of a drug will be considered acceptable if it causes one of these diseases.

Another relevant factor is whether the adverse outcome is immediate or delayed. Most individuals are less concerned about delayed risks than immediate risks. This is one of the factors that has probably slowed the success of anti-smoking efforts. In part this is a function of denial; delayed risks seem as if they may never occur. In addition, an economic concept of "discounting" plays a role here. An adverse event in the future is less bad than the same event today, and a beneficial effect today is better than the same beneficial effect in the future. Something else may occur between now and then, which could make that delayed effect irrelevant or, at least, mitigate its impact. Thus, a delayed adverse event may be worth incurring if it can bring about beneficial effects today.

It is also important whether the adverse outcome is a Type A reaction or a Type B reaction. As described in Chapter 1, Type A reactions are the result of an exaggerated but otherwise usual pharmacological effect of a drug. Type A reactions tend to be common, but they are dose-related, predictable, and less serious. In contrast, Type B reactions are aberrant effects of a drug. Type B reactions tend to be uncommon, are not related to dose, and are potentially more serious. They may be due to hypersensitivity reactions, immunologic reactions, or some other idiosyncratic reaction to the drug. Regardless, Type B reactions are the more difficult to predict or even detect. If one can predict an adverse effect, then one can attempt to prevent it. For example, in order to prevent aminophylline-induced arrhythmias and seizures, one can begin therapy at lower doses and follow serum levels carefully. For this reason, all other things being equal, Type B reactions are usually considered less tolerable.

Finally, the acceptability of a risk also varies according to how well established it is. The same adverse effect is obviously less tolerable if one knows with certainty that it is caused by a drug than if it is only a remote possibility.

CHARACTERISTICS OF THE EXPOSURE

The acceptability of a risk is very different, depending upon whether an exposure is essential or optional. Major adverse effects are much more acceptable when one is using a therapy that can save or prolong life, such as chemotherapy for malignancies. On the other hand, therapy for self-limited illnesses must have a low risk to be acceptable. Pharmaceutical products intended for use in healthy individuals, such as vaccines and contraceptives, must be exceedingly low in risk to be considered acceptable.

The acceptability of a risk is also dependent on whether the risk is from the presence of a treatment or its absence. One could conceptualize deaths from a disease that can be treated by a drug that is not yet on the market as an adverse effect from the absence of treatment. For example, the six-year delay in introducing β-blockers into the US market has been blamed for resulting in more deaths than all recent adverse drug reactions combined.[16] As a society, we are much more willing to accept risks of this type than risks from the use of a drug that has been marketed prematurely. Physicians are taught *primum non nocere*—first do no harm. This is somewhat analogous to our willingness to allow patients with terminal illnesses to die from these illnesses without intervention, while it would be considered unethical and probably illegal to perform euthanasia. In general, we are much more tolerant of sins of omission than sins of commission.

Whether any alternative treatments are available is another determinant of the acceptability of risks. If a drug is the only available treatment for a disease, particularly a serious disease, then greater risks will be considered acceptable. This was the reason zidovudine was allowed to be marketed for treatment of AIDS, despite its toxicity and the limited testing which had been performed.[4] Analogously, studies of toxic shock syndrome associated with the use of tampons were of public health importance, despite the infrequency of the disease, because consumers could choose among other available tampons that were shown to carry different risks.[15]

Whether a risk is assumed voluntarily is also important to its acceptability. We are willing to accept the risk of death in automobile accidents more than the much smaller risk of death in airline accidents, because we control and understand the former and accept the attendant risk voluntarily. Some people even accept the enormous risks of death from tobacco-related disease, but would object strongly to being given a drug that was a small fraction as toxic. In general, it is agreed that patients should be made aware of possibly toxic effects of drugs that they are prescribed. When a risk is higher than it is with the usual therapeutic use of a drug, as with an invasive procedure or an investigational drug, one usually asks the patient for formal informed consent. The fact that fetuses cannot make voluntary choices about whether or not to take a drug contributes to the unacceptability of drug-induced birth defects.

Finally, from a societal perspective, one also needs to be concerned about whether a drug will be and is used as intended or whether misuse is likely. Misuse, in and of itself, can represent a risk of the drug. For example, a drug is considered less acceptable if it is addicting and, so, is likely to be abused. In addition, the potential for overprescribing by physicians can also decrease the acceptability of the drug. For example, in the controversy about birth defects from isotretinoin, there was no question that the drug was a powerful teratogen, and that it was a very effective therapy for serious cystic acne refractory to other treatments. There also was no question about its effectiveness for less severe

Table 5.3. Annual risks of death from some selected hazards*

Hazard	Annual death rate (per 100 000 exposed individuals)
Heart disease (US, 1985)	261.4
Sport parachuting	190
Cancer (US, 1985)	170.5
Cigarette smoking (age 35)	167
Hang gliding (UK)	150
Motorcycling (US)	100
Power boat racing (US)	80
Cerebrovascular disease (US, 1985)	51.0
Scuba diving (US)	42
Scuba diving (UK)	22
Influenza (UK)	20
Passenger in motor vehicle (US)	16.7
Suicide (US, 1985)	11.2
Homicide (US, 1985)	7.5
Cave exploration (US)	4.5
Oral contraceptive user (age 25–34)	4.3
Pedestrian (US)	3.8
Bicycling (US)	1.1
Tornados (US)	0.2
Lightning (US)	0.05

* Data derived from references 18–20.

acne. However, that effectiveness led to its widespread use, including in individuals who could have been treated with less toxic therapies, and a larger number of pregnancy exposures, abortions, and birth defects than otherwise would have occurred.[17]

PERCEPTIONS OF THE EVALUATOR

Finally, much depends ultimately upon the perceptions of the individuals who are making the decision about whether a risk is acceptable. In the US, there have been more than a million deaths from traffic accidents over the past 30 years; tobacco-related diseases kill the equivalent of three jumbo jet loads every day; and 3000 children are born each year with embryopathy from their mothers' use of alcohol in pregnancy.[18] Yet, these deaths are accepted with little concern, while the uncommon risk of an airplane crash or being struck by lightning generates fear. The decision about whether to allow isotretinoin to remain on the market hinged on whether the efficacy of the drug for a small number of people who had a disease which was disfiguring but not life-threatening was worth the birth defects that would result in some other individuals. There is no way to remove this subjective component from the decision about the acceptability of risks. Indeed, much more research is needed to elucidate patients' preferences in these matters. However, this subjective component is part of what makes informed consent so important. Most people feel that the final subjective judgment about whether an individual should assume the risk of ingesting a drug should be made by that individual, after education by their physician. However, as an attempt to assist that judgment, it is useful to have some quantitative information about the risks inherent in some other activities. Some such information is presented in Table 5.3.

CONCLUSION

This chapter reviewed when pharmacoepidemiology studies should be performed. After beginning with a discussion of the various reasons why one might perform pharmacoepidemiology studies, it reviewed the difference between safety and risk. It concluded with a discussion of the determinants of one's tolerance of risk. Now that it is hopefully clear when one might want to perform a pharmacoepidemiology study, the next part of this book will provide perspectives on pharmacoepidemiology from some of the different fields that use it.

REFERENCES

1. Mattison N, Richard BW. Postapproval research requested by the FDA at the time of NCE approval, 1970–1984. *Drug Inf J* 1987; **21**: 309–29.
2. Humphries TJ, Myerson RM, Gifford LM *et al.* A unique post-market outpatient surveillance program of cimetidine: report on phase II and final summary. *Am J Gastroenterol* 1984; **79**: 593–6.
3. Joint Commission on Prescription Drug Use. *Final Report.* Washington, DC, 1980.
4. Young FE. The role of the FDA in the effort against AIDS. *Public Health Rep* 1988; **103**: 242–5.
5. Strom BL, Carson JL, Schinnar R, Sim E, Morse ML. The effect of indication on the risk of hypersensitivity reactions associated with tolmetin sodium vs. other nonsteroidal antiinflammatory drugs. *J Rheumatol* 1988; **15**: 695–9.
6. Rossi AC, Knapp DE. Tolmetin-induced anaphylactoid reactions. *N Engl J Med* 1982; **307**: 499–500.
7. Strom BL, and members of the ASCPT Pharmacoepidemiology Section. Position paper on the use of purported postmarketing drug surveillance studies for promotional purposes. *Clin Pharmacol Ther* 1990; **48**: 598.

8. Bortnichak EA, Sachs RM. Piroxicam in recent epidemiologic studies. *Am J Med* 1986; **81**: 44–8.

9. Strom BL, Carson JL, Morse ML, West SL, Soper KA. The effect of indication on hypersensitivity reactions associated with zomepirac sodium and other nonsteroidal antiinflammatory drugs. *Arthritis Rheum* 1987; **30**: 1142–8.

10. Strom BL, Berlin JA, Kinman JL, Spitz RW, Hennessy S, Feldman H *et al.* Parenteral ketorolac and risk of gastrointestinal and operative site bleeding: a postmarketing surveillance study. *JAMA* 1996; **275**: 376–82.

11. Feldman HI, Kinman JL, Berlin JA, Hennessy S, Kimmel SE, Farrar J *et al.* Parenteral ketorolac: the risk for acute renal failure. *Ann Intern Med* 1997; **126**: 193–9.

12. Hennessy S, Kinman JL, Berlin JA, Feldman HI, Carson JL, Kimmel SE *et al.* Lack of hepatotoxic effects of parenteral ketorolac in the hospital setting. *Arch Intern Med* 1997; **157**: 2510–14.

13. Rogers AS, Porta M, Tilson HH. Guidelines for decision making in postmarketing surveillance of drugs. *J Clin Res Pharmacol* 1990; **4**: 241–51.

14. Lowrance WW. *Of Acceptable Risk*. Los Altos, CA: William Kaufmann, 1976.

15. Stallones RA. A review of the epidemiologic studies of toxic shock syndrome. *Ann Intern Med* 1982; **96**: 917–20.

16. Binns TB. Therapeutic risks in perspective. *Lancet* 1987; **2**: 208–9.

17. Marwick C. FDA ponders approaches to curbing adverse effects of drug used against cystic acne. *JAMA* 1988; **259**: 3225.

18. Urquhart J, Heilmann K. *Risk Watch—The Odds of Life*. New York: Facts on File, 1984.

19. O'Brien B. *"What Are My Chances Doctor?"—A Review of Clinical Risks*. London: Office of Health Economics, 1986.

20. Silverberg E, Lubera JA. Cancer statistics. *CA Cancer J Clin* 1988; **38**: 5–22.

Part II

PERSPECTIVES ON PHARMACOEPIDEMIOLOGY

6

A View from Academia

ROBERT M. CALIFF[1] and LEANNE K. MADRE[2]

[1]Duke Clinical Research Institute, Durham, North Carolina, USA; [2]Duke University Medical Center, Durham, North Carolina, USA.

INTRODUCTION

The field of pharmacoepidemiology provides a challenge to the traditional academic community. It may be viewed as one element of a group of disciplines necessary to understand how to deliver diagnostic and therapeutic technologies in a manner that optimizes health—a field that might more broadly be called "therapeutics." A variety of forces continue to push issues of the risks and benefits of therapy into the public consciousness, while academic medicine has had difficulty accepting that the discipline should be a focus. This reticence to embrace the study of therapeutics as a priority relative to the more basic sciences is one element of a rather narcissistic stance taken by academic medical centers (AMCs) that has contributed to a backlash about the size of the public investment requested to support the research done in academia.

However, academia is fully capable of creating new approaches that can provide a basis for the discipline of therapeutics. The Centers for Education and Research on Therapeutics (CERTs) organization represents one such effort to change this dynamic by creating a consortium of academic centers linked to multiple government and private entities with a vision of serving as a trusted national resource for people seeking to improve health through the best use of medical therapies. This program, mandated by the authorization for the FDA, brings together AMCs, government agencies, the medical products industry, and consumer advocates with core funding through the Agency for Healthcare Research and Quality (AHRQ) and offers the opportunity to join government with private funding to meet the mission.[1] The mission of the CERTs is to conduct research and provide education that will advance the optimal use of drugs, medical devices, and biological products.[2] This mission is achieved through activities that develop knowledge about therapies and how best to use them, manage risk by improving the ability to measure both beneficial and harmful effects of therapies as used in practice, improve practice by advancing strategies to ensure that therapies are used always and only when they should be, and inform policy makers about the state of clinical science and effects of current and proposed policies. This multicenter effort is at least partially succeeding in bringing pharmacoepidemiology, and the study of therapeutics in general, back into the mainstream of academic medicine, and it provides insight into additional approaches that are needed.

Pharmacoepidemiology, Fourth Edition   Edited by B.L. Strom
© 2005 John Wiley & Sons, Ltd

ISSUES DRIVEN BY SUCCESS

Before launching into the "problem solving" mode, we should acknowledge the tremendous benefits that therapeutics have provided. People are living longer with less disability than ever before.[3] Whereas most previous gains came from broad public health measures, an increasing portion of the gains in disability-free life expectancy is coming from medical care. Therefore, it would be incorrect to imply that the system is a disaster. Instead, our view is that we are making steady progress in therapeutics that can be accelerated by better planning and integration of the discipline of clinical therapeutics and that can be enhanced by considering AMCs to be a fundamental building block of this system.

The basis for a growing gap between the potential and the reality of therapeutics is the confluence of multiple societal trends (Table 6.1). The United States and other postindustrial countries are experiencing a dramatic change in demographics, with an enormous increase in the proportion of the population that will be elderly. At the same time, in developing countries, progress is being made in instituting public health, economic, and educational measures that will reduce the epidemic causes of premature death. These changes will greatly increase the importance of medical therapeutics to prevent, delay, treat, and palliate chronic diseases. The two new issues on the scene, massive obesity in the young and biological terrorism, only heighten the importance of therapeutic knowledge and academic infrastructure to supply a competent and creative workforce.

These demographic and public health changes are occurring at a time when a revolution in biological knowledge is leading to previously unthinkable therapeutic possibilities. The combined research investment of the US government and the medical products industry (drugs, biologics, and

Table 6.1. Societal trends and the growing gap between the potential and the reality of therapeutics

(1) Increasing burden of disease

    (a) Aging of the population—"baby boomers"
    (b) Fattening of the younger generation leading to early chronic disease

(2) Accelerating technology availability

    (a) NIH investment in biology
    (b) Imaging/engineering

(3) Financial limitations

    (a) Competing forces of government and payer restraint and "consumerism"
    (b) Expanding understanding of therapeutics principles

devices) now exceeds $60 billion per year. Most common diseases have one or more known effective therapies, and many highly prevalent diseases such as cardiovascular disease and cancer have multiple effective therapies. The body of knowledge about each of these therapies is rapidly proliferating, while our ability to learn even more is growing faster still.[4]

The continued evolution of computing has enabled pharmacoepidemiology in particular to take an even more prominent role. Hardly a day passes without a publication or news story about a secondary analysis of a data set showing a relationship between a therapy and an outcome. The reason is that health care transactions are increasingly captured in computers, either directly or by the capture of claims data, and these data sets can be manipulated by increasingly usable and powerful statistical packages. This technological advance has also rapidly opened up cross-cultural communications, thus fostering international collaborations exemplified by the International Society for Pharmacoepidemiology (ISPE) (www.pharmacoepi.org).

All of these trends are positive, but they raise a new set of problems that must be addressed, at least partly through the efforts of AMCs. As the potential of technology continues to accelerate and our inability to provide all technologies to all people is increasingly evident, we simply need better knowledge about how to effectively apply technologies, including diagnostic devices, drugs, biologics, and therapeutic devices, to the right patient at the right time.[5]

INADEQUATE KNOWLEDGE BASE

There is a large and growing gap between the potential of therapies to ameliorate human disease and our actual base of knowledge. This gap does not emanate from lack of progression in studies of therapeutics. Rather, the problem has grown because the pace of technology development continues to accelerate relative to our ability to test and evaluate it.

Drugs and devices are still developed in relatively small studies of limited duration, often without measuring health outcomes as an endpoint and almost always without direct measures of costs. Instead we rely on biomarkers, surrogates, or partial efficacy evaluations for regulatory approval, in combination with limited safety data from short-term studies. These studies usually also exclude many patients who ultimately will receive these therapies. The excluded patients tend to be the elderly and minorities, usually with a high rate of comorbidities, particularly renal dysfunction or advanced chronic disease. The result is that many therapeutics reach the market with incomplete documentation of their use in the populations at highest risk.

The extent of this inadequate knowledge base is perhaps most glaring in the arena of pediatrics. Before the Pediatric Research Equity Act 2003, the term "therapeutic orphan" was an apt term to describe children; it had been accepted that children could not be studied in clinical trials because of the difficulties with ensuring consent. However, since the institution of patent extensions for the study of compounds already on the market and the requirement to study drugs in development if they will be used in children, clinical trials of therapeutics in children have proliferated. Most recently, a Congressional mandate has led to a concerted effort to evaluate older drugs that are no longer on patent, but which are frequently used in children. This effort is completely dependent upon a consortium of academic pediatrics programs funded by the National Institute of Child Health and Human Development (NICHD).[6,7]

In other cases, the fundamental knowledge about a problem common to multiple therapeutics is lacking. The impact of drugs on the risk of torsade de pointes, a sometimes lethal cardiac arrhythmia, is an excellent example. While outstanding work has been done on the genetic and biological basis for QT prolongation,[8] much less is known about appropriate medical decision making in the face of drugs known to cause QT interval prolongation.[9] Recent surveys of clinicians have found that the knowledge of practitioners about the details of this problem is scant.[10] Even drugs that have been used for years often have not undergone an adequate evaluation. Katchman and colleagues recently described that methadone causes QT interval prolongation[11] and sudden death.[12] This type of inquiry is unlikely to be done solely by industry and will require collaboration with academic institutions.

Devices are approved for marketing with a different set of standards from drugs[13] (see also Chapter 31). Often no randomized trials have been done. The rationale for this different set of rules emanates from the short life cycle of devices (often measured in months) and the iterative nature of device development. The myocardial laser revascularization technologies have provided an example for study. Developed to relieve angina in patients refractory to standard medical and device therapies, transmyocardial laser revascularization (TMR) was initially approved for human use based on a series of observational studies using historical controls and without blinding. The availability of the Society of Thoracic Surgeons database allowed the use of TMR to be tracked. Early in its adoption, it was surprisingly used most often off-label, and often in patients with a labeled contraindication with operative mortality

rates that were much higher than expected.[14] Further focus on this issue has led to more rational use of the device, and new clinical trials are demonstrating the appropriate role of both TMR and percutaneous myocardial revascularization (PMR).

Another excellent example is in the entire field of gout therapy. Partially effective treatments for acute gout and prophylaxis for chronic gout were developed decades ago. Unfortunately, new drugs have not been forthcoming, and the old drugs never underwent the types of outcome studies that could define the appropriate dose and approach to use in diverse populations. Accordingly, a consortium of academics and professional society members has developed a set of clinical practice guidelines for gout based on the scanty available data.[15]

These latter two projects underscore the importance of the combined resources of professional organizations and AMCs in solving major problems in therapeutics.

SUBOPTIMAL PRACTICE

The gap between the practice of health care delivery and the knowledge base that should guide that practice is vast.[16] In primary prevention and in diseases for which standards of care have evolved, demonstration of imperfect levels of adherence to practice standards abound.[17] This gap has been well demonstrated in the hospital setting, where decision making is largely up to the treating physician. Evolving data from the outpatient setting, not surprisingly, show an even larger gap.[18] The complexity of the outpatient therapeutic transaction is driven by multiple factors, most prominently the actions of the patient in adhering to the prescriber's recommendations.

The CERT at the University of Alabama has focused on inadequate practices in the area of diseases of the bones and joints. In particular, it has shown that practitioners often fall short in terms of osteoporosis treatment in all patients and in patients treated with glucocorticoids,[19] and that significant racial[20] and specialty-related differences exist in the use of coxibs for arthritis.[21] These studies of practice variation have led to substantial collaborative efforts to develop guidelines and quality indicators in rheumatology.[22]

The issue of antibiotic use in children with suspected otitis media provides another fascinating example of inadequate clinical practice. There is a widespread view that unnecessary antibiotics are frequently prescribed to children with suspected otitis media, and that this overuse problem results in an increase in antibiotic resistance in addition to an unwarranted increase in costs. Studies in the HMO Research Network have documented that the use of antibiotics is declining, but that much more work needs to be done on this issue.[23] A randomized trial has shown the benefit of educational outreach in changing this behavior,[24] and a study at the CERT at the University of Pennsylvania has shown the tension between the desire of practitioners to improve societal outcomes and their obligation to individual patients.[25] By combining the analytic and quantitative skills in academic centers and the broad desire of practitioners to improve, particularly in a managed care setting, we are seeing a national improvement in practice.

Another important therapeutic issue is the suboptimal use of therapies for coronary artery disease (CAD) and heart failure. Both in acute and chronic manifestations of heart failure and CAD, a modest number of proven beneficial therapies are available, yet they are often not used when indicated or are applied in incorrect manners to the wrong patients.[26] Studies in the Tennessee Medicaid system,[27] the HMO Research Network,[28] and North Carolina[29] have all found the same basic problems. These differences have been amplified by multicultural studies demonstrating not only differences in use of secondary preventive medications, but also differences in outcomes,[30,31] including issues related to access to therapies.[32] Often, a lack of knowledge leads to effective drugs not being prescribed. In other cases, the physician disagrees with the indication, although this is not the major factor inhibiting optimal use of therapies. Recent data from Tennessee indicated that even when the right medications were prescribed at hospital discharge, 15% of patients did not fill the prescriptions.[27] A recent analysis demonstrated that current mechanisms provide major economic disincentives to focus on adherence to therapies that save lives in heart failure patients.[33]

COUNTERPRODUCTIVE OR NONPRODUCTIVE POLICIES

At the time of the initial funding of the CERTs, numerous counterproductive policies relating to therapeutics could be cited. The prototypical case was the temporary effort in the state of New Hampshire to limit the use of prescription medications in the state Medicaid program. The result was that the emergency departments in the state were overwhelmed with acute visits from people whose chronic diseases had become uncontrolled due to lack of access to drugs.[34]

Several examples have been the topics of major CERTs studies. The group at the University of Pennsylvania evaluated the role of utilization review in prescribing[35] (see also Chapter 29). Using sophisticated epidemiological techniques, they were unable to find any benefit of the usual

state Medicaid approach with regard to prescribing errors or avoidable hospitalizations. The investigators believed that structural and functional principles probably explained the futility of these broadly applied programs: low rates of alerts, lack of linkage between alerts, the complex reasons that drugs are prescribed, and the time lags between prescription and review.[36] The ability of several academic centers to collaborate on assessing the evidence is likely to lead to further improvement in advice to policy makers.[37]

The group at Vanderbilt University evaluated the impact of switching to a fully capitated specialty "carve out" program for mental health services in the state of Tennessee.[38] These investigators documented that in patients on antipsychotics there was a clear loss of continuity in the transition. Furthermore, patients needing antipsychotic drugs were less likely to take them, a phenomenon that was most pronounced in the sickest patients. Similar problems have been described by the Harvard group.[39]

ROLE OF ACADEMIC MEDICAL CENTERS

While AMCs may be only one of many entities in the therapeutics arena, all physicians, pharmacists, and dentists are trained at AMCs, as are a large proportion of nurses. Therefore, in the long run, AMCs have the opportunity and responsibility for providing the basal national infrastructure for practitioners of therapeutics. AMCs also provide a home for the majority of clinicians who influence public sources of information and opinion. Finally, AMCs receive the bulk of funding from the US National Institutes of Health (NIH), the main source of medical research funding.[40]

IMPROVE KNOWLEDGE

While knowledge alone is not enough to correct the gap between research and practice, it is a necessary first step. Of course, this effort begins with training in nursing, pharmacy, medical, dental, and public health schools. Even assuming perfect work in the "basic training" years, however, the number of existing practitioners exceeds the number of trainees by a large margin.

Much of the work of the CERTs has been focused on improving the knowledge of therapeutics among practitioners, but AMCs have not done an adequate job of relating to practitioners, leaving much knowledge transmission to the medical products industry itself. As stated by Stephen Soumerai, a leader in the evaluation of methods intended to change prescribing behavior, when it comes to translating the knowledge into practice, "Everything works some of the time, and nothing works all of the time."

New legislation in the United States has given the opportunity to take back a large portion of continuing education into the AMC arena.[41] Professional organizations, buttressed by government regulation about using continuing medical education for advertising,[42] have produced stringent guidelines that call for independent control of programs that educate health professionals.

REINVIGORATE CLINICAL PHARMACOLOGY

The field of clinical pharmacology has been poorly supported by Federal funding sources, and for the most part AMCs have responded by decreasing the number of faculty positions. This mismatch of funding and societal need can be corrected partially by programs such as the CERTs. In addition, as the importance and scope of clinical pharmacology have expanded, several key entrepreneurial opportunities exist. The General Clinical Research Centers funded by the NIH have continued to receive excellent levels of funding. The pharmaceutical, biotechnology, and device industries are also feeling the pressure from the shortage of talent in developing the knowledge needed for successful drug development. The focus on the safety of medical products and the long-term balance of risk and benefit has created a large demand for expertise in the industry, well beyond the focus on product development. Finally, the societal focus on patient safety will require methodology developed by this field to monitor the use of drugs and devices. Further efforts are needed to link AMCs with the needs of the industry and government with regard to the postmarketing phase.

CREATE A REPOSITORY OF DATABASE RESOURCES

Increasingly, the evidence needed to guide choices at the individual and policy levels will be driven by empirical analysis of data from populations. At a national level, entities such as the CERTs can provide the opportunity for multiple parties to answer questions from databases. Multiple databases are available for interrogation with specific questions about therapeutics. However, recent concerns about privacy and the sheer size of the databases emphasize the need for facilities with experts in data management and analysis. The CERTs represent one approach to this by bringing together experts from multiple academic centers into an organization with a coordinating center charged with facilitating common projects.

In this construct the databases continue to reside with their developers, but systems are developed to enhance the sharing of portions of the databases to answer specific questions. The HMO Research Network has created a prototypical example of this "federated" approach, in which questions can be asked[43] and the system brings together elements of databases from the various health maintenance organizations to provide answers. Issues of privacy, anonymization, sharing, and scope of the data have been worked out in advance to improve the efficiency of the process of gaining access to the data.

At the local level, there is a pressing need for institutions and health systems to develop data repositories and local expertise in appropriate analysis related to quality. AMCs have the expertise to set the example by organizing data repositories and providing access to data for the purposes of improving quality and developing a generalized understanding of diagnostic and therapeutic strategies. This effort should not stop at the national level, however. Indeed, access to the UK General Practice Research Database[44] (see Chapter 22) has allowed multiple important observations to be made of direct relevance to global health.

IMPROVE PRACTICE

The case for improving practice is self-evident. Yet AMCs must question which role they should play. While AMCs train providers in their basic skills, the province of clinical practice has many entities with variable agendas and opportunities to demonstrate better approaches to the organization of health care. This larger clinical enterprise dwarfs the ability of AMCs to directly change the practice of medicine. In this regard the AMCs should seek to leverage their unique position to move national practice towards higher quality health care.

At the most fundamental level, AMCs have a responsibility to apply resources to science by evaluating therapies that are already marketed. Much has been written about the lack of incentive for the medical products industry to study its products as patent life nears the end.[45] Furthermore, rules on generics require only evidence of bioequivalence, and the profit margin on generics is not thought to justify the funding of outcome studies. A similar situation exists with regard to food additives and "alternative and complementary" therapies. There is no source to perform these evaluations other than the cadre of AMCs, ideally buttressed with Federal funding. The Clinical Research Roundtable of the Institute of Medicine has stressed the need for an elevation of funding for pragmatic clinical trials.[46]

At a basal level, AMCs also should be instilling in practitioners a fundamental understanding of the principles of therapeutics and the measurement of quality in health care delivery. Although the American Society for Clinical Pharmacology and Therapeutics has put forward a model curriculum for its particular domain, a well-defined curriculum on the broader field of therapeutics does not exist, and teaching of the fundamentals of biostatistics, probability, decision making and health care systems has not been well received, and perhaps not well executed.[47] Preliminary work by the CERTs has established the high degree of difficulty in making curriculum changes in US health education programs. The curriculum is packed, and many contingents are so adamant about not losing time that insertion of new material is seen as a zero-sum game, in which addition of anything new means elimination of something else. Nevertheless, we are seeing a gradual increase in the emphasis on skills that will improve the quality of therapeutics in undergraduate, house staff, and continuing education programs. One approach to this dilemma has been the development of focused curricula which are posted on the Internet for use in multiple settings and institutions.

AMCs also have the challenge of training and supporting the researchers who will define the field in the future. Currently, the AHRQ has scant funds for training and faculty development, and this arena has purposefully not been a focus of the NIH. The NIH Roadmap may provide the opportunity to develop a larger cadre of experts in the related fields of clinical epidemiology, biostatistics, clinical trials, health economics, health services research, and clinical pharmacology.[48]

Finally, AMCs must consider developing novel models of care delivery that improve the use of marketed products. Much of the work of the CERTs has indicated that the quality of medical care will improve most dramatically when systematic changes are made in the organization and funding of delivery.[49] The huge increase in people with chronic disease coupled with advances in effective but expensive technology[50,51] provides strong evidence that the current system, as marginal as it is today, will be nonviable in the near future. Yet, few AMCs are leading the way by testing novel approaches to team-based care delivery using advanced information technology.

INFORM CONSTITUENTS

Policy Makers

Ultimately, many issues in therapeutics can only be solved by informing policy makers to increase the chances of rational policies that provide incentives for behavior that improves the use of therapeutics. The potential to leverage expertise for benefit has never been greater as more health care resources fall to the Federal government and large payer plans.

The Public

Informing the public about the balance of risks and benefits of therapeutics is a tremendous task, about which surprisingly little is known. An increasing number of studies are showing that much information made available to the public is either biased or not understandable. Yet, at AMCs, little attention has been focused on translating medical research findings into statements that can be acted upon effectively by the public.[52]

The Press

Surveys of the public indicate that more health-related decisions are based on press reports than on doctor visits.[53] Even when the FDA wants to get a message to the public, it must use the press to get this message out. It can be argued that observational studies about the broad issue of therapeutics dominate the press reports on medicine, often with inadequate attention to the quantitative issues involved in the interpretation. Unfortunately, the role of the press in therapeutics and public health has received inadequate attention in academia. In a recent "think tank,"[54] multiple issues about the press were raised, and a research agenda has been put forward for consideration.

SPECIAL ROLE OF PUBLIC–PRIVATE PARTNERSHIPS

The dramatic effects of the aging of the population combined with the fattening of the younger generation will create an enormous societal challenge. Indeed, the problems are arguably so overwhelming that public–private partnerships may be the only way to create enough resources to find effective solutions.

The CERTs have developed a model approach to public–private partnership based on a set of principles that increase the likelihood that modest public investment will yield a larger private investment while also safeguarding the ecumenical nature of the enterprise. These principles are designed to encourage engagement of industry partners in the research enterprise under a set of rules that can be considered by the CERTs' governance and openly discussed.

The first priority of the CERTs is to tackle issues of public interest. CERTs is a major initiative to improve the rational use of therapeutics through research and education activities that are in the public interest but would not otherwise be done. Second, the CERTs are actively seeking public–private partnership, rather than avoiding it. CERTs is a public–private partnership; therefore centers seek useful, appropriate interactions with private organizations to support and enhance education, research, and demonstration projects. AHRQ works with the centers to establish appropriate agreements to optimize use and sharing of resources. Third, the issue of conflicts of interest is acknowledged and confronted. Potential conflicts of interest are likely to exist in any public–private partnership. These potential conflicts cannot be completely avoided or eliminated. The obligation is to disclose fully and manage potential conflicts in a manner that minimizes the risk of those conflicts, while maximizing progress to achieve CERTs goals. Fourth, academic integrity is paramount. As academic researchers, individuals conducting projects under the CERTs umbrella will retain final decision making about study design, analysis, conclusions, and publication and will ensure that their work complies with their respective institutions' conflict-of-interest rules.

Finally, one size does not fit all in CERTs activities. CERTs activities are defined as projects supported in whole or in part by AHRQ funds under the CERTs demonstration program. Such activities are subject to processes established for the CERTs program, such as the review of potential conflicts of interest. Individuals affiliated with the centers also conduct education and research activities outside of CERTs that are not subject to CERTs processes.

In summary, AMCs have a vital role to play in pharmacoepidemiology and therapeutics. This role includes providing a fundamental basis of training and maintenance of an academic discipline. However, it also includes creative integration with health care providers, government agencies, and the broader medical industry.

REFERENCES

1. Califf RM. The Centers for Education and Research on Therapeutics. The need for a national infrastructure to improve the rational use of therapeutics. *Pharmacoepidemiol Drug Saf* 2002; **11**: 319–27.

2. The Centers for Education and Research on Therapeutics (CERTs). Available at http://www.certs.hhs.gov. Accessed October 4, 2004.

3. Califf RM. Defining the balance of risk and benefit in the era of genomics and proteomics. *Health Aff* 2004; **23**: 77–87.

4. Califf RM, DeMets DL. Principles from clinical trials relevant to clinical practice: Part I. *Circulation* 2002; **106**: 1015–21.

5. Woosley RL. Centers for Education and Research in Therapeutics. *Clin Pharmacol Ther* 1994; **55**: 249–55.

6. Rodriguez WJ, Roberts R, Murphy D. Current regulatory policies regarding pediatric indications and exclusivity. *J Pediatr Gastroenterol Nutr* 2003; **37**(suppl 1): S40–5.

7. Pasquali SK, Sanders SP, Li JS. Oral antihypertensive trial design and analysis under the pediatric exclusivity provision. *Am Heart J* 2002; **144**: 608–14.

8. Anderson ME, Al-Khatib SM, Roden DM, Califf RM. Duke Clinical Research Institute/American Heart Journal Expert Meeting on Repolarization Changes. Cardiac repolarization: current knowledge, critical gaps, and new approaches to drug development and patient management. *Am Heart J* 2002; **144**: 769–81.

9. Al-Khatib SM, Allen LaPointe NM, Kramer JM, Califf RM. What clinicians should know about the QT interval. *JAMA* 2003; **289**: 2120–7.

10. Curtis LH, Ostbye T, Sendersky V, Hutchison S, Allen LaPointe NM, Al-Khatib SM *et al.* Prescription of QT-prolonging drugs in a cohort of about 5 million outpatients. *Am J Med* 2003; **14**: 135–41.

11. Katchman AN, McGroary KA, Kilborn MJ, Kornick CA, Manfredi PL, Woosley RL *et al.* Influence of opioid agonists on cardiac human ether-a-go-go-related gene K$^+$ currents. *J Pharmacol Exp Ther* 2002; **303**: 688–94.

12. Piguet V, Desmeules J, Ehret G, Stoller R, Dayer P. QT interval prolongation in patients on methadone with concomitant drugs. *J Clin Psychopharmacol* 2004; **24**: 446–8.

13. O'Shea JC, Kramer JM, Califf RM, Peterson ED. Results of Experts Meetings—Part I: identifying holes in the safety net. *Am Heart J* 2004; **147**: 977–84.

14. Peterson ED, Kaul P, Kaczmarek RG, Hammill BG, Armstrong PW, Bridges CR *et al.* From controlled trials to clinical practice: monitoring transmyocardial revascularization use and outcomes. *J Am Coll Cardiol* 2003; **42**: 1611–6.

15. Mikuls TR, MacLean CH, Olivieri J, Patino F, Allison JJ, Farrar JT *et al.* Quality of care indicators for gout management. *Arthritis Rheum* 2004; **50**: 937–43.

16. Lenfant C. Shattuck Lecture: Clinical research to clinical practice—lost in translation? *N Engl J Med* 2003; **349**:868–74.

17. Institute of Medicine. *Crossing the Quality Chasm: A New Health System for the 21st Century*. Washington, DC: National Academy Press, 2001.

18. Butler J, Arbogast PG, Daugherty J, Jain MK, Ray WA, Griffin MR. Outpatient utilization of angiotensin-converting enzyme inhibitors among heart failure patients after hospital discharge. *J Am Coll Cardiol* 2004; **43**: 2036–43.

19. Mudano A, Allison J, Hill J, Rothermel T, Saag K. Variations in glucocorticoid induced osteoporosis prevention in a managed care cohort. *J Rheumatol* 2001; **28**: 1298–305.

20. Mudano AS, Casebeer L, Patino F, Allison JJ, Weissman NW, Kiefe CI *et al.* Racial disparities in osteoporosis prevention in a managed care population. *South Med J* 2003; **96**: 445–51.

21. Patino FG, Allison J, Olivieri J, Mudano A, Juarez L, Person S *et al.* The effects of physician specialty and patient comorbidities on the use and discontinuation of coxibs. *Arthritis Rheum* 2003; **49**: 293–9.

22. Saag KG, Olivieri JJ, Patino F, Mikuls TR, Allison JJ, MacLean CH. Measuring quality in arthritis care: the Arthritis Foundation's quality indicator set for analgesics. *Arthritis Rheum* 2004; **51**: 337 – 49.

23. Finkelstein JA, Stille C, Nordin J, Davis R, Raebel MA, Roblin D *et al.* Reduction in antibiotic use among US children, 1996–2000. *Pediatrics* 2003; **112**: 620–7.

24. Finkelstein JA, Davis RL, Dowell SF, Metlay JP, Soumerai SB, Rifas-Shiman SL *et al.* Reducing antibiotic use in children: a randomized trial in 12 practices. *Pediatrics* 2001; **108**: 1–7.

25. Metlay JP, Shea JA, Asch DA. Antibiotic prescribing decisions of generalists and infectious disease specialists: thresholds for adopting new drug therapies. *Med Decis Making* 2002; **22**: 498–505.

26. Ansari M, Shlipak MG, Heidenreich PA, Van Ostaeyen D, Pohl EC, Browner WS *et al.* Improving guideline adherence: a randomized trial evaluating strategies to increase beta-blocker use in heart failure. *Circulation* 2003; **107**: 2799–804.

27. Butler J, Arbogast PG, BeLue R, Daugherty J, Jain MK, Ray WA *et al.* Outpatient adherence to beta-blocker therapy after acute myocardial infarction. *J Am Coll Cardiol* 2002; **40**: 1589–95.

28. Higashi T, Shekelle PG, Solomon DH, Knight EL, Roth C, Chang JT *et al.* The quality of pharmacologic care for vulnerable older patients. *Ann Intern Med* 2004; **140**: 714–20.

29. Allen LaPointe NM, Kramer JM, DeLong ER, Ostbye T, Hammill BG, Muhlbaier LH *et al.* Patient-reported frequency of taking aspirin in a population with coronary artery disease. *Am J Cardiol* 2002; **89**: 1042–6.

30. Kaul P, Newby LK, Fu Y, Mark DB, Califf RM, Topol EJ *et al.* International differences in evolution of early discharge after acute myocardial infarction. *Lancet* 2004; **363**: 511–7.

31. Pilote L, Granger C, Armstrong PW, Mark DB, Hlatky MA. Differences in the treatment of myocardial infarction between the United States and Canada. A survey of physicians in the GUSTO trial. *Med Care* 1995; **33**: 598–610.

32. Rao SV, Kaul P, Newby LK, Lincoff AM, Hochman J, Harrington RA *et al.* Poverty, process of care, and outcome in acute coronary syndromes. *J Am Coll Cardiol* 2003; **41**: 1948–54.

33. Cowper PA, DeLong ER, Whellan DJ, Allen LaPointe NM, Califf RM. Economic effects of beta blocker therapy in patients with heart failure. *Am J Med* 2004; **116**: 104–11.

34. Soumerai SB, Ross-Degnan D, Avorn J, McLaughlin T, Choodnovskiy I. Effects of Medicaid drug-payment limits on admission to hospitals and nursing homes. *N Engl J Med* 1991; **325**: 1072–7.

35. Hennessy S, Bilker WB, Zhou L, Weber AL, Brensinger C, Wang Y *et al.* Retrospective drug utilization review, prescribing errors, and clinical outcomes. *JAMA* 2003; **290**: 1494–9.

36. Hennessy S, Strom BL, Lipton HL, Soumerai SB. Drug utilization review. In: Strom BL, ed., *Pharmacoepidemiology*, 3rd edn. Chichester: John Wiley & Sons, 2000; pp. 505–24.

37. Christensen DB, Campbell WH, Fulda TR, Pugh MC, Smith DH, Lipowski EE *et al.* Evaluation of drug utilization review programs. *JAMA* 2004; **291**: 185.

38. Ray WA, Daugherty JR, Meador KG. Effect of a mental health "carve-out" program on the continuity of antipsychotic therapy. *N Engl J Med* 2003; **348**: 1885–94.

39. Soumerai S. Unintended outcomes of Medicaid drug cost-containment policies on the chronically mentally ill. *J Clin Psychol* 2003; **64**(suppl 17): 19–22.

40. Blumenthal D. Academic–industrial relationships in the life sciences. *N Engl J Med* **349**: 2452–9.

41. Moynihan R. Drug company sponsorship of education could be replaced at a fraction of its cost. *BMJ* 2003; **326**: 1163.

42. Relman AS. Defending professional independence: ACCME's proposed new guidelines for commercial support of CME. *JAMA* 2003; **289**: 2418–20.

43. Platt R, Davis R, Finkelstein J, Go AS, Gurwitz JH, Roblin D *et al.* Multicenter epidemiologic and health services research on therapeutics in the HMO Research Network Center for Education and Research on Therapeutics. *Pharmacoepidemiol Drug Saf* 2001; **10**: 373–7.

44. Lewis JD, Brensinger C, Bilker WB, Strom BL. Validity and completeness of the General Practice Research Database for studies of inflammatory bowel disease. *Pharmacoepidemiol Drug Saf* 2002; **11**: 211–8.

45. Food and Drug Administration. Innovation or stagnation? Challenge and opportunity on the critical path to new medical products. Available from: http://www.fda.gov/oc/initiatives/criticalpath/whitepaper.html/. Accessed: August 2, 2004.

46. Sung NS, Crowley WF Jr, Genel M, Salber P, Sandy L, Sherwood LM *et al.* Central challenges facing the national clinical research enterprise. *JAMA* 2003; **289**: 1278–87.

47. Rosebraugh CJ, Honig PK, Yasuda SU, Pezzullo JC, Flockhart DA, Woosley RL. Formal education about medication errors in internal medicine clerkships. *JAMA* 2001; **286**: 1019–20.

48. The NIH roadmap. Available from: http://www.nihroadmap.nih.gov/. Accessed: July 20, 2004.

49. Pearson SA, Ross-Degnan D, Payson A, Soumerai SB. Changing medication use in managed care: a critical review of the available evidence. *Am J Managed Care* 2003; **9**: 715–31.

50. Woolhandler S, Campbell T, Himmelstein DU. Costs of health care administration in the United States and Canada. *N Engl J Med* 2003; **349**: 768–75.

51. Tunis SR. Why Medicare has not established criteria for coverage decisions. *N Engl J Med* 2004; **350**: 2196–8.

52. Campbell WH, Califf RM, for the CERTs Risk Communication Workshop Participants. Improving communication about drug risks to prevent patient injury: proceedings of a workshop. *Pharmacoepidemiol Drug Saf* 2003; **12**: 183–94.

53. National Health Council. *Americans Talk about Science and Medical News: The National Health Council Report.* Washington, DC: National Health Council, 1997.

54. Mebane F. The importance of news media in pharmaceutical risk communication: proceedings of a workshop. *Pharmacoepidemiol Drug Saf* 2004; **14**(5): 297–306.

7

A View from Industry

ROBERT F. REYNOLDS, DALE B. GLASSER AND GRETCHEN S. DIECK

Pfizer Inc., New York, NY, USA.

INTRODUCTION

Over the past century, medicines and vaccines have transformed the practice of modern medicine and significantly improved the public's health, by reducing morbidity and increasing life expectancy across the globe. More than a half million pharmaceutical products are currently available in the United States,[1] and nearly 350 new medications were approved in the 1990s by the US Food and Drug Administration (FDA) to treat conditions that affect millions of people.[2–5] Despite recent challenges in the discovery and development of new medications,[5,6] 35 new medicines were approved in 2003 for the treatment of diseases such as Alzheimer's disease, cancer, and HIV infection, and more than $30 billion was invested by pharmaceutical and biotechnology companies for new drug research and development.[7]

The role of epidemiology in drug development, safety assessment, and commercialization has expanded significantly in recent years. Traditionally, the pharmaceutical industry and regulatory agencies have relied on basic science research and clinical studies of experimental design to assess the efficacy and safety of new medications prior to approval, and spontaneous reporting systems to assess the safety of medications after approval. Fifteen years ago, epidemiology was primarily used defensively in response to legal or regulatory questions. Now, however, pharmaceutical and biotechnology companies employ epidemiologists and apply observational study designs and methods in many functional areas within pharmaceutical companies.

The goal of this chapter is to provide an overview of the ways in which epidemiologic design and methods are applied within industry, with a particular focus on its uses for drug safety evaluation. The renewal of the Prescription Drug User Fee Act in 2002 (PDUFA III) resulted in the emergence of a new framework for evaluating and managing medication risks. We provide a brief overview of the potential impact of this framework on drug safety evaluation before describing the many uses of epidemiology within pharmaceutical companies. We then conclude with a discussion of the areas where epidemiology and industry

Pharmacoepidemiology, Fourth Edition   Edited by B.L. Strom
© 2005 John Wiley & Sons, Ltd

sponsorship and partnership are most likely to advance the field of pharmacoepidemiology.

THE NEW REGULATORY AND INDUSTRY FOCUS ON RISK MANAGEMENT AND EPIDEMIOLOGY

During the process of drug development and marketing, national regulatory agencies, such as the US FDA, or multinational agencies, such as the European Medicines Evaluation Agency (EMEA), regulate the pharmaceutical industry. These agencies require that a pharmaceutical manufacturer demonstrate that a new medication, device or vaccine is safe and effective before approving, and that information about the effects of these medications is communicated to patients and physicians. The manufacturer has a further obligation to evaluate the safety of products on an ongoing basis, in order to develop and maintain product labeling that ensures appropriate prescribing of drugs by physicians and safe use by patients. Implicit in this process is the need for a logical basis for drug approval, for a rational and balanced approach to both pre- and postmarketing surveillance of drug safety, and for a scientific, evidence-based regulatory environment. As such, manufacturers devote significant efforts and resources to meeting worldwide regulatory requirements for drug research and development, monitoring the postmarketing safety of medications in compliance with required spontaneous reporting systems and time frames, and in completing Phase IV commitments.

More than a decade ago, concerns were raised that the FDA was taking too long to review New Drug Applications (NDA) and make decisions on approval.[2,3] Because a thorough review of the safety and efficacy data is essential, staff shortages at the FDA may have delayed many valuable, and in some cases lifesaving, medications from being available to the large numbers of patients who could benefit. Patient advocacy groups, in particular HIV-AIDS activists, were instrumental in forcing changes to this regulatory process, and in providing patients with access to potentially life-saving medications sooner.[8] In 1992, the Prescription Drug User Fee Act (PDUFA) was passed. This enabled the FDA to hire hundreds of additional reviewers with funds provided by the sponsors (manufacturers) submitting an NDA. In return, manufacturers could expect a decision on approval within one year of submitting an NDA (6 months if the drug was approved for expedited review by the FDA). Following the introduction of PDUFA in 1992, the mean length of the approval phase decreased by more than 20%.[3,4] The Act expired in 1997 and was subsequently renewed by Congress (PDUFA II).

Since that time, there has been an increased regulatory emphasis on postmarketing surveillance, and a greater likelihood for observational studies to be required as post-approval safety commitments.[9] Regulatory agencies have long recognized the importance of continuously evaluating the risk-benefit balance of medications.[10] Recently, however, regulatory agencies and the pharmaceutical industry have placed greater importance on the development of guidelines and standard processes for recognizing and, where possible, minimizing risk.[11-14] Increased public awareness of the potential risks of medications and a greater technological ability to identify possible proxy measures of risk outcomes have undoubtedly contributed to this greater awareness. There has been a gradual shift from the traditional mode of passive risk assessment and communication (e.g., voluntary spontaneous reporting systems and information dissemination) to the use of more active forms of evaluating and managing potential medication risks, such as restrictions in use and distribution or mandatory education programs. This shift has resulted in calls for a scientifically-based process for managing medication risks.[13,14] (See also Chapter 35.)

Now, with the enactment of the 2002 rewrite of PDUFA (PDUFA III), risk management, the scientific process by which risks are identified, assessed, communicated, and minimized, has a formal role in the development, review and approval of new drugs. This legislation acknowledges that there are both risks and benefits inherent in therapeutic interventions, and that a common goal of manufacturers and the FDA is optimizing therapeutic benefit and minimizing medication risk. For the first time, under PDUFA III, revenue collected in the form of prescription drug user fees will be earmarked for certain postmarketing risk assessment activities. Further, recommendations that risk management plans be developed prior to drug approval have played a key role in moving the risk management planning process into earlier stages in drug development, even though filing of a formal pre-approval risk management plan remains voluntary at this time. The focus on risk management during the pre-approval period provides an opportunity to explore and quantify potential safety signals and to document the exploratory and decision-making process and rationale in a risk management plan, which will necessarily evolve throughout the life cycle of the drug. Risk management plans and programs will ultimately benefit the public health, resulting in earlier approval of drugs in addition to the approval of drugs with therapeutic benefits that outweigh clearly defined safety risks. (See also Chapter 35.)

Epidemiology plays a central role in risk management activities, whether through studies of the natural history of disease, disease progression/treatment pathways, and mortality and morbidity patterns, or in the design and implementation of post-approval safety studies or risk minimization programs. The emerging risk management framework, with its emphasis on scientifically based methodologies and transparent decision-making, provides a unique opportunity for epidemiologists to contribute to the development of effective and safe medications and to build the public's confidence in the actions of industry and government.

EPIDEMIOLOGY IN THE PHARMACEUTICAL INDUSTRY

Epidemiology contributes to the success of several important functions within a pharmaceutical company, including product planning, portfolio development, and the commercialization of drugs, but its greatest contribution is in the area of drug safety evaluation. The observational methods used in some functions, particularly those supporting the commercialization and marketing of new drugs, are often described by other terminology within companies (e.g., outcomes, health economics), and are discussed in more depth elsewhere in this book (see Chapters 43 and 44).

EVALUATING DRUG SAFETY

The safety profile of any drug reflects an evolving body of knowledge extending from pre-clinical investigations to the first use of the agent in humans and through the post-approval life cycle of the product. Drug manufacturers, however, have traditionally relied on two major sources for information on the safety of drugs: the clinical trials supporting the New Drug Application (NDA) and, once the drug is marketed, spontaneous reports received throughout the world. Both are useful and have a place in assessing drug safety, but have limitations that can be addressed, in part, by the proper use of observational epidemiology. Epidemiologic studies can complement these two sources of data to provide a more comprehensive and pragmatic picture of the safety profile of a drug.

There are many relevant safety issues that can only be studied through observational epidemiology. Only epidemiologic methods are practical for estimating the incidence of and risk factors for rarely occurring events in large populations exposed to a drug (see also Chapter 3), to study events with a long latency period, or to study cross-generational effects of a drug. For example, case reports of a few patients with primary pulmonary hypertension exposed to appetite suppressant drugs led to a formal epidemiologic study documenting this association and strengthened labeling for the drug.[15]

While observational epidemiology offers numerous advantages, epidemiologic studies should never be viewed in isolation from other data sources when addressing questions of a drug's safety. Results from clinical trials, spontaneous reports, epidemiologic studies, and where relevant, pre-clinical datasets, should all be evaluated for their potential to address the particular safety question raised, with close consideration given to the unique strengths and limitations of the study designs and data collection methods used.

Clinical Trials

The randomized controlled clinical trial is considered the gold standard methodology to study the safety and efficacy of a drug. However, trials are limited by the relatively small numbers of patients studied and the short time period over which patients are observed. The numbers of patients included in premarketing clinical trials are usually adequate to identify only the most common and acutely occurring adverse events. Typically, these trials have a total patient sample size up to several thousand. Using the "rule of three", where the sample size needed is roughly three times the reciprocal of the frequency of the event, at least 300 patients would be required in a trial in order to observe at least one adverse event that occurs at a rate of 1/100. Likewise, a sample of 3000 is needed to observe at least one adverse event with 95% probability if the frequency of the event is 1/1000. (See Chapter 3 for more discussion of the sample sizes needed for studies.) Thus, clinical trials are usually only large enough to detect events that occur relatively frequently, and are not intended or designed to address all potential safety issues related to a particular drug.[16]

An additional limitation of clinical trials with respect to drug safety is the strict inclusion/exclusion criteria common in these studies. Patients included in pre-approval clinical studies may be the healthiest segment of that patient population. Special groups such as the elderly, pregnant women, or children are frequently excluded from trials.[10] Patients in clinical trials also tend to be treated for well-defined indications, have limited and well-monitored concomitant drug use, and are closely followed for early signs and symptoms of adverse events which may be reversed with proper treatment. In contrast, once a drug is marketed, it is used in a "real-world" clinical context. Patients using the drug may have multiple co-morbidities for which they are being treated simultaneously. Patients may also be taking over-the-counter medications, "natural" remedies, or illicit drugs unbeknownst to the prescribing physician. The interactions of various drugs and treatments may result in a particular drug having a different safety profile in a post-marketing setting compared to the controlled premarketing environment.[17] An example is the drug mibefradil, which was voluntarily withdrawn from the market after less than a year by the manufacturer as a result of new information about multiple potentially serious drug interactions.[18] Adherence to medications also often differs between closely monitored trials and general post-approval use, as is the case with antihypertensives.[19] (See also Chapter 48.)

Spontaneous Reporting Systems

Spontaneous reporting systems are valuable for identifying relatively rare events and providing signals about potentially serious safety problems, especially with respect to new drugs (see also Chapters 11 and 12).[20] While there is currently no uniform definition, a signal is generally understood to be a higher than expected relative frequency of a drug event pair. Depending on the circumstances and the information available on background rates of events in the populations using the drug, definitions of "higher than expected" will vary by drug class, indication and over time. Ultimately, signals are used to generate hypotheses, which then may be studied through observational or interventional studies as appropriate; however, spontaneous reports must be interpreted within the context of the strengths and limitations of the particular reporting systems.[20–24] These voluntary reports are subject to many biases and external influences on reporting rates, which are unmeasured and in many cases unmeasurable. Events may be underreported and the decision as to which events get reported is potentially strongly affected by bias.[20] The effects of these biases differ among drugs and differ over time. The number of spontaneous reports received most often relates to the length of time a drug has been on the market, the initial rate of sale of the drug, secular trends in spontaneous reporting, and the amount of time a manufacturer's sales representatives spend with physicians "detailing" the product.[20] Certain types of events seem to be more likely to be reported, such as those which are serious and/or unlabeled,[25–27] events that occur rarely in the general population, those that occur acutely with drug administration, and those associated with publicity in the lay or professional media.[28–30] The frequency of reporting varies by drug class and drug company.[26] The number of reports does not equal the number of patients, since events may be reported several times. Most importantly, and a frequently misunderstood point, valid incidence rates cannot be generated from spontaneous reporting systems, since neither the true numerator nor true denominator is known, and thus relative safety cannot be assessed with any validity. Additionally, the events reported have an underlying background rate in the population, even in the absence of drug treatment, which may not be known.

Media coverage in particular has a significant effect on the timing and volume of adverse events voluntarily reported to spontaneous reporting systems. This effect has been documented for a variety of drug classes and adverse events.[28–30] For example, in a prospective study in the US, televised media was found to significantly influence the reporting of spontaneous adverse events for triazolam.[30] The investigators compared reports received four weeks before a nationally televised program on Halcion (triazolam) to reports within four weeks after the program. Nearly twice as many cases (67 compared to 37) were reported in the month following the program. Reports by consumers also increased from 46% to 60% during this period.

Another well-known example of the impact the media has on spontaneous reporting is illustrated by the spontaneous reports reported following the 1990 publication of an article suggesting that the antidepressant fluoxetine was associated with suicidal behavior and violent aggression towards others.[31] Shortly after publication of this article,[31] spontaneous reports of suicidal events associated with fluoxetine increased significantly, as did the proportion reported by consumers (see Figures 7.1 and 7.2). Notably, reporting rates for other drugs in the same class did not rise in a similar manner, suggesting that the reporting of events had been stimulated by the publication. Intense publicity contributed to loss of market share for this product although practitioners and an FDA Advisory Committee reached the conclusion that at that time there was no scientific evidence linking suicidal behavior with this agent.[32,33] The FDA Advisory Committee did suggest that the manufacturer further support the evidence of the drug's safety with prospective epidemiologic studies. Subsequent studies and re-analyses of clinical trial data did not demonstrate an increased risk of suicide or aggressive behavior associated with fluoxetine among adults, and millions of patients worldwide have benefited from this therapy.[34–37]

Notwithstanding these important limitations, spontaneous reporting systems have been successfully used in a number of circumstances to alert regulatory agencies and manufacturers to a potentially high frequency of serious adverse events in a newly launched drug. One example is temafloxacin, which was approved by the FDA in January, 1992. By June 1992, the drug was voluntarily withdrawn from the market by the manufacturer, following reports of 6 deaths and more than 70 other serious adverse events, including hemolytic

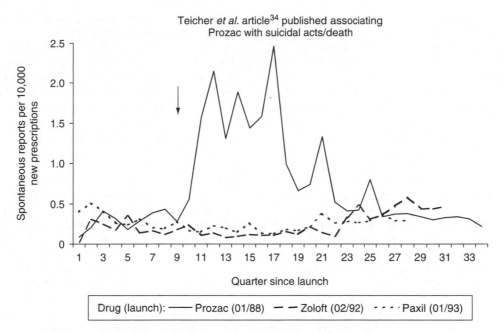

Figure 7.1. Reporting of suicidal acts/deaths associated with SSRIs following publication of Teicher *et al.* 1990 article. Data source: Spontaneous report data from FDA AERS database, new prescription data from IMS America.

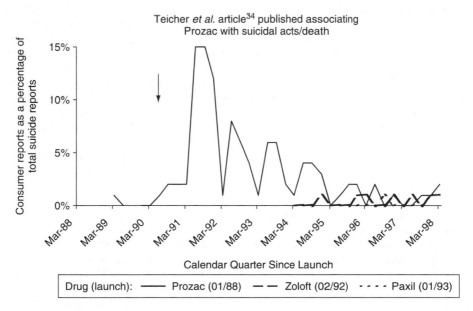

Figure 7.2. Consumer reports as a percentage of total suicide reports for SSRIs following publication of Teicher *et al.* 1990 article. Data source: Spontaneous report data from FDA AERS database.

anemia, renal failure, severe hypoglycemia, and anaphylaxis. In the first four months after marketing, an estimated 174,000 individuals took this drug,[38] allowing the rapid observation of serious adverse events occurring less frequently than those observed in clinical trials. Another example is that of mibefradil, a calcium channel blocker first marketed in the US in August 1997. Three drugs (astemizole, cisapride, and terfenadine) were listed as having an interaction with mibefradil at the time of approval. Through spontaneous reports (as well as continued clinical studies), more than 25 drugs were subsequently identified that were potentially harmful if used with mibefradil. Mibefradil had no known special benefits that could not be met with other drugs. The manufacturer and the FDA decided that the number and diversity of drugs with which it interacted could not be practically handled via the usual warnings in the label, and the risk-benefit profile was deemed to be unfavorable. The drug was voluntarily withdrawn from the US market in June 1998.[18]

In order to evaluate safety signals arising from spontaneous reporting systems, it is necessary to know as much as possible about the population using the drug. For example, knowledge about the distribution of age, gender, concomitant illnesses, and medications in users of a particular drug can provide information necessary to estimate the expected background rates of events that one might observe. A number of commercial vendors, such as NDC Health Information Services, HICA, Solucient, and IMS Health, provide extensive information about the use and sales of prescription products. Although information about actual drug ingestion is not available, assumptions can be made about the frequency of use from calculating the interval between refills in longitudinal resources. Additionally, information about the frequency of off-label use or the frequency of co-prescribing with medications that are contraindicated may be explored.

Signal Detection

Signal detection is a rapidly growing field primarily using the data collected in voluntary spontaneous reporting systems to enhance the qualitative screening capabilities of expert medical reviewers at pharmaceutical companies and regulatory agencies.[39–40] Typically, medical reviewers have relied on convincing clinical criteria and frequency of events to identify potential signals. Statistical methods have traditionally been underused in analyses of spontaneous reporting data, in large part due to the variable quality of the reports and data collection methods; however, these methods are now being employed in an attempt to identify safety signals earlier than has been possible in the past, due

to the large, and ever-increasing, volume of spontaneously-reported post-approval safety data.[40]

Three automated signal detection methods are emerging as the most commonly used by regulatory agencies, drug monitoring centers, and pharmaceutical manufacturers. The practical utility of these methods, as well as the impact of the adverse event coding dictionary used (e.g. MedDRA, WHO-ART or COSTART), is still being tested, and there is a pressing need to validate these methods before they significantly enhance decision-making about potential safety issues, relative to the standard methods of signal detection already employed.

The proportional reporting ratio (PRR) is the simplest of these methods and the easiest to understand.[41] Akin to an odds ratio, the PRR is a proportion of proportions, typically the proportional ratio of adverse event(s) for drugs of interest to the same adverse event(s) of all other drugs in the spontaneous reporting database; a PRR of 1.0 thus indicates no suspected association between the adverse event and the drug of interest, based only on information contained within the specific database being analyzed. As the PRR becomes increasingly greater than one, the statistical association between the adverse event and the drug (the "signal") increases, although this association may not be causal and due to other factors. Early detection of adverse signals can be implemented by calculating the PRR over time, a technique employed by the United Kingdom's Medicines and Healthcare products Regulatory Agency and the Drug Safety Research Unit (DSRU) at the University of Southampton.[40] The use of this method to inform regulatory decision-making has been contested, however, underscoring the need for continued investigation into the positive predictive capabilities of this method.[42]

The other two most frequently used signal detection methods are based on Bayesian statistical methods.[40,43] While Bayesian methods are less intuitive than the PRR because of their complexity, a potential advantage of these methods is that they inherently take into account the variance of the data and have commercially available computer interfaces with sophisticated graphics, which enhance signal detection capabilities. The Bayesian Confidence Propagation Neural Network (BCPNN) calculates a signal, or information component (IC), which is the weight in a neural network (akin to machine learning) that is repeatedly refined by means of Bayesian statistical methods. The Multi-item Gamma Poisson Shrinker (MGPS) calculates a reporting ratio (RR), based on observed to expected counts, for each AE-drug association under consideration; the RRs are then updated and adjusted via Bayesian methods. This method is used by the WHO

Collaborative Center for Drug Monitoring to provide alerts to regulatory authorities and pharmaceutical manufacturers.[43] Currently, a joint working group of individuals from the FDA and the pharmaceutical industry are evaluating the utility of MGPS using the FDA's spontaneous reports database.

Despite the rapid development of these methods, and in some cases implementation, all are limited by the fact that most of the signals identified using these methods are known associations or represent one or more forms of confounding (e.g., confounding by indication) that bias voluntary reporting systems. Given the uncertainty around predictive performance of these methods and the limited quality of the data collected using spontaneous reporting systems (see Chapters 11 and 12), this suggests that use of these approaches to compare between drugs or drug classes is advisable at this time. For the near future at least, signal detection using spontaneous report data will need to continue to incorporate rigorous clinical-based criteria and reviewer assessment to assess drug safety accurately.

In the future, these limits may be addressed by using prospective data collection systems for signal detection, which permit population-based estimates of medication-related adverse events and patterns of drug use (see Section IIIb). These prospective datasets have relatively complete data on individuals affected by adverse events as well as information about the population using the medication, in contrast to spontaneous reporting databases. The use of population-based data sources to identify drug-event pairs may result in an ability to detect signals more rapidly than would be possible using passive surveillance systems alone, and to apply methods developed for disease surveillance in other databases, such as the tree-based scan statistic.[44] Since the use of structured data sources for signal detection is new, significant research and validation is required in the coming years to determine how population-based surveillance systems will best contribute to pharmacovigilance.

Descriptive Epidemiology Studies

There is increasing recognition within the pharmaceutical industry that a strong epidemiology program in support of drug development is often important for the successful risk management of new medications. Epidemiologic studies conducted prior to product approval are useful for establishing the prevalence/incidence of risk factors and co-morbidity among patients expected to use the new medication; identifying patterns of health care utilization and prescribing of currently approved treatments; and quantifying background rates of mortality and serious nonfatal events.

With the wide availability of computerized health databases, it is now possible to conduct studies across diverse patient populations (e.g., private/public assistance insurance or varying geographical areas) and compare disease rates, examining the effect of differences in clinical practice or access to health care. When these data are available prior to approval, background rates of mortality and morbidity provide an important context for interpreting rare events observed in Phase III clinical trials and spontaneous reports. These data also provide the "real world" estimates necessary to design feasible postmarketing studies. Descriptive epidemiologic studies can also be conducted post-approval to describe new drug users' characteristics and patterns of use, and may also provide measurements of the drug's effectiveness at the population level.

For example, during the development of a new oral treatment for patients with migraine, eletriptan, two epidemiologic studies were conducted to better understand the risk of cardiovascular and cerebrovascular morbidities and mortality of migraine patients.[45,46] Triptans represent a major advance in the acute treatment of migraine. The triptans are believed to act, in part, by selectively constricting extracerebral, intracranial blood vessels that become dilated during a migraine attack. This activity is likely mediated through a receptor subtype present in other vascular beds, such as the coronary arteries. Triptans have only a limited potential to produce coronary artery vasoconstriction,[47] but are nonetheless contraindicated in patients with vascular disease. Although the associations of migraine and cardiovascular or cerebrovascular morbidity have been evaluated in some epidemiologic studies, at the time of eletriptan's development there were no published population-based studies assessing the risk of cardiovascular or cerebrovascular morbidity and mortality among migraine patients who are exposed or not exposed to triptans. The studies were conducted using the General Practice Research Database (GPRD) in the UK[45] (see Chapter 24) and the United HealthCare Research Database in the US (see Chapter 19).[46] Data from both studies demonstrated that the use of triptans is not associated with an increased risk of acute myocardial infarction (MI), non-MI ischemic heart disease (IHD) or unstable angina, ventricular arrhythmia, stroke/transient ischemic attack (TIA), all-cause mortality, or cardiovascular mortality. Further, the GPRD study found that triptans were less likely to be prescribed to those with cardiovascular disease risk factors, such as a history of hypertension, diabetes, heart disease, and obesity, a finding which suggests that general practitioners in the UK prescribe triptans consistent with current product labeling. The results of these studies were filed to the eletriptan NDA, providing important information on which the manufacturer and the FDA can evaluate the cardiovascular safety of eletriptan and other triptans.

Another example of the usefulness of descriptive epidemiology studies is from the epidemiology program for tiotropium, a once daily inhaled anticholinergic bronchodilator. Patients with chronic obstructive pulmonary disease (COPD) are at an increased risk of illness and death, and are at a particularly high risk for cardiovascular disease,[48] but the precise magnitude of risk has been poorly described. In order to better understand the health status of this population, three descriptive studies of patients with COPD were conducted. Results from these studies,[49] currently unpublished, revealed that persons with diagnosed and treated COPD, as identified in large medical claims databases, have higher rates of all-cause morbidity and mortality when compared to persons without COPD. Both the baseline and period prevalence of conditions such as hypertension, hyperlipidemia, and obesity were also increased in persons with COPD relative to those without COPD. With the exception of beta-blockers, which are contraindicated in obstructive lung disease, all cardiovascular drugs were used approximately twice as often in persons with COPD, and rates of mortality and hospitalizations for selected serious cardiovascular events were significantly elevated among patients with COPD compared to persons without COPD. These studies were conducted prior to tiotropium's approval in the US, and have provided important background information on the patient population to be treated as well as a context for interpreting spontaneous reports received post-approval.

In addition to the role descriptive epidemiology studies play in characterizing the background rates of morbidity and mortality, epidemiologic studies conducted before or during the clinical development program are also useful to place the incidence of adverse events observed in clinical trials in perspective. Data are often lacking on the expected rates of events in the population likely to be treated. For example, studies examining the risk factors for and rates of sudden unexplained death among people with epilepsy were able to provide reassurance that the rates observed in a clinical development program were within the expected range for individuals with comparably severe disease.[50–52]

Post-approval Safety Studies

During the premarketing phases of drug development, randomized clinical trials involve highly selected subjects and in the aggregate include at most a few thousand patients. These studies are sufficiently large to provide evidence of a beneficial clinical effect and to exclude large increases in risk of common adverse events. However, premarketing trials are rarely large enough to detect small differences in the risk of common adverse events or to reliably estimate the risk of rare events. Identification and quantification of potentially infrequent but serious risks requires larger studies that are designed to distinguish between the role of background risk factors and the effects of a particular drug on the rate of outcomes. Because of the complexity of design and cost, large controlled trials have not been widely used for the postmarketing evaluation of drugs. Recently, regulators and the medical community have communicated a desire for safety data from the populations that will actually use the drugs in "real-world" clinical practice settings. This has led to a greater emphasis on the use of observational methods to understand the safety profile of new medications after they are marketed.

An example of how observational methods can be successfully used to provide additional scientific evidence regarding the safety of a new medication is evidenced in the case of sildenafil. Sildenafil was approved for the treatment of erectile dysfunction (ED) in March 1998, followed by an approval in the EU in May 1998. Immediately following the launch of sildenafil in the US, spontaneous reports of death and myocardial infarction among users of sildenafil were received by the manufacturer and regulatory authorities. The volume of reports and proportion of consumer reports for sildenafil was unlike patterns seen for other new drugs at the time, and was unusual enough to raise regulatory concerns about the safety of sildenafil. Scientific studies conducted prior to sildenafil's approval highlighted the prevalence of cardiovascular risk factors in patients with ED and evidence that ED can be an early warning sign of cardiovascular disease,[53] but the exact risk and predictors of acute cardiovascular events that occur among men with ED who seek and receive treatment were unknown at the time. Thus, in response to concerns raised by European regulators, two post-approval safety studies were initiated to investigate the postmarketing safety of sildenafil.

To obtain data on sildenafil's postmarketing safety in a timely manner, the first study undertaken was a UK Prescription Event Monitoring (PEM) study,[54] conducted by an independent academic center, the DSRU at Southampton University in the UK (see Chapter 14). In this case, a PEM study was the only feasible data source by which results could be obtained rapidly, as it was not possible to use automated administrative or medical records databases since sildenafil was not reimbursed by these health systems. The first stage of the PEM study, in 5601 patients followed for an average of four and a half months, was completed in

2000. Results from the first stage demonstrated that the age-standardized mortality ratio for ischemic heart disease/myocardial infarction among sildenafil users was similar to that of the general male population in England.[55] The second stage of the sildenafil PEM study included more than 22,000 men and followed patients significantly longer than did cohort I, with a mean follow up of seventeen and a half months.[56] The results from this cohort were consistent with the earlier study: the age-standardized mortality ratio in men using sildenafil compared to the general English male population, indicated that mortality among sildenafil users was not elevated when compared to the 1998 rates in English men. The largest PEM study to date in the UK, with more than 28,000 patients in total, provided evidence supporting other data sources, such as clinical trials, that the incidence of death due to cardiovascular disease among men receiving a prescription for sildenafil in a clinical practice setting is similar to the rate observed in men not using sildenafil.[56] Further, and most importantly, no cardiovascular or cerebrovascular safety signals were identified from the PEM study.

In addition to the UK PEM study, a prospective observational study, the International Men's Health Study (IMHS), was initiated to assess the occurrence of cardiovascular events in men receiving sildenafil for the treatment of erectile dysfunction (ED). This cohort of more than 5000 men receiving prescriptions for sildenafil in Germany, France, Spain, and Sweden was followed for approximately eighteen months on average to assess cardiovascular risk factors, cardiovascular events, and use of ED treatments.[57] This study was unique in that the event rate for cardiovascular disease was compared for "time on treatment" relative to "time off treatment" among the cohort of sildenafil users. In part this design was chosen because sexual activity has its own inherent risk of cardiovascular morbidity and mortality,[58] and it was not possible to determine the risk of sildenafil use alone by epidemiologic methods, given the required sample size for a case-crossover design. Upon completion of this community-based study, the rates of cardiovascular disease events were found to be comparable to previously published figures from clinical trial and population-based epidemiologic data, providing further evidence supporting the cardiovascular safety of sildenafil.

These post-approval studies did not examine comparative safety, since sildenafil was the first in its class of drugs. However, epidemiologic studies can be used to examine the comparative risks associated with particular drugs within a therapeutic class, as they are actually used in clinical practice. For example, one large study determined that among anti-ulcer drugs, cimetidine was associated with the highest risk of developing symptomatic acute liver disease.[59] Other studies, examining the risk of hip fractures in users of benzodiazepines, found that users of long-acting agents were at greater risk than those using short-acting agents.[60,61]

Observational epidemiologic studies may not always be the most appropriate method of evaluating safety signals or comparing the safety profile of different medications, especially when there are concerns of confounding by indication (see Chapter 42). Confounding by indication occurs when the risk of an adverse event is related to the indication for medication use but not the use of the medication itself. The result, in observational studies, is a form of selection bias, where patients taking a particular medication are selected in a fashion that makes them at unequal risk of the outcome under study. As with any other form of confounding, one can, in theory, control for its effects if one can reliably measure the severity of the underlying illness, but in practice this is not easily or completely done (see Chapter 42). This is especially so when a drug may have specific properties affecting the type of patient it is used for within its indication. In these cases, studies using randomization, whether experimental or observational in design, may be necessary.

It is in this context that a Large Simple Trial (LST) design may be the most appropriate study design for postmarketing safety evaluation (see Chapter 41). This was the approach adopted for ziprasidone, an atypical antipsychotic for the treatment of schizophrenia launched in the US in 2001. In typical psychiatric practice, patients treated with a new medication may be systematically different from those treated with other drugs, due to prescribers' channeling of the drug to patients with more severe schizophrenia and/or comorbidities and risk factors. This possibility existed because ziprasidone was the newest of the products at that time, and most likely to be used in patients who had failed prior therapies. In addition, there were concerns that patients treated with ziprasidone might differ from those treated with other antipsychotic drugs, due to prescribers' channeling of the drug to patients with underlying cardiovascular disease or metabolic illnesses, especially given the low propensity for weight gain associated with ziprasidone.[62] Given these likely selection phenomena, random allocation of patients was the only approach providing the certainty of an unbiased comparison between groups. Randomization of treatment assignment is a key feature of an LST, which controls for confounding of outcome by known and unknown factors. Further, the large study size provides the power needed to evaluate small risks, both absolute and relative. By maintaining simplicity in study procedures, including the study's inclusion/exclusion criteria, patients' use of concomitant medications and the frequency of patient monitoring, the study approximates real life practice.

The Ziprasidone Observational Study of Cardiac Outcomes (ZODIAC) Large Simple Trial compares the cardiovascular safety of ziprasidone and olanzapine. The study, to involve some 18,000 patients, is unprecedented in psychiatric research, both in size and design. The primary objective of the study is to estimate relative non-suicide mortality among users of ziprasidone and olanzapine. The secondary objectives are to examine other causes of death, and to estimate the relative incidence of all-cause hospitalization and hospitalization for arrhythmia, myocardial infarction, or diabetic ketoacidosis, and to determine the rate of treatment discontinuation. Patients from 18 countries, the United States, Brazil, Argentina, Peru, Chile, Sweden, Hong Kong, Korea, Malaysia, Singapore, Taiwan, Thailand, Hungary, Poland, Romania, Slovakia, Uruguay, and Mexico are currently being enrolled from various treatment settings. After the enrolling physician determines a patient's eligibility and obtains informed consent, brief information, including demographics, disease severity, cardiac risk factors, and prior anti-psychotic medication use, is collected on a baseline questionnaire. Following random assignment of medication, no further study-related interventions, tests, or visits are required. Physicians and patients may change regimens and dosing of the assigned study medication, and concomitant medications are permitted. Patients are followed as clinically appropriate and outcomes are assessed for up to one year. Information on the patients' vital status and whether or not he or she has been hospitalized is being obtained through follow-up with the treating physician or other designated member of the medical care team. The study has three independent scientific committees: a Scientific Steering Committee responsible for general oversight of the study, a Data Safety Monitoring Board safeguarding study participants, and an Endpoint Committee, blinded to treatment status, and charged with assessing whether reported events meet study endpoint criteria.

The ZODIAC LST is also linking primary data collection with automated data obtained from state Medicaid programs (see Chapter 20), since many patients in the study receive their usual care from Medicaid. It was recognized shortly after initiating the study that in some cases the secondary endpoints of all-cause hospitalization, or hospitalization for arrhythmia, myocardial infarction or diabetic ketoacidosis may not be known by the enrolling physician or other treatment team members. In order to quantify the potential impact of unknown hospitalizations on the secondary analyses, the hospitalization records for patients enrolled in state Medicaid programs in the US will be linked confidentially to the information collected from the physician, if a patient has consented to this practice. The sensitivity of each hospitalization endpoint can then be estimated by using hospitalizations identified in the Medicaid inpatient records as the complete comparison group (i.e., the "gold standard"). Linking primary data collection with existing data sources is a research practice that should increase in the future, and is a method of building on the specific strengths of primary and secondary data sources.

Long Latency Outcomes

Epidemiologic methods provide the only practical way to study the association between drugs and effects with very long latency periods. Early recipients of human growth hormone (derived from human cadaveric pituitary tissue) were found to have elevated risks of Creutzfeldt-Jacob disease (CJD).[63–67] Recombinant growth hormone became available in the mid 1980s, but due to the long latent period for CJD, cases continued to be diagnosed well after that time. Another example where epidemiologic methods were used to identify longer-term adverse effects of treatment, is in the association of first-generation antipsychotics with tardive dyskinesia.[68]

Modern chemotherapy for childhood cancer has only been in use since approximately 1970 and it is only fairly recently that large numbers of children are being cured of cancer, allowing for the estimation of the long-term risks associated with the use of cytotoxic agents. Epidemiologic studies have documented the association between iatrogenic leukemia and treatment with alkylating agents or epipodo-phyllotoxins for previous cancers.[69,70] Second malignant neoplasms (of the solid tumor type) have also been associated with the use of alkylating agents and anti-tumor antibiotics.[71,72] Chemotherapy given to children prior to or during the adolescent growth spurt has been associated with slowing of skeletal growth and loss of potential height.[73–75] Decreased bone mineral density has also been documented following chemotherapeutic treatment in childhood.[76,77]

Survivors of adult cancers have also been the subjects of studies examining associations between chemotherapy and late effects. Examples include findings of decreased bone mineral density in women treated with cytotoxic agents for breast cancer[78] and in men and women treated for Hodgkin's disease,[79,80] which may be due to a direct effect of treatment on bone, a secondary effect mediated via gonadal toxicity, or a combination of the two.

Evaluating a Drug's Effects on Pregnancy and Birth Outcomes

Unless a medication is being developed specifically to treat a pregnancy-related condition, pregnant women are generally excluded from clinical trials for ethical reasons, due to potential risks to the developing fetus and newborn.[81] In addition, most clinical trials that enroll women cease study of pregnant women upon detection of pregnancy. Thus, at the time of introduction to market, the effects of many medications on pregnancy are not well known, with the foundation of drug safety during pregnancy often resting largely on animal reproductive toxicology studies. This is a significant public health consideration, particularly if the medication will be used by many women of childbearing potential, since approximately half of all pregnancies in the U.S. are unplanned.[82] While postmarketing spontaneous adverse event reporting of pregnancy outcomes may be helpful for identifying extremely rare outcomes associated with medication use during gestation, the limitations of these data are well-established (see above).

Epidemiologic methods have also been used to study cancers in individuals exposed to drugs in utero, peri-conceptually or immediately after birth and to examine possible teratologic effects of various agents (see also Chapter 34). A classic example of exposure in utero is the association between maternal use of DES and clear-cell adenocarcinoma of the vagina.[83,84] Other examples include the possible association between prenatal exposure to metronidazole and childhood cancer,[85] and childhood cancers and the use of sedatives during pregnancy.[86] A number of studies have examined the potential association between childhood cancer and exposure to vitamin K in the neonatal period.[87–90] Finally, although animal teratology testing is part of the pre-approval process of all drugs, questions about a possible relationship between a specific drug and birth defects may arise in the postmarketing period. In these cases, epidemiologic methods are necessary to gather and evaluate the information in the population actually using the drug to examine possible teratogenicity. Such studies include those examining diazepam use and oral clefts;[91] spermicide use and Down's syndrome, hypospadias, and limb reduction deformities;[92] and Bendectin[TM] use and oral clefts, cardiac defects, and pyloric stenosis.[93,94]

In certain circumstances registries are used to obtain information about the safety of new medications during pregnancy. The information provided by such registries allows health care professionals and patients to make more informed choices on whether to continue or initiate drug use during pregnancy, or provides reassurance after a pregnancy has occurred on therapy, based on a benefit-risk analysis that can be conducted for each individual.

A pregnancy exposure registry is typically prospective and observational, conducted to actively collect information about medication exposure during pregnancy and subsequent pregnancy outcome. Such registries differ from passive postmarketing surveillance systems in that they collect data from women prior to knowledge of the pregnancy outcome, proceeding forward in time from drug exposure to pregnancy outcome rather than backward in time from pregnancy outcome to drug exposure; this has the effect of minimizing recall bias. The prospective nature of properly designed pregnancy registries also allows them to examine multiple pregnancy outcomes within a single study. Ideally, a pregnancy registry will be population-based, thus increasing generalizability. It will allow for a robust cause-effect assessment between drug exposure and outcome by being prospective in nature; by collecting information on the timing of drug exposure, detailed treatment schedule, and dosing; by using standard and predefined definitions for pregnancy outcomes and malformations; and by recording these data in a systematic manner. The registry will ideally also follow offspring of medication-exposed women for a prolonged period after birth, to allow for detection of any delayed malformations in children who seem normal at birth. Finally, a pregnancy registry should also allow for effects of the medication on pregnancy outcome to be distinguished from the effects of the disease state warranting the treatment, if applicable, on pregnancy outcome. This criterion is ideally met by enrolling two comparator groups: pregnant women who are disease-free and not on the medication under study, and pregnant women with the disease who are not undergoing treatment or who are on different treatment. In practice, however, it is usually not feasible to meet these criteria because it is difficult to enroll pregnant women who are disease-free or not using medication. Thus, in many cases, only pregnant women with the disease using the drug of interest, or other treatments for the disease, are followed.

In general, when analyzing data from pregnancy registries, those cases identified prospectively, i.e., prior to knowledge of pregnancy outcomes, should be separated from those cases identified retrospectively, i.e., after pregnancy outcome has been determined by prenatal diagnosis, abortion, or birth, as the latter will be biased towards reporting of abnormalities. To minimize ascertainment bias, risk rates will ideally be calculated only from those cases identified prospectively. Also, since losses to follow-up may represent a higher proportion of normal pregnancy outcomes than abnormal pregnancy outcomes, participants in pregnancy registries should be aggressively followed to obtain complete pregnancy outcome reports.

Pregnancy exposure registries currently in existence include those that examine the effects of medications used for specific medical conditions, such as HIV infection[95] and epilepsy,[96] as well as those that investigate the pregnancy effects of specific drugs, such as bupropion for depression[97] and varicella virus vaccine for the prevention of chicken pox.[98] Pregnancy registries may be sponsored by university-based research groups, by government agencies, by pharmaceutical companies, or by collaborative efforts on the part of all three entities. While standard epidemiologic methods for estimating risks for pregnancy outcomes associated with drug exposures using data from pregnancy exposure registries have not yet been agreed upon, potential methods have been proposed and await further validation.[99] Recent release by the FDA of guidelines for establishing these important safety studies will also go a long way towards standardizing methods for pregnancy exposure registries, further increasing their utility for clinical and public health decision-making.[100]

Epidemiology and Risk Management

Epidemiology provides a major foundation in the area of risk management in its role in identifying and assessing risk (see Chapter 35). Epidemiology has been used to help understand risks inherent in the population being studied, to provide further understanding of the underlying disease, in comparing rates of disease between drugs, and even in evaluating the effectiveness of programs designed to minimize risk. The role of epidemiology is illustrated in four well-known risk management case studies presented in Figures 7.3–7.6.

PORTFOLIO PLANNING AND DEVELOPMENT

Product planning is a critical function within innovative pharmaceutical companies, because of the need for new and promising developmental drugs in product pipelines. Epidemiology plays a key role in the planning and development process. For example, basic epidemiologic techniques have been useful for defining potential markets, for determining how a drug is actually being used in the population, and for determining unmet medical and public health needs. Further, the methods of epidemiology are useful for studying high-risk groups such as the elderly, the poor, expectant mothers, providing important knowledge about the relative benefits and risks of therapy in populations rarely studied in clinical trials.

Estimating the incidence and prevalence of a disease is crucial for evaluating the current and projected future unmet medical need for drugs in development. These epidemiologic data provide critical information for decisions about which drug candidates to develop, since the potential market of a drug is an important consideration in drug and portfolio planning. This is especially relevant given that drug development takes on average eight and a half years and costs an average of $850 million.[7] Of 10,000 screened compounds, only 250 enter preclinical testing, 5 clinical testing, and one is approved by the FDA.[7,10] Successful companies thus must carefully choose which early candidates in their pipeline to progress. Information regarding the descriptive epidemiology of a condition may lead to decisions to progress a candidate drug on a "fast track" or to apply for approval under the US or EU orphan drug legislation.

Epidemiologic studies of prevalence,[118,119] the natural history of a condition,[120–123] or the frequency with which complications of a condition occur[124] are particularly important for portfolio planning long-term. The rich data resources available for public use from the US National Center for Health Statistics, the Agency for Healthcare Policy and Research, the National Institutes of Health, and similar agencies outside of the US, such as the Office of National Statistics in the UK, can be used for these studies, or alternatively, this information may be derived from population-based studies commissioned by industry using primary or secondary data sources, although the cost and time investment is considerably higher. Epidemiologic studies are also used to better understand regional prevalence and incidence of disease, especially in emerging markets where the burden of disease is often poorly characterized. An example is the InterASIA study (International Collaborative Study of Cardiovascular Disease in ASIA), a cross-sectional survey conducted in 2000–2001 among more than 20,000 men and women, to estimate the prevalence and distribution of cardiovascular disease risk factors in a nationally representative sample of the general population in China and Thailand.[125] InterASIA, independently carried out by an academic institution but funded by a pharmaceutical company, has already contributed significantly to a greater understanding of the prevalence of cardiovascular risk factors and disease in Asia.[126] In addition to prevalence, epidemiologic studies can estimate the burden (cost and disability) associated with specific conditions, providing data helpful for valuing a drug to patients and society.

PATTERNS OF MEDICATION USE AND BENEFICIAL EFFECTS OF DRUGS

Once a drug is approved, epidemiologic methods can be used to monitor its use and the type of patients who receive the drug. Observational studies may be informative as to the frequency of off-label use[127] and use of multiple medications.[128,129] Epidemiologic methods and databases such as the National Ambulatory Medical Care Survey may be used to monitor trends in the prescribing of certain pharmaceutical products, changes in the characteristics of users over time,[130,131] or to study patterns of medication use among high-risk populations, such as the elderly with cognitive impairment.[132] These methods are also used to quantify the beneficial effects of drugs (see also Chapter 42). Study endpoints may vary from outcomes such as well-being or quality-of-life (see Chapter 44) to more quantitative variables such as blood pressure level, direct and/or indirect cost savings, and utilization of the health care system. Post-approval studies of benefit are particularly relevant when the clinical trials have focused on surrogate measures of efficacy, and there is a desire for further information regarding a medication's impact on mortality or other long-term health outcomes.

Epidemiologic methods are also increasingly used to carry out economic studies (see also Chapter 43). Health economics studies are useful for marketing medications when a manufacturer can demonstrate that use of its product is equally effective but less costly than a competitor's. These studies may be used to justify inclusion of brand name products on formularies of health maintenance organizations (HMOs), hospitals, and state Medicaid programs. Recent studies include the economic advantages of the addition of selective serotonin reuptake inhibitors to speed the improvement of depression,[133] the cost-effectiveness of several agents for hypertension,[134] the investigation of cost-effectiveness of a treatment for mild to moderate Alzheimer's disease,[135] the measurement of direct and indirect costs of treating allergic rhinitis,[136] and the quality-of-life and health economic benefits, including work productivity, associated with improved glycemic control.[137]

ISSUES IN PHARMACOEPIDEMIOLOGY

RESOURCES FOR PHARMACOEPIDEMIOLOGY

In order to respond rapidly and responsibly to safety issues, high quality, valid data resources must be available. As a result of this need, the development and use of record linkage and automated databases, including hospital databases, has experienced considerable growth over the past two decades (see Chapters 15–24). These databases offer several advantages over *ad hoc* epidemiologic studies or expanding the scope of clinical trials. First, automated databases are usually large in size, ranging from hundreds of thousands to millions of patients, often with many years of "observation". A second advantage is speed; since information on study subjects is already computerized, the data can be accessed quickly rather than waiting years for results of studies in which patients are identified and followed over time. The third advantage is cost relative to prospective studies. Clinical trials or other prospective observational studies may cost millions of dollars, compared to hundreds of thousands of dollars for database studies.

Considerable progress has been made in the development of new and existing research databases containing information on drug usage and health-related outcomes. This is advantageous as a variety of data sources are necessary for research in pharmacoepidemiology. The limitations of many automated datasets are well established and need to be considered before conducting a study on a newly marketed medication. Each data source will have its own strengths and limitations, which are usually related to important factors: the reasons for collecting the data (e.g., research, monitoring clinical practice, or reimbursement); the type of data collected and its coding systems; the resources devoted to evaluating and monitoring the research quality of the data; and national or regional variations in medical practice. A common research limitation of automated data sources is that sufficient numbers of users may not yet be recorded, or the medication may not be marketed in the country where the database is located. Some data resources suffer from a considerable "lag-time" between data entry and availability for research purposes. Further, even though many health maintenance organizations have overall enrollments of hundreds of thousands of members, these numbers may be inadequate to study the risks of extremely rare events associated with a specific drug or not contained in the HMO's research database. Finally, results from these sources are often limited in their generalizability.

Many of these data collection systems were designed for administrative purposes, rather than for epidemiologic research studies. As a result, information needed to assess a specific safety issue may be unavailable and the quality of medical information may be inadequate. Often it is desirable to validate findings based solely on diagnostic or procedural codes used for reimbursement purposes through a detailed review of at least a subset of medical records, as the usefulness of this type of research to answer an important safety question may be limited if the data are not properly validated. For some databases, medical record review may not be feasible due to concerns about patient confidentiality or anonymity, especially following recently enacted legislation on the privacy of health records (HIPPA). Continuing study of the research validity of these databases is crucial, and should be pursued when feasible.[138–142]

INTERPRETING PHARMACOEPIDEMIOLOGY STUDIES

Careful, scientifically sound research carried out using resources of high quality does not guarantee that a study's findings will be appropriately interpreted. Assuming that a safety issue has been suitably addressed using appropriate data resources, the study findings may still be improperly interpreted or misused. This has implications for the pharmaceutical industry and patients who lose access to beneficial and safe medications. Regulatory agencies are also affected by having to devote scarce resources to evaluating erroneous safety issues in order to make regulatory decisions, and by the impact these interpretations have on the public's confidence in the regulatory process. Ultimately, a disservice has been carried out to the public by generating unwarranted fears, by the removal of safe and effective drugs, and by higher costs for pharmaceuticals.

The media misinterpretation of epidemiologic results may have an impact on drugs in the market resulting in useful drugs being precipitously withdrawn from the market. Bendectin™, used for nausea during pregnancy, was marketed in the US from 1956 through 1983. The manufacturer voluntarily withdrew the drug from the market in 1983 because of the cost of defending the large number of product liability lawsuits filed following extensive publicity suggesting that the drug was teratogenic. Numerous epidemiologic studies in varying settings with various designs were performed to examine this issue. The results did not support the suspicion that Bendectin™ was a teratogen.[143,144] Because of its withdrawal, this drug is no longer available to the 10–25% of all pregnant women who could potentially benefit from its use.[145] Neutel reported that, in the year following withdrawal of Bendectin™ from the market, hospitalizations for vomiting in pregnancy (per thousand live births) in Canada rose by 37% and by 50% the year after that, with similar findings in the US. Their estimates of excess hospital costs during the years immediately following withdrawal (1983–1987) were $16 million in Canada and $73 million in the US.[146]

Misinterpretation of epidemiologic studies perpetuates the impression that the discipline is weak by generating controversy over study results, while promoting needless anxiety on the part of both patients and physicians. In such circumstances, the weaknesses of these studies are emphasized and the strength of the discipline overlooked. As a result, the information that epidemiology contributes may be considered to be of questionable usefulness. Greater understanding of the strengths and limitations of epidemiology is needed by the public, the media, the government, and often by industry itself. These diverse groups have common interests and, through their joint efforts, the discipline of pharmacoepidemiology may be improved by focusing support, assessing study quality, and advancing a greater understanding of the field.

The relationship between science and industry also contributes to the misinterpretation of research results, and causes distrust of pharmaceutical companies, and increasingly the academic institutions with which they partner.[147] Academic-industry partnerships have been in place since the early twentieth century, but their primary purpose initially was developing research capabilities within the emerging pharmaceutical industry. After the second World War, and due in large part to the government's funding of biomedical research through the National Institutes of Health (NIH), these relationships declined. The 1980s witnessed a resurgence of industry funding with the flattening of growth in the NIH budget and the passage of the Bayh-Dole Act in 1980[147]. The academic-industry relationships that followed have clearly resulted in benefits to society, in particular more timely and effective technology transfer, but are plagued by concerns about researcher bias and the failure to communicate results adequately or, in some cases, at all.[147]

Academic institutions, the NIH, and companies have responded to these concerns in multiple ways.[147–149] However, the rules in place and processes used to manage potential conflicts of interest vary significantly. It is now generally recognized that there is a need for disclosure of financial interest, and often a limit on researchers having significant financial interests in a company that supports their research. In the future, conflicts of interest other than financial should also be examined, including peer or group recognition, career advancement, or political affiliations. For clinical research it is also essential to insure that appropriate processes are in place to safeguard research participants and their confidentiality. Detailed recommendations on these processes, such as when and how to convene Data Safety Monitoring Boards or guidelines for conducting research in pharmacoepidemiology, are currently available.[150,151] Further guidance is needed to assist companies, universities, and regulatory agencies in defining types of conflict of interest, particularly conflicts other than financial, and in clarifying when these conflicts are significant and reportable.

FUTURE DIRECTION OF PHARMACOEPIDEMIOLOGY

RESOURCES

Industry should play an active role in the creation and development of resources that are necessary to validly and rapidly address safety questions. Important areas for support by industry in the coming years are: the maintenance of existing data sources; the creation of new data sources; development and validation of new epidemiologic methods applied to drug epidemiology; and education and training programs in pharmacoepidemiology.

Industry support is critical to the development of new database resources. Research groups may have access to various types of information, but lack the financial resources to develop the information into a usable database. Pharmaceutical companies actively seeking new data resources should not overlook potentially valuable sources of information and, where circumstances permit, provide guidance and funding for the development of a viable data resource. Data linkage between existing databases is another area where industry support directly promotes the growth of research resources through financial support.

The development of new study designs and methods in pharmacoepidemiology must also continue, and this is an area where industry may also play a role. New methods are needed to accrue large numbers of individuals on particular therapeutic regimens rapidly and to be able to follow them prospectively to identify and quantify beneficial and adverse health outcomes associated with new medications. Exploring options for rapid cohort creation or obtaining real-time access to automated data may be costly and demands a special commitment from drug companies, private foundations, and government agencies to recognize that such an investment may ultimately be necessary to provide additional options for evaluating drug safety and effectiveness. Epidemiologists working within pharmaceutical companies should also keep abreast of new study designs or approaches to data-based methods for controlling confounding, such as propensity scores, that may offer improved methods of evaluating the risks and safety associated with pharmaceutical products. For example, recent publications have used the case-crossover design to investigate the association between road-traffic accidents and benzodiazepine use,[152] case-time-control designs to study birth defects,[153]

and new-user designs to adjust for bias associated with the inclusion of prevalent medication users in observational studies.[154]

Finally, there are a limited number of formal training programs in pharmacoepidemiology at universities, although the number and scope of these programs have increased in recent years. In order to meet the increasing needs of industry, regulatory agencies, and universities with respect to trained epidemiologists, the pharmaceutical industry should increase their role in supporting training and fellowship programs. Such support insures a sufficient number of epidemiologists with expertise in drug safety evaluation while also providing a structure for the implementation of high quality pharmacoepidemiologic research.

PROFESSIONAL ASSOCIATIONS AND COLLABORATIVE RESEARCH EFFORTS

Scientific fora for the exchange of new research results and opportunities for communication between individuals and organizations with differing perspectives are essential to advance the field of pharmacoepidemiology. A number of venues provide the opportunity for industry representatives to work together, such as the Pharmaceutical Research and Manufacturing Association (PhRMA), and to work with members of regulatory authorities worldwide on issues of mutual interest (Council for International Organizations of Medical Sciences (CIOMS)). Academic, industry, and regulatory authority based scientists also communicate research results with each other through the International Society for Pharmacoepidemiology (ISPE) and the Centers for Education and Research on Therapeutics (CERTs).[155]

Combining research efforts across pharmaceutical companies benefits companies, regulators, and the public through the creation or improvement of shared data resources and epidemiologic methods. A recent example of this type of effort is described in Figure 7.7, which outlines the history of a unique collaboration among manufacturers of antiretroviral medications for the treatment of HIV/AIDS, US and European regulatory agencies, academics, and patient advocates.

PHARMACOGENOMICS

Pharmacogenomics has the potential to transform medical practice, and pharmaceutical prescribing, by understanding how genetic variability affects the ways in which people respond to drugs.[162] Pharmacogenomics examines the gene variability (e.g., metabolic gene polymorphism) that dictates drug response and explores the ways these variations can be

The FDA approved Geodon/Zeldox (ziprasidone) for the treatment of schizophrenia in February 2001. The initial NDA for Geodon was rejected in June 1998 based on "the judgment that Geodon prolongs the QTc and that this represents a risk of potentially fatal ventricular arrhythmias that is not outweighed by a demonstrated and sufficient advantage of Geodon over already marketed antipsychotic drug products".[101] The letter of non-approval recommended that the sponsor perform an additional study to determine the QTc effect of Geodon at peak plasma concentration in comparison with other atypical antipsychotics and with several standard antipsychotics.[101]

The sponsor conducted a comparative clinical study of six antipsychotics which indicated Geodon's QTc interval at steady state was 10 milliseconds greater than that of haloperidol, quetiapine, olanzapine and risperidone and approximately 10 millisecond less than that of thioridazine; further, the results were similar in the presence of a metabolic inhibitor.[102] Following the 1998 non-approval, the sponsor also conducted descriptive and comparative epidemiologic studies to quantify the risk of mortality and cardiovascular disease among schizophrenic patients receiving pharmacotherapy, and designed an innovative postapproval study for assessing the safety of Geodon.

Descriptive Epidemiologic Studies
Numerous studies have documented that patients with schizophrenia have higher mortality rates than the general population but few have examined if these rates changed following the introduction of atypical antipsychotics. Prior to approval, and as part of the Geodon epidemiology program, the sponsor conducted two descriptive epidemiologic studies: one in the U.S. used United Healthcare's Research Database[103] and another in Canada used Saskatchewan Health's database.[104] The results confirmed that patients with schizophrenia have higher background rates of mortality and cardiovascular outcomes, regardless of treatment type.

Comparative Epidemiologic Studies
In an effort to determine the "real-world" effects of the use of QT_c prolonging drugs among schizophrenic patients, the sponsor conducted two comparative epidemiologic studies: one used data from the U.S. Medicaid system[105] and another used the General Practice Research Database from the U.K.[106] These studies compared antipsychotics with varying propensities for QTc prolongation, from lower to higher: haloperidol, risperidone, clozapine and thioridazine. The results indicate that rates of sudden death and cardiac events are similar among users of haloperidol, clozapine, risperidone and low-dose thioridazine, and that users of high-dose thioridazine have higher rates of these events.

Post-approval Safety Study: ZODIAC Large Simple Trial
The Ziprasidone Observational Study of Cardiac Outcomes (ZODIAC) is a large simple trial designed to examine the 'real-world' cardiovascular safety of ziprasidone compared to olanzapine. The defining characteristics of ZODIAC include:

- Prospective study large enough to detect small risks: 18,000 patients currently from 18 countries: USA, Sweden, Brazil, Argentina, Peru, Chile, Hong Kong, Korea, Malaysia, Singapore, Taiwan, Thailand, Hungary, Poland, Romania, Slovakia, Uruguay, and Mexico
- Control for channeling bias by using 1:1 random assignment to ziprasidone or olanzaplne
- No additional study monitoring or tests required after randomization
- Patients followed up during usual care over 12 months
- Endpoints: primary – mortality (all-cause, suicide, non-suicide, cardiovascular, sudden death); secondary -hospitalizations (all-cause, myocardial infarction, arrhythmia, diabetic ketoacidosis)

The design of ZODIAC carries several advantages over more commonly used observational postmarketing study designs. Random allocation of patients provides for an unbiased comparison between groups; the large study size provides the power needed to evaluate small risks, both absolute and relative; and the simplicity of an uncontrolled trial minimizes the artificiality imposed by controlled premarketing trials. ZODIAC began in 2002 and has so far randomized more than 10,000 patients.

Key Points:

- Descriptive epidemiologic studies can be used to establish baseline rates of disease in the patient population and comparative epidemiologic studies can quantify the adverse effects of drugs for the same indication
- Prospective epidemiologic studies, such as large simple trials, can be used to evaluate potentially small risks in a "real-world" context

Figure 7.3. Risk management case study: Geoden/Zeldox (ziprasidone).

The FDA approved Accutane (isotretinoin) for the second-line treatment of severe recalcitrant cystic acne in 1982. While the human teratogenicity of Accutane was not known at the time of the drug's introduction to market, available preclinical data suggested that teratogenicity might be a safety issue. Thus, a black box warning was included in the label, specifying that Accutane not be used during pregnancy and recommending contraception for women of child-bearing potential.[107]

Spontaneous reports of congenital abnormalities in infants of Accutane users following launch clearly established the human teratogenicity of the drug.[13] These spontaneous reports suggested the current labeling alone was not effective at preventing contraindicated individuals from using Accutane. Following a 1988 meeting of the Dermatologic Drugs Advisory Committee, the FDA decided a Pregnancy Prevention Program (PPP) should be implemented, targeting physicians identified as prescribers of Accutane and their patients, and providing them with the following:

- Guidelines for prescribing Accutane, including pregnancy tests
- A patient qualification checklist
- A patient information brochure
- Information about contraceptives
- Details regarding a patient reimbursement program for contraception referrals
- A patient consent form

The effectiveness of the PPP was evaluated by an ongoing survey of women treated with Accutane, which monitored pregnancy rates and outcomes, patients' awareness of risks, and patient behavior. A tracking study of physicians prescribing Accutane was also performed in parallel, to follow physician behavior. Furthermore, in 1989, Accutane's sponsor began distributing the medication exclusively in 10-capsule blister packs including red and black warnings, along with a drawing of a malformed baby and the "Avoid Pregnancy" symbol.

Despite implementation of the PPP and packaging modifications to Accutane, pregnancy exposures continued. In addition, reports of reduced efficacy of oral contraceptives among women taking Accutane prompted the FDA to recommend a label change in 1994, emphasizing that women of childbearing potential taking Accutane should use two forms of reliable contraception (e.g. oral contraceptive plus barrier method) simultaneously.

Results published in 1995 from the ongoing PPP patient survey showed that the pregnancy rate among female patients was substantially lower than the rate among women of childbearing potential. However, more recent data from this survey and the physician tracking study also showed a high percentage of physicians and women were not complying with the core components of the PPP.[108] In response to these findings, a meeting of the Dermatologic and Ophthalmic Drugs Advisory Committee was convened in 2000, at which the FDA requested a strengthened form of the PPP, the System to Manage Accutane-Related Teratogenicity (SMART).

SMART requires physicians who prescribe Accutane to study the "Guide to Best Practices" and return a "Letter of Understanding" certifying their understanding of the material; only after doing so can they obtain the self-adhesive Accutane Qualification Stickers that must be attached to all new prescriptions. Physicians may also obtain the stickers by completing a half-day continuing medical education course. The stickers indicate to pharmacists that the patient meets five specified criteria and is, thus, "qualified" to receive Accutane. SMART also requires pharmacists to dispense Accutane only upon presentation of a written prescription with an Accutane Qualification Sticker attached and dispensings may be of no more than a one month supply within seven days from the date of "qualification." Pharmacists must also provide a Medication Guide to all patients.

The SMART program is currently being evaluated by epidemiologic analyses of data collected for the ongoing patient survey, the results of which were the subject of a 2004 joint meeting of FDA's Drug Safety & Risk Management and Dermatologic & Ophthalmic Drugs Advisory Committees.

Key Points:

- A medication with risks can be made available to patients by implementing a comprehensive risk management program given a favorable benefit–risk balance.
- Risk management programs must be continually evaluated to determine whether they are preventing the undesired outcome, using epidemiologic research methods where appropriate.
- Further research to determine whether programs such as SMART can be implemented, or are effective in managing risk to patients while ensuring appropriate access to new medications, is needed.

Figure 7.4. Risk management case study: Accutane (isotretinoin).

used to predict how a patient will respond to a drug. By knowing how patients who share certain gene profiles will respond to a drug it will be possible to customize drug therapies for specific populations or even individuals. In the future, based on scientific knowledge and appropriate labeling about which medicine to prescribe, a doctor may be able to administer a genetic test that will indicate the appropriate medication according to the patient's profile. Although this science is still in its infancy, the development of pharmacogenomics groups within industry provides an

---

The FDA approved Lotronex (alosetron) for diarrhea-predominant irritable bowel syndrome (IBS) in women in February 2000. The medication achieved rapid market acceptance, with 130,000 prescriptions filled for the medication by the end of May 2000.

By June 2000, the accumulation of spontaneous reports of serious adverse events for Lotronex, including four reports of serious complications of constipation, five reports of ischemic colitis, and two reports of hepatic abnormalities,[109] prompted the FDA to convene a Gastrointestinal Drugs Advisory Committee meeting to review the approval of Lotronex. At this meeting, there was a lack of epidemiologic data on the background risk of complications of constipation and ischemic colitis in IBS patients making it difficult to provide a context for the observed spontaneous reports.[13] The FDA stated that only 20% of women with diarrhea-predominant IBS were likely to benefit directly from Lotronex and strongly recommended that the drug be targeted only to those women most likely to respond to treatment.[13] The sponsor proposed a risk management plan for Lotronex, consisting of the following three components:

- A risk definition dimension, including conduct of epidemiologic, clinical and mechanistic studies to evaluate and quantify risks and identify risk factors for adverse events
- A communications program targeted to physicians, pharmacists and patients
- An evaluation of the communications program coupled with monitoring of prescribing via an HMO database

Following the June 2000 meeting, a "Medication Guide" for patients was developed, to help ensure that women using Lotronex would understand the rare but serious risks of Lotronex and how they could recognize those risks and act early to prevent serious complications. The Lotronex label for health professionals was also modified to more strongly indicate the potential side effects of the treatment as well as to attempt to specify those patients who were more likely to benefit from the drug. "Dear Health Care Professional" and "Dear Pharmacist" letters were sent out by the sponsor to highlight these label changes.[110]

Despite these risk management efforts, by November 2000, 49 cases of ischemic colitis and 21 cases of severe constipation had been reported for Lotronex, with ten cases requiring surgery and three cases resulting in death. In response, the FDA convened another advisory committee meeting in November 2000. Unable to agree on a feasible risk management plan with FDA, the sponsor withdrew Lotronex from the market in late November 2000.[111]

Over the next year, IBS patients who had successfully used Lotronex and their healthcare professionals lobbied the FDA and the sponsor with letters requesting reintroduction of Lotronex. Following discussions with the FDA, the sponsor filed a supplemental new drug application for Lotronex in December 2001 for the approval of Lotronex for limited marketing to women with diarrhea-predominant IBS who were treatment refractory with other therapy. The FDA approved the reintroduction of Lotronex under these restricted conditions in June 2002, provided the sponsor agreed to implement a new risk management plan, comprised of five components:

- A physician prescribing program
- A comprehensive education program for physicians, pharmacists, and patients
- A reporting and collection system for serious adverse events associated with Lotronex use
- Conduct of epidemiologic studies to more clearly define risks for gastrointestinal adverse events in Lotronex users
- A plan to evaluate the effectiveness of the Lotronex risk management program, utilizing epidemiologic research

Key Points:

- Medications removed from the market can be reintroduced if the benefits of the medication outweigh the risks for a subset of the population, and the risks to patients are appropriately managed through a comprehensive risk management program.
- Epidemiologic research to characterize the populations or subpopulation(s) that might benefit most from a medication should be conducted during development and prior to approval whenever possible.

Figure 7.5. Risk management case study: Lotronex (alosetron).

opportunity for epidemiologists with expertise in genetics to significantly contribute to the earliest stages of drug development. (See also Chapter 39.)

CONCLUSIONS

Epidemiology makes a significant contribution to the development and marketing of safe and effective pharmaceutical products worldwide. It facilitates the regulatory process and provides a rational basis for drug safety evaluation, particularly in the post-approval phase. Like any other discipline, it must be properly understood and appropriately utilized. Industry has an opportunity to contribute to the development of the field and the responsibility to do so in a manner that expands resources while assuring scientific validity. Achieving this goal requires financial and intellectual support as well as a better understanding of the nature of the discipline and its uses. With the passage of the PDUFA III legislation, the need for scientists with training and research experience in pharmacoepidemiology has never been greater. Epidemiologists within industry have an opportunity to build on the successes of the last twenty years by advancing the methods of drug safety evaluation and risk management, and applying epidemiologic designs and methods to new areas within industry.

The FDA approved Propulsid (cisapride) for the treatment of nocturnal heartburn associated with gastroesophageal reflux disease (GERD) in August 1993. Uptake of the drug was rapid, with approximately 5 million outpatient prescriptions written by 1995.[13] During the same time period, the FDA received 34 spontaneous reports of torsades de pointes, 23 of QT interval prolongation, including four deaths, among patients using Propulsid.[112]

In response, the FDA added a "black box" warning to the label in 1995, cautioning against use of contraindicated medications due to risk of potentially fatal cardiac arrhythmias. The manufacturer followed with a "Dear Healthcare Professional" letter explaining the label change.[112]

Despite these efforts, spontaneous reports of cardiac abnormalities associated with Propulsid continued to mount, resulting in four actions:[113,114]

- An expansion of the "black box" warning in 1998; use of Propulsid was now contraindicated in patients using medications that could prolong the QT interval and in patients with known heart disease or conditions associated with cardiac arrhythmias.
- An FDA "talk paper" to announce the label change.
- A "Dear Healthcare Professional" letter distributed to twice as many individuals as received the first mailing.
- A letter to pharmacy chains and groups providing safety information to announce the label change.

These actions also failed to reduce inappropriate prescribing and the number of adverse event reports increased. Another label change, instituted in January 2000, recommended that physicians perform electrocardiograms and blood tests prior to prescribing Propulsid.[115] In March 2000, one month prior to a scheduled meeting of the FDA Gastrointestinal Drugs Advisory Committee, the manufacturer voluntarily withdrew Propulsid from the market.[116]

Several epidemiologic analyses have retrospectively examined patterns in contraindicated Propulsid use. One found only a two percent reduction in all contraindicated Propulsid use after the 1998 regulatory actions.[112] Another found the 1998 actions were followed by a substantial decline in Propulsid prescriptions codispensed with contraindicated drugs while the 1995 actions, which were accompanied by less publicity, had little effect.[113] Among contraindicated coprescriptions of Propulsid, a third study found fifty percent were written by the same physician and 89 percent were dispensed by the same pharmacy.[117]

Key Points:

- More research is needed regarding the effectiveness of label changes and "Dear Doctor" letters in changing physicians' prescribing behavior.
- Epidemiologic methods and data sources are useful to elucidate the prescribing and dispensing behavior of physicians and pharmacists.
- In cases where the risk(s) are defined and information needs to be communicated to physicians, targeted educational interventions may be needed.

Figure 7.6. Risk management case study: Propulsid (cisapride).

The HAART OC was formed in response to a request by the European Medicines Agency for the Evaluation of Medicinal Products (EMEA) for more information regarding short and long-term complications of antiretroviral medications, with particular emphasis on heart attacks and strokes. Although labeling changes for protease inhibitors describing a general warning of possible morphologic and metabolic abnormalities had already been adopted, this unique collaborative working group was established in 1999 to determine and support the most robust methods for investigating the effects of antiretroviral therapy on metabolic complications.

The HAART OC currently consists of representatives from eight pharmaceutical manufacturers of HIV antiretroviral medications (Abbott Laboratories, Boehringer Ingelheim, Bristol-Myers Squibb, Gilead Sciences, GlaxoSmithKline, Hoffmann-La Roche, Merck & Co., and Pfizer), as well as academic, regulatory and community representatives from both the US and Europe.

Collectively, pharmaceutical company members of the committee have committed over seven million dollars to sponsor the following collaborative studies of antiretroviral medications:

- **Lipodystrophy Case Definition Study** – a case-control study of 1,081 male and female HIV-positive outpatients from clinics worldwide conducted to develop a case definition of HIV lipodystrophy[156]
- **D:A:D: Multi-Cohort Prospective Epidemiologic Study of Cardiovascular Morbidity** – a prospective observational study of over 20,000 participants from several patient cohorts in the U.S., Australia, and 11countries throughout Europe to look for increases in rates of heart attacks, strokes, and diabetes[157–159]
- **Retrospective Cohort Analysis of Cardiovascular Morbidity and Mortality: Review of the Veterans Administration (VA) database** – a retrospective cohort study using automated data from the USVA system to determine whether there was a significant increase in the rate of heart attacks and strokes following the introduction of HAART[160]
- **Meta-analysis of Existing Collaborative Cohort Studies Regarding Relative Incidences of Metabolic Abnormalities** – a meta-analysis of recently initiated metabolic studies of major clinical trial networks and other related studies

Research proposals were peer-reviewed before they were approved and funded by the HAART OC. Each study is conducted by an academic researcher and has its own Steering Committee. The HAART OC receives regular status reports and critically evaluates progress on the individual studies. Each of the sponsored studies represents a collaborative effort at multiple levels, as exemplified by the combining of databases (e.g., the prospective observational study combines data from a large number of existing HIV research cohorts, some of which normally compete for research resources and patients) and investigators (e.g., principal investigators of large metabolic studies from several research networks are collaborating to harmonize the data collected in each study, laying the groundwork for future meta-analyses).

In an April 2003 statement the EMEA indicated "the available results from the [cohort] studies clearly demonstrate that the benefit risk balance of anti-retroviral treatment remains strongly positive."[161]

Key Points:

- The HAART OC is a unique combination of industry, academia, regulators, and advocacy groups, formed to collaboratively investigate challenging safety issues.
- The committee has funded and produced rigorous research that might not have otherwise been funded by any single sponsor and continues to work collaboratively to standardize methods for investigating safety questions common to all antiretroviral products.

Figure 7.7. Industry, academia, regulator, and patient advocate collaboration: the Oversight Committee for the Evaluation of Metabolic Complications of Highly Active Antiretroviral Therapy (HAART OC).

DISCLAIMER

The views expressed are those of the authors, which are not necessarily those of Pfizer, Inc.

REFERENCES

1. Vuckovic N, Nichter M. Changing patterns of pharmaceutical practice in the United States. *Soc Sci Med* 1997; **44**: 1285–1302.
2. Kaitin KI, Manocchia M, Seibring M, Lasagna L. The new drug approvals of 1990, 1991, and 1992: trends in drug development. *J Clin Pharmacol* 1994; **34**: 120–7.
3. Kaitin KI, Manocchia M. The new drug approvals of 1993, 1994, and 1995: trends in drug development. *Am J Therapeutics* 1997; **4**: 46–54.
4. Kaitin KI, Healy EM. The new drug approvals of 1996, 1997, and 1998: drug development trends in the user fee era. *Drug Inf J* 2000; **34**: 1–14.
5. Kaitin KI, Cairns C. The new drug approvals of 1999, 2000, and 2001: Drug development trends a decade after passage of the Prescription Drug User Fee Act of 1992. *Drug Inf J* 2003; **37**: 357–71.
6. Kermani F, Bonacossa P. Patent issues and future trends in drug development. *J Comm Biotechnol* 2003; **9**: 332–8.
7. Pharmaceutical Research and Manufacturers of America (PhRMA). *Pharmaceutical Industry Profile 2003*. Washington DC: PhRMA; 2003.

8. Drews J. *In Quest of Tomorrow's Medicines*. New York: Springer; 1999.

9. Food and Drug Administration. *Report to Congress: Report on Postmarketing Studies*. Washington DC: FDAMA 130; US FDA.

10. Food and Drug Administration. *From Test Tube to Patient: Improving Health Through Human Drugs*. Washington DC: US FDA CDER; 1999.

11. Food and Drug Administration. *Managing the Risk from Medical Product Use: Creating a Risk Management Framework*. Washington DC: US FDA; 1999.

12. Hyslop DL, Read HA, Masica DN, Kotsanos JG. Pharmaceutical risk management: a call to arms for pharmacoepidemiology. *Pharmacoepidemiol Drug Saf* 2002; **11**: 417–20.

13. Andrews E, Dombeck M. The role of scientific evidence of risk and benefits in determining risk management policies for medications. *Pharmacoepidemiology Drug Saf*. In press.

14. Perfetto EM, Ellison R, Ackermann S, Sherr M, Zaugg AM. Evidence-based risk management: how can we succeed? *Drug Inf J* 2003; **37**: 127–34.

15. Abenhaim L, Moride Y, Brenot F, Rich S, Benichou J, Kurz X, *et al*. Appetite-suppressant drugs and the risk of primary pulmonary hypertension. International Primary Pulmonary Hypertension Study Group. *N Engl J Med* 1996; **335**: 609–16.

16. Faich GA, Lawson DH, Tilson HH Walker AM*l*. Clinical trials are not enough: drug development and pharmacoepidemiology. *J Clin Res Drug Dev* 1987; **1**: 75–8.

17. Rogers AS. Adverse drug events: identification and attribution. *Drug Intell Clin Pharm* 1987; **21**: 915–20.

18. Food and Drug Administration. *Roche laboratories announces withdrawal of Posicor from the market*. FDA Talk Paper, June 8, 1998.

19. Andrade SE, Walker AM, Gottlieb LK, Hollenberg NK, Testa MA, Saperia GM *et al*. Discontinuation of anti-hyperlipidemic drugs – do rates reported in clinical trials reflect rates in primary care settings? *NEJM* 1995; **332**: 1125–31.

20. Goldman SA. Limitations and strengths of spontaneous reports data. *Clin Ther* 1998; **20**: C40–4.

21. Edwards IR, Olsson S. WHO Programme – Global Monitoring. In: Mann R, Andrews E, eds., *Pharmacovigilance*. New York: Wiley; 2002. p. 169–82.

22. Davis S, Raine JM. Spontaneous Reporting – UK. In: Mann R, Andrews E, eds., *Pharmacovigilance*. New York: Wiley; 2002. p. 195–208.

23. Moore N, Kreft-Jais C, Dahnani A. Spontaneous Reporting – France. In: Mann R, Andrews E, eds., *Pharmacovigilance*. New York: Wiley; 2002. p. 209–18.

24. Graham DJ, Ahmad SR, Piazza-Hepp T. Spontaneous Reporting – USA. In: Mann R, Andrews E, eds., *Pharmacovigilance*. New York: Wiley; 2002. p. 219–28.

25. Moride Y, Haramburu F, Requejo AA, Begaud B. Under-reporting of adverse drug reactions in general practice. *Br J Clin Pharmacol* 1997; **43**: 177–81.

26. Alvarez-Requejo A, Carvajal A, Begaud B, Moride Y, Vega T, Martin Arias LH. Under-reporting of adverse drug reactions. Estimate based on a spontaneous reporting scheme and a sentinel system. *Eur J Clin Pharmacol* 1998; **54**: 483–8.

27. Brewer T, Colditz GA. Postmarketing surveillance and adverse drug reactions: current perspectives and future needs. *JAMA* 1999; **281**: 824–9.

28. Lasagna L. The Halcion story: trial by media. *Lancet* 1980; **1**: 815–6.

29. Rossi AC, Hsu JP, Faich GA. Ulcerogenicity of piroxicam: an analysis of spontaneously reported data. *BMJ* 1987; **294**: 147–50.

30. Meinzinger MM, Barry WS. Prospective study of the influence of media on reporting medical events. *Drug Inf J* 1990; **24**: 575–7.

31. Teicher MH, Glod C, Cole J. Emergence of intense suicidal preoccupation during fluoxetine treatment. *Am J Psychiatry* 1990; **147**: 207–10.

32. Ahmad SR. USA: Fluoxetine "not linked to suicide". *Lancet* 1991; **338**: 875–6.

33. FDA Psychopharmacologic Drugs Advisory Committee Meeting. September 21, 1991.

34. Heiligenstein JH, Beasley CM Jr, Potvin JH. Fluoxetine not associated with increased aggression in controlled clinical trials. *Int Clin Psychopharmacol* 1993; **8**: 277–80.

35. Coccaro EF, Kavoussi RJ. Fluoxetine and impulsive aggressive behavior in personality-disordered subjects. *Arch Gen Psych* 1997; **54**: 1081–8.

36. Warshaw MG, Keller MB. The relationship between fluoxetine use and suicidal behavior in 654 subjects with anxiety disorders. *J Clin Psych* 1996; **57**: 158–66.

37. Leon AC, Keller MB, Warshaw MG, Mueller TI, Solomon DA, Coryell W, Endicott J. Prospective study of fluoxetine treatment and suicidal behavior in affectively ill subjects. *Am J Psych* 1999; **156**: 195–201.

38. Finch RG. The withdrawal of Temafloxacin: are there implications for other quinolones? *Drug Saf* 1993; **8**: 9–11.

39. Clark JA, Klincewicz SL, Stang PE. Spontaneous adverse event signaling methods: classification and use with health care treatment products. *Epidemiol Rev* 2001; **23**: 191–210.

40. Hauben M. A brief primer on automated signal detection. *Ann Pharmacother* 2003; **37**.

41. Evans SJW, Waller PC, Davis S. Use of proportional reporting ratios (PRRs) for signal generation from spontaneous adverse drug reaction reports. *Pharmacoepidemiol Drug Saf* 2001; **10**: 483–6.

42. Moore N, Hall G, Sturkenboom M, Mann R, Lagnaoui R, Begaud B. Biases affecting the proportional reporting ratio (PRR) in spontaneous reports pharmacovigilance databases: the example of sertindole. *Pharmacoepidemiol Drug Saf* 2003; **12**: 271–81.

43. Edwards RI, Lindquist M, Bate A. Data Mining. In: Mann R, Andrews E, eds., *Pharmacovigilance*. New York: Wiley; 2002. p. 291–300.

44. Kulldorff M, Fang Z, Walsh SJ. A tree-based scan statistic for database disease surveillance. *Biometrics* 2003; **59**: 323–331.

45. Hall GC, Brown MM, Mo J, MacRae KD. Triptans in migraine: the risks of stroke, cardiovascular disease, and death in practice. *Neurology* 2004; **62**: 563–8.

46. Velentgas P, Cole JA, Mo J, Sikes CR, Walker AM. Severe vascular events in migraine patients. *Headache* 2004; **44**: 7.

47. VanDenBrink AM, van den Broek RWM, de Vries R, Bogers AJJC, Avezaat CJJ, Saxena PR. Craniovascular selectivity of eletriptan and sumatriptan in human isolated blood vessels. *Neurology* 2000; **55**: 1524–30.

48. Petty TL. Scope of the COPD problem in North America: early studies of prevalence and NHANES III data: basis for early identification and intervention. *Chest* 2000; **117**: S326–31.

49. de Luise C, Lanes SF, Curkendall SM, Jones JK, Lanza L, Sidney S. Cardiovascular morbidity and mortality among person with Chronic Obstructive Pulmonary Disease. Oral presentation at ISPE Annual Conference, August 2004, Bordeaux, France.

50. Tennis P, Cole TB, Annegers JF, Leestma JE, McNutt M, Rajput A. Cohort study of incidence of sudden unexplained death in persons with seizure disorder treated with antiepileptic drugs in Saskatchewan, Canada. *Epilepsia* 1995; **36**: 29–36.

51. Derby LE, Tennis P, Jick H. Sudden unexplained death among subjects with refractory epilepsy. *Epilepsia* 1996; **37**: 931–5.

52. Leestma JE, Annegers JF, Brodie MJ, Brown S, Schraeder P, Siscovick D, *et al.* Sudden unexplained death in epilepsy: observations from a large clinical development program. *Epilepsia* 1997; **38**: 47–55.

53. Jackson G. Erectile Dysfunction and Cardiovascular Disease. *IJCP* 1999; **53**: 363–8.

54. Mann RD. Prescription event monitoring – recent progress and future horizons. *Br J Clin Pharmacol* 1998; **46**: 195–201.

55. Shakir SA. Wilton LV. Boshier A. Layton D. Heeley E. Cardiovascular events in users of sildenafil: results from first phase of prescription event monitoring in England. *BMJ* 2001; **322**: 651–2.

56. Boshier A, Wilton LV, Shakir SAW. Evaluation of the safety of sildenafil for male erectile dysfunction: experience gained in general practice use in England in 1999. *BJU International* 2004; **93**: 7.

57. Pfizer, Inc. Pfizer announces early end of European cardio-vascular (CV) study: No CV concerns with Viagra. Vienna, Austria: Press Release 2004 (www.pfizer.com).

58. Muller JE, Mittleman A, Maclure M, Sherwood JB, Toffler GH. Triggering myocardial infarction by sexual activity. Low absolute risk and prevention by regular physical exertion. Determinants of Myocardial Infarction Onset Study. *JAMA* 1996; **275**: 1405–9.

59. Garcia Rodriguez LA, Wallander MA, Stricker BH. The risk of acute liver injury associated with cimetidine and other acid-suppressing anti-ulcer drugs. *Br J Clin Pharmacol* 1997; **43**: 183–8.

60. Ray WA, Griffin MR, Downey W. Benzodiazepines of long and short elimination half-life and the risk of hip fracture. *JAMA* 1989; **262**: 3303–7.

61. Cummings SR, Nevitt MC, Browner WS, Stone K, Fox KM, Ensrud KE, *et al.* Risk factors for hip fracture in white women: Study of Osteoporotic Fractures Research Group. *N Engl J Med* 1995; **332**: 767–73.

62. Data on file. Pfizer, Inc., New York, New York.

63. Mills JL, Fradkin J, Schonberger L, Gunn W, Thomson RA, Piper J, *et al.* Status report on the US Human Growth Hormone Recipient Follow-Up Study. *Horm Res* 1990; **33**: 116–9.

64. Fradkin JE, Schonberger LB, Mills JL, Gunn WJ, Piper JM, Wysowski DK, *et al.* Creutzfeldt-Jakob Disease in pituitary growth hormone recipients in the United States. *JAMA* 1991; **265**: 880–4.

65. Huillard d'Aignaux J, Alperovitch A, Maccario J. A statistical model to identify the contaminated lots implicated in iatrogenic transmission of Creutzfeldt-Jakob disease among French human growth hormone recipients. *Am J Epidemiol* 1998; **147**: 597–604.

66. Billette de Villemeur T, Deslys JP, Pradel A, Soubrie C, Alperovitch A, Tardieu M, *et al.* Creutzfeldt-Jakob disease from contaminated growth hormone extracts in France. *Neurology* 1996; **47**: 690–5.

67. Buchanan CR, Preece MA, Milner RD. Mortality, neoplasia, and Creutzfeldt-Jakob disease in patients treated with human pituitary growth hormone in the United Kingdom. *BMJ* 1991; **302**: 824–8.

68. Correll CC, Leucht S, Kane JM. Lower risk for tardive dyskinesia associated with second-generation antipsychotics: a systematic review of 1-year studies. *Am J Psychiatry* 2004; **161**: 414–25.

69. Tucker MA, Meadows AT, Boice JD, Stovall M, Oberlin O, Stone BJ, *et al.* Leukemia after therapy with alkylating agents in childhood cancer. *J Natl Cancer Inst* 1987; **78**: 459–64.

70. Hawkins MM, Kinnier-Wilson LM, Stovall MA, Marsden HB, Potok MHN, Kingston JE, *et al.* Epipodophyllotoxins, alkylating agents, and radiation and risk of secondary leukaemia after childhood cancer. *BMJ* 1992; **304**: 951–8.

71. deVathaire F, Francois P, Hill C, Schweisguth O, Rodary C, Sarrazin D, *et al.* Role of radiotherapy and chemotherapy in the risk of second malignant neoplasms after cancer in childhood. *Br J Cancer* 1989; **59**: 792–6.

72. Tucker MA, D'Angio GJ, Boice JD, Strong LC, Li FP, Stovall M, *et al.* Bone sarcomas linked to radiotherapy and chemotherapy in children. *N Engl J Med* 1987; **317**: 588–93.

73. Glasser DB, Duane K, Lane JM, Healey JH, Caparros-Sison B. The effect of chemotherapy on growth in the skeletally immature individual. *Clin Orthop* 1991; **262**: 93–100.

74. Roman J, Villaizan CJ, Garcia-Foncillas J, Salvador J, Sierrasesumaga L. Growth and growth hormone secretion in children with cancer treated with chemotherapy. *J Pediatr* 1997; **131**: 105–21.

75. Mohnike K, Dorffel W, Timme J, Kluba U, Aumann V, Vorwerk P, *et al.* Final height and puberty in 40 patients after

antileukaemic treatment during childhood. *Eur J Pediatr* 1997; **156**: 272–6.

76. Brennan BM, Rahim A, Adams JA, Eden OB, Shalet SM. Reduced bone mineral density in young adults following cure of acute lymphoblastic leukaemia in childhood. *Br J Cancer* 1999; **79**: 1859–63.

77. Arikoski P, Komulainen J, Voutilainen R, Riikonen P, Parviainen M, Tapanainen P, *et al*. Reduced bone mineral density in long-term survivors of childhood acute lymphoblastic leukemia. *J Pediatr Hematol Oncol* 1998; **20**: 234–40.

78. Bruning PF, Pit JM, deJong-Bakker M, van den Ende A, Hart A, van Enk A. Bone mineral density after adjuvant chemotherapy for premenopausal breast cancer. *Br J Cancer* 1990; **61**: 308–10.

79. Redman JR, Bajorunas DR, Wong G, McDermott K, Gnecco C, Schneider R, *et al*. Bone mineralization in women following successful treatment of Hodgkin's disease. *Am J Med* 1988; **85**: 65–72.

80. Holmes SJ, Whitehouse RW, Clark ST, Crowther DC, Adams JE, Shalet SM. Reduced bone mineral density in men following chemotherapy for Hodgkin's disease. *Br J Cancer* 1994; **70**: 371–5.

81. Mastroianni AC, Faden R, Federmen, eds., *Women and Health Research: Ethical and Legal Issues of Including Women in Clinical Trials*. Washington DC: National Academy of Science Press; 1994.

82. Colley GB, Brantley MD, Larson MK. *Family Planning Practices and Pregnancy Intention*. Atlanta: CDC; 1997.

83. Herbst AL, Ulfelder H, Poskanzer DC. Association of maternal stilbestrol therapy with tumor appearance in young women. *N Engl J Med* 1971; **284**: 878–81.

84. Herbst AL, Kurman RJ, Scully RE, Poskanzer DC. Clear-cell adenocarcinoma of the genital tract in young females. *N Engl J Med* 1972; **287**: 1259–64.

85. Thapa PB, Whitlock JA, Brockman Worrell KG, Gideon P, Mitchel EF Jr, Roberson P, *et al*. Prenatal exposure to metronidazole and risk of childhood cancer: a retrospective cohort study of children younger than 5 years. *Cancer* 1998; **83**: 1461–8.

86. Kinnier-Wilson LM, Kneale GW, Stewart AM. Childhood cancer and pregnancy drugs. *Lancet* 1981; **2**: 314–5.

87. Olsen JH, Hertz H, Blinkenberg K, Verder H. Vitamin K regimens and incidence of childhood cancer in Denmark. *BMJ* 1994; **308**: 895–6.

88. Parker L, Cole M, Craft AW, Hey EN. Neonatal vitamin K administration and childhood cancer in the north of England: retrospective case-control study. *BMJ* 1998; **316**: 189–93.

89. McKinney PA, Juszczak E, Findlay E, Smith K. Case-control study of childhood leukaemia and cancer in Scotland: findings for neonatal intramuscular vitamin K. *BMJ* 1998; **316**: 173–7.

90. von Kries R, Gobel U, Hachmeister A, Kaletsch U, Michaelis J. Vitamin K and childhood cancer: a population based case-control study in Lower Saxony, Germany. *BMJ* 1996; **313**: 199–203.

91. Rosenberg L, Mitchell AA, Parsells JL, *et al*. Lack of relation of oral clefts to diazepam use during pregnancy. *N Engl J Med* 1983; **309**: 1282–5.

92. Louik C, Mitchell AA, Werler MM, Hanson JW, Shapiro S. Maternal exposure to spermicides in relation to certain birth defects. *N Engl J Med* 1987; **317**: 474–8.

93. Mitchell AA, Rosenberg L, Shapiro S, Slone D. Birth defects related to Bendectin use in pregnancy: I. Oral clefts and cardiac defects. *JAMA* 1981; **245**: 2311–14.

94. Mitchell AA, Schwingl PJ, Rosenberg L, Louik C, Shapiro S. Birth defects in relation to Bendectin use in pregnancy: II. Pyloric stenosis. *Am J Obstet Gynecol* 1983; **147**: 737–42.

95. Covington DL, Tilson H, Elder J, Doi PA, for APR Steering Committee. Assessing teratogenicity of antiretroviral drugs: monitoring and analysis plan of the antiretroviral pregnancy registry. *Pharmacoepidemiol Drug Saf* 2002; **11**: S137.

96. Beghi E, Annegers JF for Collaborative Group for the Pregnancy Registries in Epilepsy. Pregnancy registries in epilepsy. *Epilepsia* 2001; **42**: 1422–25.

97. Reiff-Eldridge R, Heffner CR, Ephross SA, Tennis PS, White AD, Andrews EB. Monitoring pregnancy outcomes after prenatal drug exposure through prospective pregnancy registries: a pharmaceutical company commitment. *Am J Obstet Gynecol* 2000; **182**: 159–63.

98. Shields KE, Galil K, Seward J, *et al*. Varicella vaccine exposure during pregnancy: data from the first 5 years of the pregnancy registry. *Obstet Gynecol* 2001; **98**: 14–19.

99. Goldstein DJ, Sundell KL, DeBrota DJ, Offen WW. Determination of pregnancy outcome risk rates after exposure to an intervention. *Clinical Pharmacol Ther* 2001; **69**: 7–13.

100. Food and Drug Administration. *Guidance for industry: establishing pregnancy exposure registries*. Rockville: FDA; 2002.

101. http://www.fda.gov/ohrms/dockets/ac/00/transcripts/3619t1.rtf/. Accessed February 24, 2004.

102. Harrigan EP, Miceli JJ, Anziano R, Watsky E, Reeves KR, Cutler NR et al. A randomized evaluation of the effects of six antipsychotic agents on QTc, in the absence and presence of metabolic inhibition. *J Clin Psychopharmacol* 2004; **24**: 62–9.

103. Enger C, Weatherby L, Reynolds RF, Glasser DB, Walker AM. Serious cardiovascular events and mortality among patients with schizophrenia. *J Nerv and Ment Disease* 2004; **192**: 19–27.

104. Curkendall S, Mo Jingping, Glasser DB, Jones J. Cardiovascular disease in patients with schizophrenia, Saskatchewan, Canada. *J Clin Psych*. 2004; **192**: 19–27.

105. Hennessey S, Bilker WB, Knauss JS, Margolis DJ, Kimmel SE, Reynolds RF *et al*. Cardiac arrest and ventricular arrhythmia in patients taking antipsychotic drugs: cohort study using administrative data. *BMJ* 2002; **325**: 1070–4.

106. Hennessey S, Bilker WB, Knauss JS, Margolis DJ, Kimmel SE, Reynolds RF *et al*. Comparative cardiac safety of low-dose

thioridazine and low-dose haloperidol. *Br J Clin Phamacol.* 2004; **58**: 81–87.

107. http://www.fda.gov/ohrms/dockets/ac/accutane/1782t2a.pdf/. Accessed February 23, 2004.

108. http://www.fda.gov/ohrms/dockets/ac/00/transcripts/3639t1a.pdf/. Accessed February 23, 2004.

109. http://www.fda.gov/ohrms/dockets/ac/00/transcripts/3627t2a.pdf/. Accessed February 23, 2004.

110. http://www.fda.gov/bbs/topics/NEWS/NEW00734.html/. Accessed February 23, 2004.

111. http://www.gsk.com/press_archive/press_06072002.htm/. Accessed February 23, 2004.

112. Smalley W, Shatin S, Wysowski DK. Contraindicated use of cisapride: impact of Food and Drug Administration regulatory action. *JAMA* 2000; **284**: 3036–9.

113. Weatherby LB, Walker AM, Fife D, Vervaet P, Klausner MA. Contraindicated medications dispensed with cisapride: temporal trends in relation to the sending of 'Dear Doctor' letters. *Pharmacoepidemiol Drug Saf* 2001; **10**: 211–18.

114. http://www.fda.gov/bbs/topics/ANSWERS/ANS00882.html/. Accessed February 23, 2004.

115. http://www.fda.gov/bbs/topics/ANSWERS/ANS00999.html/. Accessed February 23, 2004.

116. http://www.fda.gov/bbs/topics/ANSWERS/ANS01007.html/. Accessed February 23, 2004.

117. Jones JK, Fife D, Curkendall S, Goehring E, Guo JJ, Shannon M. Coprescribing and codispensing of cisapride and contraindicated drugs. *JAMA* 2001; **286**: 1607–9.

118. Chute CG, Panser LA, Girman CJ, Oesterling JE, Guess HA, Jacobsen SJ, *et al.* The prevalence of prostatism: a population-based survey of urinary symptoms. *J Urol* 1993; **150**: 85–9.

119. Sagnier PP, Girman CJ, Garraway M, Kumamoto Y, Lieber MM, Richard F, *et al.* International comparison of the community prevalence of symptoms of prostatism in four countries. *Eur Urol* 1996; **29**: 15–20.

120. Chute CG, Stephenson WP, Guess HA, Lieber M. Benign Prostatic Hyperplasia: a population-based study. *Eur Urol* 1991; **20**: 11–17.

121. Jacobsen SJ, Girman CJ, Guess HA, Rhodes T, Oesterling JE, Lieber MM. Natural history of prostatism: longitudinal changes in voiding symptoms in community dwelling men. *J Urol* 1996; **155**: 595–600.

122. Roberts RO, Jacobsen SJ, Rhodes T, Girman CJ, Guess HA, Lieber MM. Natural history of prostatism: impaired health states in men with lower urinary tract symptoms. *J Urol* 1997; **157**: 1711–17.

123. Rhodes T, Girman CJ, Jacobsen SJ, Roberts RO, Guess HA, Lieber MM. Longitudinal prostate growth rates during 5 years in randomly selected community men 40 to 79 years old. *J Urol* 1999; **161**: 1174–9.

124. Jacobsen SJ, Jacobson DJ, Girman CJ, Roberts RO, Rhodes T, Guess HA, Lieber MM. Natural history of prostatism: risk factors for acute urinary retention. *J Urol* 1997; **158**: 481–7.

125. He J, Neal B, Gu D, Suriyawongpaisal P, Xin X, Reynolds R *et al.* International Collaborative Study of Cardiovascular Disease in Asia (InterASIA): Design and Rationale. *Ethn Dis.* 2004; **14**: 260–268.

126. Dongfeng G, Reynolds K, Wu ZX, Chen J, Duan X, Munter P *et al.* Prevalence, awareness, treatment, and control of hypertension in China. *Hypertension* 2002; **40**: 920–7.

127. Turner S, Longworth A, Nunn AJ, Choonara I. Unlicensed and off label drug use in paediatric wards: prospective study. *BMJ* 1998; **316**: 343–5.

128. Simons LA, Tett S, Simons J, Lauchlan R, McCallum J, Friedlander Y, Powell I. Multiple medication use in the elderly. Use of prescription and non-prescription drugs in an Australian community setting. *Med J Aust* 1992; **57**: 242–6.

129. Millar WJ. Multiple medication use among seniors. *Health Rep.* 1998; **9**: 11–7.

130. Sclar DA, Robinson LM, Skaer TL, Galin RS. Trends in the prescribing of antidepressant pharmacotherapy: office-based visits, 1990–1995. *Clin Ther* 1998; **20**: 870–84.

131. Martinez M. Agusti A. Arnau JM. Vidal X. Laporte JR. Trends of prescribing patterns for the secondary prevention of myocardial infarction over a 13-year period. *Eur J Clin Pharmacol* 1998; **54**: 203–8.

132. Schmader KE, Hanlon JT, Fillenbaum GG, Huber M, Pieper C, Horner R. Medication use patterns among demented, cognitively impaired and cognitively intact community-dwelling elderly people. *Age Ageing* 1998; **27**: 493–501.

133. Tome MB, Isaac MT. Cost-benefit & cost-effectiveness analysis of the rapid onset of selective serotonin reuptake inhibitors by augmentation. *Int J Psychiatry Med* 1997; **27**: 377–90.

134. Andersson F, Kartman B, Andersson OK. Cost-effectiveness of felodipine-metoprolol (Logimax) and enalapril in the treatment of hypertension. *Clin Exp Hypertens* 1998; **20**: 833–46.

135. Neumann PJ, Hermann RC, Kuntz KM, Araki SS, Duff SB, Leon J, *et al.* Cost-effectiveness of donepezil in the treatment of mild or moderate Alzheimer's disease. *Neurology* 1999; **2**: 1138–45.

136. Santos R, Cifaldi M, Gregory C, Seitz P. Economic outcomes of a targeted intervention program: the costs of treating allergic rhinitis patients. *Am J Man Care* 1999; **5**: S225–34.

137. Testa MA. Simonson DC. Health economic benefits and quality of life during improved glycemic control in patients with type 2 diabetes mellitus: a randomized, controlled, double-blind trial. *JAMA* 1998; **280**: 1490–6.

138. Glynn RJ, Monane M, Gurwitz JH, Choodnovskiy I, Avorn J. Agreement between drug treatment data and a discharge diagnosis of diabetes mellitus in the elderly. *Am J Epidemiol* 1999; **49**: 541–9.

139. Melfi CA, Croghan TW. Use of claims data for research on treatment and outcomes of depression care. *Med Care* 1999; **37**: AS77–80.

140. Lewis JD, Brensinger C, Bilker WB, Strom BL. Validity and completeness of the General Practice Research Database for studies of inflammatory bowel disease. *Pharmacoepidemiol Drug Saf* 2002; **11**: 211–18.

141. Metlay JP, Hardy C, Strom BL. Agreement between patient self-report and a Veterans Affairs national pharmacy database for identifying recent exposures to antibiotics. *Pharmacoepidemiol Drug Saf* 2003; **12**: 9–15.

142. Hennessey S, Bilker WB, Weber A, Strom BL. Descriptive analyses of the integrity of a US Medicaid claims database. *Pharmacoepidemiol Drug Saf* 2003; **12**: 103–11.

143. Brent RR. The Bendectin saga: another American tragedy. *Teratology* 1983; **27**: 283–6.

144. Brent RL. Bendectin: review of the medical literature of a comprehensively studied human nonteratogen and the most prevalent tortogen-litigen. *Reprod Toxicol* 1995; **9**: 337–49.

145. Holmes LB. Teratogen update: Bendectin. *Teratology* 1983; **27**: 277–81.

146. Neutel CI, Johansen HL. Measuring drug effectiveness by default: the case of Bendectin. *Can J Public Health* 1995; **86**: 66–70.

147. Blumenthal D. Academic-industrial relationships in the life sciences. *NEJM* 2003; **349**: 2452–2459.

148. Zuger A. How tightly do ties between doctor and drug company bind? *New York Times* July 27, 2004.

149. Steinbrook R. Financial conflicts of interest and the NIH. *NEJM* 2004; **350**: 327–330.

150. International Society for Pharmacoepidemiology (ISPE). 1996. Guidelines for Good Epidemiology Practices for Drug, Device and Vaccine Research in the United States. (http://www.pharmacoepi.org/resources/goodprac.cfm, Accessed August 5, 2004).

151. Ellenberg SS, Fleming TR, DeMets DL. Data Monitoring Committee in Clinical Trials. New York: John Wiley, 2003.

152. Barbone F, McMahon AD, Davey PG, Morris AD, Reid IC, McDevitt DG, *et al*. Association of road-traffic accidents with benzodiazepine use. *Lancet* 1998; **352**: 1331–6.

153. Hernandez-Diaz S, Hernan MA, Meyer K, Werler MM, Mitchell AA. Case-crossover and case-time-control designs in birth defects epidemiology. *Am J Epi* 2003; **158**: 385–91.

154. Ray WA. Evaluating medication effects outside of clinical trials: new-user designs. *Am J Epi* 2003; **158**: 915–20.

155. Califf RM. The need for a national infrastructure to improve the rational use of therapeutics. *Pharmacoepidemiol Drug Saf* 2002; **11**: 319–27.

156. Carr A, Emery SE, Law M, Puls R, Lundgren JD, Powderly WG. An objective case definition of lipodystrophy in HIV-infected adults. *Lancet* 2003; **361**: 726–35.

157. Law M, Friis-Moller N, Weber R, Reiss P, Thiebaut R, Kirk O *et al*. Modelling the three year risk of myocardial infarction among participants in the DAD study. *HIV Med* 2003; **4**: 1–10.

158. Friis-Moller N, Weber R, Reiss P, Thiebaut R, Kirk O, Monforte A *et al*. Cardiovascular risk factors in HIV patients – association with antiretroviral therapy. Results from the DAD study. *AIDS* 2003; **17**: 1179–93.

159. The DAD Study Group. Combination antiretroviral therapy and the risk of myocardial infarction. *NEJM* 2003; **349**: 1993–2003.

160. Bozzette SA, Ake C, Tam HK, Chang SC, Louis TA. Cardiovascular and cerebrovascular events in patients treated for Human Immunodeficiency Virus infection. *NEJM* 2003; **348**: 702–10.

161. The European Agency for the Evaluation of Medicinal Products. CPMP Public Statement: *Metabolic and cardiovascular complications of antiretroviral combination therapy in HIV-infected patients*. Doc Ref.: EMEA/CPMP/2383/03. 2003.

162. Johnson JA. Drug target pharmacogenomics: an overview. *Am J Pharmacogenomics* 2001; **1**: 271–81.

8

A View from Regulatory Agencies

PETER ARLETT[1], JANE MOSELEY[2] and PAUL J. SELIGMAN[3]

[1] Pharmaceuticals Unit, DG Enterprise and Industry, European Commission, Brussels, Belgium; [2] Medicines and Healthcare Products Regulatory Agency, London, UK; [3] FDA, Center for Drug Evaluation and Research, Rockville, Maryland, USA.

INTRODUCTION

Pharmacoepidemiology is changing the way medicines are regulated. The balance of benefits and risks of a medicine changes through the life of a medicine, and pharmacoepidemiology impacts at all stages, from drug discovery and development, through medicines licensing, to safety monitoring and pharmacoeconomics of marketed products. Governments regulate medicines to protect public health. The public is protected from poor quality, ineffective, or unsafe products. In our quest to better regulate medicines, pharmacoepidemiology is proving an ever more essential tool. It allows us to make decisions based on data that are more robust, gives us choices when previously we had none, and in some cases allows, as an aid to risk minimization, medicines with established safety problems to be used in the marketplace safely.

This chapter outlines some key principles in pharmacoepidemiology relevant to drug regulation and describes the context in which epidemiology may be applied. The chapter is organized by describing how pharmacoepidemiology may be relevant, and how it may be applied, at each step in the life of a medicine.

PHARMACOEPIDEMIOLOGY IN DRUG REGULATION: DEFINITIONS, SCOPE, AND SOME KEY PRINCIPLES

DEFINITIONS

It is important to ensure that we have a common understanding of some key terminology used in pharmacoepidemiology as applied to drug regulation. Box 8.1 provides definitions for essential terms, particularly those peculiar to drug regulation. In most cases, the definitions provided are internationally agreed upon. For example, the definition of pharmacovigilance is that provided by the World Heath Organization (WHO). In contrast, other commonly used terms, such as risk management, have no widely accepted definitions, therefore we have suggested pragmatic definitions of our own.

Pharmacoepidemiology, Fourth Edition   Edited by B.L. Strom
© 2005 John Wiley & Sons, Ltd

Adverse drug event (ADE)   An adverse event is any untoward medical occurrence in a patient administered a medicinal product and which does not necessarily have to have a causal relationship with this treatment. An adverse event can therefore be any unfavorable and unintended sign (for example, an abnormal laboratory finding), symptom, or disease temporally associated with the use of a medicinal product, whether or not considered related to this medicinal product.

Adverse drug reaction (ADR)   Adverse drug reactions, as established by regional regulations, guidance, and practices, concern noxious and unintended responses to a medicinal product. The phrase "responses to a medicinal product" means that a causal relationship between a medicinal product and an adverse event is at least a reasonable possibility. A reaction, in contrast to an event, is characterized by the fact that a causal relationship between the drug and the occurrence is suspected. For regulatory reporting purposes, if an event is spontaneously reported, even if the relationship is unknown or unstated, it meets the definition of an adverse drug reaction.

Approval   In the United States, the word approval is used for medicines licensing and originates in the statutory language of the Federal Food, Drug, and Cosmetic Act.

Authorization   Term used in the EU for the process of licensing a medicine. Authorization results in a Marketing Authorization (i.e., the legal document).

Demonstrating safety*   Active or systematic surveillance of an exposed population to preset milestones defined as patient exposure rather than calendar time such that a predefined unacceptable risk can be excluded with a given degree of confidence.

Efficacy   The property that enables drugs to produce beneficial responses under ideal conditions (usually applied to randomized controlled clinical trials).

Impact analysis*   A quantitative tool for prioritizing signals, the purpose of which is to focus further, detailed, signal evaluation on those for which the strongest evidence exists and those most likely to have an impact on public health.

Marketing Authorization   The term used for the license to market a drug in the EU.

Orphan medicine or drug   Term applied by relevant legislation (e.g. US Orphan Drug Act) to a medicine designated as an orphan medicine under that legislation. The medicine is for the diagnosis, prevention, or treatment of a rare disease, rare being further defined in the relevant legislation.

PASS   Post-approval safety studies are studies or trials conducted after a medicine is marketed to provide additional details about the medicine's safety profile.

Pharmacovigilance   The science and activities relating to the detection, assessment, understanding, and prevention of adverse effects or any other drug-related problems.

Pharmacovigilance plan   Based on the safety specification, the pharmacovigilance plan proposes measures to monitor the safety of a drug once marketed.

PIL   Patient Information Leaflet is the EU term for the part of the Marketing Authorization providing information about the medicine to the patient. By law it should be provided to the patient when the medicine is dispensed or administered.

Process audit*   This term is generally used in pharmacovigilance to describe the audit of the different steps in the pharmacovigilance process.

Renewal   In the EU new Marketing Authorizations are only valid for an initial 5 years, at which time the efficacy and, particularly, safety of the product are reviewed and the Marketing Authorization is updated and renewed.

Risk management*   The US FDA has proposed that risk management is the overall and continuous process of minimizing risks throughout a product's life cycle to optimize its benefit/risk balance. Risk management is a continuous process of learning about and interpreting a product's benefits and risks, evaluating interventions in the light of new knowledge that is acquired over time, and revising interventions when necessary.

Risk minimization*   This can be considered to be a subset of risk management, comprising interventions to minimize the risks associated with the use of a medicine and evaluation of the effectiveness of those interventions.

Risk quantification*   Assessment of the frequency, severity and seriousness of a risk.

Risk reduction*   A synonym for risk minimization.

Safety specification   The safety specification is a summary of the identified risks of a drug, the potential for important unidentified risks, the populations potentially at risk, and situations that have not been adequately studied.

Signal   A drug safety signal has been defined by the WHO as "reported information on a possible causal relationship between an adverse event and a drug, the relationship being unknown or incompletely documented previously. Usually more than a single report is required to generate a signal, depending upon the seriousness of the event and the quality of the information".

Solicited report Those reports derived from organized data collection systems, which include clinical trials, registries, post-approval named patient use programs, other patient support and disease management programs, surveys of patients or health care providers, or information gathering on efficacy or patient compliance.

SPC Summary of Product Characteristics is the term used to signify the part of the European Marketing Authorization that contains information about the product to help prescribers and dispensers use the medicine safely and effectively.

Spontaneous ADR report An unsolicited communication by a health care professional or consumer to a company, regulatory authority or other organization (e.g. WHO, Regional Centre, Poison Control Center) that describes one or more adverse drug reactions in a patient who was given one or more medicinal products and that does not derive from a study or any organized data collection scheme.

* In most cases, the definitions provided are internationally agreed upon. In contrast, other commonly used terms, such as risk management, have no widely accepted definitions. This can and has resulted in confusion. Therefore, for these terms we have suggested a pragmatic definition of our own.

Box 8.1. Definitions for essential terms and some commonly used abbreviations.

SCOPE OF PHARMACOEPIDEMIOLOGY IN DRUG REGULATION

Before considering detail, it is well worth gaining an overview of the scope of pharmacoepidemiology in drug regulation. Table 8.1 provides such an overview. It mirrors the structure and content of this chapter and may help to orient you as you navigate your way through.

SOME KEY PRINCIPLES

The protection of public health is central to decision making by pharmaceutical regulators. Given this public health-oriented approach, several key concepts underscore the regulatory process.

Regulators have obligations to ensure that medicines on the market are of acceptable safety, quality, and efficacy. We approach this by taking evidence-based decisions, balancing risk and benefits from a population perspective at different stages of the product life cycle. Pharmacoepidemiology can make important contributions to these decisions, decisions which impact on a wide range of people, particularly the end-user of medicines. Regulators also need to respond when study results of potential public health importance are published, adopting critical evaluation and taking any regulatory action if necessary.

When making these decisions, a wide range of study designs, broadly divided into descriptive and analytic studies, are employed. The concept of an "evidence hierarchy" based on study designs is helpful. The hierarchy reflects the

Table 8.1. Scope of pharmacoepidemiology in drug regulation

Stage in life cycle	Examples of possible applications of pharmacoepidemiology
Drug discovery	Identification of potential markets through study of disease distribution and medicines utilization
Drug development	Estimation of potential market size, unmet medical needs, demonstration of efficacy and safety. Selection of likely co-prescribed medicines for interaction studies. Planning safety data collection strategy for the development and post-licensing phases
Orphan drugs	Estimation of prevalence of disease, providing information on other treatments, demonstration of efficacy and safety, demonstrating significant benefit
Licensing	Information on the disease to be treated, existing therapies, safety profile of alternative therapies, demographics of toxicities associated with the medicine. Planning of safety monitoring post-licensing and risk minimization strategies
Post-licensing: pharmacovigilance	An aid to all steps in the pharmacovigilance process: signal detection and evaluation, benefit/risk assessment, measurement of the health effects of action taken to reduce risk
Variation, renewal, reclassification	Evaluation of benefits and risks in new indications. Re-evaluation of benefits and risks when new data are available regarding an established indication. Estimation of market size and use of existing therapies when considering a move to use without prescription
Pharmacoeconomics	Estimation of costs of therapy and benefits in economic terms to support reimbursement or inclusion in formularies

robustness of the data available. Descriptive studies, which include single case reports, case series, and uncontrolled cohorts or registries, limit the inferences that we make about causality. While largely hypothesis generating, these studies are most frequently the basis of post-licensing regulatory actions when time and resources do not permit more thorough analytic studies. Analytical studies include comparators and have the ability to test specific hypotheses. These include case–control studies, cohort studies, nested case–control studies, and case–crossover analyses, as well as randomized clinical trials. It is accepted that randomized controlled trials offer greater control of bias in the study design and are at a higher level in the evidence hierarchy than observational analytical studies. Meta-analyses offer methods of amalgamating data scientifically from different studies.

When we consider the safety of medicines, we have a complex interaction of regulatory medicine, medicines' safety, and pharmacoepidemiology. This interaction can be better understood by considering three axes (see Figure 8.1). While it is clear that safety concerns can arise at any time in the medicine's life cycle (axis 1), data elements from different sources in the evidence hierarchy (axis 2) fulfill different roles in the evolution of safety concerns (axis 3), from generation of data on safety, to evaluation, to hypothesis testing.

It is worth noting that, in the context of a major safety concern, observational, descriptive, and analytical studies are only a subset of all the available data; all available information should be considered for relevance. Conventional pharmacoepidemiologic data are based on observational, descriptive, and analytical studies in humans, including randomized clinical trials. However, in addition to these data sources there is a wealth of other data that should be considered in an overall assessment, for example, of a medicine safety issue. These include data based on pharmacodynamic and pharmacokinetics studies and nonclinical studies, including *in vitro* and animal studies.

From the public health perspective, there are a number of key concerns in relation to the nature and use of pharmacoepidemiologic data. These include the nature of the hypothesis, the aims and objectives posed, the details of methodology, ethical considerations, and the quality of the data. The UK Medicines and Healthcare products Regulatory Agency (MHRA) Excellence in Pharmacovigilance model outlines two main global aims in pharmacovigilance: the detection of harm and the demonstration of safety. The first is heavily dependent on spontaneous ADR reporting systems to flag previously unrecognized rare safety signals, including unusual patterns or excessive numbers of anticipated risks. To demonstrate safety post-licensing, the

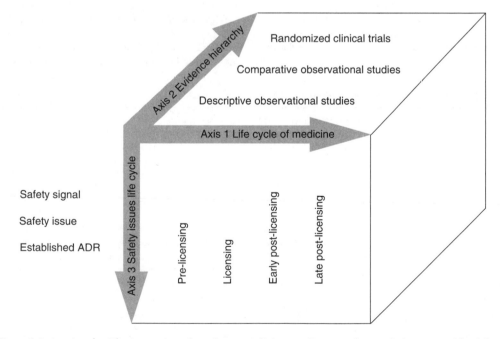

Figure 8.1. Jane's cube: The interaction of regulatory medicine, medicines' safety, and pharmacoepidemiology.

evaluation of safety requires planned collection of outcome and exposure data on a sample of the newly exposed population until preset milestones of patient exposure are met. Active surveillance earlier in the life cycle of the marketed medicine than is frequently conducted at present serves this need.[1]

Pharmacoepidemiologic data are used to ensure the maximum benefit at the minimum risk for the end-user of the medicine. The goal of analyzing spontaneous ADR reports is to maximize the detection of unrecognized safety issues and to minimize the chance of missing a safety signal. The patient and public health perspective is central to assessment of the impact of a given report of a suspected ADR on the medicine's benefit/risk profile. The development of clear surveillance case definitions in building a case series is essential in ensuring that the initial evaluation of a safety concern includes all possible cases that may be drug-related.

The highest professional standards must be applied in the design and conduct of post-licensing studies. A protocol with clear objectives, an independent advisory committee, and ethical review will help ensure that these studies generate useful safety data and dispel the concern of patients and health professionals that some post-licensing safety studies are principally for promotional purposes.

DRUG LIFE CYCLE

PRE-LICENSING

Epidemiology Informs Key Milestones in Medicines Development

In drug regulation, pharmacoepidemiology has, to date, been most used as an aid to pharmacovigilance. However, there are also numerous applications of epidemiological methodologies long before a medicine is licensed and used in the marketplace. When a pharmaceutical company is selecting potential disease targets to pursue and at key milestones during medicines development, epidemiologic techniques can be used to estimate and measure potential market size, the demographics of the diseased population, unmet medical needs, and how existing therapies are used in treatment. Such techniques can also be applied to further evaluate risk factors associated with adverse events observed during this period. For example, longitudinal patient databases such as the UK General Practice Research Database (GPRD) can be utilized (see Chapter 22). If considering developing a new medicine to treat diabetes mellitus, the GPRD can be used to measure disease incidence and prevalence in a population of defined size, and therefore the size of the potential UK market can be extrapolated. By knowing the age and sex distribution of the target population, together with the common co-pathologies, clinical trials can be designed that are both feasible (do not try to recruit 50% men for a disease affecting 90% women) and relevant to the likely clinical use of the product.

The GPRD records treatments, as well as diagnoses so a detailed analysis of existing drug use can be made. This may inform decisions about potential market size, possible niches in the market, how the developmental medicine might best be used, and what other drugs are likely to be used concomitantly. This information has the potential to be used in making decisions about which medicines should be studied for interactions and on the inclusion and exclusion criteria of trials.

During medicines development, the traditional way to learn about the safety of a product is through the systematic collection of adverse event data during randomized, comparative clinical trials. However, epidemiologic techniques, including more descriptive methods, can supplement clinical trial data. For example, after the randomized period of a clinical trial, patients often continue on study therapy in an unblinded "extension phase." Although the adverse event data are less robust than those from the randomized study, they provide useful additional information on the product's safety, including valuable long-term exposure data. Comparisons can be made to adverse events during the randomized part of the study, perhaps with patients serving as their own controls or between patients continuing on active treatment and those opting to stop treatment. Similar descriptive safety analyses can be conducted when patients receive an investigational medicine on a "compassionate use" or "named patient" basis. Indeed, some regulatory authorities will only allow such use if protocols are put in place for the systematic collection of adverse event data. In the global medicines market, a medicine may be investigational in one country or region and already licensed and marketed in others. In this situation, safety data, such as spontaneously reported ADRs originating from the region where the medicine is marketed, can supplement the randomized data from the region where the medicine remains investigational. When adverse events are observed during clinical trials, epidemiologic techniques, such as nested case–control studies, can be used to understand better the risk factors associated with the adverse events. Such information can inform companies and regulators about populations at risk that can be used to more effectively manage risks post-licensing. Finally, while randomized studies are conducted, epidemiologic studies of the disease being treated and its existing therapy can be conducted.

Epidemiologic techniques can also be used to collect and analyze efficacy data. In some situations, for example when a disease is very rare or when conducting comparator trials may be judged unethical, the only possible way to collect efficacy data may be through epidemiologic techniques.

When considering the role of pharmacoepidemiology in the assessment of a medicine's efficacy and safety, the importance of confounding by the indication must always be borne in mind in the analysis and interpretation of such studies (see Chapter 40). When comparing treated patients with untreated patients, treated patients will have a higher rate of any disease that the medicine is intended to treat, although studies of the medicine's effectiveness may be considered in some situations where effects are so dramatic that no comparator group is required.[2,3] Randomization operates to control confounding in the study of intended effects.[4]

Safety Assessment

To be licensed, the balance of benefits and risks of a medicine has been judged acceptable for the indications granted. However, regulators are often questioned on how or why major medicine safety issues arise subsequently. To understand why our knowledge of safety at licensing is provisional, this section will consider the extent and nature of the pre-licensing drug safety assessment, the limitations of clinical trials, and situations where a more extensive safety database may be needed.

Individual clinical trials are generally powered to answer specific efficacy questions with tight inclusion and exclusion criteria and they are usually of limited duration. Although the rate of common ADRs can also be estimated, such trials are unlikely to observe rare ADRs or reactions that only follow longer-term exposure (see Chapter 3). Furthermore, just because nothing goes wrong, this does not necessarily mean that everything is all right; if none of n patients experienced an adverse event, then the upper 95% confidence limit is at most approximately $3/n$.[5] One study has shown that the average human safety database for new medicine applications contained an average of 1480 subjects.[6] This gives us an idea of the reaction frequency detectable in clinical trials.

Assessment of clinical trial safety data must be undertaken with the aim of minimizing the risk to future trial participants and patients. This assessment should take carefully considered case definitions and time dependency into account. A single case report of a suspected unexpected serious adverse drug reaction (SUSAR) from a clinical trial may prompt the use of analytic tools such as data mining and other signal detection strategies on these data.[7] Sophisticated analysis tools with graphical displays are also being developed that take the denominator and other data into account.[8]

Good clinical risk assessment depends on adequately designed and conducted preclinical studies, clinical pharmacology studies, and clinical trials programs to ensure that sufficient safety data are generated to allow for licensing of the product. The size of the human safety database needed pre-authorization depends on many factors, including the product, the population, the indication, the duration of use of the drug, and the results of the preclinical and clinical pharmacology programs.[9]

Safety data, ideally, should be comparator-controlled safety data, including long-term safety data, to allow for comparisons of event rates and for accurate attribution of adverse events. Data should be available extending over a range of doses and in a diverse population. Risk assessment should address potential interactions (both drug–food and drug–drug interactions), demographic subpopulations, and effects of comorbid diseases. Risk assessment needs to be tailored to the medicine in question; issues may arise such as special developmental safety concerns in the pediatric population, less obvious or insidious ADRs that may not normally be reported, or special biologic safety problems. In some cases a large simple safety study is needed where serious safety signals have arisen that cannot be addressed using the existing data (see Chapter 39).

ICH guideline E1[10] outlines the size of the human database needed for licensing a medicine for non-life-threatening conditions. It recommends that data on at least 1500 patients be available when chronic/recurrent treatments for non-life-threatening diseases are considered, with 300–600 exposed for more than 6 months and 100 for more than 12 months. A larger database is needed when other concerns arise (see Table 8.2).

While all drugs are assessed for safety during their development, there is no consistent or agreed standard for a specific safety development plan. The Council for International Organizations of Medical Sciences (CIOMS) VI working group is drafting practical guidance on the process of developing and implementing a pharmacovigilance plan during development of a medicine. The planning of safety data

Table 8.2. Factors that may increase the required size of the pre-licensing human database

- Need to further estimate a specific rare ADR based on preclinical, pharmacological, class, or other data
- Benefit is small, benefit is experienced by a fraction of the treated population, or benefit is uncertain
- High morbidity/mortality condition
- Healthy population (e.g. vaccines)
- Safe alternatives already available

collection and promotion of the importance of safety data during development will assist in risk identification, assessment, and decision making, will better protect clinical trial subjects, and will form the basis of the safety specification and plan required at the time of licensing. The guidance will give consideration to responsibilities within companies, when a safety development plan should be developed, how it should be maintained, and what its structure might be.[11]

The Role of Scientific (Regulatory) Advice During a Medicine's Development

In both the EU and the US, systems exist for pharmaceutical companies to obtain scientific and regulatory advice during their development of a medicine. In the US, the FDA encourages frequent interactions and scientific dialog with application sponsors throughout a product's life cycle. The FDA is currently performing a formal, comprehensive assessment of the added value, costs, and impact of even more extensive feedback during drug development. In the EU, scientific and regulatory advice is given at the request of companies to answer specific questions on the design of studies or on the preparation of a license application. To date, it has been relatively rare for companies to seek or obtain advice on epidemiologic studies to be conducted during product development or in the post-licensing period. However, such advice is both available and highly recommended to improve the quality of license applications and the conduct of pharmacovigilance and therefore to better serve the public by maximizing a medicine's chance of success at the time of license application and minimizing risks once it is on the market. Scientific advice from regulators is also available regarding risk minimization strategies. When planning pharmacoepidemiology studies, seeking the best advice from regulators and outside experts in epidemiology should improve the quality of the study and make clear the outcomes and expectations of such an endeavor.

The Relevance of Pharmacoepidemiology to Orphan Medicines

An orphan disease is a rare disease and an orphan medicine is therefore (logically) a medicine to diagnose, prevent, or treat a rare disease (examples of designated orphan medicines in the EU can be found at http://www.pharmacos.eudra.org/F2/register/orphreg.htm). The 1983 US Orphan Drug Act[12] guarantees the developer of an orphan-designated product several incentives: 7 years of market exclusivity following US market approval in the same indication, tax credits for

clinical research in the product's development, and available funding from the US orphan products grant program. In addition, orphan-designated products have exemption from application fees for US FDA approval. This legislation has been very effective in bringing products for rare diseases to the market. During the 10 years before the Orphan Drug Act the American pharmaceutical industry developed approximately 10 orphan medicines. In contrast, between 1983 and 2003, 242 orphan-designated products have received FDA marketing approval. Furthermore the US legislation has formed the basis for similar incentive-based orphan laws in other regions, notably the EU and Japan.[13]

Pharmacoepidemiology plays a central role in the consideration of orphan medicines, first in designating a medicine as an orphan product and second in supporting the collection of data demonstrating the safety and efficacy of the product needed to license it.

In the US legislation, a rare disease or condition is defined as any disease or condition that affects fewer than 200 000 people in the US. In the EU Regulation on Orphan Medicinal Products,[14] the definition of rare is given as "not more than five in 10 thousand persons in the Community." In applying for orphan designation, companies have to substantiate that the disease to be diagnosed, prevented, or treated has a prevalence below the legal threshold. Such substantiation usually requires the application of pharmacoepidemiologic techniques. For example, a company could use a longitudinal patient database in a locality where they are trying to establish prevalence and search the database for all cases of a particular condition. The number of cases in the entire country or region can then be calculated if one knows the total population covered by the database and the total population of the country or region. Surveys of specialist treatment centers have sometimes been used to establish estimates of prevalence for very rare diseases, and for some rare diseases, national or regional registries exist which can form the basis of the prevalence calculation. These may be particularly useful if the disease is so rare that even very large databases, such as the UK GPRD, are unlikely to contain cases. As a general rule, the expert committees responsible for orphan designation require a greater level of precision in the prevalence estimate the closer it is to the threshold for designation (i.e., 5 in 10 000 in the EU).

In the EU Regulation on Orphan Medicinal Products, designation also requires that "there exists no satisfactory method of diagnosis, prevention or treatment of the condition in question . . . or if such method exists, that the medicinal product will be of significant benefit to those affected by that condition." Herein lie two further opportunities for the pharmacoepidemiologist: to establish that no satisfactory methods of treatment exist, or to establish that the product will be of significant benefit (further defined as "a clinically relevant advantage or a major contribution to patient care"). How might these be established? A reasonable starting point might be the longitudinal patient database. A search of such a database for existing cases of the disease followed by a search for each patient with that disease for prescriptions or medical interventions may provide all the information required.

The three pillars of drug regulation are quality, safety, and efficacy. Epidemiology may have a role to play in establishing the safety and efficacy of orphan medicines. The licensing criteria applied to orphan medicines are the same as those applied to any other medicine. However, the rarity of patients and their dispersal over a large area may make the conduct of a randomized study impractical, or even impossible. Randomized, parallel, double-blind controlled trials may be extremely difficult, especially if there is no current treatment available and the condition is life-threatening. If such a study design is not possible then alternative designs will have to be employed. If existing regulatory guidance on study design is not being followed then it is strongly advised to seek protocol advice from the relevant regulatory authorities before starting to enroll patients. Some of the alternative trial designs that have been used to study orphan medicines are described below.[13]

Open protocol trials, which allow patients to be added to ongoing studies, were considered the only option with very rare diseases in the earliest days of the US Orphan Drug Act.[13] However, their use is now discouraged as, when they are used, it is virtually impossible to return to controlled studies. In a *randomized withdrawal trial* all patients receive the study drug in an open-label phase and then responders are randomized to either continue treatment or placebo, which can then be compared. This design is not suitable for life-threatening diseases, for drugs with a long half-life, or for diseases with variable signs and symptoms. In *historical control clinical trials*, patients given the investigational medicine are compared with the known history of the disease. As they have no placebo arm it may be easier to recruit patients. The results of such studies can be very difficult to interpret unless the new treatment has a major effect and the course of the disease was severe, relentless, and well established. Biases include interpretation of the condition and temporal bias. The role for the pharmaco-epidemiologist in documenting the known history of the disease is clear. *Open label studies* have also been employed, both investigator and patient knowing the identity of the medicine. Bias is likely in such trials and difficulties may well occur in the evaluation of efficacy of the product. However, such studies may significantly add to knowledge on a product's safety. In a *crossover design trial* each group of patients receives each treatment twice during the trial. Recruitment may be easier as all patients know that they will (at some stage) receive the new treatment. These studies are well suited to small groups of patients with a rapidly responding disease, since the same patient may serve as both treatment and control subject. Difficulties will occur when the washout period for patients to return to baseline is too long (e.g., the drug has a long half-life) or washout is impossible because of the progressive nature of the disease being treated.

LICENSING A MEDICINE

Before a medicine can be marketed it is necessary to obtain a product license. The term "Marketing Authorization" now replaces "license" in the EU, and in the US the term "approval" is used for drugs and the term "license" is used for biologics. In this chapter we have chosen to use the terms "license" and "licensing" as synonymous with these other terms as they are generally familiar to readers. The licensing of a medicine is a key step in a product's life and the licensing system is the main tool that regulators have to protect public health, ensuring that only medicines meeting strict criteria of quality, safety, and efficacy reach the market. To obtain a product license, pharmaceutical companies have to submit detailed documentation relating to the product and its development. Application dossiers are organized in a pyramidal hierarchy of detail. At the top of the hierarchy are summary reports bringing together the key information on the safety, quality, and efficacy of the product, together with an overall assessment of the balance of benefits and risks of the product. Below these in the hierarchy are individual reports documenting all the results from the numerous pharmaceutical, preclinical, and clinical studies that provide the evidence to support the quality, safety, and efficacy of the product. At the base of the hierarchy sit the data from the individual studies.

The Common Technical Document (CTD) is the internationally agreed format for applications for licenses. The ICH M4E guideline provides very valuable guidance on the clinical section of the CTD.[15] The CTD (section 2.5.5) requests an "Overview of Safety." This should be a concise critical analysis of the safety data, noting how results support and justify proposed prescribing information. A critical analysis of safety should consider adverse effects characteristic of the pharmacological class and approaches taken to monitor for similar effects, special approaches to monitoring for particular adverse events (e.g., ophthalmic, QT interval prolongation), relevant animal toxicology, and product quality information. Findings that affect or could affect the evaluation of safety in clinical use should be considered with the nature of the patient population and the extent of exposure, both for test drug and control treatments. Limitations of the safety database, e.g., related to inclusion/exclusion criteria and study subject demographics, should be considered, and the implications of such limitations with respect to predicting the safety of the product in the marketplace should be explicitly discussed. Other relevant sections of the CTD critical to safety include section 2.7.4 "Summary of clinical safety," which is a summary of data relevant to the safety in the intended population, integrating the results of individual clinical study reports. Section 5.3.5 of the CTD should contain the reports of individual efficacy and safety studies, conducted by the sponsor, or otherwise available, including all completed and all ongoing studies of the medicine in both the proposed and non-proposed indications. Guideline ICH E3 describes the contents of a full report for a study contributing evidence pertinent to both safety and efficacy.[16]

Regulatory authorities assess the dossiers and, supported by expert committees, make decisions on whether a medicine can be licensed. As well as making decisions on the overall balance of benefits and risks of the medicine (and therefore whether a license can be granted), the regulatory authorities must also make decisions on how the product should be used in the marketplace, including its indications and contraindications for use. The license includes regulated information about the product aimed at the medicine's users. In the EU this information is called the Summary of Product Characteristics and Patient Information Leaflet. In the US this information is contained in the package insert. The primary audience for the package insert is physicians, pharmacists, and other health care professionals (the package insert is sometimes called "professional labeling"). Many US products also come with patient labeling, which (as its name implies) is written to be readily understandable by patients, consumers, and other "lay" persons.

Epidemiologic studies or work conducted during the development of the product should, where relevant, be included in the dossier submitted to support the license application. However, the epidemiologist's role in the licensing process goes further than this. More and more, regulatory authorities are requiring that the measures to monitor the safety of the product once on the market and measures to minimize the risks to patients from the product are documented, assessed, and agreed on during the licensing process.

The ICH E2E guideline "Pharmacovigilance Planning" provides a structured method for summarizing the risks associated with a drug and for presenting a pharmacovigilance plan for when the product is marketed.[17] The guideline is intended to aid industry and regulators in planning pharmacovigilance activities, especially in preparation for the early postmarketing period of a new medicine. The ICH guideline uses the term "safety specification," first coined in a pharmacovigilance strategy project by the UK regulatory authority,[1] for a document presenting the identified risks of a medicine, the potential for important unidentified risks, and the potentially at-risk populations and situations that have not been studied pre-licensing. Box 8.2 provides a

---

Nonclinical
Nonclinical safety concerns not resolved by clinical data (e.g., concerns from animal toxicity studies, general pharmacology studies, and drug interaction studies).

Clinical
Limitations of the human safety database (e.g., related to the size of the study population, and the study inclusion and exclusion criteria) should be considered and the implications of such limitations with respect to predicting the safety of the product in the marketplace should be discussed.

Populations not studied in the pre-licensing phase (e.g., children, the elderly, pregnant or lactating women, patients with hepatic or renal disorders, subpopulations with genetic polymorphisms, and patients of different ethnic origins) and the implications of this to predicting the safety of the product in the marketplace.

Adverse events and adverse drug reactions: this section should list the important identified and potential risks, including those that require further characterization or evaluation.

Identified and Potential Interactions
Epidemiology of the indication and important adverse events: to help understand the safety profile of the medicine and to put any adverse events seen in clinical trials into context, it is important to describe the epidemiology of the indication (disease to be treated by the drug) and the important adverse events in the target population. The incidence, prevalence, and mortality should be discussed, where possible, stratified by age, sex, and ethnic origin.

Pharmacological Class Effects

Summary: Ongoing Safety Issues

Box 8.2. The safety specification: summary of structure.

summary of the proposed structure of the safety specification. The safety specification is intended to help identify the need for specific data collection in the post-licensing period and also to facilitate the construction of the pharmacovigilance plan. The pharmacovigilance plan is based on the safety specification. It sets out the proposed methods for monitoring the safety of the product, including both "routine pharmacovigilance," i.e., the methodologies such as spontaneous reporting and periodic safety update reports that are required of companies by law, and any specific studies planned as a result of risks or potential risks identified in the safety specification. Box 8.3 provides a summary of the proposed structure of the pharmacovigilance plan. Some regulatory authorities are likely to require safety specifications and pharmacovigilance plans as part of applications for licenses for new chemical entities and biotechnology-derived products. In addition, they may be required for applications for significant changes in established products (e.g., new dosage form, new route of administration, or new manufacturing process of a biotechnology-derived product) and for established products that are to be introduced to

new populations or in significant new indications. From reference to Boxes 8.2 and 8.3 it is clear that the epidemiologist has a central role in the construction of the safety specification and pharmacovigilance plan.

Whereas the ICH guideline "Pharmacovigilance Planning" provides a structured method for documenting the risk profile of the product and planned safety monitoring, it does not deal with how to minimize risks to patients (other than through effective safety monitoring). As previously stated, regulatory authorities are encouraging and in some instances requiring that measures to minimize the risks to patients from the product are documented, assessed, and agreed on during the licensing process (see also Chapter 33). Here again, the epidemiologist can play a central role. The FDA has issued draft guidance on designing risk minimization plans and how these should be presented to the FDA for approval.[18,19] Before describing some of the key concepts included in the FDA guidance, it is worth considering for a moment some of the terminology used (see also Box 8.1). Terminology is used differently in different regions and this can cause confusion. For example, the term risk management has been used to mean "the overall and continuing process of minimizing risks throughout a product's life cycle to optimize its benefit/risk balance."[18] Given that the WHO definition of pharmacovigilance is "the science and activities relating to the detection, assessment, understanding and *prevention* of adverse effects or any other drug related problems," it can be seen that the scope of the terms risk management and pharmacovigilance overlap. For this reason, we prefer to use the broad definition of pharmacovigilance as proposed by the WHO while avoiding the term risk management altogether. For interventions which aim to reduce risk we prefer the term "risk minimization."

In terms of risk minimization (see also Chapter 33), the draft FDA guidance recommends that companies consider submitting risk reduction plans to the FDA for discussion and agreement as appropriate. Such plans might be submitted during product development, at the time of licensing assessment, or in the post-licensing phase (particularly in the event of an emerging or changing drug safety issue). An ideal submission to a regulator on risk minimization would provide the background of the risk reduction goals and rationale for the approach, the targeted goals and objectives, the proposed tools, a rationale to support them and an implementation plan, and an evaluation plan. The draft FDA guidance on risk minimization contains some key concepts important to the epidemiologist. The draft FDA guidance proposes that the sponsor for products should consider how to minimize risks from its product's use. Risk minimization planning might encompass product labeling, risk assessment,

---

Summary of Ongoing Safety Issues
Including the important identified risks, potential risks, and missing information.

Routine Pharmacovigilance Practices
Those pharmacovigilance practices that are common to all products should be described, including collection of spontaneous ADR reports, expedited reporting of ADR reports, reporting of periodic safety update reports, signal detection, issue evaluation, updating of labeling, and liaison with regulatory authorities. Some regulators may require an overview of the company's organization and practices for conducting pharmacovigilance.

Safety Action Plan for Specific Issues/Important Missing Information
For each risk issue the following should be presented (and justified): what is the issue, objective of the proposed action, proposed action, rationale for the action, oversight of the issue and the action, milestones for evaluation and reporting. Outline protocols for specific studies may be presented.

Summary of Actions to be Completed, Including Milestones
An overall pharmacovigilance plan for the product, bringing together the actions for all the individual risk issues and missing information, should be presented.

Box 8.3. The pharmacovigilance plan: summary of structure.

collecting data on suspected ADRs, and special medicine safety studies and interventions. For many products with well-recognized and non-serious ADRs, risk minimization may simply include product labeling and careful postmarketing surveillance (collecting safety data and assessment of those data). However, for other products, perhaps those with a poorly defined safety profile, serious ADRs, or emerging safety issues, a more formal risk minimization plan should be developed and agreed upon with the regulators. Risk minimization programs should have one or more risk reduction goals as endpoints. The best risk reduction goals would be tailored to specific risks of concern and, ideally, evidence-based methods would be used to target the achievement of critical processes, behaviors, and human factors to increase safety. The risk minimization goals are translated into individual risk minimization programs or protocols. A risk minimization plan or program would be an evolving plan, constantly evaluated for success, and amended if goals were not met or safety problems changed or emerged. In general, tools that facilitate or constrain prescribing, dispensing, or use of a product to the most appropriate situations or patient populations should be employed only when such an approach is necessary to achieve the goals of the program. Table 8.3, based on the FDA guidance,[18] illustrates some of the risk minimization tools currently in use.

The epidemiologist can play a central role in the selection of risk minimization tools to meet specific goals. Tools should have a high likelihood of achieving their objective based on evidence of effectiveness in other settings. Factors to consider in selecting tools might include input from stakeholders on the feasibility and acceptability of tools, consistency with tools already in use, documented effectiveness in achieving a specific objective, and the degree of variability, validity, and reproducibility of the tool and/or result. Several studies have documented that previous risk communication and risk minimization interventions to reduce safety problems have been variably effective.[20–22] Evaluation of risk minimization, both before and after implementation, is therefore crucial in order to make ongoing efforts to minimize risks to patients and to remedy problems or failures. More than one method of evaluation may be necessary to assess a risk minimization intervention, and trade-offs may be necessary between validity, accuracy, timeliness, representativeness, biases, societal impositions, and costs. Ideally, evaluation measures will be of actual health outcomes; the measure would capture the outcome itself rather than a surrogate. If a process measure is chosen rather than actual outcome, it is important to review the evidence supporting the link between the process and the ultimate outcome of interest.

Table 8.3. Some possible risk minimization tools

(1) Generalized education and outreach to health professionals and patients (beyond the US package insert or EU product information):

  (a) Health care professional letters
  (b) Training programs
  (c) Continued medical education
  (d) Public notices (communications from the regulatory authorities)
  (e) Medication guides

(2) Systems that guide the circumstances of individual prescribing, dispensing, or use:

  (a) Patient agreements/informed consent
  (b) Certification programs for practitioners
  (c) Enrolment of doctors/pharmacists/patients in a safety program
  (d) Limited supply or refills of product
  (e) Specialized product packaging
  (f) Systems to attest that safety measures (e.g., liver function testing)have been satisfied (e.g., stickers on prescriptions, physician attestation of capabilities)

(3) Restricted access systems designed to enforce individual compliance with program elements:

  (a) Prescribing only by registered physicians
  (b) Dispensing only by registered pharmacies or practitioners
  (c) Dispensing only to patients with evidence of safe-use conditions (e.g., lab test results)

(4) Product withdrawal (specific measures depend on the legal framework in different regions):

  (a) Suspension of marketing and use
  (b) Suspension of the license
  (c) Revocation of the license

POST-LICENSING

At the time of licensing, due to the limitations of clinical trials in simulating the complexities of "real-world" use, we generally have incomplete knowledge about the safety of a new medicine. For most medicines, following launch onto the market, the exposure to a medicine increases from a few hundred or thousands of patients exposed during the development program, to tens or hundreds of thousands or even millions of patients. With the increasing globalization of the pharmaceutical industry, this mass exposure can occur within months of a product launch. Furthermore, the controlled way the medicine was used during development switches to the relative anarchy of everyday prescribing, dispensing, and usage of medicines. With the general availability of the product, we learn about the effects of a medicine in everyday practice, including rare ADRs and ADRs that only occur after prolonged use, as well as ADRs associated with co-prescribing with other medications and those unique to or enhanced by comorbidities in the treated population. The additional knowledge of the safety profile in normal clinical use must be systematically managed and evaluated for the protection of patients.

The epidemiologist's role is much better established in the post-licensing phase of a medicine's life: the epidemiologist plays a central role in pharmacovigilance, but may also be involved in the variation, renewal, and reclassification of medicines (see Table 8.1). In addition, governments are increasingly requiring data on cost-effectiveness (see Chapter 41) and relative effectiveness prior to including a new medicine in formularies for use or prior to agreeing to reimburse patients for the cost of the medicine. Here again the epidemiologist may play a role in the collection, analysis, or presentation of data.

Pharmacovigilance

The monitoring of the safety of marketed medicines is known as pharmacovigilance, defined by the WHO as "the science and activities relating to the detection, assessment, understanding and prevention of adverse effects or any other drug related problems." In most regions of the world, pharmaceutical legislation places specific responsibilities on pharmaceutical companies to conduct pharmacovigilance for their products. For example, according to EU law,[23,24] companies holding a Marketing Authorization (license) for a product have to have a system of pharmacovigilance in place, including a "qualified person" responsible for the conduct of pharmacovigilance, a system to collect and report suspected ADRs, and the production and submission to regulators of periodic safety update reports.[25] In some countries there are also legal obligations on certain health care professionals to report suspected ADRs to the regulatory authorities (e.g., in France). To understand the practice of pharmacovigilance it is helpful to break it down into process steps. Table 8.4 provides such a breakdown. The subsequent sections describe these steps in more detail with particular emphasis on aspects relevant to the epidemiologist.

Table 8.4. Pharmacovigilance process steps

- Data collection
- Data management
- Signal (safety issue) detection
- Risk assessment and quantification
- Benefit/risk assessment and decision making
- Action to reduce risk or increase benefit
- Communication of risks or interventions
- Audit (measurement of outcome of interventions)

Data Collection and Management

Data on drug safety from all available sources needs to be collected and managed systematically in order to be able to detect possible drug safety hazards as effectively as possible. The subsequent assessment of emerging data enables us to detect and judge the severity of previously unrecognized safety issues, as well as changes in the frequency of, severity of, or risk factors for known safety issues. These aspects of pharmacovigilance, known as signal detection and signal evaluation, are described in a specific section later.

Pharmaceutical companies have obligations to collect all data relevant to the safety of their products and to submit such data to regulators in line with guidance and legislation. Regulators monitor these data for signals but also collect and screen safety data on medicinal products for signal detection independently of pharmaceutical companies. Safety data collection is carried out throughout the post-licensing lifetime of the product, until the product is discontinued or withdrawn, as new safety issues can and have emerged at any time, even with well-established products.

The collection and management of data has to be systematic, incorporating quality assurance and control measures, utilizing necessary resource, skills, and equipment to ensure timely access to the data for signal detection. The processes have evolved and been harmonized in the knowledge that pre-licensing and post-licensing clinical safety reporting concepts and practices are interdependent and that reports need to be transferred efficiently to different parties. The result is that there are widely agreed definitions, standards, contents, and conditions for case reporting, including for electronic transmission for individual case reports. Projects are establishing electronic communication standards to ensure the integrity of information and data exchange between pharmaceutical companies and authorities. There are also agreed standards, content, and format for periodic safety update reports (PSURs) for companies which are submitted to regulators at fixed time points from licensing. Other safety data and potential safety signals will come to the attention of regulators through processes involving applications to change product licenses (variations), post-licensing commitments and follow-up measures (agreed at the time of licensing), regular screening of the published literature, communication among regulators, and patient and health professional enquiries.

The breadth of medicines in use means that different mechanisms are required to gather relevant safety and exposure data across a range of domains, including prescription and non-prescription settings and different care settings (such as emergency care, hospitals, primary care, private, military, palliative care, contraceptive services, residential care homes, psychiatric services, emergency wards). Herbal and traditional medicines may pose safety concerns where data standards and availability are particularly limited.[26]

Regulation and Ethics in Research

The EU pharmacovigilance guidance[27] provides guidance on the essential principles to be applied in a variety of situations regarding the conduct of studies that evaluate the safety of licensed products and are sponsored or partly sponsored by the pharmaceutical industry. The extent and objectives of post-licensing safety studies, design, conduct, liaison with regulatory authorities, promotion of medicines, doctor participation, and payment and ethical issues are addressed. In the US, the FDA has published a guidance for industry entitled "Good Clinical Practice: Consolidated Guidance." Good clinical practice (GCP) is an international ethical and scientific quality standard for designing, conducting, recording, and reporting trials that involve the participation of human subjects, applicable to both clinical trials and postmarketing studies. Compliance with this standard provides public assurance that the rights, safety, and well-being of trial subjects are protected, consistent with the principles that have their origin in the Declaration of Helsinki, and that the clinical trial data are credible. The FDA has developed a website[28] that addresses matters related to human subject protection and provides guidance for conducting clinical trials with investigational drugs and information for compliance with the regulations of the FDA. The website contains links to the GCP guidance referenced above, as well as appropriate regulations.

For prospectively conducted post-licensing studies, regulations require that the highest possible standards of professional conduct and confidentiality must always be maintained and any relevant national legislation on data protection should be followed (see also Chapter 38). The patient's right to confidentiality is paramount. The patient's identity in the study documents should be codified, and only authorized persons should have access to identifiable personal details if data verification procedures demand inspection of such details. Identifiable personal details must always be kept in confidence. Reference to an ethics committee is required if patients are to be approached for information, additional investigations are to be performed, or if it is proposed to allocate patients systematically to treatments. Since May 2004, in the EU, interventional studies fall under the EU Clinical Trials Directive.[7] Post-licensing safety studies that are randomized clinical trials or observational studies where interventions over and above normal clinical practice occur are subject to the requirements in this legislation. In the US, the Belmont Report is the basic foundation on which current standards for the protection of human subjects rest. Much of the biomedical research conducted in the US is governed either by the rule entitled "Federal Policy for the Protection of Human Subjects" (also known as the "Common Rule," which is codified for HHS at subpart A of Title 45 CFR Part 46) and/or the FDA Protection of Human Subjects Regulations at 21 CFR Parts 50 and 56. FDA has additional human subject protection regulations, which apply to research involving products regulated by the FDA. Although these human subject regulatory requirements, which apply to most Federally funded and to some privately funded research, include protections to help ensure the privacy of subjects and the confidentiality of information, the intent of the Privacy Rule, among other things, is to supplement these protections by requiring covered entities to implement specific measures to safeguard the privacy of individually identifiable health information. Patient confidentiality is also a recurring theme in the previously referenced US GCP guidance.

Research conducted on existing medical records must also consider data protection, anonymization, consent, and confidentiality. The 1998 Data Protection Act, the UK's implementation of the relevant European Union directive,[29] emphasized the need for consent by those from whom data originate. The UK General Medical Council followed earlier statements on confidentiality with guidance that express consent is usually needed before the disclosure of identifiable information for purposes such as research and epidemiology. Where it is not practicable for the person who holds the records either to obtain express consent to disclosure or to anonymize records, data may be disclosed for research, provided participants have been given information about access to their records, and about their right to object. Any objection must be respected. Usually such disclosures will be made to allow a person outside the research team to anonymize the records, or to identify participants who may be invited to participate in a study.[30]

In the UK there is also the system of "Caldicott guardians": a key responsibility of whom is to agree and review internal protocols for the protection and use of identifiable information obtained from patients. Operating in a strategic and advisory role, guardians need to be satisfied that these protocols address the requirements of national guidance/policy and law and that their operation is monitored.[31] In the UK, the Health and Social Care Act 2001 included a clause that allowed Regulations to be made to allow disclosure of information for specified purposes (that have been approved by an independent statutory body, the

Patient Information Advisory Group). This provides a secure basis in law for disclosures where it is not practicable to obtain patients' consent.

The view of the UK Data Protection Commissioner is that any personal data which has been encoded remains personal data in the sense of the Data Protection Act 1998, provided that the key for decoding it remains in existence. Thus, coded data falls within the scope of the Data Protection Act even if the key for decoding it is not accessible to the researcher. The view of some researchers is that these interpretations, if widely held and enforced, would compromise many surveillance activities essential for protection of the health of individuals and the public overall.[32] Researchers also consider that there is a need to find a balance between facilitating important research and protecting the confidentiality of patients, and that interpretation of the Data Protection Act 1998 and how it affects the delivery of health care and epidemiologic research requires further clarification.[33–35] In the US, researchers conducting retrospective reviews of medical records must also take steps to ensure patient privacy and the protection of associated medical records. See Chapter 38 for more information on ethical issues in conducting pharmacoepidemiologic research.

Signal Detection

A signal is defined by the WHO as "reported information on a possible causal relationship between an adverse event and a drug, the relationship being unknown or incompletely documented previously. Usually more than a single report is required to generate a signal, depending upon the seriousness of the event and the quality of the information."[36] Volume IX of the rules governing Medicinal Products for Human and Veterinary Use in the EU considers a signal to be "a potentially serious safety problem associated with a product indicated by a series of unexpected or serious ADRs or changes in severity, characteristics or frequency of expected adverse effects."[27] Historically, most medicine safety signals have come from spontaneously reported suspected ADRs. However, major safety issues may be detected from any of the data sources relevant to a medicine's safety. For example, newly conducted toxicity studies on old established drugs have led to important regulatory action. One example is carcinogenicity with the stimulant laxative danthron.[37] New randomized clinical trials have also raised safety questions about established products. For example, the ALLHAT study that compared different antihypertensives showed higher mortality, particularly from cardiac failure, in the group receiving one therapy compared to the comparator

treatments.[38] Examples could be given from any of the data sources discussed in this chapter.

Spontaneous Reports

The signal detection methodologies in common use by regulatory agencies based on spontaneous reports of suspected ADRs must be considered in the context of the strengths and weaknesses of such a monitoring system (see also Chapters 9 and 10). Used to generate information about rare and previously unknown ADRs, spontaneous reports are collected largely through passive surveillance systems where reporting of suspected ADRs to regulatory authorities is voluntary for health professionals (in most countries) but statutory for license holders. In some countries, notably the US, suspected ADR reports are also accepted directly from patients.

Spontaneous ADR reports are most useful where the reaction is unusual and unexpected in the indication being treated and where the ADRs occur in a close temporal relationship with the start of treatment or following a dose increment. From the regulatory viewpoint, these are reports of *suspected* ADRs and the unique feature of spontaneous reporting systems is that the suspicion of the reporter has been captured. An assessment of individual ADR reports may indicate whether there could be alternative explanations for the observed reaction other than the medicine. Poor quality and/or incomplete information in the case report often makes interpretation of the causal relationship between the product and the observed reaction, as well as wider generalization, difficult. The number of ADR cases reported may not be a good indicator of a signal as channeling of high-risk patients to newer therapies also leads to increased reporting with a newer agent. ADRs are less likely to be suspected and reported spontaneously where the reaction has an insidious onset, the reactions occur only following long-term treatment, or where the disease being treated has a high incidence of similar outcomes. In addition, those ADRs which are caused by a lack of efficacy may not be considered as ADRs and therefore not reported. Spontaneous ADR reports are voluntary for health professionals in most countries. Underreporting is a feature of all such reporting systems. The frequency of reporting for a given medicine varies over time, with time from first marketing, and with periods of media activity surrounding the product.[39]

A comparison of Prescription-Event Monitoring (PEM) (see Chapter 12) study results for a sample of 10 drugs in the UK with suspected ADR reports on the UK regulatory safety database (ADROIT) indicated that up to 32.1% of serious unlabeled reactions were reported to regulators compared to 6.5% for non-serious labeled reactions. Serious unlabeled and non-serious unlabeled reactions were significantly more likely to be reported than were non-serious labeled reactions.[40] This study has been recently updated for 15 newly marketed medicines; 53% of events classified as serious ADRs had been reported spontaneously to the UK authorities.[41]

A similar pattern of reporting was observed in France, although the underreporting appeared greater.[42] Reasons for underreporting included lack of time, lack of report forms, and the misconception that absolute confidence that the medicine caused an event is important in the decision to send in a report.[43] Given the variability in reporting and the numerous factors that affect reporting, it is well accepted that reporting rates cannot be used to reliably estimate incidence rates and that comparison of reporting rates between medicines or countries may not be reliable or informative. The UK Committee on Safety of Medicines (CSM) has been cautious in using spontaneous ADR reports alone as a basis for major regulatory activity unless the evidence has been compelling and cannot be explained by factors other than increased toxicity.[44,45]

Generally, spontaneous ADR reports are examined by systematic manual review of every report received. As an aid to signal detection, screening algorithms based on automated signal detection systems have been explored. Such methods have been referred to as data mining. Although the methodologies of approaches differ, the automated systems using quantitative signal detection in pharmacovigilance assess the extent to which the number of observed cases differs from the number of expected cases as a measure of disproportionality. Comparisons between the WHO method of data mining (Bayesian confidence propagation neural network (BCPNN) information component) and reporting odds ratios, proportional reporting ratios (PRR), Yule's Q, Poisson probability, and chi-square test showed that these different measures were broadly comparable when four or more cases per drug–reaction combination had been collected. The aim of these statistical aids is to provide the means of comparing the frequency of a medicine–event combination with all other such combinations in the database under consideration, with the potential for early detection of signals of potential medicine–event associations. Any such signals must be confirmed by detailed evaluation by skilled clinicians and epidemiologists of the case reports that generated the signal.[46] Detailed descriptions of the PRR, the empirical Bayes geometric mean, the BCPNN information component, and other methods have been published.[47–55]

With data mining, signals are generated without external exposure data, adverse event background information, or medical information on ADRs. Further detailed evaluation of relevant data is needed. The systems cannot distinguish between already known associations and new associations, so the reviewers must filter these known reactions. Medicine interactions and ADR syndromes, and signals among subgroups defined by gender or by age are refinements that may enhance sensitivity. Overall, these quantitative methods are an additional tool, but the impact of false positives and false negatives needs to be considered in the context of the public health function of pharmacovigilance. True signals may not be detectable above the statistical threshold where the database contains large numbers of a particular drug–ADR combination.[56] Furthermore, the choice of threshold criteria when data mining will directly impact on the numbers of potential signals identified.

Coding systems and retrieval may also affect signal detection patterns. For example, in drug regulation, a medical dictionary called MedDRA is used that was developed specifically for the purpose of coding adverse events and reactions. However, signal detection requires knowledge of the dictionary and its structure. MedDRA is organized in a hierarchical structure with lower level terms (LLTs) collected together under preferred terms (PTs), which in turn are grouped together under higher level terms (HLTs), eventually reaching the highest level in the hierarchy, the system organ classes (SOCs). Signal detection at PT level may dilute potential signals by searching the database for only one of a number of clinically related terms. In contrast, the combinations of PTs brought together at higher levels in the hierarchy may limit the ability to detect signals, as PTs that represent different medical concepts or conditions that differ greatly in their clinical importance may be grouped together, particularly at the highest levels in the hierarchy.[57,58]

The concept of critical terms (e.g., Stevens–Johnson syndrome, aplastic anemia) has also been employed in signal detection, where these terms are often indicative of serious medicine-associated toxicity; reports including critical terms require special attention and should be singled out for special attention, irrespective of data mining results or numbers of reports received.

Prioritization: Impact Analysis Concepts

Detailed signal evaluation using all the relevant data is complex and resource intensive. Regulators therefore need to prioritize signals. The potential impact of a safety issue on public health is the foundation for regulators' prioritization but, to date, the judgment of impact has been based on qualitative and subjective criteria. Such criteria include "SNIP": regulators would prioritize relatively **S**trong signals that are judged to be **N**ew, clinically **I**mportant, and have the potential for **P**revention.[59]

UK regulators have developed and piloted a new, quantitative tool for prioritizing signals, the purpose of which is to focus further detailed signal evaluation on those issues for which there is the strongest evidence and those where action is most likely to have an impact on public health. These two dimensions of evidence—strength and public health impact—are scored on the basis of various components. The components for the evidence strength score are: (i) the PRR applied to spontaneous reporting data and its lower 95% confidence limit (this is a means of taking into account both the magnitude of the signal and the degree of precision of the estimate), (ii) the strengths/weaknesses of the case series being considered, and (iii) the biological plausibility of the putative reaction based on the number of factors supporting plausibility. The components of the public health impact score are: (i) the number of cases of the ADR in the population per year since the first ADR was reported for the medicine, (ii) the potential health consequences of the ADR (fatal and nonfatal), and (iii) the order of magnitude of the reporting rate for the medicine–reaction combination during the previous year. A cross-classification of strength of evidence with public health impact can provide assistance in prioritizing signals. The numerical results of the six variables have been categorized into four groups with suggested consequential actions (Figure 8.2). The scoring tables and cut-off points have been derived empirically. While additional factors supporting plausibility such as class effects or postulated mechanisms are helpful if present, their absence

does not preclude signals scoring a high priority. A sensitivity analysis tests the robustness of the categorization in relation to each of the six input variables.

Signal Evaluation and Risk Quantification

The initial steps of evaluation of a potential medicine safety issue will focus on causality assessment, identification of any other possible causes of the adverse events being reported, and assessing the risk to both individuals and the public, in terms of both frequency and seriousness of the reactions.

When a signal of a suspected ADR arises from spontaneous reports, any other similar cases reported previously, forming a case series, should also be evaluated. Developing a case definition and determining the dictionary hierarchy level to be used are essential to the identification of additional cases. From a regulatory perspective, surveillance case definitions should favor sensitivity over specificity. Search strategies should be reproducible in view of the dynamic nature of the reporting database. Reporting rates, the number of ADR reports received divided by the estimated usage (exposure) to the product, can be useful for hypothesis generation. However, they are subject to many limitations. Numerators are subject to known variability and under-ascertainment. The choice of denominator should be dictated by the medicine safety question; for example, all use of a particular route of administration or all use in children. The CIOMS Working Group V report "Current challenges in pharmacovigilance: pragmatic approaches" gives a good description of the factors in selection, and the limitations of the different denominator formats such as number of packs, number of units, number of person-treatment days, number of patients, or number of prescriptions.[60] The ideal choice of denominator, such as number of patients, may not be readily available for all sectors of the market, such as hospital-based, primary care, or non-prescription use. Matching the numerator and denominator means taking at least the time period and geographical location into account. While further stratification by age, sex, or other covariates is desirable, it is often impossible where only data on volume sold are available.[60] (See also Chapter 27.)

Ideally, systematic studies should be reviewed in order to estimate the incidence of an ADR and the confidence interval around the estimate. The calculation of frequency estimates using patient-time as the denominator assumes that the rate of a hazard is constant; three models of hazard function (the instantaneous incidence rate) are summarized. In the peak-shaped hazard model, the hazard increases rapidly over an initial period and then drops to baseline

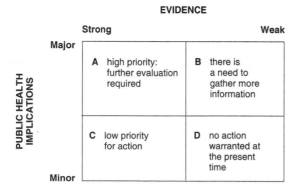

Figure 8.2. Impact analysis of safety signals based on spontaneous reports.

level (e.g., clozapine-induced agranulocytosis). In the constant hazard model the rate reaches a plateau shortly after the beginning of treatment (e.g., upper gastrointestinal bleeding associated with NSAIDs). Lastly, in the increasing hazard rate model the hazard continues to increase over time (e.g., HRT and breast cancer). Additionally, using the upper one-sided 95% confidence interval reflects the uncertainty in the data and gives a worst-case scenario. The FDA has also drafted a concept paper *Risk Assessment of Observational Data: Good Pharmacovigilance Practices and Pharmacoepidemiological Assessment*, which focuses on the quality of case reporting, the approaches to signal interpretation, and the conduct of observational studies,[61] and more recently its risk guidances, discussed in more detail in Chapter 33.

Evaluation of spontaneous reports should consider demographic factors such as age, gender, race, or other subgroups, the effects of exposure dose, duration, the effects of time (as calendar time, or product life cycle), the effects of other drugs, comorbid conditions, and/or the target population. Owing to the nature of the data, spontaneous ADR reports generally do not permit a direct conclusion on the association between a particular ADR and the medicine in the population. However, some factors in case reports that strengthen the association include the presence of a positive re-challenge, positive de-challenge, and a clear absence of alternative causes. Classifications have been derived for assessment of the likelihood of causality in individual spontaneous reports.[36] (Causality assessment is dealt with in detail in Chapter 36.) If a safety issue warrants detailed assessment, the evaluation must be widened to consider all available data, including preclinical, clinical pharmacology, clinical trials, pharmacoepidemiology studies, and class effects.

The Assessment of Data from Non-Spontaneous Sources

Data employed in a regulatory risk assessment are critically reviewed, bearing in mind limitations of data derived from sources at different levels of the evidence hierarchy.[62] The pharmacoepidemiologic data sources (other than spontaneous reports), and their strengths and weaknesses for risk assessment, are considered below.

Active Surveillance

Spontaneous reporting of suspected ADRs and intensified reporting of suspected ADRs through facilitation using online systems or reminders built into prescribing or dispensing systems are forms of "passive" surveillance. Full ascertainment of the exposure experience of an enumerated population is not available. Where full ascertainment of

drug utilization in a defined population is available, rates of ADRs can readily be determined for the group under consideration. PEM attempts to carry out such population-based *active* surveillance (see Chapter 12). The Drug Safety Research Unit (DSRU) is the center for PEM in England. PEM studies are general practitioner (community)-based and exposure is based on dispensed prescription data in England. Following dispensing of prescriptions of the study medicine, general practitioners are sent questionnaires to ascertain adverse events in the exposed population. The mean cohort size of DSRU PEM studies is approximately 11 000 patients. PEM produces incidence rates for events reported during treatment. Response rates for questionnaires are in the range of 60%.[63,64] Variations on this process are now carried out by Japan and New Zealand.[65,66]

Registries

Registries are a systematic collection of defined events or product exposures in a defined patient population for a defined period of time. Registries also require protocols detailing objectives, background, research methods, patient recruitment and follow-up, projected sample size, and methods for data collection, management, and analysis. Registries can serve a number of functions. Registries are most commonly used as an information gathering and hypothesis generating tool, particularly on exposure to medicines during pregnancy and for orphan medicines, where information may be severely limited pre-licensing. They can also act as the population basis for linkage studies (by linking medical records to municipal population registers, patient movement and mortality can be tracked anonymously) or as the provider of denominator data in the exposed population (for example the Australian Childhood Immunization Register).[67] Early registration of exposed pregnancies, before knowledge of pregnancy outcome, allows prospective evaluation of pregnancy outcomes in relation to exposures, and examples are to be found in relation to asthma, rheumatoid arthritis, and epilepsy treatments.[68–71] Potential limitations of registry data are recognized. These include the size and representativeness of the sample. However, these types of registry reports can be a valuable and cost-effective way to collect data regarding the use of medicines during pregnancy when other data collection methods (e.g., cohort studies) are not appropriate or feasible.[72] Population-based birth defects registries also exist but may suffer from underascertainment.[73] An example of a registry of medicine-induced events is the registry of medicine-induced cardiac arrhythmias.[74] The information collected by the registry will be used to develop detailed profiles of people most at risk for medicine-induced arrhythmias and to determine whether a genetic test can be developed that can identify at-risk patients prospectively.[74] Another example of a registry of medicine-induced events is the US National Registry of Drug-Induced Ocular Side Effects.[75]

Registries have also been used as a hypothesis testing tool, for example looking at the increased risk of malignancies in transplant patients and then assessing for possible risk factors,[76,77] and in the investigation of the effect of hormone replacement therapy on colorectal cancer.[78]

In addition to disease and exposure registries, potentially useful information for the assessment of medicine safety can exist in registers of clinical trials (e.g., www.trialscentral.org and www.controlled-trials.com), safety studies (MHRA safety study register), and vaccine trials.[79] Registries can also be used as a risk minimization tool. Clozapine registries were created to minimize the risk of potentially fatal agranulocytosis secondary to treatment. The registration of patients and linking of blood test results to the dispensing of the medicine helps prevent inappropriate re-treatment in patients previously suffering bone marrow suppression or in patients with a current low white blood cell count. In one clozapine registry, agranulocytosis dropped to 0.38% from a pre-registry rate of between 1% and 2%.[80,81] In an effort to prevent fetal exposures to thalidomide, a registry-based program has been set up to regulate prescription, dispensing, and use of the medicine. This requires registration of all participating prescribers, pharmacies, and patients.[82]

Comparative Observational Studies

Comparative observational studies may be carried out for a number of reasons. For example, a company may conduct an observational cohort study to evaluate the general safety profile of its product in normal conditions of use. Specific safety studies may be commissioned or undertaken to address a specific medicine-related safety issue. In such a situation the objective is to evaluate the risk compared to different exposure or no exposure. In the past, such studies have usually been carried out in response to an identified safety concern. Companies may also be required to carry out general or specific comparative observational studies to quantify known risks or expand the safety database as a condition of licensing of the product. Companies are not the only parties involved in conducting such studies; academics and regulators may also commission or conduct studies.

The time scale and quality of studies are important considerations for regulators when making decisions. Regulators face a major challenge in the need to address potential major public health concerns urgently; good quality population-based data are extremely useful when

available or if it is feasible to obtain them within a short time frame. The use of validated automated medical record or claims databases offers relatively fast ways of testing hypotheses on a population basis (see Chapters 13–22). It is recognized that proper utilization of these databases requires powerful computers and skilled and experienced epidemiologists and analysts. It should be noted that the primary purpose of these databases is patient care or insurance, the database population is constantly changing, and, because of the administrative nature of the database, it may not contain the information needed to answer questions about drug exposures and medical outcomes.[83–87]

The principal designs and advantages and disadvantages of various comparative study types, such as cohort and case–control studies, are covered in Chapter 3, and will not be addressed here. However, there are a number of concerns which merit mention from the regulatory perspective. All of these studies, either field-based or using existing medical records, specific or general comparative studies, should be carefully designed and carried out to a high quality. General safety studies have been criticized previously because of poor recruitment and use as marketing tools. These studies should have detailed protocols outlining aims and measurable objectives, background, sample size implications, rationale, and definitions of source populations, study population and study base, outcome and exposure definition, and analysis plans. Issues such as bias and confounding (particularly channeling of patients) and appropriate comparator groups need very detailed consideration at the study design stage.

When assessing the findings of a pharmacoepidemiology study, various factors need to be considered. These include how the study deals with new users and existing/prevalent users,[88] those cases with "alternate proximate cause," or subjects with contraindications.[89,90] Other issues to be assessed include design, sample representativeness, data source and quality, measurement and reliability, diagnosis, comparison groups, outcome, missing subjects/bias testing, dose, duration and/or other variations in exposure, covariates, age/period/cohort effects, and statistical techniques.[91–94] Confounding by indication is a particular concern when interpreting a study. If the indication is a medical disorder that predisposes to the event under study, any imbalance in the underlying risk profile between treated and comparison groups can generate biased results.[95,96] Newer study methods that employ techniques such as case series analyses, case-crossover, or case–time control may be appropriate depending on the research question being addressed.[97–102] (See Chapter 48.)

Not all drug safety issues are currently amenable to study using formal epidemiologic techniques. This may occur where both outcome and exposure are rare, as in possible fibrosis with ergot derivatives (e.g., pergolide). Better and larger data linkage of prescribing in both primary and secondary care is needed.

Recent comparative studies that have contributed to regulatory decision making include the Million Women Study in HRT,[103] phenylpropanolamine and stroke,[104] antipsychotics and QT prolongation,[105] and vitamin K and childhood cancer.[106]

Clinical Trials, Large Simple Safety Trials, and Meta-analyses

A large simple safety study, which is a clinical study designed to assess relatively few safety outcomes in a large number of patients, has a role to play both pre- and post-licensing (see Chapter 39). Pre-licensing, a large simple safety trial may be indicated where a safety signal of concern in the clinical trial database has arisen that is not otherwise well addressed or where the medicine is intended as a preventative product in asymptomatic individuals. Post-licensing, clinical trials provide sources of signals of safety concerns, for example when clinical trials are conducted for the purpose of extending the indications for treatment. Other large trials may be conducted with the express purpose of examining a specific safety issue. Regulatory guidance on medical, statistical, and design issues in clinical trials is outlined in ICH guidelines.[107–112] Meta-analyses can also provide useful syntheses of data, when assessing a medicine safety concern (see Chapter 44). These are also subjected to rigorous assessment by regulators.[113]

Hypotheses

Equivalence testing can also be applied to pharmacoepidemiology. The aim may be to test the risk of a given substance with a known risk or with another medicine.[114] To demonstrate that the test product is not meaningfully different from the reference product, the largest difference that is clinically acceptable, such that a difference greater than this would matter in practice, is prespecified as Δ. For the two risks to be considered equivalent, the two-sided 95% confidence interval of the difference between the two products should lie entirely within $+\Delta$ and $-\Delta$. This approach allows the conclusion of equivalence, rather than the commonly used approach of difference testing and concluding equivalence when the null hypothesis of equality is not rejected. The equivalence approach had not been widely employed in pharmacovigilance. Factors to consider are the prespecification of equivalence limits and what constitutes an acceptable threshold value of relative risk or risk difference, sensitivity, and size of the study.

If a study does not demonstrate a difference on the basis of conventional hypothesis testing, this does not necessarily mean that the risks are the same; the nature of pharmacoepidemiologic data may predispose to finding no difference given "noise" such as non-differential misclassification, which operates to bias results to the null. Most regulators assessing studies will be circumspect on the interpretation of results that include the null value, noting these as inconclusive or due to limited data. However, when interpreting studies we must ask the question: "is this evidence of absence or absence of evidence?" Rothman and Greenland[115] provide some advice on this question, noting that the precision of the confidence interval illustrates what size of effect the data are consistent with and suggesting the use of P value functions.

Other Data Sources

There is considerable interest in how pharmacoepidemiologic and pharmacogenetic research can be used to explain the observed variability in drug response in patient populations with known polymorphisms in their genetic profile (see Chapter 37). The ultimate utility of this is maximizing the benefit/risk balance for patients on an individual basis for a given substance.[116,117]

The Hill set of criteria reminds us to look outside the index evidence when assessing possible causal associations. As examined in Rothman and Greenland,[115] careful attention to these criteria is necessary.

Background studies in the target disease (morbidity and mortality) and drug utilization (covariates associated with exposure) will also furnish a regulator with important information when assessing a safety issue.

Benefit/Risk Assessment

Assessment of the balance of benefit and risk is conducted throughout the life of a medicine, through medicine development, at the time of license application, and then continuously in the post-licensing phase. The principles underlying benefit/risk assessment are the same at all stages. However, the data that may be available will differ substantially. Every year products are withdrawn from various markets around the world for safety reasons.[118] In the past, however, regulators and companies have often used different methods of benefit/risk assessment and reached very different conclusions.[119] These differences have even occurred among different regulators in different countries. Examples include withdrawal from the European market of tolcapone, troglitazone, and trovafloxacin, while in the US the use of these products was initially restricted and monitoring was introduced. These differences clearly suggest a different assessment of the balance of benefits and risks in these two regions. The lack of standardization of benefit/risk assessment led CIOMS to set up a working group to produce guidelines on standardized benefit/risk assessment.[120]

In the post-licensing phase, once a safety issue has been identified, and evaluation has resulted in a judgment that the medicine may be a significant threat to public health, it is important to proceed next to a thorough benefit/risk assessment. Benefit/risk assessment can be made robust by following a systematic plan and ensuring that all relevant data are considered. The key parts of the assessment are given in Table 8.5.[121]

The *disease being treated* by the medicine under investigation will have a major impact on the balance of benefits and risks. For example, if the disease is self-limited, such as influenza in an otherwise healthy young adult, serious ADRs would have a considerable negative impact on the balance of benefits and risks. In contrast, with a disease with a high mortality, serious ADRs may still be outweighed by the benefits afforded by the drug. In addition to describing the natural history of the disease, it is also important to describe the demography of the disease, including its incidence and prevalence. This allows all the patient groups likely to be exposed to be considered, as well as the public health impact of benefits and risks to be judged.

The *population being treated* also needs to be considered. When used in normal clinical practice, a medicine may not be used within the confines of the licensed indication. For example, a medicine may be used in children despite only having an indication in adults. It is important to consider the

Table 8.5. Key elements of benefit/risk assessment

(1) Description of the target disease
(2) Description of the populations being treated
(3) Description of the purpose of the intervention
(4) Documentation of alternative therapies and their benefits and risks
(5) Evaluation of the degree of efficacy
(6) Evaluation of the type of risk
(7) Quantification of the risk and identification of risk factors
(8) Impact of the risk on individuals and populations
(9) Comparison of benefits and risks with alternative therapies/no treatment
(10) Consideration of all benefits and risks by indication and population
(11) Judgment on the balance of benefits and risks and ways to maximize benefit and reduce risk

balance of benefit and risk in all populations being treated. Differences may occur in how medicines are handled by different populations, for example, reduced metabolism in the elderly and in some ethnic groups. Efficacy may also differ among groups, an example being the efficacy of ACE inhibitors in lowering blood pressure in different ethnic groups.

Just as the nature of the disease being treated is important, the *purpose of the intervention* should also be described. Medicines may be used for prevention, treatment, as part of a procedure, or for diagnosis. These factors will impact on the balance of benefits and risks. For example, a medicine used to prevent disease in an otherwise healthy individual must have a very well-established safety profile, particularly if the disease being prevented is rare or non-serious.

The *therapeutic alternatives* to the medicine being evaluated should be identified. For some conditions no specific treatment may be a viable alternative. For the majority of diseases, however, there will be alternative medicines available and, in some, surgical intervention may be effective, for example, surgery for a prolapsed intervertebral disc as an alternative to long-term analgesics. For some conditions, particularly psychological and chronic conditions, complementary medicines and psychological therapies may be established alternatives. Once the main alternatives to the treatments under evaluation have been identified, their benefit and risk profiles should be considered.

The term "efficacy" is normally used to mean benefit within a clinical trial setting, whereas "effectiveness" is usually used to mean benefit under normal conditions of use. For most medicines, an *evaluation of benefits* in normal clinical use has not been conducted and therefore clinical trial efficacy has to be used as a "surrogate" of benefit. The robustness of premarketing efficacy data is often far superior to that available for risk, as clinical trials are designed first and foremost to demonstrate the efficacy of the product. Another important consideration when assessing benefit is whether efficacy has been demonstrated in terms of clinical outcomes. For example, when many of the antiretroviral agents were licensed to treat HIV infection and AIDS, only surrogate markers of clinical endpoints were available, such as increases in CD4 lymphocyte count and reduction of HIV RNA viral load. Only subsequently have morbidity and mortality data confirmed the major benefit of these medicines in terms of morbidity and mortality in the treatment of HIV-infected individuals. When a major safety issue occurs for a medicine where robust data on clinical benefit are available, the judgment on the balance of benefits and risks might be different from that for a medicine where only data using surrogates of clinical endpoints exist.

The longevity of the effect of a medicine should also be taken into account. For chronic disease, the initial efficacy may be marked, but if this is not sustained the overall benefit of the medicine may be very limited. This may be due to tachyphylaxis or, for infectious diseases, the development of resistance.

Another factor to consider is whether the medicine being evaluated is to be used as *first or second line therapy*. For example, a medicine that is used as a first line chemo-therapeutic agent where alternatives exist might be judged to have a different balance of benefits and risks from a chemotherapeutic agent which is only indicated in patients who had failed all other treatments. This concept of first and second line therapy is often used when restricting the use of medicines with a major safety issue.

The *degree of efficacy* needs to be documented for each indication (whether licensed or not) and each population treated. For example, ACE inhibitors are indicated for post-myocardial infarction prophylaxis, cardiac failure, hyper-tension, and to prevent renal damage in patients with diabetes mellitus. Convincing mortality data exist showing a benefit of ACE inhibitors in some but not all of these indications. Therefore if a major safety issue arose, the balance of benefits and risks might be different for the different indications.

Once causality has been established between the adverse event and the medicinal product, assessment of its seriousness and severity will help in the judgment of the individual and population *impact of the risk* being considered. Whereas seriousness usually relates to the outcome of an ADR (e.g., the reaction had a fatal outcome or resulted in hospitalization), severity is also important. For example, a small rise in liver function tests is unlikely to be indicative of major liver pathology whereas a rise ten times the upper limit of normal may well be a marker of major disease. Neither of these suspected reactions may be considered serious by traditional definitions. However, the latter, being severe, may constitute an important health risk. In order to identify ways to reduce risk, it is essential to try to investigate whether the risk is associated with a particular patient group, particular dosage, results from an interaction, or whether there is an early warning sign. Table 8.6 outlines how these factors may allow risk to be reduced and how the balance of benefits and risks of the medicine may be favorably maintained.

The *frequency of the adverse reaction* must be assessed. Frequency will impact on the benefit/risk balance for an individual, as well as the impact of the medicine's toxicity on populations. As well as considering the new toxicity that has led to the benefit/risk assessment, it is also important to consider the overall *adverse reaction profile* of the medicine. It would be unusual for a medicine to have only one recognized ADR and clearly the overall risk from the medicine will depend on both the new ADR being evaluated and the known safety issues with that medicine.

As well as documenting what the alternative therapies are, it is helpful when assessing risks to select one comparator medicine, possibly of the same class and indication, for a direct head-to-head comparison. This may be difficult, however, as there may not be a clear comparator and even if one exists, the evidence of benefit and risk may differ both quantitatively and qualitatively. If a comparator can be selected then both the benefits and risks should be compared between the two medicines in all indications and populations.

Having described the target disease and population being treated, the purpose of the intervention and alternative ther-apies, and evaluated the benefits and risks, it is then neces-sary to try to judge the *overall balance of risks and benefits* of the medicine. Benefits and risks for all indications and populations need to be taken into consideration. The overall balance may be very difficult to judge: the type of evidence available for benefit may be very different from that available for risk. The concepts of *number needed to treat* for benefit and *number needed to harm* for risk can help to quantify and may therefore aid in the comparison.[122–124] However, whenever possible, some estimate of the number

Table 8.6. Possible safeguards to minimize risk

Factor	Safeguard
At risk patients	ADR only occurs in specific patient groups, e.g., elderly, cardiac failure. Use of the medicine in this group can be contraindicated
Dosage	ADR only occurs at higher doses or is most serious at higher doses: reducing the maximum authorized dose should reduce risk (but consider implications of reduced efficacy on benefit/risk balance)
Interactions	If the risk is increased or only occurs following a pharmacodynamic or pharmacokinetic interaction, then contraindicating concomitant use of the interacting medicine should reduce the risk
Early warning signs	For many adverse reactions, detecting the reaction early can avert a serious outcome, so reducing risk. Examples include monitoring liver enzymes with hepatotoxic medicines and renal function with nephrotoxic medicines

of serious ADRs that would occur for a given positive outcome should be attempted. For example, when evaluating
the balance of benefits and risks of a thrombolytic agent in
the treatment of acute myocardial infarction, an estimate of
the number of serious cases of hemorrhage per infarct
prevented could be calculated.

Peer review of any assessment is an important step in
ensuring its quality, and involving a range of additional
experts in the judgment should result in a more balanced
decision. In the UK, expert advice is usually sought from
the Committee on Safety of Medicines, the Government's
independent, expert scientific advisory committee on medicines.
At an EU level, the Committee for Human Medicinal Products
is consulted. The FDA has a number of "advisory committees,"
which provide advice to the FDA on matters relating to the
safety and effectiveness of the products it regulates. One of
these committees, the Drug Safety and Risk Management
(DSaRM) advisory committee, was chartered specifically to
provide guidance on matters related to drug safety and risk
management. DSaRM is comprised of physicians, pharmacists,
and others with expertise in a variety of areas, including
pharmacoepidemiology, pharmacotherapy, medical cognition,
health policy and consumer safety issues, risk management,
and medication errors.

Formal decision analysis techniques can be employed to
support judgments and should help those responsible for
decisions to think through the implications of different
options for regulatory action.

Action to Reduce Risk or Increase Benefit and Communication

Following the benefit/risk assessment it will usually be
necessary to take action either to increase the benefit of the
medicine by improving its rational use or to reduce the risk
by improving the manner in which it is used, which usually
involves educating practitioners and consumers, but on
occasion requires restricting its use.

The term "regulatory action" is usually used to refer to
action taken in relation to licenses. However, here we use
a broader definition covering all measures that could be
taken by regulators or companies to improve the benefit/
risk balance. Regulatory action may be voluntary, where
for example a company voluntarily submits a variation or
cancels a license. In contrast, the regulatory authority
may take compulsory action. Whenever possible the
desired regulatory outcome should be achieved through
voluntary action. Compulsory action is more likely to
lead to litigation and should be reserved for major public
health threats where agreement for voluntary action with
the company cannot be reached.

When taking decisions on the appropriate regulatory
action, certain guiding principles should be remembered:

- Objectivity: assessment and decision making should be
  evidence based and free from any conflict of interest.
- Equity: there should be equity of regulatory action on
  products if the risk assessment and particularly the benefit/
  risk assessment is the same for different products.
- Accountability: decision makers are accountable for decisions
  and regulatory action taken.
- Transparency: within the confines of regional laws on
  commercial confidentiality and data protection, decision
  making and action taken should be transparent to
  stakeholders.

If the overall balance of benefits and risks is judged to be
negative, then the product will be withdrawn unless risk
minimization strategies can be identified which would swing
the balance away from risk or towards benefit. Table 8.6
gives some examples of how risks might be minimized and
Table 8.7 gives examples of what regulatory action might
be considered.

Effective communication about safety issues is essential
if ADRs are to be prevented. Communications about a
safety issue need to be planned and a communication team
will normally need to be established. The messages to be
conveyed should be targeted, understandable, open, informative, and balanced. In the past, communication documents
have often been written by those medicines safety specialists
responsible for evaluating the safety issue. However, in
order to ensure that messages are clear, concise, and understandable, it is wise to involve communications specialists
in writing documents and, if time permits, to user-test
messages prior to distribution. Different but compatible
messages may be required for health care professionals,
patients, and the media. The method chosen to distribute the
message will depend on the urgency of communication and
the target audience. Timing communications, particularly
for urgent safety issues such as product withdrawals, is
essential. If the media carry a major medicine safety issue
that leads to patients consulting their health care professionals
and those professionals have not been briefed in advance,
then the regulators and pharmaceutical companies will be
judged to have failed both professionals and patients. This
can be a major challenge but must be our aim when
planning safety communications. For those interested in the
topic, a fuller discussion can be found elsewhere.[125] It is
very easy for non-specialists to misquote and misrepresent
data, including epidemiologic data, in communication
documents, and the epidemiologist has a role in checking
such documents for accuracy. In addition, by advising on

Table 8.7. Putting safeguards into action in response to a risk

Action	Comment
Continued passive surveillance	May be appropriate for non-serious ADRs where causality is not established
Actively collect further data	If causality not established, mechanism unclear, or risk factors not identified
Add warning to product information	For less serious reactions, particularly those that are unavoidable, warning health care professionals and patients may be the only action necessary. Changes may be made to any of the following sections of the product information: warnings, interactions, pregnancy and lactation, adverse reactions, preclinical
Changes to product information to reduce risk	Restrict indication, reduce maximum dose, contraindicate use in those at high risk, advise monitoring, etc. See Table 8.6
Suspension of the license	Urgent threat to public health and preliminary assessment suggests balance of benefits and risks is negative. However, further evaluation or study is required prior to final decision. Ideally, companies will be persuaded to voluntarily guarantee that all marketing and use of the product will stop rather than using compulsory powers
Suspension of marketing and use	As suspension of the license, but named patient use considered to also present an unacceptable hazard. Again, companies will ideally be persuaded to voluntarily guarantee that all marketing and use of the product will stop
Revocation of the license	Further evaluation is not considered useful and the balance of benefits and risks cannot be made favorable. Ideally, companies will be persuaded to voluntarily cancel licenses
Change in legal status	If restricting availability of the product to specific health care professionals may reduce risks or increase benefits
Specific risk minimization program	In exceptional circumstances (notably where a product has exceptional benefit but also major risks) it may be justified to develop a specific, detailed risk reduction program. This may involve education programs, registries, patient consent forms, restricted distribution, etc. See Table 8.3

data collection, including survey methods, the epidemiologist may have a role in verifying that information has been received, understood, and followed.

Audit (Measurement of the Outcome of Interventions)

It was stressed in the section that described the FDA's current thinking on risk minimization planning that evaluation of the success of risk minimization plans is crucial to public health protection. Equally, evaluation (audit) of the success or impact of regulatory action taken in response to a specific safety issue is an essential duty of companies and regulators to the public. The main objective of most actions is to inform and change behavior, be it prescribing or dispensing behavior or the habits of the public. These objectives can be very difficult to achieve and this is why we cannot assume that our actions have been effective. The epidemiologist has a central role in measuring and judging the impact of regulatory interventions, and for this reason an entire separate chapter is dedicated to this topic (see Chapter 33).

Other Regulatory Activities

In addition to pharmacovigilance, there are other roles for the epidemiologist in the post-licensing phase of a medicine's life. For many medicines the initial licensed therapeutic use is just the first of an expanding range of uses. Further uses may be in different populations with the same disease (for example children, the elderly, or individuals with comorbidity), in populations with the same disease but of a different severity or at a different stage in the disease's evolution, in the same disease but as part of a different treatment regimen, or even to treat a completely different disease.

The epidemiologist may have a role in identifying potential new uses for the medicine. By studying the disease, the demographics of the populations affected, the current treatment, and natural history of the disease, additional potential uses may be identified. In addition to seeking expert opinion and understanding the pharmacology of the medicine, use of longitudinal patient databases can be very informative in identifying potential new uses. Just as with initial licensing, to obtain a licensed new indication, a company will need to obtain data supporting the safe and effective use of the medicine in the new disease area or population. In the EU, a regulatory process known as variation of the license is the usual method of adding new therapeutic indications, although companies may choose to obtain a separate new license. The process of variation is used not only for changing the license with regard to new indications but for any changes, be they related to the quality (e.g., storage), safety, or efficacy.

In some regions of the world a license is only valid for a set period of time. For example, in the EU, after 5 years a license has to be renewed. On occasion, this is only an administrative process. However, more and more, regulators are using this regulatory tool to conduct a full safety and efficacy review of the product and, particularly if major safety issues have emerged during the preceding 5 years, to conduct a full benefit/risk assessment. During the 5 years, in addition to new safety issues emerging, the evolution of the disease may have changed (think of HIV infection in the 1980s compared to the late 1990s) or new, safer, or more effective therapies may be available (again, think of HIV), which may have a major impact on the use and possibly benefit/risk balance of the medicine. The epidemiologist may play a role in documenting the current natural history of the disease, the current use of the medicine, and of alternative therapies, and in collecting data to support the continued use of the medicine (possibly in a different way).

An additional regulatory measure is the control of the distribution of the medicine, including whether it can be obtained only with a prescription from a registered doctor, whether it can be dispensed by a pharmacist without a prescription, or whether it can be bought without the intervention of any health care professional. Different classifications of prescription status are in use in different regions of the world (and in the EU among different countries). However, most countries control the distribution of medicines by use of some prescription classification. Companies need to apply to the regulatory authorities to change the prescription status; in some countries this is referred to as reclassification. Companies may wish to have their medicine used without prescription, as this may increase sales, but only certain types of conditions, symptoms, or diseases are appropriate for non-prescription treatment. Disease factors include whether it is easily diagnosable without the intervention of a doctor and whether misdiagnosis could have serious consequences. The main factors related to the medicine itself are whether it is safe (and the safety profile is well established) and simple to take. It should also be remembered that the profile of the population receiving the medicine may change dramatically when the intervention of a doctor is excluded. The epidemiologist may play a role in establishing that a medicine can be used safely and effectively without the intervention of a doctor. For example, the epidemiologist may collect data on how a disease is diagnosed and the population's ability to self-diagnose, or likely comorbidities present in those who might obtain the medicine and co-treatments they may use (which might interact with the

newly reclassified medicine). If a medicine is reclassified to non-prescription use, new safety issues may emerge and renewed vigilance in safety monitoring will usually be required. This may be particularly challenging, as, in many countries, doctors remain the main reporters of suspected ADRs. Examples of previously prescription-only medicines that are now available without prescription (in some countries) include stomach acid suppressing drugs like cimetidine and ranitidine, nonsteroidal anti-inflammatory drugs like ibuprofen, some topical corticosteroids, some topical anti-virals like acyclovir, and both topical and oral antifungals including fluconazole.

CONCLUSIONS

This chapter presents the combined views of three regulators operating in different regions with different approaches to the use of pharmacoepidemiology in drug regulation. We have taken a broad scope and tried to consider all of the many and varied interfaces between the two. Our guiding principle has been the role of pharmacoepidemiology throughout the life cycle of a medicine, from development, through licensing, to marketing for general use. We have explored the impact of different types of data on regulation. Pharmacoepidemiology has a central and increasingly recognized role in the regulation of medicines, its use underpinning more and more regulatory decisions. A major challenge ahead is improving the robustness and richness of the pharmacoepidemiologic data upon which decisions are based. The technical, scientific, and legal issues are challenging, including the need for rapid data access and analysis (for urgent safety issues), statistical power, dealing with bias and confounding, obtaining data from sectors of the health market where currently they are lacking, and consent and confidentiality (protecting the individual but not at the expense of harming the public). Despite these challenges, we believe the use of pharmacoepidemiology is making an important contribution to better regulation and better protection of public health.

DISCLAIMER

This review does not constitute formal regulatory advice and in all cases relevant pharmaceutical legislation and formal guidance should be consulted for pharmaceutical obligations for license holders or applicants. Furthermore, the opinions expressed are those of the authors and do not necessarily represent the opinions of the organizations for which the authors work.

REFERENCES

1. Waller PC, Evans SJW. A model for the future conduct of pharmacovigilance. *Pharmacoepidemiol Drug Saf* 2003; **12**: 17–29.
2. McMahon AD. Approaches to combat with confounding by indication in observational studies of intended drug effects. *Pharmacoepidemiol Drug Saf* 2003; **12**: 551–8.
3. Lasagna L. Are drug benefits also part of pharmacoepidemiology? *J Clin Epidemiol* 1990; **43**: 849–50.
4. Miettinen OS. The need for randomization in the study of intended effects. *Stat Med* 1983; **2**: 267–71.
5. Handley JA, Lippman-Hand A. If nothing goes wrong, is everything all right? Interpreting zero numerators. *JAMA* 1983; **249**: 1743–5.
6. Rawlins MD, Jefferys DB. Study of United Kingdom product licence applications containing new active substances, 1987–9. *BMJ* 1991; **302**: 223–5.
7. Directive 2001/20/EC of the European Parliament and of the Council of 4 April 2001 on the approximation of the laws, regulations and administrative provisions of the Member States relating to the implementation of good clinical practice in the conduct of clinical trials on medicinal products for human use. *Off J Eur Commun* 2001; **121**: 34–44.
8. Szarfman A, Talarico VL, Levine J. Analysis and risk assessment of hematological data from clinical trials. In: Bloom JC, ed., *Comprehensive Toxicology*, vol. 4: *Toxicology of the Hematopoietic System*. New York: Elsevier Science, 1997; pp. 363–79.
9. FDA Center for Drug Evaluation and Research. Concept Paper: Premarketing Risk Assessment. March 3, 2003. Available from http://www.fda.gov/cder/meeting/riskManageI.htm. Accessed March 2004.
10. International Conference on Harmonisation of Technical Requirements for Registration of Pharmaceuticals for Human Use (ICH). E1: The Extent of Population Exposure to Assess Clinical Safety for Drugs Intended for Long-Term Treatment of Non-Life-Threatening Conditions. ICH, 1994. Available at: http://www.ich.org. Accessed March 2004.
11. Council for International Organizations of Medical Sciences (CIOMS), http://www.cioms.ch.
12. Orphan Drug Act of 1983, 21 USC § 360aa-360ee, Pub. L. No. 97-414, 96 Stat. 2049, 1983, amended by Pub.L. 99-91, 99 Stat. 387, 1985 and Pub.L. 105-115, 111 Stat. 2325, 1997.
13. Haffner ME. The current environment in orphan drug development. *Drug Inf J* 2003; **37**: 373–9.
14. Regulation (EC) No 141/2000 of the European Parliament and of the Council of 16 December 1999 on orphan medicinal products. *Off J Eur Commun* L18/1 22.1.2000. Available at: http://europa.eu.int/eur-lex/pri/en/oj/dat/2000/l_018/l_01820000122en00010005.pdf.
15. International Conference on Harmonisation of Technical Requirements for Registration of Pharmaceuticals for Human Use (ICH). M4: The Common Technical Document. Available at: http://www.ich.org. Accessed March 2004.
16. International Conference on Harmonisation of Technical Requirements for Registration of Pharmaceuticals for Human Use (ICH). E3: Structure and Content of Clinical Study Reports. ICH, 1995. Available at: http://www.ich.org. Accessed: March 2004.
17. International Conference on Harmonisation of Technical Requirements for Registration of Pharmaceuticals for Human Use (ICH). E2E: Pharmacovigilance Planning. ICH, 2003. Available at: http://www.ich.org. Accessed March 2004.
18. FDA Center for Drug Evaluation and Research. Concept Paper: Risk Management Programs, March 3, 2003. Available at: http://www.fda.gov/cder/meeting/riskManageII.htm. Accessed: March 2004.
19. FDA Center for Drug Evaluation and Research Draft Guidance for Industry: Development and Use of Risk Minimization Action Plans, April 2004. Available at: http://www.fda.gov/cder/guidance/index.htm.
20. Graham DJ, Drinkard CR, Shatin D, Tsong Y, Burgess ML. Liver enzyme monitoring in patients treated with troglitazone. *JAMA* 2001; **286**: 831–3.
21. Smalley W, Shatin D, Wysowski D, Durwitz J, Andrade S, Goodman M *et al.* Contraindicated use of cisapride: impact of Food and Drug Administration Regulatory Action. *JAMA* 2000; **284**: 3036–9.
22. Weatherby LB, Nordstrom BL, Fife D, Walker AM. The impact of wording in "Dear Doctor" letters and in black box labels. *Clin Pharmacol Ther* 2002; **72**: 735–42.
23. Arlett PR, Harrison P. Compliance in European pharmacovigilance: a regulatory view. *Pharmacoepidemiol Drug Saf* 2001; **10**: 301–2.
24. Council Regulation (EEC) No 2309/93 of 22 July 1993 laying down Community procedures for the authorization and supervision of medicinal products for human and veterinary use and establishing a European Agency for the Evaluation of Medicinal Products. *Off J Eur Commun* 1993; **L214**: 1–21. Available at: http://europa.eu.int/eur-lex/en/consleg/pdf/1993/en_1993R2309_do_001.pdf.
25. Directive 2001/83/EC of the European Parliament and of the Council of 6 November 2001 on the Community code relating to medicinal products for human use. *Off J Eur Commun* 2001; **L311**: 67–128. Available at: http://europa.eu.int/eur-lex/pri/en/oj/dat/2001/l_311/l_31120011128en00670128.pdf.
26. Henderson L, Yue QY, Bergquist C, Gerden B, Arlett P. St John's wort (*Hypericum perforatum*): drug interactions and clinical outcomes. *Br J Clin Pharmacol* 2002; **54**: 349–56.
27. European Commission. *The Rules Governing Medicinal Products in the European Union*, vol. 9: *Pharmacovigilance: Medicinal Products for Human use and Veterinary Medicinal Products*. Available at: http://pharmacos.eudra.org/F2/eudralex/vol-9/pdf/Vol9_10-2004.pdf.
28. FDA, http://www.fda.gov/cder/about/smallbiz/clinical_investigator.htm. Accessed March 2004.
29. Directive 95/46/EC of the European Parliament and of the Council of 24 October 1995 on the protection of individuals with regard to the processing of personal data and on the free movement of such data. *Off J Eur Commun* 1995; **38**: 31–55.

30. General Medical Council. *Research: The Role and Responsibilities of Doctors*. London: General Medical Council, February 2002. Available at: http://www.gmc-uk.org/standards/research.htm.

31. NHS Executive. *Protecting and Using Patient Information: A Manual for Caldicott Guardians*. Leeds: NHS Executive, 1999. Available at: http://www.dh.gov.uk/PublicationsAndStatistics/Publications/PublicationsPolicyAndGuidance/PublicationsPolicyAndGuidanceArticle/fs/en?CONTENT_ID=4068134&chk=MYBgCq.

32. Verity C, Nicoll A. Consent, confidentiality, and the threat to public health surveillance. *BMJ* 2002; **324**: 1210–13.

33. Strobl J, Cave E, Walley T. Data protection legislation: interpretation and barriers to research. *BMJ* 2000; **321**: 890–2.

34. Coleman MP, Evans BG, Barrett G. Confidentiality and the public interest in medical research—will we ever get it right? *Clin Med* 2003; **3**: 219–28.

35. Higgins J. The Patient Information Advisory Group and the use of patient-identifiable data. *J Health Serv Res Policy* 2003; **8** (suppl 1): 8–11.

36. The Uppsala Monitoring Centre, WHO Collaborating Centre for International Drug Monitoring, http://www.who-umc.org.

37. Committee on Safety of Medicines and Medicines Control Agency. Danthron restricted to constipation in the terminally ill. *CSM/MCA Curr Prob Pharmacovigilance* May 2000: **26**; 4. Available at: http://medicines.mhra.gov.uk/ourwork/monitorsafequalmed/currentproblems/cpmay2000.pdf.

38. Ball SG. Discontinuation of doxazosin arm of ALLHAT. Antihypertensive and Lipid-Lowering Treatment to Prevent Heart Attack. *Lancet* 2000; **355**: 1558.

39. Castel JM, Figueras A, Pedros C, Laporte JR, Capella D. Stimulating adverse drug reaction reporting: effect of a drug safety bulletin and of including yellow cards in prescription pads. *Drug Saf* 2003; **26**: 1049–55.

40. Martin RM, Kapoor KV, Wilton LV, Mann RD. Underreporting of suspected adverse drug reactions to newly marketed ("black triangle") drugs in general practice: observational study. *BMJ* 1998; **317**: 119–20.

41. Heeley E, Riley J, Layton D, Wilton LV, Shakir SA. Prescription-event monitoring and reporting of adverse drug reactions. *Lancet* 2001; **358**: 1872–3.

42. Moride Y, Haramburu F, Requejo AA, Begaud B. Under-reporting of adverse drug reactions in general practice. *Br J Clin Pharmacol* 1997; **43**: 177–81.

43. Belton KJ, Lewis SC, Payne S, Rawlins MD, Wood SM. Attitudinal survey of adverse drug reaction reporting by medical practitioners in the United Kingdom. *Br J Clin Pharmacol* 1995; **39**: 223–6.

44. Rawlins MD. Spontaneous reporting of adverse drug reactions. II: Uses. *Br J Clin Pharmacol* 1988; **26**: 7–11.

45. Waller P. Dealing with uncertainty in drug safety: lessons for the future from sertindole. *Pharmacoepidemiol Drug Saf* 2003; **12**: 283–90.

46. Gould AL. Practical pharmacovigilance analysis strategies. *Pharmacoepidemiol Drug Saf* 2003; **12**: 559–74.

47. Meyboom RH, Lindquist M, Egberts AC, Edwards IR. Signal selection and follow-up in pharmacovigilance. *Drug Saf* 2002; **25**: 459–65.

48. Purcell P, Barty S. Statistical techniques for signal generation: the Australian experience. *Drug Saf* 2002; **25**: 415–21.

49. Bright RA, Nelson RC. Automated support for pharmacovigilance: a proposed system. *Pharmacoepidemiol Drug Saf* 2002; **11**: 121–5.

50. Szarfman A, Machado SG, O'Neill RT. Use of screening algorithms and computer systems to efficiently signal higher-than-expected combinations of drugs and events in the US FDA's spontaneous reports database. *Drug Saf* 2002; **25**: 381–92.

51. van Puijenbroek E, Diemont W, van Grootheest K. Application of quantitative signal detection in the Dutch spontaneous reporting system for adverse drug reactions. *Drug Saf* 2003; **26**: 293–301.

52. Egberts AC, Meyboom RH, van Puijenbroek EP. Use of measures of disproportionality in pharmacovigilance: three Dutch examples. *Drug Saf* 2002; **25**: 453–8.

53. van Puijenbroek EP, Bate A, Leufkens HG, Lindquist M, Orre R, Egberts AC. A comparison of measures of disproportionality for signal detection in spontaneous reporting systems for adverse drug reactions. *Pharmacoepidemiol Drug Saf* 2002; **11**: 3–10.

54. Evans SJ, Waller PC, Davis S. Use of proportional reporting ratios (PRRs) for signal generation from spontaneous adverse drug reaction reports. *Pharmacoepidemiol Drug Saf* 2001; **10**: 483–6.

55. Lindquist M, Stahl M, Bate A, Edwards IR, Meyboom RH. A retrospective evaluation of a data mining approach to aid finding new adverse drug reaction signals in the WHO international database. *Drug Saf* 2000; **23**: 533–42.

56. Gogolak VV. The effect of backgrounds in safety analysis: the impact of comparison cases on what you see. *Pharmacoepidemiol Drug Saf* 2003; **12**: 249–52.

57. Brown EG. Methods and pitfalls in searching drug safety databases utilising the Medical Dictionary for Regulatory Activities (MedDRA). *Drug Saf* 2003; **26**: 145–58.

58. Brown EG. Effects of coding dictionary on signal generation: a consideration of use of MedDRA compared with WHO-ART. *Drug Saf* 2002; **25**: 445–52.

59. Waller PC, Lee EH. Responding to drug safety issues. *Pharmacoepidemiol Drug Saf* 1999; **8**: 535–52.

60. *Current Challenges in Pharmacovigilance: Pragmatic Approaches*. Report of CIOMS Working Group V. Geneva: 2001.

61. FDA Center for Drug Evaluation and Research. Concept Paper: Risk Assessment of Observational Data: Good Pharmacovigilance Practices and Pharmacoepidemiologic Assessment, March 3, 2003. Available at: http://www.fda.gov/cder/meeting/riskManageIII.htm. Accessed: March 2004.

62. Oxford Centre for Evidence-Based Medicine. Levels of Evidence and Grades of Recommendation. Available at: http://www.cebm.net/levels_of_evidence.asp. Accessed: March 2004.

63. Mackay FJ. Post-marketing studies: the work of the Drug Safety Research Unit. *Drug Saf* 1998; **19**: 343–53.

64. Mann RD. Prescription-event monitoring—recent progress and future horizons. *Br J Clin Pharmacol* 1998; **46**: 195–201.

65. Kubota K. Prescription-event monitoring in Japan (J-PEM). *Drug Saf* 2002; **25**: 441–4.

66. Coulter DM. Signal generation in the New Zealand Intensive Medicines Monitoring Programme: a combined clinical and statistical approach. *Drug Saf* 2002; **25**: 433–9.

67. Lawrence G, Menzies R, Burgess M, McIntyre P, Wood N, Boyd I *et al*. Surveillance of adverse events following immunisation: Australia, 2000–2002. *Commun Dis Intell* 2003; **27**: 307–23.

68. Scialli AR. The Organization of Teratology Information Services (OTIS) registry study. *J Allergy Clin Immunol* 1999; **103**: S373–6.

69. Lipani JA, Strand V, Johnson K, Woodworth T, Furst D, Singh G *et al*. A proposal for developing a large patient population cohort for longterm safety monitoring in rheumatoid arthritis. OMER-ACT Drug Safety Working Party. *J Rheumatol* 2001; **28**: 1170–3.

70. Armenti VT, Moritz MJ, Davison JM. Drug safety issues in pregnancy following transplantation and immunosuppression: effects and outcomes. *Drug Saf* 1998; **19**: 219–32.

71. A North American Registry for Epilepsy and Pregnancy, a unique public/private partnership of health surveillance. *Epilepsia* 1998; **39**: 793–8.

72. White AD, Andrews EB. The Pregnancy Registry program at Glaxo Wellcome Company. *J Allergy Clin Immunol* 1999; **103**: S362–3.

73. Fox DJ, Druschel CM. Estimating prevalence of fetal alcohol syndrome (FAS): effectiveness of a passive birth defects registry system. *Birth Defects Res Part A Clin Mol Teratol* 2003; **67**: 604–8.

74. The University of Arizona Center for Education and Research on Therapeutics. Registry of medicine-induced cardiac arrhythmias. Available at: http//www.qtdrugs.org. Accessed: December 2003.

75. Fraunfelder FT, Meyer SM. The national registry of drug-induced ocular side effects. *Aust J Ophthalmol* 1984; **12**: 129–31.

76. Vial T, Descotes J. Immunosuppressive drugs and cancer. *Toxicology* 2003; **185**: 229–40.

77. Jarlbaek L, Andersen M, Kragstrup J, Hallas J. Cancer patients' share in a population's use of opioids. A linkage study between a prescription database and the Danish cancer registry. *J Pain Symptom Manage* 2004; **27**: 36–43.

78. Csizmadi I, Collet JP, Benedetti A, Boivin JF, Hanley JA. The effects of transdermal and oral oestrogen replacement therapy on colorectal cancer risk in postmenopausal women. *Br J Cancer* 2004; **90**: 76–81.

79. Sorensen HT, Fonager KM. Myocarditis and inflammatory bowel disease. A 16-year Danish nationwide cohort study. *Dan Med Bull* 1997; **44**: 442–4.

80. Honigfeld G, Arellano F, Sethi J, Bianchini A, Schein J. Reducing clozapine-related morbidity and mortality: 5 years of experience with the Clozaril National Registry. *J Clin Psychiatry* 1998; **59** (suppl 3): 3–7.

81. Pascoe SJ. The adjunctive use of a centralised database in the monitoring of clozapine-related neutropenia. *Pharmacoepidemiol Drug Saf* 2003; **12**: 395–8.

82. Lary JM, Daniel KL, Erickson JD, Roberts HE, Moore CA. The return of thalidomide: can birth defects be prevented? *Drug Saf* 1999; **21**: 161–9.

83. Lawrenson R, Williams T, Farmer R. Clinical information for research; the use of general practice databases. *J Public Health Med* 1999; **21**: 299–304.

84. Jick SS, Kaye JA, Vasilakis-Scaramozza C, Garcia Rodriguez LA, Ruigomez A, Meier CR *et al*. Validity of the general practice research database. *Pharmacotherapy* 2003; **23**: 686–9.

85. Garcia Rodriguez LA, Perez Gutthann S. Use of the UK General Practice Research Database for pharmacoepidemiology. *Br J Clin Pharmacol* 1998; **45**: 419–25.

86. Rathmann W. Data safety and drug safety in Germany: a closing gap? *Pharmacoepidemiol Drug Saf* 2001; **10**: 625–30.

87. Hallas J. Conducting pharmacoepidemiologic research in Denmark. *Pharmacoepidemiol Drug Saf* 2001; **10**: 619–23.

88. McMahon AD, MacDonald TM. Design issues for drug epidemiology. *Br J Clin Pharmacol* 2000; **50**: 419–25.

89. Rothman KJ, Ray W. Should cases with a "known" cause of their disease be excluded from study? *Pharmacoepidemiol Drug Saf* 2002; **11**: 11–4.

90. Garbe E, Boivin JF, LeLorier J, Suissa S. Selection of controls in database case–control studies: glucocorticoids and the risk of glaucoma. *J Clin Epidemiol* 1998; **51**: 129–35.

91. Bartko JJ, Carpenter WT Jr, McGlashan TH. Statistical issues in long-term follow up studies. *Schizophr Bull* 1988; **14**: 575 87.

92. Shapiro S. Bias in the evaluation of low-magnitude associations: an empirical perspective. *Am J Epidemiol* 2000; **151**: 939–45.

93. Hertz-Picciotto I. Shifting the burden of proof regarding biases and low-magnitude associations. *Am J Epidemiol* 2000; **151**: 946–50.

94. Kaye JA, Vasilakis-Scaramozza C, Jick SS, Jick H. Pitfalls of pharmacoepidemiology. *BMJ* 2000; **321**: 1528–9.

95. Signorello LB, McLaughlin JK, Lipworth L, Friis S, Sorensen HT, Blot WJ. Confounding by indication in epidemiologic studies of commonly used analgesics. *Am J Ther* 2002; **9**: 199–205.

96. Jick H, Garcia Rodriguez LA, Perez-Gutthann S. Principles of epidemiological research on adverse and beneficial drug effects. *Lancet* 1998; **352**: 1767–70.

97. Gargiullo PM, Kramarz P, DeStefano F, Chen RT. Principles of epidemiological research on drug effects. *Lancet* 1999; **353**: 501.

98. Donnan PT, Wang J. The case-crossover and case-time-control designs in pharmacoepidemiology. *Pharmacoepidemiol Drug Saf* 2001; **10**: 259–62.

99. Suissa S. The case-time-control design: further assumptions and conditions. *Epidemiology* 1998; **9**: 441–5.

100. Maclure M. Case-crossover design: a method for studying transient effects on the risk of acute events. *Am J Epidemiol* 1991; **133**: 144–53.

101. Farrington CP. Relative incidence estimation from case series for vaccine safety evaluation. *Biometrics* 1995; **51**: 228–35.

102. Farrington CP, Nash J, Miller E. Case series analysis of adverse reactions to vaccines: a comparative evaluation. *Am J Epidemiol* 1996; **143**: 1165–73.

103. Beral V, Million Women Study Collaborators. Breast cancer and hormone-replacement therapy in the Million Women Study. *Lancet* 2003; **362**: 419–27.

104. Kernan WN, Viscoli CM, Brass LM, Broderick JP, Brott T, Feldmann E *et al.* Phenylpropanolamine and the risk of hemorrhagic stroke. *N Engl J Med* 2000; **343**: 1826–32.

105. Reilly JG, Ayis SA, Ferrier IN, Jones SJ, Thomas SH. QTc-interval abnormalities and psychotropic drug therapy in psychiatric patients. *Lancet* 2000; **355**: 1048–52.

106. Fear NT, Roman E, Ansell P, Simpson J, Day N, Eden OB, United Kingdom Childhood Cancer Study.Vitamin K and childhood cancer: a report from the United Kingdom Childhood Cancer Study. *Br J Cancer* 2003; **89**: 1228–31.

107. International Conference on Harmonisation of Technical Requirements for Registration of Pharmaceuticals for Human Use (ICH). E6: Good Clinical Practice: Consolidated Guideline. ICH, 1996. Available at: http://www.ich.org. Accessed March 2004.

108. International Conference on Harmonisation of Technical Requirements for Registration of Pharmaceuticals for Human Use (ICH). E7: Studies in Support of Special Populations: Geriatrics. ICH, 1993. Available at: http://www.ich.org. Accessed March 2004.

109. International Conference on Harmonisation of Technical Requirements for Registration of Pharmaceuticals for Human Use (ICH). E8: General Considerations for Clinical Trials. ICH, 1997. Available at: http://www.ich.org. Accessed: March 2004.

110. International Conference on Harmonisation of Technical Requirements for Registration of Pharmaceuticals for Human Use (ICH). E9: Statistical Principles for Clinical Trials. ICH, 1998. Available at: http://www.ich.org. Accessed March 2004.

111. International Conference on Harmonisation of Technical Requirements for Registration of Pharmaceuticals for Human Use (ICH). E10: Choice of Control Group and Related Issues in Clinical Trials. ICH, 2000. Available at: http://www.ich.org. Accessed March 2004.

112. International Conference on Harmonisation of Technical Requirements for Registration of Pharmaceuticals for Human Use (ICH). E11: Clinical Investigation of Medicinal Products in the Pediatric Population. ICH, 2000. Available at: http://www.ich.org. Accessed March 2004.

113. Moher D, Cook DJ, Eastwood S, Olkin I, Rennie D, Stroup DF. Improving the quality of reports of meta-analyses of randomised controlled trials: the QUOROM statement. QUOROM Group. *Br J Surg* 2000; **87**: 1448–54.

114. Tubert-Bitter P, Manfredi R, Lellouch J, Begaud B. Sample size calculations for risk equivalence testing in pharmacoepidemiology. *J Clin Epidemiol* 2000; **53**: 1268–74.

115. Rothman KJ, Greenland S. *Modern Epidemiology*, 2nd edn. Philadelphia, PA: Lippincot-Raven, 1998.

116. Maitland-van der Zee AH, de Boer A, Leufkens HG. The interface between pharmacoepidemiology and pharmacogenetics. *Eur J Pharmacol* 2000; **410**: 121–30.

117. Jones JK. Pharmacogenetics and pharmacoepidemiology. *Pharmacoepidemiol Drug Saf* 2001; **10**: 457–61.

118. Jefferys DB, Leakey D, Lewis JA, Payne S, Rawlins MD. New active substances authorised in the United Kingdom between 1972 and 1994. *Br J Clin Pharmacol* 1998; **45**: 151–6.

119. Lumkin MM. International pharmacovigilance: developing cooperation to meet the challenges of the 21st century. *Pharmacol Toxicol* 2000; **86** (suppl 1), 20–2.

120. Council for International Organizations of Medical Sciences (CIOMS). *Benefit–Risk Balance for Market Drugs: Evaluating Safety Signals*, Report of the CIOMS Working Group IV. Geneva: CIOMS, 1998.

121. Arlett PR. Risk benefit assessment. *Pharmaceutical Physician* 2001: **12**: 12–7.

122. Bjerre LM, LeLorier J. Expressing the magnitude of adverse effects in case–control studies: "the number of patients needed to be treated for one additional patient to be harmed." *BMJ* 2000; **320**: 503–6.

123. Altman DG. Confidence intervals for the number needed to treat. *BMJ* 1998; **317**: 1309–12.

124. Smeeth L, Haines A, Ebrahim S. Numbers needed to treat derived from meta-analyses—sometimes informative, usually misleading. *BMJ* 1999; **318**: 1548–51.

125. Waller PC, Arlett P. Responding to signals. In: Mann R, Andrews E, eds, *Pharmacovigilance*. Chichester: John Wiley & Sons, 2002; pp. 105–28.

Part III

SOURCES OF DATA FOR PHARMACOEPIDEMIOLOGY STUDIES

Part IIIa

Ad Hoc Data Sources Available for Pharmacoepidemiology Studies

9

Spontaneous Reporting in the United States

SYED RIZWANUDDIN AHMAD[1], ROGER A. GOETSCH[2] and NORMAN S. MARKS[1]

[1] Office of Drug Safety/DDRE, Silver Spring, Maryland, USA; [2] Office of Drug Safety/DSRCS, Rockville, Maryland, USA.

INTRODUCTION

The United States Food and Drug Administration (FDA) is the Federal public health agency that has regulatory responsibility for ensuring the safety of all marketed medical products, including pharmaceuticals (i.e., drugs and biologics) (see also Chapter 8). In order to ensure that safe and effective pharmaceuticals are available, the FDA relies on both the recognition, and *voluntary* reporting, of serious adverse events (AEs) by health care providers and their patients and the *mandatory* reporting of AEs by manufacturers as required by law and regulation.

All unsolicited reports from health care professionals or consumers, received by the FDA via either the voluntary or mandatory route, are called *spontaneous* reports. A spontaneous report is a clinical observation that originates outside of a formal study.[1] The individual spontaneous reports of adverse drug reactions (ADRs), medication errors, and product quality problems, sent directly to the FDA through the MedWatch program (see below) or to the manufacturer and then indirectly from the manufacturer to the FDA, combined with data from formal clinical studies and from the medical and scientific literature, comprise the primary data source upon which postmarketing surveillance depends. In the US,

a large majority of reports, between 70% and 75%, are submitted either directly or indirectly by health care professionals as voluntary reports, with consumer/patient reports comprising about 15% of reports.[2,3]

In addition to this passive process for safety surveillance, the FDA continues to explore the use of new active surveillance methodologies for collecting reports of adverse effects and evaluating adverse events. The FDA may also explore drug safety questions in large population-based claim databases that link prescriptions with adverse outcomes.[4]

When the FDA approves a pharmaceutical product for prescribing and dispensing by health care providers in the United States, the agency has conducted a rigorous, science-based, multidisciplinary review of controlled clinical trials sponsored and conducted by a pharmaceutical company. The FDA has determined that the product's benefits outweigh any known or anticipated risks for the general population when the product is used as indicated in the approved prescribing information. However, the limitations inherent in the controlled clinical trial setting in the identification of rare, but clinically important, adverse events inevitably insure that uncertainties will remain about the safety of the pharmaceutical once it is marketed and used in a wider population, over longer periods of time, in patients with

Pharmacoepidemiology, Fourth Edition   Edited by B.L. Strom
© 2005 John Wiley & Sons, Ltd

comorbidities and concomitant medications, and for "off-label" uses not previously evaluated.[5]

Given these recognized and accepted limitations in the pre-approval New Drug Application (NDA) process, the agency relies on the public, both health care professionals and their patients, for the voluntary reporting of suspected, serious, and unlabeled ADRs, medication errors, and product quality problems observed during the use of the pharmaceutical in the "real-world" setting, in order to manage the risk of product use and reduce the possibility of harm to patients.

Harm to patients from pharmaceutical use may occur due to four types of risk (Figure 9.1).[6] Most injuries and deaths associated with the use of medical products result from their *known side effects*, some unavoidable but others able to be prevented or minimized by careful product choice and use. It is estimated that more than half the side effects of pharmaceuticals are avoidable.[7]

Other sources of preventable adverse events are *medication errors*, which may occur when the product is administered incorrectly or when the wrong drug or dose is administered.

Injury from *product quality problems* is of interest to the FDA, which has regulatory responsibility for oversight of product quality control and quality assurance during the manufacturing and distribution process.

The final category of potential risk, those risks most amenable to identification by an effective voluntary reporting system, involves the *remaining uncertainties* about a product. These uncertainties include unexpected and rare AEs, long-term effects, unstudied uses and/or unstudied populations, unanticipated medication errors due to name confusion or packaging format, and product quality defects during the manufacturing process.

This chapter reviews the history of AE reporting in the United States, its terminology, and its regulatory aspects. The strengths, limitations, and applications of the FDA's Adverse Event Reporting System (AERS) are discussed, as are future plans.

DESCRIPTION

HISTORY OF US PHARMACEUTICAL SAFETY REGULATION

The FDA is the first US consumer protection agency. Its predecessor, the Bureau of Drugs, was established in order to implement the Biologics Control Act of 1902. Subsequent drug regulatory laws, in 1906, 1938, and 1962, have all resulted from widespread public concern about drug safety and demands that the US Congress address a perceived crisis that threatened the health and lives of children. Each law or amendment incrementally strengthened the FDA's capability to effectively monitor the postmarketing safety of drugs and other medical products.

The 1902 Act was passed by the US Congress in reaction to the public outrage from hundreds of cases of post-vaccination tetanus and the deaths of several dozen children due to tetanus-contaminated diphtheria antitoxin. This first drug safety law required annual licensing of manufacturers and distributors and the labeling of all products with the name of the manufacturer. Neither the premarketing safety and efficacy nor the postmarketing safety of these products were regulated by the government.[8]

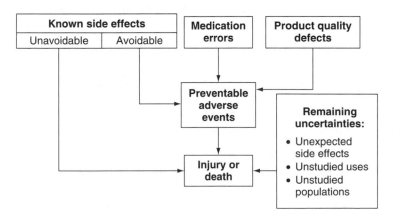

Figure 9.1. Sources of risk from medical products.

The Pure Food and Drug Act of 1906 prohibited interstate commerce of mislabeled and adulterated drugs and foods.[9] Again, the safety of drugs after consumption was not addressed. For example, in 1934 the Agency began investigations on products containing dinitrophenol, a component in diet preparations that increased metabolic rate to dangerous levels, and was responsible for many deaths and injuries. However, the Office of Drug Control could not seize the products, and was limited to posting warnings. The safety of drugs after consumption was not addressed until the 1930s and unfortunately it was again a disaster that prompted Congress to act.[10]

These continuing problems with dangerous drugs that fell outside the controls of the Pure Food and Drug Act finally received national attention with the elixir of sulfanilamide disaster in 1937. The S.E. Massengill Co. introduced a flavorful oral dosage form of the new anti-infective "wonder drug" by using an untested solvent, the antifreeze diethylene glycol. By the time the FDA became aware of the problem and removed the product from pharmacy shelves and medicine cabinets, the preparation had caused 107 deaths, including many children. Even though the toxic effects of diethylene glycol were well documented by 1931, with no drug safety regulations in place, the only charge that could be brought under the 1906 Act was misbranding the product, since there was no alcohol in the "elixir," as implied by the name.

In June 1938, the Federal Food, Drug and Cosmetic Act was passed by the US Congress. The law required new drugs to be tested for safety before marketing, the results of which would be submitted to the FDA in an NDA. The law also required that drugs have adequate labeling for safe use. Again, no postmarketing safety monitoring was mandated by this new law.

During the 1950s, there was a rapid expansion of the pharmaceutical industry and an increase in the number of new products. A new broad spectrum antibiotic, chloramphenicol, was approved by the FDA in early 1949 as "safe and effective when used as indicated" (the standard for approval in the 1938 Act). However, the small number of patients exposed to chloramphenicol during pre-approval clinical trials was not adequate to observe serious but rare adverse events that would occur in fewer than 1 in 1000 patients. Within six months of approval, reports in the medical literature in the US and Europe suggested the association of fatal aplastic anemia with chloramphenicol use.

In late June 1952, in order to gather the necessary data to evaluate this issue, the FDA ordered the staff in all 16 district offices to contact every hospital, medical school, and clinic in cities with populations of 100 000 or more to collect information on any cases of aplastic anemia or other blood dyscrasias attributed to chloramphenicol. Within four days of field contacts, an additional 217 cases of chloramphenicol-associated blood dyscrasias had been identified.[11]

The delay in identification of and regulatory action on reports of aplastic anemia associated with chloramphenicol use demonstrated the necessity for monitoring adverse events following the approval and marketing of new drugs. In response to this need the American Medical Association (AMA) established a Committee on Blood Dyscrasias, which began collecting case reports of drug-induced blood-related illness in 1954. At that time, the AMA had a potential information source of over 7000 hospitals and 250 000 physicians. The AMA's program was expanded in 1961 to a more comprehensive "Registry on Adverse Reactions." The program was discontinued in 1971 because of parallel efforts by the FDA.[12]

In 1956, the FDA piloted its own drug ADR surveillance program in cooperation with the American Society of Hospital Pharmacists (the predecessor of the American Society of Health-System Pharmacists), the national association of medical records librarians, and the AMA.[13] The reporting program began with 6 hospitals and by 1965 had grown to over 200 teaching hospitals which reported to the FDA on a monthly basis. In addition, reports were sent to the FDA from selected Federal hospitals (Department of Defense, Veterans Administration, Public Health Service) and published reports were culled from the medical literature and received from the World Health Organization.[14]

The 1962 Kefauver–Harris Amendments to the Food, Drug, and Cosmetic Act of 1938 required proof of efficacy before drug approval and marketing. For the first time, this law also mandated that pharmaceutical manufacturers must report AEs to the FDA for any of their products having an NDA, the vast majority of prescription products introduced since 1938.

The FDA began to computerize the storage of its AE reports in 1967, and by early 1968 received, coded, and entered all data from the FDA Form 1639 Drug Experience Reports into the Spontaneous Reporting System (SRS).[15] The SRS was replaced in November 1997 with the Adverse Event Reporting System (AERS), a computerized information database that supports the FDA's postmarketing safety surveillance program for all approved drug and therapeutic biologic products. AERS is an internationally compatible system designed as a pharmacovigilance tool for storing and analyzing safety reports.

By 1991, there were five different forms for manufacturers and health professionals to report medical product problems to the agency. In 1993, then-FDA Commissioner David A. Kessler, MD, citing confusion with the multiple forms, launched the FDA's MedWatch Adverse Event Reporting Program. A single-page voluntary reporting form, FDA form 3500 (The "MedWatch" form) was introduced to report adverse events associated with all medical products except vaccines, and the FDA form 3500A was provided for use by mandatory reporters (see Figures 9.2 and 9.3). The MedWatch program was charged with the task of facilitating, supporting, and promoting the voluntary reporting process. Since 1993, over 200 000 voluntary reports have been received from health care professionals and consumers, coded, and entered into the FDA AERS database (see Figure 9.4).

REGULATORY REPORTING REQUIREMENTS

In the US, AE reporting by individual health care providers and consumers is voluntary. However, manufacturers, packers, and distributors of FDA-approved pharmaceuticals (drugs and biologic products) all have mandatory reporting requirements governed by regulation. Historically, only nonbiologic pharmaceutical products with approved NDAs (i.e., all prescription and some over-the-counter drugs) were subject to mandatory reporting requirements. In 1994, this requirement was expanded to include biologic products.[16]

It should be emphasized that these regulations are aimed at pharmaceutical manufacturers, but also provide a useful framework for reporting by practitioners to either the FDA and/or the manufacturer. In the US, most health professionals and consumers report AEs to the manufacturer rather than directly to the FDA. This pattern is not seen in many other countries, where consumers and health professionals report directly to a governmental public health agency.

CURRENT REQUIREMENTS

The main objective of the FDA postmarketing reporting requirement is to provide early prompt detection of signals about potentially serious, previously unknown safety problems with marketed drugs, especially with newly marketed drugs. To understand the regulatory requirements, one first needs to define several terms. These definitions are revisions that became effective in April 1998.[17]

An *adverse experience* is any AE associated with the use of a drug or biologic product in humans, whether or not considered product related, including the following: an AE occurring in the course of the use of the product in professional practice, an AE occurring from overdose of the product, whether accidental or intentional, an AE occurring from abuse of the product, an AE occurring from withdrawal of the product, and any failure of expected pharmacologic action.

An *unexpected adverse experience* means any AE that is not listed in the current labeling for the product. This includes events that may be symptomatically and pathophysiologically related to an event listed in the labeling, but differ from the event because of greater severity or specificity.

A *serious adverse experience* is any AE occurring at any dose that results in any of the following outcomes: death, a life-threatening AE, inpatient hospitalization or prolongation of existing hospitalization, a persistent or significant disability/incapacity, or congenital anomaly/birth defect. Important medical events that may not result in death, may not be life-threatening, or may not require hospitalization may be considered a serious AE when, based upon appropriate medical judgment, they may jeopardize the patient or subject and may require medical or surgical intervention to prevent one of the outcomes listed in this definition. Examples of such medical events include allergic bronchospasm requiring intensive treatment in an emergency room or at home, blood dyscrasias or convulsions that do not result in inpatient hospitalization, or the development of drug dependency or drug abuse.

Table 9.1 outlines the US mandatory reporting requirements regarding pharmaceuticals. By regulation, companies are required to report to the FDA *all* adverse events of which they become aware and to provide as complete information as possible. Although pharmaceutical reporting is mandated, it still relies primarily on information provided to them by health professionals through both voluntary reporting and the scientific literature.

In the case of over-the-counter (OTC) drugs, reports are only required on OTC products marketed under an approved NDA, including those prescription drugs that undergo a switch to OTC status. Reports are not currently required for other OTC drugs (i.e., older drug ingredients which are marketed without an NDA), although voluntary reporting is encouraged for serious events.

Both prescription and OTC drugs require FDA safety and efficacy review prior to marketing, unlike dietary supplements (which include vitamins, minerals, amino acids, botanicals, and other substances used to increase total dietary intake). By law,[18] the manufacturers of these latter products do not have to prove safety or efficacy, but that same law places the responsibility on the FDA to demonstrate that a particular product is unsafe or presents a potentially serious risk to public health. In addition, manufacturers of these products do not have to report AEs to the FDA. As a result, direct-to-FDA voluntary reporting by health professionals and their patients of serious adverse events associated with and possibly causally linked to dietary supplements is particularly

U.S. Department of Health and Human Services

MEDWATCH

The FDA Safety Information and
Adverse Event Reporting Program

**For VOLUNTARY reporting of
adverse events and product problems**

Page ___ of ___

Form Approved: OMB No. 0910-0291, Expires: 03/31/05
See OMB statement on reverse.

FDA USE ONLY
Triage unit sequence #

A. PATIENT INFORMATION

1. Patient Identifier
2. Age at Time of Event:
   or _____
   Date of Birth:
3. Sex
   ☐ Female
   ☐ Male
4. Weight
   _____ lbs
   or
   _____ kgs

In confidence

B. ADVERSE EVENT OR PRODUCT PROBLEM

1. ☐ Adverse Event   and/or   ☐ Product Problem (e.g., defects/malfunctions)

2. Outcomes Attributed to Adverse Event (Check all that apply)
   ☐ Death: _____ (mo/day/yr)
   ☐ Life-threatening
   ☐ Hospitalization – initial or prolonged
   ☐ Disability
   ☐ Congenital Anomaly
   ☐ Required Intervention to Prevent Permanent Impairment/Damage
   ☐ Other: _____

3. Date of Event (mo/day/year)

4. Date of This Report (mo/day/year)

5. Describe Event or Problem

6. Relevant Tests/Laboratory Data, Including Dates

7. Other Relevant History, Including Preexisting Medical Conditions (e.g., allergies, race, pregnancy, smoking and alcohol use, hepatic/renal dysfunction, etc.)

PLEASE TYPE OR USE BLACK INK

C. SUSPECT MEDICATION(S)

1. Name (Give labeled strength & mfr/labeler, if known)
   #1
   #2

2. Dose, Frequency & Route Used
   #1
   #2

3. Therapy Dates (If unknown, give duration) from/to (or best estimate)
   #1
   #2

4. Diagnosis for Use (Indication)
   #1
   #2

5. Event Abated After Use Stopped or Dose Reduced?
   #1 ☐ Yes ☐ No ☐ Doesn't Apply
   #2 ☐ Yes ☐ No ☐ Doesn't Apply

6. Lot # (if known)
   #1
   #2

7. Exp. Date (if known)
   #1
   #2

8. Event Reappeared After Reintroduction?
   #1 ☐ Yes ☐ No ☐ Doesn't Apply
   #2 ☐ Yes ☐ No ☐ Doesn't Apply

9. NDC # (For product problems only)
   ___ - ___ - ___

10. Concomitant Medical Products and Therapy Dates (Exclude treatment of event)

D. SUSPECT MEDICAL DEVICE

1. Brand Name

2. Type of Device

3. Manufacturer Name, City and State

4. Model #
   Catalog #
   Serial #

Lot #
Expiration Date (mo/day/yr)
Other #

5. Operator of Device
   ☐ Health Professional
   ☐ Lay User/Patient
   ☐ Other: _____

6. If Implanted, Give Date (mo/day/yr)

7. If Explanted, Give Date (mo/day/yr)

8. Is this a Single-use Device that was Reprocessed and Reused on a Patient?
   ☐ Yes ☐ No

9. If Yes to Item No. 8, Enter Name and Address of Reprocessor

10. Device Available for Evaluation? (Do not send to FDA)
    ☐ Yes ☐ No ☐ Returned to Manufacturer on: _____ (mo/day/yr)

11. Concomitant Medical Products and Therapy Dates (Exclude treatment of event)

E. REPORTER (See confidentiality section on back)

1. Name and Address   Phone #

2. Health Professional? ☐ Yes ☐ No

3. Occupation

4. Also Reported to:
   ☐ Manufacturer
   ☐ User Facility
   ☐ Distributor/Importer

5. If you do NOT want your identity disclosed to the manufacturer, place an "X" in this box: ☐

Mail to: **MEDWATCH**   -or-   FAX to:
5600 Fishers Lane   1-800-FDA-0178
Rockville, MD 20852-9787

FDA

FORM FDA 3500 (12/03)   Submission of a report does not constitute an admission that medical personnel or the product caused or contributed to the event.

Figure 9.2. MedWatch voluntary reporting form (FDA Form 3500).

ADVICE ABOUT VOLUNTARY REPORTING

Report adverse experiences with:

- Medications *(drugs or biologics)*
- Medical devices *(including in-vitro diagnostics)*
- Special nutritional products *(dietary supplements, medical foods, infant formulas)*
- Cosmetics
- Medication errors

Report product problems – quality, performance or safety concerns such as:

- Suspected counterfeit product
- Suspected contamination
- Questionable stability
- Defective components
- Poor packaging or labeling
- Therapeutic failures

Report SERIOUS adverse events. An event is serious when the patient outcome is:

-Fold Here-

- Death
- Life-threatening *(real risk of dying)*
- Hospitalization *(initial or prolonged)*
- Disability *(significant, persistent or permanent)*
- Congenital anomaly
- Required intervention to prevent permanent impairment or damage

Report even if:

- You're not certain the product caused the event
- You don't have all the details

How to report:

- Just fill in the sections that apply to your report
- Use section C for all products except medical devices
- Attach additional blank pages if needed
- Use a separate form for each patient
- Report either to FDA or the manufacturer *(or both)*

Confidentiality: The patient's identity is held in strict confidence by FDA and protected to the fullest extent of the law. FDA will not disclose the reporter's identity in response to a request from the public, pursuant to the Freedom of Information Act. The reporter's identity, including the identity of a self-reporter, may be shared with the manufacturer unless requested otherwise.

If your report involves a serious adverse event with a device and it occurred in a facility outside a doctor's office, that facility may be legally required to report to FDA and/or the manufacturer. Please notify the person in that facility who would handle such reporting.   -Fold Here-

Important numbers:

- 1-800-FDA-0178 – To FAX report
- 1-800-FDA-1088 – To report by phone or for more information
- 1-800-822-7967 – For a VAERS form for vaccines

To Report via the Internet:
http://www.fda.gov/medwatch/report.htm

The public reporting burden for this collection of information has been estimated to average 30 minutes per response, including the time for reviewing instructions, searching existing data sources, gathering and maintaining the data needed, and completing and reviewing the collection of information. Send comments regarding this burden estimate or any other aspect of this collection of information, including suggestions for reducing this burden to:

 Department of Health and Human Services *Please DO NOT*
 Food and Drug Administration   *RETURN this form*
 MedWatch; HFD-410   *to this address.*
 5600 Fishers Lane
 Rockville, MD 20857

OMB statement:
"An agency may not conduct or sponsor, and a person is not required to respond to, a collection of information unless it displays a currently valid OMB control number."

U.S. DEPARTMENT OF HEALTH AND HUMAN SERVICES
Food and Drug Administration

FORM FDA 3500 (12/03) (Back)   Please Use Address Provided Below – Fold in Thirds, Tape and Mail

**DEPARTMENT OF
HEALTH & HUMAN SERVICES**

Public Health Service
Food and Drug Administration
Rockville, MD 20857

Official Business
Penalty for Private Use $300

BUSINESS REPLY MAIL
FIRST CLASS MAIL PERMIT NO. 946 ROCKVILLE MD

POSTAGE WILL BE PAID BY FOOD AND DRUG ADMINISTRATION

MED**W**ATCH
The FDA Safety Information and Adverse Event Reporting Program
Food and Drug Administration
5600 Fishers Lane
Rockville, MD 20852-9787

Figure 9.2. (Continued).

Form Approved: OMB No. 0910-0291, Expires: 03/31/05
See OMB statement on reverse.

U.S.Department of Health and Human Services

MEDWATCH

The FDA Safety Information and
Adverse Event Reporting Program

**For use by user-facilities,
importers, distributors and manufacturers
for MANDATORY reporting**

Page ____ of ____

Mfr Report #

UF/Importer Report #

FDA Use Only

A. PATIENT INFORMATION

1. Patient Identifier	2. Age at Time of Event: or ————— Date of Birth:	3. Sex ☐ Female ☐ Male	4. Weight ————— lbs or ————— kgs
In confidence			

B. ADVERSE EVENT OR PRODUCT PROBLEM

1. ☐ Adverse Event   and/or   ☐ Product Problem *(e.g., defects/malfunctions)*

2. Outcomes Attributed to Adverse Event *(Check all that apply)*
☐ Death: _____ *(mo/day/yr)*
☐ Life-threatening
☐ Hospitalization – initial or prolonged

☐ Disability
☐ Congenital Anomaly
☐ Required Intervention to Prevent Permanent Impairment/Damage
☐ Other: _____

3. Date of Event *(mo/day/year)*

4. Date of This Report *(mo/day/year)*

5. Describe Event or Problem

6. Relevant Tests/Laboratory Data, Including Dates

7. Other Relevant History, Including Preexisting Medical Conditions *(e.g., allergies, race, pregnancy, smoking and alcohol use, hepatic/renal dysfunction, etc.)*

PLEASE TYPE OR USE BLACK INK

C. SUSPECT MEDICATION(S)

1. Name *(Give labeled strength & mfr/labeler, if known)*
#1
#2

2. Dose, Frequency & Route Used
#1
#2

3. Therapy Dates *(If unknown, give duration) from/to (or best estimate)*
#1
#2

4. Diagnosis for Use *(Indication)*
#1
#2

5. Event Abated After Use Stopped or Dose Reduced?
#1 ☐ Yes ☐ No ☐ Doesn't Apply
#2 ☐ Yes ☐ No ☐ Doesn't Apply

6. Lot # *(if known)*
#1
#2

7. Exp. Date *(if known)*
#1
#2

8. Event Reappeared After Reintroduction?
#1 ☐ Yes ☐ No ☐ Doesn't Apply
#2 ☐ Yes ☐ No ☐ Doesn't Apply

9. NDC # *(For product problems only)*
— —

10. Concomitant Medical Products and Therapy Dates *(Exclude treatment of event)*

D. SUSPECT MEDICAL DEVICE

1. Brand Name

2. Type of Device

3. Manufacturer Name, City and State

4. Model # Catalog # Serial #	Lot # Expiration Date *(mo/day/yr)* Other #	5. Operator of Device ☐ Health Professional ☐ Lay User/Patient ☐ Other:

6. If Implanted, Give Date *(mo/day/yr)*

7. If Explanted, Give Date *(mo/day/yr)*

8. Is this a Single-use Device that was Reprocessed and Reused on a Patient?
☐ Yes   ☐ No

9. If Yes to Item No. 8, Enter Name and Address of Reprocessor

10. Device Available for Evaluation? *(Do not send to FDA)*
☐ Yes   ☐ No   ☐ Returned to Manufacturer on:_____ *(mo/day/yr)*

11. Concomitant Medical Products and Therapy Dates *(Exclude treatment of event)*

E. INITIAL REPORTER

1. Name and Address

Phone #

2. Health Professional? ☐ Yes ☐ No

3. Occupation

4. Initial Reporter Also Sent Report to FDA
☐ Yes ☐ No ☐ Unk.

FDA

Submission of a report does not constitute an admission that medical personnel, user facility, importer, distributor, manufacturer or product caused or contributed to the event.

FORM FDA 3500A (9/03)

Figure 9.3. MedWatch mandatory reporting form (FDA Form 3500A).

Medication and Device Experience Report *(Continued)*

Refer to guidelines for specific instructions.

Submission of a report does not constitute an admission that medical personnel, user facility, importer, distributor, manufacturer or product caused or contributed to the event.

U.S. DEPARTMENT OF HEALTH AND HUMAN SERVICES
Public Health Service • Food and Drug Administration

FDA USE ONLY

Page ____ of ____

F. FOR USE BY USER FACILITY/IMPORTER *(Devices Only)*

1. Check One
☐ User Facility ☐ Importer

2. UF/Importer Report Number

3. User Facility or Importer Name/Address

4. Contact Person

5. Phone Number

6. Date User Facility or Importer Became Aware of Event *(mo/day/yr)*

7. Type of Report
☐ Initial
☐ Follow-up # _____

8. Date of This Report *(mo/day/yr)*

9. Approximate Age of Device

10. Event Problem Codes *(Refer to coding manual)*

Patient Code ____ - ____ - ____
Device Code ____ - ____ - ____

11. Report Sent to FDA?
☐ Yes _____
☐ No *(mo/day/yr)*

12. Location Where Event Occurred
☐ Hospital
☐ Home
☐ Nursing Home
☐ Outpatient Treatment Facility
☐ Outpatient Diagnostic Facility
☐ Ambulatory Surgical Facility
☐ Other: _____ *(Specify)*

13. Report Sent to Manufacturer?
☐ Yes _____
☐ No *(mo/day/yr)*

14. Manufacturer Name/Address

G. ALL MANUFACTURERS

1. Contact Office – Name/Address *(and Manufacturing Site for Devices)*

2. Phone Number

3. Report Source *(Check all that apply)*
☐ Foreign
☐ Study
☐ Literature
☐ Consumer
☐ Health Professional
☐ User Facility
☐ Company Representative
☐ Distributor
☐ Other: _____

4. Date Received by Manufacturer *(mo/day/yr)*

5.
(A)NDA # _____
IND # _____
PLA # _____
Pre-1938 ☐ Yes
OTC Product ☐ Yes

6. If IND, Give Protocol #

7. Type of Report *(Check all that apply)*
☐ 5-day ☐ 15-day
☐ 10-day ☐ Periodic
☐ Initial ☐ Follow-up # _____

8. Adverse Event Term(s)

9. Manufacturer Report Number

H. DEVICE MANUFACTURERS ONLY

1. Type of Reportable Event
☐ Death
☐ Serious Injury
☐ Malfunction
☐ Other: _____

2. If Follow-up, What Type?
☐ Correction
☐ Additional Information
☐ Response to FDA Request
☐ Device Evaluation

3. Device Evaluated by Manufacturer?
☐ Not Returned to Manufacturer
☐ Yes ☐ Evaluation Summary Attached
☐ No *(Attach page to explain why not)* or provide code: _____

4. Device Manufacture Date *(mo/yr)*

5. Labeled for Single Use?
☐ Yes ☐ No

6. Evaluation Codes *(Refer to coding manual)*

Method ____ - ____ - ____ - ____
Results ____ - ____ - ____ - ____
Conclusions ____ - ____ - ____ - ____

7. If Remedial Action Initiated, Check Type
☐ Recall ☐ Notification
☐ Repair ☐ Inspection
☐ Replace ☐ Patient Monitoring
☐ Relabeling ☐ Modification/ Adjustment
☐ Other: _____

8. Usage of Device
☐ Initial Use of Device
☐ Reuse
☐ Unknown

9. If action reported to FDA under 21 USC 360i(f), list correction/removal reporting number:

10. ☐ **Additional Manufacturer Narrative** and/or **11.** ☐ **Corrected Data**

The public reporting burden for this collection of information has been estimated to average one hour per response, including the time for reviewing instructions, searching existing data sources, gathering and maintaining the data needed, and completing and reviewing the collection of information. Send comments regarding this burden estimate or any other aspect of this collection of information, including suggestions for reducing this burden to:

Department of Health and Human Services
Food and Drug Administration
MedWatch; HFD-410
5600 Fishers Lane
Rockville, MD 20857

OMB Statement:
"An agency may not conduct or sponsor, and a person is not required to respond to, a collection of information unless it displays a currently valid OMB control number."

FORM FDA 3500A (9/03) (Back)

Please DO NOT RETURN this form to this address

Figure 9.3. (Continued).

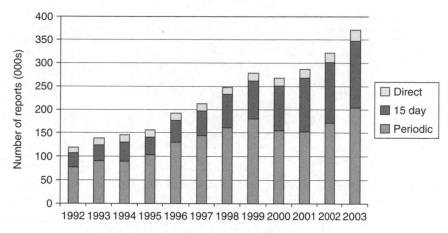

Figure 9.4. ADE reports by year and type, 1992–2003.

Table 9.1. Mandatory AE reporting requirements for pharmaceuticals

15-day "Alert Reports"	All serious and unexpected AEs, whether foreign or domestic, must be reported to the FDA within 15 calendar days
15-day "Alert Reports" follow-up	The manufacturer must promptly investigate all AEs that are the subject of a 15-day Alert Report and submit a follow-up report within 15 calendar days
Periodic AE reports	All non-15-day, domestic, AE reports must be reported periodically (quarterly for the first 3 years after approval, then annually). Periodic reports for products marketed prior to 1938 are not required. Periodic reporting does not apply to AE information obtained from postmarketing studies or from reports in the scientific literature
Scientific literature	A 15-day Alert Report based on information from the scientific literature (case reports or results from a formal clinical trial). A copy of the published article must accompany the report, translated into English if foreign
Postmarketing studies	No requirement for a 15-day Alert Report on an AE acquired from a postmarketing study *unless* manufacturer concludes a reasonable possibility that the product caused the event

important. To help promote reporting and tracking of adverse events associated with dietary supplements, the FDA's Center for Food Safety and Nutrition (CFSAN) launched its CFSAN Adverse Event Reporting System (CAERS) in the summer of 2003.[19]

The specific regulations governing postmarketing AE reporting by pharmaceutical companies are listed in Table 9.2. Accompanying separate guidances for drugs and biologics were made available in 1992[20] and 1993,[21] respectively. As can be seen, the regulations have each been amended numerous times.

Many of the proposed rules, draft guidance documents, and a docket memo (in various stages of development) encourage electronic AE reporting. Electronic reporting is an important step because reports are available for review more quickly. Further, electronic reporting reduces data entry costs, allowing the Center for Drug Evaluation and Research (CDER) to use its resources for additional pharmacovigilance efforts. The proposed rules, draft guidances, and docket memo and their associated statutes are as follows:

• The proposed rule on Adverse Event Reporting and guidance on electronic submissions are currently being finalized.
• A draft Guidance for Industry, "Providing Regulatory Submissions in Electronic Format—Postmarketing Expedited Safety Reports," was released in May 2001.

Table 9.2. Federal regulations regarding postmarketing adverse event reporting

21 CFR 310.305 Prescription drugs not subject to premarket approval	[July 3, 1986 (51 FR 24779), amended October 13, 1987 (52 FR 37936); March 29, 1990 (55 FR 1578); April 28, 1992 (57 FR 17980); June 25, 1997 (62 FR 34167); October 7, 1997 (62 FR 52249); March 4, 2002 (67 FR 9585)]
21 CFR 314.80 Human drugs with approved new drug applications (NDAs)	[February 22, 1985 (50 FR 7493) and April 11, 1985 (50 FR 14212), amended May 23, 1985 (50 FR 21238); July 3, 1986 (51 FR 24481); October 13, 1987 (52 FR 37936); March 29, 1990 (55 FR 11580); April 28, 1992 (57 FR 17983); June 25, 1997 (62 FR 34166, 34168); October 7, 1997 (62 FR 52251); March 26, 1998 (63 FR 14611); March 4, 2002 (67 FR 9586)]
21 CFR 314.98 Human drugs with approved abbreviated new drug applications (ANDAs)	[April 28, 1992 (57 FR 17983), amended January 5, 1999 (64 FR 401)]
21 CFR 600.80 Biological products with approved product license applications (PLAs)	[October 27, 1994 (59 FR 54042), amended June 25, 1997 (62 FR 34168); October 7, 1997 (62 FR 52252); March 26, 1998 (63 FR 14612); October 20, 1999 (64 FR 56449)]

- A memo entitled, "Postmarketing Expedited Safety Reports—15-Day Alert Reports," was added to public Docket 92S-0251 on May 22, 2002. This memo allows for voluntary electronic reporting of 15-day (expedited) safety reports with no paper submissions required.
- A draft Guidance for Industry entitled, "Providing Regulatory Submissions in Electronic Format—Postmarketing Periodic Adverse Drug Experience Reports," was published on June 24, 2003.

As of the end of 2003, nearly 20% of all expedited reports were submitted electronically, and the FDA encourages firms to participate in this voluntary process, replacing MedWatch (3500A) reports. To facilitate this effort, the FDA hosts a meeting twice yearly with representatives from major pharmaceutical firms. The purpose of this meeting is to discuss electronic AE reporting, including ways to stimulate increased electronic reporting within the industry. A description of the process of how the FDA handles these reports will be provided in a later section of this chapter.

Recent Changes

In recent years, there has been a significant international effort to standardize the pharmaceutical regulatory environment worldwide through the auspices of the International Conference on Harmonisation (ICH) of Technical Requirements for Registration of Pharmaceuticals for Human Use. These efforts toward international harmonization have a direct impact on how the FDA is currently rewriting regulations on AE reporting. AERS was launched in November 1997 and is an internationally compatible system in full accordance with the ICH initiatives.

The initiatives that directly affect postmarketing surveillance are:

- M1 IMT (International Medical Terminology): AERS uses the Medical Dictionary for Regulatory Activities (MedDRA) as its coding tool for reported adverse reaction/adverse event terms via individual case safety reports.
- M2 ESTRI (Electronic Standards for the Transfer of Regulatory Information): AERS uses ESTRI standards for submission of individual case safety reports in electronic form via the electronic data interchange (EDI) gateway.
- E2B(M) (Data Elements for Transmission of Individual Case Safety Reports): AERS has implemented the E2B data format into its database, and will use the E2B as the standard for electronic submissions.
- E2C PSUR (Periodic Safety Update Reports): defines a standard format for clinical safety data management for PSURs for marketed drugs. Initially, PSURs will be submitted on paper, and the FDA has published guidance to allow these summaries to be sent in electronically to the electronic Central Document Room (eCDR).

The Agency has undertaken a major effort in implementation of the electronic reporting of Individual Case Safety Reports (ICSRs) based on the ICH E2B(M), M1 (MedDRA), and M2 standards, and to clarify and revise its regulations regarding pre- and postmarketing safety reporting requirements for human drug and biologic products. In the *Federal Register* of October 7, 1997 (62 FR 52237), the FDA published a final rule amending its regulations for expedited safety reporting. This final rule implements the ICH E2A initiative on clinical safety data management. Based on E2A, the final rule provides an internationally accepted definition of "serious," requires the submission of the MedWatch 3500A for paper submissions, requires expedited reports in a 15 calendar rather than working day time frame, and harmonizes procedures for reporting pre- and postmarketing as well as international and domestic reporting. With regard to the postmarketing safety reporting regulations for human drug and licensed biologic products, the Agency published a proposed rule in the *Federal Register* of October 27, 1994 (59 FR 54046), to amend these requirements, as well as others, to implement international standards, and to facilitate the reporting of adverse experiences.

To help the pharmaceutical manufacturers understand the new requirements, on August 27, 1998 the FDA published an interim guidance for industry, "Postmarketing Adverse Experience Reporting for Human Drugs and Licensed Biological Products: Clarification of What to Report."

In the *Federal Register* of November 5, 1998 (63 FR 59746), the Agency published an Advanced Notice of Proposed Rulemaking to notify manufacturers that it is considering preparing a proposed rule that would require them to submit individual case reports electronically using standardized medical terminology, standardized data elements, and electronic transmission standards as recommended by ICH in the M1, M2, and E2B(M) initiatives. The FDA published a Public Docket 92A-0251, "Electronic Submission of Postmarketing Expedited Periodic Individual Case Safety Reports," which allows pharmaceutical companies to submit reports to the FDA electronically.

In March 2001, the Agency issued a "Guidance for Industry: Postmarketing Safety Reporting for Human Drug and Biological Products Including Vaccines," which superceded the March 1992 document.

The November 2001 Guidance for Industry "Electronic Submission of Postmarketing Expedited Safety Reports," describes how pharmaceutical companies may submit ICSRs using EDI gateway and physical media (e.g., CD-ROM) and attachments to ICSRs using only physical media.

In May 2002, the FDA issued a Guidance for Industry "Providing Regulatory Submissions in Electronic Format— Postmarketing Periodic Adverse Drug Experience Reports," which describes how pharmaceutical companies may submit periodic ICSRs with and without attachments and descriptive information (including PSURs) using physical media.

In September 2003, the FDA issued a Guidance for Industry "Providing Regulatory Submissions in Electronic Format— Annual Reports for NDAs and ANDAs," which describes how pharmaceutical companies may submit descriptive information (including PSURs) using physical media.

On October 1, 2003, the FDA transferred certain product oversight responsibilities from the Center for Biologics Evaluation and Research (CBER) to the CDER. This consolidation provides greater opportunities to further develop and coordinate scientific and regulatory activities between CBER and CDER, leading to a more efficient and consistent review program for human drugs and biologics. The FDA believes that as more drugs and biologic products are developed for a broader range of illnesses, such interaction is necessary for both efficient and consistent agency action. Under the new structure, the biologic products transferred to CDER will continue to be regulated as licensed biologics.

PROPOSED MODIFICATIONS

At the current time, the FDA is working on further modifications to the postmarketing safety reporting requirements. A Serious Adverse Drug Reaction (SADR) Reporting Proposed Rule is expected to be published in the near future, that focuses on report quality, standardizes terminology to "Adverse Drug Reaction," and encourages active query by health care professional at the company who speaks directly with the initial reporter of the serious adverse reaction report. This entails, at a minimum, a focused line of questioning designed to capture clinically relevant information, follow-up, and determination of seriousness, and defines the minimum data set for safety reports. The proposed rule will also implement the ICH E2C: International PSUR, which contains marketing status, core labeling (company core data sheet (CCDS); company core safety information (CCSI) is safety information in CCDS), changes in safety status since last report, exposure data, clinical explanation of cases, data line (narrative summary of the individual case safety reports which provide demographic, drug, and event information) listings and tables, status of postmarketing surveillance safety studies, overall critical analyses, and assessments. The earlier October 27, 1994 proposed amendments to the postmarketing periodic AE reporting requirements will be reproposed in this current Proposed Rule, based on a guidance on this topic developed by ICH.[22]

As noted previously, OTC products without an NDA are not subject to reporting. To bring these products into the postmarketing safety net, the FDA plans to publish an OTC ADR Reporting Proposed Rule. Consideration is being given to the requirement for ADR reporting for OTC monograph drugs, since most marketed OTC drugs lack an approved NDA. The FDA's review of marketed OTC drugs without approved NDAs (ANDAs) has been accomplished through rulemaking establishing conditions in OTC drug monographs for drugs within therapeutic classes (e.g., laxatives). An OTC drug monograph specifies the conditions (i.e., ingredients and concentrations, testing procedures, dosage, labeling, and mode of administration) under which an OTC drug is generally recognized as safe and effective and is not misbranded.

In an effort to expand the Agency's ability to monitor and improve the safe use of human and biologic products both during clinical trials and once the products are on the market, the FDA on March 14, 2003 published a proposed rule, titled "Safety Reporting Requirements for Human Drug and Biological Products" (*"The Tome"*), which would require companies to file expedited reports of suspected ADRs unless the company is certain the product did not cause the reaction.

The Tome recommended the replacement of periodic drug adverse experience reports (21 CFR 314.80) with PSURs. Currently, CDER encourages industry to submit a waiver to allow submission of PSURs instead of periodic drug adverse experience reports. PSURs are in the format proposed by the ICH of Technical Requirements for Registration of Pharmaceuticals for Human Use, Topic E2C. The PSUR summarizes the safety data received by a sponsor for an application from worldwide sources for a specific time frame. The number of PSURs received is dependent on the number of NDAs/ANDAs marketed. The PSUR format enhances postmarketing drug and therapeutic biologic safety because it requires additional information and analyses (such as patient exposure data) not required in the periodic adverse drug experience report. These additional data enhance our review of postmarketing safety.

DATA COLLECTION: THE MEDWATCH PROGRAM

An effective national postmarketing surveillance system depends on voluntary reporting of adverse events, medication errors, and product quality problems by health professionals and consumers to the FDA, either directly or via the manufacturer. Neither individual health professionals nor hospitals are required by Federal law or regulation to submit AE reports on pharmaceuticals, although Federal law does require hospitals and other "user facilities" to report deaths and serious injuries that occur with medical devices.[23]

Many health care organizations recommend and promote the reporting of AEs to the FDA. Adverse event monitoring by hospitals is included in the Joint Commission on the Accreditation of Health Care Organizations (JCAHO) standards for patient safety issued in 2003. In order to maintain full accreditation, JCAHO requires each health care organization to monitor for adverse events involving pharmaceuticals and devices, with medication monitoring to be a continual collaborative function. JCAHO standards indicate that medical product AE reporting should be done per applicable law/regulation, including those of state/Federal bodies.[24]

The FDA encourages all health care providers (physicians, pharmacists, nurses, dentists, and others) to consider adverse event reporting to the FDA as part of their professional responsibility. The American Society of Health-System Pharmacists has issued guidelines on ADR monitoring and reporting.[25]

The American Medical Association and American Dental Association advocate physician and dentist participation in adverse event reporting systems as an obligation.[26,27] Since 1994, The *Journal of the American Medical Association* has instructed its authors that adverse drug or device reactions should be reported to the appropriate government agency, in addition to submitting such information for publication.[28] The International Committee of Medical Journal Editors have revised the "Uniform Requirements for Manuscripts Submitted to Biomedical Journals" to also encourage timely reporting of urgent public health hazards.[29]

Given the vital importance of postmarketing surveillance, MedWatch, the FDA Safety Information and Adverse Event Reporting Program, was established in 1993.[30,31] While the FDA's longstanding postmarketing surveillance program predates MedWatch, this outreach initiative to health care professionals and patients was designed to promote and facilitate the voluntary reporting process by both health care providers and their patients.

The MedWatch program has four goals. The first is to increase awareness of drug, device, and other medical product-induced disease and the importance of reporting. Health professionals are taught that no drug or other medical product is without risk and are encouraged to consider medical products as possible causes when assessing a clinical problem in a patient. This goal is accomplished through educational outreach, which includes professional presentations, publications, and a continuing education program.[32]

The second goal of MedWatch is to clarify what should be reported. Health professionals and their patients are encouraged to limit reporting to serious AEs, enabling the FDA and the manufacturer to focus on the most potentially significant events. Causality is not a prerequisite for reporting; suspicion that a medical product may be related to a serious event is sufficient reason to notify the FDA and/or the manufacturer.

The third goal is to make it convenient and simple to submit a report of a serious AE, medication error, or product quality problem directly to the FDA. A single-page form is used for reporting suspected problems with all human-use medical products (except vaccines) regulated by the Agency—drugs, biologics, medical devices, special nutritionals (e.g., dietary supplements, medical foods, infant formulas), and cosmetics. There are two versions of the form (see Figures 9.2 and 9.3). The FDA form 3500 is used for voluntary reporting, while the FDA form 3500A is used for mandatory reporting. Both forms are available on the FDA MedWatch website (http://www.fda.gov/medwatch) and may be downloaded as fillable forms for saving and printing. The postage-paid FDA 3500 form may be returned to the FDA by mail or by fax to 1-800-FDA-0178.

In 1998, the MedWatch program implemented an online version of the voluntary FDA 3500 form for reporting via the Internet (see www.fda.gov/medwatch). In 2003, about 40% of the direct (voluntary) reports received from providers and consumers were sent to the FDA via this online application. In addition, MedWatch provides a toll-free 800 phone number, 1-800-FDA-1088, for reporters who wish to submit a report verbally to a MedWatch health professional.

Vaccines are the only FDA-regulated human-use medical products that are not reported on the MedWatch reporting form. Reports concerning vaccines are sent to the vaccine adverse event reporting system (VAERS) on the VAERS-1 form, available by calling 1-800-822-7967 or from the VAERS website at www.fda.gov/cber/vaers/vaers.htm. VAERS is a joint FDA/Center for Disease Control and Prevention program for mandatory reporting by physicians of vaccine-related adverse events (see also Chapter 30).

The FDA recognizes that health professionals have concerns regarding their confidentiality as reporters, and that of the patients whose cases they report. In order to encourage reporting of adverse events, FDA regulations offer substantial protection against disclosure of the identities of both reporters and patients. In 1995, a regulation went into effect strengthening this protection against disclosure by preempting state discovery laws regarding voluntary reports held by pharmaceutical, biological, and medical device manufacturers.[33] In addition, the Health Insurance Portability and Accountability Act (HIPAA) Privacy Rule (see www.fda.gov/medwatch/hipaa.htm) specifically permits pharmacists, physicians, or hospitals to continue to report adverse events and other information related to the quality, effectiveness, and safety of FDA-regulated products (see also Chapter 38).

Manufacturers who participate in the FDA "MedWatch to Manufacturer" program (MMP) are provided with copies of serious reports submitted directly to the FDA for new molecular entities (see www.fda.gov/medwatch). To facilitate obtaining follow-up information, health professionals who report directly to the FDA are asked to indicate whether they prefer that their identity not be disclosed through the MMP to the manufacturer of the product involved in the case being reported. When such a preference is indicated, this information will not be shared.

The fourth goal of MedWatch is to provide timely and clinically useful safety information on all FDA-regulated medical products to health care professionals and their patients. The FDA's interest in informing health professionals about new safety findings is not only to enable them to incorporate new safety information into daily practice, but also to demonstrate that voluntary reporting has a definite clinical impact.

As new information becomes available through "Dear Health Professional Letters," public health advisories and safety alerts, it is posted on the MedWatch website and immediate notification of the posting is sent by email to subscribers of the MedWatch listserve. This listserve reaches health care professionals, consumers, and the media. In 2004, MedWatch disseminated new safety information on over 45 drug or therapeutic biologic products as "safety alerts" to over 45 000 individual subscribers. One can subscribe to the MedWatch listserve by visiting the website (http://www.fda.gov/medwatch/elist.htm).

MedWatch also has a network of more than 160 health care professional, health care consumer and health care media organizations that have allied themselves with the FDA as MedWatch Partners. Each of these organizations works with MedWatch to promote voluntary reporting and disseminate safety information notifications to their members or subscribers by using their websites, email distribution lists, and publications such as bulletins and journals.

SAFETY ASSESSMENT: THE ADVERSE EVENT REPORTING SYSTEM (AERS)

AERS is a client–server, Oracle-based relational database system that contains all AE reports on pharmaceuticals submitted to the Agency either directly or via the manufacturer. The mission of AERS is to reduce adverse events related to FDA-regulated products by improving postmarketing surveillance and helping to prevent adverse outcomes related to medical errors.

AERS was designed and implemented with the following concepts in mind:

- friendly screen layout and help function;
- enhanced search capabilities, quality control features and electronic review of reports;
- improve the operational efficiency, effectiveness, and quality control of the process for handling AEs;
- improve the accessibility of AE information to all safety evaluators and medical officers within the FDA;
- implement and maintain compatibility with ICH standards;
- build the capability to receive electronic submissions of AEs using ICH standards;
- provide automated signal generation capabilities and improved tools for the analysis of potential AE signals.

Pharmaceutical manufacturers submit paper AE reports to the FDA central document room, where they are tracked and forwarded to the Office of Drug Safety (ODS) in the FDA's CDER. Reports submitted by individuals are mailed, faxed, sent via the Internet, or phoned into MedWatch, and are triaged to the appropriate FDA Center(s) (i.e., CDER, CBER, Center for Devices and Radiological Health (CDRH), Center for Veterinary Medicine (CVM), and CFSAN).

When received by the ODS, these incoming 3500 and 3500A reports are assigned a permanent report number (individual safety report), imaged, and stored in a Retrieval-Ware Imaging System; subsequently they are entered verbatim into the AERS database. Data entry has a number of sequential steps involving comparative entry, quality comparison of critical entry fields, and coding and quality control into standardized international medical terminology using MedDRA. Direct and 15-day expedited reports receive priority handling and are entered into AERS within 14 days.

Automated quality control is performed to review reports for timeliness, completeness, and accuracy of coding. Statistical samples are also used to spot check manufacturer performance in providing accurate and timely reports, which can be used for compliance functions.

Although the bulk of the data entry into AERS is currently done through manual coding, AERS is designed for electronic submission of ICH E2B(M) standardized, MedDRA precoded individual case safety reports. This design concept incorporates the ICH standards for content, structure, and transmittal of individual case safety reports. To prepare for full-scale implementation of electronic submissions, a step-by-step pilot program was in place. The pilot moved into full production in 2002 for capturing ICSRs.

Copies of all reports in the AERS database are available to the public through the FDA Freedom of Information Office, with all confidential information redacted (e.g., patient, reporter, institutional identifiers). The AERS database, in non-cumulative quarterly updates, can be obtained from the National Technical Information Service (www.NTIS.gov) or from the FDA website (www.fda.gov/cder/aers/extract.htm).

A variety of technology-assisted features in the AERS augment the AE review by the ODS's safety evaluators. Safety evaluators have the following pharmacovigilance tools available for AE report screening to generate signals:

- *Primary triage*: the program screens incoming reports and alerts safety evaluators to serious and unlabeled events, and serious medical events known to be drug-related (e.g., *torsade de pointes*, agranulocytosis, toxic epidermal necrolysis, etc.).

- *Secondary triage/surveillance*: provides a tool for signal identification based on overall specific counts for each risk category associated with all ADR reports received for a given drug.
- *Periodic (canned) reports*: enables periodic reviews of the AERS database, including all new actions in a time period.
- *Active (canned and/or ad hoc) query*: represents active investigation of case series signals found from any of the above levels of screening.

The AERS maximizes the ability of the Agency to identify and assess signals of importance in the spontaneous reporting system. Starting in 2004 and over a 5-year period, these upgrades will occur in what we are calling AERS II. AERS will be upgraded to handle the FDA's processing of post-marketing adverse event reports related to human drugs and therapeutic biologics over the next 5 years. It will be web based, accept electronic submissions, meet ICH, HL7, E2B(M), eXtensible Markup Language (XML), and Tagged Image File Format (TIFF) requirements; handle multiple product coding schemes (bar codes), interface to industry and other government systems, and include a reporting repository providing pre-tailored reports and an ad hoc feature for specialized needs.

FDA EVALUATION OF REPORTS OF ADVERSE EVENTS

Every single workday, the FDA receives nearly one thousand spontaneous reports of adverse events either directly or through the industry. The ODS in CDER employs about 25 postmarketing safety evaluators and over a dozen epidemiologists.

The primary duty of safety evaluators is to review adverse event reports. Most of the safety evaluators are clinical pharmacists who are assigned specific groups or classes of drugs or therapeutic biologic products based on their past training and/or experience. These safety evaluators work under the tutelage and guidance of about half a dozen team leaders who have considerable experience in the evaluation and assessment of adverse event reports, substantial knowledge of the drug or therapeutic biologic agent, and awareness of the limitations of the AERS data. Every serious labeled or unlabeled adverse event report or reports describing important medical events such as liver failure, cardiac arrhythmias, renal failure, and rhabdomyolysis are electronically transferred into the computer inbox of the safety evaluators, who monitor these events daily. The safety evaluators try to identify a potential "signal," which is defined as a previously unrecognized or unidentified serious adverse event.

Epidemiologists within the ODS are medical/clinical epidemiologists with MDs/MPHs or PhDs. Medical epidemiologists help in the "signal" development by evaluation of potential adverse event case reports (numerator data) and identification of risk factors/confounders. Epidemiologists are frequently asked to quantify and describe the exposed population (denominator data). Epidemiologists also critique published and unpublished epidemiologic studies, and participate in the design and development of protocols for epidemiologic studies submitted by drug companies in areas of regulatory interest.

The essential elements of a case report include drug name, concise description of the adverse event, date of onset of the event, drug start/stop dates, if applicable, baseline patient status (comorbid conditions, use of concomitant medications, presence of risk factors), dose and frequency of administration, relevant laboratory values at baseline and during therapy, biopsy/autopsy reports, patient demographics, de-challenge (event abates when the drug is discontinued) and re-challenge (event recurs when drug is restarted), and information about confounding drugs or conditions where available. For example, in a report describing hepatotoxicity, baseline information about liver status and information about liver enzyme monitoring would be considered essential.[34]

If a "signal" is noted, the safety evaluator may try to find additional cases by querying the AERS database, doing literature searches, contacting foreign regulatory agencies directly, or collecting cases through the World Health Organization (WHO) Uppsala Monitoring Centre in Sweden. If the report is poorly documented, the safety evaluator may contact the reporter or the manufacturer for follow-up information. A case definition may be developed in collaboration with an epidemiologist and refined as new cases are identified. After a case series is assembled, the safety evaluator may look for common trends, potential risk factors, or any other items of importance. Meanwhile, with the help of drug utilization specialists in the ODS, drug usage data is obtained for the relevant drug or class of drugs or drugs within the same therapeutic category. Drug usage data are used in a variety of ways, including to obtain demographic information on the population exposed to pharmaceutical products, average duration and dose of dispensed prescription, and the specialty of the prescribing physicians. These data allow the FDA to examine how long non-hospitalized patients stay on prescription medication therapy and to learn drug combinations that may be prescribed to the same patients concurrently. These data are also used in association with AERS data to understand the context within which ADEs occur. Additionally, one or more epidemiologists may be consulted to find the background incidence of the adverse outcome in question and to estimate the reporting rates of the adverse outcome, and compare it with the background rate at which the same event occurs in the population. Simply stated, a reporting rate is the number of reported cases of an adverse event of interest divided by some measure of the suspect drug's utilization, usually the number of dispensed prescriptions.[35] If the issue is of regulatory importance, it may be brought to the attention of others within the ODS by presentation at one of the two in-house ODS forums, the Safety Evaluator Forum and the Epi Forum. At these forums relevant personnel from the review divisions in the CDER Office of New Drugs may be invited since they are ultimately responsible for regulatory actions involving the marketing status of the product. The review division may request manufacturer-sponsored postmarketing studies to further evaluate the issue. Simultaneously, epidemiologists in the ODS may explore the feasibility of conducting pharmacoepidemiology studies in one or more large claims database(s) that link prescriptions with medical records. The FDA has funded extramural researchers through a system of cooperative agreement for more than a decade. These investigators have access to large population-based databases and the FDA utilizes their resources to answer drug safety questions and to study the impact of regulatory decisions.

After confirmation of a "signal" the FDA can initiate various regulatory actions, the extent and rigor of which depend on the seriousness of the adverse event, the availability, safety, the acceptability of alternative therapy, and the outcome of previous regulatory interventions.[4] Regulatory interventions to manage the risk include labeling change such as a boxed warning, restricted use or distribution of the drug, name or packaging change(s), a "Dear Health Care Professional" letter, or, rarely, possible withdrawal of a medical product from the market (see Table 9.3 and also Chapter 33).

The time between the first identification of a safety risk and the implementation of a regulatory action may take several months to years depending on the nature of the problem and the public health impact. For example, several years elapsed between the time when dangerous drug interactions with cisapride and a number of other drugs were identified and when the drug was ultimately removed from the market for general use. Similarly, severe liver failure in association with the use of the antidiabetic drug troglitazone was noted a few months after marketing but it took a few years before the drug was removed from the market. In the examples of both cisapride and troglitazone, a variety of regulatory interventions, such as repeated labeling changes and "Dear Health Care Professional" letters, were applied over the years

Table 9.3. Recent safety-based drug withdrawals

Drug name	Year approved/year withdrawn
Phenylpropanolamine	—/2000 (never approved by FDA)
Fenfluramine	1973/1997
Terfenadine	1985/1998
Astemizole	1988/1999
Cisapride	1993/2000
Dexfenfluramine	1996/1997 (not an NME)
Bromfenac	1997/1998
Cerivastatin	1997/2001
Grepafloxin	1997/1999
Mibefradil	1997/1998
Troglitazone	1997/2000
Rapacuronium	1999/2001
Rofecoxib	1999/2004
Alosetron*	2000/2000
Valdecoxib	2001/2005

* Returned to market in 2002 with restricted distribution.

to manage the risk before these products were removed from the market. These regulatory interventions did not achieve meaningful improvement in prevention of contraindicated drug use or in liver enzyme testing, respectively.[36,37]

To notify health professionals of important new safety information discovered after marketing, the FDA often requests that the manufacturer send a "Dear Health Care Professional" letter to warn providers of particular safety issues. This is done in combination with a labeling change, although only a small proportion of labeling changes result in such letters. Frequently, the change in labeling may be accompanied by issuance of a press release (also known as a Talk Paper) or public health advisory. Additionally, FDA scientists may disseminate new drug safety information through publications in professional journals[38–65] and presentations at professional meetings.

There were 43 drug or biologic letters/safety notifications posted in 2002 and 36 in 2003. In 2003, safety-related labeling changes were approved by the FDA for 20–45 drug products each month. "Dear Health Care Professional" letters and other safety notifications, and summaries of safety-related labeling changes approved each month, can be found on the MedWatch website (www.fda.gov/medwatch/safety.htm). Table 9.4 lists some examples of recent "Dear Health Care Professional" letters.

The FDA can seek to restrict or limit the use of a drug product through labeling if the adverse reaction associated with the drug has severe consequences. For example, the labeling for the new arthritis/pain drug valdecoxib was strengthened with new warnings following postmarketing

reports of serious adverse effects, including life-threatening risks related to skin reactions—including Stevens–Johnson Syndrome, and anaphylactoid reactions. The labeling now advises people who start valdecoxib and experience a rash to discontinue the drug immediately and also the drug is contraindicated in patients allergic to sulfa-containing products. The drug has recently been removed from the market.

Drug safety problems can also lead to the removal of a drug from the market. Fortunately, such product withdrawals are very uncommon; there have been only 22 drugs taken off the US market since 1980; drugs withdrawn recently are listed in Table 9.3.

In addition to the technology used in current adverse event reporting, including sophisticated relational databases and network connections for electronic transfer, new methods to evaluate and assess spontaneous reports are being explored to take advantage of the sheer volume of data. Aggregate analysis tools and data mining techniques are currently being developed by ODS, WHO,[66] and others, to systematically screen large databases of spontaneous reports.

Since 1998, the FDA has explored automated and rapid Bayesian data mining techniques to enhance its ability to monitor the safety of drugs, biologics, and vaccines after they have been approved for use.[67] In May 2003, the FDA announced the establishment of a Cooperative Research and Development Agreement (CRADA) with a private software development company. The CRADA is expected to improve the utility of safety data mining technology. The FDA's CDER and CBER will work with this private company to develop new and innovative ways for extracting information related to drug safety and risk assessment. To this end, a desktop data mining software tool, called WebVDME, has been developed and is currently being piloted.

Data mining is a technique for extracting meaningful, organized information from large complex databases. In data mining the strategy is to use a computer to identify potential signals in large databases that might be overlooked, for a variety of reasons, in a manual review on a case-by-case basis. Drug–AE signals are generated by comparing the frequency of reports with what would be expected if all drugs and AEs were assumed to follow certain patterns. The goal is to distinguish the more important or stronger signals to facilitate identification of combinations of drugs and events that warrant more in-depth follow-up. Data mining is a tool best suited for generation of possible signals and it cannot replace or override the meticulous hands-on review by safety evaluators. Further, whether it has any advantage over the hands-on review,

Table 9.4. Recent FDA MedWatch safety alerts/"Dear Health Care Professional" letters, 2003

Drug	Details
Topamax® (topiramate)	Revised the WARNINGS and PRECAUTIONS to notify health care professionals that Topamax causes hyperchloremic, non-anion gap metabolic acidosis (decreased serum bicarbonate). Measurement of baseline and periodic serum bicarbonate during topiramate treatment is recommended.
Permax® (pergolide mesylate)	Revised the WARNINGS and PRECAUTIONS sections to inform health care professionals of the possibility of patients falling asleep while performing daily activities, including operation of motor vehicles, while receiving treatment with Permax®. Many patients who have fallen asleep have perceived no warning of somnolence.
Arava® (leflunomide)	In postmarketing experience worldwide, rare, serious hepatic injury, including cases with fatal outcome, have been reported during treatment with Arava. Most cases occurred within 6 months of therapy and in a setting of multiple risk factors for hepatotoxicity.
Viread® (tenofovir disoproxil fumarate)	Notified health care professionals of a high rate of early virologic failure and emergence of nucleoside reverse transcriptase inhibitor resistance associated mutations in a clinical study of HIV-infected treatment-naive patients receiving a triple regimen of didanosine, lamivudine and tenofovir disoproxil fumarate.
Lariam® (mefloquine hydrochloride)	Notified health care professionals of the Lariam Medication Guide developed in collaboration with the FDA to help travelers better understand the risks of malaria, the risks and benefits associated with taking Lariam to prevent malaria, and the potentially serious psychiatric adverse events associated with use of the drug.
Prandin® (repaglinide)	Revised the PRECAUTIONS/Drug Interaction section to inform health care professionals of a drug–drug interaction between repaglinide and gemfibrozil. Concomitant use may result in enhanced and prolonged blood glucose-lowering effects of repaglinide.
Serevent Inhalation Aerosol® (salmeterol xinafoate)	New labeling includes a boxed warning about a small, but significant, increased risk of life-threatening asthma episodes or asthma-related deaths observed in patients taking salmeterol in a recently completed large US safety study.
Ziagen® (abacavir)	High rate of early virologic non-response observed in a clinical study of therapy-naive adults with HIV infection receiving once-daily three-drug combination therapy with lamivudine (Epivir, GSK), abacavir (Ziagen, GSK), and tenofovir (Viread, TDF, Gilead Sciences).
Genotropin® (somatropin [rDNA origin] for injection)	Fatalities have been reported with the use of growth hormone in pediatric patients with Prader–Willi syndrome with one or more of the following risk factors: severe obesity, history of respiratory impairment or sleep apnea, or unidentified respiratory infection.
Topamax® (topiramate) tablets/ sprinkle capsules	Oligohidrosis (decreased sweating) and hyperthermia have been reported in topiramate-treated patients. Oligohidrosis and hyperthermia may have potentially serious sequelae, which may be preventable by prompt recognition of symptoms and appropriate treatment.
Risperdal® (risperidone)	Cerebrovascular adverse events (e.g., stroke, transient ischemic attack), including fatalities, were reported in patients in trials of risperidone in elderly patients with dementia-related psychosis.
Avonex® (Interferon beta-1a)	Postmarketing reports of depression, suicidal ideation and/or development of new or worsening of pre-existing psychiatric disorders, including psychosis, and reports of anaphylaxis, pancytopenia, thrombocytopenia, autoimmune disorders of multiple target organs, and hepatic injury.

and the degree to which it generates false signals, remain to be evaluated.

STRENGTHS

LARGE-SCALE AND COST-EFFECTIVE

Two vital advantages of surveillance systems based on spontaneous reports are that they potentially maintain ongoing surveillance of all patients, and are relatively inexpensive.[68] Spontaneous reporting systems are the most common method used in pharmacovigilance to generate signals on new or rare adverse events not discovered during clinical trials.[69]

GENERATION OF HYPOTHESES AND SIGNALS

Making the best possible use of the data obtained through monitoring underlies postmarketing surveillance.[70] Toward that goal, the great utility of spontaneous reports lies in *hypothesis generation*,[71] with need to explore possible explanations for the adverse event in question. By raising suspicions,[72] spontaneous report-based surveillance programs perform an important function, which is to generate *signals* of potential problems that warrant further investigation.

Assessment of the medical product–adverse event relationship for a particular report or series of reports can be quite difficult. Table 9.5 lists factors that are helpful in evaluating the strength of association between a drug and a reported adverse event.[73]

The stronger the drug–event relationship in each case and the lower the incidence of the adverse event occurring spontaneously, the fewer case reports are needed to perceive causality.[74] It has been found that for rare events, coincidental drug–event associations are so unlikely that they merit little concern, with greater than three reports constituting a signal requiring further study.[75] In fact, it has been suggested that a temporal relationship between medical product and adverse event, coupled with positive de-challenge and re-challenge,

Table 9.5. Useful factors for assessing causal relationship between drug and reported adverse events

---

- Chronology of administration of agent, including beginning and ending of treatment and adverse event onset
- Course of adverse event when suspected agent stopped (de-challenge) or continued
- Etiologic roles of agents and diseases in regard to adverse event
- Response to readministration (re-challenge) of agent
- Laboratory test results
- Previously known toxicity of agent

---

can occasionally make isolated reports conclusive as to a product–event association.[76] Biological plausibility and reasonable strength of association aid in deeming any association as causal[77] (see also Chapter 36).

However, achieving certain proof of causality through adverse event reporting is unusual. Confirmation of an association between a drug and an adverse reaction usually requires further additional studies.[78] Attaining a prominent degree of suspicion is much more likely, but still may be considered a sufficient basis for regulatory decisions.[74]

OPPORTUNITY FOR CLINICIAN CONTRIBUTIONS

The reliance of postmarketing surveillance systems on health professional reporting enables an individual to help improve public health. This is demonstrated by one study that found direct practitioner participation in the FDA spontaneous reporting system was the most effective source of new ADR reports that led to changes in labeling.[76] Ensuring that the information provided in the adverse event report is as complete and in-depth as possible further enhances postmarketing surveillance. Thus, while possessing inherent limitations, postmarketing surveillance based on spontaneous reports data is a powerful tool for detecting adverse event signals of direct clinical impact.

WEAKNESSES

There are important limitations to consider when using spontaneously reported adverse event information. These limitations include difficulties with adverse event recognition, underreporting, biases, estimation of population exposure, and report quality.

ADVERSE EVENT RECOGNITION

The attribution of AEs (or any other medical product-associated adverse event) may be quite subjective and imprecise.[79] While an attribution of association between the medical product and the observed event is assumed by the reporters with all spontaneously reported events, every effort is made to rule out other explanations for the event in question. It is well known that placebos[80] and even no treatment[81] can be associated with adverse events. In addition, there is almost always an underlying background rate for any clinical event in a population, regardless of whether there was exposure to a medical product.

Reaching a firm conclusion about the relationship between exposure to a medical product and the occurrence of an adverse event can be difficult. In one study, clinical pharmacologists and treating physicians showed complete agreement less than half the time when determining whether medication, alcohol or "recreational" drug use had caused hospitalization.[82]

Such considerations emphasize the crucial need for careful, thoughtful review of adverse event reports upon their receipt by the FDA or the manufacturer. It is through this process that causality, or at least a high degree of suspicion for a product–adverse event association, is put to the test (see also Chapter 36). Ultimately, formal pharmacoepidemiology studies are usually needed to strengthen the observed association.

UNDERREPORTING

Another major concern with any spontaneous reporting system is underreporting of adverse events.[71, 77] The extent of underreporting is unknown and may be influenced by the severity of the event, the specialty of the reporter, how long the drug has been on the market, whether the event is labeled, and whether the drug is prescription or non-prescription.[83] It has been estimated that rarely more than 10% of serious ADRs, and 2–4% of non-serious reactions, are reported to the British spontaneous reporting program.[77] A similar estimate is that the FDA receives by direct report less than 1% of suspected serious ADRs.[84] This means that cases spontaneously reported to any surveillance program, which comprise the numerator, generally represent only a small portion of the number that have actually occurred. The impact of underreporting can be somewhat lessened if submitted reports, irrespective of number, are of high quality.

BIASES

Spontaneously reported information is subject to the influence of a number of biases. These include the length of time a product has been on the market, size of sponsors' detail force, target population, health care providers' awareness, the quality of the data, and publicity effects.[85–89]

In addition, it has been observed that spontaneous reporting of adverse events for a drug tends to peak at the end of the second year of marketing and reporting declines thereafter (Weber effect).[90]

In addition to these biases, it is possible that reported cases might differ from nonreported cases in characteristics such as time to onset or severity.[75]

ESTIMATION OF POPULATION EXPOSURE

Compounding these limitations is the lack of denominator data, such as user population and drug exposure patterns,[75] that would provide an estimate of the number of patients exposed to the medical product, and thus at risk for the adverse event of interest. Numerator and denominator limitations make incidence rates computed from spontaneously reported data problematic,[75] if not completely baseless. However, even if the exposed patient population is not precisely known, estimation of the exposure can be attempted through the use of drug utilization data.[91]

This approach, whose basic methodologies are applicable to medical products in general, can be of utility. Major sources of data on the use of drugs by a defined population include market surveys based on sales or prescription data, third-party payers or health maintenance organizations, institutional/ambulatory settings, or specific pharmacoepidemiology studies.[91] Cooperative agreements and contracts with outside researchers enable the FDA to use such databases in its investigations (see Part IIIb). Care must be taken in interpreting results from studies using these databases. That drug prescribing does not necessarily equal drug usage,[91] and the applicability of results derived from a specific population (such as Medicaid recipients) to the population at large, need to be weighed carefully.

REPORT QUALITY

The ability to assess, analyze, and act on safety issues based on spontaneous reporting is dependent on the quality of information submitted by health professionals in their reports. A complete adverse event report should include the following:

- product name (and information such as model and serial numbers in the case of medical devices);
- demographic data;
- succinct clinical description of the adverse event, including confirmatory/relevant test/laboratory results;
- confounding factors such as concomitant medical products and medical history;
- temporal information, including the date of event onset and start/stop dates for use of medical product;
- dose/frequency of use;
- biopsy/autopsy results;
- de-challenge/re-challenge information;
- outcome.

SUMMARY

The major limitations of the FDA's AE reporting system reflect the fact that the data are generated in an uncontrolled and incomplete manner. Although manufacturers are legally required to submit AE reports to the FDA and some of those reports are based on formal studies, the majority of AEs originate with practicing physicians who may or may not notify the manufacturer or the FDA when they observe an AE in one of their patients. It appears that they generally do not choose to report AEs, and the number of reports that the FDA receives is not representative of the extent of adverse events that occur in the United States. The number of reports in the system is also influenced by a variety of other factors, such as the extent and quality of the individual manufacturer's postmarketing surveillance activities, the nature of the event, the type of drug, the length of time it has been marketed, and publicity in the lay or professional press. Because of these limitations, AE reports are primarily useful for hypothesis generating, rather than hypothesis testing. Ironically, the scientifically uncontrolled nature of AE reporting creates its greatest advantage—the ability to detect and characterize AEs occurring across a broad range of medical practice—as well as its most serious limitations.

PARTICULAR APPLICATIONS

OVERALL

The FDA's AERS contains almost 3 million reports, with the earliest dating back to 1969. While reporting levels remained fairly constant during the 1970s—about 18 000 reports were entered into the database in 1970, and slightly over 14 000 reports were added in 1980—reporting increased dramatically after 1992, as can be seen in Figure 9.4. By 1992, the annual number of reports had risen to 120 000, and in 2003 was over 370 000. Forty percent of these reports were serious and unexpected (i.e., 15-day).

As noted earlier, the AERS contains reports from a variety of sources. Reports may be from the United States or other countries. The suspected AEs may have been observed in the usual practice of medicine or during formal studies; case reports from the literature are also included. Reports come to the FDA either directly from health professionals or consumers, or from pharmaceutical manufacturers. The vast majority (over 90%) of adverse drug event reports are received by the FDA through the manufacturer, with the remainder received directly from health care professionals or consumers.

In 2003, of all voluntary reports sent directly to the FDA, 68% involved drugs, 14% medical devices, 12% drug quality problems, 3% biologics, and 3% dietary supplements. The sources were: 59% from pharmacists, 15% from physicians, 9% from nurses, and 6% from non-health professionals (with 11% source not given).

SPECIFIC EXAMPLES

Temafloxacin (Omniflox®): Withdrawn from Market

This oral antibiotic was first marketed in February 1992. During the first three months of its use, the FDA received approximately 50 reports of serious adverse events, including three deaths. These events included hypoglycemia in elderly patients as well as a constellation of multi-system organ involvement characterized by hemolytic anemia, frequently associated with renal failure, markedly abnormal liver function tests, and coagulopathy. When approved by the FDA, temafloxacin was already being used in Argentina, Germany, Italy, Ireland, Sweden, and the United Kingdom. However, the FDA's experience with this drug demonstrates the critical importance of postmarketing surveillance and the timely reporting of adverse events. Prior to FDA approval, slightly more than 4000 patients had received the drug in clinical trials, and temafloxacin was considered to have a side effect profile similar to other quinolone antibiotics. In its first three months of commercial marketing, many thousands of patients received the drug. Only after this much broader clinical experience did the serious side effects described above become apparent. Less than four months after its introduction into the marketplace, the drug was withdrawn.[92]

Linezolid (Zyvox®): Serious, Unlabeled ADR Noted Shortly After Approval

Linezolid (Zyvox®), a synthetic antibacterial agent of the oxazolidinone class, was approved for use in April 2000. It is indicated for the treatment of adult patients with the following infections caused by susceptible strains of designated microorganisms: vancomycin-resistant *Enterococcus faecium*, including cases with concurrent bacteremia; nosocomial pneumonia; complicated and uncomplicated skin and skin structure infections; and community-acquired pneumonia, including cases with concurrent bacteremia.

At the time of approval, safety data were limited, based primarily on its use in controlled clinical trials. The most serious adverse event noted in the initial product labeling was thrombocytopenia, mentioned in the Precautions section and the Laboratory Changes subsection of the Adverse Reactions section.

As reported in the Animal Pharmacology section of the product labeling, linezolid had caused dose- and time-dependent myelosuppression, as evidenced by bone marrow hypocellularity, decreased hematopoiesis, and decreased levels of circulating erythrocytes, leukocytes, and platelets in animal studies.

Within the first six months the drug was on the market, four cases of red cell aplasia associated with its use were received by the FDA. In addition, six other cases suggestive of myelosuppression had been submitted, as well as two cases of sideroblastic anemia.

With the increasing number of cases being received by the FDA, an in-depth review of this problem was undertaken. AERS was searched for reports of hematologic toxicity associated with linezolid and a total of 27 reports were retrieved through September 20, 2000. These reports were reviewed to find any that may have been suggestive of myelosuppression but were not necessarily reported as such (e.g., reductions in white blood count, hemoglobin and hematocrit, and platelets). In addition to the four red cell aplasia cases, six additional cases suggestive of myelosuppression were identified:

- A bone marrow transplant recipient who had a delayed engraftment that was thought to be due to linezolid myelosuppression.
- Three cases reported as routine complete blood counts (CBC), revealing decreased white blood cells (WBC), hemoglobin and hematocrit, and platelets. Personal communication with the reporters in these three cases found no further follow-up such as bone marrow biopsy, nor progression to more serious disease.
- Two cases were received as direct reports; one described as bone marrow suppression and thrombocytopenia in a 65-year-old male and the other as pancytopenia in a 51-year-old female.

Because of the rapidity with which these cases were reported to the FDA in the short time linezolid had been on the market, and the relatively small estimated number of courses of therapy sold, the FDA and the manufacturer agreed to the addition of prominent warnings to be included in the labeling concerning the development of myelosuppression. Changes were made to the Warnings and Precautions sections to recommend to clinicians that:

Myelosuppression (including anemia, leukopenia, pancytopenia, and thrombocytopenia) has been reported in patients receiving linezolid. In cases where the outcome is known, when linezolid was discontinued, the affected hematologic parameters have risen toward pretreatment levels. Complete blood counts should be monitored weekly in patients who receive linezolid, particularly in those who receive linezolid for longer than two weeks, those with pre-existing myelosuppression, those receiving concomitant drugs that produce bone marrow suppression, or those with a chronic infection who have received previous or concomitant antibiotic therapy. Discontinuation of therapy with linezolid should be considered in patients who develop or have worsening myelosuppression.

Valproic Acid (Depakote®): Increased Severity of Labeled ADR Noted After Many Years of Use

Valproic acid products, including Depakote®, Depakene®, and Depacon®, have been used in clinical care since FDA approval in 1978. Although pancreatitis was first listed in the package inserts of valproate products in 1981, as with most drugs, there was limited safety data on this product at the time of approval. In clinical trials, there were 2 cases of pancreatitis without alternative etiology in 2416 patients, representing 1044 patient-years experience.

Initially, these drugs were indicated for a narrow labeled use and a limited population. Over two decades, the product was used for a wider range of both on-label and off-label indications, and the population exposed to the drug included a broader population than that exposed during the pre-approval clinical trials. With this increased use, the FDA received a number of voluntary reports through the MedWatch spontaneous reporting system of more severe forms of pancreatitis, often hemorrhagic, sometimes fatal, and with a number of cases occurring in infants and adolescent children. Although this ADR, pancreatitis, was "labeled" or known, the increased severity of the condition prompted the ODS postmarketing surveillance staff and the review division to initiate an epidemiological investigation and the development of a case series. This evaluation demonstrated that the rate based upon the reported cases exceeded that expected in the general population and there were cases in which pancreatitis recurred after re-challenge with valproate. With the agreement of the manufacturer, the FDA approved new safety labeling changes to the Warnings and Precautions sections and modified a black box warning to inform clinicians and their patients:

Pancreatitis: cases of life-threatening pancreatitis have been reported in both children and adults receiving valproate. Some of the cases have been described as hemorrhagic with rapid progression from initial symptoms to death. Cases have been reported shortly after initial use as well as after several years of use. Patients and guardians should be warned that abdominal pain, nausea, vomiting, and/or anorexia can be symptoms of pancreatitis that require prompt medical evaluation. If pancreatitis is diagnosed, valproate should ordinarily be discontinued. Alternate treatment for the underlying medical condition should be initiated as clinically indicated (see warnings and precautions).

THE FUTURE

The systematic collection and evaluation of postmarketing reports of serious ADRs by the FDA has come a long way since its inception about 50 years ago. The May 1999 report to the FDA Commissioner *Managing the Risks from Medical Product Use: Creating a Risk Management Framework*[6] found that the postmarketing surveillance program currently in place performed well for the goal it was designed to achieve—the rapid detection of unexpected serious AEs. Yet, it should be remembered that spontaneous reporting, although invaluable, is only one tool used in managing medical product risk. The report recognized that the FDA's programs are not designed to evaluate the rate, or impact, of known adverse events. The report proposed several options for improving risk management, including expanding the use of automated systems for reporting, monitoring, and evaluating AEs, and increasing the Agency's access to data sources that would supplement and extend its spontaneous reporting system. This could include use of large-scale medical databases from health maintenance organizations to reinforce, support, and enhance spontaneous signals and provide background rates and descriptive epidemiology.

Since the 1999 report, the FDA has continued to work with academia and industry to address these recommendations. In recognition of the increasing importance of postmarketing surveillance and risk assessment in the regulatory setting, a variety of initiatives are under way within the FDA. In 2002, the ODS was created within the CDER, with its three divisions focusing on improved identification and epidemiologic evaluation of ADRs, the evaluation of medication errors, and further research and implementation of risk communication activities directed toward both health care professionals and patients. The recent reauthorization of the Prescription Drug Users Fee Act (PDUFA) in 2002 will, for the first time, allow the FDA to apply user fee funds to the postmarketing activities of the Agency. In anticipation of these expanded efforts the FDA has published several guidance documents on postmarketing risk evaluation, risk communication, and risk management (see www.fda.gov/bbs/topics/news/2004/NEW01059.html).

In 2003, the ODS initiated a formal, competitive process of direct access to longitudinal, patient-level, electronic medical record data which can be used to study ADRs. Acquisition of this resource will directly enhance the ODS's ability to achieve one of the FDA's strategic goals, i.e., improving patient and consumer safety. In addition, online access to this data resource will allow the ODS to conduct drug safety studies in large population-based settings.

The FDA's current and future efforts include the following: increasing the quality of incoming reports of adverse events with a focus on making the AERS more efficient; establishing global reporting standards; promoting speed of reporting and assessment through electronic reporting; exploring new assessment and data visualizing methodologies; and, finally, exploring tools beyond spontaneous reporting. The last initiatives involve identification and assessment of linked databases and registries which can be accessed to expand surveillance, provide confirmatory evidence for signals, assess regulatory impact of labeling changes through studies, and, in general, build on the known strengths of spontaneous reporting—signal generation of potentially important events.

In addition, the ODS will refine current techniques to assess drug risks through the development and evaluation of risk management programs. We will continue to consider appropriate risk communication tools in order to clearly articulate drug safety information to both health professionals and patients in a timely manner. Our goals for the next 3–5 years include plans to develop and establish "best practices" for risk management plans and to develop quantitative approaches to the review of postmarketing safety data.

In summary, spontaneous reporting of AEs provides an important cornerstone for pharmacovigilance in the US. Regulators and manufacturers of medical products worldwide are moving forward the "single safety message transmission" with global harmonization for data standards and data transmission, improvements in relational database systems, the development of new risk assessment methodologies, and increased access to other data resources, including computerized medical records, to improve our overall ability to manage risk from pharmaceuticals.

DISCLAIMER

The opinions expressed are those of the authors and do not necessarily represent the views of the FDA or the US Government.

REFERENCES

1. Faich GA. Adverse-drug-reaction monitoring. *N Engl J Med* 1986; **314**: 1589–92.

2. Faich GA, Milstien JB, Anello C, Baum C. Sources of spontaneous adverse drug reaction reports received by pharmaceutical manufacturers. *Drug Info J* 1987; **21**: 251–5.

3. Knapp DE, Perry ZA. *Annual Adverse Drug Reaction Report: 1989*. Report of Surveillance Section, Surveillance and Data Processing Branch, Division of Epidemiology and Surveillance, Office of Epidemiology and Biostatistics, Center for Drug Evaluation and Research, FDA.

4. Ahmad SR. Adverse drug event monitoring at the Food and Drug Administration. *J Gen Intern Med* 2003; **18**: 57–60.

5. Laughren T. Premarketing studies in the drug approval process: understanding their limitations regarding the assessment of drug safety. *Clin Ther* 1998; **20** (suppl C): C12–19.

6. FDA. *Managing the Risks from Medical Product Use*. Report to the FDA Commissioner from the Task Force on Risk Management. Rockville, MD: Food and Drug Administration, May 1999.

7. Bates DW, Leape LL, Petrycki S. Incidence and preventability of adverse drug events in hospitalized adults. *J Gen Intern Med* 1993; **8**: 289–94.

8. Hilts PJ. *Protecting America's Health: The FDA, Business, and One Hundred Years of Regulation*. New York: Knopf, 2003.

9. FDA Consumer. The Long Struggle for the 1906 Law, June 1981. Available at: http://www.cfsan.fda.gov/~lrd/history2.html.

10. Jackson CO. *Food and Drug Legislation in the New Deal*. Princeton, NJ: Princeton University Press, 1970.

11. Maeder T. *Adverse Reactions*. New York: Morrow, 1994.

12. Moser RH. The obituary of an idea. *JAMA* 1971; **216**: 2135–6.

13. Kerlan I. Reporting adverse reactions to drugs. *Bull Am Soc Hosp Pharm* 1956; **13**: 311–14.

14. FDA. *Monthly Report: Adverse Reactions to Drugs and Therapeutic Devices*. Report of Adverse Reaction Branch, Division of Medical Information, Bureau of Medicine, August 1965.

15. FDA. *Semi-Monthly Adverse Reaction Alert Report and Reactions of Clinical Significance*. Report of Division of Drug Experience, October 1968.

16. Adverse experience reporting requirements for licensed biological products: final rule. *Fed Regist* 1994; **59**: 54034–44.

17. Expedited safety reporting requirements for human drug and biological products: final rule. *Fed Regist* 1997; **62**: 52237–53.

18. Dietary Supplement Health and Education Act (DSHEA) of 1994, Public Law 103–417, 103rd Congress.

19. Bren L. FDA's response to food, dietary supplement, and cosmetic adverse events. *FDA Consumer* July/August, 2003.

20. FDA Center for Drug Evaluation and Research. *Guidelines for Postmarketing Reporting of Adverse Drug Experiences*. Rockville, MD: CDER, 1992.

21. FDA Center for Drug Evaluation and Research. *Guideline for Adverse Experience Reporting for Licensed Biological Products*. Rockville, MD: CDER, 1993.

22. FDA. Guideline on Clinical Safety Data Management: Periodic Safety Update Reports for Marketed Drugs, May 19, 1997 *Fed Regist* 1997; **62**: 27470–6.

23. Safe Medical Devices Act of 1990. Public Law 101–629. *Stat* 1990; **104**: 4511.

24. JCAHO. Available at: http://www.hosp.uky.edu/pharmacy/departpolicy/PH03–02.pdf.

25. American Society of Health-System Pharmacists. ASHP Guidelines on Adverse Drug Reaction Monitoring and Reporting. Available at: http://www.ashp.org/bestpractices/MedMis/MedMis_Gdl_ADR.pdf.

26. American Medical Association. Reporting adverse drug and medical device events: report of the AMA's Council on Ethical and Judicial Affairs. *Food Drug Law J* 1994; **49**: 359–66.

27. American Dental Association. *Advisory Opinion 5.D.1, Reporting Adverse Reactions*. Principles of Ethics and Code of Professional Conduct, January 2004.

28. Anonymous. JAMA instructions for authors. *JAMA* 2004; **291**: 125–30.

29. Glass RM. Reporting of public health hazards or major advances—revision of uniform requirements. *JAMA* 1998; **280**: 2035.

30. Kessler DA. Introducing MedWatch: a new approach to reporting medication and device adverse effects and product problems. *JAMA* 1993; **269**: 2765–829.

31. Ahmad SR. MedWatch. *Lancet* 1993; **341**: 1465.

32. FDA MedWatch. Clinical therapeutics and the recognition of drug-induced disease, MedWatch continuing education article. Available at: http://www.fda.gov/medwatch/articles/dig/ceart.pdf.

33. Protecting the identities of reporters of adverse events and patients: preemption of disclosure rules. *Fed Regist* 1995; **60**: 16962–8.

34. Ahmad SR, Freiman JP, Graham DJ, Nelson RC. Quality of adverse drug experience reports submitted by pharmacists and physicians to the FDA. *Pharmacoepidemiol Drug Saf* 1996; **5**: 1–7.

35. Graham DJ, Ahmad SR, Piazza-Hepp T. Spontaneous Reporting—USA. In: Mann R, Andrews E, eds, *Pharmacovigilance*. Chichester: John Wiley & Sons, 2002; pp. 219–27.

36. Smalley W, Shatin D, Wysowski DK, Gurwitz J, Andrade SE, Goodman M *et al*. Contraindicated use of cisapride: impact of food and drug administration regulatory action. *JAMA* 2000; **284**: 3036–9.

37. Graham DJ, Drinkard CR, Shatin D, Tsong Y, Burgess MJ. Liver enzyme monitoring in patients treated with troglitazone. *JAMA* 2001; **286**: 831–3.

38. Brinker AD, Mackey AC, Prizont R. Tegaserod and ischemic colitis (letter). *N Engl J Med* 2004; **351**: 1361–4.

39. Bonnel RA, Graham DJ. Peripheral neuropathy in patients treated with leflunomide. *Clin Pharm Therapeutics* 2004; **75**: 580–5.

40. Griffin MR, Stein CM, Graham DJ, Daugherty JR, Arbogast PG, Ray WA. High frequency of use of rofecoxib at greater

than recommended doses: cause for concern. *Pharmacoepidemiol Drug Saf 2004*; **13**: 339–43.

41. Brinker A, Johnston M. Acute pulmonary edema in association with amiodarone. *Chest* 2004; **125**: 1591–2.

42. Wysowski DK, Farinas E. Finasteride and benign prostatic hyperplasia. *N Engl J Med* 2004; **350**: 1359.

43. Fraunfelder FW, Fraunfelder FT, Goetsch RA. Adverse ocular effects and OTC lice shampoo. *Arch Ophthalmol* 2003; **121**: 1790–1.

44. Phelan K, Mosholder A, Lu S. Lithium interaction with the cyclooxygenase 2 inhibitors rofecoxib and celecoxib and other nonsteroidal antiinflammatory drugs. *J Clin Psychiatry* 2003; **64**: 1328–34.

45. Chang JT, Green L, Beitz J. Renal failure with the use of zoledronic acid. *N Engl J Med* 2003; **349**: 1676–8.

46. Ahmad SR, Graham DJ. Pneumonitis with antiandrogens. *Ann Intern Med* 2003; **139**: 3–4.

47. Flowers C, Racoosin J, Lu S, Beitz J. Pergolide-associated valvular heart disease. *Mayo Clin Proc* 2003; **78**: 730–1.

48. Beck P, Wysowski DK, Downey W, Butler-Jones D. Statin use and the risk of breast cancer. *J Clin Epidemiol* 2003; **56**: 280–5.

49. Graham DJ, Green L, Senior JR, Nourjah P. Troglitazone-induced liver failure: a case study. *Am J Med* 2003; **114**: 299–306.

50. Bonnel RA, La Grenade L, Karwoski CB, Beitz J. Allergic contact dermatitis from topical doxepin: Food and Drug Administration's postmarketing surveillance experience. *J Am Acad Dermatol* 2003; **48**: 294–6.

51. Manda B, Drinkard CR, Shatin D, Graham DJ. The risk of esophageal obstruction associated with an anti-allergy medication (Claritin-D 24-Hour—original formulation). *Pharmacoepidemiol Drug Saf* 2004; **13**: 29–34.

52. Graham DJ, Drinkard CR, Shatin D. Incidence of idiopathic acute liver failure and hospitalized liver injury in patients treated with troglitazone. *Am J Gastroenterol* 2003; **98**: 175–9.

53. O'Connell KA, Wilkin JK, Pitts M. Isotretinoin (Accutane) and serious psychiatric adverse events. *J Am Acad Dermatol* 2003; **48**: 306–8.

54. Brinker A, Staffa J. Concurrent use of selected agents with moxifloxacin: an examination of labeling compliance within 1 year of marketing. *Arch Intern Med* 2002; **162**: 2011–2.

55. Kornegay CJ, Vasilakis-Scaramozza C, Jick H. Incident diabetes associated with antipsychotic use in the United Kingdom General Practice Research Database. *J Clin Psychiatry* 2002; **63**: 758–62.

56. Thambi L, Kapcala LP, Chambers W, Nourjah P, Beitz J, Chen M *et al*. Topiramate-associated secondary angel-closure glaucoma: a case series. *Arch Ophthal* 2002; **120**: 1108.

57. Bonnel RA, Villaba ML, Karwoski CB, Beitz J. Deaths associated with inappropriate intravenous colchicine administration. *J Emergency Med* 2002; **22**: 385–7.

58. Ahmad SR, Kortepeter C, Brinker A, Chen M, Beitz J. Renal failure associated with the use of celecoxib and rofecoxib. *Drug Saf* 2002; **25**: 537–44.

59. Shaffer D, Singer S, Korvick J, Honig P. Concomitant risk factors in reports of torsades de pointes associated with macrolide use: review of the United States Food and Drug Administration Adverse Event Reporting System. *Clin Infect Dis* 2002; **35**: 197–200.

60. Wysowski DK, Honig SF, Beitz J. Uterine sarcoma associated with tamoxifen use. *N Engl J Med* 2002; **346**: 1832–3.

61. Wysowski DK, Farinas E, Swartz L. Comparison of reported and expected deaths in sildenafil (Viagra) users. *Am J Cardiol* 2002; **89**: 1331–4.

62. Brinker A, Bonnel R, Beitz J. Abuse, dependence, or withdrawal associated with tramadol. *Am J Psychiatry* 2003; **159**: 881.

63. Kortepeter C, Chen M, Knudsen JF, Dubitsky GM, Ahmad SR, Beitz J. Clozapine and venous thromboembolism. *Am J Psychiatry* 2002; **159**: 876–7.

64. Bonnel RA, Villalba ML, Karwoski CB, Beitz J. Aseptic meningitis associated with rofecoxib. *Arch Intern Med* 2002; **162**: 713–5.

65. Staffa JA, Chang J, Green L. Cerivastatin and reports of fatal rhabdomyolysis. *N Engl J Med* 2002; **346**: 539–40.

66. Bate A, Lindquist M, Edwards IR, Orre R. A data mining approach for signal detection and analysis. *Drug Saf* 2002; **25**: 393–7.

67. Szarfman A, Machado SG, O'Neill RT. Use of screening algorithms and computer systems to efficiently signal higher-than-expected combinations of drugs and events in the US FDA's spontaneous reports database. *Drug Saf* 2002; **25**: 381–92.

68. Fletcher AP. Spontaneous adverse drug reaction reporting vs event monitoring: a comparison. *J R Soc Med* 1991; **84**: 341–4.

69. Alvarez-Requejo A, Carvajal A, Begaud B, Moride Y, Vega T, Arias LH. Under-reporting of adverse drug reactions: estimate based on a spontaneous reporting scheme and a sentinel system. *Eur J Clin Pharmacol* 1988; **54**: 483–8.

70. Finney DJ. The detection of adverse reactions to therapeutic drugs. *Stat Med* 1982; **1**: 153–61.

71. Strom BL, Tugwell P. Pharmacoepidemiology: current status, prospects, and problems. *Ann Intern Med* 1990; **113**: 179–81.

72. Finney DJ. Statistical aspects of monitoring for dangers in drug therapy. *Methods Inf Med* 1972; **10**: 1–8.

73. Standardization of definitions and criteria of causality assessment of adverse drug reactions: drug-induced liver disorders: report of an international consensus meeting. *Int J Clin Pharmacol Ther Toxicol* 1990; **28**: 317–22.

74. Auriche M, Loupi E. Does proof of causality ever exist in pharmacovigilance? *Drug Saf* 1993; **9**: 230–5.

75. Begaud B, Moride Y, Tubert-Bitter P, Chaslerie A, Haramburu F. False-positives in spontaneous reporting: should we worry about them? *Br J Clin Pharmacol* 1994; **38**: 401–4.

76. Temple RJ, Jones JK, Crout JR. Adverse effects of newly marketed drugs. *N Engl J Med* 1979; **300**: 1046–7.

77. Rawlins MD. Pharmacovigilance: paradise lost, regained or postponed? The William Withering Lecture 1994. *J R College Physicians Lond* 1995; **29**: 41–9.

78. Meyboom RH, Hekster YA, Egberts AC, Gribnau FW, Edwards IR. Causal or casual? The role of causality assessment in pharmacovigilance. *Drug Saf* 1997; **17**: 374–89.

79. Koch-Weser J, Sellers EM, Zacest R. The ambiguity of adverse drug reactions. *Eur J Clin Pharmacol* 1997; **11**: 75–8.

80. Green DM. Pre-existing conditions, placebo reactions, and "side effects." *Ann Intern Med* 1964; **60**: 255–65.

81. Reidenberg MM, Lowenthal DT. Adverse nondrug reactions. *N Engl J Med* 1968; **279**: 678–9.

82. Karch FE, Smith CL, Kerzner B, Mazzullo JM, Weintraub M, Lasagna L. Adverse drug reactions—a matter of opinion. *Clin Pharmacol Ther* 1976; **19**: 489–92.

83. Rogers AS, Israel E, Smith CR. Physician knowledge, attitudes, and behavior related to reporting adverse drug events. *Arch Intern Med* 1988; **148**: 1589–92.

84. Scott HD, Rosenbaum SE, Waters WJ, Colt AM, Andrews LG, Juergens JP *et al*. Rhode Island physicians' recognition and reporting of adverse drug reactions. *R I Med J* 1987; **70**: 311–16.

85. Goldman SA. Limitations and strengths of spontaneous reports data. *Clin Ther* 1998; **20** (suppl C): C40–4.

86. Sachs RM, Bortnichak EA. An evaluation of spontaneous adverse drug reaction monitoring systems. *Am J Med* 1986; **81** (suppl 5B): 49–55.

87. Bhasin S, Reyburn H, Steen J, Waller PC. The effects of media publicity on spontaneous adverse reaction reporting with mefloquine in the UK. *Pharmacoepidemiol Drug Saf* 1997; **6** (suppl 2): 32.

88. Rossi AC, Hsu JP, Faich GA. Ulcerogenicity of piroxicam: analysis of spontaneously reported data. *BMJ* 1987; **294**: 147–50.

89. Tsong Y. Comparing reporting rates of adverse events between drugs with adjustment for year of marketing and secular trends in total reporting. *J Biopharm Stat* 1995; **5**: 95–114.

90. Weber JCP. Epidemiology of adverse reactions to nonsteroidal antiinflammatory drugs. In: Rainsford KD, Velo GP, eds, *Advances in Information Research*, vol. 6. New York: Raven, 1984; pp. 1–7.

91. Serradell J, Bjornson DC, Hartzema AG. Drug utilization study methodologies: national and international perspectives. *Drug Intell Clin Pharm* 1987; **21**: 994–1001.

92. Blum MD, Graham DJ, McCloskey CA. Temafloxacin syndrome: review of 95 cases. *Clin Infect Dis* 1994; **6**: 946–50.

10

Global Drug Surveillance: The WHO Programme for International Drug Monitoring

I. RALPH EDWARDS, STEN OLSSON, MARIE LINDQUIST and BRUCE HUGMAN
WHO Collaborating Centre for International Drug Monitoring (Uppsala Monitoring Centre), Uppsala, Sweden.

INTRODUCTION

The general awareness that modern drugs could carry unexpected hazards was triggered by a letter to the editor of the *Lancet* published on the 16th of December 1961.[1] In this historical document of fifteen lines, Dr McBride from Australia reported that he had noted an increased frequency of limb malformations among babies, and that a common denominator seemed to be the intake of a new hypnotic drug—thalidomide—by their mothers.

In the wake of the public health disaster that then unraveled, governments in many countries arranged procedures for the systematic collection of information about suspected adverse drug reactions (ADRs). These systems were based on the spontaneous reporting of suspected ADRs by physicians. They were first organized in Australia, Canada, Czechoslovakia, Ireland, the Netherlands, New Zealand, Sweden, the UK, the US, and West Germany. They were initiated between 1961 and 1965. Similar systems now operate in more than 70 countries. Many of the principles which are still important in pharmacovigilance were elaborated in these early days, mainly by Finney.[2–4]

In 1968, ten countries from Australasia, Europe, and North America agreed to pool all reports that had been sent to their national monitoring centers in a WHO-sponsored international drug monitoring project. The aim was to identify even very rare but serious reactions as early as possible. The scheme was set up at WHO headquarters in Geneva in 1970. The economic and operational responsibilities were transferred to Sweden in 1978 with the establishment of the WHO Collaborating Centre for International Drug Monitoring in Uppsala (now known as the Uppsala Monitoring Center, UMC). The formal responsibility for and the coordination of the program, however, remained with WHO headquarters. Today, 73 countries participate in the program as full members and a further 12 as associate members (Figure 10.1), annually contributing approximately 200 000 suspected ADR reports to the WHO database in Uppsala. This database holds nearly three million case reports to date. There are guidelines covering all aspects of reporting, and defaults are actively followed up. National centers should report at a minimum monthly frequency, with preliminary reports if full details and evaluations are incomplete. The data are,

Pharmacoepidemiology, Fourth Edition   Edited by B.L. Strom
© 2005 John Wiley & Sons, Ltd

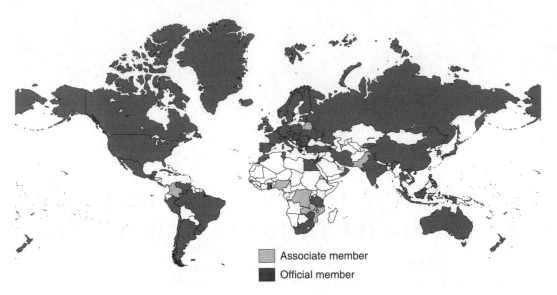

Figure 10.1. Map of countries in the WHO program.

however, heterogeneous and subject to all kinds of influences, and the WHO program has agreed on the following caveat to be used by all who produce analyses based on the data:

> interpretations of adverse reactions data, and particularly those based on comparisons between pharmaceutical products, may be misleading. The information tabulated in the accompanying printouts is not homogeneous with respect to the sources of information or the likelihood that the pharmaceutical product caused the suspected adverse reaction. Some describe such information as "raw data". Any use of this information must take into account at least the above.

Spontaneous reporting systems are still most frequently used for the detection of new drug safety signals. In developing countries they are also used for the detection of substandard and counterfeit drugs. In all countries about half the adverse reactions that take patients to hospitals have been judged to be avoidable. Now, therefore, there is also a need to consider medical error as a signal that there is a problem with a medical product.

A new trend in spontaneous reporting is the growing number of reports directly from consumers rather than health professionals. Just as health professionals' reports tell of their concerns about drugs, so do consumer reports and from a different and important perspective.

In all these dimensions, spontaneous reports generate data about possible ADRs, or about broader problems with drugs; they provide the basis for further analysis or for hypotheses for systematic studies. The next steps are:

- to prove or refute these hypotheses;
- to estimate the incidence, relative risk, and excess risk of the ADRs;
- to explore the mechanisms involved;
- to identify special risk groups.

In some unusual circumstances, spontaneous reporting can be used to provide valuable information for these latter tasks as well, but each case requires its own analysis and the exercise of expert clinical judgment.

A recent WHO publication[5] highlights the new challenges for pharmacovigilance:

> Within the last decade, there has been a growing awareness that the scope of pharmacovigilance should be extended beyond the strict confines of detecting new signals of safety concerns. Globalization, consumerism, the explosion in free trade and communication across borders, and increasing use of the Internet have resulted in a change in access to all medicinal products and information on them.

Internationally there is confusion over what is meant by a "Signal." The WHO definition is:

Reported information on a possible causal relationship between an adverse event and a drug, the relationship being unknown or incompletely documented previously. (note) Usually more than a single report is required to generate a signal, depending upon the seriousness of the event and the quality of the information.[5]

This definition is neutral in terms of action that might be taken. The view that a signal should be seen as a first hint that there is a need to look more closely at a drug and a reported ADR was presaged by Finney in 1974: "a signal is a basis of communication between WHO and national centres; only rarely will it carry the force of a proven danger" and "Signals are intended to arouse suspicions and to stimulate deeper investigation."[4]

Amery in 1999 also echoed this sentiment: "a signal may be defined as new information pointing to a previously unknown causal relationship between an adverse event, or its incidence, and a drug: the information must be such that, if confirmed, it may lead to action regarding the medicine" and "Thus signal generation aims at timely identification of previously unsuspected adverse effects, but any signals require further evaluation as they themselves do not prove that there is a safety problem."[6]

The current European Medicines Evaluation Agency (EMEA) consideration of signals is found in Procedures for Transmission and Management of Detected Signals as "a potentially serious safety problem (e.g. a series of unexpected or serious ADRs or an increase in the reporting rate of a known ADR report)."[7] Another definition by Meyboom *et al.*[8] refers to a signal as a "set of data constituting a hypothesis that is relevant to the rational and safe use of a drug in humans," with the addition "such data are usually clinical, pharmacological, pathological or epidemiological in nature." Both these statements carry with them the implication that some action should be taken to alert others to the signal. It is the issue of when to take a signal forward for others to consider it, or for the broader health professions or the public to know about a signal, that is often the subject of intense debate, given both the implications for the future of the drug and for the safety of patients. The Meyboom definition gives a wider view of the information used to detect signals and also usefully uses the term "hypothesis," which again underlines the tentative nature of a signal.

Even if all the above statements/definitions are clear that a signal is provisional the issue is further confused by the fact that some use the term "alert" as an alternative for "signal". Others use "alert" to be the warning that is sent out concerning a signal. Thus not only are the two terms used interchangeably, they are used in the opposite senses by different authorities.

Box 10.1. Definition of "signal."

These changes have given rise to new kinds of safety concerns, such as:

- illegal sale of medicines and drugs of abuse over the Internet;
- increasing self-medication practices;
- irrational and potentially unsafe donation practices;
- widespread manufacture and sale of counterfeit and substandard medicines;
- increasing use of traditional medicines outside the confines of the traditional culture of use;
- increasing use of traditional and herbal medicines with other medicines with potential for adverse interactions.

According to the same publication, the specific aims of pharmacovigilance are to:

- improve patient care and safety in relation to the use of medicines and all medical and paramedical interventions;
- improve public health and safety in relation to the use of medicines;
- contribute to the assessment of benefit, harm, effectiveness and risk of medicines, encouraging their safe, rational and more effective (including cost-effective) use;
- promote understanding, education, and clinical training in pharmacovigilance and its effective communication to the public.

As pharmacovigilance has evolved, the scope of the WHO Collaborating Centre has been extended accordingly, as reflected in the Centre's new vision and goals, and the introduction in the mid-1990s of a new working name, the Uppsala Monitoring Centre (UMC).

DESCRIPTION

OVERVIEW OF ADR REPORTING SCHEMES

ADR reporting schemes differ in a number of dimensions. There are two parallel more or less global systems.

1. The medical literature: many journals publish case reports of patients who experience possible ADRs.
2. National pharmacovigilance systems: case reports of suspected ADRs are collected by national pharmacovigilance centers.

The focus of this chapter is on the second of these (though case reports from the literature are included in some of the national systems). In this second category there are now two international systems:

1. One under the auspices of WHO in which data on all suspected ADRs are pooled and coordinated by the UMC in Sweden.
2. The European Union (EU) pharmacovigilance system.

In the latter, all Member States and the EMEA are connected via secure intranet (Eudranet) for the exchange of pharmacovigilance information. A database, Eudrawatch, is under development for the collation and analysis of reports of serious ADRs associated with products authorized through the EU centralized procedure. It should be noted that all European countries also belong to, and report to, the WHO system and that the EMEA has access to the WHO database information.

Information on various national pharmacovigilance centers has been compiled.[9] In the future this publication will be updated on the UMC's website (www.who-umc.org). National systems themselves are organized in many different ways. Most are centralized, but an increasing number are decentralized. For most of the national systems the reporting of ADRs is voluntary, but for some it is mandatory. Most national systems receive their reports directly from health practitioners. Some, however, receive most of their reports from health practitioners via pharmaceutical manufacturers, including the largest national system, that of the US (see Chapter 9).

Most centers review each report on an individual basis using a clinical diagnostic and decision-making approach, making judgments about each case as to how likely it is that the drug caused the adverse event (see also Chapter 36). However, others use mainly an aggregate or epidemiological approach to the analysis of the reports (see Chapter 9). Finally, the national centers differ dramatically in how they interact with reporters of ADRs. Some treat their reporters anonymously, providing feedback only in the form of regulatory actions or occasional published papers. Others provide very direct feedback—verbal, written, and/or published—to maximize the dialog between the reporters and the center. Guidelines are available on setting up and running a pharmacovigilance center.[10]

ORGANIZATION, AFFILIATION, AND TASKS OF NATIONAL MONITORING CENTERS

In most countries, the monitoring center is part of the drug regulatory authority.

- In some, The Philippines and New Zealand, for example, the functions are carried out jointly by the drug control authority and a university institution. The latter receive the initial reports and perform analyses for consideration by the regulatory authority.
- In Germany, the ADR monitoring program was originally organized by the Drug Commission of the German Medical Profession. In 1978 the responsibility for the evaluation of drug-induced risks was transferred to the National Institute of Health (Bundesgesundheitsamt), and in 1993 a new agency was formed for control of medicines and devices (BfArM). The Drug Commission still collects and evaluates ADR reports from physicians and pharmacists, which then are relayed to the health authorities.
- In France, the French Medicines Agency has taken up duties formerly carried out by the Ministry of Health. It also serves as a coordinating and executive body for a network of 31 regional centers that are connected to major regional university hospitals. Each center is responsible for ADR monitoring in its region. The evaluated reports are fed into a central database. The regional centers are co-sponsored by the agency, the hospitals, and the universities. Other public or even private sources of support can be used as well, provided they are ethical, receive reports, and are authorized by the agency.
- Argentina, Canada, Spain, Sweden, and Thailand also have developed decentralized systems, in parts similar to that of the French.
- In the United Kingdom there are four selected regional centers connected to university hospitals, which have a special responsibility for stimulating ADR reporting in their particular areas.

Regional systems have the advantage that good communication and personal relationships may be established between the staff of the monitoring center and the reporting professionals. They are, however, demanding in the number of staff needed and, unless the reports are fed directly into a central database, can result in delays in the flow of information.

In Morocco, Tanzania, and some other countries the national centers also function as Poison Information Centers, or are closely related to drug information services. These may serve as useful models for other countries, since intoxication and adverse reactions are often related. Also, requests for drug information are often about adverse drug reactions, which may be well known or rare and unexpected. This may further add to the value of a center, as the local physicians then feel that they not only feed in reports of ADRs, but in return receive clinically useful information.

Some regional centers, e.g., in Barcelona (Spain), Bordeaux (France), and those in Sweden, are also engaged in formal pharmacoepidemiology studies to follow up potential signals created by the spontaneous reports.

In many countries ADR monitoring starts within a hospital or academic setting, and may also continue that way. The original activities of the Boston Collaborative Drug Surveillance were a prime example of such an approach. Several other countries, including India and Thailand, as well as some mentioned below, have strong individual hospital monitoring. See Chapter 35 for more on hospital pharmacoepidemiology.

REPORTING REQUIREMENTS

The greatest need for information on undesirable and unexpected drug effects relates to drugs that are newly marketed. Thus, most countries emphasize the need to report even trivial reactions to new drugs, while for established medicines only serious reactions are usually requested.

Some countries have clearly identified which new drugs they want observed most closely. In the United Kingdom such drugs are marked with a black triangle in the British National Formulary. The Marketing Authorization Holders (MAHs) are encouraged to include it in all other product information and advertisements. This system is voluntary and in particular cannot be enforced for centralized products (i.e., those approved by the EMEA for use in the European Union).

In Denmark and Sweden, a list of drugs of special interest for monitoring is published in the national medical journal. In New Zealand and Ireland, some selected new drugs are put in an intensive reporting program. In New Zealand, the Intensive Medicines Monitoring Programme monitors cohorts of all patients taking selected new drugs and specifically requests that all clinical events be reported, not just suspected ADRs. Most countries, however, issue rather general recommendations as to what type of reactions should be reported to national centers.

In at least ten countries, it is mandatory for physicians and dentists to report cases of suspected serious adverse reactions to the regulatory authority. Both the Council for International Organizations of Medical Sciences (CIOMS) and the International Conference on Harmonisation (ICH) have worked on good pharmacovigilance practices, which set guidelines for the proper management of individual cases and case series.[11,12] (See also www.ich.org, safety topics.) The US is working on such guidelines as well (see Chapters 8 and 9).

In some 25 countries, including the EU, Japan, and the US, it is obligatory for pharmaceutical companies (or MAHs in the EU) to submit to the regulatory authority cases of suspected adverse reactions that have become known to them (clinical events that might have been caused by the drug, and sometimes those where no such attribution has been made).

SOURCES OF REPORTS

The regulatory status and organization of a national drug monitoring program also determines the sources and the type of information that will be received. Three main groups of countries can be identified:

- Countries obtaining a substantial contribution of reports directly from physicians in hospitals and general practice, such as Australia, France, Ireland, the Netherlands, New Zealand, the nordic countries, Spain, Thailand, and the United Kingdom.
- Countries receiving a vast majority of their information via the pharmaceutical industry, such as Germany, Italy, and the US.
- Countries mainly dependent on information from hospital physicians only, such as Japan, India, Romania, and Bulgaria.

The contribution from dentists is generally small. Some countries accept reports from pharmacists, nurses, and consumers.

HANDLING AND EVALUATION OF REPORTS

When a report reaches a national center a physician or a pharmacist normally reads it. (In some countries pharmacists at the national centers have access to medical consultants.) A judgment is made about whether the information provided is sufficient as the basis for an opinion on the correctness of the diagnosis and causality, or if more data should be requested. In a majority of countries participating in the WHO scheme, the medical officer makes an assessment of each case with regard to the probability of a causal relationship between the clinical event and the drug(s) administered. In many countries an advisory committee of clinical experts helps the national center in making the final causality assessment and the evaluation of the clinical importance of the cumulative reports. The WHO has a system of classifying the summary reports it holds according to their content: a "Quality Grading" based on a publication by Edwards *et al.*[13]

In recent years there has been an international effort to harmonize the terms used to describe the adverse events and to set criteria and definitions for at least the major serious types of reactions. Similarly, there have been efforts to harmonize the way data are stored and communicated internationally. The main agencies involved in this work have been the WHO, CIOMS, ICH, and the EU. For example, internationally agreed criteria and definitions have been published for reactions frequently reported to the WHO database[14,15] and by some other groups involved with ADR monitoring.[16–19] The Medical Dictionary for Regulatory Activities (MedDRA) is becoming more and more used throughout the world, and the ICH E2B format, which is a guideline for the transmission format for information to be included on an adverse reaction case report, and the corresponding IT message specification for transmission, ICH ICSR DTD (Individual Case Safety Reports Document Type Definition), are on the way to being the global data storage and transfer standards for the world.

No common standard for the detailed operational assessment of causal relationship between drug and ADR has been agreed internationally. Most experts agree about which factors should be taken into account in the assessment, but how much weight should be given to each of the factors is the subject of continuing scientific debate (see Chapter 36).[20] A number of more or less complicated and comprehensive algorithms for the assessment of causality have been constructed.[21,22] When tested by their inventors, these algorithms have, in general, been found to decrease variability among ratings produced by different individuals.[23–25] This has not, however, always been the case when independent groups have tested the algorithms.[26,27] Moreover, it has not been possible to test whether the assessments reached by the use of algorithms have been more valid than those reached without them. No algorithm has yet been constructed that can cope with the wide varieties of exposure-event categories seen by a national center and yet is simple enough to be used when evaluating a large number of cases on a routine basis.

The only country today using an algorithm on a routine basis for the assessment of causality in ADR reports is France, where the existence of 31 different regional centers necessitates some standardization.[28] Some national centers are of the opinion that causality rating of each single case as submitted introduces bias, and that it is an unacceptable allocation of resources. It is therefore better to use the term "relationship" since this does not imply a value judgment. However, an international agreement has recently been reached among the countries participating in the WHO drug monitoring scheme on common definitions of the terms most often used to describe relationships in a semi-quantitative way (Table 10.1). Methods for assessing relationships in case reports are discussed in more detail in Chapter 36.

An apparent causal relationship in a single case, or even a series, is not the only issue in comprehensive early signal detection. Many case reports with limited information might be excluded from serious consideration, but a case record that does not allow for remote assessment of the relationship between drug and ADR does not mean that the original observer was incorrect, only that the observation cannot be confirmed. Thus quantity, as well as quality, of

Table 10.1. Terminology for causality assessment

Certain. A clinical event, including laboratory test abnormality, occurring in a plausible time relationship to drug administration, and which cannot be explained by concurrent disease or other drugs or chemicals. The response to withdrawal of the drug (de-challenge) should be clinically plausible. The event must be definitive pharmacologically or phenomenologically, using a satisfactory re-challenge procedure if necessary.

Probable/likely. A clinical event, including laboratory test abnormality, with reasonable time sequence to administration of the drug, unlikely to be attributed to concurrent disease or other drugs or chemicals, and which follows a clinically reasonable response on withdrawal (de-challenge). Re-challenge information is not required to fulfill this definition.

Possible. A clinical event, including laboratory test abnormality, with a reasonable time sequence to administration of the drug, but which could also be explained by concurrent disease or other drugs or chemicals. Information on drug withdrawal may be lacking or unclear.

Unlikely. A clinical event, including laboratory test abnormality, with a temporal relationship to drug administration which makes a causal relationship improbable, and in which other drugs, chemicals, or underlying disease provide plausible explanations.

Conditional/unclassified. A clinical event, including laboratory test abnormality, reported as an adverse reaction, about which more data is essential for a proper assessment or the additional data are under examination.

Unassessable/unclassifiable. A report suggesting an adverse reaction that cannot be judged because information is insufficient or contradictory, and which cannot be supplemented or verified.

reports of associations is valuable. The use of "poor quality" reports as a trigger for a signal should be taken seriously if the clinical event is serious.[13] Early warning is the goal, and a signal based on doubtful evidence should promote the search for better.

There also may be certain items of information within a set of reports that trigger consideration of a signal other than just the medicinal product and clinical event: the apparent over-representation of higher doses of the relevant drug, or concomitant treatment, or certain patient characteristics may be of interest for the safe use of the drug product.

The above are just some of the common issues for consideration during the evaluation of an early signal. There are many others, such as the finding of a problem with one medicinal product, which triggers a search into products with similar effects. What is clear is that there are very complex interacting patterns of information, which may trigger ideas and concerns.

Many national regulatory authorities systematically review and evaluate information from a variety of sources, in addition to spontaneous ADR reports, to identify new ADRs or changing ADR profiles on the basis of which action should be initiated to improve the safe use of medicines. The web and review journals such as *Reactions Weekly* (ADIS International) are useful in this respect. (*Reactions Weekly* also links its literature findings to those of the WHO database where relevant.)

FEEDBACK TO REPORTERS

Some form of feedback from the national center must be arranged for clinicians to feel that they are involved in an iterative and progressive process. In many countries, each reporter receives a personal acknowledgment, often including a preliminary evaluation of the case. Adverse reaction bulletins are produced regularly in many countries and then distributed to the medical profession. Sometimes the information is included in a local medical journal or a drug information bulletin.

This is, perhaps, the central point at which effective communications are essential for the success of pharmacovigilance. Once physicians know of their national reporting system, believe reporting is important, know where to find their reporting form, and feel motivated to act (all major communications and motivational challenges in themselves), they must feel that their efforts have some reward (recognition, at least) and some effect on medical knowledge and practice.[29]

DETECTION AND EVALUATION OF SIGNALS

Spontaneous adverse drug reaction reporting is principally a method of identifying the previously unrecognized hazards of marketed medicines. Within the WHO program a "signal" concerns information regarding a possible relationship between a drug and an adverse event or drug interaction. In trying to detect signals from international data it should be understood that a signal is an early hypothesis, and that it simply calls for further work to be performed on that hypothesis.

In the early days of pharmacovigilance, when reports were relatively few, signals were looked for manually or through checking, for example, quarterly lists of submitted case reports sorted in various ways to help review (e.g., all deaths, new-to-the-system). Profiles based on the proportion of reports regarding different system organ classes were compared and differences in the proportion of reactions reported were used as prompts for further analyses.[30–32] Later, differences in such proportions were tested by statistical significance tests. A published signal, for example, based on such a test was the higher proportion of serum sickness-like reactions to cefaclor, in comparison with other cephalosporins and ampicillin.[33]

The French "case–non case" method is based on the same principle, comparing the proportion of, for example, hypoglycemia reported for acetylcholinesterase (ACE) inhibitors with that reported for other cardiovascular drugs.[34]

The human brain is excellent at finding significant patterns in data: humans would not have survived if that were not so! It is a complex process to examine large numbers of case reports for new factors that may impact upon the safe use of the drug or drugs concerned, especially when for each case report there is a considerable amount of information. Being able to remember the adverse reaction terms used on different reports, how they might be interrelated, and their time trend of reporting is just a hint of such complexity. The vast volume of data in drug safety today cannot be given effective attention, let alone held in the human memory for analysis. Although many important signals have had their origin in open-minded clinical review of data, some presorting is now necessary for the reasons stated above. Also, in order not to miss possible important signals there is a place for subjecting the data to analysis in ways that allow us to see patterns without our preconceptions blinding us to possibilities outside our conditioned experience.

It is true that in looking for significant patterns by sifting through data, something which *looks* probable may turn up by chance: data "dredging" or "trawling" or a "fishing expedition" is bound to catch something, but not necessarily much that is useful. Data dredging should be used as a pejorative term for unstructured fiddling about with data, or worse, the application of a structure to data to make it fit a biased hypothesis in a way to give added credibility to the result.

Formal *data mining*, or "knowledge finding/detection," on the other hand, is not a random rummaging through data in an aimless fashion, which is what the term "dredging" implies. Data mining/knowledge finding should be considered as a term for the application of a tool or tools to analyze large amounts of data in a transparent and unbiased fashion, with the aim of highlighting information worth closer consideration.

It is certainly true that the involvement of the variables and the characterization of any of their relationships in advanced pattern recognition is "unsupervised" in data mining, in that a predetermined logic for finding patterns is allowed to run free of human interference. However, in signaling methods using data mining, the level of flexibility and the kind of logic that is applied to data is systematic and transparent.

Data mining approaches to signal detection may use different methodologies but they have in common that they look for "disproportionalities" in data, i.e., a relationship or pattern standing out from the database background experience.[35]

Two of the advantages of these approaches are:

- no external data are needed and the limitations of such data (including delay in receipt) do not apply;
- they may be expected to counteract some of the biases related to variable reporting. For example, if the overall level of reporting is high because of new drug bias, this will not necessarily affect the proportion of all reactions for the drug; while the high overall reporting rate can be related to the extent of drug use, a specific adverse reaction may still be disproportionally reported if it is common.

One possible disadvantage is that, as the background data changes for all drugs in the data set, so does the expectedness (disproportionality) for the drug–ADR combination in question. Stratification will also have the same effect by altering the background data included. This can, however, be taken into account during analysis. It is clear that in a large database the addition of new information to the background will have relatively less influence.

Two approaches to knowledge finding are described below, in some detail, as examples: one for identifying complex patterns in data, and the other for looking at relatively simple relationships.

A Bayesian Approach Using Neural Networks as Implemented for the WHO Database

Description

The main use of the WHO program's international database is to find novel drug safety signals: new information. One begins to see the problem as looking for the proverbial "needle in a haystack."[36] As noted above, if important signals are not to be missed, the first analysis of information should be free from preconception.[37,38]

With this in mind, the UMC has developed a signal detection system that combines a data mining tool for screening of raw data with the subsequent application of different filtering algorithms. This quantitative filtering of the data is intended to focus clinical review on the most potentially important drug–ADR combinations, which can be likened to a clinical triage system for guiding clinical review towards areas of first concern.[39,40] The resulting "priority package" is scrutinized by independent experts on an international review panel. Based on evaluations of the available evidence and expert opinion, hypotheses of potential drug-induced problems are formulated as "signals." These are circulated to all national centers participating in the WHO program for consideration of public health implications.

The first step towards this new signaling process was the development of a data mining tool for the WHO database. The Bayesian Confidence Propagation Neural Network (BCPNN) methodology,[41] was designed to identify statistically significant disproportionalities in a large data set, with a high performance, to allow for automated screening of all combinations of drugs and adverse reactions in the WHO database (Box 10.2).

The BCPNN provides an efficient computational model for the analysis of large amounts of data and combinations of variables, whether real, discrete, or binary. It is robust and relevant results can still be generated despite missing data. The missing data do not prevent the identification of disproportionally reported drug–ADR or other combinations; only the uncertainty is greater and denoted by wider confidence limits. If required, it is also possible to impute values, and to create best-case, worst-case information. This is advantageous as most reports in the database contain some empty fields. The results are reproducible, making validation and checking simple. The BCPNN is easy to train; it only takes one pass across the data, which makes it highly time-efficient. Only a small proportion of all

The BCPNN methodology aims to identify unexpectedly strong dependencies between variables (e.g., drugs and adverse reactions) within the WHO database, and how dependencies change with addition of new data. The dependencies are selected using a measure of disproportionality called the information component (*IC*):

$$IC = \log_2 \frac{p_{xy}}{p_x p_y}$$

where:

p_x = probability of a specific drug being listed on a case report
p_y = probability of a specific ADR being listed on a case report
p_{xy} = probability that a specific drug–adverse reaction combination is listed on a case report.

Thus, the *IC* value is based on:

• the number of case reports with drug X (c_x);
• the number of case reports with ADR Y (c_y);
• the number of reports with the specific combination (c_{xy});
• the total number of reports (C).

Positive *IC* values indicate that the particular combination of variables is reported to the database more often than statistically expected from reports already in the database. The higher the value of the *IC*, the more the combination stands out from the background.

From the distribution of the *IC*, expectation and variance values are calculated using Bayesian statistics. Estimates of precision (credibility intervals) are provided for each point estimate of the *IC*, thus both the point estimate of unexpectedness as well as the certainty associated with it can be examined. The credibility for each *IC* provides a measure of the robustness of the value. The higher the c_x, c_y, and c_{xy} levels are, the narrower becomes the credibility interval. If a positive *IC* value increases over time and the credibility interval narrows, this shows a likelihood of a positive quantitative association between the studied variables. Recently, work has allowed for modifications of the method to take into account problems of non-normal distribution of data at low count values as well as a modification of the Bayesian prior assumptions that were originally taken as being non-association of drug and ADR.

Box 10.2. The BCPNN methodology.

possible drug–adverse reaction combinations are actually non-zero in the database. Thus, use of a sparse matrix method makes searches through the database quick and efficient.

The BCPNN is a neural network where learning and inference are done using the principles of Bayes' law. Bayesian statistics fit intuitively into the framework of a neural network approach as both build on the concept of adapting on the basis of new data.

The new signaling system uses the BCPNN to scan incoming ADR reports and to compare them statistically with what is already stored in the database, before clinical review. Every three months, the complete WHO database is scanned to produce the combinations database. This is a table that contains frequency counts for each drug, for each ADR, and for each drug–ADR combination for which the UMC has received case reports during the last quarter. Only combinations where the drug has been reported as "suspected" are included. For each drug–adverse reaction combination, statistical figures generated by the BCPNN are also given. The figures from the previous quarter are also included and the data are provided to all national pharmacovigilance centers in an electronic format.

The neural network architecture allows the same framework to be used both for data mining/data analysis as well as for pattern recognition and classification. Pattern recognition by the BCPNN does not depend upon any *a priori* hypothesis, as an unsupervised search and detection approach is used. For the regular routine output the BCPNN is used as a one-layer model, although it has been extended to a multilayer network. To find complex dependencies that have not necessarily been considered before, a recurrent network is used for investigations of combinations of several variables in the WHO database. Two important applications based on BCPNN that the UMC is developing are syndrome detection and identification of possible drug interactions. Other possibilities include finding age profiles of drug–adverse reactions, determining at-risk groups, and searching for dose–response relationships.

Naturally, changes in patterns such as patient groups, drug classes, organ systems, and drug doses may also be important. However, as with any subdivision of data, a very large overall amount is necessary initially to attain statistical significance in subsets. This is a major advantage of using the large, pooled WHO database, and the UMC is trying to maximize this potential.

Stratification of data has the same problem of needing a large data set as well as the problem of deciding in advance what strata may be relevant in any particular situation, although it may be valuable in removing the effects of confounders. Stratification is, therefore, done after signals have been found, as deemed necessary.[42]

"Validation" of the BCPNN Data Mining Approach

Critics of data mining can reasonably suggest that, with all the possible relationships in a huge database, many medicine–adverse reaction associations will occur by chance, even though they seem to be significantly associated. The BCPNN methodology used by the UMC does take account of the size of the database in assigning probabilities. It is clear that national centers and reviewers must not be provided with what amounts to a huge amount of useless probabilistic information. On the other hand, it is clear that the process of finding signals early will entail some false positives.

Determining the performance of the BCPNN is a difficult task because there is no gold standard for comparison and there are different definitions of the term signal. According to the definition used in the WHO program, a signal is essentially a hypothesis together with data and arguments, and is not only uncertain but also preliminary in nature: the status of a signal may change substantially over time, as new knowledge is gained.

Two main studies of the performance of the BCPNN have been reported in a single paper.[43]

One study concerned a retrospective test of the BCPNN predictive value in new signal detection as compared with reference literature sources (Martindale's Extra Pharmacopoeia, and the US Physicians Desk Reference). The BCPNN method detected signals with a positive predictive value of 44% and the negative predictive value was 85%.

The second study was a comparison of the BCPNN with the results of the former signaling procedure, which was based on clinical review of summarized case data. Six out of ten previously identified signals were also identified by the BCPNN. These combinations all showed a substantial subsequent reporting increase. The remaining four drug–ADR combinations that were not identified by the BCPNN had a small, or no, increase in the number of reports, and were not listed in the reference sources seven years after they had been circulated as signals.

Of course, the use of the selected literature sources as a gold standard is open to debate. The literature is not intended as an early signaling system, and uses many sources for its information other than the WHO database: the biases affecting inclusion and exclusion of ADR information therefore may be very different. Factors such as those affecting the differential reporting to WHO and the inclusion of new information in the reference sources will have an effect which is independent of the performance of the BCPNN.

The BCPNN is run every quarter by the UMC, and just one quarter was selected: since the BCPNN is used in continuous analysis, the specificity and sensitivity are subject to necessary time-dependent changes in classification of "positives" and "negatives." It is difficult to consider something as a "non-association" because of this time dependency, and it is clear that there is an asymmetry in the effect of time on the results.

An assumption was made that a substantial increase in the number of reports of an association over the period indicated ongoing clinical interest in an association. More reports may be seen as a support for the validity of the associations, though there is often a tendency for ADRs that are becoming well known to be more reported anyway.

Another obvious limitation is that the BCPNN method for signal detection is dependent on the terminology used for recording of adverse reactions. Very little work has been done on any of the medical terminologies in use or proposed to determine their relative value in searching for new drug signals.

Although the UMC found that the use of the BCPNN gave a 44% positive predictive value, and a high negative predictive value of 85%, the usual approaches for assessing the power of a method are difficult to apply, because of the reasons outlined above. Further, and importantly, negative predictive value will always be high when the *a priori* probability is low. Thus, an 85%, negative predictive value may not even be perceived as high in this situation. It is for these reasons that "validation" is placed in quotation marks in the title of this section.

The BCPNN (or indeed any other data mining method) is not a panacea for drug safety monitoring. It is important to be aware of the limitations of the BCPNN and that it cannot replace expert review.[40] However, it may be a very useful tool in preliminary analysis of complex and large databases.

Proportional Reporting Ratios

This is an approach pioneered in the UK[44] but now widely used because of its simplicity. The proportion of all reactions to a drug that represent a particular medical condition of interest is compared with the same proportion for all drugs in the database. The resulting statistic is called a proportional reporting ratio (PRR). Judgments about signals may then be made using the PRR, along with the associated value of chi-squared and the absolute number of reports.

As with the other methods, this approach uses the total number of reports for the drug as a denominator to calculate the proportion of all reactions that are the type of interest (e.g., hepatitis). This proportion may be compared with the value for other drugs. It is also possible to compare complete profiles of ADR reporting for drugs of different types of reactions, where differences in the profile may represent potential signals. The result of such a calculation is also called a PRR, where the PRR is $a/(a+b)$ divided by $c/(c+d)$ in the following two-by-two table:

	Reaction(s) of interest	All other reactions
Drug of interest	a	b
All other drugs in database	c	d

The result of the PRR, as well as the other methods described below, is to highlight drug–ADR combinations with a disproportionally high reporting rate: the mathematics involved are different but the principles are similar.[45]

The expected or null value for a PRR is 1.0 and the numbers generated are measures of association that behave in a fashion similar to relative risks. Measures of statistical association for each value are calculated using standard methods for significance (see below). The higher the PRR, the more the disproportionality stands out statistically. Examination of changes in PRRs over time may help to demonstrate how disproportionalities can be identified as early as possible.

PRRs have advantages over calculation of reporting rates, since they are simple in concept and calculation, and enjoy the merits of data mining in general. However, and importantly, this does not take into account clinical relevance and the effects of biases including confounding, selective underreporting, and the effects of summarizing report information.

It is again important to recognize that PRRs are not a substitute for detailed review of cases, but an aid to deciding which series of cases most warrant further review.

Also, PRRs and chi-square values are measures of association and not causality. The result of a PRR provides a signal; it does not prove causation. Testing of the resulting hypothesis usually requires formal study in more structured data.

There are a number of possible extensions to the method that are being evaluated further, for example by Professor Stephen Evans in the UK, using the differences in observed and expected reporting rates (sequential probability ratio test) as a way of highlighting the more important possible signals (personal communication). Also, PRR calculations could be restricted to particular groups of drugs, to serious or fatal reports, or to particular age groups.

Other Data Mining Approaches for Signal Detection

Data mining approaches have been adopted by several national pharmacovigilance centers, including the Netherlands, the UK, and the US.[44,46,47] and also by some pharmaceutical companies. A recent paper analyzed the concordance among different measures (PRR, reporting odds ratios (ROR), and the IC).[45] The different methods all use the principle of finding disproportionality as described for the PRR, but the mathematical theory behind them is different, for example, a Bayesian approach and information theory underpinning the BCPNN. The result of the comparative study was that no clear differences were present, except for when there were fewer than four reports per drug–ADR combination, though this depends on the Bayesian prior probability used in those methods using Bayes' theory. The methods all have their somewhat different advantages and disadvantages. Before a partially automated signal detection system is implemented, it is therefore recommended that careful consideration be given to the possible alternatives in looking for the most practical and appropriate in a given setting.

QUANTITATIVE ASPECTS OF REPORTING

Case reports are submitted by national centers to the UMC for inclusion in the WHO database.[48] Figure 10.2 depicts the cumulative number of reports stored in the database. In most countries reporting has gradually increased over time. It usually takes some 5–10 years of operation before reporting reaches a stable level. The number of reports relayed to the UMC is often less than that received in the country, for various technical reasons. In France, reports received by the national agency from the manufacturers (50%) are not sent to the UMC, nor are reports on drugs that are marketed only in France. Also, reports evaluated as unclassifiable or reactions due to overdoses are omitted

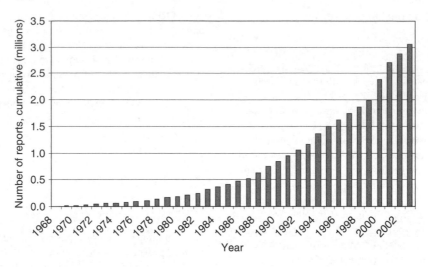

Figure 10.2. Cumulative number of reports in the WHO database, 1968–2003.

from some but not all countries. The US situation is special in this regard and is described separately (see Chapter 9). (The issue is also discussed further below; see "Limitations".)

INTERNATIONAL REPORTING STANDARDS

There is no international standard for good pharmacovigilance practice but some useful publications give advice regarding some aspects.[12,49,50]

In recent years there has been an increasing tendency among regulators to demand that manufacturers report suspected ADRs occurring in other countries directly to them, in spite of the fact that most of such reports are already available to them through the WHO system. At first, these requirements also meant that the manufacturers had to report these cases on several different forms, according to different rules and time schedules.

In order to decrease the workload of manufacturers and increase the cost-effectiveness of international reporting, an initiative was started in 1986 to harmonize the rules for international reporting of single cases under the auspices of CIOMS, which is affiliated to the WHO. This initiative, called "CIOMS I,"[11] is now accepted in most countries and by most manufacturers, and has been accepted by the ICH as a guideline for use in Japan, the European Union, and the US. This system has definitely decreased the diversity of rules in international reporting, although national variation still exists even in the ICH member countries. There is also

a CIOMS guideline on electronic reporting of adverse reactions internationally.[51]

Both inside and outside ICH, many of the smaller drug control agencies felt that they did not have the capacity to cope with the massive increase in the number of reports that the CIOMS I initiative produced. They preferred periodic safety updates, including the evaluation of the safety situation at large by the company. In some countries such safety updates were mandatory, but again there were differences in the rules, formats, and time schedules. Therefore, a second CIOMS project—"CIOMS II"—was initiated to harmonize the contents, format, and time schedule for periodic safety updates.[52] Some novel features of this scheme were:

- the creation of an international "birth date" for each drug product, which was the day of first approval in any country;
- the inclusion of drug exposure data and experience from both pre- and postmarketing studies;
- the principle that the manufacturer should write an overall safety evaluation of the product.

The CIOMS II safety updates are now unofficially accepted by ICH countries and have been made into a guideline followed by the EU, the US, and Japan. Many more countries accept periodic safety updates according to the CIOMS/ICH format, although again there are some variations in demands by regulatory authorities, which frustrates the concept of complete global standardization that the pharmaceutical industry seeks in order to reduce the administrative burden.

The European Parliament adopted a regulation in 1995 creating the EMEA, which is located in London, UK. According to this regulation, any serious suspected adverse reaction that is reported to an MAH by a health professional must be reported to the health authority of the country in which it occurred within 15 days. Health authorities must also report to the EMEA and to the MAH within 15 days. MAHs are also required to report ADRs occurring outside the EU as well as from the world literature that are both serious and unexpected (known as *unlabeled*: not fully covered in the Summary of Product Characteristics package insert which accompanies the drug product). Similar regulations exist in the US, described in Chapter 8, and in some other countries.[12] This "15-day reporting" certainly has the advantage of getting prompt warnings of new signals of adverse drug reactions, but needs to be considered against the need for follow-up reports and the possible errors and duplications, which seem to have been difficult to avoid so far.

The problems of managing and distributing large numbers of ADR reports within 15 days has led to a commitment from many countries to communicate data electronically. However, standardization of data sets and terminology is required for this to be implemented effectively. The MedDRA[53] and Electronic Standards for the transfer of Regulatory Information were introduced to the ICH (M1 and M2 topics) in 1994. Both are applicable to the pre- and postmarketing phases of the regulatory cycle (see www.ich.org).

MedDRA was based on the terminology developed by the Medicines Control Agency (now the Medicines and Healthcare products Regulatory Agency; MHRA) in the UK. It provides greater specificity of data entry (more terms) than previously used adverse reaction terminologies and hierarchical data retrieval categories. However, it does not contain specific definitions of the terms to be used. In this regard, the CIOMS initiative is relied upon. Its use for ADR reporting will be mandated in some countries, but other countries, especially small and developing countries, have expressed doubts since their computer resources are limited and their number of reports is small.

STRENGTHS

Spontaneous reporting systems are relatively inexpensive to operate, although their true total costs to the health care system, including the substantial investment by the pharmaceutical industry in their maintenance, is unknown. They remain the only practical means of covering whole populations and all drugs. They allow significant concerns of health professionals and patients to be expressed, pooled, and acted upon to form hypotheses of drug risks. One physician, one pharmacist, and a secretary can usually manage between one and two thousand reports a year, depending on the amount of scrutiny, follow-up, feedback, and other activities that are part of the program. The basic technical equipment needed is also a relatively minor investment. Together with other qualities (Table 10.2), some of which are unique, this makes a spontaneous reporting system one of the essential, basic ingredients in a comprehensive system for the postmarketing surveillance of drug-induced risks.

A spontaneous reporting system has the potential to cover the total patient population. It does not exclude patients treated for other concomitant diseases or those who are using other drug products. Moreover, the surveillance can start as soon as a drug is approved for marketing and has no inherent time limit. Thus, it is potentially the most cost-effective system for the detection of new ADRs that occur rarely, mostly in special subgroups, like the elderly, or in combination with other drugs.

In an early analysis of how important ADRs were first suspected and then verified, Venning[54] found that 13 out of 18 reactions were first signaled by an anecdotal report made by a physician with an open and critical mind. The fact that these reports were published in medical journals led the author to conclude that spontaneous reporting systems were of little value in the signaling process. However, the majority of these reactions actually were detected before most

Table 10.2. Strengths and limitations of spontaneous reporting systems

Strengths
Inexpensive and simple to operate
Covers all drugs during their whole life cycle
Covers the whole patient population, including special
  subgroups, such as the elderly
Does not interfere with prescribing habits
Can be used for follow-up studies of patients with severe
  ADRs, to study mechanisms

Limitations
The amount of clinical information available is often too limited
  to permit a thorough case evaluation
Underreporting decreases sensitivity and makes the systems
  sensitive to selective reporting
The reporting rate is seldom stable over time
No direct information on incidence

spontaneous reporting systems were operational. In later analyses of where the first suspicion that a new drug could cause agranulocytosis and Stevens–Johnson syndrome appeared, it was found that, for the vast majority, the first report appeared in the WHO database more than six months before it was published.[55,56] The opposite situation was found in only a few cases. Some of these signals were published. In most cases, however, a spontaneous reporting system needs to be supplemented by other sources of information, as described in the section on "Particular applications," below.

LIMITATIONS

Spontaneous reporting systems are mainly intended to produce signals about potential new ADRs. To fulfill this function properly, it must be recognized that a number of false signals will be produced and, therefore, that each signal must be scrutinized and verified before it can be accepted and acted upon. Preferably a signal should be followed up using an analytic epidemiologic study design and one or more of the data resources described in Chapters 11–24. Signals might be of rare reactions, however, so the constraints of any epidemiologic study are an important consideration. Quite often it is not easily possible to create even a case–control study that will answer questions about rare serious reactions. In such instances, it seems reasonable to qualify the result by a statement such as: "spontaneous reports have suggested adverse reaction x, but further studies have been unable to confirm this at an incidence more frequent than . . . ."

A more serious disadvantage is that not all reactions are reported and that the proportion that is reported in any specific situation is hard to estimate. A basic requirement for the generation of a report is that a physician suspects that a drug may be causing the signs and/or symptoms of his/her patient. This is relatively easy when the inherent pharmacological actions or chemical properties of the drug can predict the reaction. There are also some diseases that are considered as "typically" drug-induced reactions, such as agranulocytosis and severe skin reactions, so that the basic level of suspicion is high. It is, however, very hard to make the mental connection between a drug therapy and a medical event if the event simulates a common, spontaneously occurring disease or other untoward event, which has never previously been described as drug-induced. Some examples of this include the first cases of the oculomucocutanous syndrome, Guillain–Barré syndrome, and changes in the body fat distribution, structural heart valve changes, and visual field defects with a specific pattern. It is also hard to make the mental connection between a drug and a medical event if there is a long time lag between exposure and disease.

Even if the physician suspects the signs and symptoms of his or her patient to be drug-induced, ignorance of the value of ADR reporting or of the reporting rules, and overwork, have been given as reasons for not reporting. Increased information and feedback by national agencies, medical schools, pharmaceutical manufacturers, and professional journals in collaboration could rectify these inadequacies. The health care authorities also have a clear role here. It is their responsibility to monitor the quality of health care and to build ADR reporting practices in their quality assurance systems, as well as in continuing medical education.

Besides delaying the detection of new ADRs, underreporting creates two other important problems. First, it will underestimate the frequency of the ADR and, thereby, underestimate the importance of the problem. This may not be so serious as long as one recognizes that the reported frequency is likely to be a minimum level of incidence. More important is that underreporting may not be random but selective, which may introduce serious bias.

The effect of selective reporting becomes potentially disastrous if the number of reports of an ADR for different drugs is compared in an uncritical way. There are many possible reasons for apparent differences. The overall rate of reporting has increased over the years, and reporting is often higher during the first years a new drug is on the market (the "Weber effect"[57]). Finally, a drug that is claimed to be very safe may first be tried on patients who do not tolerate the previous drug products (channeling bias). Furthermore, there may be reporting distortions if there are suspicions or rumors circulated about a drug.

Another interesting example of biased reporting is the four-fold difference in reports of hemorrhagic diarrheas in relation to sales of the two penicillin-v products Calciopen® and Kåvepenin® in Sweden. An analysis of the situation failed to reveal any differences in the two products. They were produced in the same factory from the same batch and only the form, product name, and MAH differed. There were, however, differences in the use of the products. The older product was used to a larger extent by older physicians, by ear, nose, and throat specialists, and private practitioners, groups who traditionally do not report ADRs. This could not, however, totally explain the apparent difference in ADR rate, as the reporters were seldom the prescribers, but other health care professionals who managed the patients' illness. The most important explanation was probably that the newer product was more commonly recommended and used in "high reporting" areas. A similar situation arose when minocycline was found to have a higher reporting rate for the lupus syndrome and hepatic injury, both together and separately, than other tetracyclines. This difference in rate is probably due, at least in part, to the much more protracted use of minocycline in the management of young people with acne, as compared with the shorter-term use of the other tetracyclines to treat infection.[58]

PARTICULAR APPLICATIONS

WITHOUT THE ADDITION OF OTHER DATA

It is rarely possible to use spontaneous reports to establish more than a suspicion of a causal relationship between an adverse event and a drug, unless:

1. there is at least one case with a positive re-challenge and some other supportive cases which do not have known confounding drugs or diseases, or
2. there is an event which is phenomenologically very clearly related to single drug exposure, such as anaphylaxis, or
3. there is a cluster of exposed cases reported, the background incidence of the adverse event is close to zero, and there is no confounding.

Even the reappearance of an adverse event when a drug is given again is certainly no proof of causality,[59] unless this is done in tightly controlled circumstances, which may be unethical. Thus, re-exposure to a drug that has caused an ADR is often accidental. In practice, however, one is reassured that there is strong evidence for a causal relationship if there is a cluster of cases with good clinical information, in which the same event has reappeared with repeated exposure at least once in each patient. This is only possible if the medical event in question is of a type that would diminish or disappear after withdrawal of the drug and not reappear spontaneously. Thus, the observation of five cases of aseptic meningitis that reappeared within hours after again taking the antibiotic trimethoprim for urinary tract infections,[60] will convince most clinicians that this drug can and did cause such a reaction. For typical "hit and run" effects like thromboembolic diseases and for diseases that can be cyclic, information on re-challenge, however, can be misleading. For example, one unpublished case report involved a young boy who developed agranulocytosis three times in connection with infections treated with ampicillin. It was not until after the fourth time, when agranulocytosis

developed *before* ampicillin was given, that his cyclic neutropenia was discovered. Contrast this with a patient who three times developed the Guillain–Barré syndrome after tetanus vaccination. Such unpublished material has influenced policy.[61]

Information on re-challenge is relatively uncommon in most spontaneous reporting systems. Planned re-challenge may be dangerous, is seldom warranted from a clinical point of view, and can be unethical. However, information on a positive re-exposure was available in as many as 13% of 200 consecutive nonfatal cases reported in the nordic countries.[62] In the French pharmacovigilance database, re-exposure is reported in 8.5% of reports, positive in 6%.[63]

An example of comparing rates of a cluster of events with the known background occurred with the cardiovascular drug aprindine. Four cases of agranulocytosis were reported in the first two years the drug was marketed. As the background incidence of agranulocytosis is only five to eight per million inhabitants per year,[64] this made a strong case for a causal relationship.[65] Similarly, there were 25 confirmed cases of motor and sensory neuropathy following meningitis A vaccination in 130 000 children, which was much higher than the likely background incidence.[66]

These examples show some ways in which spontaneous ADR reports can lead to firm conclusions being made, and such reports may be the only information available, particularly during the early marketing of a product. It should not be necessary to emphasize that reports should be of good quality when they are the only evidence used!

WITH THE ADDITION OF DENOMINATOR DATA

Today, most drug regulatory authorities in industrialized countries and pharmaceutical manufacturers collate information that can be used to estimate both the size and the characteristics of the exposed population and the background incidence of diseases. In many countries there are national statistics on drug sales and/or prescribing (see Chapter 27). In many countries information on drug sales and prescribing is confidential, but in the nordic countries this information is published periodically.[67]

IMS Health is a unique source of information on pharmaceutical sales and prescribing habits in a large number of countries (see Chapters 23 and 27). The data are collected continuously on nearly all drug products. The prescription data are obtained from rolling panels of prescribers in each country, constituted to reflect the national mix of medical specialists and medical practice type. These data are not without the usual drawbacks of continuous routine data collection, yet their use has provided many important insights into drug safety issues. For example, data from several countries have been combined with ADR information from the WHO database to provide rough incidence estimates of certain drug-induced problems, and perspectives on possible reasons for differences of ADR reporting have also proved useful.[68,69]

WITH THE ADDITION OF NUMERATOR DATA

If the rate of reporting is known, the numerator can be inferred with some accuracy. From studies using registers of hospital discharge diagnoses, it has been possible to calculate reporting rates for some areas, for ADRs, and for selected periods of time. Considering serious reactions such as blood dyscrasias, thromboembolic disease, and Stevens–Johnson syndrome, between 20% and 40% of the patients discharged with these diagnoses have been found to be reported.[70] By identifying all positive BCG cultures in bacteriology laboratories, it was found that almost 80% of all children who developed an osteitis after BCG vaccination had been reported.[71] However, reporting rates probably cannot be generalized. The magnitude of underreporting is important to know when evaluating the data, but should not be used to correct for underreporting in the calculations since the reporting rate is time-, problem-, drug-, and country-specific.

EXAMPLES OF USING SPONTANEOUS REPORTS TO ESTIMATE RISK

If information from an efficient spontaneous reporting system can be combined with information on drug sales and prescription statistics, it is possible to start to consider reporting rates as a rough estimate of the frequency or incidence rate of an ADR. Such estimates can never reach the accuracy of those derived from clinical trials or formal epidemiologic studies. However, they can serve as a first indicator of the size of a potential problem, and certainly an indicator of health professionals' concerns about a problem. For very rare reactions, they may actually be the only conceivable measure.

With knowledge of the number of defined daily doses (DDDs) sold and the average prescribed daily dose (PDD) (see Chapter 27), it is possible to get a rough estimate of the total person-time of exposure for a particular drug. The number of cases reported per patient "exposure time" might then be a very rough, preliminary guide to minimum incidence.[12,72] If prescription statistics are available, the number of prescriptions may be a better estimate of drug use among outpatients than the number of treatment-weeks calculated from sales data, especially where drug use is mostly short term and doses and treatment times may vary with patient age and indication.

If the background incidence of a disease is known or can be estimated from other sources, it is sometimes also possible to calculate rough estimates of relative risks and excess risks from spontaneously reported data on ADRs plus sales and prescription statistics. For example, single cases of aplastic anemia in patients taking acetazolamide (a carbonic anhydrase inhibiting diuretic which is used mainly for the treatment of glaucoma) have been reported since the drug was introduced in the mid-1950s.[73] There are no estimates of the incidence of this reaction, but it was certainly thought to be very rare, probably rarer than aplastic anemia occurring after the use of chloramphenicol. Between 1972 and 1988, 11 cases were reported to have occurred in Sweden.[74] Based on sales and prescription data, it could be estimated that the total exposure time was 195 000 patient-years during the same period of time, yielding a reported incidence of about 1 in 20 000 prescriptions, or 50 per million patient-years. From a population-based case–control study of aplastic anemia in which Sweden participated,[75] it could be estimated that the total yearly incidence of aplastic anemia in the relevant age groups was about 6 per million exposed persons. In the case–control study it was not possible to estimate the relative risk for the association between acetazolamide and aplastic anemia, because there were no exposed controls. However, if the spontaneously reported incidence of aplastic anemia among persons exposed to acetazolamide is compared with the total incidence of aplastic anemia from the case–control study, the relative risk could be estimated to be around 10.

Several potential sources of errors in this study must be considered. The degree of underreporting in this example is unknown. However, in one study the reporting rate for aplastic anemia was found to be 30%,[76] and since then reporting in general has doubled. There is no known association between glaucoma and aplastic anemia that could act as a confounder, but some of the reported patients had taken other drugs during the six months before the detection of their aplastic anemia. There were only two patients who had been treated with drugs that, on clinical pharmacological grounds, seemed to be reasonable alternative possibilities as causal agents. However, it is a clear limitation that multiple drug exposures cannot be corrected for in a rough analysis such as this.

In some instances it has been possible to compare risk estimates from a formal epidemiologic case–control study with those derived from the Swedish drug monitoring system.

The relative risks for agranulocytosis induced by cotrimoxazole and sulphasalazine were astonishingly alike.[77]

USING SPONTANEOUS REPORTING DATA TO IDENTIFY MECHANISMS AND RISK GROUPS

As soon as it has been established that a drug can induce a certain adverse reaction, it becomes important to identify the mechanisms involved, and whether any group of patients is at a particularly increased risk, and if any measure could be taken at the patient and/or the population level to reduce the risk. Usually a multitude of different methods must be applied, both in the laboratory and at a population level. A good spontaneous reporting system can be of value in this work in certain circumstances, if the data can be compared to sales and prescription data or if the patients can be subjected to special investigations.

For example, in one study of the characteristics of patients developing hypoglycemia during treatment with glibenclamide (an oral antidiabetic drug), the distribution of prescribed daily doses was similar in patients with episodes of severe hypoglycemia and in the general population. However, patients hospitalized because of severe hypoglycemia were older and were more likely to have had a previous episode of cerebrovascular disease.[78]

In studies published on oral contraceptives and thromboembolic disease, it was found that women who were reported to have developed deep vein thrombosis while taking oral contraceptives were deficient in Leiden factor V more often than would have been expected from the general population.[79,80]

Another study[81] investigated patients reported to have developed lupoid reactions while taking hydralazine for hypertension. A much higher percentage of these patients were slow acetylators than the 40% expected from the distribution of this phenotype in the population at large.

In a more sophisticated study, Strom and colleagues used spontaneously reported cases of suprofen-induced "acute flank pain syndrome" in a case–control study designed to identify patient-specific risk factors for the development of the syndrome.[82] Patients who were reported to have developed the syndrome were compared to a random sample of patients who had taken the drug without problems. Risk factors identified were, among others, male sex, hay fever and asthma, participation in exercise, and alcohol consumption. Most of these factors are consistent with the postulated pathogenic mechanism of acute diffuse crystallization of uric acid in the renal tubules.

CONTEMPORARY ISSUES: AN EXAMPLE

The monograph CIOMS IV entitled *Benefit–Risk Balance for Marketed Drugs* (which should really have been *Effectiveness and Risk Balance*!)[83] promotes the idea that the positive side of drug action and the negative side can both be reduced to similar terms to allow comparison between therapies for the same indication. At the first signal of a problem with a drug the first question should be, "How does this drug compare with others?" Most often there is no information on the relative effectiveness of drugs in real-life practice, only some premarketing efficacy data, in highly selected patients. For this reason, comparisons at the signal stage are often for the safety side only.

Another major thrust of CIOMS IV was that all similar drugs reasonably used for a particular target indication should be compared and that analysis should consider *the whole safety profile* of the drugs, not just a target adverse reaction. Because the safety profiles of drugs are usually made of a multiplicity of adverse reaction terms, CIOMS IV suggested reducing the comparison to a few: some of those most frequently reported ADRs and the most serious, the latter being assessed using clinical judgment and irrespective of reporting rate.

Following a signal that the lipid lowering statin, cerivastatin, was associated with rhabdomyolysis, the UMC carried out a preliminary assessment in 2000. The CIOMS logic was used in this study, but no data on effectiveness were considered. Even given these limitations, the comparison was interesting.[84]

All the statin drugs classified as similar in the WHO Anatomic–therapeutic Chemical Classification (ATC group C10AA)[85] were selected from the WHO database. Gemfibrozil was specifically included as well because it was very strongly implicated as an interacting drug. IMS Health worldwide sales figures for the years 1989–2000 were obtained for the same drugs and from nearly the same countries (IMS does not have data from the Netherlands, Iran, Costa Rica, and Croatia, but these countries contribute a relatively very small number of ADR reports). IMS data are difficult to obtain prior to that date and therefore missed the launch of the first statin on the market by two years. The IMS data were converted to million patient-years and, since the mean dosages used equate closely with dosage forms, these were used as a rate denominator in all subsequent work. The rates are shown in Table 10.3.

Also, IMS Health data on co-prescription between statins and gemfibrozil and fibrates was used, together with age and gender breakdowns of statin prescriptions in the US.

Table 10.3. Sales denominators for statin drugs, 1989–2000

Drug name	Million patient-years
Atorvastatin	22.49
Cerivastatin	3.92
Fluvastatin	8.44
Lovastatin	20.51
Pravastatin	46.55
Simvastatin	44.97

All critical ADR terms (WHO Critical Terms List) associated with the statins were inspected by a clinician, who selected the ADR terms with the most serious clinical import in terms of possible lethal outcome or permanent disability. They were then grouped, resulting in 13 ADR groups:

- disseminated intravascular coagulation
- neuroleptic malignant syndrome
- cardiomyopathy
- anaphylactic shock
- death
- serious hepatic damage
- rhabdomyolysis
- pulmonary fibrosis
- Stevens–Johnson syndrome
- renal failure
- myopathy
- pancreatitis
- serotonin syndrome.

Because of the small numbers, anaphylactic shock, disseminated intravascular coagulation, and neuroleptic malignant syndrome were not evaluated further, and it was considered that the overall report profiles were qualitatively similar.

There were, however, some quantitative differences. Of rates above 1 per million patient-years, the rates that stood out were: cardiomyopathy, myopathy, renal failure, rhabdomyolysis, and death with cerivastatin, and myopathy for lovastatin. This caused the study to focus on the issues of rhabdomyolysis, myopathy, and renal failure as reasonable in comparing and differentiating the safety profiles of the drugs.

The various other analyses that were done can be found in WHO Drug Information[84] (http://www.who.int/druginformation). The following is a summary of some of the study's conclusions:

This signal was known for two years before the drug was taken off the market and attempts were made to warn the medical profession of the very important risk of interaction. The result of repeated "Dear Doctor" letters was only a 2% change in prescribing behavior. It was and is clear that the communication of these key messages must be improved and that monitoring impact is an all important practice.

Based on an analysis of spontaneous reports there appears to be a strong link between cerivastatin and rhabdomyolysis and renal failure (possibly related) which was quantitatively greater than with the other statins. Since cerivastatin is the most recently marketed this may increase the overall reporting rate relatively. The Weber effect was not a complete explanation for the rhabdomyolysis reporting.

Disproportionality of the combination cerivastatin/gemfibrozil and cerivastatin/clopidogrel against their use strongly suggests interaction with both drugs. This almost entirely affects muscle ADRs. This effect of the combination was not seen as strikingly with the other drugs, though it was obvious with lovastatin. Disproportionality of cerivastatin reports of rhabdomyolysis and its use in older women suggests they may be a risk group, though lovastatin was relatively highly used in older women and seemed less likely to cause rhabdomyolysis in this group.

There were clear problems of case definition. The link between myopathy and death on older reports suggests misclassification under the broader, more neutral term. The need for case definition when the ADR involves a rare disease is important and may delay and confuse positive action. It is certainly possible that the profile of lovastatin and muscle disorder and death was not very different to cerivastatin. The availability of rhabdomyolysis as a used term since the mid 90s probably resulted in lower numbers of reports of rhabdomyolysis with older drugs, particularly lovastatin. Reports of myopathy are high for lovastatin after the first years of launch. Lovastatin has been on the market longest and there may be a depletion effect.

The purpose of giving this example study here is not to promote or endorse any of its conclusions, but to indicate the range of issues that are raised. It seems unlikely that the above issues could be answered without very extensive studies, because of the rarity of rhabdomyolysis, but this is an important issue because of the wide and increasing use of the statins. It is just one example of the safety management problems with "blockbuster drugs," and the need for risk management planning.[86] The failure of repeated communications about the interaction between cerivastatin and gemfibrozil raises the need for a much greater attention to communications of risk and their impact.[87] This subject is dealt with elsewhere (see Chapter 33), and has been the topic of two international workshops, both of which resulted in monographs.[88,89]

THE FUTURE

In western countries, the population is growing progressively older and, thus, we can expect a steady increase in the chronic use of medications. Even if the drugs to be used are more sophisticated and "targeted," they are also likely to be more pharmacologically active and hence may be more difficult to use. With the continued development of clinical trial methodology, adverse reactions that are caused by pharmacologic mechanisms will probably be better known both as to range and incidence when new medicines are approved. However, there will still be the classical idiosyncratic reactions, which cannot be predicted and which are too rare to be detected in the clinical premarketing trials.

At the same time, there is increasing commercial pressure for the pharmaceutical industry to find "blockbuster" drugs that will be marketed globally to maximize profit in the shortest possible time. Other changes in the industry—shortened times for drug development and increasing outsourcing of functions—make for an environment where some premarketing safety issues may go unnoticed. The increasing challenge to pharmacovigilance is not only to be able to find early signals of drug problems, but to rapidly determine true effectiveness and risk during regular clinical use.

Pharmacovigilance programs are now being established also in developing countries, from which there has been little information in the past. It is likely that the monitoring of populations with other patterns of morbidity and different nutritional status will reveal different types of adverse reactions than what we have learned to expect from populations in the industrialized world, even from established medicines. The influence of co-medication with traditional medicines, and the unexpected failure of efficacy because of substandard or counterfeit medicines, will have to be covered by the pharmacovigilance systems. The developing countries have some diseases that are not seen in the so-called developed world. Malaria is one example only, but this scourge and others are being treated by new chemical entities within large public health programs. Pharmacovigilance and pharmacoepidemiology must be employed alongside such programs if drug-related risk is to be detected early and limited.

The role of spontaneous reporting in the future will be of even more central importance if it can be developed further. The basic requisite for its enhanced effectiveness is an increased flow of information, both in quantitative and qualitative terms. For example, to increase the reporting of classical, rare ADRs such as blood dyscrasias, toxic epidermal necrolysis, and liver and kidney damage, the automatic collection of information about all patients who have been hospitalized with these conditions could be instituted. This could be accomplished through case–control surveillance of rare diseases that are often elicited by drugs. Alternatively, manual retrieval of case summaries, providing high quality information, or alternatively through automated transfer of computerized hospital discharge diagnoses, could be used to study case series. Of course, in such automated systems, one would lose the important screening impact of the provider who thought the adverse outcome was due to the drug. Periodically it may be beneficial to focus on certain new drug classes to clarify their ADR spectrum as soon as possible (the HIV ADR reporting scheme in the UK is an example).

However, the detection of the totally unexpected will most probably continue to rely on the capacity of the alert human mind for the foreseeable future. Therefore, it is essential to enhance the practicing clinician's awareness of and cooperation with ADR reporting. Here a regional system with mutual benefits, like the French system, seems promising.

WHO and the UMC have taken several initiatives to promote the importance of effective communications.[88,89] Another publication on crisis management in pharmacovigilance also deals with communications issues,[90] and the publication *Viewpoint* is aimed at explaining some of the issues involved in pharmacovigilance to the general public.[91] Alongside the development of scientific excellence, while the core of pharmacovigilance is the discovery of knowledge about drug safety, its achievements are of little value if they do not actively affect clinical practice and the wisdom and compliance of patients. The basic aim of encouraging reporting requires more than scientific confidence: it demands all the advanced skills of persuasion, motivation, and marketing. Some countries have shown great imagination and creativity in this area, but the impact of the science on public health will depend heavily on a much more committed and professional approach to making information relevant and meaningful and to influencing behavior.

Medical therapy becomes ever more complex. Multiple drug use may result in adverse interactions. Not only is there polypharmacy caused by a single physician treating multiple disease processes, but with increasing specialization, more than one doctor may be prescribing without others' knowledge. Moreover, there are the drugs which the patient may use from an ever-increasing selection of over-the-counter drugs and herbals, made available in increasingly sophisticated societies. Treating complex diseases also requires consideration of the interaction between concomitant diseases and drugs used for the target illness.

It is clear that there is more and more pressure on doctors and health professionals in general. The increasing technical and professional complexity of their work is apparent, and we must add to that the increasing administrative and bureaucratic load they have, as well as their gross work overload in many countries. Undergraduate medical training does not give sufficient time to adverse reactions as a most important cause for morbidity; postgraduate education is too frequently concerned with the latest therapy and the importance of being up-to-date in the scholarly rather than the practical sense. There is unending pressure on doctors, including the threat of litigation for even the most genuine of errors by the most careful of doctors. Patients are increasingly informed on medical matters and encouraged, rightly, to understand their therapy and to be active partners rather than passive objects in its management. Unfortunately, the reliability of information sources is very variable, including that massive amount on the Internet. This involves doctors in an increasing need to justify their advice on therapy and even to undo confusion because of conflicting information.

Good communication practices and the best use of information technology should be very high on the agenda of everyone committed to drug safety improvement. This offers the only way of ensuring that health professionals can easily express their concerns over the safety of drug products to an agency that can collate, analyze, and use the information for focused communication back to health professionals and their patients in ways that can be useful in daily practice, and not be seen merely to add to information overload.

The problem is not just that there is more information to assimilate, but that it is currently provided as isolated, unfocused messages. What we need is focused, relevant messages available at the critical points of need: when doctors are prescribing, pharmacists are dispensing, and patients are being treated.

ACKNOWLEDGMENTS

We gratefully acknowledge the work of Dr Mary Couper in the review of this chapter and her many helpful comments. She has made many of the recent developments within the WHO program possible by her great energy and insights into what needs to be done.

We also acknowledge the work and ideas which come from very many colleagues from the, currently, 73 countries around the world who constantly enliven us with new perspectives and insights.

REFERENCES

1. McBride WG. Thalidomide and congenital abnormalities. *Lancet* 1961; **2**: 1358.
2. Finney DJ, Sadusk J. The scientific group on monitoring adverse drug reactions report to the Director General, report PA/d.65 Geneva: World Health Organization, 1964.
3. Finney DJ. The design and logic of a monitor of drug use. *J Chronic Dis* 1965; **18**: 77–98.
4. Finney DJ. Systematic signalling of adverse reactions to drugs. *Methods Inf Med* 1974; **13**: 1–10.
5. WHO. *The Importance of Pharmacovigilance. Safety Monitoring of Medicinal Products*. Geneva: World Health Organization, 2002.
6. Amery W. Signal generation from spontaneous adverse event reports. *Pharmacoepidemiol Drug Saf* 1999; **8**: 147–50.
7. EMEA. *Note for Guidance on Procedure for Competent Authorities on the Undertaking of Pharmacovigilance Activities*. London: The European Agency for the Evaluation of Medicinal Products, 1999.
8. Meyboom RH, Egberts AC, Edwards IR, Hekster YA, de Koning FH, Gribnau FW. Principles of signal detection in pharmacovigilance. *Drug Saf* 1997; **16**: 355–65.
9. Olsson S, ed. *National Pharmacovigilance Systems*, 2nd edn. Uppsala: Uppsala Monitoring Centre, 1997.
10. UMC. *Safety Monitoring of Medicinal Products*. Uppsala: Uppsala Monitoring Centre, 2000.
11. CIOMS. *International Reporting of Adverse Drug Reactions*. Geneva: CIOMS, 1990.
12. CIOMS. *Current Challenges in Pharmacovigilance: Pragmatic Approaches*. Geneva: CIOMS, 2001.
13. Edwards IR, Lindquist M, Wiholm BE, Napke E. Quality criteria for early signals of possible adverse drug reactions. *Lancet* 1990; **336**: 156–8.
14. Benichou C. Criteria of drug-induced liver disorders. Report of an international consensus meeting. *J Hepatol* 1990; **11**: 272–6.
15. Benichou C, Solal-Celigny P. Standardization of definitions and criteria for causality assessment of adverse drug reactions. Drug-induced blood cytopenias: report of an international consensus meeting. *Nouv Rev Fr Hematol* 1991; **33**: 257–62.
16. CIOMS. Basic requirements for the use of terms for reporting of drug reactions. *Pharmacoepidemiol Drug Saf* 1992; **1**: 39–45.
17. CIOMS. Basic requirements for the use of terms for reporting of drug reactions (II). *Pharmacoepidemiol Drug Saf* 1992; **1**: 133–7.
18. CIOMS. Harmonizing the use of adverse drug reactions and minimum requirements for their use: respiratory disorders and skin disorders. *Pharmacoepidemiol Drug Saf* 1997; **6**: 115–27.

19. CIOMS. Basic requirements for the use of terms for reporting adverse drug reactions (VIII): renal and urinary system disorders. *Pharmacoepidemiol Drug Saf* 1997; **6**: 203–11.

20. Meyboom RH, Hekster YA, Egberts AC, Gribnau FW, Edwards IR. Causal or casual? The role of causality assessment in pharmacovigilance. *Drug Saf* 1997; **17**: 374–89.

21. Herman RL. Drug–event association: perspectives, methods and uses. *Drug Inf J* 1984; **18**: 195–337.

22. Venulet J, Berneker G-C, Ciucci AG, eds, *Assessing Causes of Adverse Drug Reactions*. London: Academic Press, 1982.

23. Karch FE, Lasagna L. Toward the operational identification of adverse drug reactions. *Clin Pharmacol Ther* 1977; **21**: 247–54.

24. Kramer MS, Leventhal JM, Hutchinson TA, Feinstein AR. An algorithm for the operational assessment of adverse drug reactions. I. Background, description, and instructions for use. *JAMA* 1979; **242**: 623–32.

25. Naranjo CA, Busto U, Sellers EM, Sandor P, Ruiz I, Roberts EA *et al*. A method for estimating the probability of adverse drug reactions. *Clin Pharmacol Ther* 1981; **30**: 239–45.

26. Louik C, Lacouture PG, Mitchell AA, Kauffman R, Lovejoy FH, Jr, Yaffe SJ *et al*. A study of adverse reaction algorithms in a drug surveillance program. *Clin Pharmacol Ther* 1985; **38**: 183–7.

27. Pere JC, Begaud B, Haramburu F, Albin H. Computerized comparison of six adverse drug reaction assessment procedures. *Clin Pharmacol Ther* 1986; **40**: 451–61.

28. Moore N, Biour M, Paux G, Loupi E, Begaud B, Boismare F *et al*. Adverse drug reaction monitoring: doing it the French way. *Lancet* 1985; **2**: 1056–8.

29. Biriell C, Edwards IR. Reasons for reporting adverse drug reactions—some thoughts based on an international review. *Pharmacoepidemiol Drug Saf* 1997; **6**: 21–6.

30. Weber JCP. Epidemiology in the United Kingdom of adverse drug reactions from nonsteroidal anti-inflammatory drugs. In: Rainsford KD, Velo GP, eds, *Side Effects of Anti-Inflammatory Drugs*. Lancaster: MTP Press, 1986; pp. 27–36.

31. Holmberg L, Boman G, Bottiger LE, Eriksson B, Spross R, Wessling A. Adverse reactions to nitrofurantoin. Analysis of 921 reports. *Am J Med* 1980; **69**: 733–8.

32. Wiholm B-E, Myrhed M, Ekman E. Trends and patterns in adverse drug reactions to nonsteroidal anti-inflammatory drugs reported in Sweden. In: Rainsford KD, Velo GP, eds, *Side Effects of Anti-Inflammatory Drugs*. Lancaster: MTP Press, 1986; pp. 55–62.

33. Stricker BH, Tijssen JG. Serum sickness-like reactions to cefaclor. *J Clin Epidemiol* 1992; **45**: 1177–84.

34. Moore N, Kreft-Jais C, Haramburu F, Noblet C, Andrejak M, Ollagnier M *et al*. Reports of hypoglycaemia associated with the use of ACE inhibitors and other drugs: a case/non-case study in the French pharmacovigilance system database. *Br J Clin Pharmacol* 1997; **44**: 513–18.

35. Egberts AC, Meyboom RH, van Puijenbroek EP. Use of measures of disproportionality in pharmacovigilance: three Dutch examples. *Drug Saf* 2002; **25**: 453–8.

36. Edwards IR. Adverse drug reactions: finding the needle in the haystack. *BMJ* 1997; **315**: 500.

37. Bate A. *The Use of a Bayesian Confidence Propagation Neural Network in Pharmacovigilance*. Umeå: Umeå University, 2003.

38. Bate A, Lindquist M, Edwards IR, Olsson S, Orre R, Lansner A *et al*. A Bayesian neural network method for adverse drug reaction signal generation. *Eur J Clin Pharmacol* 1998; **54**: 315–21.

39. Lindquist M. *Seeing and Observing in International Pharmacovigilance—Achievements and Prospects in Worldwide Drug Safety*. Nijmegen: University of Nijmegen, 2003.

40. Lindquist M, Edwards IR, Ståhl M, Brown EG, Bate A, Kiuru A. The effect of different strategies of signal finding in WHO international ADR data. *Proceedings of ISoP Conference 2001*, abstract L14.

41. Bate A, Orre R, Lindquist M, Edwards IR. Explanation of data mining methods. Available at: http://www.bmj.bmjjournals.com/cgi/content/full/322/7296/1207/DC1/.

42. Bate AJ, Lindquist M, Edwards IR, Orre R. Understanding quantitative signal detection methods in spontaneously reported data. *Pharmacoepidemiol Drug Saf* 2002; **11** (suppl 1): 214–15.

43. Lindquist M, Stahl M, Bate A, Edwards IR, Meyboom RH. A retrospective evaluation of a data mining approach to aid finding new adverse drug reaction signals in the WHO international database. *Drug Saf* 2000; **23**: 533–42.

44. Evans SJ, Waller PC, Davis S. Use of proportional reporting ratios (PRRs) for signal generation from spontaneous adverse drug reaction reports. *Pharmacoepidemiol Drug Saf* 2001; **10**: 483–6.

45. van Puijenbroek EP, Bate A, Leufkens HG, Lindquist M, Orre R, Egberts AC. A comparison of measures of disproportionality for signal detection in spontaneous reporting systems for adverse drug reactions. *Pharmacoepidemiol Drug Saf* 2002; **11**: 3–10.

46. van Puijenbroek EP, van Grootheest K, Diemont WL, Leufkens HG, Egberts AC. Determinants of signal selection in a spontaneous reporting system for adverse drug reactions. *Br J Clin Pharmacol* 2001; **52**: 579–86.

47. DuMouchel W. Bayesian data mining in large frequency tables, with an application to the FDA spontaneous reporting system. *Am Stat* 1999; **53**: 177–90.

48. Edwards IR, Olsson, S. The WHO International Drug Monitoring Programme—vision and goals of the Uppsala Monitoring Centre. In: Aronson JK, ed., *Side Effects of Drugs*, Annual 26. Amsterdam: Elsevier Science, 2003; pp. 548–57.

49. Meyboom RHB. Good practice in the postmarketing surveillance of medicines. *Pharm World Sci* 1997; **4**: 19.

50. Meyboom RHB. The case for good pharmacovigilance practice. *Pharmacoepidemiol Drug Saf* 2000; **9**: 335–6.

51. CIOMS. *Harmonization of Data Fields for Electronic Transmission of Case-Report Information Internationally*, public report. Geneva: CIOMS, 1995.

52. CIOMS. *International Reporting of Periodic Drug Safety Update Summaries*. Geneva: CIOMS, 1992.

53. Wood KL, Wood SM. The new international medical terminology for regulatory activities: a tool to improve the utilisation of regulatory data and to support its communication within and between organisations. In: Mitchard M, ed., *Electronic Communication Technologies: A Practical Guide for Healthcare Manufacturers*. Buffalo, NY: Interpharm Press, 1998; pp. 299–331.

54. Venning GR. Identification of adverse reactions to new drugs II. How were 18 important adverse reactions discovered and with what delay? *BMJ* 1983; **286**: 289–92.

55. Wiholm B-E, Lindquist M. The detection and evaluation of drug induced agranulocytosis by spontaneous reports. Abstract. In: *III World Conference on Clinical Pharmacology and Therapeutics*, Stockholm, 1986.

56. Li D, Lindquist M, Edwards IR. Evaluation of early signals of drug-induced Stevens–Johnson Syndrome in the WHO ADR data base. *Pharmacoepidemiol Drug Saf* 1992; **1**: 11–9.

57. Weber JCP. Epidemiology of adverse reactions to nonsteroidal antiinflammatory drugs. *Adv Inflam Res* 1984; **6**: 1–7.

58. Edwards IR, Fletcher AP, Lindquist M, Pettersson M, Sanderson GH, Schou JS. *The ADR Signal Analysis (ASAP), final report*. EU-funded technical report, 1997.

59. Rothman KJ. Causal inference in epidemiology. In: *Modern Epidemiology*. Boston, MA: Little, Brown, 1986; pp. 7–21.

60. Carlson J, Wiholm B-E. Trimethoprim associated aseptic meningitis. *Scand J Infect Dis* 1987; **19**: 687.

61. Stratton KR, Howe CJ, Johnston RB Jr. Adverse events associated with childhood vaccines other than pertussis and rubella. Summary of a report from the Institute of Medicine. *JAMA* 1994; **271**: 1602–5.

62. Nordic Council on Medicines. *Drug Monitoring in the Nordic Countries. An Evaluation of Similarities and Differences*, report no. 25. Uppsala: Nordic Council on Medicines, 1989.

63. Moore N, Noblet C, Kreft-Jais C, Lagier G, Ollagnier M, Imbs JL. [French pharmacovigilance database system: examples of utilisation]. *Therapie* 1995; **50**: 557–62.

64. The International Agranulocytosis and Aplastic Anemia Study. Risks of agranulocytosis and aplastic anemia. A first report of their relation to drug use with special reference to analgesics. *JAMA* 1986; **256**: 1749–57.

65. van Leeuwen R, Meyboom RH. Agranulocytosis and aprindine. *Lancet* 1976; **2**: 1137.

66. Hood DA, Edwards IR. Meningococcal vaccine—do some children experience side effects? *N Z Med J* 1989; **102**: 65–7.

67. Nordic Council on Medicines. *Nordic Statistics on Medicines 1975–1977*, part II. Uppsala: Nordic Council on Medicines, 1978.

68. Lindquist M, Pettersson M, Edwards IR, Sanderson JH, Taylor NF, Fletcher AP *et al*. How does cystitis affect a comparative risk profile of tiaprofenic acid with other non-steroidal antiinflammatory drugs? An international study based on spontaneous reports and drug usage data. ADR Signals Analysis Project (ASAP) team. *Pharmacol Toxicol* 1997; **80**: 211–17.

69. Stahl MM, Lindquist M, Pettersson M, Edwards IR, Sanderson JH, Taylor NF *et al*. Withdrawal reactions with selective serotonin re-uptake inhibitors as reported to the WHO system. *Eur J Clin Pharmacol* 1997; **53**: 163–9.

70. Wiholm B-E. Spontaneous reporting of ADR. In: *Detection and Prevention of Adverse Drug Reactions*, Skandia International Symposia. Stockholm, Sweden: Almqvist and Wiksell, 1983; pp. 152–67.

71. Bottiger M, Romanus V, de Verdier C, Boman G. Osteitis and other complications caused by generalized BCG-itis. Experiences in Sweden. *Acta Paediatr Scand* 1982; **71**: 471–8.

72. Bottiger LE, Boman G, Eklund G, Westerholm B. Oral contraceptives and thromboembolic disease: effects of lowering oestrogen content. *Lancet* 1980; **1**: 1097–101.

73. Fraunfelder FT, Meyer SM, Bagby GC, Jr, Dreis MW. Hematologic reactions to carbonic anhydrase inhibitors. *Am J Ophthalmol* 1985; **100**: 79–81.

74. Mortimer O, Wiholm B-E. Acetazolamid-pancytopenia: the Swedish Adverse Drug Reactions Advisory Committee 46, 1985.

75. The International Agranulocytosis and Aplastic Anemia Study. Incidence of aplastic anemia: the relevance of diagnostic criteria. *Blood* 1987; **70**: 1718–21.

76. Bottiger LE, Westerholm B. Drug-induced blood dyscrasias in Sweden. *BMJ* 1973; **3**: 339–43.

77. Keisu M, Ekman E, Wiholm BE. Comparing risk estimates of sulphonamide-induced agranulocytosis from the Swedish Drug Monitoring System and a case–control study. *Eur J Clin Pharmacol* 1992; **43**: 211–14.

78. Asplund K, Wiholm BE, Lithner F. Glibenclamide-associated hypoglycaemia: a report on 57 cases. *Diabetologia* 1983; **24**: 412–17.

79. Bloemenkamp KW, Rosendaal FR, Helmerhorst FM, Buller HR, Vandenbroucke JP. Enhancement by factor V Leiden mutation of risk of deep-vein thrombosis associated with oral contraceptives containing a third-generation progestagen. *Lancet* 1995; **346**: 1575–82.

80. Legnani C, Cini M, Cosmi B, Poggi M, Boggian O, Palareti G. Risk of deep vein thrombosis: interaction between oral contraceptives and high factor VIII levels. *Haematologica* 2004; **89**: 1347–51.

81. Strandberg I, Boman G, Hassler L, Sjoqvist F. Acetylator phenotype in patients with hydralazine-induced lupoid syndrome. *Acta Med Scand* 1976; **200**: 367–71.

82. Strom BL, West SL, Sim E, Carson JL. The epidemiology of the acute flank pain syndrome from suprofen. *Clin Pharmacol Ther* 1989; **46**: 693–9.

83. CIOMS. *Benefit–Risk Balance for Marketed Drugs: Evaluating Safety Signals*, 1st edn. Geneva: World Health Organization, 1998.

84. WHO International Drug Monitoring. *Cerivastatin and Gemfibrosil*, report no. 16(1). Geneva: World Health Organization, 2002.

85. WHO Collaborating Centre for Drug Statistics Methodology. *Guidelines for ATC classification and DDD Assignment*, 3rd edn. Oslo, 2000.

86. Edwards IR. The accelerating need for pharmacovigilance. *J R Coll Physicians Lond* 2000; **34**: 48–51.

87. Edwards IR, Hugman B. The challenge of effectively communicating risk–benefit information. *Drug Saf* 1997; **17**: 216–27.

88. UMC. *Dialogue in Pharmacovigilance—More Effective Communication*. Uppsala: Uppsala Monitoring Centre, 2002.

89. UMC. *Effective Communications in Pharmacovigilance*. Uppsala: Uppsala Monitoring Centre, 1998.

90. UMC. *Expecting the Worst—Crisis Management*. Uppsala: Uppsala Monitoring Centre, 2002.

91. UMC. *Viewpoint*. Uppsala: Uppsala Monitoring Centre, 2002.

11

Case–Control Surveillance

LYNN ROSENBERG, PATRICIA F. COOGAN and JULIE R. PALMER
Slone Epidemiology Center, Boston University, Boston, Massachusetts, USA.

INTRODUCTION

There is no assurance that medications are safe at the time they are released to the market, because premarketing trials for safety and efficacy are too small to detect any but common adverse effects and too brief to detect effects that occur after long latent intervals or durations of use.[1] Indeed, as described in Chapter 1, numerous drugs have been removed from the market, sometimes many years after approval.[2–5] Postmarketing surveillance serves not only to document unintended adverse effects of medications, but also to document beneficial effects unrelated to the indications for use. Documentation of long-term safety is also important, particularly for drugs that are widely used by healthy individuals. Since drugs used for chronic conditions tend to be taken regularly and for long periods, there may well be unintended health effects. On the other hand, removal of a drug from the market because of concerns that turn out to be unfounded would not serve the public's health.

The need for surveillance of prescription medications is clear. However, non-prescription drugs can also have serious adverse effects and unintended benefits. More and more drugs previously available only by prescription, such as ibuprofen, naproxen, and cimetidine, are being approved for over-the-counter sales, and the change from prescription to non-prescription sales often results in large increases in use.[6] Until recently, most over-the-counter medications were used for acute self-limiting conditions. However, therapeutic areas that are currently under consideration by pharmaceutical companies for changes from prescription to non-prescription sales include hypercholesterolemia, osteoporosis, hypertension, and depression.[7]

The use of dietary supplements, including herbal supplements, has increased dramatically in recent years. In the Slone Survey, an ongoing survey of a random sample of the US population conducted by the Slone Epidemiology Center, each of 10 supplements had been taken in the preceding week by at least 1% of the population during the years 1998 to 2001.[8] Dietary supplements are often self-prescribed for many of the same reasons that "traditional" prescription and non-prescription drugs are used. Supplements are sold over-the-counter and they do not have to be shown to be efficacious or safe before being marketed.[9] In view of their widespread use, their potential to act as carcinogens,[9–13] and their possible influence on estrogen action and metabolism,[14–18] dietary supplements should be monitored

Pharmacoepidemiology, Fourth Edition   Edited by B.L. Strom
© 2005 John Wiley & Sons, Ltd

for unanticipated effects on the occurrence of cancer and other illnesses.

Cohort studies, such as linkage studies of pharmacy data with outcome data, figure prominently among the postmarketing strategies currently in use.[19–24] These studies are useful for monitoring prescription drugs but generally lack information on non-prescription medications and dietary supplements. They are also problematic for the documentation of carcinogenic effects that may occur long after the initiation of drug use. We have developed a surveillance system, Case–Control Surveillance (CCS), which uses case–control methodology to systematically evaluate and detect effects of medications and other exposures on the risk of serious illnesses, principally cancers. CCS includes monitoring of non-prescription drugs and dietary supplements as well as prescription drugs. CCS also includes a biologic component that allows for the assessment of whether genetic polymorphisms modify the effect of a medication or supplement on the risk of the illness.

DESCRIPTION

OVERVIEW

CCS began in 1976 when the US Food and Drug Administration (FDA) provided funding for the monitoring of nonmalignant and malignant illnesses in relation to medication use. Because of concerns about the effects of medications on cancer risk (e.g., postmenopausal female hormone use on risk of endometrial cancer),[25] we sought funding to continue CCS, with a focus on cancers. The National Cancer Institute has provided funding for that purpose since 1988.

In CCS, multiple case–control studies are conducted simultaneously. Individuals with recently diagnosed cancer or nonmalignant conditions are interviewed in a set of participating hospitals. Information is obtained by standard interview on lifetime history of regular medication use and factors that might confound or modify drug–disease associations. Inpatient drug use is generally not recorded. The discharge summary is obtained for all patients, and the pathology report for patients with cancer. A biologic component was added in 1998: participants provide cheek cell samples from which DNA is extracted and stored. Since the beginning of the study, over 70 000 patients have been interviewed, of whom about 25 000 had recently diagnosed primary cancers of various sites.

The CCS database is used for hypothesis testing and discovery. In-depth analyses of the data are carried out to investigate hypotheses that arise from a variety of sources.

The data are also "screened" periodically by means of multiple comparisons to discover new associations. Institutional review board approval has been obtained from all collaborating institutions, and the study complies with all Health Insurance Portability and Accountability Act (HIPAA) requirements. All participants provide written informed consent separately for the interview and for the buccal cell sample.

METHODS

Case and Control Identification and Accrual

The collaborating institutions, located in several geographic areas, have changed over time. The current network, supervised by Dr Brian Strom, consists of seven teaching and community hospitals in Philadelphia. Hospitals in Baltimore, Boston, New York, and other areas have participated in the past.

Specially trained nurse-interviewers employed by CCS interview adult patients aged 21–79 years in collaborating hospitals. The interviewers enroll patients with recently diagnosed cancers or recently diagnosed nonmalignant disorders; the latter serve as a pool of potential controls in case–control analyses, and from time to time a control diagnosis may itself be of interest as the outcome (e.g., cholecystitis,[26] pelvic inflammatory disease[27]). Patients with conditions of acute onset (e.g., traumatic injury, appendicitis) are suitable controls in many analyses, and they are selectively accrued. For more chronic conditions (e.g., orthopedic disorders, kidney stones), recruitment is confined to patients whose diagnosis was made within the previous year. Only patients living in areas within about 50 miles of the hospital are eligible; the interviewers have a list of acceptable ZIP codes and only patients residing in those areas are interviewed. To accrue cases of special interest, the interviewers selectively seek out patients with particular diagnoses according to a priority list. The interviewers find cases through a variety of methods, including checking admissions lists and patient charts. If the interviewer has a choice of interviewing a patient with a priority cancer and a patient with a cancer of another site, the priority cancer will be chosen. The interviewers try to interview all new cases but hospital stays are short and patients are often occupied with having tests, treatments, and visitors. Thus, in practice, the interviewers enroll all patients who are available. Patients are recruited without knowledge of their exposure status. Written informed consent is obtained before interviews are conducted. The interview setting—a hospital or clinic room—is similar for cases and controls. The interviewers are unaware if the patient is a "case" or "control" because many diseases and hypotheses are assessed, and cases in one analysis may be controls in another.

Participation rates in CCS exceeded 90% before the inclusion of the collection of cheek cell samples. After the addition of this biologic component, about 20% of patients have refused to participate. Currently, among the 80% of patients who agree to be interviewed, about 95% provide a cheek cell sample. Patients who agree to provide a biologic sample in addition to the interview are similar in age and sex to those who participate only in the interview; white patients are slightly more likely to participate in the biologic component than black patients.

Table 11.1 shows the numbers of patients with newly diagnosed cancer of various sites that have been accrued in CCS since 1976 in the four largest centers in which CCS has operated—Baltimore, Boston, New York City, and Philadelphia. All subsequent tables refer to the same four areas. CCS currently includes 7160 patients with breast cancer, about 2700 with large bowel cancer, at least 1000 each with lung cancer, malignant melanoma, prostate cancer, or ovarian cancer, and at least 500 each with endometrial cancer, leukemia, bladder cancer, pancreatic cancer, non-Hodgkin's lymphoma, or renal cancer.

Table 11.2 lists the more common diagnoses among patients admitted for nonmalignant conditions. These patients serve

Table 11.1. Cases of incident cancer of selected sites accrued in CCS since 1976; Baltimore, Boston, New York City, and Philadelphia

Cancer	No.
Breast	7160
Large bowel	2700
Lung	1770
Malignant melanoma	1495
Prostate	1375
Ovary	1000
Endometrium	870
Leukemia	815
Bladder	600
Pancreas	575
Non-Hodgkin's lymphoma	530
Kidney/kidney pelvis	525
Testis	420
Hodgkin's disease	310
Stomach	345
Esophagus	240
Gallbladder	135
Choriocarcinoma	50
Liver	60
Small intestine	40

Table 11.2. Patients with nonmalignant conditions accrued in CCS since 1976; Baltimore, Boston, New York City, and Philadelphia

Nonmalignant Condition	No.
Fracture	2750
Other injury	2700
Uterine fibroid	1700
Benign neoplasm	1520
Cholecystitis	1460
Displacement of intervertebral disc	1360
Ovarian cyst	1350
Hernia	1080
Appendicitis	930
Cholelithiasis	890
Calculus of kidney and ureter	720
Pelvic inflammatory disease	700
Benign prostatic hypertrophy	610
Ectopic pregnancy	470
Diverticulitis	420
Endometriosis	390
Cellulitis	380
Pancreatitis	290
Spinal stenosis	250
Bowel obstruction	250

as a pool of controls for analyses of various cancers, although in some instances nonmalignant diagnoses themselves have been assessed as the outcome of interest. Among the most common nonmalignant diagnoses are traumatic injury (e.g., fractured arm), benign neoplasms, acute infections (e.g., appendicitis), orthopedic disorders (e.g., disc disorder), gallbladder disease, and hernias.

Interview Data

Drug Information

It is not feasible to ask specifically about thousands of individual drug entities. Instead, histories of medication use are obtained by asking about use for 43 indication or drug categories, e.g., headache, cholesterol lowering, oral contraception, menopausal symptoms, herbals/dietary supplements. The drug name and the timing, duration, and frequency of use are recorded for each episode of use. The drug dose is recorded when it is part of the brand name, e.g., for oral contraceptives and conjugated estrogens, the brand name sometimes indicates the dosage.

Thousands of different specific medications have been reported. Table 11.3 shows the prevalence of reported use of selected medications and drug classes for which there

Table 11.3. Use of selected drugs and drug classes in CCS, 1976–2003 and 1998–2003; Baltimore, Boston, New York City, and Philadelphia

Category	1976–2003 (n=61 672) (%)	1998–2003 (n=4317) (%)
Aspirin-containing drugs	47.5	30.5
Oral contraceptives (women only)	42.0	55.5
Acetaminophen-containing drugs	38.9	55.3
Conjugated estrogens (women aged 50+)	23.7	34.6
Benzodiazepines	20.8	12.3
Thiazide diuretics	14.2	9.2
Ibuprofen	13.7	32.7
Phenylpropranolamine	9.6	2.7
Beta-adrenergic blockers	8.7	11.8
Histamine H_2 antagonists	7.4	16.4
Phenothiazines	4.2	2.6
Calcium channel blockers	3.9	13.0
Oral anticoagulants	3.9	6.7
Phenolphthalein laxatives	3.8	0.7
Aromatic anticonvulsants	3.7	2.5
Naproxen	3.3	8.1
Phenobarbital	2.6	1.0
Indomethacin	2.5	1.1
Insulin	2.3	4.1
Statins	1.6	13.2
Selective serotonin uptake inhibitors	1.3	9.5

Table 11.4. Use of selected drugs in CCS, 1976–2003; Baltimore, Boston, New York City, and Philadelphia

Drug name	%
Aspirin	32
Acetaminophen	29
Ascorbic acid	20
Diazepam	14
Ibuprofen	14
Tocopherol acetate	13
Iron	13
Tetracycline	8
Ampicillin	7
Erythromycin	6
Aluminum hydroxide gel	6
Hydrochlorothiazide	6
Cortisone	6
Prednisone	6
Guaifenesin	5
Furosemide	5
Vitamin B complex	4
Synalgos	4
Propranolol HCl	4
Bufferin®	4
Cimetidine	4
Calcium	4
Triamterene/hydrochlorothiazide	4
Miconazole nitrate	4
Chlordiazepoxide HCl	3
Vitamin A	3
Ranitidine HCl	3
Levothyroxine sodium	3
Warfarin sodium	3
Propoxyphene HCl	3
Norinyl	3
Oxycodone/APAP	3
Aluminum hydroxide/magnesium hydroxide	3
Methyldopa	3
Cyanocobalamin	3
Percodan®	3
Acetaminophen with codeine	3
Midol®	3
Diphenhydramine HCl	2
Indomethacin	2
Psyllium hydrophilic colloid	2
Codeine	2
Pseudoephedrine HCl	2
Potassium chloride	2
Chlorpheniramine maleate	2
Nitroglycerin	2
Contoz®	2
Sulfisoxazole	2
Digoxin	2
Yellow phenolphthalein	2
Nyquil®	2
Diphenoxylate HCl/atropine SO_4	2
Milk of magnesia	2
Thyroid	2
Fiorinal®	2
Trimethoprim/sulfamethoxazole	2
Excedrin®	2

have been marked changes in the prevalence of use over time. The left-hand column shows the prevalence among CCS patients interviewed during 1976–2003, and the right-hand column the prevalence among patients interviewed during 1998–2003. There were large increases in recent years in the use of acetaminophen, various nonsteroidal anti-inflammatory drugs, histamine H_2 antagonists, calcium channel blockers, statins, and selective serotonin reuptake inhibitors. Some of these increases were attributable in part to changes from prescription to over-the-counter sales; for example, those for the histamine H_2 antagonist cimetidine, and the nonsteroidal anti-inflammatory drug ibuprofen.

In recent years, CCS patients have increasingly reported the use of dietary supplements. In 2000–2003, use of glucosamine was reported by 1.5%, ginkgo biloba by 1.3%, echinacea by 1.2%, and ginseng by 0.9%.

Tables 11.4 and 11.5 show the frequency of use of the most commonly reported drugs and drug classes by CCS participants from 1976 to 2003.

Table 11.5. Use of selected drug classes in CCS, 1976–2003; Baltimore, Boston, New York City, and Philadelphia

Drug Class	%
Vitamins/minerals	62
Aspirin-containing drugs	47
Acetaminaphen-containing drugs	39
Iron	36
Oral contraceptives	26
Folic acid	26
Antihistamines	24
Estrogens	22
Benzodiazepines	21
Corticosteroids	17
Narcotic pain formulas	16
Vitamin A	15
Antacids	15
Thiazides	14
Diazepam	14
Ibuprofen	14
Sulfonamides	13
Laxatives	11
Folic acid antagonists	10
Tetracyclines	10
Phenylpropanolamine	10
Calcium salts	10
Beta-adrenergic blockers	9
Ampicillin/amoxicillin	8
Phenacetin	8
Pseudoephedrine	8
Histamine H_2 antagonists	7
Macrolide antibiotics	7
Codeine	6
Conjugated estrogens	6
Antifungals	6
Barbiturates	6
Thyroid supplements	6
Guaifenesin	6
Antidepressants	5
Furosemide	5
Phenothiazines	4
Docusate salts	4
Calcium channel blockers	4
Oral anticoagulants	4
Hypnotics and tranquilizers	4
Cephalosporins	4
Aromatic anticonvulsants	4
Tricyclic antidepressants	4
Naproxen	3
Methyldopa	3
Antimalarials	3
Sulfonylureas	3
Nitrates	3
ACE inhibitors	3
Xanthines (excludes caffeine)	3
Phenobarbital	3
Cardiac glycosides	2
Indomethacin	2
Digitalis	2
Insulin	2
Meprobamate	2
Heparin	2
Statins	2
Other anti-hyperlipidemics	2
Aminoglycosides	2

Information on Factors Other Than Drugs

Information on many factors that may confound or modify drug–disease associations is routinely collected: descriptive characteristics (e.g., age, height, current weight, weight 10 years ago, weight at age 20, years of education, marital status, racial/ethnic group), habits (cigarette smoking, alcohol consumption, coffee consumption), gynecologic and reproductive factors (age at first birth, parity, age at menarche and menopause, and type of menopause), medical history (cancer, hypertension, diabetes, other serious illnesses, vasectomy, hysterectomy, oophorectomy), family history of cancer, use of medical care (e.g., number of visits to a physician in each of the previous two years). These factors may be of interest in their own right as risk factors.

Information from the Hospital Record

A copy of the discharge summary is obtained for every patient enrolled in the study and the pathology report for all patients with cancer. These are reviewed and abstracted in the central office by the study nurse-coordinator, blind to exposure category, in order to properly classify the diagnosis.

Buccal Cell Samples

The collection of buccal cell samples from patients in CCS began in 1998. Patients who agree to provide samples rub the inside of each cheek with a brush (two samples per patient[28]). This method of DNA collection is suitable for hospital patients because it is noninvasive. The samples are mailed to the collaborating laboratory for extraction and storage of the DNA. Samples collected in this manner have been analyzed successfully for the NAT2-341 gene polymorphism, attesting to the quality and quantity of the extracted DNA.[29]

The stored DNA serves as a resource to identify subgroups that may be at increased risk of particular outcomes related to particular exposures by virtue of inherited genotype, and to elucidate mechanisms of carcinogenesis. The metabolism of environmental carcinogens, including drugs, likely involves genes that regulate phase I monooxygenation and phase II conjugation of potential carcinogens.[30–36]

Drug Dictionary

Our research group has for many years maintained a drug dictionary. The dictionary is a computerized linkage system composed of individual medicinal agents and multi-component products, each assigned a specific code number. All combination products are linked to their individual components. Thus, groupings (coalitions) of drugs that contain a particular entity can be easily formed. For example, "Tylenol" is contained in some 50 products coded in our drug dictionary. The constituents of the products can be obtained from the dictionary; e.g., Tylenol Cold Effervescent Formula contains acetaminophen, chlorpheniramine maleate, and phenylpropanolamine HCl. Tylenol products and all other products containing acetaminophen are contained in the acetaminophen coalition, a total of over 450 products. Coalitions of many other types of drugs have also been formed, e.g., selective serotonin reuptake inhibitors, calcium channel blockers, tricyclic antidepressants, thiazide diuretics, benzodiazepines, and beta-adrenergic blockers. The dictionary is continuously maintained and updated by research pharmacists who determine the components of newly encountered products, assign code numbers, and update coalitions. The dictionary currently contains over 15 000 single agent and 7900 multicomponent product codes linked to some 23 000 commercial products, including dietary supplements.

DATA ANALYSIS

Hypothesis Testing

Case and Control Specification

For each analysis, the case series is defined, e.g., women with invasive primary breast cancer diagnosed less than a year before admission and documented in the pathology report. Proper control selection is essential for validity. For the particular exposure at issue, appropriate controls should have been admitted for conditions that are not caused, prevented, or treated by that exposure.[37–39] Our approach is to select three or four appropriate diagnostic categories with sufficient numbers to allow for examination of uniformity of the exposure of interest across the categories. If our judgment about control selection is correct, the prevalence of that exposure will be uniform across the diagnostic categories selected for that analysis.

Aspects of Drug Use

We assess use that began at least a year before admission because use of more recent onset could not have antedated the onset of the cancer. Depending upon the hypothesis, different categories of drug use are of interest. For example, for breast cancer, analyses may focus on drug use at potentially vulnerable times during reproductive life (e.g., soon after menarche, before the birth of the first child, in the recent past). The particular drug or drug regimen may also be relevant, e.g., the risk of endometrial cancer is increased by unopposed estrogen supplements, but little or not at all by combined use of estrogen with a progestogen.

The observation of greater effects for more frequent or long duration use provides support for a causal role. Some drugs, particularly non-prescription drugs such as aspirin, other NSAIDs, and acetaminophen, are often used sporadically. Sporadic use in the past cannot be reported accurately. Furthermore, regular use is more likely to play an etiologic role than sporadic use. Thus, our greatest reliance is placed on regular use (e.g., at least 4 times a week for at least 3 months), and particularly on regular use for several years or more.

The timing of use may also be relevant. In our analysis of CCS data on nonsteroidal anti-inflammatory drugs and large bowel cancer,[40] we found that use that had ceased at least a year previously was unrelated to risk, whereas use that continued into the previous year was associated with a reduced odds ratio. The latter relationship had been suggested by the animal data. In addition, there was no excess of cases among past users, suggesting that cessation of use, possibly due to symptoms, did not explain the inverse association with use that continued into the previous year. "Latent interval" analyses may focus on whether an effect appears long after use. For example, analyses in our assessment of a non-drug exposure, vasectomy, in relation to the risk of 10 cancer sites considered the interval between vasectomy and the occurrence of the cancer.[41] Also of interest is how long an increased or reduced odds ratio persists after an exposure has occurred. For example, in our assessment of the risk of ovarian cancer in relation to oral contraceptive use, the reduction in users persisted for 15–19 years after cessation of use,[42] extending the previous period, which had been estimated to be about 10–15 years.

The dose of drugs used in the past is difficult to study because of inaccurate recall.[43] For example, women generally use several different brands of oral contraceptives and they have difficulty remembering the brand (with dosage) accurately.[44–48] Therefore, we do not ask for the dose of the drug used, although the medication name sometimes indicates the dose. For all drugs, the frequency of use and duration provide a useful measure of the intensity of exposure.

Control of Confounding Factors

Odds ratios (and 95% confidence intervals) are estimated from multiple logistic regression analysis.[38] We first identify potential confounding factors, i.e., risk factors for the disease of interest that are related to use of the drug of interest among the controls. Potential confounding factors are controlled in the regression models if their inclusion materially alters the odds ratio, e.g., by 10% or more.

Effect Modification

Certain subgroups may be particularly vulnerable to or particularly protected by an exposure. Effect modification is assessed by examining exposure–disease associations in subgroups and by statistical modeling, such as the use of interaction terms in logistic regression. For example, in our analysis of estrogen supplements in relation to risk of breast cancer, the overall findings were null but supplement use was associated with increased risk of breast cancer among thin women,[49] as observed elsewhere.[50,51] We generally test for interactions specified *a priori* on the basis of results of previous studies or biologic plausibility.

Statistical Power

CCS has excellent statistical power for the detection of associations that are of public health importance. Table 11.6 shows the sample sizes needed for 80% power to detect a range of odds ratios for a range of exposure prevalences.

Drug/Genotype Analyses

Whether an association between a drug exposure and a cancer is modified by inherited genotype is assessed in two ways: by examining the relation of use of the drug to cancer risk within strata of those with and without the genotype of interest, and by the inclusion of an exposure–genotype interaction term in the logistic regression model.[52]

Discovery of Unsuspected Associations

Animal data may lead to the identification of new associations in CCS data. For example, experiments in rodents suggested that nonsteroidal anti-inflammatory drugs might reduce the occurrence of large bowel cancer. An analysis of CCS data revealed an inverse association of large bowel cancer with aspirin use,[40] an association

Table 11.6. Estimated number of cases for detection of various odds ratios, given various drug exposure prevalences in the controls*

Exposure prevalence in controls (%)	Odds ratio			
	1.5	2	3	4
15	380	115	40	25
10	520	150	50	30
5	950	270	85	45
3	1520	425	130	70
2	2235	620	185	100
1	4395	1205	360	185
0.5	8710	2385	700	360
0.25	17 340	4740	1390	710

* Power = 80%, α = 0.05 (two-tailed); control-to-case ratio = 4 : 1.

that has since been confirmed in many subsequent studies.[53–57]

Associations are also identified by systematic "screening" of the data, in which the prevalence of use of a particular drug or drug class (standardized for age, sex, and hospital) among patients with a particular cancer or other illness of interest is compared with the prevalence among patients with other illnesses. Often significant associations ($p < 0.05$) seen in a screen disappear once further cases and controls are enrolled in CCS, or after analyses in which there is careful specification of the case and control groups and control for confounding factors other than age, sex, and study center. We carry out in-depth analyses of new associations if the association is replicated in data collected in CCS in subsequent years, is explained by a highly plausible mechanism, or is of public health importance. Non-drug factors are also screened, and it was in the course of such a screen that we observed an unexpected association between alcohol use and breast cancer.[58] Examples of other unexpected associations from screening are oral contraceptive use with choriocarcinoma[59] and with Crohn's disease.[60] All of these associations have received independent confirmation.[61–65] Further evidence for the validity of the screen findings is the appearance of many known associations that were discovered previously, such as the increased risks of myocardial infarction and venous thromboembolism associated with oral contraceptive use.

Associations that arise in the course of multiple comparisons may of course be due to chance. Even if associations are not due to chance, the magnitude of the association will tend to "regress to the mean" in subsequent studies.[41] For these reasons, new associations are presented with the utmost caution.

STRENGTHS

ASSESSMENT OF NON-PRESCRIPTION MEDICATIONS AND DIETARY SUPPLEMENTS AS WELL AS PRESCRIPTION MEDICATIONS

CCS can be used to test hypotheses concerning use of all reported prescription medications from any source. Monitoring systems that rely on pharmacy data can assess only those medications that are prescribed within the system; prescriptions obtained elsewhere (e.g., family planning clinics, friends, and relatives) cannot be assessed. Sometimes prescribed medications are not taken, which is a disadvantage of relying on prescription data.

CCS is the only surveillance system that systematically assesses use of non-prescription products, both non-prescription medications and dietary supplements. The prevalence of dietary supplement use has become high enough that assessment of their effects on disease occurrence is of public health importance.

CCS has documented adverse effects of medications, such as increased risk of liver cancer[66] and breast cancer[67,68] associated with oral contraceptive use, and increased risk of localized and advanced endometrial cancer associated with postmenopausal estrogen supplement use.[25] Protective effects have also been documented with CCS data, e.g., oral contraceptive use related to reduced risks of ovarian[42] and endometrial cancer,[69] and aspirin use associated with reduced risks of colorectal cancer[40] and stomach cancer.[70] CCS has often documented the safety of drugs after alarms were raised about adverse effects. For example, in experiments in rodents given phenolphthalein, an agent used in non-prescription laxatives, there were increased risks of several cancers.[71] The FDA called for human data on this question.[72] CCS responded and found no increased risk.[73] A small cohort study suggested that calcium channel blockers increased the risk of several cancers;[74,75] results from the much larger CCS database refuted that finding.[76] Animal data raised the concern that benzodiazepines increased the risk of several cancers; data from CCS were null.[77–79] Animal data raised the possibility of increased risks of cancer associated with hydralazine use; CCS results were null.[80,81]

Many case–control or cohort studies have reported on selected medications, such as noncontraceptive estrogens or oral contraceptives, but comprehensive information on a wide variety of drugs is not routinely collected. The effects of many drugs have not been well assessed. CCS has provided data on the risk of various outcomes in relation to a wide range of medications, including ACE inhibitors, acetaminophen, antidepressants, antihistamines, aspirin and other NSAIDs, benzodiazepines, beta-androgenic blockers, calcium channel blockers, female hormone supplements, hydralazine, oral contraceptives, phenolphthalein-containing laxatives, phenothiazines, rauwolfia alkaloids, selective serotonin reuptake inhibitors, statins, thiazides, and thyroid supplements (see the list of publications in the Appendix).

DISCOVERY OF UNSUSPECTED ASSOCIATIONS

Because CCS obtains data on many exposures and many outcomes, the system has the capacity for discovery of unsuspected associations. For example, an inverse association between aspirin use and risk of colorectal cancer was documented in CCS. The publication of the finding[40] provoked many subsequent studies, which confirmed the association.[53–57] The National Cancer Institute found the findings to be of sufficient potential public health importance to support a randomized trial of aspirin as a preventive of colonic polyps. Other associations discovered in CCS are positive associations of long-term oral contraceptive use with gestational trophoblastic disease[59] and with Crohn's disease,[60] and of alcohol consumption with increased risk of breast cancer.[58] These associations have been confirmed in subsequent studies.[61–65]

ASSESSMENT OF EFFECTS AFTER LONG INTERVALS OR DURATIONS OF USE

Because the effects of drugs, particularly carcinogenic effects, may become evident only after many years, the capacity for a surveillance system to assess long latent intervals or long durations of use is important. The case–control design used by CCS is efficient for assessing the effects of exposures that occurred in the distant past or after long durations of exposure. For example, CCS documented that the adverse effect of estrogen supplements on risk of endometrial cancer persisted for 15–19 years after cessation of use.[25] Cohort studies are ill suited for these assessments unless the study has been collecting information for many years.[37]

CONTROL OF CONFOUNDING

In observational research, control of confounding is crucial for validity. Drug use is a health-related activity and is associated with factors such as medical history that are in turn strongly associated with disease risk. CCS systematically collects detailed information on important potential confounding factors. These include demographic characteristics, aspects of medical history, reproductive and gynecologic history, family history of cancer, use of tobacco and alcohol, and use of medical care, in addition to use of prescription and non-prescription drugs and dietary supplements. Thus, it is possible to control for these factors in multivariable analyses.

ACCURATE OUTCOME DATA

For all patients, CCS collects information from the hospital record. Pathology reports are obtained for all patients with cancer. CCS is therefore able to accurately classify the diagnosis for which the patient was admitted.

HIGH STATISTICAL POWER

CCS has accrued a large database, with large numbers of patients with cancers of various sites and other illnesses (Table 11.1). Many drugs or drug classes have been taken by at least 1% of the population (Tables 11.4 and 11.5). CCS has high statistical power relative to cohort studies, with excellent power to assess the effects of exposures of public health importance. As shown in Table 11.6, small odds ratios associated with uncommon drug exposures can be detected for common cancers.[38] For less common cancers, odds ratios associated with more common exposures can be detected. For very rare cancers, only relatively large effects can be detected for relatively common exposures. However, an appreciable number of cases of a rare cancer will be attributable to the exposure only when the odds ratio is large and the exposure common.

BIOLOGIC COMPONENT

Unanticipated adverse or beneficial effects of medications may be confined to vulnerable subgroups. CCS has the capacity to assess whether those subgroups are defined by genetic polymorphisms, i.e., whether genetic polymorphisms modify drug–disease associations. This can serve both to identify vulnerable populations and to elucidate mechanisms.

PRODUCTIVITY AND SUBSTANTIVE FINDINGS

CCS has been highly productive: 79 papers have been published (see Appendix). Some of the associations assessed have been briefly described in this chapter.

WEAKNESSES

POTENTIAL FOR BIAS

Selection Bias

When feasible, population-based case–control studies are optimal. Population-based CCS is infeasible for logistic and budgetary reasons. Even in population-based data, however, biased selection of cases and controls may occur because of non-participation. In CCS, the high participation rates reduce the potential for selection bias due to non-participation. In addition, the cases in CCS are persons with various cancers admitted to the hospitals under surveillance, and they define a secondary base which comprises members of the population at large who would be admitted to the same hospitals were they to develop cancer.[82–84] Enrollment is limited to cases and controls who live within approximately 50 miles of the hospital. The purpose is to include only persons from the secondary base and to exclude referrals from outside that base. Of course, referral patterns for different cancers could be different.

In the analysis of the risk of a particular cancer, we often select a control group of patients with other cancers judged to be unrelated to the exposure; such controls are probably representative of the same base as the cases. A second control group admitted for nonmalignant conditions guards against the possibility that the exposure may cause all cancers. We check for uniformity of the exposure of interest across the various control categories; uniformity suggests the absence of selection bias.

As another check for bias, a disease unrelated to the drug exposure at issue may be included in the assessment of the relation of that drug to the outcome of interest. For example, in our assessment of acetaminophen in relation to risk of transitional cell cancers, we also assessed renal cell cancer because the latter outcome had not been associated with acetaminophen use.[85]

Recall Bias

It would be desirable to obtain exposure data based on complete and accurate records, with the caveat that people often do not fill prescriptions or take the drugs prescribed.

Validation studies of self-reported prescription drug use are generally difficult in the US because people get drugs from many sources, records are often absent, and participation rates may be suboptimal. Because we believe that recent or long-term use is best remembered, we focus on these categories. The literature on validation of drug use indicates that recent and long-term use of oral contraceptives and female hormone supplements is reported with acceptable accuracy; the product names are less well reported.[43–48,86–88] The relatively few validation studies of other prescription drugs have yielded variable results, with the best agreement for drugs used on a long-term basis, such as those for diabetes and hypertension.[43,89,90] A review of validation studies[43] concluded that reporting is affected by the type of medication and drug use patterns (e.g., better reporting for chronically used prescriptions) and by the design of data collection. (See also Chapter 45.) For non-prescription drugs and dietary supplements, validation is infeasible because records of use do not exist.

CCS reduces reporting bias (i.e., differential reporting by cases and controls) by using the same highly structured interview and similar interview settings for cases and controls. Patients are asked about 43 indications for drug use and drug classes. This approach masks hypotheses about particular drugs. Furthermore, control patients admitted for a serious nonmalignant condition are as likely to carefully search their memories as case patients admitted for a cancer. As a check for reporting bias, we may assess a drug or drug class unrelated to the outcome. For example, beta-blockers and ACE inhibitors were assessed in our analysis of cancer risk in relation to calcium channel blockers, because the former drug classes had not been linked to cancer risk.[76]

Nondifferential Misclassification

Nondifferential underascertainment of drug use will weaken observed associations. As an example, the effect on "true" odds ratios of 3, 2, and 1.5 of 30% underascertainment of drug use among cases and controls for a range of "true" exposure prevalences in the controls is given in Table 11.7. While the effect of nondifferential underascertainment is for the estimate to move towards the null, the changes are small, no more than about 10% in the worst case. Effects are of course smaller if underascertainment of drug use is less than 30%. Thus, nondifferential misclassification likely has only small effects on odds ratios estimated for exposures of interest in CCS.

Table 11.7. Observed odds ratio given 30% underascertainment of drug use in cases and controls

True prevalence of drug use in controls

	True odds ratio		
	3.0	2.0	1.5
	Observed odds ratio		
15%	2.7	1.9	1.5
10%	2.8	1.9	1.5
5%	2.9	2.0	1.5
1%	3.0	2.0	1.5

The ultimate test of validity of CCS results is whether they are confirmed by well-conducted studies that use different methods. CCS results have repeatedly passed that test.

PARTICULAR APPLICATIONS

CCS has the capacity to assess the risk of illnesses in relation to use of prescription drugs, non-prescription drugs, and dietary supplements reported by participants. As described in previous sections, CCS has documented increased risk, decreased risk, and absence of risk. In addition, CCS has generated important new hypotheses, probably the most important of which are the positive association of alcohol with breast cancer and the inverse association of nonsteroidal anti-inflammatory drugs with large bowel cancer. Now that dietary supplement use has become widespread, CCS will assess the unintended health effects of these agents. When particular issues arise, the system can be steered to selectively accrue cases of the disease of interest, but extremely rare diseases are beyond the scope of CCS and other routine monitoring systems.

The scope of CCS is broad, with major contributions having been made to the evaluation of the health effects of a wide range of medications in relation to a range of illnesses. In recent years, there has been a particular focus on non-prescription medications, such as the widely used nonsteroidal anti-inflammatory drugs, mostly obtained over-the-counter. The diseases assessed include breast cancer, ovarian cancer, endometrial cancer, choriocarcinoma, prostate cancer, large bowel cancer and other gastrointestinal cancers, lung cancer, melanoma, liver cancer, pelvic inflammatory disease, cholecystitis, and venous thromboembolism. The drugs and drug classes assessed include ACE inhibitors, acetaminophen, antidepressants, antihistamines, aspirin and other NSAIDs, benzodiazepines, beta-blockers, calcium channel blockers, female hormone supplements, hydralazine, oral contraceptives, phenolphthalein, phenothiazines, rauwolfia alkaloids, statins, thiazides, and thyroid supplements. CCS has also made contributions to assessment of the health effects of non-drug factors, such as the tar and nicotine content of cigarettes, menthol cigarette smoking, alcohol and coffee consumption, and vasectomy.

THE FUTURE

Medication use in the US is widespread and increasing, spurred in part by direct marketing to consumers. New prescription drugs continue to be introduced to the market. Until medications and supplements have been used by appreciable numbers of people for appreciable periods, their health effects cannot and will not have been adequately monitored.

CCS will continue to monitor the effects of prescription drugs. The switch from prescription to over-the-counter sales has increased in recent years, and the use of dietary supplements has become widespread. CCS will carry out the monitoring of new and older over-the-counter medications, and of dietary supplements.

Several medications are of particular interest. Statins, the first of which was introduced to the market in 1987, are among the most widely used drugs in the US. Data from in vitro experiments suggest that the statins may have chemopreventive potential at various sites,[91–101] but there is also concern about a potential to increase cancer risk.[102,103] Selective serotonin reuptake inhibitors are also widely used, often by healthy persons. A recent report of three cases of breast neoplasia among men who took SSRIs[104] raises the concern that these drugs may affect breast cancer incidence. Histamine H_2 antagonists may have a stimulatory effect on the immune system.[105,106] It has been suggested that cimetidine could prevent prostate cancer,[107] but there are also concerns about possible increases in risk of breast cancer.[108,109] Nonsteroidal anti-inflammatory drugs also require continuing attention because of their widespread use, and because of the introduction of new agents. The inverse association of use with risk of colon cancer has raised interest in assessment of potential effects at other cancer sites. The health effects of dietary supplements are almost entirely unknown; CCS will devote considerable attention to their relation to the risk of cancer.

Knowledge about the actions of genetic polymorphisms has increased greatly in recent years. Genes with allelic variability that regulate the metabolism of drugs are likely candidates for modification of drug–cancer relationships.[31–35] CCS will have the capacity to assess plausible hypotheses that arise in the future about modification of drug effects on cancer risk by genetic polymorphisms.

ACKNOWLEDGMENTS

CCS was originated in 1975 by Dr Samuel Shapiro and the late Dr Dennis Slone. It was originally supported by contracts from the US Food and Drug Administration. Since 1988, CCS has been supported by the National Cancer Institute (CA45762). Additional support for data analyses has been provided by various pharmaceutical companies, which are acknowledged in the papers that relied on their support.

APPENDIX: CASE–CONTROL SURVEILLANCE PUBLICATIONS

1. Rosenberg L, Shapiro S, Kaufman DW, Slone D, Miettinen OS, Stolley PD. Patterns and determinants of conjugated estrogen use. *Am J Epidemiol* 1979; **109**: 676–86.
2. Kaufman DW, Shapiro S, Rosenberg L, Monson RR, Miettinen OS, Stolley PD *et al.* Intrauterine contraceptive device use and pelvic inflammatory disease. *Am J Obstet Gynecol* 1980; **136**: 159–62.
3. Kaufman DW, Slone D, Rosenberg L, Miettinen OS, Shapiro S. Cigarette smoking and age at natural menopause. *Am J Pub Health* 1980; **70**: 420–2.
4. Shapiro S, Kaufman DW, Slone D, Rosenberg L, Miettinen OS, Stolley PD *et al.* Recent and past use of conjugated estrogens in relation to adenocarcinoma of the endometrium. *N Engl J Med* 1980; **303**: 485–9.
5. Rosenberg L, Shapiro S, Slone D, Kaufman DW, Miettinen OS, Stolley PD. Thiazides and acute cholecystitis. *N Engl J Med* 1980; **303**: 546–8.
6. Shapiro S, Kaufman DW, Slone D, Rosenberg L, Miettinen OS, Stolley PD *et al.* Use of thyroid supplements in relation to breast cancer. *JAMA* 1980; **244**: 1685–7.
7. Kaufman DW, Shapiro S, Slone D, Rosenberg L, Miettinen OS, Stolley PD *et al.* Decreased risk of endometrial cancer among oral contraceptive users. *N Engl J Med* 1980; **303**: 1045–7.
8. Rosenberg L, Slone D, Shapiro S, Kaufman DW, Helmrich SP, Miettinen OS *et al.* Breast cancer and alcoholic-beverage consumption. *Lancet* 1982; **i**: 267–70.

9. Kaufman DW, Shapiro S, Slone D, Rosenberg L, Helmrich SP, Miettinen OS *et al*. Diazepam and the risk of breast cancer. *Lancet* 1982; **i**: 537–9.

10. Rosenberg L, Shapiro S, Slone D, Kaufman DW, Helmrich SP, Miettinen OS *et al*. Epithelial ovarian cancer and the use of combination oral contraceptives. *JAMA* 1982; **247**: 3210–12.

11. Helmrich SP, Slone D, Shapiro S, Rosenberg L, Kaufman DW, Bain C *et al*. Risk factors for breast cancer. *Am J Epidemiol* 1983; **117**: 35–45.

12. Kaufman DW, Watson J, Rosenberg L, Helmrich SP, Miller DR, Miettinen OS *et al*. The effect of different types of intrauterine device upon the risk of pelvic inflammatory disease. *JAMA* 1983; **250**: 759–62.

13. Rosenberg L, Schwingl PJ, Kaufman DW, Miller DR, Helmrich SP, Stolley PD *et al*. Breast cancer and cigarette smoking. *N Engl J Med* 1984; **310**: 92–4.

14. Rosenberg L, Miller DR, Kaufman DW, Helmrich SP, Stolley PD, Schottenfeld D *et al*. Breast cancer and oral contraceptive use. *Am J Epidemiol* 1984; **119**: 167–76.

15. Helmrich SP, Rosenberg L, Kaufman DW, Miller DR, Schottenfeld D, Stolley PD *et al*. Lack of an elevated risk of malignant melanoma in relation to oral contraceptive use. *J Natl Cancer Inst* 1984; **72**: 617–20.

16. Shapiro S, Parsells JL, Rosenberg L, Kaufman DW, Stolley PD, Schottenfeld D. Risk of breast cancer in relation to the use of rauwolfia alkaloids. *Eur J Clin Pharmacol* 1984; **26**: 143–6.

17. Kaufman DW, Miller DR, Rosenberg L, Helmrich SP, Stolley PD, Schottenfeld D *et al*. Noncontraceptive estrogen use and the risk of breast cancer. *JAMA* 1984; **252**: 63–7.

18. Rosenberg L, Miller DR, Helmrich SP, Kaufman DW, Shapiro S. Breast cancer and coffee drinking. *Banbury Report 17: Coffee and Health*. Cold Spring Harbor, NY: 1984, pp. 189–95.

19. Miller DR, Rosenberg L, Helmrich SP, Kaufman DW, Shapiro S. Ovarian cancer and coffee drinking. *Banbury Report 1: Coffee and Health*. Cold Spring Harbor, NY: 1984, pp. 157–65.

20. Lesko SM, Rosenberg L, Kaufman DW, Helmrich SP, Miller DM, Strom B *et al*. Cigarette smoking and the risk of endometrial cancer. *N Engl J Med* 1985; **313**: 593–6.

21. Rosenberg L, Miller DR, Helmrich SP, Kaufman DW, Schottenfeld D, Stolley PD *et al*. Breast cancer and the consumption of coffee. *Am J Epidemiol* 1985; **122**: 391–9.

22. Lesko SM, Kaufman DW, Rosenberg L, Helmrich SP, Miller DR, Stolley PD *et al*. Evidence of increased risk of Crohn's disease in oral contraceptive users. *Gastroenterology* 1985; **89**: 1046–9.

23. Shapiro S, Parsells JL, Rosenberg L, Kaufman DW, Helmrich SP, Rosenshein N *et al*. Risk of localized and widespread endometrial cancer in relation to recent and discontinued use of conjugated estrogens. *N Engl J Med* 1985; **313**: 969–72.

24. Miller DR, Rosenberg L, Kaufman DW, Schottenfeld D, Stolley PD, Shapiro S. Breast cancer risk in relation to early contraceptive use. *Obstet Gynecol* 1986; **68**: 863–8.

25. Miller DR, Rosenberg L, Kaufman DW, Helmrich SP, Schottenfeld D, Lewis J *et al*. Epithelial ovarian cancer and coffee drinking. *Int J Epidemiol* 1987; **16**: 13–17.

26. Helmrich SP, Rosenberg L, Kaufman DW, Strom B, Shapiro S. Venous thromboembolism in relation to oral contraceptive use. *Obstet Gynecol* 1987; **69**: 91–5.

27. Kaufman DW, Kelly JP, Rosenberg L, Stolley PD, Schottenfeld D, Shapiro S. Hydralazine and breast cancer. *J Natl Cancer Inst* 1987; **78**: 243–6.

28. Schatzkin A, Palmer JR, Rosenberg L, Helmrich SP, Miller DR, Kaufman DW *et al*. Risk factors for breast cancer in black women. *J Natl Cancer Inst* 1987; **18**: 213–17.

29. Rosenberg L, Lesko SM. Cigarette smoking and endometrial cancer. In: Rosenberg MJ, ed., *Smoking and Reproductive Health*. Littleton, MA: PSG, 1987; pp. 160–6.

30. Levy M, Miller D, Kaufman D, Siskind V, Schwingl P, Rosenberg L *et al*. Major upper gastrointestinal bleeding and the use of aspirin and other nonnarcotic analgesics. *Arch Intern Med* 1988; **148**: 281–5.

31. Rosenberg L, Palmer JR, Kaufman DW, Strom BL, Schottenfeld D, Shapiro S. Breast cancer in relation to the occurrence and timing of induced and spontaneous abortion. *Am J Epidemiol* 1988; **127**: 981–9.

32. Miller DR, Rosenberg L, Kaufman DW, Stolley P, Warshauer ME, Shapiro S. Breast cancer before age 45 and oral contraceptive use: new findings. *Am J Epidemiol* 1989; **129**: 269–80.

33. Kaufman DW, Palmer JR, Rosenberg L, Stolley P, Warshauer E, Shapiro S. Tar content of cigarettes in relation to lung cancer. *Am J Epidemiol* 1989; **129**: 703–11.

34. Kaufman DW, Kelly JP, Rosenberg L, Stolley PD, Warshauer ME, Shapiro S. Hydralazine use in relation to cancers of the lung, colon, and rectum. *Eur J Clin Pharmacol* 1989; **36**: 259–64.

35. Rosenberg L, Palmer JR, Shapiro S. Gestational trophoblastic disease and oral-contraceptive use. *Am J Obstet Gynecol* 1989; **161**: 1087–8.

36. Rosenberg L, Werler MM, Palmer JR, Kaufman DW, Warshauer ME, Stolley PD *et al*. The risks of cancers of the colon and rectum in relation to coffee consumption. *Am J Epidemiol* 1989; **130**: 895–903.

37. Palmer JR, Rosenberg L, Kaufman DW, Warshauer ME, Stolley P, Shapiro S. Oral contraceptive use and liver cancer. *Am J Epidemiol* 1989; **130**: 878–82.

38. Kaufman DW, Kelly JP, Welch WR, Rosenberg L, Stolley PD, Warshauer ME *et al*. Noncontraceptive estrogen use and epithelial ovarian cancer. *Am J Epidemiol* 1989; **130**: 1142–51.

39. Kelly JP, Rosenberg L, Kaufman DW, Shapiro S. Reliability of personal interview data in a hospital-based case–control study. *Am J Epidemiol* 1990; **131**: 79–90.

40. Kaufman DW, Werler MM, Palmer JR, Rosenberg L, Stolley PD, Warshauer ME *et al*. Diazepam use in relation to breast cancer: results from two case–control studies. *Am J Epidemiol* 1990; **131**: 483–90.

41. Rosenberg L, Palmer JR, Zauber AG, Warshauer ME, Stolley PD, Shapiro S. Vasectomy and the risk of prostate cancer. *Am J Epidemiol* 1990; **132**: 1051–5.

42. Austin KL, Palmer JR, Seddon JM, Glynn RJ, Rosenberg L, Gragoudas ES *et al*. Case control study of idiopathic retinal detachment. *Int J Epidemiol* 1990; **19**: 1045–9.

43. Miller DR. Breast cancer and early oral contraceptive use: studies from the Slone Epidemiology Unit. In: Mann RD, ed., *Oral Contraceptives and Breast Cancer*. Park Ridge, NJ: Parthenon, 1990; pp. 137–57.

44. Rosenberg L, Palmer JR, Shapiro S. Oral contraceptive use in relation to the risk of breast cancer: the data of Slone Epidemiology Unit in women aged 45–59 years. In: Mann RD, ed., *Oral Contraceptives and Breast Cancer*. Park Ridge, NJ: Parthenon, 1990; pp. 159–68.

45. Palmer JR. Oral contraceptive use and gestational choriocarcinoma. *Cancer Detect Prev* 1990; **15**: 45–8.

46. Rosenberg L, Palmer JR, Zauber AG, Warshauer ME, Stolley PD, Shapiro S. A hypothesis: NSAIDs reduce the incidence of large bowel cancer. *J Natl Cancer Inst* 1991; **83**: 355–8.

47. Lesko SM, Rosenberg L, Kaufman DW, Stolley PD, Warshauer ME, Lewis JL *et al*. Endometrial cancer and age at last delivery: evidence of an association. *Am J Epidemiol* 1991; **133**: 554–9.

48. Palmer JR, Rosenberg L, Clarke EA, Stolley PD, Warshauer ME, Zauber AG *et al*. Breast cancer and cigarette smoking: a hypothesis. *Am J Epidemiol* 1991; **134**: 1–13.

49. Johannes CB, Kaufman DW, Rosenberg L, Palmer JR, Stolley PD, Lewis JL Jr *et al*. Side of origin of epithelial ovarian cancer. *Br Med J* 1992; **304**: 27–8.

50. Kaufman DW, Palmer JR, de Mouzon J, Rosenberg L, Stolley PD, Warshauer E *et al*. Estrogen replacement therapy and the risk of breast cancer: results from the case–control surveillance study. *Am J Epidemiol* 1991; **134**: 1375–85.

51. Palmer JR, Rosenberg L, Strom BL, Harlap S, Zauber AG, Warshauer ME *et al*. Oral contraceptive use and risk of cutaneous malignant melanoma. *Cancer Causes Control* 1992; **3**: 547–54.

52. Kaufman DW, Palmer JR, Rosenberg L, Shapiro S. Oestrogen replacement therapy and breast cancer: new results from the Slone Epidemiology Unit's Case–Control Surveillance Study. In: Mann RD, ed., *Hormone Replacement Therapy and Breast Cancer Risk*. Park Ridge, NJ: Parthenon, 1992; pp. 173–84.

53. Shapiro S. Case–control surveillance. In: Strom BL, ed., *Pharmacoepidemiology*, 2nd edn. Chichester: John Wiley & Sons, 1994; pp. 301–22.

54. Rosenberg L, Palmer JR, Zauber AG, Warshauer ME, Lewis JL Jr, Strom BL *et al*. A case–control study of oral contraceptive use and invasive epithelial ovarian cancer. *Am J Epidemiol* 1994; **139**: 654–61.

55. Rosenberg L, Palmer JR, Zauber AG, Warshauer ME, Strom BL, Harlap S *et al*. The relation of vasectomy to the risk of cancer. *Am J Epidemiol* 1994; **140**: 431–8.

56. Rosenberg L. NSAIDs and cancer. *Prev Med* 1995; **24**: 107–9.

57. Palmer JR, Rosenberg L, Harlap S, Strom BL, Warshauer ME, Zauber AG *et al*. Adult height and risk of breast cancer among US black women. *Am J Epidemiol* 1995; **141**: 845–9.

58. Rosenberg L, Palmer JR, Zauber AG, Warshauer ME, Strom BL, Harlap S *et al*. The relation of benzodiazepine use to the risk of selected cancers: breast, large bowel, malignant melanoma, lung, endometrium, ovary, non-Hodgkin's lymphoma, testis, Hodgkin's disease, thyroid and liver. *Am J Epidemiol* 1995; **141**: 1153–60.

59. Palmer JR, Rosenberg L, Rao RS, Strom BL, Warshauer ME, Harlap S, Zauber A *et al*. Oral contraceptive use and breast cancer risk among African-American women. *Cancer Causes Control* 1995; **6**: 321–3.

60. Rosenberg L, Palmer JR, Rao RS, Zauber AG, Strom BL, Warshauer ME *et al*. Case–control study of oral contraceptive use and risk of breast cancer. *Am J Epidemiol* 1996; **143**: 25–37.

61. Zhang Y, Rosenberg L, Colton T, Couples A, Palmer JR, Strom BL *et al*. Adult height and risk of breast

cancer among white women in a case–control study. *Am J Epidemiol* 1996; **143**: 1123–8.

62. Palmer JR, Rosenberg L, Rao RS, Zauber A, Strom BL, Warshauer ME *et al*. Induced and spontaneous abortion in relation to risk of breast cancer (United States). *Cancer Causes Control* 1997; **8**: 841–9.

63. Rosenberg L, Rao RS, Palmer JP, Strom BL, Zauber AG, Warshauer ME *et al*. Transitional cell cancer of the urinary tract and renal cell cancer in relation to acetaminophen use. *Cancer Causes Control* 1998; **9**: 83–8.

64. Rosenberg L, Rao RS, Palmer JR, Strom BL, Stolley PD, Zauber AG *et al*. Calcium channel blockers and the risk of cancer. *JAMA* 1998; **279**: 1000–4.

65. Rosenberg L, Stephenson WP, Rao RS, Palmer JR, Strom BL, Shapiro S. The diagnosis of renal cell cancer in relation to hypertension (United States). *Cancer Causes Control* 1998; **9**: 611–14.

66. Shapiro S. Case–control surveillance. In: Strom BL, ed., *Pharmacoepidemiology*, 3rd edn. Chichester: John Wiley & Sons, 2000; pp. 209–30.

67. Coogan PF, Rao RS, Rosenberg L, Palmer JR, Strom BL, Zauber AG *et al*. The relationship of nonsteroidal anti-inflammatory drug use to the risk of breast cancer. *Prev Med* 1999; **29**: 72–6.

68. Kelly JP, Rosenberg L, Palmer JR, Rao RS, Strom BL, Stolley PD *et al*. Risk of breast cancer according to use of antidepressants, phenothiazines, and antihistamines. *Am J Epidemiol* 1999; **150**: 675–82.

69. Coogan PF, Rosenberg L, Palmer JR, Strom BL, Zauber AG, Stolley PD *et al*. Nonsteroidal anti-inflammatory drugs and risk of digestive cancers at sites other than the large bowel. *Cancer Epidemiol Biomark Prev* 2000; **9**: 119–23.

70. Coogan PF, Rosenberg L, Zauber AG, Stolley PD, Strom BL, Shapiro S. NSAIDs and risk of colorectal cancer according to presence or absence of family history of disease. *Cancer Causes Control* 2000; **11**: 249–55.

71. Rosenberg L, Palmer JR, Rao RS, Coogan PF, Strom BL, Zauber AG *et al*. A case–control study of analgesic use and ovarian cancer. *Cancer Epidemiol Biomarkers Prev* 2000; **9**: 933–7.

72. Coogan PF, Rosenberg L, Palmer JR, Strom BL, Stolley PD, Zauber AG *et al*. Risk of ovarian cancer according to use of antidepressants, phenothiazines, and benzodiazepines. *Cancer Causes Control* 2000; **11**: 839–45.

73. Coogan PF, Rosenberg L, Palmer JR, Strom BL, Zauber AG, Stolley PD *et al*. Phenolphthalein laxatives and risk of cancer. *J Natl Cancer Inst* 2000; **92**: 1943–4.

74. Kaufman DW, Rosenberg L, Mitchell AA. Signal generation and clarification: use of case–control data. *Pharmacoepidemiol Drug Saf* 2001; **10**: 197–203.

75. Coogan PF, Rosenberg L, Palmer JR, Strom BL, Zauber AG, Shapiro S. Statin use and the risk of breast and prostate cancer. *Epidemiology* 2002; **13**: 262–7.

76. Blackman JA, Coogan PF, Rosenberg L, Strom BL, Zauber AG, Palmer JR *et al*. Estrogen replacement therapy and risk of lung cancer by cell type. *Pharmacoepidemiol Drug Saf* 2002; **11**: 561–7.

77. Coogan P, Rosenberg L. Response to Etminan letter Re: Statin use and the risk of breast and prostate cancer [letter]. *Epidemiology*, 2002; **13**: 607–8.

78. Brooks DR, Palmer JR, Strom BL, Rosenberg L. Menthol cigarettes and risk of lung cancer. *Am J Epidemiol* 2003; **158**: 609–16.

79. Zhang Y, Coogan PF, Palmer JR, Strom BL, Rosenberg L. Cigarette smoking and increased risk of mucinous epithelial ovarian cancer. *Am J Epidemiol* 2004; **159**: 133–9.

REFERENCES

1. Brewer T, Colditz G. Postmarketing surveillance and adverse drug reactions: current perspectives and future needs. *JAMA* 1999; **281**: 824–9.

2. Lasser KE, Allen PD, Woolhandler SJ, Himmelstein DV, Wolfe SM, Bor DH. Timing of new black box warnings and withdrawals for prescription medications. *JAMA* 2002; **287**: 2215–20.

3. FDA. List of drug products that have been withdrawn or removed from the market for reasons of safety or effectiveness. 21 CFR Part 216. Docket No. 98N-0655. *Fed Regist* 1998; **63**: 54082–9.

4. FDA issues voluntary removal of drugs with phenylpropanolamine. Release #00B-139, November, 2000.

5. Bayer Corporation. Market withdrawal of Baycol. August 8, 2001. Available at: www.baycol-rhabdomyolysis.com/baycol_recall.

6. Soller RW. OTCS 2000: Achievements and challenges. *Drug Inf J* 2000; **34**: 693–701.

7. Francesco International. Potential government high priority therapeutic areas for OTC. SWITCH® Newsletter, SwitchTrends. Available at: http://www.rxtootcswitch.com. Accessed January 14, 2004.

8. Kaufman DW, Kelley JP, Rosenberg L, Anderson TE, Mitchell AA. Recent patterns of medication use in the US: the Slone Survey. *JAMA* 2002; **287**: 337–44.

9. Kessler DA. Cancer and herbs. *N Engl J Med* 2000; **342**: 1762–3.

10. Newall CA, Anderson LA, Philpson JD. *Herbal Medicine: A Guide for Healthcare Professionals*. London: The Pharmaceutical Press, 1966.

11. Nortier JL, Martinez MC, Schmeiser HH, Arlt VM, Bieler A, Petein M *et al*. Urothelial carcinoma associated with the use of a Chinese herb (*Aristolochia fangchi*). *N Engl J Med* 2000; **342**: 1686–92.

12. Czeczot H, Tudek B, Kusztelak J, Szynczyk T, Dobrowolska B, Glinkowska G *et al*. Isolation and studies of mutagenic activity in the Ames test of flavonoids naturally occurring in medical herbs. *Mutat Res* 1990; **240**: 209–16.

13. Kapadia GJ, Chung EB, Ghosh B, Shukla YN, Besak SP, Morton JF *et al*. Carcinogenicity of some folk medicinal herbs in rats. *J Natl Cancer Inst* 1978; **60**: 683–6.

14. Shin HR, Kim JY, Yun TK, Morgan G, Vainio H. The cancer-preventive potential of Panax ginseng: a review of human and experimental evidence. *Cancer Causes Control* 2000; **11**: 565–76.

15. Eagon PK, Elm MS, Hunter DS. Medicinal herbs: modulation of estrogen action. Era of Hope Meeting for the Department of Defense Breast Cancer Research Program; Jun 8–11, 2000, Atlanta, Georgia.

16. Dixon-Shanies D, Shaich N. Growth inhibition of human breast cancer cells by herbs and phytoestrogens. *Oncol Rep* 1999; **6**: 1383–7.

17. Gurley BJ, Gardner SF, Hubbard MA. Clinical assessment of potential cytochrome P450-mediated herb–drug interactions. AAPS Annual Meeting and Exposition, presentation #3460; Oct 9–Nov 2, 2000, Indianapolis, Indiana.

18. Budzinski JW, Foster BC, Vandenhoek S, Arnason JT. An in vitro evaluation of human cytochrome P450 3A4 inhibition by selected commercial herbal extracts and tinctures. *Phytomedicine* 2000; **7**: 273–82.

19 Royal College of General Practitioners. *Oral Contraceptives and Health*. An interim report from the oral contraceptive study of the Royal College of General Practitioners. New York: Pitman Medical, 1974.

20. Friedman GD. Kaiser Permanente medical care program: Northern California and other regions. In: Strom BL, ed., *Pharmacoepidemiology*, 2nd edn. Chichester: John Wiley & Sons, 1994; pp. 187–98.

21. Saunders KW, Stergachis A, Von Korff M. Group Health Cooperatives of Puget Sound. In: Strom BL, ed., *Pharmacoepidemiology*, 2nd edn. Chichester: John Wiley & Sons, 1994; pp. 171–86.

22. Carson JL, Strom BL. Medicaid databases. In: Strom BL, ed., *Pharmacoepidemiology*, 2nd edn. Chichester: John Wiley & Sons, 1994; pp. 199–216.

23. Sharpe CR, Collet J-P, McNutt M, Belzile E, Boivin J-F, Hanley JA. Nested case–control study of the effects of non-steroidal anti-inflammatory drugs on breast cancer risk and stage. *Br J Cancer* 2000; **83**: 112–20.

24. Jick H, Jick S, Derby LE, Vasilakis C, Myers MW, Meier CR. Calcium channel blockers and risk of cancer. *Lancet* 1997; **349**: 525–8.

25. Shapiro S, Kelly JP, Rosenberg L, Kaufman DW, Helmrich SP, Rosenshein NB *et al*. Risk of localized and widespread endometrial cancer in relation to recent and discontinued use of conjugated estrogens. *N Engl J Med* 1985; **313**: 969–72.

26. Rosenberg L, Shapiro S, Slone D, Kaufman DW, Miettinen OS, Stolley PD. Thiazides and acute cholecystitis. *N Engl J Med* 1980; **303**: 546–8.

27. Kaufman DW, Shapiro S, Rosenberg L, Monson RR, Miettinen OS, Stolley PD *et al*. Intrauterine contraceptive device use and pelvic inflammatory disease. *Am J Obstet Gynecol* 1980; **136**: 159–62.

28. Garcia-Closas M, Egan K, Abruzzo J, Newcomb PA, Titus-Ernstoff L, Franklin T *et al*. Collection of genomic DNA from adults in epidemiologic studies by buccal cytobrush and mouthwash. *Cancer Epidemiol Biomarkers Prev* 2001; **10**: 687–96.

29. Cozier YC, Palmer JR, Rosenberg L. Comparison of methods of collection of DNA samples by mail in the Black Women's Health Study. *Ann Epidemiol*. 2004; **14**: 117–22.

30. Rebbeck T, Walker AH, Phelan CM, Godwin AK, Buetow KH, Garber JE *et al*. Defining etiologic heterogeneity in breast cancer using genetic markers. *Prog Clin Biol Res* 1997; **396**: 53–61.

31. Nebert DW. Role of genetics and drug metabolism in human cancer risk. *Mutat Res* 1991; **247**: 267–81.

32. Daly AK, Cholerton S, Gregory W, Idle JR. Metabolic polymorphisms. *Pharmacol Ther* 1993; **57**: 129–60.

33. Idle JR. Is environmental carcinogenesis modulated by host polymorphism? *Mutat Res* 1991; **247**: 259–66.

34. Kato S, Shields PG, Caporaso NE, Sugimura H, Trivers GE, Tucker MA *et al*. Analysis of cytochrome P450 2E1 genetic polymorphisms in relation to human lung cancer. *Cancer Epidemiol Biomarkers Prev* 1994; **3**: 515–18.

35. Poulsen HE, Loft S. The impact of genetic polymorphisms in risk assessment of drugs [review]. *Arch Toxicol* 1994; **16**(suppl): 211–22.

36. Koop DR, Tierney DJ. Multiple mechanisms in the regulation of ethanol-inducible cytochrome P45011E1. *Bioessays* 1990; **12**: 429–35.

37. Rothman KJ. *Modern Epidemiology*. Boston, MA: Little, Brown, 1986; p. 60.

38. Schlesselman SS. *Case–Control Studies: Design, Conduct, Analysis*. New York: Oxford University Press, 1982.

39. Miettinen OS. Valid sampling in the context of a base secondary to the cases. In: *Theoretical Epidemiology. Principles of Occurrence Research in Medicine*. New York: John Wiley & Sons, 1985: pp. 79–82.

40. Rosenberg L, Palmer JR, Zauber AG, Warshauer ME, Stolley PD, Shapiro S. A hypothesis: NSAIDs reduce the incidence of large bowel cancer. *J Natl Cancer Inst* 1991; **83**: 355–8.

41. Rosenberg L, Palmer JR, Zauber AG, Warshauer ME, Strom BL, Harlap S *et al*. The relation of vasectomy to the risk of cancer. *Am J Epidemiol* 1994; **140**: 431–8.

42. Rosenberg L, Palmer JR, Zauber AG, Warshauer ME, Lewis JL Jr, Strom BL *et al*. A case–control study of oral contraceptive use and invasive epithelial ovarian cancer. *Am J Epidemiol* 1994; **139**: 654–61.

43. West SL, Strom BL. Validity of pharmacoepidemiology drug and diagnosis data. In: Strom BL, ed., *Pharmacoepidemiology*, 2nd edn. Chichester: John Wiley & Sons, 1994; pp. 199–216.

44. Nischan P, Ebeling K, Thomas DB, Hirsch U. Comparision of recalled and validated oral contraceptive histories. *Am J Epidemiol* 1993; **138**: 697–703.

45. Glass R, Johnson B, Vessey M. Accuracy of recall of histories of oral contraceptive use. *Br J Prev Soc Med* 1974; **28**: 273–5.

46. Rosenberg MJ, Layde PM, Ory HW, Strauss LT, Rooks JB, Rubin GL. Agreement between women's histories of oral contraceptive use and physician records. *Int J Epidemiol* 1983; **12**: 84–7.

47. Stolley PD, Tonascia JA, Sartwell PE, Tockman MS, Tonascia S, Rutledge A *et al*. Agreement rates between oral contraceptive users and prescribers in relation to drug use histories. *Am J Epidemiol* 1978; **107**: 226–35.

48. van Leeuwen FE, van Duijn CM, Camps MH, Kempers BA, Mentjens MF, Mulder HB *et al*. Agreement between oral contraceptive users and prescribers: implications for case–control studies. *Contraception* 1992; **45**: 399–408.

49. Kaufman DW, Palmer JR, de Mouzon J, Rosenberg L, Stolley PD, Warshauer E *et al*. Estrogen replacement therapy and the risk of breast cancer: results from the case–control surveillance study. *Am J Epidemiol* 1991; **134**: 1375–85.

50. Schairer C, Lubin J, Troisi R, Sturgeon S, Brinton L, Hoover R. Menopausal estrogen and estrogen–progestin replacement therapy and breast cancer risk. *JAMA* 2000; **283**: 485–91.

51. Magnusson C, Baron JA, Correia N, Bergstrom R, Adami HO, Persson I. Breast cancer risk following long-term estrogen and estrogen–progestin-replacement therapy. *Int J Cancer* 1999; **81**: 339–44.

52. Garcia-Closas M, Lubin JH. Power and sample size calculations in case–control studies of gene–environmental interactions: comments on different approaches. *Am J Epidemiol* 1999; **149**: 689–92.

53. Thun MJ, Namboodiri MM, Heath CW Jr. Aspirin use and reduced risk of fatal colon cancer. *N Engl J Med* 1991; **325**: 1593–6.

54. Gann PH, Manson JE, Glynn RJ, Buring JE, Hennekens CH. Low-dose aspirin and incidence of colorectal tumors in a randomized trial. *J Natl Cancer Inst* 1993; **35**: 1220–4.

55. Giovannucci E, Egan KM, Hunter DJ, Stampfer MJ, Colditz GA, Willett WC *et al*. Aspirin and the risk of colorectal cancer in women. *N Engl J Med* 1995; **333**: 609–14.

56. Thun MS, Namboodiri MM, Calle EE, Flanders MD, Heath CW Jr. Aspirin use and risk of fatal cancer. *Cancer Res* 1993; **53**: 1322–7.

57. Rosenberg L, Louik C, Shapiro S. Nonsteroidal antiinflammatory drug use and reduced risk of large bowel carcinoma. *Cancer* 1998; **82**: 2326–33.

58. Rosenberg L, Slone D, Shapiro S, Kaufman DR, Helmrich SP, Miettinen OS *et al*. Breast cancer and alcoholic-beverage consumption. *Lancet* 1982; **i**: 267–70.

59. Rosenberg L, Palmer JR, Shapiro S. Gestational trophoblastic disease and oral-contraceptive use. *Am J Obstet Gynecol* 1989; **161**: 1087–8.

60. Lesko SM, Kaufman DW, Rosenberg L, Helmrich SP, Miller DR, Stolley PD *et al*. Evidence of increased risk of Crohn's disease in oral contraceptive users. *Gastroenterology* 1985; **89**: 1046–9.

61. Rosenberg L, Metzger LS, Palmer JR. Epidemiology of breast cancer. Alcohol consumption and risk of breast cancer: a review of the evidence. *Epidemiol Rev* 1993; **15**: 133–44.

62. Willett W, Stampfer MJ, Colditz GA, Rosner BA, Hennekens CH, Speizer FE. Moderate alcohol consumption and the risk of breast cancer. *N Engl J Med* 1987; **316**: 1174–80.

63. Schatzkin A, Jones DY, Hoover RN, Taylor PR, Brinton LA, Ziegler RG *et al*. Alcohol consumption and breast cancer in the epidemiologic follow-up study of the First National Health and Nutrition Examination Survey. *N Engl J Med* 1987; **316**: 1169–73.

64. Palmer JR, Driscoll SD, Rosenberg L, Berkowitz RS, Lurain JR, Soper J *et al*. Oral contraceptive use and risk of gestational trophoblastic tumors. *J Natl Cancer Inst* 1999; **91**: 635–40.

65. Ramcharan S, ed. *The Walnut Creek Contraceptive Drug Study: A Prospective Study of the Side Effects of Oral Contraceptives*, vol. III. Washington, DC: US Government Printing Office, 1981.

66. Palmer JR, Rosenberg L, Kaufman DW, Warshauer ME, Stolley P, Shapiro S. Oral contraceptive use and liver cancer. *Am J Epidemiol* 1989; **130**: 878–82.

67. Rosenberg L, Miller DR, Kaufman DW, Helmrich SP, Stolley PD, Schottenfeld D *et al*. Breast cancer and oral-contraceptive use. *Am J Epidemiol* 1984; **119**: 167–76.

68. Rosenberg L, Palmer JR, Rao RS, Zauber AG, Strom BL, Warshauer ME *et al*. Case–control study of oral contraceptive use and risk of breast cancer. *Am J Epidemiol* 1996; **143**: 25–37.

69. Kaufman DW, Shapiro S, Slone D, Rosenberg L, Miettinen OS, Stolley PD *et al*. Decreased risk of endometrial cancer among oral contraceptive users. *N Engl J Med* 1980; **303**: 1045–7.

70. Coogan PF, Rosenberg L, Palmer JR, Strom BL, Zauber AG, Stolley PD *et al*. Nonsteroidal anti-inflammatory drugs and risk of digestive cancers at sites other than the large bowel. *Cancer Epidemiol Biomarkers Prev* 2000; **9**: 119–23.

71. National Toxicology Program. Technical report on the toxicology and carcinogenesis studies of phenolphthalein (CAS no. 77-09-8). In: *F344/N Rats and B6C3F, Mice (Feed Studies) NTP TR 465*. NIH Publication no. 95-3390, 1995.

72. Associated Press. Study ordered on ingredients of laxatives. *New York Times* May 24, 1996.

73. Coogan PF, Rosenberg L, Palmer JR, Strom BL, Zauber AG, Stolley PD *et al*. Phenolphthalein laxatives and risk of cancer. *J Natl Cancer Inst* 2000; **92**: 1943–4.

74. Pahor M, Guralnik JM, Salive ME, Corti M-C, Carbonin P, Havlik RJ. Do calcium channel blockers increase the risk of cancer? *Am J Hypertens* 1996; **9**: 695–9.

75. Pahor M, Guralnik JM, Corti M-C, Salive ME, Cerhan JR, Wallace RB *et al*. Calcium-channel blockade and incidence of cancer in aged populations. *Lancet* 1996; **348**: 493–7.

76. Rosenberg L, Rao RS, Palmer JR, Strom BL, Stolley PD, Zauber AG *et al*. Calcium channel blockers and the risk of cancer. *JAMA* 1998; **279**: 1000–4.

77. Kaufman DW, Shapiro S, Slone D, Rosenberg L, Helmrich SP, Miettinen OS *et al*. Diazepam and the risk of breast cancer. *Lancet* 1982; **i**: 537–9.

78. Kaufman DW, Werler MM, Palmer JR, Rosenberg L, Stolley PD, Warshauer ME *et al*. Diazepam use in relation to breast cancer: results from two case–control studies. *Am J Epidemiol* 1990; **131**: 483–90.

79. Rosenberg L, Palmer JR, Zauber AG, Warshauer ME, Strom BL, Harlap S *et al*. The relation of benzodiazepine use to the risk of selected cancers: breast, large bowel, malignant melanoma, lung, endometrium, ovary, non-Hodgkin's lymphoma, testis, Hodgkin's disease, thyroid and liver. *Am J Epidemiol* 1995; **141**: 1153–60.

80. Kaufman DW, Kelly JP, Rosenberg L, Stolley PD, Schottenfeld D, Shapiro S. Hydralazine and breast cancer. *J Natl Cancer Inst* 1987; **78**: 243–6.

81. Kaufman DW, Kelly JP, Rosenberg L, Stolley PD, Warshauer ME, Shapiro S. Hydralazine use in relation to cancers of the lung, colon, and rectum. *Eur J Clin Pharmacol* 1989; **36**: 259–64.

82. Wacholder S, McLaughlin JK, Silverman DT, Mandel JS. Selection of controls in case–control studies. I. Principles. *Am J Epidemiol* 1992; **135**: 1019–28.

83. Wacholder S, McLaughlin JK, Silverman DT, Mandel JS. Selection of controls in case–control studies. II. Types of controls. *Am J Epidemiol* 1992; **135**: 1029–41.

84. Wacholder S, McLaughlin JK, Silverman DT, Mandel JS. Selection of controls in case–control studies. III. Design options. *Am J Epidemiol* 1992; **135**: 1042–50.

85. Rosenberg L, Rao RS, Palmer JP, Strom BL, Zauber AG, Warshauer ME *et al*. Transitional cell cancer of the urinary tract and renal cell cancer in relation to acetaminophen use. *Cancer Causes Control* 1998; **9**: 83–8.

86. Spengler RF, Clarke EA, Woolever CA, Newman AM, Osborn RW. Exogenous estrogens and endometrial cancer: a case–control study and assessment of potential biases. *Am J Epidemiol* 1981; **114**: 497–506.

87. Goodman MT, Nomura AMY, Wilkens LR, Kolonel LN. Agreement between interview information and physician records on history of menopausal estrogen use. *Am J Epidemiol* 1990; **131**: 815–25.

88. Persson I, Bergkvist L, Adami H-O. Reliability of women's histories of climacteric oestrogen treatment assessed by prescription forms. *Int J Epidemiol* 1987; **16**: 222–8.

89. Paganini-Hill A, Ross RK. Reliability of recall of drug usage and other health-related information. *Am J Epidemiol* 1982; **116**: 114–22.

90. Harlow SD, Linet MS. Agreement between questionnaire data and medical recall: the evidence of accuracy of recall. *Am J Epidemiol* 1989; **129**: 233–48.

91. Keyomarsi K, Sandoval L, Band V, Pardee A. Synchronization of tumor and normal cells from G1 to multiple cell cycles by lovastatin. *Cancer Res* 1991; **51**: 3602–9.

92. Inano H, Suzuki K, Onoda M, Wakabayashi K. Anti-carcinogenic activity of simvastatin during the promotion phase of radiation-induced mammary tumorigenesis of rats. *Carcinogenesis* 1997; **18**: 1723–7.

93. Addeo R, Altucci L, Battista T, Bonapace IM, Cancemi M, Cicatiello L *et al*. Simulation of human breast cancer MCF-7 cells with estrogen prevents cell cycle arrest by HMG-CoA reductase inhibitors. *Biochem Biophys Res Commun* 1996; **220**: 864–70.

94. Ghosh PM, Ghosh-Choudhury N, Moyer Ml, Mott GE, Thomas CA, Foster BA *et al*. Role of RhoA activation in the growth and morphology of a murine prostate tumor cell kine. *Oncogene* 1999; **18**: 4120–30.

95. Lee SJ, Ha MJ, Lee J, Nguyen P, Choi YH, Pirnia F *et al*. Inhibition of the 3-hydroxy-3methylglutarlyl-coenzyme A reductase pathway induces p53-independent transcriptional regulation of p21 (WAF1/CIP1) in human prostate carcinoma cells. *J Biol Chem* 1998; **273**: 10618–23.

96. Marcelli M, Cunningham GR, Haidacher SK, Padayatty SJ, Sturgis L, Kagan C *et al*. Caspase-7 is activated during lovastatin-induced apoptosis of the prostate cancer cell line LNCaP. *Cancer Res* 1998; **58**: 76–83.

97. Carlberg M, Dricu A, Blegen H, Wang M, Hjertman M, Zickert P *et al*. Mevalonic acid is limiting for *n*-linked glycosylation and translocation of the insulin-like growth factor-1 receptor to the cell surface. *J Biol Chem* 1996; **271**: 17453–62.

98. Agarwal B, Rao CV, Bhendwal S, Ramey WR, Shirin H, Reddy BS *et al*. Lovastatin augments sulindac induced apoptosis in colon cancer cells and potentiates chemopreventive effects of sulindac. *Gastroenterology* 1999; **117**: 838–47.

99. Agarwal B, Bhendwal S, Halmos B, Moss F, Ramey WG, Holt PR. Lovastatin augments apoptosis induced by chemotherapeutic agents in colon cancer cells. *Clin Cancer Res* 1999; **5**: 2223–9.

100. Rao S, Porter DC, Chen X, Herliczek T, Lowe M, Keyomarsi K. Lovastatin-mediated G1 arrest is through inhibition of the proteasome, independent of hydroxymethyl glutaryl-CoA reductase. *Proc Natl Acad Sci USA* 1999; **96**: 7797–802.

101. Hawk MA, Cesen KT, Siglin JC, Stoner GD, Ruch RJ. Inhibition of lung tumor cell growth in vitro and mouse lung tumor formation by lovastatin. *Cancer Lett* 1996; **109**: 217–22.

102. Newman TB, Hulley SB. Special communication. Carcinogenicity of lipid-lowering drugs. *JAMA* 1966; **275**: 55–60.

103. Sacks FM, Pfeffer MA, Moye LA, Rouleau JL, Rutherford JD, Cole TG *et al*. The effect of pravastatin on coronary events after myocardial infarction in patients with average cholesterol levels. *N Engl J Med* 1996; **335**: 1001–9.

104. Wallace WA, Balsitis M, Harrison BJ. Male breast neoplasms in association with selective serotonin re-uptake inhibitor therapy: a recent report of three cases. *Eur J Surg Oncol* 2001; **27**: 429–31.

105. Hellstrand K, Asea A, Hermodsson S. Role of histamine in natural killer cell-mediated resistance against tumor cells. *J Immunol* 1990; **145**: 4365–70.

106. Hellstrand K, Hermodsson S, Naredi P, Mellqvist UH, Brune M. Histamine and cytokine therapy. *Acta Oncol* 1998; **37**: 347–53.

107. Feldman M, Burton ME. Histamine2-receptor antagonists. Standard therapy for acid-peptic diseases. *N Engl J Med* 1990; **323**: 1672–80.

108. Galbraith RA, Michnovicz JJ. The effects of cimetidine on the oxidative metabolism of estradiol. *N Engl J Med* 1989; **321**: 269–74.

109. Michnovicz JJ, Galbraith RA. Cimetidine inhibits catechol estrogen metabolism in women. *Metabolism* 1991; **40**:170–4.

12

Prescription-Event Monitoring

SAAD A.W. SHAKIR

Drug Safety Research Unit, Southampton, UK.

INTRODUCTION

The thalidomide disaster, which caused the development of phocomelia in nearly 10 000 children whose mothers took thalidomide during pregnancy,[1] was the stimulus for the establishment of systems to monitor suspected adverse drug reactions (ADRs) and the development of modern pharmacovigilance. The reasons for monitoring postmarketing drug safety were summarized in 1970 in a report of the Committee on Safety of Drugs in the UK (which later became the Committee on Safety of Medicines, CSM):

> No drug which is pharmacologically effective is entirely without hazard. The hazard may be insignificant or may be acceptable in relation to the drug's therapeutic action. Furthermore, not all hazards can be known before a drug is marketed; neither tests in animals nor clinical trials in patients will always reveal all the possible side effects of a drug. These may only be known when the drug has been administered to large numbers of patients over considerable periods of time.[2]

Premarketing clinical trials are effective in studying the efficacy of medicines. However, while they define many aspects of the safety profiles of medicines, premarketing clinical trials have limitations in defining the clinically necessary safety profiles of drugs. These limitations include:

- the small numbers of patients, in epidemiologic terms, included in premarketing clinical trial programs;[3]
- the large numbers of patients in these programs who receive the study products for short durations (many only receive a single dose); this limits the power of premarketing clinical trials to detect rare ADRs or ADRs with long latency;
- premarketing development programs are dynamic; doses and formulations can change during drug development; in some programs, large numbers of patients studied receive lower doses or different formulations from those eventually marketed;
- the exclusion from clinical trials of special populations such as the young, the old, women of childbearing age, and patients with concurrent diseases, eliminates many patients who may be at higher risk for developing ADRs, limiting the generalizability of the results of such trials.

Therefore, there has been general agreement for more than 30 years that the clinically necessary understanding of drug safety depends on postmarketing monitoring and postmarketing safety studies. This has resulted in not only the establishment

Pharmacoepidemiology, Fourth Edition   Edited by B.L. Strom
© 2005 John Wiley & Sons, Ltd

of voluntary systems for reporting suspected ADRs (see Chapters 9 and 10) but the development of a range of other methods to monitor and study postmarketing drug safety.

Soon after the establishment of spontaneous reporting systems, it was recognized that, while such systems have many real advantages for detecting and defining ADRs, particularly rare ADRs, they also have limitations.[4]

The theoretical basis for establishing a system to monitor events regardless of relatedness to drug exposure was proposed by Finney in 1965.[5] This and the limited contribution of the spontaneous reporting system in detecting hazards such as the oculomucocutaneous syndrome with practolol led Inman to establish the system of Prescription-Event Monitoring (PEM) at the Drug Safety Research Unit (DSRU) at Southampton in 1981.[6] Subsequently the CSM, wishing to consider monitoring the postmarketing safety of medicines, established a committee under the chairmanship of Professor David Grahame-Smith. The committee reported in June 1983 and again in July 1985, and in these reports showed an appreciation of the need for prescription-based monitoring. It also specifically recommended that postmarketing surveillance (PMS) studies should be undertaken "on newly-marketed drugs intended for widespread long-term use."[7] PEM is one form of pharmacovigilance that, with the development and harmonization of drug regulation in the European Community, has its basis in Directives 65/65 and 75/319, and in Regulation 2309/93.

DESCRIPTION

The PEM process is summarized in Figure 12.1. In the UK, virtually all patients are registered with a National Health Service (NHS) general practitioner (GP), who provides primary medical care and acts as a gateway to specialist and hospital care. The file notes in general practice in the UK include not only information obtained in primary care but data about all contacts with secondary and tertiary care, such as letters from specialist clinics, hospital discharge summaries, and results of laboratory and other investigations. It is a lifelong record; when a patient moves to a new area, all his notes are sent to his new GP.

The GP issues prescriptions for the medicines he/she considers medically warranted. The patient takes the prescription to a pharmacist, who dispenses the medication and then sends the prescription to a central Prescription Pricing Authority (PPA) for reimbursement. The DSRU is, under longstanding and confidential arrangements, provided with electronic copies of all those prescriptions issued throughout England for the drugs being monitored. Products that are selected for study by PEM are new drugs which are expected to be widely used by GPs; in some cases the DSRU is unable to study suitable products because of limited resources. In addition, the DSRU conducts studies on established products when there is a reason to do so, for example, a new indication

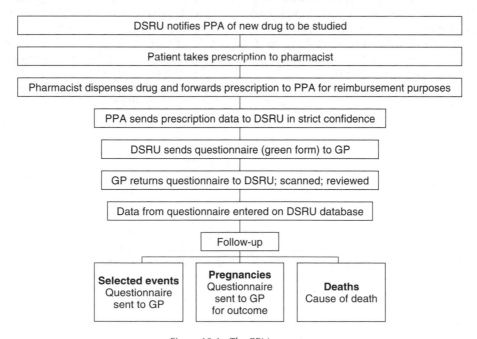

Figure 12.1. The PEM process.

or extending usage to a new population. Collection of the exposure data usually begins immediately after the new drug has been launched. These arrangements operate for the length of time necessary for the DSRU to collect the first 50 000 prescriptions that identify 20 000–30 000 patients given the new drug being monitored. For each patient in each PEM study, the DSRU prepares a computerized longitudinal record in date order of the use of the drug. Thus, in PEM, the exposure data are national in scope and provide information on the first cohort to receive the drug being monitored after it has been launched into everyday clinical usage. The exposure data are of drugs both prescribed and dispensed, but there is no measure of compliance.

After an interval of 3–12, but usually 6, months from the date of the first prescription for each patient in the cohort, the DSRU sends to the prescriber a "green form" questionnaire seeking information on any "events" that may have occurred while the patient was taking the drug or in the months that followed. This takes place on an individual patient basis. To limit the workload of GPs, no doctor is sent more than four green forms in any one month. The green form, illustrated in Figure 12.2, is intended to be simple. It requests information

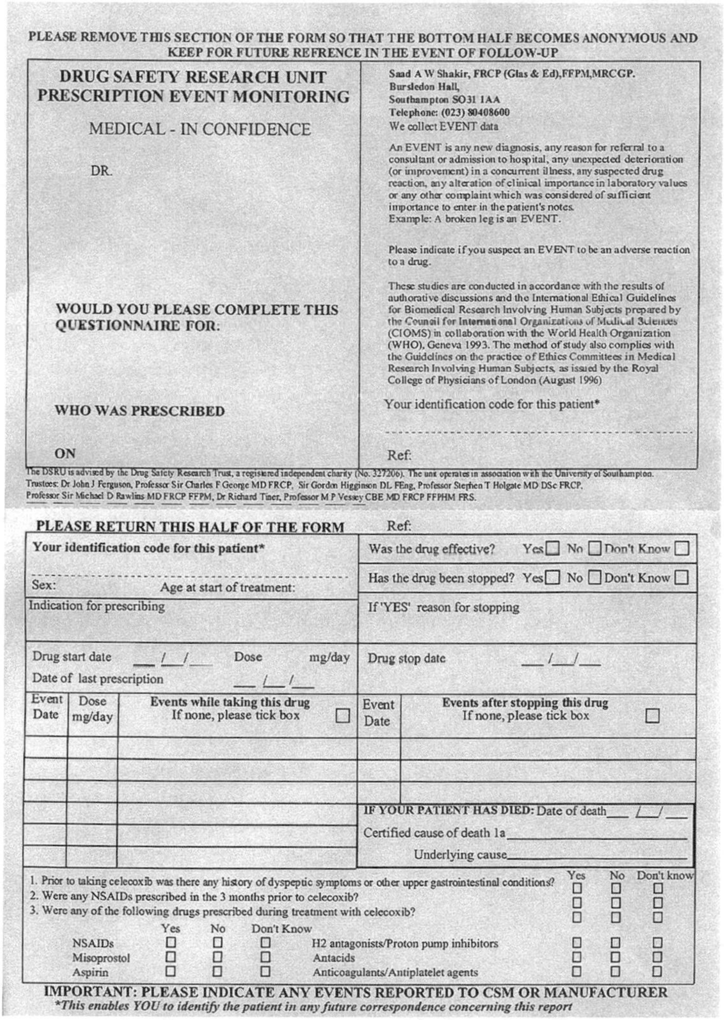

PLEASE REMOVE THIS SECTION OF THE FORM SO THAT THE BOTTOM HALF BECOMES ANONYMOUS AND KEEP FOR FUTURE REFRENCE IN THE EVENT OF FOLLOW-UP

DRUG SAFETY RESEARCH UNIT
PRESCRIPTION EVENT MONITORING

MEDICAL - IN CONFIDENCE

DR.

WOULD YOU PLEASE COMPLETE THIS QUESTIONNAIRE FOR:

WHO WAS PRESCRIBED

ON

Saad A W Shakir, FRCP (Glas & Ed),FFPM,MRCGP.
Bursledon Hall,
Southampton SO31 1AA
Telephone: (023) 80408600
We collect EVENT data

An EVENT is any new diagnosis, any reason for referral to a consultant or admission to hospital, any unexpected deterioration (or improvement) in a concurrent illness, any suspected drug reaction, any alteration of clinical importance in laboratory values or any other complaint which was considered of sufficient importance to enter in the patient's notes.
Example: A broken leg is an EVENT.

Please indicate if you suspect an EVENT to be an adverse reaction to a drug.

These studies are conducted in accordance with the results of authorative discussions and the International Ethical Guidelines for Biomedical Research Involving Human Subjects prepared by the Council for International Organizations of Medical Sciences (CIOMS) in collaboration with the World Health Organization (WHO), Geneva 1993. The method of study also complies with the Guidelines on the practice of Ethics Committees in Medical Research Involving Human Subjects, as issued by the Royal College of Physicians of London (August 1996)

Your identification code for this patient*

Ref:

The DSRU is advised by the Drug Safety Research Trust, a registered independent charity (No. 327206). The unit operates in association with the University of Southampton.
Trustees: Dr John J Ferguson, Professor Sir Charles F George MD FRCP, Sir Gordon Higginson DL FEng, Professor Stephen T Holgate MD DSc FRCP, Professor Sir Michael D Rawlins MD FRCP FFPM, Dr Richard Tiner, Professor M P Vessey CBE MD FRCP FFPHM FRS.

PLEASE RETURN THIS HALF OF THE FORM Ref:

Your identification code for this patient*

Sex: Age at start of treatment:

Indication for prescribing

Was the drug effective? Yes ☐ No ☐ Don't Know ☐

Has the drug been stopped? Yes ☐ No ☐ Don't Know ☐

If 'YES' reason for stopping

Drug start date __/__/__ Dose mg/day

Date of last prescription __/__/__

Drug stop date __/__/__

Event Date	Dose mg/day	**Events while taking this drug** If none, please tick box ☐	Event Date	**Events after stopping this drug** If none, please tick box ☐

IF YOUR PATIENT HAS DIED: Date of death __/__/__
Certified cause of death 1a ______
Underlying cause ______

	Yes	No	Don't know
1. Prior to taking celecoxib was there any history of dyspeptic symptoms or other upper gastrointestinal conditions?	☐	☐	☐
2. Were any NSAIDs prescribed in the 3 months prior to celecoxib?	☐	☐	☐
3. Were any of the following drugs prescribed during treatment with celecoxib?	☐	☐	☐

	Yes	No	Don't Know		Yes	No	Don't know
NSAIDs	☐	☐	☐	H2 antagonists/Proton pump inhibitors	☐	☐	☐
Misoprostol	☐	☐	☐	Antacids	☐	☐	☐
Aspirin	☐	☐	☐	Anticoagulants/Antiplatelet agents	☐	☐	☐

IMPORTANT: PLEASE INDICATE ANY EVENTS REPORTED TO CSM OR MANUFACTURER
This enables YOU to identify the patient in any future correspondence concerning this report

Figure 12.2. Green form for the PEM study on Celebrex (celecoxib).

on age, indication for treatment, dose, starting date and stopping date (duration of treatment), reasons for stopping therapy, all events which have occurred since the start of treatment, and the cause(s) of death if applicable. The green form includes the definition of an "event," which is: "any new diagnosis, any reason for referral to a consultant or admission to hospital, any unexpected deterioration (or improvement) in a concurrent illness, any suspected drug reaction, any alteration of clinical importance in laboratory values or any other complaint which was considered of sufficient importance to enter in the patient's notes."

A recent development in the PEM process is the inclusion of a small number of "additional" questions in the green forms. Such questions aim to examine aspects such as confounding by indication, concurrent illnesses, and concomitant medications. For example, the green forms in the PEM studies of the COX-2 inhibitors, e.g., celecoxib, included questions regarding previous history of dyspeptic conditions, and the green forms for the PEM studies of PDE5 inhibitors for erectile dysfunction, such as sildenafil, included questions about history of cardiovascular disease.

The GP is not paid to provide information to the DSRU, which is provided, under conditions of medical confidence, in the interest of drug safety. The system provides good contact with the GPs and facilitates the collection of any follow-up or additional data considered necessary by the research scientists/ physicians monitoring each study and working within the DSRU. Table 12.1 includes a list of the categories of medical events for which follow-up is sought by research fellows. Table 12.2 lists the medically serious events that have been associated with the use of medicines; follow-up information is sought for these too. All pregnancies reported during treatment or within three months of stopping the drug are followed up to determine the outcome.

PEM collects event data and does not ask the doctor to determine whether any particular event represents an ADR.

Table 12.1. Events for which follow-up information is sought from GPs

- Medically important adverse events reported during premarketing development
- Medically important events reported during postmarketing in other countries (for products launched elsewhere before the UK)
- Medically important events considered to be possibly associated with the product during the PEM
- All pregnancies
- Any deaths for which the cause is not known or which may be related to the medication
- Reports of overdose and suicide

Table 12.2. Rare serious adverse events that have been associated with the use of medicines

Agranulocytosis
Alveolitis
Anemia aplastic
Anaphylaxis
Angioneurotic edema
Arrhythmia
Bone marrow abnormal
Congenital abnormality
Dermatitis exfoliative
Disseminated intravascular coagulation
Erythema multiforme
Erythroderma
Guillain–Barré syndrome
Hepatic failure
Hepatitis
Jaundice
Leukopenia
Multiorgan failure
Nephritis
Nephrotic syndrome
Neuroleptic malignant syndrome
Neutropenia
Pancreatitis
Pancytopenia
Pseudomembranous colitis
Renal failure acute
Retroperitoneal fibrosis
Stevens–Johnson syndrome
Sudden unexpected death
Thrombocytopenia
Torsade de pointes
Toxic epidermal necrolysis
Any event for which there is a positive re-challenge

This list is based on a similar list used by the Medicines Control Agency (MCA), UK.

If, however, an event is considered to be an ADR or has been reported by means of the "yellow card" scheme, then the doctor is asked to indicate this on the green form.

Each green form is seen by the medical or scientific officer monitoring the study in the DSRU. This initial review aims to identify possible serious ADRs or events requiring action, e.g., external communications or expedited follow-up.

Events are coded and entered into a database using a hierarchical dictionary, arranged by system–organ class with specific "lower" terms grouped together under broader "higher" terms. The DSRU dictionary has been developed over the past 20 years and contains 11 640 doctor summary terms (as near as possible to the term used by the reporting doctor, e.g., crescendo angina) and 1720 lower-level terms mapped to 1185 higher-level terms, within 27 system–organ classes.

Interim analyses of the computerized data are usually undertaken every 2500 patients in each study and contacts are, whenever possible, maintained with the company holding the product license, so that the pharmaceutical companies (although the study is independent of them) can comply with the drug safety reporting procedures of the regulatory authorities.

Based on data from 88 PEM studies conducted to date, the GP response rate (percentage of green forms returned) has been 56.0% ± SD 8.3%. The mean cohort size has been 10 942 patients. The collection periods (the time for which it has been necessary to collect prescriptions yielding a finished cohort size averaging over 10 000 patients) vary markedly depending on the usage of the drug.

The DSRU is an independent registered medical nonprofit organization associated with the University of Portsmouth. The Unit is extensively supported by donations and grants from the pharmaceutical industry. The drugs to be monitored are chosen by the DSRU, preference being given to innovative medicines intended for widespread use. A list of all completed PEM studies is available on the DSRU's website (www.dsru.org).

STRENGTHS

PEM has a number of important strengths. First, as indicated above, the method is non-interventional in nature and does not interfere with the treatment the doctor considers as most appropriate for the individual patient. Information is collected after the prescribing decision has been made and implemented. This means that in PEM, data are collected on patients who would receive the drug in question in everyday clinical practice and not upon some highly selected group of patients who may be nonrepresentative of the "real-world" population. In this way, the system avoids the problem of generalizability inherent in randomized clinical trials, including many postmarketing safety clinical trials.

Second, the method is national in scale and provides "real-world" data showing what actually happens in everyday clinical practice. It largely overcomes the problem of making clinical trial data truly representative of the whole population that will receive the drug. For example, PEM studies include unlicensed and unlabelled prescribing, e.g., unlicensed prescribing for children.

Third, as indicated above, PEM exposure data are derived from dispensed prescriptions. Considering the large number of patients who do not get a prescription dispensed,[8] this is an advantage compared to pharmacoepidemiologic databases that rely on prescription data.

Fourth, because the data are concerned with events, the method could detect adverse reactions or syndromes that none of the reporting doctors suspect to be due to the drug.[5] The database allows the study of diseases as well as drugs.[5,10] Both of these advantages are in line with the early proposals of Finney on event reporting.[5]

Fifth, the method allows close contact between the research staff in the DSRU and the reporting doctors. This facilitates follow-up of important events, pregnancies, deaths, etc. (Tables 12.1 and 12.2), and allows for the maximum clinical understanding of confounders and biases, and the natural history of ADRs.

Sixth, the method prompts the doctor to fill in the green form and does not rely on the clinician taking the initiative to report. This "prompting" effect of PEM is most important; two studies have demonstrated that ADR reporting is more complete in PEM than in spontaneous ADR reporting systems, such as the yellow card system in the UK.[12,13]

Seventh, the method has been shown to be successful in regularly producing data on 10 000 or more patients given newly marketed drugs which, by virtue of their success in the marketplace, involve substantial patient exposure. It fulfills, therefore, the original objective of providing a prescription-based method of postmarketing surveillance of new drugs intended for widespread, long-term use.

Eighth, the method identifies patients with adverse drug reactions who can be studied further, for example, in nested case–control studies to examine risk factors for ADRs including pharmacogenetic risk factors (see Chapter 37). Relatedly, while information on some co-prescribed drugs can be obtained in the initial green form, more detailed information about concomitant medications can be obtained for selected cases, e.g., important medical events, during follow-up.

Ninth, the large number of completed PEM studies allows comparisons of the safety profiles of drugs in the same therapeutic groups.[14–17] It is also possible to conduct comparisons with external data.[18,19]

Finally, pharmacoepidemiologic methods are complementary. PEM can evaluate signals generated in other systems or databases. Similarly, it provides a technique that can generate signals or hypotheses which can themselves be refuted or confirmed by other pharmacoepidemiologic methods.

WEAKNESSES

Like all pharmacoepidemiologic methods, of course PEM has weaknesses. First, not all of the green forms are returned and this could induce a selection bias.

Second, PEM depends on reporting by doctors. As such, it can be as good as but no better than the clinical notes of the GPs and depends on the accuracy and thoroughness of the doctors in completing the green forms. Underreporting, including underreporting of serious and fatal adverse events, is possible in PEM.

Third, PEM is currently restricted to general practice. Drugs which are mainly used in hospitals cannot be studied with the current method of PEM.

Fourth, while studying exposure by dispensing rather than prescribing is an advantage, there is no measure of compliance using dispensed prescriptions, i.e., it is not known whether the patient actually took the dispensed medication.

Finally, detection of rare ADRs is not always possible even with cohorts of 10 000–15 000 patients.[20]

PARTICULAR APPLICATIONS

SEARCHING FOR SIGNALS

Signal detection and evaluation is the primary concern of pharmacovigilance. Several methods are applied for signal detection in PEM.

Assessment of Important Adverse Events

The initial evaluation is conducted by manual examination by research fellows of newly received green forms for adverse events that may possibly be related to drug exposure. The assessments of individual reports or clusters of reports take into consideration a number of points, including:

- the temporal relationship (time to onset);
- the clinical and pathological characteristics of the event;
- the pharmacological plausibility based on previous knowledge of the drug and the therapeutic class if appropriate;
- whether the event was previously reported as an adverse reaction in clinical trials or postmarketing in the UK or in other countries;
- any possible role of concomitant medications or medications taken prior to the event;
- the role of the underlying or concurrent illnesses;
- the effect of de-challenge or dose reduction;
- the effect of re-challenge or dose increase;
- patient's characteristics, including previous medical history, such as history of drug allergies, presence of renal or hepatic impairment, etc.;
- the possibility of drug interactions.

In this activity, PEM is functioning in a manner very similar to spontaneous reporting systems (see Chapters 9, 10, and 36), although with much higher rates of reporting. An example

of a safety signal generated in PEM as a result of careful clinical evaluation is the visual field defects with the anti-epileptic drug vigabatrin.[21]

Medically Important Events

As mentioned above, special consideration is given to the categories and events listed in Tables 12.1 and 12.2.

Reasons for Stopping the Drug

The green form questionnaire asks the doctor to record the reason why the drug was withdrawn if, in fact, it was withdrawn. Clinical reasons for stopping a drug are ranked according to numbers received in a list, which is very informative because it includes possible adverse reactions which the doctor and/or the patient considered serious or sufficiently troublesome to stop the medication. The clinical reasons for withdrawal are ranked according to the number of reports of each event and are used to generate signals. For example, PEM has identified drowsiness/sedation, and weight gain with the antidepressant mirtazapine and assessed the strengths of signals generated by other methods in PEM.[22]

Analysis of Events During the Study/Events While on Drug

Table 12.3 shows the first page of a table that summarizes all reports received throughout a typical PEM study, whether or not the patient was still on the drug. Denominators are given (in terms of patient-months of observation) for each month of the study, and for each of the 1700 or so events in the DSRU dictionary. The number of events reported is shown for each month of the study. Table 12.4 provides similar data but is restricted to events reported between the date of starting and stopping the drug being monitored. Each of these tables shows events grouped into organ–system class and displayed as higher and lower terms where the dictionary has been divided in this way. Each table also shows the total number of reports for each event, the total over the first six months of observation, and the number of events where the date of event was unknown. Comparison of these two tables (and a third table listing off-drug events of unknown date) indicates the number of reports for each event when the patients were not receiving the drug being monitored. This allows on-drug/off-drug comparisons (although the period after the drug being monitored has been withdrawn may be a period in which some other (and unknown) drug was being given in individual patients).

These tables can generate signals: the total for an event may be unusually high and this can be confirmed or refuted

Table 12.3. All events reported on green forms for meloxicam (summarizing all reports received throughout a typical PEM study, whether or not the patient was still on the drug)

Event	Total	Mth 1	Mth 2	Mth 3	Mth 4	Mth 5	Mth 6	Mths 1–6	Not known
Denominator total*	130 615	19 083	19 075	19 068	19 063	19 054	19 046		
Denominator male	41 711	6 172	6 167	6 166	6 164	6 160	6 158		
Denominator female	86 690	12 586	12 583	12 577	12 574	12 568	12 562		
Skin									
Acne	13	1	1	1	3	1	3	10	—
Acne	8	1	—	1	1	—	3	6	—
Acne rosacea	5	—	1	—	2	1	—	4	—
Alopecia	1	—	—	—	1	—	—	1	—
Cyst sebaceous	14	4	3	2	1	1	1	12	—
Dermatitis	43	8	6	2	3	5	4	28	—
Dermatitis contact	4	2	—	—	1	1	—	4	—
Dry skin	21	5	3	2	3	2	1	16	—
Eczema	91	14	12	10	13	7	9	66	—
Eczema	71	10	9	8	9	5	7	48	—
Eczema atopic	1	1	—	—	—	—	—	1	—
Intertrigo	16	2	3	1	4	2	2	14	—
Pompholyx	3	1	—	1	—	—	—	2	—
Eczema varicose	11	2	2	1	1	1	2	9	—
Eruption bullous	8	—	2	1	1	1	1	6	—
Blister	7	—	2	1	1	—	1	5	—
Pemphigoid	1	—	—	—	—	1	—	1	—
Erythema	3	1	1	—	—	—	—	2	—
Erythema multiforme	1	—	1	—	—	—	—	1	—
Folliculitis	6	—	1	1	2	—	2	6	—
Granuloma	1	1	—	—	—	—	—	1	—
Granulomatosis	1	—	—	—	—	1	—	1	—
Haematoma nail	1	—	—	—	—	—	1	1	—
Hair loss	8	1	1	2	—	—	1	5	—
Herpes simplex, skin	4	—	1	—	1	1	—	3	—
Herpes zoster	42	7	4	7	6	8	6	38	—
Hyperkeratosis	6	—	3	1	—	1	—	5	—
Hyperkeratosis	2	—	1	—	—	1	—	2	—
Pityriasis	4	—	2	1	—	—	—	3	—
Infection skin, unspecified/local baterial	188	29	21	27	30	25	22	154	—
Abscess skin	31	3	—	4	12	6	3	28	—
Cellulitis	73	17	9	11	9	8	6	60	—
Erysipelas	2	—	1	—	—	1	—	2	—
Impetigo	6	—	—	1	—	1	1	3	—
Infection skin	59	7	8	10	8	6	7	46	—
Paronychia	17	2	3	1	1	3	5	15	—
Lice	1	—	—	—	—	—	—	—	—
Lichen planus	1	—	1	—	—	—	—	1	—
Lupus discoid	1	—	—	—	1	—	—	1	—

* Patient-months of observation.

by comparisons across the database of all 88 drugs that have been studied to date, or by comparison with drugs of the same therapeutic group on with the same indication for use. The trend of reports over the months of observation may be informative: Type A side effects (pharmacologically related) tend to occur early in the study (although this period may also be affected by carryover effects from previous medication), or the number of reports may rise as time passes (as with long latency adverse reactions). Again, formal trend analysis can be used to explore, on a comparative basis, such apparent signals. An example is weight gain with the atypical antipsychotic olanzapine.[23]

Table 12.4. Events reported on green forms during treatment with meloxicam (summarizing all reports received throughout a typical PEM study, restricted to events reported between the date of starting and stopping the drug being monitored)

Event	Total	Mth 1	Mth 2	Mth 3	Mth 4	Mth 5	Mth 6	Mths 1–6	Not known
Denominator total*	74 948	15 382	10 812	9 497	8 676	8 036	7 560		
Denominator male	23 711	4 895	3 384	2 979	2 723	2 528	2 377		
Denominator female	50 185	10 245	7 282	6 392	5 840	5 403	5 084		
Skin									
Acne	10	1	1	—	3	1	1	7	—
Acne	5	1	—	—	1	—	1	3	—
Acne rosacea	5	—	1	—	2	1	—	4	—
Alopecia	1	—	—	—	1	—	—	1	—
Cyst sebaceous	9	3	3	1	1	—	1	9	—
Dermatitis	27	8	3	2	2	2	1	18	—
Dermatitis contact	3	2	—	—	—	1	—	3	—
Dry skin	17	5	3	—	3	1	1	13	—
Eczema	59	11	11	8	8	3	2	43	1
Eczema	44	7	8	6	5	3	2	31	1
Eczema atopic	1	1	—	—	—	—	—	1	—
Intertrigo	11	2	3	1	3	—	—	9	—
Pompholyx	3	1	—	1	—	—	—	2	—
Eczema varicose	6	2	—	1	1	—	1	5	—
Eruption bullous	4	—	1	1	1	—	—	3	—
Blister	4	—	1	1	1	—	—	3	—
Pemphigoid	—	—	—	—	—	—	—	—	—
Erythema	2	1	1	—	—	—	—	2	—
Erythema multiforme	1	—	1	—	—	—	—	1	—
Folliculitis	4	—	—	1	2	—	1	4	—
Granuloma	1	1	—	—	—	—	—	1	—
Granulomatosis	—	—	—	—	—	—	—	—	—
Haematoma nail	1	—	—	—	—	—	1	1	—
Hair loss	5	1	1	1	—	—	—	3	—
Herpes simplex, skin	1	—	1	—	—	—	—	1	—
Herpes zoster	28	7	3	4	5	6	1	26	—
Hyperkeratosis	3	—	1	1	—	1	—	3	—
Hyperkeratosis	2	—	1	—	—	1	—	2	—
Pityriasis	1	—	—	1	—	—	—	1	—
Infection skin, unspecified/local baterial	124	25	13	16	16	19	13	102	—
Abscess skin	17	2	—	1	5	6	2	16	—
Cellulitis	52	16	5	9	5	6	4	45	—
Erysipelas	2	—	1	—	—	1	—	2	—
Impetigo	3	—	—	1	—	1	—	2	—
Infection skin	38	5	5	5	5	3	4	27	—
Paronychia	12	2	2	—	1	2	3	10	—
Lice	—	—	—	—	—	—	—	—	—
Lichen planus	1	—	1	—	—	—	—	1	—
Lupus discoid	—	—	—	—	—	—	—	—	—

* Patient-months of observation.

Ranking of Incidence Density and Reasons for Withdrawal

The incidence density (ID) for a given time period t is calculated, for each event in the dictionary, in the usual way:

$$ID_t = \frac{N_t}{D_t} \times 1000$$

where N_t is the number of reports of the event during treatment for period t, D_t is the number of patient-months of treatment for period t, and the results are given in terms of 1000 patient-months of exposure. These results are then ranked in order of the estimate of ID_1 (the incidence density for the event in question in the first month of exposure). The incidence densities in the second to sixth months of treatment are also routinely calculated (ID_2).

Table 12.5 shows the first page of such a report of ranked incidence densities from a typical PEM study. For each event, the table presents the value of ID_1 minus ID_2 and the 99% confidence intervals around this difference. This difference can itself generate signals, which require confirmation or refutation by further evaluation or another study. The

basis for this is that most pharmacologically-related ADRs occur soon after initial exposure. However, for ADRs with long latency the comparison can be reversed, e.g., comparing the ID in month 6 with the ID in months 1–5.

The ranked reasons for withdrawals can be compared with the ranked incidence density estimates, and this comparison

Table 12.5. Incidence densities (IDs) ranked for meloxicam in order of ID_1 per 1000 patient months

	Event	N_1	N_2	ID_1	ID_2	$ID_1 - ID_2$	99% CI min.	99% CI max.	N_A	ID_A
1	Condition improved	903	1015	58.7	22.8	35.9	30.6	41.3	2067	27.6
2	Dyspepsia	435	379	28.3	8.5	19.8	16.1	23.5	903	12.0
3	Respiratory tract infection	214	387	13.9	8.7	5.2	2.5	7.9	675	9.0
4	Nausea, vomiting	189	136	12.3	3.1	9.2	6.8	11.6	351	4.7
5	Pain abdomen	146	163	9.5	3.7	5.8	3.7	8.0	357	4.8
6	Diarrhea	118	110	7.7	2.5	5.2	3.3	7.1	251	3.3
7	Dose increased	106	206	6.9	4.6	2.3	0.4	4.2	353	4.7
8	Headache, migraine	81	82	5.3	1.8	3.4	1.8	5.0	192	2.6
9	Minor surgery	75	100	4.9	2.2	2.6	1.1	4.2	198	2.6
10	Hospital referrals no admission	74	144	4.8	3.2	1.6	0.0	3.2	270	3.6
11	Edema	74	96	4.8	2.2	2.7	1.1	4.2	195	2.6
12	Dizziness	68	70	4.4	1.6	2.9	1.4	4.3	152	2.0
13	Gastrointestinal unspecified	66	64	4.3	1.4	2.9	1.4	4.3	144	1.9
14	Pain joint	57	143	3.7	3.2	0.5	−0.9	1.9	236	3.1
15	Malaise, lassitude	56	81	3.6	1.8	1.8	0.5	3.2	153	2
16	Constipation	56	57	3.6	1.3	2.4	1	3.7	119	1.6
17	Hospital referral paramedical	51	55	3.3	1.2	2.1	0.8	3.4	111	1.5
18	Cough	48	73	3.1	1.6	1.5	0.2	2.7	140	1.9
19	Asthma, wheezing	48	46	3.1	1	2.1	0.9	3.3	107	1.4
20	Rash	46	90	3	2	1	−0.03	2.2	151	2
21	Nonsurgical admissions	45	59	2.9	1.3	1.6	0.4	2.8	127	1.7
22	Noncompliance	42	61	2.7	1.4	1.4	0.2	2.5	113	1.5
23	Hypertension	42	57	2.7	1.3	1.5	0.3	2.6	119	1.6
24	Intolerance	42	21	2.7	0.5	2.3	1.1	3.4	71	0.9
25	Urinary tract infection	39	99	2.5	2.2	0.3	−0.9	1.5	163	2.2
26	Depression	38	76	2.5	1.7	0.8	−0.4	1.9	139	1.9
27	Pain back	29	87	1.9	2	−0.1	−1.1	1	142	1.9
28	Dyspnoea	29	38	1.9	0.9	1	0.1	2	73	1
29	Fall	26	77	1.7	1.7	0	−1	1	115	1.5
30	Infection skin, unspecified	25	77	1.6	1.7	−0.1	−1.1	0.9	124	1.7
31	Malignancies	25	33	1.6	0.7	0.9	0	1.8	68	0.9
32	Unspecified side effects	25	13	1.6	0.3	1.3	0.5	2.2	42	0.6
33	Pain in chest, tight chest	24	60	1.6	1.3	0.2	−0.7	1.2	94	1.3
34	Pain	24	48	1.6	1.1	0.5	−0.4	1.4	84	1.1
35	Ischemic heart disease	24	43	1.6	1	0.6	−0.3	1.5	78	1
36	Cardiac failure	24	29	1.6	0.7	0.9	0	1.8	58	0.8
37	Pruritus	22	50	1.4	1.1	0.3	−0.6	1.2	84	1.1
38	Ulcer, mouth	21	43	1.4	1	0.4	−0.5	1.3	71	0.9
39	Hematological tests	20	39	1.3	0.9	0.4	−0.4	1.3	65	0.9
40	Palpitation	20	22	1.3	0.5	0.8	0	1.6	46	0.6
41	Orthopaedic surgery	19	95	1.2	2.1	−0.9	−1.8	0	139	1.9
42	Osteoarthritis	17	53	1.1	1.2	−0.1	−0.9	0.7	83	1.1
43	Micturition disorder	16	39	1	0.9	0.2	−0.6	0.9	61	0.8
44	Anxiety	16	34	1	0.8	0.3	−0.5	1	58	0.8

Table 12.6. Most frequently reported events

Reason	Number
Not effective	2989
Condition improved	1834
Dyspepsia	539
Nausea, vomiting	209
Pain abdomen	171
Noncompliance	117
Gastrointestinal unspecified	104
Diarrhea	103
Orthopedic surgery	87
Effective	81
Headache, migraine	72
Hospital referrals no admission	69
Rash	64
Dizziness	60
Intolerance	59
Malaise, lassitude	58
Patient request	50
Edema	49
Minor surgery	45
Hospital referral paramedical	38
Nonsurgical admissions	36
Pain	33
Unspecified side effects	33
Constipation	31
Asthma, wheezing	30
Ulcer, mouth	23
Indication for meloxicam changed	21
Pruritus	20
Nonformulary	18
Dyspnea	16
Hemorrhage gastrointestinal, unspecified	16
Surgery, unspecified	16
Tinnitus	16
Distension, abdominal	12
Drowsiness, sedation	12
Hemorrhage gastrointestinal upper	12
Pain in chest, tight chest	12
Anemia	11
Pain, joint	11
Hemorrhage rectal	10

can also generate signals. There is usually a good correlation, in terms of the most frequently reported events, and an example of this is given in Table 12.6; other examples have been published elsewhere.[24,25]

Comparison of Event Rates and Adjusted Rates

Rate comparisons can be helpful in exploring apparent associations. An example occurred when looking at the

gastrointestinal events of celecoxib (a COX-2 inhibitor) compared with the NSAID meloxicam.[14]

Analysis showed that the adjusted rate ratio of symptomatic upper gastrointestinal events or complicated upper gastrointestinal conditions (perforations/bleeding) for rofecoxib compared with meloxicam were 0.77 (95% CI 0.69, 0.85) and 0.56 (95% CI 0.32, 0.96), respectively.

Examples of other signals and comparisons that have been explored include deaths from cardiac arrhythmias and suicide with atypical antipsychotics,[15] sedation with non-sedating antihistamines,[16] and bleeding with SSRIs.[17]

Automated Signal Generation

The DSRU is exploring the application of automated signal generation as a possible additional tool in PEM. Feasibility studies apply comparisons of incidence rate ratios (IRRs). The exploratory work included confirming historical signals, e.g., Stevens–Johnson syndrome with the anti-epileptic product lamotrigine,[26] and new signals such as exacerbation of colitis with rofecoxib.[27] There are a number of methodological issues which need to be further examined with automated signal generation such as the selection of comparator(s) and the level of dictionary terms used, i.e., higher- or lower-level terms, because both factors may influence whether a signal is generated or its strength.[26] However, with refinement, automated signal generation is likely to prove useful in spontaneous reporting, clinical trials, and pharmacoepidemiologic studies.

Long Latency Adverse Reactions

Special interest attaches to reactions that emerge only on prolonged treatment and may be missed in the premarketing trials, many of which are frequently of short duration. An example occurred in the PEM study of finasteride,[20] a product used for the treatment of benign prostatic hypertrophy, when it was shown that reports of impotence/ejaculatory failure and decreased libido were received in relation to the first and all subsequent months of treatment, but reports of gynecomastia were only rarely received before the fifth month of therapy. A further important example has occurred in relation to visual field defects in patients receiving long-term treatment with vigabatrin.[21,28,29] The initial PEM study showed three cases of bilateral, irreversible peripheral field defects, whereas no similar reports occurred with other anti-epileptic drugs or in any of the other drugs already monitored by PEM. A follow-up exploration with a repeat questionnaire, sent to the doctors whose patients had received vigabatrin for over six months, has shown that the incidence of this serious event is much higher and that many of the relevant patients have objective evidence of visual field defects.

Comparison with External Data

With 88 completed PEM studies to date, there are increasing opportunities to conduct comparisons among PEM studies.[14–17] However, it is not always possible to identify suitable comparators. Therefore, external comparators are sought where necessary and appropriate. For example, there were concerns about cardiovascular safety when sildenafil (the first PDE5 inhibitor marketed for erectile dysfunction) was launched in the UK in 1998. Mortality from ischemic heart disease in users of sildenafil in the PEM study was compared with external epidemiologic data for men in England. The standardized mortality ratio (SMR) for deaths reported to have been caused by ischemic heart disease was not higher for sildenafil users, SMR 69.9 (95% CI, 42.7–108.0).[18] Similarly, death from ischemic heart disease in the bupropion PEM (when used for smoking cessation) was compared with external data and showed no difference in the SMR.[19] Obviously there is higher potential for bias when using external comparators than comparisons undertaken between PEM studies; results of external comparisons must be considered very carefully.

Outcomes of Pregnancy

Special interest attaches to determining the proportion and nature of congenital anomalies in babies born to women exposed to newly marketed drugs during the first trimester. PEM studies have shown that from 831 such pregnancies, 557 infants were born, of whom 14 (2.5%) had congenital anomalies.[30] Projects are underway to compare pregnancy outcomes following drug exposure between PEM studies or between PEM studies and external comparators. The comparisons within the PEM database include comparing pregnancy outcomes for women who continue to take a particular drug with women who stop taking the drug. It is important that studying pregnancy outcomes continues in order to exclude, to the greatest extent possible, teratogenic effects of medicines.

Studies to Examine Hypotheses Generated by Other Methods

In addition to examining signals generated in PEM, the database provides a resource that is being used increasingly to evaluate signals and hypotheses generated by other methods. An example of such studies is the comparison of mortality and rates of cardiac arrhythmias with atypical antipsychotic drugs.[31]

STUDIES OF BACKGROUND EFFECTS AND DISEASES

Background Effects

The PEM database allows the study of diseases as well as drugs. An example includes a study of the prevalence of Churg–Strauss syndrome and related conditions in patients with asthma. The study defined the period prevalence rate for this condition, 6.8 (95% CI, 1.8–17.3) per million patient-year of observation, and demonstrated a much higher period prevalence rate in patients receiving asthma medications compared to other PEM cohorts.[10] In another study, the PEM database was used to define age- and gender-specific asthma deaths in patients using long-acting beta-2 agonists.[32]

Study of the database also shows some of the characteristics of ADR reporting. Doctors are asked to note on the green form if they have previously reported an event spontaneously as an ADR (in a patient being monitored by PEM). Two studies compared events that were considered as ADRs by doctors reported in PEM, with spontaneous reports sent by the same doctors to the regulatory authority. The studies[12,13] showed that reporting of suspected spontaneous ADRs to the UK regulatory authority was 9% (95% CI, 8.00–10.00) and 9% (95% CI, 8–9.8), respectively. In the more recent study, published in 2001,[13] it was shown that, of 4211 ADRs reported on the PEM green form questionnaires, only 376 (9.0%) had also been reported on yellow cards to the CSM. It is of interest that a higher proportion of serious reactions were reported to the CSM by doctors, which suggests that doctors use the spontaneous adverse reaction reporting scheme more energetically when reporting those serious reactions that worry them most.

It is possible to study in PEM general patterns of ADRs. Our studies in this area have also shown that, in general practice in England, suspected ADRs to newly marketed drugs are recorded more often in adults aged between 30 and 59 years and are 60% more common in women than in men.[33]

THE FUTURE

In the future, PEM aims to utilize improvements in information technology, application of additional study designs such as nested case–control studies, and the application of new biological developments such as pharmacogenetics to enhance the PEM process. Modification of the PEM method is sometimes necessary to examine specific drug safety questions. In addition, it is possible to modify the PEM process to examine questions related to risk management of marketed medicinal products.

NESTED CASE–CONTROL STUDIES

PEM cohorts provide opportunities to conduct nested case–control studies, for example, for patients who develop selected ADRs and matched patients who receive the same drug without developing ADRs. A nested case–control study is planned to study patients who were reported to have had ischemic cardiac events in the cohort of users of the PDE5 inhibitor tadalafil and matched controls, to examine the risk factors for events such as hypertension, smoking, etc. There are plans to broaden the scope for the application of nested case–control studies to PEM.

PHARMACOGENETICS

There is increasing interest in understanding the role of pharmacogenetics in the efficacy and safety of medicines (see Chapter 37). Given the interest in understanding the roles of polymorphic genotypes of receptors, protein carriers, and metabolizing enzymes of drugs, there are many opportunities in PEM to study the genotypes of patients who develop selected ADRs compared to patients who do not develop such ADRs. Moreover, there are opportunities to study the genotypes of patients who do not respond to some drugs. Nested case–control pharmacogenetic studies of both types are under way in PEM.

MODIFIED PEM STUDIES

In some cases, it is considered necessary to modify PEM methodology to answer specific safety question(s) regarding the safety of a particular product. A study is underway to examine specific eye events (discoloration of the iris and lengthening of eye lashes) that have been reported following the use of an ophthalmic product used for the treatment of glaucoma. The length of the PEM follow-up and details of the outcome questionnaires were modified in order to answer the specific research questions.

RISK MANAGEMENT

Risk management is attracting immense interest in pharmacovigilance (see Chapter 33). The management of risk of medicines requires identification, measurement, and assessment of risk, followed by risk/benefit evaluation, then taking actions to eliminate or reduce the risk, followed by methods to monitor that the actions taken achieve their objectives. PEM does not only contribute to the identification and measurement of risks of medicines but, with some additions, can examine how the risks of medicines are being managed

in real-world clinical settings. Two studies are underway on two new antidiabetic agents, rosiglitazone and pioglitazone, where detailed questionnaires are sent to doctors who reported selected adverse events such as liver function abnormalities or fluid retention to study how these events were detected and managed, as well as their outcomes. Another study is to monitor the introduction of carvedilol for the treatment of cardiac failure. The product (combined alpha- and beta-adrenergic blocker) has been used for the treatment of angina and hypertension for some time, but there was concern about its appropriate use for cardiac failure in the community. The aim of the modified PEM study is to monitor how the product is being managed in the community, for example what investigations were undertaken prior to starting the drug, who supervised the dose titration, etc. The design includes sending an eligibility questionnaire followed by up to three detailed questionnaires for a period of up to two years.

CONCLUSION

PEM contributes to the better understanding of the safety of medicines. Both signals generated by PEM and those generated in other systems and studied further by PEM have been useful to inform the debates on the safety of medicines, including supporting public health and regulatory decisions. In addition, the breadth of the PEM database provides opportunities for research on disease epidemiology and risk management of adverse drug reactions. Like all scientific methods, PEM is evolving, aiming to reduce its weaknesses and enhance its strengths. New methodological modifications and additions include more effective utilization of information technology and statistics, as well as the application of new study designs such as nested case–control and pharmacogenetic studies. Pharmacovigilance and pharmacoepidemiology are emerging and exciting disciplines with evolving study methods. PEM continues to contribute to the progress of these important scientific and public health disciplines.

ACKNOWLEDGMENTS

PEM is a team effort and I am only one member of a large team. The DSRU is most grateful to the thousands of doctors across England who provide the Unit, free of charge, with the safety information which makes its public health work possible. The Unit is equally grateful to the PPA; PEM would not be possible without their immense support.

I am most grateful to previous and current staff of the DSRU; this chapter is based on their work! Special gratitude goes to

Professor Ron Mann for allowing me to use material from the previous edition, which he wrote, and to Georgina Spragg and Lesley Flowers, who helped in locating research material and typing the manuscript.

REFERENCES

1. McBride WG. Thalidomide and congenital abnormalities. *Lancet* 1961; **2**: 1358.
2. Committee on Safety of Drugs. Cited in: Mann RD, ed., *Modern Drug Use—An Enquiry on Historical Principles*. Lancaster, PA: MTP Press–Kluwer, 1984; p. 619.
3. Rawlins MD, Jefferys DB. Study of United Kingdom product licence applications containing new active substances, 1987–9. *BMJ* 1991; **302**: 223–5.
4. Rawlins MD, Mann RD. Monitoring adverse events and reactions. In: Mann RD, Rawlins MD, RM Auty, eds, *A Textbook of Pharmaceutical Medicine, Current Practice*. Carnforth: Parthenon, 1993; p. 319.
5. Finney DJ. The design and logic of a monitor of drug use. *J Chron Dis* 1965; **18**: 77–98.
6. Inman WHW, Weber JCP. Post-marketing surveillance in the general population. In: Inman WHW, Gill EP, eds, *Monitoring for Drug Safety, 2nd edn*. Lancaster: MTP, 1985; p. 13.
7. Committee on Safety of Medicines. Cited in: Mann RD, ed., *Adverse Drug Reactions*. Carnforth: Parthenon, 1987; pp. 62–3.
8. Beardon PHG, Brown SV, McGilchrist MM, McKendick AD, McDevitt DG, MacDonald TM. Primary non-compliance with prescribed medication in primary care. *BMJ* 1993; **307**: 846–8.
9. Martin RM, Wilton LV, Mann RD. Prevalence of Churg–Strauss syndrome, vasculitis, eosinophilia and associated conditions: retrospective analysis of 58 prescription-event monitoring cohort studies. *Pharmacoepidemiol Drug Saf* 1999; **8**: 179–89.
10. Layton D, Key C, Shakir SA. Prolongation of the QT interval and cardiac arrhythmias associated with cisapride: limitations of the pharmacoepidemiological studies conducted and proposals for the future. *Pharmacoepidemiol Drug Saf* 2003; **12**: 31–40.
11. Martin RM, Kapoor KV, Wilton LV, Mann RD. Underreporting of suspected adverse drug reactions to newly marketed ("black triangle") drugs in general practice: observational study. *Br Med J* 1998; **317**: 119–20.
12. Heeley E, Riley J, Layton D, Wilton LV, Shakir S. Prescription-event monitoring and reporting of adverse drug reactions. *Lancet* 2001; **356**: 1872–3.
13. Layton D, Hughes K, Harris S, Shakir SAW. Comparison of the incidence rates of selected gastrointestinal events reported for patients prescribed celecoxib and meloxicam in general practice in England using prescription-event monitoring (PEM) data. *Rheumatology (Oxford)* 2003; **42**; 1332–41.
14. Wilton LV, Heeley EL, Pickering RM, Shakir SAW. Comparative study of mortality rates and cardiac dysrhythmias in post-marketing surveillance studies of sertindole and two other atypical antipsychotic drugs, risperidone and olanzapine. *J Psychpharmacol* 2001; **15**: 120–6.
15. Mann RD, Pearce GL, Dunn N, Shakir S. Sedation with "non-sedating" antihistamines: four prescription-event monitoring studies in general practice. *BMJ* 2000; **320**: 1184–6.
16. Layton D, Clark D, Pearce G, Shakir SAW. Is there an association between selective serotonin reuptake inhibitors and risk of abnormal bleeding? Results from a cohort study based on prescription event monitoring in England. *Eur J Clin Pharmacol* 2001; **57**: 167–76.
17. Shakir S, Wilton LV, Heeley E, Layton D. Cardiovascular events in users of sildenafil: results from first phase of prescription-event monitoring in England. *BMJ* 2001; **322**: 651–2.
18. Boshier A, Wilton LV, Shakir SA. Evaluation of the safety of bupropion (Zyban) for smoking cessation from experience gained in general practice use in England in 2000. *Eur J Clin Pharmacol* 2003; **59**: 767–73.
19. Wilton L, Pearce G, Edet E, Freemantle S, Stephens MDB, Mann RD. The safety of finasteride used in benign prostatic hypertrophy: a non-interventional observational cohort study in 14 772 patients. *Br J Urol* 1996; **78**: 379–84.
20. Wilton LV, Stephens MDB, Mann RD. Visual field defect associated with vigabatrin: observational cohort study. *BMJ* 1999; **319**: 1165–66.
21. Biswas PN, Wilton LV, Shakir SAW. The pharmacovigilance of mirtazapine: results of a prescription event monitoring study on 13,554 patients in England. *J Psychopharmacol* 2003; **17**; 121–6.
22. Biswas PN, Wilton LV, Pearce GL, Freemantle S, Shakir SA. The pharmacovigilance of olanzapine: results of a post-marketing surveillance study on 8858 patients in England. *J Psychopharmacol* 2001; **15**; 265–71.
23. Layton D, Shakir SAW. Safety profile of rofecoxib as used in general practice in England: results of a prescription-event monitoring study. *Br J Clin Pharmacol* 2003; **55**: 166–74.
24. Wilton LV, Key C, Shakir SAW. The pharmacovigilance of pantoprazole: the results of postmarketing surveillance on 11,541 patients in England. *Drug Saf*. 2003; **26**; 121 32.
25. Heeley E, Wilton LV, Shakir SA. Automated signal generation in prescription-event monitoring. *Drug Saf* 2002; **25**: 423–32.
26. Layton D, Heeley E, Shakir SAW. Identification and evaluation of a possible signal of exacerbation of colitis during rofecoxib treatment, using Prescription-Event Monitoring (PEM) data. *J Clin Pharm Ther* 2004; 29: 171–81.
27. Stephens MDB, Wilton LV, Pearce G, Mann RD. Visual field defects in patients taking vigabatrin. *Pharmacoepidemiol Drug Saf* 1997; **6** (suppl 2): S18.
28. Wilton LV, Stephens MDB, Mann RD. Visual field defects in patients on long term vigabatrin therapy. *Pharmacoepidemiol Drug Saf* 1999; **8** (suppl 2): 5108.
29. Wilton LV, Pearce GL, Martin RM, Mackay FJ, Mann RD. The outcomes of pregnancy in women exposed to newly marketed drugs in general practice in England. *Br J Obstet Gynaecol* 1998; **105**: 882–9.

30. Wilton LV, Heeley EL, Pickering RM, Shakir SA. Comparative study of mortality rates and cardiac dysrhythmias in post-marketing surveillance studies of sertindole and two other atypical antipsychotic drugs, risperidone and olanzapine. *J Psychopharmacol* 2001; **15**: 120–6.

31. Martin RM, Shakir S. Age- and gender-specific asthma death rates in patients taking long-acting beta2-agonists: prescription event monitoring pharmacosurveillance studies. *Drug Saf* 2001; **24**: 475–81.

32. Martin RM, Biswas PN, Freemantle SN, Pearce GL, Mann RD. Age and sex distribution of suspected adverse drug reactions to newly marketed drugs in general practice in England: analysis of 48 cohort studies. *Br J Clin Pharmacol* 1998; **46**: 505–30.

Part IIIb

Automated Data Systems Available for Pharmacoepidemiology Studies

13

Overview of Automated Databases in Pharmacoepidemiology

BRIAN L. STROM

University of Pennsylvania School of Medicine, Philadelphia, Pennsylvania, USA.

INTRODUCTION

Once hypotheses are generated, usually from spontaneous reporting systems (see Chapters 9 and 10), techniques are needed to test these hypotheses. Usually between 500 and 3000 patients are exposed to the drug during Phase III testing, even if drug efficacy can be demonstrated with much smaller numbers of patients. Studies of this size have the ability to detect drug effects with an incidence as low as 1 per 1000 to 6 per 1000 (see Chapter 3). Given this context, postmarketing studies of drug effects must then generally include at least 10 000 exposed persons in a cohort study, or enroll diseased patients from a population of equivalent size for a case–control study. A study of this size would be 95% certain of observing at least one case of any adverse effect that occurs with an incidence of 3 per 10 000 or greater (see Chapter 3). However, studies this large are expensive and difficult to perform. Yet, these studies often need to be conducted quickly, to address acute and serious regulatory, commercial, and/or public health crises. For all of these reasons, the past two decades have seen a growing use of computerized databases containing medical care data,

so called "automated databases," as potential data sources for pharmacoepidemiology studies.

Large electronic databases can often meet the need for a cost-effective and efficient means of conducting postmarketing surveillance studies. To meet the needs of pharmacoepidemiology, the ideal database would include records from inpatient and outpatient care, emergency care, mental health care, all laboratory and radiological tests, and all prescribed and over-the-counter medications, as well as alternative therapies. The population covered by the database would be large enough to permit discovery of rare events for the drug(s) in question, and the population would be stable over its lifetime. Although it is normally preferable for the population included in the database to be representative of the general population from which it is drawn, it may sometimes be advantageous to emphasize the more disadvantaged groups that may have been absent from premarketing testing. The drug(s) under investigation must of course be present in the formulary and must be prescribed in sufficient quantity to provide adequate power for analyses.

Other requirements of an ideal database are that all parts are easily linked by means of a patient's unique identifier, that the records are updated on a regular basis, and that the records are verifiable and are reliable. The ability to conduct medical chart review to confirm outcomes is also a necessity for most studies, as diagnoses entered into an electronic database may include rule-out diagnoses or interim diagnoses and recurrent/chronic, as opposed to acute, events. Information on potential confounders, such as smoking and alcohol consumption, may only be available through chart review or, more consistently, through patient interviews. With appropriate permissions and confidentiality safeguards in place, access to patients is sometimes possible and useful for assessing compliance with the medication regimen, as well as for obtaining information on other factors that may relate to drug effects. Information on drugs taken intermittently for symptom relief, over-the-counter drugs, and drugs not on the formulary must also be obtained directly from the patient.

These automated databases are the focus of this section of the book. Of course, no single database is ideal. In the current chapter, we introduce these resources, presenting some of the general principles that apply to them all. In Chapters 14–22, we present more detailed descriptions of those databases that have been used in a substantial amount of published research, along with the strengths and weaknesses of each.

DESCRIPTION

So-called automated databases have existed and been used for pharmacoepidemiologic research in North America since 1980, and are primarily administrative in origin, generated by the request for payments, or claims, for clinical services and therapies. In contrast, in Europe, medical record databases have been developed for use by researchers, and similar databases have been developed in the US more recently.

CLAIMS DATABASES

Claims data arise from a person's use of the health care system (see Figure 13.1). When a patient goes to a pharmacy and gets a drug dispensed, the pharmacy bills the insurance carrier for the cost of that drug, and has to identify which medication was dispensed, the milligrams per tablet, number

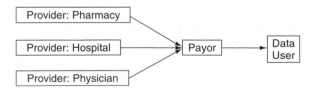

Figure 13.1. Sources of claims data.

of tablets, etc. Analogously, if a patient goes to a hospital or to a physician for medical care, the providers of care bill the insurance carrier for the cost of the medical care, and have to justify the bill with a diagnosis. If there is a common patient identification number for both the pharmacy and the medical care claims, these elements could be linked, and analyzed as a longitudinal medical record.

Since drug identity and the amount of drug dispensed affect reimbursement, and because the filing of an incorrect claim about drugs dispensed is fraud, claims are often closely audited, e.g., by Medicaid (see Chapter 18). Indeed, there have also been numerous validity checks on the drug data in claims files that showed that the drug data are of extremely high quality, i.e., confirming that the patient was dispensed exactly what the claim showed was dispensed, according to the pharmacy record. In fact, claims data of this type provide some of the best data on drug exposure in pharmacoepidemiology (see Chapter 45).

The quality of disease data in these databases is somewhat less perfect. If a patient is admitted to a hospital, the hospital charges for the care and justifies that charge by assigning International Classification of Diseases—Ninth Revision—Clinical Modification (ICD-9-CM) codes and a Diagnosis Related Group (DRG). The ICD-9-CM codes are reasonably accurate diagnoses that are used for clinical purposes, based primarily on the discharge diagnoses assigned by the patient's attending physician. (Of course, this does not guarantee that the physician's diagnosis is correct.) The amount paid by the insurer to the hospital is based on the DRG, so there is no reason to provide incorrect ICD-9-CM codes. In fact, most hospitals have mapped each set of ICD-9-CM codes into the DRG code that generates the largest payment.

In contrast, however, outpatient diagnoses are assigned by the practitioners themselves, or by their office staff. Once again, reimbursement does not usually depend on the actual diagnosis, but rather on the procedures administered during the outpatient medical encounter, and these procedure codes indicate the intensity of the services provided. Thus, there is no incentive for the practitioner to provide incorrect ICD-9-CM diagnosis codes, but there is also no incentive for them to be particularly careful or complete about the diagnoses provided. For these reasons, the outpatient diagnoses are the weakest link in claims databases.

MEDICAL RECORD DATABASES

In contrast, medical record databases are a more recent development, arising out of the increasing use of computerization in medical care. Initially, computers were used in medicine primarily as a tool for literature searches. Then, they were used for billing. Now, however, there is increasing use of computers to record medical information itself. In many instances, this is replacing the paper medical record as the primary medical record. As medical practices increasingly become electronic, this opens up a unique opportunity for pharmacoepidemiology, as larger and larger numbers of patients are available in such systems. The best-known and most widely used example of this approach is the General Practice Research Database, described in Chapter 22.

Medical record databases have unique advantages. Important among them is that the validity of the diagnosis data in these databases is better than that in claims databases, as these data are being used for medical care. When performing a pharmacoepidemiology study using these databases, there is no need to validate the data against the actual medical record, since one is analyzing the data from the actual medical record. However, there are also unique issues one needs to be concerned about, especially the uncertain completeness of the data from other physicians and sites of care. Any given practitioner provides only a piece of the care a patient receives, and inpatient and outpatient care are unlikely to be recorded in a common medical record.

STRENGTHS

Computerized databases have several important advantages. These include their potential for providing a very large sample size. This is especially important in the field of pharmacoepidemiology, where achieving an adequate sample size is uniquely problematic. In addition, these databases are relatively inexpensive to use, especially given the available sample size, as they are by-products of existing administrative systems. Studies using these data systems do not need to incur the considerable cost of data collection, other than for those subsets of the populations for whom medical records are abstracted and/or interviews are conducted. The data can be complete, i.e., for claims databases, information is available on all medical care provided, regardless of who the provider was. As indicated above, this can be a problem though for medical records databases. In addition, these databases can be population-based, they can include outpatient drugs and diseases, and there is no opportunity for recall and interviewer bias, as they do not rely on patient recall or interviewers to obtain their data.

WEAKNESSES

The major weakness of such data systems is the uncertain validity of diagnosis data. This is especially true for claims databases, and for outpatient data. It is less problematic for inpatient diagnoses (see Chapters 14–21 and Chapter 45) and for medical record databases (see Chapter 22).

In addition, such databases can lack information on some potential confounding variables. For example, in claims databases there are no data on smoking, alcohol, date of menopause, etc., all of which can be of great importance to selected research questions. This argues that one either needs access to patients or to physician records, if they contain the data in question, or one needs to be selective about the research questions that one seeks to answer through these databases, avoiding questions that require such data on variables which may be important potential confounders that must be controlled for.

A major other disadvantage of claims-based data is the instability of the population due to job changes, employers' changes of health plans, and changes in coverage for specific employees and their family members. The opportunity for longitudinal analyses is thereby hindered by the continual enrollment and dis-enrollment of plan members. However, strategies can be adopted for selecting stable populations within a specific database, and for addressing compliance, for example, by examining patterns of refills for chronically used medications.

Further, by definition, such databases only include illnesses severe enough to come to medical attention. In general, this is not a problem, since illnesses that are not serious enough to come to medical attention and yet are uncommon enough for one to seek to study them in such databases, are generally not of importance.

Finally, some results from studies that utilize these databases may not be generalizable, e.g., on health care utilization. This is especially relevant for databases created by data from a population that is atypical in some way, e.g., US Medicaid data (see Chapter 18).

PARTICULAR APPLICATIONS

Based on these characteristics, one can identify particular situations when these databases are uniquely useful or uniquely problematic for pharmacoepidemiologic research. These databases are useful in situations:

1. when looking for uncommon outcomes because of the need for a large sample size;
2. when a denominator is needed to calculate incidence rates;
3. when one is studying short-term drug effects (especially when the effects require specific drug or surgical therapy that can be used as validation of the diagnosis);

4. when one is studying objective, laboratory-driven
   diagnoses;
5. when recall or interviewer bias could influence the
   association;
6. when time is limited;
7. when the budget is limited.

Uniquely problematic situations include:

1. illnesses that do not reliably come to medical attention;
2. inpatient drug exposures that are not included in some of
   these databases;
3. outcomes that are poorly defined by the ICD-9-CM coding
   system, such as Stevens–Johnson syndrome;
4. descriptive studies, since the population might be
   skewed;
5. delayed drug effects, wherein patients can lose eligibility
   in the interim;
6. important confounders about which information cannot
   be obtained without accessing the patient, such as cigarette
   smoking, occupation, menarche, menopause, etc.

THE FUTURE

Given the frequent use of these data resources for pharmacoepidemiologic research in the recent past, we have already
learned much about their appropriate role. Inasmuch as it
appears that these uses will be increasing, we are likely to
continue to gain more insight in the coming years. However,
care must be taken to ensure that all potential confounding
factors of interest are available in the system or addressed
in some other way, diagnoses under study are chosen
carefully, and medical records can be obtained to validate
the diagnoses. In this part of the book, in Chapters 14–22,
we review the details of a number of these databases. The
databases selected for detailed review have been chosen
because they have been the most widely used in published
research. They are also good examples of the different types
of data that are available. There are multiple others like
each of them (see Chapter 23) and undoubtedly many more
will emerge over the ensuing years. Each has its advantages
and disadvantages, but each has proven it can be useful in
pharmacoepidemiology studies.

14

Group Health Cooperative

KATHLEEN W. SAUNDERS[1], ROBERT L. DAVIS[2] and ANDY STERGACHIS[3]

[1] Center for Health Studies, Group Health Cooperative, Seattle, Washington, USA; [2] Center for Health Studies, Group Health Cooperative, and Departments of Pediatrics and Epidemiology, University of Washington, Seattle, Washington, USA; [3] Departments of Epidemiology and Pharmacy, University of Washington, Seattle, Washington, USA.

INTRODUCTION

Traditional group and staff model health maintenance organizations (HMOs) employ a defined set of providers to deliver comprehensive health care services to a defined population of patients for a fixed, prepaid annual fee. HMO enrollees typically receive their health care services within these integrated systems through a uniform benefit package.[1] Care is usually provided within a defined geographic area that allows for, among other things, large comparable groups of subjects for public health research.[1]

Several of the unique features of traditional group and staff model HMOs have adapted as a result of market force pressures as the majority of employed Americans are now covered by some type of managed health care plan. Managed health care characterizes health plans that use mechanisms to monitor and control the cost, quality, and use of health services generally delivered by a specified network of health care providers.

While the term "managed care" was once synonymous with traditional HMOs, it now encompasses new organizational forms such as network model HMOs and individual practice associations (IPAs).[1] Most of these new models feature insurance organization contracts with physicians' groups to provide care for enrollees, as opposed to fully integrated delivery systems.[1] In order to compete with these new health care models, staff model HMOs are using more mixed models of care, creating their own networks and IPAs.[1] Pressure is also mounting to offer a wider selection of benefit options, such as point-of-service plans, which allow enrollees to seek care wherever they want.[1] "One-size-fits-all" benefit packages that used to be the rule in HMOs have been transformed into individualized plans that may number in the hundreds. Managed care organizations often use pharmacy benefits management (PBM) companies to perform some or all of the management of prescription drug benefits. Thus, while traditional HMOs continue to play an important role in public health research, including postmarketing drug

Pharmacoepidemiology, Fourth Edition   Edited by B.L. Strom
© 2005 John Wiley & Sons, Ltd

surveillance, it is important to keep in mind the market trends that threaten some of the unique features of these organizations.

Some of these trends are evident at Group Health Cooperative (GHC). While this chapter emphasizes the advantages of conducting postmarketing drug surveillance in a predominantly closed staff model HMO, it also acknowledges the implications of an organization moving toward a more mixed model of care.

There has been longstanding interest in the use of data from HMOs to study the effects of marketed drugs. Since the time of the report of the Joint Commission on Prescription Drug Use in 1980, recommendations have been made on the use of HMO records for postmarketing drug surveillance.[2] There are several advantages to conducting research in an HMO setting.[3] Because every HMO has an identifiable population base, it is possible to determine denominators for epidemiologic research, enabling investigators to calculate incidence and prevalence rates. Other key features of HMOs relevant to the conduct of postmarketing drug surveillance include the availability of:

1. a relatively stable population base;
2. accessible and complete medical records for each enrollee;
3. in many instances, computerized databases.

Such computerized databases are an important feature of GHC. In general, these automated files contain information recorded during the routine delivery of health services. At GHC, such data have been used extensively to evaluate drug usage and the adverse and beneficial effects of marketed drugs and medical procedures.

In 1983, GHC made explicit its commitment to research and evaluation by establishing the Center for Health Studies. The mission of the Center for Health Studies is to develop GHC as a setting for population-based and intervention research, through its own program of research and through collaborative ties with other scientists, including those affiliated with the University of Washington, the Fred Hutchinson Cancer Research Center, and the HMO Research Network. The HMO Research Network is a group of 14 HMOs that was formed in order to facilitate health services and epidemiologic research in managed care organizations (see Chapter 16). All of these HMOs have dedicated research units with active, full time academically oriented research personnel.[4]

This chapter reviews the characteristics of the GHC setting and databases, the advantages and disadvantages of GHC data resources for postmarketing drug surveillance, selected methodologic issues pertaining to postmarketing drug surveillance that arise in an HMO setting like GHC, the implications of the new Health Insurance Portability and Accountability Act (HIPAA) regulations, and expected future directions for research with the GHC databases.

DESCRIPTION

GROUP HEALTH COOPERATIVE

GHC, a nonprofit consumer-directed HMO established in 1947, currently provides health care on a prepaid basis to approximately 562 000 persons in Washington State. About three-quarters of these enrollees are part of the "staff model"—that is, they receive outpatient care at GHC facilities, with the exception of specific services not provided by GHC providers (e.g., temporomandibular care). In the latter case, GHC contracts with selected community providers to whom enrollees are referred. Approximately 25% of enrollees deviate from the staff model in that they receive care from non-GHC provider networks located in geographic areas not served by GHC medical centers.

Included among these 562 000 enrollees are 114 000 enrollees who belong to Group Health Options, Inc., a wholly owned subsidiary of GHC established in 1990. These "point-of-service" enrollees—members of either the Options or Alliant plans—can receive care from Group Health providers or GHC provider networks at greater benefit coverage, or from other, out-of-network community providers with slightly more out-of-pocket costs. In 2003, 11% of GHC Options' enrollees' health care costs were incurred through these out-of-network community providers.

Approximately 10% of State of Washington residents were enrolled in GHC in 2003. The majority of GHC enrollees receive health benefits through their place of employment (i.e., group enrollees). In addition, as of September 2003 GHC had arrangements for providing services to approximately 58 500 Medicare, 30 000 Medicaid, and 18 000 Washington Basic Health Plan recipients. The Basic Health Plan is a state-subsidized program that provides medical insurance to low income, uninsured residents who earn too much to qualify for Medicaid.

Historically, GHC has offered comprehensive health care coverage for outpatient care, inpatient services, emergency care, mental health services, and prescribed drugs. However, changes are occurring in this approach to comprehensive coverage. Beginning in 1993, Medicare enrollees new to GHC did not receive drug coverage, but could purchase prescription drugs from GHC pharmacies at prices competitive with the rest of the community. Also, in an effort to attract new enrollees, the Cooperative is offering a wider range of coverage choices. For example, in 2003 individuals and families could purchase catastrophic coverage that featured a $1500 deductible and no prescription drug or maternity benefits. Even with comprehensive coverage, nearly all benefit plans required small copayments for services, such as prescriptions, nonpreventive care outpatient visits, and emergency treatment. Coverage policies for outpatient drugs are controlled by GHC's drug formulary, guided by its Pharmacy and Therapeutics Committee.

GHC's facilities consist of 1 hospital, 24 primary care clinics, and 5 specialty centers. GHC operated two hospitals until the Cooperative formed a strategic alliance with Virginia Mason Medical Center in 1993, which resulted in the closure of one GHC hospital as a full-service, tertiary facility. The two organizations contract with each other for hospital services. GHC plans to operate its one remaining hospital (Eastside) until 2007, after which inpatient services in that area will be provided by another hospital (Overlake) as part of a strategic partnership between Group Health and Overlake Hospital Medical Center.

GHC contracts with Group Health Permanente, a partnership of physicians responsible for providing medical services at the Cooperative's facilities. In 2003, this Permanente Medical Group consisted of 1087 staff, including physicians and other practitioners. Among the physician group, the following percentages are board certified: 89% primary care; 94% pediatric; 100% ob/gyn; 89% other specialties—compared to a national average of 89%. The distribution of patients to primary care providers' practices is based on a panel system in which each primary care provider (family practice physician, pediatrician, or internist) has responsibility for managing and coordinating the care of a panel or caseload of patients. Upon enrollment in GHC, patients are offered a choice of primary care physicians and may change primary care physicians at any time during their tenure in the plan. Historically, the GHC primary care physician has played a "gatekeeper" role, serving as the source of patients' referrals to specialists. Beginning in 2003, it became possible for enrollees to "self-refer" to many types of medical specialists.

As shown in Table 14.1, compared to other Seattle–Tacoma–Bremerton area residents, GHC enrollees have slightly higher educational attainment but are quite similar in age, gender, and racial/ethnic composition. GHC enrollees have similar median income, but there is less representation within the highest extreme of income distribution. Differences noted between the GHC population and the US population

(fewer blacks, higher educational level, less representation within the lowest extreme of income distribution among GHC enrollees) primarily reflect differences between the demographic composition of Seattle–Tacoma–Bremerton and the US population as a whole.

DATABASES AT GHC

GHC's automated and manual databases serve as major resources for many epidemiologic studies, in part because individual records can be linked through time and across data sets by the unique consumer number assigned to each enrollee. Once assigned, the consumer number remains with an enrollee, even if the individual dis-enrolls and rejoins GHC at a later date.

Table 14.2 lists the research data sets that have been developed from GHC's databases. Data are available in SAS format on several different platforms such as an MVS mainframe, a UNIX system, and the Center for Health Studies' Data Warehouse on an NT server. For relational database purposes, much of these data, and some additional data not listed in Table 14.2, are available in a Sybase Data Warehouse on a UNIX system. Files are updated in real time, daily, weekly, monthly, quarterly, or semi-annually, using data from clinical and administrative computer systems. Every file contains the unique patient identifier common to all of the data sets. Physician identifiers are also unique across all files. It should be noted that as part of a statewide consolidation effort, data from Central and Eastern Washington enrollees are gradually being incorporated into these databases. As of 2003, automated pharmacy data were available statewide. Historically, however, studies based on automated data were limited to western Washington enrollees.

A brief description of each of GHC's data files follows.

Enrollment

Group Health maintains a variety of enrollment and demographic files. Current enrollment files contain records for every person presently enrolled in GHC, some 562 000 enrollees. They contain person-based information on selected patient characteristics such as patient consumer number, subscriber number (used to aggregate family members on the same contract), date of birth, sex, primary care provider, plan, assigned clinic, patient address, and telephone number. (Note that information on race, years of education, and income, as presented in Table 14.1, is not routinely

Table 14.1. Demographic characteristics of Group Health Cooperative enrollees

Characteristic	Percentage of total population		
	GHC enrollees	Seattle–Tacoma–Bremerton area	United States
Age (years)[a]			
<25	33	34	35
25–64	55	56	53
65+	12	10	12
Sex[a]			
Male	47	50	49
Female	53	50	51
Race or ethnicity[b]			
White	90	88	82
Black	3	4	11
Asian or Pacific Islander	4	6	3
American Indian, Eskimo or Aleut	1	1	1
Other	2	1	3
Years of education[c]			
<12	9	10	20
12	23	23	29
13–15	31	34	27
>15	37	32	24
Annual household income[d]			
<$15 000	17	17	24
$15–30 000	28	24	26
$30–45 000	26	23	21
$45–60 000	16	15	13
>$60 000	13	20	17

[a] Age and sex for Group Health are based on 2002 Group Health enrollment data. Age and sex for the Seattle–Tacoma–Bremerton area and the United States are based on 2000 census data for Seattle–Tacoma–Bremerton, WA CMSA and the US, respectively.

[b] Race for Group Health is based on two random samples of Group Health enrollees surveyed in 1990: 1308 enrollees aged 18–64[5] and 2513 enrollees aged 65 and over.[6] Race for adults aged 18 and over for the Seattle–Tacoma–Bremerton area and the US is based on 1990 census data for the Seattle–Tacoma, WA CMSA and the US, respectively. Race data from 2000 are not reported because the census question was changed, resulting in a much larger proportion of "other" responses. This change made it difficult to compare these data to Group Health data on race.

[c] Years of education for Group Health enrollees aged 25 and over are based on a random sample of 1133 enrollees surveyed in 1984.[7] Years of education for adults aged 25 and over for the Seattle–Tacoma–Bremerton area and the US are based on 2000 Census data.

[d] Annual household income for Group Health enrollees is based on a random sample of 1133 enrollees surveyed in 1984,[7] with income figures corrected for inflation between 1984 and 1989 and stated in 1989 dollars. Income figures for the Seattle–Tacoma–Bremerton area and the US are based on 1990 Census data.

collected, but was obtained through special surveys from random samples of enrollees.) This file is often used to select probability samples of current GHC enrollees. GHC also maintains historical enrollment files. For example, the consumer file contains a record for everyone who has either sought care or been enrolled at Group Health. A derivative data set includes a person's estimated original enrollment date (not available for all persons). Another historical data set contains all enrollment periods (up to five) for the approximately two million persons who have been enrolled at GHC at any time since 1980.

Pharmacy

The pharmacy file includes data on each prescription dispensed at GHC-owned outpatient pharmacies since March 1977. A computerized record is created for every medication at the time the prescription is filled. As shown in

Table 14.2. Automated databases organized for analytic studies at GHC

Database	Years Available
Enrollment	1980–present
Pharmacy	March 1977–present
Hospitalization	January 1972–present
Laboratory	January 1986–present
Radiology	January 1986–present
Outpatient visits without diagnosis	July 1984–December 1991
Outpatient visits with diagnosis	January 1992–present
Cancer surveillance system	January 1974–present
Cause of death	January 1977–present
Community health services	June 1989–present
Cost information system	June 1989–present
Claims from non-GHC providers	June 1989–present
Breast cancer screening program	January 1985–present
Immunization	February 1991–present (with historical and non-GHC information backfilled from patient report)

Table 14.3. Selected variables available from automated drug files on all prescriptions dispensed from GHC outpatient pharmacies, 1977 to present

Patient data
Consumer #
Birth date
Sex
Group coverage
Copay status

Drug data
Drug number
Therapeutic class
Drug form and strength
Date dispensed
Quantity dispensed
Cost to GHC
Refill indicator
Number of days supply dispensed

Prescriber or pharmacy data
Prescribing physician
Pharmacy location

Table 14.3, each record contains selected information about the patient, the prescription, and the prescriber. An additional variable, days supply, was added to the pharmacy database in 1996. This field, motivated by the Cooperative's

need to charge the appropriate one-, two-, or three-month patient copayment amount, indicates the number of days the medication should last. Examples of studies that utilized this data file are cited in the section on "Particular applications."

Hospital

The hospitalization databases contain records of every discharge, including newborn and stillborn infants, from GHC-owned hospitals since January 1972. The Commission on Professional Hospital Activities—Professional Activity Study (CPHA-PAS) provided hospital discharge information from January 1972 through December 1984. Since January 1985, GHC's hospital information system (HIS) has included information for discharges from GHC-owned hospitals. The information in the hospitalization database includes patient characteristics, diagnoses, procedures, diagnostic related group (DRG), and discharge disposition. Virtually all hospitalizations not captured in HIS are included in GHC's outside claims files. To facilitate evaluation of hospital costs and utilization, all records of discharges from GHC and non-GHC hospitals since June 1989 have been combined into an annual utilization data set.

Laboratory

Automated laboratory data are available from January 1986. The online laboratory system interconnects all GHC laboratories, including inpatient settings, and contains patient-specific information on all laboratory tests. Specific variables contained in the research file include the name of the test ordered, the date ordered, the specimen source, the results, and the date of the results. This database has been used in studies of acyclovir safety[8] and studies of the epidemiology of *Chlamydia trachomatis* infection.[9] Recent studies have used the laboratory database to examine the effect of improvement in hemoglobin A1c levels on health care utilization and costs among patients with diabetes[10] and to assess whether diabetes alters the risk of acute urinary tract infections among postmenopausal women.[11] Researchers have also used this database to assess the reliability of self-reported screening by fecal occult blood testing, finding that self-reported testing rates exceeded rates based on automated data by 13.9%.[12]

Radiology

This system, established in 1986, contains records of all radiographic studies performed at GHC facilities, including CT and MRI scans. Radiology records were maintained in a separate database through June 1995; since then these records have been combined with those in the outpatient visits file.

Outpatient Visits

The GHC outpatient registration system was initiated in mid-1984 and includes selected information about each outpatient visit. The database includes a record of the date of visit, the provider seen, the provider's specialty, and the location of care. Beginning in 1991, and fully operational in 1992, diagnosis and procedure data have been incorporated in the registration database. This information was not available in automated form before that time. This database has been used to examine ambulatory utilization patterns related to quitting smoking,[13] ambulatory utilization patterns of children of smokers,[14] and back-pain-related visit utilization following randomization to one of three treatments for low back pain.[15] Outpatient visit data have been particularly useful in studies of antibiotic usage among GHC children, because the majority of pediatric antibiotic use occurs in the context of outpatient ambulatory visits.[16]

Cancer Surveillance System and Other Registries

Since 1974, GHC has participated in the National Cancer Institute's Surveillance, Epidemiology, and End Results (SEER) program. As part of this program, the Center for Health Studies periodically receives data files with information on all newly diagnosed cancers among GHC enrollees from the Cancer Surveillance System (CSS) at the Fred Hutchinson Cancer Research Center, one of 13 SEER population-based registries in the United States.[17] The CSS reporting area consists of the 13 contiguous counties of northwest Washington State. The database, which currently covers the period 1974 through mid-2003, contains information for each newly diagnosed cancer case, including patient demographics, anatomical site, stage at diagnosis, and vital status at follow-up, which is ongoing for all surviving cases in the register. This database has been used to evaluate GHC's Breast Cancer Screening Program[18] and mammography performance.[19,20]

GHC has also developed several electronic disease-specific registries that identify relevant populations of patients. Examples include registries of patients with diabetes, depression, and heart disease.

Cause of Death

Using data from the State of Washington vital statistics files, a file of deaths among GHC enrollees between the years 1977 to the present has been developed. The death file was produced through record linkages between the State of Washington's death certificate database and the GHC membership files.

Community Health Services System

GHC's Community Health Services department operates visiting nurse, hospice, respite, and geriatric nurse practitioner programs, a nursing home rounding system, and numerous other community-based service programs. Computerized information from this department, available since mid-1989, includes type of provider, type of procedure, diagnosis, location of service, and price and billing information.

Utilization Management/Cost Management Information System

Due to a growing need for utilization and cost information, the Utilization Management/Cost Management Information System (UM/CMIS) was developed at GHC in 1989. This system uses information from other systems (e.g., registration, pharmacy) to assign both direct and indirect costs to individual encounters based on the units of service utilized. Thus, it is possible to use UM/CMIS data to estimate an individual's total health care costs, as well as the costs of individual components of care, such as primary care visits, pharmacy prescriptions, mental health services, and inpatient stays. These data have been used to study the health care costs associated with several conditions or diseases, including asthma in children,[21] depression,[22] breast cancer,[23] bipolar disorder,[24] smoking,[25] and diagnosed domestic violence.[26] A new costing system was introduced in January 2004.

Immunizations Database

The immunizations database was initially developed as part of the Vaccine Safety Datalink (VSD), a CDC-collaborative study with GHC and seven other HMOs nationwide[27] (see Chapter 30). This database contains immunization records from February 1991 to the present for GHC enrollees 0–6 years of age, while immunizations for GHC members of all ages have been included since 1995. GHC also receives a regular feed of immunization data from Washington State for all children enrolled in GHC at the time. This feed includes historical data on immunizations, including those received when the child was not a Group Health enrollee (if applicable), thereby preventing a loss of immunization information when children change health plans or providers.

The immunization database has been used in several studies of vaccine safety. One study examined the relationship between the diphtheria and tetanus toxoids and whole-cell pertussis (DTP) vaccine and measles, mumps, and rubella (MMR) vaccine and the risk of a first seizure, subsequent seizures, and neurodevelopmental disability in children.[28] Another case–control study found no association between the MMR vaccine and inflammatory bowel disease.[29] And another study examined the risk of anaphylaxis after vaccination of children and adolescents.[30] The immunization database has also been used in studies of the utility of immunization tracking systems.[31,32] In a study of the effectiveness of the pneumococcal polysaccharide vaccine among people aged 65 years and older, Jackson and colleagues found that receipt of the vaccine was associated with a reduced risk of pneumococcal bacteremia but that the vaccine did not reduce the risk of pneumonia among older adults.[33]

Claims Database

The claims databases record information on health care services that GHC purchases from non-GHC providers. These databases contain a record of each bill received by GHC for outside services since 1989, such as inpatient and emergency care and referrals to non-GHC providers. These claims databases have become even more critical as traditional HMOs have shifted to more mixed models of care, because they provide a means of giving a full accounting of an individual's medical care. For example, they capture bills from network providers who have contracted to provide care to GHC enrollees in outlying areas and for prescriptions filled at community pharmacies in outlying areas.

Other Databases

Important data are also being generated from an ongoing program on breast cancer screening. All GHC women aged 40 years or older are being mailed questionnaires that solicit information on factors associated with the incidence of breast cancer. Approximately 85% of the women complete the questionnaires. Programmatically, the information from this database is being used to ascertain individual level of risk for breast cancer, with a woman's risk group determining the frequency of screening mammography. Included in the breast cancer screening database are items pertaining to lifetime smoking history, use of estrogens, and reproductive history.

A variety of manually maintained outpatient and inpatient medical records, clinical logs, and registries are often employed in research. Many research studies include direct patient contact through in-person interviews, surveys, or clinical examinations and tests.

STRENGTHS

The advantages of the GHC databases derive from their size, the accessibility and quality of their data, and the feasibility of linking patients to a primary care provider in a staff model HMO. GHC serves a moderately large population, currently over 562 000 persons, and this allows the study of relatively uncommon adverse events. The GHC population is well defined in terms of age, sex, geographic location, and duration of GHC membership. Turnover in membership at GHC is estimated to be approximately 15% per year. This relative stability facilitates long-term follow-up. For example, recent Center for Health Studies' longitudinal studies of patients with back pain and depression have obtained follow-up data for more than 80% of the original cohort after a one-year period. Typically, such studies are successful in following persons by telephone whether or not they remain GHC enrollees.

A single patient identification number permits following the records of individuals across time. The unique patient consumer number is assigned to each enrollee upon initial enrollment at GHC and remains with the individual even if dis-enrollment and re-enrollment occur.

An obvious advantage to the GHC setting for research is the extensive use of computer technology. As previously noted, numerous automated databases are available at GHC and can be utilized for postmarketing drug and vaccine safety surveillance. Because the data are collected in an ongoing manner as a by-product of health care delivery, there is no requirement for individual patient contact. Thus, the high cost and potential for recall bias that would otherwise be associated with primary data collection are minimized or avoided. However, GHC has mechanisms for contacting patients directly for primary data collection, as appropriate. Examples include interview-based case–control studies, health surveillance activities, and clinical research studies. In addition, manual medical records and registries are also available for use. The manual medical records are retained for at least 10 years following dis-enrollment (or until a child is 10 years past majority, whichever is later), permitting studies of very long-term outcomes.

Another advantage to GHC as a research setting is the longevity of the plan. In existence for more than 50 years, Group Health has a subset of enrollees whose tenure in the Cooperative spans decades. This longevity facilitates studies that require very long-term follow-up. Such long-term follow-up was crucial, for example, in the study mentioned previously that examined a hypothesized relationship between inflammatory bowel disease (IBD) and measles vaccination. The onset of IBD often occurs in late adolescence or early adulthood, yet the immunization of interest (MMR vaccine) is delivered in the second year of life. This long lag between exposure and outcome necessitated the creation of a data set of members born into GHC as far back as 1958 who remained enrolled until at least 1972. Medical records (both hospitalization and outpatient) were used to confirm the diagnosis of IBD, and, since these records extended back to birth, were also used to collect information on childhood immunizations.[29]

The many advantages GHC has as a setting for pharmacoepidemiological research are only strengthened by Group Health's participation in the HMO Research Network (see Chapter 16). Such participation permits the examination of practice patterns and health care delivery and quality among geographically distinct populations in many different parts of the United States.

Another benefit of these collaborative projects is the ability to study rare events. Since specific exposures such as medications or vaccinations are easily identifiable by automated data routinely collected for billing purposes, studies of rare events following these exposures can often be performed in a more efficient and less biased fashion than otherwise possible. For example, in the Vaccine Safety Datalink project, immunization tracking systems within HMOs were linked with automated medical care utilization data on seizures evaluated in clinics, emergency departments, or hospitals in order to study the risk for seizures following vaccination.[28] Such events would otherwise be too rare to study within most individual HMOs. Similarly, using automated pharmaceutical files to track medication usage, studies can be done of rare adverse events following use of specific medications or among subjects with specific conditions.

WEAKNESSES

LOGISTIC AND OPERATIONAL

Despite the large size of the GHC databases, most marketed drugs are used by a relatively small proportion of a population. Thus, the GHC databases still may be too small to detect associations between drug exposures and rare outcomes. The detection of rare adverse events requires combining data from multiple health care delivery systems, as has been done in the case of the Centers for Education and Research on Therapeutics (CERT) (see "Strengths") (see Chapter 16).

The data presently available in automated files do not include some potentially important confounding variables. The lack of information on confounding factors such as race,[34] smoking, and alcohol consumption may lead to challenges in the study and interpretation of drug-associated health effects. Confounding by indication occurs when the underlying diagnosis or other clinical features that trigger use of a certain drug also predict patient outcome in their own right. For example, in a study of β-blockers and the risk of coronary heart disease among persons with hypertension, confounding by indication was a concern because β-blockers are also used to treat angina pectoris and are avoided in cases of congestive heart failure, each of which may be an early manifestation of coronary heart disease.[35] Analytic studies must consider alternative methods of obtaining the necessary information on confounding factors, such as medical record abstraction and patient interview. It should be noted that GHC's new Clinical Information System, EpicCare (see "The Future"), may help solve some of these problems. Also, automated information on inpatient drugs and on outpatient diagnoses were not available until relatively recently, an important disadvantage for some retrospective studies.

Use of automated data to determine health outcomes is not always reliable without a review of medical records. In the Vaccine Safety Datalink study of seizures following vaccination, it would have been optimal to rely on computerized seizure-related diagnosis codes. However, the investigators found that these codes often identified visits of children with seizure conditions who were being seen for follow-up or well-child care. They concluded that for chronic conditions such as seizure disorders, medical record review is often necessary to distinguish acute events from follow-up or routine visits.[28] In another study, researchers evaluated the accuracy of computerized diagnostic and procedure data to identify complications and comorbidities of diabetes by comparing the automated data to chart data. The scientists concluded that automated data are useful in identifying potential diabetic complications, but that the automated data require confirmation if used for research purposes.[36]

In addition, "rule-out" diagnoses can be misleading. In reviewing the medical records of a subset of people receiving a computerized diagnosis of rheumatoid arthritis, one researcher found that it was not uncommon for the diagnosis of rheumatoid arthritis to have been subsequently ruled out by further medical tests (personal communication with Teresa McCann).

The present competitive environment in the health care industry has resulted in a growing number of mixed-model benefit plans (e.g., non-GHC provider networks and point-of-service plans) being offered by GHC, which may impact the completeness of databases of health services utilization. For example, results of laboratory tests administered outside of Group Health are not presently available in electronic form. Another threat to database completeness is the movement away from "one size fits all" comprehensive benefit packages. This has resulted in varying coverage arrangements for different groups (e.g., State employees, Basic Health Plan enrollees). For example, since 1994, GHC has not provided prescription drug coverage to new Medicare enrollees (see "Methodologic issues pertaining to use of the GHC pharmacy database"). While using automated data to assess current coverage arrangements is possible, albeit complicated, the data are not structured to facilitate retrospective inquiries into coverage. Thus, it is very difficult to track changes in coverage over time, changes that could have serious ramifications for health care utilization. It should be noted that out-of-plan use of prescription drugs has been the subject of several validity studies, and the outpatient pharmacy database has been found to be generally complete for prescription drugs (see "Methodologic issues pertaining to use of the GHC pharmacy database").

In some populations, even when individuals are part of the "staff model" and have comprehensive coverage, they may choose to receive some of their care out-of-plan. For example, one study found that a large proportion of GHC adolescents used out-of-plan care, and those using out-of-plan care were more likely to have sexually transmitted diseases and other health problems than those who solely used in-plan services.[37] Aside from jeopardizing continuity of care, this out-of-plan use limits the completeness of automated databases. Increased competition may also lead to increased patient turnover in HMOs, resulting in decreases in follow-up time for cohort studies.

The GHC formulary limits the study of many newly marketed drugs, since GHC may decide not to add a new agent or may adopt a new drug only after it has been on the market for some time. GHC often maintains only one brand of a legend drug on the drug formulary at a time, thereby preventing investigations of many direct drug-to-drug comparisons of relative toxicity and effectiveness. In particular, drugs that offer little demonstrated therapeutic advantage or value over alternative agents may be excluded from the GHC formulary. If nonformulary drugs are commonly purchased outside the GHC pharmacy system, as may have been the case with drugs for impotence and some drugs for weight loss, there is the potential for an inaccurate determination of the prevalence of usage, or even of the risk of use. Furthermore, this situation (outside procurement of nonformulary drugs) prevents GHC from proactively contacting enrollees if new information emerges concerning the potential risks or dangers of medication.

Studies of some medications that are solely (or primarily) administered as over-the-counter (OTC) products are limited since such OTC data is not routinely captured by the GHC pharmacy database. So, for example, studies that are interested in the relationship between specific OTC medications (such as acetaminophen) and their risk for certain adverse events such as liver failure, or their protective effect against febrile seizures following vaccination, must rely on other ways of collecting data on acetaminophen use. Since OTC use is typically not well documented in the medical record, the only way this information can be gathered is retrospectively by interview, thereby introducing the potential for recall bias or misclassification of exposure. In this situation, then, the benefits of the automated routine collection of pharmaceutical information are lost.

The elderly and the poor have tended to be underrepresented in HMOs,[1] leading to concerns about representativeness of studies. However, a Medicare managed care plan has been offered since 1985. GHC's enrollment of people aged 65 years and older is comparable to that of the Seattle–Tacoma–Bremerton Metropolitan area (see Table 14.1). Group Health's involvement in Healthy Options, Washington State's Medicaid managed care program, resulted in a large increase in Medicaid enrollment between 1993 and 2003. However, due to financial considerations, the Cooperative decided to reduce its Healthy Options enrollment beginning in 2004.

PARTICULAR APPLICATIONS

EXAMPLES OF USE OF GHC DATA

The principal use of the pharmacy database for epidemiologic research has been to ascertain drug exposures, often for evaluating the effectiveness or toxicity of specific medications. Examples of questions addressed by case–control studies include:

1. Do β-blockers reduce the incidence of coronary heart disease in patients with high blood pressure?[38]
2. Are thiazide diuretics associated with hip fracture?[39]
3. Is the use of hormone replacement therapy associated with an increased risk of stroke in postmenopausal women?[40]
4. Are hypertensive patients treated with calcium channel blockers at increased risk of a first myocardial infarction?[41]

The pharmacy database has also been used in retrospective and prospective cohort studies of specific medications. Examples include studies of the medical outcomes and costs associated with pentoxifylline treatment of patients with peripheral arterial disease,[42] the perinatal effects of acyclovir,[8] and suicide risk during treatment with lithium and divalproex among patients with bipolar disorder.[43] The pharmacy database has also been used to study patterns of drug use, in one case to examine patterns of asthma therapy in the 5 years following dissemination of national guidelines[44] and in others to assess compliance with antidepressants[45] and hormone replacement therapy.[46]

Physician prescribing practices are also of interest, with one study examining prescribing frequency for hormone replacement therapy.[47] In an ongoing study, CERT and Cancer Research Network (CRN) investigators together are studying patterns of hormone replacement therapy use following the termination of the Women's Health Initiative trial of combined estrogen–progestin therapy due to an increased risk of breast cancer, heart attack, and stroke. This study is being conducted in collaboration with the Cancer Research Network, another HMO Network endeavor funded by the National Cancer Institute.

The pharmacy database is increasingly used as a sampling frame. In some instances, medication use is the primary sampling criterion, as in the case of studies restricted to hypertensive patients treated with medication.[48] In other cases, medication use has been used to identify patients with particular diseases or conditions. For example, patients prescribed insulin or oral hypoglycemic agents in the last 3 years are presumed to be diabetic and are included on the diabetes registry.

In two recent studies, investigators have developed innovative methods for identifying people with potential new infections based on prescriptions for antibiotics[49] and antimicrobials[50] recorded in the pharmacy database. Researchers have also used the pharmacy database as a tool to recruit high-risk patients into special influenza clinics for vaccinations. The scientists characterized adults as "high-risk" for influenza if they, among other things, had prescriptions for steroids, insulin, or oral hypoglycemic agents; children were defined as high-risk if they were prescribed steroids or autonomic inhalers (or were enrolled in the asthma registry).[51] Other uses of the database include controlling for potential confounding represented by the use of certain kinds of drugs,[39,52] drug utilization review activities,[53–55] and studying the effect of various levels of prescription drug copayments on overall drug utilization.[56]

The pharmacy database is also used for postmarketing drug surveillance. For example, CERT investigators are using automated pharmacy databases to conduct postmarketing surveillance of Lotronex, a selective antagonist of the 5HT3 serotonin type receptors used for irritable bowel syndrome that was withdrawn from the US market in 2000 and then reintroduced in 2002 with restrictions and modified conditions of use.

Below are some detailed examples of how the GHC pharmacy database has been used for epidemiologic and health services research.

A 2002 article published in the *American Journal of Psychiatry* assessed the effects on offspring of antidepressant use by pregnant women.[57] While this issue had been examined in previous studies, uncertainty remained as to the effect of antidepressants on the embryo and fetus. This cohort study compared the perinatal outcomes, congenital malformations, and early growth and development of infants with and without prenatal exposure to antidepressants. The first step was to use hospital discharge records to identify all live births between January 1, 1986 and December 31, 1998. The newborn's discharge record could be linked to that of the mother. To ensure that paper medical records and computerized data were available, the researchers required that mothers be enrolled at medical centers owned by GHC.

The next step was to use the computerized pharmacy database to identify all tricyclic and serotonin reuptake inhibitor (SSRI) antidepressant prescription fills for the mothers during the 360 days prior to delivery. Women who had no antidepressant prescriptions in the 360 days preceding delivery were defined as "unexposed." Mothers who had at least one antidepressant prescription during the 270 days before delivery were considered "exposed." Those who fell somewhere in between (e.g., they had a fill in the period between 270 and 360 days before delivery) were excluded from the analyses. Again, to ensure completeness of information on exposure (e.g., antidepressant use), the researchers required that the mothers be enrolled continuously at GHC for the 360 days before delivery.

Infants who, according to the above definition, were exposed to antidepressants were frequency matched to infants who were unexposed. The frequency matching was based on the following maternal characteristics (all derived from automated data): age, year of delivery, lifetime number of antidepressant fills, lifetime history of outpatient psychiatric treatment, lifetime history of inpatient psychiatric treatment, and length of enrollment at GHC. Chart reviewers blinded to the infant's exposure status reviewed paper medical records for information pertaining to perinatal outcomes, congenital malformations, and developmental delay.

The researchers found no evidence that infants exposed to tricyclic antidepressants ($N = 209$) or SSRIs ($N = 185$) during pregnancy were at an increased risk for congenital malformations or developmental delay. Exposure to SSRIs during the third trimester of pregnancy was associated with lower Apgar scores. Infants exposed to SSRIs at any time during pregnancy were at an increased risk for premature delivery and lower birth weight than those infants not exposed to SSRIs. The investigators did not find any significant association between tricyclic antidepressants and premature delivery, lower birth weights, or lower Apgar scores.

While these findings do not provide a definitive answer as to the safety of using antidepressants during pregnancy, the results provide information that may help women make a difficult decision. Although SSRI use during pregnancy was associated with premature delivery, the absolute risk was only 10%. The authors concluded that women considering use of SSRIs during pregnancy may weigh "any greater risk of premature delivery against the risk of persistent or recurrent depression and the availability and acceptability of alternative treatments."

Another study published in a 2001 issue of the *Journal of the American Medical Association* examined the effects of initiation, discontinuation, and continued use of hormone replacement therapy (HRT) on breast density in postmenopausal women.[58] While prior studies had demonstrated that HRT initiation increased breast density,[59,60] little was known about what effect the continuation or discontinuation of HRT had on breast density. This is an important question because mammography has been shown to be less accurate when performed on dense versus fatty breasts.[20]

Eligible subjects for this cohort study were GHC postmenopausal women who had had two breast screening examinations between January 1996 and December 1998. The two screening exams, each of which consisted of a two-view mammogram and a clinical breast exam, were required to occur at least 11 months, and no more than 25 months, apart. Women were excluded if they were younger than 40 years and, according to computerized survey data collected through the Breast Cancer Screening Program, had any of the following:

- hysterectomy;
- history of breast cancer;
- diagnosis of cancer prior to either screening mammogram;
- breast augmentation.

The researchers turned to GHC's computerized pharmacy database to assess HRT use. For the purposes of this study,

HRT was defined as either estrogens alone or estrogens plus progestin, administered orally or by patch. The scientists relied on the strength of the pill or patch (e.g., 0.625 mg), and text instructions for use (e.g., 1 pill per day) to arrive at an estimated duration in days for each prescription and an average daily dose. Women were assumed to begin taking HRT the day following the date of their prescription, with refills considered to be extensions of HRT use.

The researchers used the date of HRT fills and the estimated duration of the prescription to classify women as users or nonusers prior to each of the two screening mammograms. Users were defined as those women filling an HRT prescription that lasted for 30 days or more and was due to run out no more than 6 weeks before the screening mammogram. Nonusers were those women who either did not fill an HRT prescription in the year before the screening mammogram, or who filled a prescription that was due to run out more than 24 weeks before the screening mammogram. Women who were not classified as either users or nonusers before each screening mammogram (e.g., their HRT fill was due to run out between 6 weeks and 24 weeks prior to the mammogram) were not included in the analysis. To ensure the completeness of data on HRT use, women were required to be continuously enrolled at GHC for the one year prior to each of the two screening exams.

According to the definitions above, women could be placed into one of the four following groups:

1. Nonusers: women who did not use HRT before either screening mammogram.
2. Discontinuers: women who used HRT before the first mammogram, but not the second.
3. Initiators: women who used HRT before the second mammogram, but not the first.
4. Continuing users: women who used HRT before each of the screening mammograms.

Breast density at each exam was rated by radiologists on a 1 to 4 scale, with 4 being the densest, and was captured using an automated reporting system. For analytic purposes, the researchers dichotomized density into low and high. Similar to the HRT use categorization described above, women could be placed into four distinct "change in breast density" categories, depending on the combination of their density ratings prior to the two exams. Because age at first screening and changes in body mass index are associated with changes in breast density, analyses controlled for these two factors. Weight and height data were available from the computerized BCSP survey data.

The scientists found that among this cohort of 5212 post-menopausal women, discontinuation of HRT was associated with subsequent decreases in breast density. Continuation of HRT was associated with sustained higher density. Consistent with previous research, this study found that initiation of HRT was associated with increases in breast density.

The researchers concluded that changes in breast density associated with HRT use are dynamic: "HRT increases breast density but these increases are potentially reversible with cessation of HRT." Given that prior studies have shown that increased breast density, as well as HRT use, adversely impact mammography accuracy, the current study's findings have important implications for breast cancer screening.

Because of the high cost of obtaining health status information through survey or medical record review, there has been interest in developing automated measures of health status.[61] To that end, Center for Health Studies researchers have used the pharmacy database to develop a Chronic Disease Score (CDS) for adults, a weighted sum of medications used for management of significant chronic diseases. There have been several iterations of the chronic disease score over time.[62–64] The latest methodology assigns empirically derived weights to classes of medications used to treat specific diseases. An individual's CDS is calculated by summing the weights of all classes of medications used (not prescriptions filled) in a one-year period, in addition to weights assigned to his or her age group and gender, and an intercept term. The CDS predicts future outpatient visit frequency, health care costs, hospitalization, and mortality, after controlling for age and gender. Several studies have used the CDS as a proxy measure of health status.[6,65] A pediatric CDS has also been developed.[66]

METHODOLOGIC ISSUES PERTAINING TO USE OF THE GHC PHARMACY DATABASE

The following sections describe methodologic problems that have been addressed by researchers using the GHC pharmacy database.

Completeness of the Database

An important issue when using GHC's outpatient pharmacy database for postmarketing drug surveillance research is the completeness of the database—that is, what proportion of prescriptions written to GHC enrollees are filled at GHC pharmacies. This issue has become more salient over time because in 1994 Group Health no longer offered prescription medication coverage to Medicare enrollees new to the Cooperative. In 2003, it was estimated that 50% of Medicare

enrollees did not have pharmacy coverage. Another factor that could potentially affect the completeness of the database over time is copayments, because reimbursement policies may influence patients' decisions on where they fill prescriptions or obtain health care services. Copayments were introduced for some plans at GHC in 1985, and by 1993 nearly all plans required modest copayments for visits and drugs. Another cause for concern is the increase in the percentage of enrollees who do not have traditional "staff model" plans. These enrollees receive their prescriptions at community pharmacies. Assuming the enrollee has drug coverage, the community pharmacy then has to bill Group Health in order for the Cooperative to be informed of the fill.

Scientists in the Cardiovascular Health Research Unit regularly ask subjects about the percentage of GHC prescriptions that they purchase at GHC pharmacies. Of about 1959 control subjects interviewed before 1994, 97% reported that they bought all or almost all (90–100%) of their prescription medications at GHC pharmacies (personal communication with Bruce Psaty). This percentage remained about the same (95.5%) when asked of 3146 control subjects interviewed between 1994 and August 2003. Thus, even in a time period (post-1993) when almost all enrollees had requirements for pharmacy copayments, the pharmacy database appeared to be very complete. Furthermore, Psaty and colleagues were able to examine completeness rates among senior enrollees (65 years of age and older) before and after January 1, 1994, the date GHC implemented its policy to no longer cover drugs for new Medicare enrollees. Among control subjects 65 years and older, 97.5% filled all or almost all of their prescription medicines at a GHC pharmacy before 1994 compared with 96.1% from January 1, 1994 on.

Other survey data also provide information on the completeness of the pharmacy database. Among 762 study subjects treated with antidepressant medications in 1996–1997, only 1.5% reported obtaining antidepressants from a non-GHC pharmacy in the prior 3 months (personal communication with Terry Bush). According to a survey of pain patients in 1989–1990, more than 90% of prescription medications used for pain management, such as opioids, sedatives/muscle relaxants, and anti-inflammatory drugs, were always filled at GHC pharmacies. However, the same survey revealed that pain patients often obtained OTC medicines, such as aspirin and acetaminophen at places other than GHC pharmacies.[67]

Indication for Use

Because there is no variable for disease or symptom indication for prescription in the pharmacy database, the medical record has often been used for this purpose.[38,42] This brings up two points:

1. To what extent are drugs identified from the pharmacy database documented in the medical record?
2. To what extent are indications for prescription recorded?

Regarding documentation of drugs, studies have found agreement rates ranging from 89% to 100% between the automated and manual sources.[39,42,68,69] One of these studies assessed whether indication for a one-time NSAID prescription was recorded in the medical record and found that 7% of the charts ($N = 501$) contained missing or vague diagnoses. There was a correlation between incomplete drug documentation and absence of an indication.[69]

With the availability of outpatient diagnoses, it became possible to assess the indication for prescription through automated means. For example, investigators wanted to identify primary care patients who were prescribed antidepressant medications for depression (antidepressants are also commonly prescribed for pain and sleep disturbance). They accomplished this by linking the antidepressant prescription record with visit records in the 120-day period preceding the prescription and in the several weeks following the fill, selecting only those prescriptions accompanied by a diagnosis of depression.[70] This method is far less expensive than chart review.

In a study of antibiotic use at GHC (in collaboration with Harvard Pilgrim Health Plan in Boston, Massachusetts), investigators were able to calculate disease-specific antibiotic use rates by linking the pediatric antibiotic prescription to the diagnosis for the most recent ambulatory visit within the preceding three days. For this purpose, the investigators developed an algorithm to assign a primary diagnosis to each patient when more than one diagnosis existed for a single visit.[71]

In Group Health's new Clinical Information System (see "The Future"), indication for prescription will be entered. It should be noted that, as is the case with the outpatient visit file, rule-out diagnoses will not be flagged. That is, the indication for prescription can be a diagnosis that is eventually ruled out by the provider.

Impact of HIPAA

In April 2003, the Health Insurance Portability and Accountability Act's (HIPAA) privacy rule went into effect. This portion of the Federal law deals with the privacy and confidentiality of patients' protected health care information (PHI). PHI is broadly defined—it is essentially anything that could potentially identify an individual, including names, dates, and medical record numbers. HIPAA applies to "covered entities," which covers most providers, clearing houses, and health plans, including most clinical research sites. Therefore, researchers at GHC must comply with HIPAA.

In many studies that involve direct patient contact, patients are asked to sign a HIPAA authorization form that informs the patient of the following:

1. information that will be used, including PHI, and things such as laboratory test results;
2. the people or organizations who will use or disclose the information and who will receive the information;
3. the purpose of the use or disclosure of information;
4. a date or event after which the information will no longer be used;
5. the patient's right to refuse to sign the authorization;
6. the patient's right to revoke authorization.

In many studies, it is not possible to obtain individual permission to use and disclose PHI and other information. In these cases, a waiver of authorization must be obtained from the institution's institutional review board (IRB). While waivers were required at GHC pre-HIPAA, the new Act specifies additional elements necessary to justify a waiver.

In studies wherein individual authorization is not obtained for use and disclosure of PHI and other information, HIPAA holds researchers to the "minimum necessary" standard—that is, researchers and staff must make a reasonable effort to use or disclose the minimum amount of patient information that is necessary to do their jobs. Limiting the type of patient information that is able to be transferred outside the covered entity has had major implications for multisite studies, where data are collected at multiple sites and then sent to a centralized location.

In response to HIPAA, some studies (especially multisite) must implement extensive procedures to ensure that PHI does not leave the individual sites. For example, in the CERT HMO Research Network, the centralized data repository (Data Center) contains only de-identified data that cannot be traced back to an individual. Data are pulled at the 10 individual sites according to standardized specifications, resulting in identical data sets at each site. At this point, site analysts run programs that have previously been passed through the Data Center. The Data Center ensures that the programs produce standardized final data sets that contain no information that can be traced back to an individual (aside from a study number), either by aggregating data across individuals or by removing any PHI. For example, the data set might contain the age of the patient at the time of a particular diagnosis, rather than the patient's birth date, which is PHI according to HIPAA.

Where individual-level data are required, the centralized programs assign study numbers that will be used at each site. However, the "crosswalk" that links a study number with a patient identifier, such as his or her consumer number, resides only at the individual sites. Further, study numbers are reassigned for each individual CERT study, thereby precluding any chance of linking individuals across studies and potentially arriving at a profile so specific that an individual could be identified.

One step removed from the de-identified data sets used in the CERT are "limited" data sets. While excluding direct patient identifiers such as name or address, these limited data sets can contain information such as diagnosis date, birth date, or zip code, that in combination with other information, could potentially be used to re-identify an individual. When limited data sets are shared with individuals or organizations outside of the covered entity in the absence of written permission from the individuals, the recipient must sign a data use agreement. The purpose of this agreement is to define the proper uses of the limited data set and to ensure that there is little chance that a patient will be re-identified.

THE FUTURE

In the second half of 2003, Group Health began implementation of a new clinical information system, EpicCare. Scheduled to be complete by the end of 2005, EpicCare has the potential to have a major impact on patient care, provider practice, and pharmacoepidemiologic research.

The six major elements of EpicCare are:

1. Clinical data repository. The clinical data repository consists of all the electronic information about a patient's health care, including the medical problem list, lab results, prescription medications, provider notes, blood pressure, weight, etc.
2. Clinical messaging. Clinical messaging allows clinicians to create, send, or forward secure clinical information and messages to other providers. This aspect of EpicCare enhances providers' ability to coordinate a patient's care.
3. Order entry. This aspect of EpicCare enables the provider to enter an order for medications, lab tests, procedures, etc. electronically. An obvious advantage is avoiding errors caused by illegible handwriting. Order entry encompasses other features, such as text completion matching and

"pick lists," to reduce errors and to make the provider's life easier. One change that will aid researchers is the association of a diagnosis with an order—for example, the order will specify that an antidepressant was prescribed for sleep, rather than depression.
4. Decision support. "Built-in" decision support rules seek to improve patient care by automatically checking information in EpicCare and issuing reminders. For example, EpicCare can check that a patient with coronary heart disease is on an antiplatelet agent.
5. Clinical documentation. The major method of documentation supported by EpicCare is direct entry. This feature enhances coordination of care because the information is immediately available to other providers, compared to the delays inherent in a system based on dictated notes. A number of features exist to facilitate entry, including the ability to insert standardized text blocks into a note.
6. MyGroupHealth functionality. MyGroupHealth refers to GHC's web-based program that allows patients to email members of their practice team and to refill medications online. With the implementation of EpicCare, patients will have access (with some restrictions) to their own electronic medical record. This means they can view their problem list, normal laboratory test results, and health reminders such as those for immunizations or screening tests.

The successful implementation of these six elements should improve clinical practice and patient care. However, it is a complex enterprise. Clinical information systems in general, and EpicCare specifically, provide data for research, especially that related to pharmacoepidemiology.

Related to the clinical information system, web-based interventions will play an increasing role in the future. The Center for Health Studies hired an informatics investigator in 2003 to help further this line of research. Prior to joining the Center, this physician–scientist conducted research on web-based support for the care of patients with type 2 diabetes.[72] Patients involved in this research project worked closely with their care team through electronic communications over the web. Patients also had self-management support tools, including access to their complete electronic medical record and the ability to upload and view their blood glucose levels alongside dietary and exercise data.

In the increasingly competitive health care industry, mergers and business changes will probably become more commonplace. GHC's alliance with Virginia Mason Medical Center for hospital care is an example of a business arrangement that has already affected patients, providers, and researchers. Another example is GHC's "statewide" initiative, whereby data on encounters occurring in eastern and western Washington, both within and outside the staff model, will be combined into a "one-stop-shopping" visits database.

GHC automated data on prescription medicine use and related health care utilization have been used extensively in studies of the effectiveness, adverse effects, utilization, and costs of drugs for over 20 years. New databases, developed in response to marketplace challenges and quality improvement initiatives, hold additional promise for expanding this field. Collaborations allow for the study of rare (and common) events possibly associated with drug use, or drug use patterns across many geographic sites.

REFERENCES

1. Fishman P, Wagner EH. Managed care data and public health: the experience of Group Health Cooperative of Puget Sound. *Annu Rev Public Health* 1998; **19**: 477–91.
2. US Senate Committee on Labor and Human Resources, Subcommittee on Health and Scientific Affairs. *Final Report of the Joint Commission on Prescription Drug Use*. Washington, DC: Government Printing Office, 1980.
3. Wagner EH. Should HMOs do research? *HMO Pract* 1987; **1**: 34–7.
4. Platt R, Davis R, Finkelstein J, Go AS, Gurwitz JH, Roblin D *et al*. Multicenter epidemiologic and health services research on therapeutics in the HMO Research Network Center for Education and Research on Therapeutics. *Pharmacoepidemiol Drug Saf* 2001; **10**: 373–7.
5. Curry SJ, McBride CM, Grothaus LC, Louie D, Wagner EH. A randomized trial of self-help materials, personalized feedback and telephone counseling with nonvolunteer smokers. *J Consult Clin Psychol* 1995; **63**: 1005–14.
6. Durham M, Beresford S, Diehr P, Grembowski D, Hecht J, Patrick D. Participation of higher users in a randomized trial of Medicare reimbursement for preventive services. *Gerontologist* 1991; **31**: 603–6.
7. Pearson DC, Grothaus L, Thompson RS, Wagner EH. Smokers and drinkers in a health maintenance organization population: lifestyles and health status. *Prev Med* 1987; **16**: 783–95.
8. Andrews EB, Stergachis A, Hecht JA. Evaluation of alternative methods of assessing pregnancy outcomes using automated indicators of pregnancy. *J Clin Res Drug Dev* 1989; **3**: 201.
9. Stergachis A, Scholes D, Heidrich FE, Sherer DM, Holmes KK, Stamm WE. Selective screening for *Chlamydia trachomatis* in a primary care population of women. *Am J Epidemiol* 1993; **138**:143–53.
10. Wagner E, Sandhu N, Newton K, McCulloch D, Ramsey S, Grothaus L. Effect of improved glycemic control on health care costs and utilization. *JAMA* 2001; **285**: 182–9.
11. Boyko E, Fihn S, Scholes D, Chen C, Normand E, Yarbro P. Diabetes and the risk of acute urinary tract infection among postmenopausal women. *Diabetes Care* 2002; **25**: 1778–83.
12. Mandelson M, LaCroix A, Anderson L, Nadel M, Lee N. Comparison of self-reported fecal occult blood testing with automated laboratory records among older women in a health maintenance organization. *Am J Epidemiol* 1999; **150**: 617–21.
13. Wagner E, Curry SJ, Grothaus L, Saunders K, McBride CM. The impact of smoking and quitting on health care utilization. *Arch Intern Med* 1995; **155**: 1789–95.
14. McBride CM, Lozano P, Curry SJ, Rosner D, Grothaus L. Use of health services by children of smokers and nonsmokers in a Health Maintenance Organization. *Am J Public Health* 1998; **88**: 897–902.
15. Cherkin D, Deyo R, Battie M, Street J, Barlow W. A comparison of physical therapy, chiropractic manipulation and provision of an education booklet for the treatment of patients with low back pain. *New Engl J Med* 1998; **339**: 1021–9.
16. Davis RL, Chu S. Antibiotic use patterns and antibiotic-resistant bacteria at Group Health Cooperative, Seattle, WA. Presented at the HMO Research Network Conference, Minneapolis, MN, May 1996.
17. National Cancer Institute. *Surveillance, Epidemiology, and End Results: Incidence and Mortality Data, 1973–1977*, National Cancer Institute Monograph 57. Bethesda, MD: National Cancer Institute, 1981.
18. Taplin SH, Taylor V, Montano D, Chinn R, Urban N. Specialty difference and the ordering of screening mammography by primary care physicians. *J Am Board Fam Pract* 1994; **7**: 375–86.
19. Taplin SH, Mandelson MT, Anderman C, White E, Thompson RS, Timlin D *et al*. Mammography diffusion and trends in late stage breast cancer: risk-based guideline implementation in a managed care setting. *Cancer Epidemiol Biomarkers Prev* 1997; **6**: 625–31.
20. Mandelson M, Oestreicher N, Porter P, White D, Finder CA, Taplin SH *et al*. Breast density as a predictor of mammographic detection: comparison of interval- and screen-detected cancers. *J Natl Cancer Inst* 2000; **92**: 1081–7.
21. Grupp-Phelan J, Lozano P, Fishman P. Health care utilization and cost in children with asthma and selected comorbidities. *J Asthma* 2001; **38**: 363–73.
22. Simon G, Von Korff M, Barlow W. Health care costs of primary care patients with recognized depression. *Arch Gen Psychiatry* 1995; **52**: 850–6.
23. Taplin SH, Barlow W, Urban N, Mandelson MT, Timlin DJ, Ichikawa L *et al*. Stage, age, comorbidity, and direct costs of colon, prostate, and breast cancer care. *J Natl Cancer Inst* 1995; **87**: 417–26.
24. Simon G, Unutzer J. Health care utilization and costs among patients treated for bipolar disorder in an insured population. *Psychiatr Serv* 1999; **50**: 1303–8.
25. Fishman P, Khan Z, Thompson E, Curry S. Health care costs among smokers, former smokers, and never smokers in an HMO. *Health Serv Res* 2003; **38**: 733–49.

26. Ulrich Y, Cain K, Sugg N, Rivara F, Rubanowice D, Thompson R. Medical care utilization patterns in women with diagnosed domestic violence. *Am J Prev Med* 2003; **24**: 9–15.

27. Chen RT, Glasser JW, Rhodes PH *et al*. Vaccine Safety Datalink Project: a new tool for improving vaccine safety monitoring in the United States. *Pediatrics* 1997; **99**: 765–73.

28. Barlow W, Davis RL, Glasser J, Rhodes PH, Thompson RS, Mullooly JP *et al*. The risk of seizures after receipt of whole-cell pertussis or measles, mumps, and rubella vaccine. *N Engl J Med* 2001; **345**: 656–61.

29. Davis R, Kramarz P, Bohlke K, Benson P, Thompson RS, Mullooly J *et al*. Measles–mumps–rubella and other measles-containing vaccines do not increase the risk for inflammatory bowel disease: a case–control study from the Vaccine Safety Datalink project. *Arch Pediatr Adolesc Med* 2001; **155**: 354–9.

30. Bohlke K, Davis R, Marcy S, Braun MM, DeStefano F, Black SB *et al*. Risk of anaphylaxis after vaccination of children and adolescents. *Pediatrics* 2003; **112**: 815–20.

31. Davis RL, Vadheim C, Black S, Shinefield H, Chen R, and the Vaccine Safety Datalink Workgroup. Utility of immunization tracking systems for self assessment, improvement, research and evaluation, and linkage with statewide networks: experience of the CDC Vaccine Safety Datalink sites. *HMO Pract* 1997; **11**: 13–17.

32. Payne T, Kanvik S, Seward R, Beeman D, Salazar A, Miller Z *et al*. Development and validation of an immunization tracking system in a large health maintenance organization. *Am J Prev Med* 1993; **9**: 96–100.

33. Jackson L, Neuzil K, Yu O, Benson P, Barlow WE, Adams AL *et al*. Effectiveness of pneumococcal polysaccharide vaccine in older adults. *N Engl J Med* 2003; **348**: 1747–55.

34. Ford M, Hill D, Nerenz D, Hornbrook M, Zapka J, Meenan R *et al*. Categorizing race and ethnicity in the HMO Cancer Research Network. *Ethn Dis* 2002; **12**: 135–40.

35. Psaty BM, Koepsell TD, Siscovick D, Wahl P, Wagner EH. An approach to several problems in the use of large databases for population-based case–control studies of the therapeutic efficacy and safety of anti-hypertensive medicines. *Stat Med* 1991; **10**: 653–62.

36. Newton K, Wagner E, Ramsey S, McCulloch D, Evans R, Sandhu N *et al*. The use of automated data to identify complications and comorbidities of diabetes: a validation study. *J Clin Epidemiol* 1999; **52**: 199–207.

37. Civic D, Scholes D, Grothaus L, McBride C. Adolescent HMO enrollees' utilization of out-of-plan services. *J Adolesc Health* 2001; **28**: 491–6.

38. Psaty BM, Koepsell TD, LoGerfo JP, Wagner EH, Inui TS. Beta-blockers and primary prevention of coronary heart disease in patients with high blood pressure. *JAMA* 1989; **261**: 2087–94.

39. Heidrich F, Stergachis A, Gross K. Diuretic drug use and the risk for hip fracture. *Ann Intern Med* 1991; **115**: 1–6.

40. Lemaitre R, Heckbert S, Psaty B, Smith N, Kaplan R, Longstreth W. Hormone replacement therapy and associated risk of stroke in postmenopausal women. *Arch Intern Med* 2002; **162**: 1954–60.

41. Psaty BM, Heckbert SR, Koepsell TD, Siscovick DS, Raghunathan TE, Weiss NS *et al*. The risk of myocardial infarction associated with anti-hypertensive drug therapies. *JAMA* 1995; **274**: 620–5.

42. Stergachis A, Sheingold S, Luce BR, Psaty BM, Revicki DA. Medical care and cost outcomes after pentoxifylline treatment for peripheral arterial disease. *Arch Intern Med* 1992; **152**: 1220–4.

43. Goodwin F, Fireman B, Simon G, Hunkeler E, Lee J, Revicki D. Suicide risk in bipolar disorder during treatment with lithium and divalproex. *JAMA* 2003; **290**: 1467–73.

44. Donahue J, Fuhlbrigge A, Finkelstein J, Fagan J, Livingston JM, Lozano P *et al*. Asthma pharmacotherapy and utilization by children in 3 managed care organizations. The Pediatric Asthma Care Patient Outcomes Research Team. *J Allergy Clin Immunol* 2000; **106**: 1108–14.

45. Simon G, Lin EHB, Katon W, Saunders K, Von Korff M, Walker E *et al*. Outcomes of "inadequate" antidepressant treatment in primary care. *J Gen Intern Med* 1995; **10**: 663–70.

46. Hill DA, Weiss NS, LaCroix AZ. Adherence to postmenopausal hormone therapy during the year after the initial prescription: a population-based study. *Am J Obstet Gynecol* 2000; **182**: 270–6.

47. Newton K, LaCroix A, Buist D, Anderson L, Delaney K. What factors account for hormone replacement therapy prescribing frequency? *Maturitas* 2001; **39**: 1–10.

48. McCloskey LW, Psaty BM, Koepsell TD, Aagaard GN. Level of blood pressure and the risk of myocardial infarction among treated hypertensives. *Arch Intern Med* 1992; **152**: 513–20.

49. Leveille S, Gray S, Black D, LaCroix AZ, Ferrucci L, Volpato S *et al*. A new method for identifying antibiotic-treated infections using automated pharmacy records. *J Clin Epidemiol* 2000; **53**: 1069–75.

50. Boudreau D, Leveille S, Gray S, Black DJ, Guralnik JM, Ferrucci L *et al*. Risks for frequent antimicrobial-treated infections in postmenopausal women. *Aging Clin Exp Res* 2003, **15**: 12–18.

51. Pearson D, Jackson L, Winkler B, Foss B, Wagener B. Use of an automated pharmacy system and patient registries to recruit HMO enrollees for an influenza campaign. *Eff Clin Pract* 1999; **2**: 17–22.

52. Stergachis A, Shy K, Grothaus L, Wagner EH, Hecht JA, Anderson G *et al*. Tubal sterilization and the long-term risk of hysterectomy. *JAMA* 1990; **264**: 2893–8.

53. Christensen DB, Campbell WH, Madsen S, Hartzema AG, Nudelman PM. Documenting outpatient problem intervention activities of pharmacists in an HMO. *Med Care* 1981; **19**: 104–17.

54. Hartzema AG, Christensen DB. Nonmedical factors associated with the prescribing volume among family practitioners in an HMO. *Med Care* 1983; **21**: 990–1000.

55. Stergachis A, Fors M, Wagner EH, Sims DD, Penna P. Effect of clinical pharmacists on drug prescribing in a primary-care clinic. *Am J Hosp Pharm* 1987; **44**: 525–9.

56. Harris B, Stergachis A, Ried LD. The effect of drug copayments on the use and cost of pharmaceuticals in a health maintenance organization. *Med Care* 1990; **28**: 907–17.

57. Simon G, Cunningham M, Davis R. Outcomes of prenatal antidepressant exposure. *Am J Psychiatry* 2002; **159**: 2055–61.

58. Rutter C, Mandelson M, Laya M, Seger D, Taplin S. Changes in breast density associated with initiation, discontinuation, and continuing use of hormone replacement therapy. *JAMA* 2001; **285**: 171–6.

59. Greendale GA, Reboussin BA, Sie A, Singh HR, Olson LK, Gatewood O *et al.* Effects of estrogen and estrogen–progestin on mammographic parenchymal density. *Ann Intern Med* 1999; **130**: 262–9.

60. Lundstrom E, Wilczek B, von Palffy Z, Soderqvist G, Von Schoultz B. Mammographic breast density during hormone replacement therapy: differences according to treatment. *Am J Obstet Gynecol* 1999; **181**: 348–52.

61. Ereth J, Diehr P, Durham M, Hecht J. A tool for administrative decision-making: predicting health status from MIS data. *J Ambulatory Care Manage* 1992; **15**: 30–9.

62. Von Korff M, Wagner EH, Saunders K. A chronic disease score from automated pharmacy data. *J Clin Epidemiol* 1992; **45**: 197–203.

63. Clark DO, Von Korff M, Saunders K, Baluch B, Simon G. A chronic disease score with empirically derived weights. *Med Care* 1995; **33**: 783–95.

64. Fishman P, Goodman M, Hornbrook M, Meenan RT, Bachman DJ, O'Keefe-Rosetti MC. Risk adjustment using automated ambulatory pharmacy data: the RxRisk model. *Med Care* 2003; **41**: 84–99.

65. Wagner EH, LaCroix AZ, Grothaus LC, Hecht J. Responsiveness of health status measures to change among older adults. *J Am Geriatr Soc* 1993; **41**: 241–8.

66. Fishman P, Shay D. Development and estimation of a pediatric chronic disease score using automated pharmacy data. *Med Care* 1999; **37**: 874–83.

67. Saunders KW, Davis RL, Stergachis A. Group Health Cooperative of Puget Sound. In: Strom BL, ed., *Pharmacoepidemiology*, 3rd edn. Chichester: John Wiley & Sons, 2000; pp. 247–62.

68. Holt V, Daling J, McKnight B, Moore D, Stergachis A, Weiss NS. Functional ovarian cysts in relation to the use of monophasic and triphasic oral contraceptives. *Obstet Gynecol* 1992; **79**: 529–33.

69. West SL, Strom BL, Freundlich B, Normand E, Koch G, Savitz DA. Completeness of prescription recording in outpatient medical records from a health maintenance organization. *J Clin Epidemiol* 1994; **47**: 165–71.

70. Lin E, Katon W, Simon G, Von Korff M, Bush T, Walker E *et al.* Low-intensity treatment of depression in primary care: is it problematic? *Gen Hosp Psychiatry* 2000; **22**: 78–83.

71. Finkelstein JA, Metlay J, Davis RL, Rifas S, Dowell SF, Platt R. Antimicrobial use in defined populations of infants and young children. *Arch Pediatr Adolesc Med* 2000; **154**: 395–400.

72. Goldberg H, Ralston J, Hirsch I, Hoath J, Ahmed K. Using an Internet comanagement module to improve the quality of chronic disease care. *Jt Comm J Qual Saf* 2003; **29**: 443–51.

15

Kaiser Permanente Medical Care Program

JOE V. SELBY[1], DAVID H. SMITH[2], ERIC S. JOHNSON[2], MARSHA A. RAEBEL[3],
GARY D. FRIEDMAN[1] and BENTSON H. McFARLAND[2]

[1] Division of Research, Kaiser Permanente Northern California, Oakland, California, USA; [2] Center for Health Research,
Kaiser Permanente Northwest Region, Portland, Oregon, USA; [3] Clinical Research Unit, Kaiser Permanente of Colorado,
and University of Colorado School of Pharmacy, Denver, Colorado, USA.

INTRODUCTION

The Kaiser Permanente (KP) Medical Care Program, with approximately 8.2 million subscribers nationally, is by far the largest and also one of the oldest prepaid, group model health care systems in the United States. The KP program is divided administratively into eight regions, seven of which have research departments (Table 15.1) that conduct public domain research (i.e., research funded and conducted with the understanding that results will be published and disseminated outside the organization). With approval from regional institutional review boards, researchers in each center access a host of administrative and clinical databases, paper medical records dating back as much as 50 years, and member populations through interviews, surveys, and direct clinical examinations. Within KP, each center is a distinct entity and each uses only the databases maintained within its region. Across regions, researchers are affiliated through KP's National Research Council. Most regional centers also participate along with other health maintenance organization (HMO)-based research units in the HMO Research Network,[1] which sponsors a variety of collaborative, multicenter projects, including pharmacoepidemiology studies.

Pharmacoepidemiology studies have been prominent for many years[2,3] in the research portfolios of two research centers, the Division of Research in the Northern California region and the Center for Health Research in the Northwest region (Portland, Oregon/southern Washington). More recently, newer KP research centers have joined in multiregional and other multicenter pharmacoepidemiology studies. A hallmark of these studies is the ability to use computerized databases to identify patients exposed to pharmaceuticals of interest as well as appropriate unexposed comparison groups, and to measure and adjust for many confounding differences between these groups.

Pharmacoepidemiology, Fourth Edition   Edited by B.L. Strom
© 2005 John Wiley & Sons, Ltd

Table 15.1. Characteristics of Kaiser Permanente regions and regional research centers

	KP Colorado	KP Georgia	KP Hawaii	KP Mid-Atlantic[a]	KP Northern California	KP Northwest[b]	KP Southern California
Year research center established	1990	1998	1999	1999	1961	1964	1978
Total members (May 2004)	417 553	265 323	234 068	498 767	3 150 793	443 986	2 967 838
% Age 65+	15	6	12	8	13	12	10
Race/ethnicity (%)							
African American	4	32	1	37	8	2	9
Asian/Pacific Islander	3	4	72	6	22	2	10
Hispanic/Latino	15	3	2	5	19	4	38
Non-Hispanic white	70	58	24	49	50	88	40
Other/unknown	8	3	1	3	1	4	3

[a] District of Columbia, Virginia, Maryland.
[b] Oregon, southern Washington State.

DESCRIPTION

Within KP, essentially all primary and specialty care and the vast majority of emergency and hospital care are delivered by providers belonging to a single medical group and working within a single care system for patients of a single health plan. All clinical information from each encounter is therefore captured accurately in clinical databases shared by providers, the health plan, and researchers. Each KP subscriber in every region receives a unique medical record number that is used for all encounters with the program. This makes it straightforward to link patient records across databases (e.g., pharmacy records with hospitalizations, outpatient laboratory results, or claims received from non-KP providers) and across time.

THE KP MEMBERSHIP

KP member populations within each region are diverse, representative of the communities from which they are drawn, and quite stable. Although race/ethnicity is not routinely collected in any region, various sources, including member surveys and certain medical records, provide estimates that demonstrate rich racial and ethnic diversity of the membership in nearly every region (Table 15.1). Unlike many for-profit, network model health plans, the proportions of KP members aged 65 years and above are close to population proportions, a fact that is important when studying drugs used for chronic illnesses. KP member populations have been directly compared with their surrounding communities. In Northern California, KP members appear to be remarkably similar to the general population in terms of race/ethnicity in comparisons based on the residential addresses of members and census block group data from the 1990 and 2000 US census (Table 15.2). KP members slightly underrepresent those at the extremes of household income.[4] Slightly fewer KP members (8.6% versus 10%) are estimated to live in households with incomes below the poverty level.

Health status of KP members is also thought to be similar to that of the general population. More than 90% of commercial subscribers along with their covered family members join KP through employer groups, with no pre-qualification screenings required, and the majority of KP members with Medicare (approximately 12% of all members) "age in" to Medicare coverage from commercial KP coverage. These membership features help to reduce potential differences in health status between members and non-members.

Table 15.2. Comparisons of race/ethnicity and household income: Kaiser Permanente Northern California membership versus general population

	KP–NC (%)	Population (%)
Race/ethnicity[a]		
African American	8.3	7.1
Asian	16.5	15.9
Hispanic	19.4	21.5
Pacific Islander	5.3	5.4
Non-Hispanic white	50.5	50.3
Household income[b]		
<$30 000	5.2	6.8
$30–49 000	21.8	21.6
$50–69 000	33.8	30.1
$70–89 000	25.0	24.1
$90 000+	14.2	17.4

[a] Population data based on 2000 US Census data for the 14-county area served by KP; KP data based on geocoded linkage of residential addresses for KP members with census tract block group characteristics.
[b] Population data from 2000 US Census data for Alameda County; KP data based on geocoded linkage of residential addresses for KP members living in Alameda County with census tract block group characteristics.

KP members tend to remain in KP for long periods, especially after the first 1–2 years of membership, making this population attractive for studies that require long-term follow-up (or follow-back in case–control studies). This is, in part, because KP physicians are not accessible except through KP health insurance; patients must remain within KP to maintain relationships with their personal physician. By contrast, patients in network model HMOs often have to switch health plans to remain with the same physician. Within KP Northern California, approximately 12% of all members depart within 1 year and 20% leave within 2 years. Thereafter, fewer than 5% leave per year, so that at 10 years follow-up, more than 50% of the initial cohort remains enrolled and under observation. Retention is much higher for older patients and for those with chronic illness. In a recent study of hormone replacement therapy and myocardial infarction in women with diabetes, Ferrara et al.[5] found that only 7.5% of cohort members left the plan during an average of more than 3 years' follow-up. Similarly, Go et al.[6] found that only 4.6% of patients with atrial fibrillation left follow-up during 2.4 years' follow-up. In the Northwest region, McFarland and colleagues[7] showed that members with severe mental disorders maintained enrollment longer than comparison subjects, and had enrollment tenure similar to members with diabetes.

Although dropout due to departures from the health plan may be modestly greater than that in epidemiologic cohorts of volunteer patients, it is also important to note that over 90% of plan dropout results from loss of access to KP membership due to changes in employment or employers' decisions to discontinue KP coverage, rather than from active decisions by members to drop out of KP. This decreases risks that dropout is related in some way to risks for outcomes (i.e., informative censoring).

THE DIVISION OF RESEARCH, KP NORTHERN CALIFORNIA

The mission of KP's oldest research center is to conduct, publish, and disseminate high-quality epidemiologic and health services research to improve the health and medical care of KP members and the society at large. Division of Research (DOR) investigators access data from an enrolled population of approximately 3.1 million members in a 14-county area that includes the San Francisco Bay and Sacramento metropolitan areas, the northern San Joaquin Valley, and Sonoma, Napa, and Fresno counties. Members represent approximately 30% of the population in these counties. More than 10 million individual members have been enrolled at some point during Northern California KP's

58-year history, and the majority of these are represented in at least some KP databases. DOR investigators include individuals with expertise in epidemiology, biostatistics/biometrics, applied behavioral science, data management, and numerous clinical specialties. Close collaborative ties also exist with researchers at local universities and departments of health. DOR investigators have made contributions in pharmacoepidemiologic research for more than 30 years.

CENTER FOR HEALTH RESEARCH, KP NORTHWEST

The Center for Health Research (CHR) was founded in 1964. A program of drug-related health services research began soon after and continues today. CHR investigators work primarily with data generated in KP's Northwest region, which provides prepaid care to more than 440 000 current members in the Portland, Oregon–Vancouver, Washington metropolitan area. As is the case in all KP regions, Northwest Permanente physicians provide nearly all medical care for these members with the exception of a few specialized services that are performed under contract in the community. Records of the small percentages of emergency care delivered at non-KP facilities as well as out-of-area events are captured in the organization's claims databases. The Northwest Region also operates KP's only prepaid group practice dental care program, which currently enrolls about 190 000 members and has provided data for a number of studies of dental health and health services.[8]

OTHER KP RESEARCH CENTERS

As illustrated in Table 15.1, five other KP regions now have research centers. Space does not allow detailed description of each of these newer centers. However, each is now able to participate in pharmacoepidemiologic studies and each accesses databases similar to those described below. Work from two of these centers (KP Southern California and KP Colorado) is discussed in some detail elsewhere in this chapter.

KP CLINICAL AND ADMINISTRATIVE DATABASES

Administrative and clinical data sets are maintained in every region and are used for clinical care, payment, and operational purposes. These are described in Table 15.3. These data sets vary somewhat in content and length of implementation by region. Because of the size of the KP membership, these databases provide remarkably large and

Table 15.3. Kaiser Permanente clinical, administrative, and research databases

Database	Content	Comments
(1) Clinical/administrative databases—available in most/all KP regions		
Membership databases	Monthly health plan enrollment status, benefit structure, source of insurance	Allows follow-up and censoring on a monthly basis; insured subscribers and their covered spouses and dependents can be easily linked
Demographic databases	Members' names, birthdates, sex, physical disabilities, preferred language, addresses, and contact information	Contains information on all past and present members; allows identification of denominators by age, gender, geographic location; contact information updated at each patient visit; high quality contact data contributes to high study response rates
Hospitalizations	Hospital discharge database (UB-92), with ICD-9 codes for primary discharge diagnosis, 15 secondary diagnoses, 11 procedures; level of care, times of discharge, race/ethnicity	Major initial source of outcomes (e.g., new MI, stroke, cancer, re-hospitalizations); provides cohorts of patients with these diagnoses. Highly accurate for most diagnoses; and serves as a source of case-mix adjustment variables
Outside referrals and claims	Encounter and cost data for services authorized by Kaiser but supplied by non-KP vendors; reason for referral; ICD-9 and CPT-4 codes; billed and paid amounts	Captures hospitalizations and emergency department care outside of KP. Adds approximately 10% to total number of hospitalizations
Outpatient visits	Encounter form-based data set with date, time of each visit, ICD-9-CM and CPT-4 diagnosis and procedure codes completed by provider; department and subdepartment involved; includes provider and type of provider seen	Key source of disease prevalence data for registry building, and for comorbidity measurement. Sensitivity varies by diagnosis depending on importance and length of ascertainment window. Captures blood pressure levels (since 2000); BMI (since 2002)
Laboratory use and results	Nearly 100% of all chemistry, hematology, microbiology, pathology use, with results, dates, times, ordering physician	These are the same data reported to clinicians and included in electronic medical records
Prescriptions	Drug name, NDC code, dosage and therapeutic class; dates, dispensing and refills; prescribing physician; prescription cost	More than 90% of all prescriptions filled by Kaiser members are captured; for the 94% of members who have drug benefit, nearly 100% of prescriptions captured
Immunization	All adult and pediatric inoculations, including skin tests, occurring in KP facilities	Starting point for studies of vaccine safety, efficacy studies, as well as quality of care studies
Service costs	Fully loaded service costs for each patient encounter and service; uses an activity-based costing methodology. Fixed and variable components of cost are broken out	Costs are calculated by member, by physician, or by facility. Has been used in a number of cost of illness studies; ideal for comparison studies (e.g., clinical trials)
(2) Disease registries available in multiple regional research centers		
Cancer registries	Databases maintained by at least four KP research centers, containing a total of more than 500 000 incident cancers dating back 20 or more years. SEER-compatible data, including stage at diagnosis, treatment, and survival	Have been used in more than 200 cohort and case–control studies of predictors of incident cancers; used increasingly for studies of quality-of-life, survival with cancer. Rapid case ascertainment methods have been developed for studies that need this feature
Diabetes registries	Rich, regularly updated clinical data on more than 400 000 current members with diabetes (and a much greater number who have been enrolled and identified in past 10 years). Data typically include all medications, lab results, complications, utilization, and costs of care	These registries have extremely high sensitivity and specificity (>98% for each). In some regions they are used for provision of care as well as research. These registries have generated numerous publications, including pharmacoepidemiology studies in several regions

(3) Additional research databases at Division of Research, KP Northern California

Multiphasic health checkup (MHC)	Rich clinical examination, laboratory, X-ray and ECG data, extensive self-report questionnaire data on behaviors, beliefs, comorbidities from more than 1 million voluntary multiphasic health checkups in more than 500 000 members, 1964–1984	By linkage with other KP databases, a remarkable cohort that has generated over 200 scientific publications; still in active use for cancer, heart disease, stroke, diabetes, and dementia research. Frozen sera stored on more than 160 000 MHC-takers from 1964 to 1970
Member health survey	Triennial mailed survey of 40 000 adult members; sociodemographic characteristics, health status, behaviors, lifestyle risk factors, use of complementary/alternative therapies, opinions about illness care, preventive services	Overall survey response rates range from 48% (in 2002), to 60% (1993) but have been above 70% in those aged 65 and over at each survey. Used to provide membership level data on race/ethnicity, behaviors, health status
KP Northern California HIV/AIDS registry	Chart-review validated data on 15 000 Kaiser Permanente members who have had HIV/AIDS since 1985, including 4775 active members with HIV/AIDS in the registry. Includes hospital, lab, pharmacy, and outpatient diagnoses	Similar registries are being developed in other KP regions
Neonatal minimum data set	Chart review, automated data on >25 000 admissions to all neonatal intensive care units in KP Northern California. Captures birth weight, gestational age, diagnoses, severity of illness score (SNAP-II), multiple process measures (e.g., length of assisted ventilation). Linked to maternal hospitalization records, State birth/death records, subsequent hospitalizations, outpatient diagnoses, and costs of care	Captures >98% of all Kaiser Permanente babies admitted to any NICU, including 100% of the admissions to and transfers into Kaiser Permanente's six level III NICUs
Acute coronary syndromes registry	>20 000 patients who have been discharged with a diagnosis of acute myocardial infarction from a Kaiser hospital since 1999 and chart reviewed for validation, collection of enzyme, ECG, and complications data	Initiated to contribute data to National Registry of Myocardial Infarction (NRMI); became independent in 2002. The registry forms the basis for outcomes reports and reports on quality of MI care
Linked mortality database	Vital status and ICD-9/10 coded cause of death for all KPNC members based on annual linkage with California State and US Social Security Administration records. Probabilistic linkage scores are enhanced with additional data available only to KP (e.g., most recent residence, usual site of care)	These linked records allow researchers to ascertain vital status and ICD-coded cause of death for our current and past enrolled population. They are particularly useful for providing endpoints in ongoing cohort studies
2000 geocode database	Links home address for more than 95% of KP members to 2000 (geocoded) to block group level data from US Census	Block group data provides proxy information on race/ethnicity and socioeconomic status. Useful for comparing user groups and particularly for pharmacoeconomic studies

Table 15.3. (Continued)

Database	Content	Comments
Neurodegenerative disease registry	Contains data on all incident cases of Parkinson's disease, amyotrophic lateral sclerosis, and multiple sclerosis.Case identification based on redundancy of diagnoses, physician specialty, pharmaceutical treatment, and laboratory or radiology testing and results	
Linked birth database	Links records for all live births occurring in KPNC or allied hospitals to State birth certificate information	
(4) Additional research databases available at Center for Health Research, KP Northwest		
EpicCare®	An electronic medical record, EpicCare® captures outpatient care with coded diagnoses, procedures, and orders for pharmacy, lab tests, etc. EpicCare® includes the full text of providers' clinical notes, which can be searched by computer or manually abstracted. EpicCare® has been used at all KPNW clinics since January 1997 and describes >900 000 unique members through December 2003	EpicCare served as the prototype for Kaiser Permanente's plan-wide HealthConnect electronic medical record. Because EpicCare is updated daily for research, patients can be identified for prospective studies or surveys soon after they present with an episode of illness
Adverse and allergic drug event reporting database	The database captures suspected adverse events spontaneously reported by providers. Reports are sent to the KPNW Formulary and Therapeutics Committee	The reports are also submitted to the Food and Drug Administration's Adverse Events Reporting System through MedWatch
Immunization database	As of 1985, the database captured immunizations for all members regardless of age. Documentation has been more complete since 1998, which marked the introduction of the KATS immunization database	The database has been instrumental in conducting studies with the CDC-funded Vaccine Safety Data Link Project, a consortium of seven HMOs
Genetics registry	The Genetics Registry captures screening and testing data from KPNW (including KP Hawaii), as well as KP Northern California and KP Southern California. The Registry began in 1986	KPNW also maintains a breast cancer registry, which includes women who received genetic counseling for inherited susceptibility
Dental administration and clinical tracking system (TEAM)	TEAM has captured office visits for dental care at KPNW since 1987. It describes the dental services that were provided	KPNW is the only KP region to cover dental services and describe them in a research database. Compared with other dental care databases, TEAM is valuable because it is possible to link dental services with patients' medical records and pharmacy records
(5) Additional research databases available at Clinical Research Unit, KP Colorado		
Operational data store	Daily extract from KP Colorado's electronic medical record; available since 1999; in addition to standard clinical data, includes vital signs, weight, height, procedure orders, referrals, smoking status and exposure, and complaints	Unique availability of vital signs data enhances ability to case-mix adjust for disease severity; procedure orders useful in studies of patient safety and patient adherence

Health risk appraisal database	Contains self-reported health risk information collected from mailed questionnaires for approximately 60% of KP Colorado members	Valuable for conducting automated analyses that require adjustment for confounding variables, particularly behaviors
Perinatal database	Contains information for over 99% of deliveries and infants born since 1992. Includes 273 variables about the mother and infant (e.g., race, gravida, birth weight, gestational age at delivery, history of cigarette or alcohol use, and infant Apgar score)	Both infant and maternal files contain unique identifiers used to merge with files containing subsequent health care experience

well-characterized study populations for addressing a host of pharmacoepidemiologic questions. Membership databases allow identification and follow-up of patient cohorts by age, sex, and area of residence and immediate censoring of individuals should they leave the health plan (and study observation). Linkage of these data to census data (geocoding) can provide proxy measures of race/ethnicity and socio-economic status.[4]

Pharmacy databases capture the vast majority of all prescription drug use in KP members, since well over 90% have pharmacy prescription coverage. For example, a recent survey found that only 3.3% of members with diabetes and pharmacy coverage reported obtaining any prescription outside of KP during the previous year (A. Karter, personal communication), although of course the proportion may be different for people with other conditions. It may be advisable to exclude these very small numbers of members without a pharmacy benefit from pharmacoepidemiology studies, particularly when quantification of exposure over time or measurement of patient adherence is required. In two regions (KP Northwest and KP Colorado), prescriptions can be identified at the time they are ordered. In all other regions, capture does not occur until the prescription is filled.

Uniform hospital discharge records are available in each region and have been used as a source of outcomes data for many years in KP studies.[5,6,9–11] For endpoints not already studied and validated, chart review is often performed to confirm diagnoses.

Laboratory tests with CPT-4 procedure codes and results are valuable for assessing disease severity, physician laboratory monitoring practices, and dosage modification in the presence of laboratory abnormalities. They may also be useful for identifying certain endpoints (e.g., new liver function test abnormalities) in patients on specific medications. However, because tests are not performed routinely and regularly in clinical practice, data for specific tests will be missing for significant fractions of most populations.

Outpatient visit counts, by department and type of provider, are useful in studies of utilization patterns and costs of care associated with use of specific medications. Outpatient diagnoses are the most important data source for identifying patients with a disease and for measuring and adjusting for levels of comorbidity (case-mix). However, the validity of outpatient diagnostic data is not as well documented as for inpatient diagnoses. Several studies indicate that, when present, these diagnoses are highly indicative of the presence of the stated illness,[12,13] but there is little information on the sensitivity of these databases. For this reason, outpatient diagnoses have been used relatively rarely as a source of outcomes.

Research staff in three regions routinely track mortality for all persons who have ever been enrolled as KP members. In both Northern and Southern California, data for past and present members are linked to California death certificates using the following identifiers: SSN, name, date of birth, ethnicity, and place of residence. Linkage programs assign probabilistic weights to each purported match, allowing users to choose how conservative to be in accepting matches as valid.[14] Researchers at the CHR also link member data with state vital statistics (e.g., birth and death) records for both Oregon and Washington. In each region, these data are valuable for studies of cause-specific and total mortality. They may also help in estimating potential differences in general health status of users and nonusers of a study drug in prospective studies of other outcomes.

ADDITIONAL RESEARCH DATABASES FOUND IN ONE OR MORE KP RESEARCH CENTERS

Individual KP research centers have developed a variety of additional databases for research studies, including many condition-specific disease registries. Many of these databases are described in Table 15.3. Most are updated regularly and can provide efficient approaches for studying questions related to the natural history of these conditions, the effectiveness or adverse effects of medications, and treatment patterns.

Complete cancer incidence data for KP members are captured in registries maintained by the research departments in at least four regions. In both California regions, registries are linked to the California State Cancer Registry. In the Northwest and Colorado regions, SEER-compatible registries have been approved by the National Cancer Institute for research purposes. Data are collected in a standardized format no later than six months post-diagnosis. Key steps include verification of patient identifiers, consolidation of data across encounters, linkage of multiple primaries, follow-up for outcomes over the life of the patient, and matching to death certificate information.

Diabetes registries are also available in at least these same four regions and have been in place for 10 years or longer. The Northern California registry has been shown to have a sensitivity of 99% and a positive predictive value of 98%. The Northwest and Colorado regions' registries may be even more accurate because they are actively used for population disease management as well as research and are regularly corrected with input from clinicians. In each region, data identifying patients are merged with ongoing data on treatments, laboratory values, complications, and health care utilization. Together, these four registries count more than 400 000 currently enrolled diabetic patients.

The KP Northern California HIV/AIDS registry captures data on all members that meet diagnostic criteria for HIV infection. Verification and collection of additional information by medical record review is then performed for each potential case. This registry contains, but is not limited to, date and facility of HIV diagnosis, date of AIDS diagnosis and facility for cases that have progressed to AIDS. Similar registries are now being developed in several other KP regions.

The KP geocoded membership database for Northern California links residential addresses for 2 658 488 members who were active and had mailing addresses in the primary 14-county catchment area of Northern California as of January 1, 2000 with US Census block group data on socio-economic status and race/ethnicity. These data can be used as adjusters for socioeconomic status in comparisons of outcomes for users versus nonusers of drugs of interest.

The multiphasic health checkup was a physical examination and extensive interview administered to more than 500 000 KP members at two Northern California medical centers between 1964 and 1984.[15] Interview responses and physiological and laboratory results were computer stored and have provided a rich database on a cohort that included over 60% of adult members enrolled at the two centers. This database, often linked with subsequent outcomes provided by other data sources, has been the source of well over 200 publications over the past 35 years, and remains useful as a source of baseline information in retrospective cohort studies, particularly of older medications.

A cost-accounting database in KP Northern California provides estimates of fully allocated costs by clinical department and by unit of service by integrating utilization databases with the program's general ledger. These data are very useful for comparing total utilization and costs of care between patient groups.

KP Northwest was the first region to implement an electronic medical record, EpicCare®, covering all outpatient care since 1997. EpicCare® describes the clinical care of more than 900 000 unique KP Northwest members through December 2003. EpicCare® served as the prototype for HealthConnect®, the electronic medical record now being implemented across the entire program (see below). It supports many studies not possible with conventional linked clinical databases by capturing types of encounters not included in these databases (e.g., telephone consults), and by including more detail, such as provider orders for prescriptions or laboratory tests, regardless of whether patients decide to act on the order. This feature can provide insight in studying questions of the quality of care and of safety in large populations. EpicCare also captures full-text clinical notes, which can then be searched by visual chart abstraction, computerized search for text words, or computerized search using natural language processing algorithms to identify more complex patterns. Because EpicCare is updated daily, incident disease can be identified rapidly for administration of surveys or telephone interviews in studying episodes of illness or natural history of disease.

This list of research databases is by no means exhaustive and omits some features of the linked databases that could be used to create other population-based registries. For example, KP Northwest maintains a separate field that efficiently links mothers and their babies.

STRENGTHS

KP's considerable strengths as a site for pharmacoepidemiology studies have been detailed extensively in this chapter. By virtue of the size, diversity, representativeness, and relative stability of its membership and the increasing richness of its computerized clinical data, KP is an appealing site for conducting epidemiologic studies. The KP membership or selected patient subgroups can often be thought of as cohorts with very rich clinical information. The key computerized databases—membership, pharmacy utilization, laboratory results, and outpatient diagnoses—cover essentially the entire enrolled populations and have now been in place for at least 10 years. Thus, cohort studies with considerable follow-up (and case–control studies with similar lengths of follow-back) are now feasible.

WEAKNESSES

Several weaknesses, including member dropout rates that are somewhat higher than those in studies of volunteers, have also been reviewed. Other limitations are considered here. The first is the absence of complete, standard information on race/ethnicity or other indicators of socioeconomic status for all members. Certain databases, including hospital discharge data and cancer and HIV/AIDS registries, routinely collect race/ethnicity. Data sets constructed by primary data collection in previous studies also contain this information. These data sources sometimes can provide cohorts with complete data and sufficient size to address certain research questions.

A continuing limitation of outpatient diagnostic databases is incomplete capture of all outpatient diagnoses, particularly for those not listed on specialty-specific encounter forms. This concern is reflected in the absence of studies using these databases as the primary source of outcomes. However, these outpatient databases remain extremely useful for initial construction of patient cohorts to study treatment/outcome associations and for case-mix adjustment.

Although records of prescriptions filled may provide more accurate measures of exposure over time than patient self-reports, they are not perfect measures of drug consumption. Nor do they provide full information on what was prescribed, since not all prescriptions are filled by patients. As with most managed care formularies, KP formularies are somewhat restrictive, with one or two agents from a particular drug class being used almost exclusively. Newer agents may also be somewhat slower to achieve widespread use than in the fee-for-service environment. This hampers head-to-head comparisons of related drugs for effectiveness and toxicity.

SPECIFIC APPLICATIONS

METHODOLOGIC ISSUES IN CONDUCTING PHARMACOEPIDEMIOLOGY STUDIES WITH KP DATA

Data derived from the provision of clinical care raise serious methodologic challenges for research, regardless of the setting. Medications are not prescribed at random to patients.

They are prescribed only to patients with specific diagnoses, and among those with the diagnosis, considerable discretion is applied in making the choice of medication to be used. Presence of comorbid conditions and greater severity of the illness for which treatment is being considered affect the choice of medications used. Notably, newer or more costly medications are often reserved for patients with more severe illness and for those in whom standard therapies have failed. These differences can be extremely potent sources of bias in observational studies and are often referred to as confounding by indication.[16] Full measurement and adjustment can rarely be assured.

Self-selection biases are similarly potent and difficult to measure,[17] as evidenced by the discrepancy between clinical trial and observational findings with respect to hormone replacement therapy and coronary heart disease.[18] Patients who continue to fill prescriptions and take recommended medications over long periods are not representative of all patients to whom the medications are prescribed. Better adherence to therapeutic recommendations may reflect better self-care practices in general as well as the ability to tolerate and avoid early adverse consequences of the study drug. Most observational studies disproportionately capture persons who are successful in remaining on medications for longer periods of time, thereby giving more weight to the exposure experience of these patients.[19]

Laboratory testing, even if recommended by the manufacturer of a study drug, is rarely done in 100% of patients. Those who are tested tend to be older, sicker, higher utilizers of health services in general, and/or those perceived by physicians to be at greater risk for complications. The use of such clinical data to identify outcomes risks bias due to incomplete ascertainment unless the outcome is an event that is captured reliably in all patients, such as cancers or other serious illnesses that uniformly come to medical attention.

The increasing automation of clinical records in health systems such as KP and the ready access to patients and their complete medical records afford many opportunities to examine and control at least in part for these biases (Table 15.4). For addressing confounding by indication, a first approach is to restrict the study sample to those from a single stratum of the confounder. Restriction to patients with the specific acute or chronic illness for which the drug is prescribed reduces possibilities of confounding by indication if the disease in question is related to the study outcome independent of the study drug. It also increases the precision and efficiency of the study by eliminating collection and analysis of non-informative data from persons who were not at risk for exposure to the drug. (See also Chapter 40.) The various disease registries described above are ideal for these

Table 15.4. Methodologic approaches to overcoming biases in KP clinical databases

Bias	Analytic Strategy	Data Sources Used
Confounding by indication	Restriction of study cohort to single stratum of confounder	Disease registries Outpatient diagnostic databases
	Restriction of study cohort to new initiators of medications	Pharmacy databases
	Adjustment of analyses for comorbidities	Hospital discharge databases Outpatient diagnostic databases Pharmacy databases
	Adjustment of analyses for disease severity	Hospital discharge databases Outpatient diagnostic databases Pharmacy databases Laboratory results databases Patient surveys Medical record review[a]
Confounding by self-selection	Adjustment for comorbidities Adjustment for disease severity Adjustment for patient behaviors	Same as above Same as above Outpatient diagnostic databases Patient surveys Medical record reviews[a]
Ascertainment bias	Restriction to severe outcomes likely to have full ascertainment	Hospital discharge databases Cancer registries
	Restriction to patients in whom outcome has been clearly measured	Laboratory results databases

[a] Because of the costs of full-text medical record review, these studies are typically performed using nested case–control methods.

applications, but *ad hoc* cohorts can also be readily constructed from clinical databases for many diseases not covered by ongoing registries.

An important strategy in studies of chronically used medications is to restrict the study to new initiators of medications,[20] whether the study drug or alternative therapy. Karter *et al.*[21,22] have shown that among persons with diabetes, those who initiate a new diabetes medication during a period of time have more severe diabetes with higher levels of glycemia, longer duration of disease, and a greater prevalence of prior complications than those not initiating or changing medications. Longitudinal pharmacy data in defined cohorts allows clear distinction of new from ongoing medication use.

Clinical databases also serve to identify and exclude patients who are not at risk for exposure because of clear contraindications to the study drug or its comparator. In a study of the beneficial and adverse effects of warfarin anticoagulation in persons with atrial fibrillation, Go *et al.*[6] were able to identify and exclude more than 2000 patients from a cohort of 13 559 patients with atrial fibrillation who had contraindications to warfarin use, including many with prior hemorrhagic events. Inclusion of these higher risk

patients in the unexposed group would likely have led to a biased assessment (underestimation) of hemorrhagic consequences of warfarin therapy.

Computerized pharmacy and/or outpatient diagnostic data allow for construction of a variety of comorbidity indices for adjusting comparisons between users and nonusers of agents under study for possible differences in total prevalence of comorbid conditions. These indices have been found to predict both mortality and future health services utilization. Several diagnosis-based indices, including diagnosis-related clusters[23] and the Charlson index,[24,25] have been used to incorporate prior inpatient and outpatient diagnostic data in recent analyses. Other frequently used indices[26,27] are built entirely from prior prescription use.

Aspects of disease severity are also captured in KP's computerized databases. Stage of diagnosis, subsequent treatments, and records of relapse are routinely available in cancer registry data. History of prior coronary artery disease, a potent measure of risk for subsequent cardiovascular events, can be identified in hospital and ambulatory diagnostic databases. Intensity of therapy in diseases such as diabetes[28] is a strong indicator of future risk for many complications. Laboratory results, such as serum lipoprotein, creatinine, and liver enzyme levels, as well as blood pressure values, are generally available in diagnosed patients and may serve to stratify patients with disease on the basis of its severity.

Factors related to self-selection are more difficult to capture in computerized clinical data. Cigarette smoking is a major behavioral confounder in pharmacoepidemiologic research because of its associations with use of a variety of medications and, independently, with many potential outcomes. Historically, determination of smoking history at KP has required either patient surveys or meticulous medical chart review. In some KP-based studies, questionnaire data originally collected for other purposes, most notably KP's multiphasic health checkup database,[15] have provided sufficiently large patient samples with smoking histories to conduct pharmacoepidemiology studies.

In the past several years, managed care systems such as KP have begun routine measurement and entry of current smoking status into computerized databases in response to new data requirements of the National Committee on Quality Assurance (NCQA) for health plan accreditation. These data are collected at all ambulatory visits, but their quality has not been carefully evaluated. In 2003, computerized data on current smoking status (current smoker: yes/no) were recorded at least once for 75% of all members aged 19 and above in KP Northern California. In a comparison of these data with data obtained from random sample member surveys, prevalence of smoking in the diagnostic database was approximately 50% higher. This discrepancy could reflect selection bias if smokers are more likely to have visits, or underreporting of smoking by survey respondents. However, it is also possible that providers may be more likely to enter smoking status for smokers than for non-smokers, leaving more non-smokers in the "missing" category. Although these data may prove useful for identifying large groups of smokers, for assessing associations of smoking with drug use, and for crude efforts to adjust other drug–outcome associations, they are unlikely to suffice when careful quantification of smoking exposure is needed.

When more detailed measurement of smoking, other behaviors, health status, or attitudes is needed, patient surveys are a relatively efficient means of collecting standardized data. Though samples are restricted to survey respondents, participation rates are typically high within KP. Karter and colleagues obtained an 85% response rate in a mailed survey with telephone follow-up of the entire KP Northern California diabetes registry membership in 1995–96. Information on race/ethnicity, duration of diabetes, height and weight, physical activity, and nutritional patterns have subsequently been used in several pharmacoepidemiology studies.

Review of paper medical records has been used extensively in the past within KP research centers to validate outcomes and to collect detailed information on exposures and confounding factors. Ready access to complete paper medical records, even when spread across several offices or medical centers, remains a strength of KP research. With the advent of computerized pharmacy, laboratory, and outpatient diagnostic data, the need for manual review of medical records has decreased, but chart review may still be important for validating outcomes where complex diagnostic criteria are required (e.g., acute hepatic failure) or for full characterization of disease severity, treatments, or other potential confounders. Because of the expense of medical record review, studies that require them usually employ case–control designs, often nested within patient cohorts.

Most pharmacoepidemiology studies within KP can be designed and analyzed as cohort studies, either retrospective or prospective, because of the richness of computerized data. Monthly membership data and mortality data allow calculation of person-time denominators and multivariate time-to-event (proportional hazards) analyses. Chart review, if needed at all, may be restricted to validation of study endpoints or to confirmation of exposure or disease status in relatively small samples of the cohort.

APPLICATIONS AT THE NORTHERN CALIFORNIA DIVISION OF RESEARCH

The first pharmacoepidemiology studies at the Division of Research were initiated during the late 1960s, when Dr Morris F. Collen (director at that time) received a contract from the US Food and Drug Administration to develop one of the first computerized systems for monitoring adverse drug reactions in both inpatients and outpatients.[29,30] Although the project was relatively short-lived, due mainly to technological limitations of computer systems of that era, it succeeded in compiling databases containing virtually all outpatient diagnoses and all prescriptions dispensed to more than 217 000 members who used KP's San Francisco medical center over the 4-year period from 1969 to 1973.[30]

Early analytic efforts included exploration of methodologic aspects of adverse event surveillance.[2,30,31] In evaluating the potential of these data for identifying adverse reactions, suspicions were confirmed that the outpatient diagnosis database was quite incomplete, particularly for minor and/or short-lived conditions, likely leading to underestimation of incidence and possibly to biased estimation of relative risks for exposures. This concern persists with modern ambulatory diagnosis databases.

Subsequently, a two-phase surveillance program was developed and funded by the National Cancer Institute in 1977 to monitor possible carcinogenic effects of drugs. These analyses used both hospital discharge and KP cancer registry data, each a much more reliable and complete source of outcomes data than the outpatient diagnosis database. After exposure to a carcinogen, the induction period for cancer is often many years, even decades. Extended follow-up is needed to ensure that cancer risk is not increased. In the hypothesis seeking phase of this still ongoing study, the 143 574-person cohort with pharmacy exposure data has now been followed for more than 20 years. Four publications[32–35] of surveillance results have reported findings from biennial screening analyses during this follow-up. In exploratory analyses, incidence of 56 types of cancer are assessed in age- and sex-adjusted comparisons of users with nonusers of each of 215 drugs or drug groups. As expected, large numbers of associations are nominally statistically significant simply by chance. Many others result from the absence of data on and inability to control for known or suspected confounders. In the second or hypothesis testing phase of this study, selected associations are re-examined using more detailed data collection methods, typically in case–control designs.

One positive finding of interest since the initial screening analyses has been an association of barbiturate use with lung cancer.[36,37] The absence of smoking history data in this cohort left the question of possible confounding by greater smoking in barbiturate users unanswered. By linking the cohort to data from KP's multiphasic health checkup database, self-reported lifetime smoking data were obtained for approximately half the cohort. Using these data and as much as 23 years' follow-up, a modest increase in risk persists after adjustment for smoking history. Phenobarbital is a known cancer promoter in experimental animals.[38] Thus, this association has biological plausibility and remains of interest.

This data source has also been an important source of evidence for lack of association with cancer incidence for drugs suspected of causing cancer, including metronidazole with any cancer,[39] digitalis with breast cancer,[40] and rauwolfia and breast cancer in women over age 50 who take it for at least five years.[41]

The computerized prescription databases introduced during the past 10 to 15 years now provide nearly complete drug exposure information for all enrolled members. Retrospective studies of longer-term outcomes such as cancers using these databases are just now becoming feasible. Many studies of shorter-term outcomes (Table 15.5) have already been completed, typically by linking the pharmacy data with other computerized records or with patient surveys or chart reviews. Several studies illustrating advantages of the KP setting or important methodologic approaches are described here.

Two studies involving the recently introduced thiazolidinedione class of oral antidiabetic medications illustrate key pharmacoepidemiologic points.[21,51] This new class of hypoglycemic agents represents a novel and important new approach to controlling blood glucose in diabetes. Shortly after introduction of the first thiazolidinedione, troglitazone, in 1997 spontaneous reports of acute hepatic failure, including death, in users of this agent began to appear. As the number of reports increased, the US Food and Drug Administration and the drug's manufacturer agreed to withdraw the drug from the market in 1999. No controlled epidemiologic studies were available at the time of this decision to help quantify the absolute or relative increase in risk associated with troglitazone. Diabetes itself, particularly when poorly controlled, is known to increase risk for hepatic failure. Thus it was essential to compare risk in troglitazone users with that of other diabetic patients. Collaborating with investigators from four other members of the HMO Research Network (HealthPartners, Fallon Community Health Plan, Harvard Pilgrim Health Care, and Lovelace Foundation), researchers at the Division of Research created a cohort of more than 170 000 adult diabetic patients, characterized drug exposure over a 3-year period, identified and chart-reviewed more than 1200 possible incident events, sent 109 cases to a panel of hepatology specialists for blinded adjudication, and ultimately identified 35 cases of acute hepatic injury or failure that did not have a probable cause other than diabetes medications. The cohort included over 9600 troglitazone users. Risk in troglitazone users was not found to differ from that of other diabetic patients. However, the entire diabetes cohort was at increased risk compared with the general population. This study strongly suggests that any troglitazone-related increase in risk was much smaller than the 20–25-fold increase suggested by spontaneous reports data.[52]

Several anecdotal reports and one controlled study from another large managed care organization[53] suggested an increased risk of congestive heart failure in users of two newer thiazolidinediones. Diabetic patients are known to be at increased risk for heart failure,[54] and poor glycemic control is an added risk factor in these patients.[55] This controlled study[53] had compared patients using thiazolidinediones with all other diabetic enrollees. Most of the thiazolidinedione users initiated the medication during the study period. Most of the comparison group were on stable therapeutic regimens. Karter et al.[21] conducted a study in the KP Northern California

Table 15.5. Selected recent pharmacoepidemiology studies at Kaiser Permanente

Reference	Study association	Design and study population	Findings	Comment
Ferrara et al.[5]	Hormone replacement therapy and risk of myocardial infarction in women with diabetes	Retrospective cohort study with time-dependent covariates; 24 420 women from KPNC diabetes registry, followed for average of 3 years	Slight decrease in risk for first MI in users of lower estrogen doses (RR: 0.88), but not with higher doses, not in first year of treatment; increased risk for MI recurrence	Diabetes registry survey provided data on race/ethnicity, duration of diabetes, smoking, education, alcohol consumption, BMI
Li et al.[42]	Use of nonsteroidal anti-inflammatory agents before and during pregnancy with risk for miscarriage	Prospective cohort study with telephone interview shortly after first positive pregnancy test; 1055 KP members	NSAID and aspirin use associated with increased risk for miscarriage (HR 1.8, 95% CI 1.0–3.2), especially use near time of conception	Analyses conducted as part of a larger cohort study of exposure to electromagnetic fields and miscarriage
Habel et al.[43]	Aspirin use and risk of prostate cancer	Retrospective cohort study; 90 100 men who took at least one multiphasic health checkup, 1964–73	Modest protective effect of aspirin with higher doses of aspirin (OR: 0.76, 95% CI 0.60–0.98)	Aspirin use and several covariates obtained from multiphasic database
Karter et al.[44]	Possible protective effect of antibiotic use for myocardial infarction in patients with diabetes	Nested case–control study in KPNC diabetes registry; 1401 MI cases, 5604 matched controls	No association of any antibiotic use with MI risk during the 24 months before MI occurred	Close matching accomplished using registry data; also allowed for time matching
Sidney et al.[45]	Effects of specific gene mutations on oral contraceptive-related risk of venous thromboembolic disease	Population-based case–control study with clinical exam, interview, and DNA collection; 196 cases, 746 controls	Strong interactions of oral contraceptive use with three candidate polymorphisms: mutations of Factor V Leiden, prothrombin, and MTHFR	Pharmacogenomic study conducted in KP Northern California and KP Southern California
Brown et al.[46]	Antidiabetic drug treatment failure and person-years of glycemic burden >8%	Population-based retrospective cohort study nested in the KPNW registry with 4889 courses of oral antidiabetic drug therapy	The average patient accumulated almost five years of excess glycemic burden (HbA1c>8%) before switching to insulin	Comprehensive longitudinal linkage of computerized laboratory results from a central laboratory with prescription data

Table 15.5. (Continued)

Reference	Study association	Design and study population	Findings	Comment
Mullooly et al.[47]	Varicella vaccination program and the incidence of varicella	Population-based retrospective cohort study in KPNW children and adolescents. A total of 3514 episodes of varicella were identified from 1996 to 1999	During the study period, overall varicella vaccine coverage increased from 3% (January 1996) to 21% (December 1999); the increase coincided with a 50% reduction in the incidence of varicella	Electronic medical record used to capture telephone consults for varicella (58% of all varicella), which would have been missed by a coded claims database
Brown et al.[48]	Background incidence of lactic acidosis before metformin was marketed in the US	Population-based retrospective cohort study; members with T2 diabetes from 3 KP regions: Northwest, Hawaii, Georgia. Seven confirmed or possible cases identified in 41 000 person-years follow-up	Background incidence of definite/possible lactic acidosis was comparable to that of metformin users. Of the 75 potential cases reviewed, only 4 were confirmed—a rate of 10 per 100 000 person-years	Kaiser Permanente's access to outpatient and hospital charts for case confirmation reduced the false positive rate that would occur through a claims-only database study
Johnson et al.[49]	Discontinuation of lithium and the risk of psychiatric hospitalization	Population-based retrospective cohort study among 1594 lithium users at KPNW between 1986 and 1991	Patients discontinuing lithium were 2.5 times more likely to experience an emergency department visit or psychiatric hospitalization compared to patients using lithium continuously (RR = 2.5; 95% CI, 2.0–3.0)	Chart abstraction was performed in a 5% random sample to supplement the coded information, for example, by identifying the specific indication for lithium
Weiss et al.[50]	Use of antidepressants or antihistamines and the occurrence of cancer	Population-based retrospective, nested case–control studies among a cohort of KPNW patients (n = 1467) with breast or cclon cancer or melanoma; 95 patients suffered a recurrence (cases) and 5 controls were matched to each	Antidepressants and antihistamines did not increase the risk of recurrence: OR = 0.97; 95% CI, 0.52–1.78)	The study is one example of drug safety investigations funded by an FDA cooperative agreement to evaluate psychotropic medications at KPNW

diabetes registry that was restricted to 18 652 new initiators of diabetes pharmacotherapy. Using this design, he found that initiators of pioglitazone were not at increased risk for developing congestive heart failure when compared to initiators of any other diabetes therapy.

Go et al.[6] identified a cohort of more than 13 000 patients with nonvalvular atrial fibrillation using inpatient and outpatient diagnostic records and computerized ECG data. After excluding 2033 patients with contraindications to warfarin therapy, the authors measured the benefits and adverse consequences of warfarin in the real-world setting of clinical practice within KP. Using propensity scores[56] modified for time-dependent survival analyses to adjust for potentially confounding variables, warfarin use was associated with a 51% reduction in incidence of thromboembolic stroke, very similar to findings in clinical trials. Risk for intracranial hemorrhage, the major adverse consequence of warfarin use, was increased (relative risk=2.0) but the absolute risk remained very low, at less than 1 per 200 person-years of exposure. Risk of non-intracranial hemorrhage was not increased at all.

Suicide is a frequent complication in bipolar disorder. Concern has been expressed regarding the relative effectiveness of current therapeutic options for reducing suicide risk in this condition. In a cohort study of 20 638 patients with diagnosed bipolar disorder conducted at KP Northern California and Group Health Cooperative in Seattle,[57] risk in lithium users was found to be substantially and significantly lower than that for users of divalproex, a treatment that has been increasing in use despite lack of careful evaluation for this complication. Findings persisted with adjustment for comorbidities and other current treatments. Interestingly, the authors also identified the increased risk for suicide in those persons initiating a new therapy, whether switching from lithium to divalproex or vice versa.

KP databases are also used frequently to examine patterns of drug prescribing and adherence,[58,59] and to look at utilization, costs, and cost-effectiveness associated with use of specific therapeutics.[60,61]

APPLICATIONS AT THE CENTER FOR HEALTH RESEARCH

As part of its pharmacoepidemiology activities, the Center for Health Research maintained cooperative agreements with the Food and Drug Administration (FDA) from 1991 through 1998. One of the authors (BHM) was the Burroughs-Wellcome (BW) Pharmacoepidemiology Scholar from 1989 through 1994. The FDA and BW programs focused on pharmacoepidemiology of psychotropic drugs. Data from KPNW were used to describe utilization of anti-psychotic,[62] antidepressant,[63] mood stabilizing,[64] and anxiolytic medications.[65] These data, in turn, had impact on regulatory decisions such as labeling changes for triazolam.[66] In addition, the program generated important methodology for use in pharmacoepidemiology.[67,68]

The Safety in Prescribing (SIP) project is an ongoing evaluation of the effects of real-time medication safety alerts delivered at the time of prescribing via the EpicCare® electronic medical record (EMR). Funded by the Agency for Health Care Research and Quality (AHRQ), the alerts target prescribing for the elderly, renal dosing, and drug interactions, and allow prescribing clinicians to change medication orders to a preferred agent. The study includes a randomized intervention measuring the incremental effect (in addition to the alerts) of a group academic detailing effort, wherein clinicians were randomized to receive an educational session on medication safety. Clinician attendance at the detailing sessions was 85%. The alerts and detailing efforts were informed by preliminary qualitative work assessing clinician barriers to using EMR-based alerts, and preferred modes of education.[68]

Another quality improvement study led by investigators at the Center for Health Research examines persistence of use of β-blocker medication after acute myocardial infarction (AMI). This AHRQ-funded study is a collaboration of several members of the HMO Research Network (KP Northwest, Health Partners, Harvard Pilgrim Health Care, and KP Georgia). While rates of β-blocker therapy initiation are quite high (>90%) in HMO settings, preliminary data from this work and from the literature suggest that persistence of use is much lower (~60%) at one year.[69] In this project, a direct-to-patient mailed intervention aims to increase the long-term use of β-blockers. In contrast to many multifaceted programs, which can be difficult to interpret, this study evaluates a single inexpensive mailed intervention. Patients identified as having had a recent myocardial infarction were randomized at the clinic level to intervention or usual care. Outcomes of persistency of use were ascertained directly from pharmacy data. Preliminary focus groups with post-AMI patients were used to elicit preferences and examine attitudes and barriers in planning the mailed educational intervention.

To quantify the use of anti-thrombotic agents in patients with atherosclerotic cardiovascular disease, including both prescription and over-the-counter drugs, Brown et al.[70] mailed a survey during 1999 to a random sample of 2500 KP Northwest members whose outpatient or hospital records indicated cardiovascular disease. Of the 72% who responded to the survey, 84% reported currently using an anti-thrombotic agent: 72% aspirin; 12% prescription anti-thrombotic agent.

Predictors of current use included prior physician advice to use aspirin or prior education about aspirin's benefits in preventing heart attack or stroke. The survey also captured several milder adverse effects possibly attributable to aspirin that could not be ascertained from clinical databases.

Keith and colleagues[71,72] used computerized laboratory results to identify a patient population with chronic kidney disease (CKD) based on the National Kidney Foundation's staging guidelines. Most of the patients identified did not have a diagnosis of chronic kidney disease listed in their medical record. Patients with CKD identified by the lab test results were found to have health care costs twice that of age- and sex-matched patients without CKD. Potential undertreatment was identified in this population in that, even in the most severe stage of disease, only about half of those with anemia were treated (blood transfusion or erythropoetin).

APPLICATIONS AT CLINICAL RESEARCH UNIT, KP COLORADO

An important area of research within the Clinical Research Unit is vaccine safety and effectiveness. In a recently completed study, Ritzwoller et al.[73] assessed the effectiveness of the 2003–2004 influenza vaccine among children and adults in Colorado. During the 2003–2004 influenza season, the circulating strain of influenza A was antigenically different from strains in the vaccine and reports of severe illness were common, particularly in children. Separate analyses were conducted in children and adults. The Clinical Research Unit participated in the study in children. The KP immunization tracking system was used to provide a time-varying measure of immunization status. Outcomes included ICD-9 coded visits for influenza-like illnesses or pneumonia and influenza among 5139 children 6–23 months of age. Chronic medical conditions, age, and sex were noted and controlled for in the analysis. The estimated hazard ratios were 0.75 (95% CI=0.56–1.00) for influenza-like illness and 0.51 (95% CI=0.29–0.91) for pneumonia and influenza, indicating that the vaccine had some effectiveness against preventing influenza, despite the mismatch between the vaccine and the circulating virus strain.

Periodic laboratory monitoring is recommended for marketed drugs that carry a risk of organ system toxicity or electrolyte imbalance (e.g., digoxin, diuretic agents, metformin). Limited published information exists about adherence to these recommendations. KP Colorado researchers are currently leading a study in collaboration with researchers from three other KP regions and six additional members of the HMO Research Network. The study will describe laboratory monitoring among patients dispensed these medications and evaluate the patient correlates of laboratory monitoring. All dispensings for a large group of drugs carrying these risks and recommendations have been identified for over 338 500 individuals. Results for initial laboratory evaluation at the start of drug therapy have been assessed.[74] Fully 39% of individuals beginning therapy with one of these medications in the time frame of the study did not have indicated baseline laboratory monitoring. Medical record reviews documented that the administrative records are accurate in the majority of situations (i.e., 72%–89%). This study demonstrates the utility of linking pharmacy and laboratory administrative databases to evaluate a quality of care question.

THE FUTURE

In 2002, KP leadership determined that the organization would implement a full electronic medical record, including physician order entry and clinical decision support systems, as well as scheduling and billing software for all inpatient and outpatient settings. A contract for these systems has been signed with Epic Systems Corporation, Madison, WI, and implementation has begun in several regions (Colorado, Georgia, Northwest, Hawaii, and Southern California). Full implementation is expected throughout the program by 2006. This system will preserve the present capabilities described in this chapter, but will also bring greater uniformity to much of the data across KP's eight regions, making cohort identification and pooling of follow-up experience across regions more complete and efficient. The increased detail of clinical information, particularly that collected during hospitalizations and ambulatory visits, and including the ability to scan free text in chart notes and imaging and procedure reports, will enhance identification of endpoints, characterization of disease severity and studies of physician practices and patient adherence.

REFERENCES

1. Vogt TM, Elston Lafata J, Tolsma D, Greene SM. The role of research in integrated health care systems: the HMO Research Network. Am J Manag Care 2004; 10: 643–8.
2. Friedman GD, Collen MF, Harris LE, Van Brunt EE, Davis LS. Experience in monitoring drug reactions in outpatients: the Kaiser-Permanente Drug Monitoring System. JAMA 1971; 217: 567–72.

3. Corelle C, Bennett M, Johnson RE, McFarland B. Using SAS software in pharmacoepidemiologic research: identifying episodes of drug use and determining average daily dose. In: *Proceedings of the Eighteenth Annual SAS Users Group International Conference 1993*. Cary, NC: SAS Institute Inc., 1993; pp. 549–51.

4. Krieger N. Overcoming the absence of socioeconomic data in medical records: validation and application of a census-based methodology. *Am J Public Health* 1992; **82**: 703–10.

5. Ferrara A, Quesenberry CP, Karter AJ, Njoroge CW, Jacobs AS, Selby JV. Current use unopposed estrogen and estrogen plus progestin and the risk of acute myocardial infarction among women with diabetes: the Northern California Kaiser Permanente Diabetes Registry 1995–1998. *Circulation* 2003; **107**: 43–8.

6. Go AS, Hylek EM, Chang Y, Phillips KA, Henault LE, Capra AM *et al*. Anticoagulation therapy for stroke prevention in atrial fibrillation: how well do randomized trials translate into clinical practice? *JAMA* 2003; **290**: 2685–92.

7. McFarland BH, Johnson RE, Hornbrook MC. Length of enrollment, service use, and costs of care for severely mentally ill members of a health maintenance organization. *Arch Gen Psychiatry* 1996; **53**: 938–44.

8. Phipps KR, Stevens VJ. Relative contribution of caries and periodontal disease in adult tooth loss for an HMO dental population. *J Public Health Dent* 1995; **55**: 250–2.

9. Petitti DB, Sidney S, Bernstein A, Wolf S, Quesenberry CP, Ziel HK. Stroke in users of low dose oral contraceptives. *N Engl J Med* 1996; **335**: 8–15.

10. Sidney S, Petitti DB, Quesenberry CP, Klatsky AL, Ziel HK, Wolf S. Myocardial infarction in users of low-dose oral contraceptives. *Obstet Gynecol* 1996; **88**: 939–44.

11. Sidney S, Petitti DB, Quesenberry CP Jr. Myocardial infarction and the use of estrogen and estrogen/progestogen therapy in postmenopausal women. *Ann Intern Med* 1997; **227**: 501–8.

12. Levin TR, Schmittdiel JA, Kunz K, Henning JM, Henke CJ, Colby CJ *et al*. Costs of acid-related disorders to a health maintenance organization. *Am J Med* 1997; **103**: 520–8.

13. Go AS, Hylek EM, Borowsky LH, Phillips KA, Selby JV, Singer DE. Warfarin use among ambulatory patients with nonvalvular atrial fibrillation: the anticoagulation and risk factors in atrial fibrillation (ATRIA) study. *Ann Intern Med* 1999; **131**: 927–34.

14. Arellano MG, Petersen GR, Petitti DB, Smith RE. The California Automated Mortality Linkage System (CAMLIS). *Am J Public Health* 1984; **74**: 1324–30.

15. Collen MF, Davis LF. The multitest laboratory in health care. *J Occup Med* 1969; **11**: 355–60.

16. Salas M, Hofman A, Stricker BH. Confounding by indication: an example of variation in the use of epidemiologic terminology. *Am J Epidemiol* 1999; **149**: 981–3.

17. Coronary Drug Project Research Group. Influence of adherence to treatment and response of cholesterol on mortality in the Coronary Drug Project. *N Engl J Med* 1980; **303**: 1038–41.

18. Writing Group for the WHI Investigators. Risk and benefits of estrogen plus progestin in healthy postmenopausal women: principal results from the Women's Health Initiative randomized controlled trial. *JAMA* 2002; **288**: 321–33.

19. Herrington DM. Hormone replacement therapy and heart disease: replacing dogma with data. *Circulation* 2003; **107**: 2–4.

20. Ray WA. Evaluating medication effects outside of clinical trials: new-user designs. *Am J Epidemiol* 2003; **158**: 915–20.

21. Karter AJ, Ahmed AT, Liu J, Moffet HH, Parker MH. Pioglitazone and subsequent congestive heart failure among patients initiating new diabetes therapies. *Diabet Med* in press.

22. Karter AJ, Ahmed AT, Liu J, Moffet HH, Parker MM, Ferrara A *et al*. Use of thiazolidinediones and risk of heart failure in people with type 2 diabetes: a retrospective cohort study: response to Delea *et al*. *Diabetes Care* 2004; **27**: 850–1.

23. Schneeweiss R, Rosenblatt RA, Cherkin DC, Kirkwood CR, Hart G. Diagnosis clusters: a new tool for analyzing the content of ambulatory medical care. *Med Care* 1983; **21**: 105–22.

24. Charlson ME, Pompei P, Ales KL, MacKenzie CR. A new method of classifying prognostic comorbidity in longitudinal studies: development and validation. *J Chronic Dis* 1987; **40**: 373–83.

25. Deyo RA, Cherkin DC, Ciol MA. Adapting a clinical comorbidity index for use with ICD-9-CM administrative databases. *J Clin Epidemiol* 1992; **45**: 613–19.

26. Clark DO, von Korff M, Saunders K, Baluch WM, Simon GE. A chronic disease score with empirically derived weights. *Med Care* 1995; **33**: 783–95.

27. Fishman PA, Goodman MJ, Hornbrook MC, Meenan RT, Bachman DJ, O'Keeffe Rosetti MC. Risk adjustment using automated ambulatory pharmacy data: the rxrisk model. *Med Care* 2003; **41**: 84–99.

28. Selby JV, Karter AJ, Ackerson LM, Ferrara A, Liu J. Developing a prediction rule from automated clinical data bases to identify high risk patients in a large population with diabetes. *Diabetes Care* 2001; **24**: 1547–55.

29. Davis LS, Collen MF, Rubin L, Van Brunt EE. Computer-stored medical record. *Comput Biomed Res* 1968; **1**: 452–69.

30. Friedman GD, Collen MF. A method of monitoring adverse drug reactions. In: LeCam LM, Neyman J, Scott EL, eds, *Proceedings of the Sixth Berkeley Symposium on Mathematical Statistics and Probability*, vol. VI. Berkeley, CA: University of California Press, 1972; pp. 367–82.

31. Friedman GD, Gerard MJ, Ury HK. Clindamycin and diarrhea. *JAMA* 1976; **236**: 2498–500.

32. Friedman GD, Ury HK. Initial screening for carcinogenicity of commonly used drugs. *J Natl Cancer Inst* 1980; **65**: 723–33.

33. Friedman GD, Ury HK. Screening for possible drug carcinogenicity: second report of findings. *J Natl Cancer Inst* 1983; **71**: 1165–75.

34. Selby JV, Friedman GD. Screening prescription drugs for possible carcinogenicity: eleven to fifteen years of follow-up. *Cancer Res* 1989; **49**: 5736–47.

35. Van Den Eeden SK, Friedman GD. Prescription drug screening for subsequent carcinogenicity. *Pharmacoepidemiol Drug Saf* 1995; **4**: 275–87.

36. Friedman GD. Barbiturates and lung cancer in humans. *J Natl Cancer Inst* 1981; **67**: 291–5.

37. Friedman GD, Habel LA. Barbiturates and lung cancer: a re-evaluation. *Int J Epidemiol* 1999; **28**: 375–9.

38. Olsen JH, Wallin H, Boice JD Jr, Rask K, Schulgen G, Fraumeni JF Jr. Phenobarbital, drug metabolism, and human cancer. *Cancer Epidemiol Biomarkers Prev* 1993; **2**: 449–52.

39. Friedman GD. Cancer after metronidazole. *N Engl J Med* 1980; **302**: 519.

40. Friedman GD. Digitalis and breast cancer. *Lancet* 1984; **2**: 875.

41. Friedman GD. Rauwolfia and breast cancer: no relation found in long-term users age fifty and over. *J Chronic Dis* 1983; **36**: 367–70.

42. Li DK, Liu L, Odouli R. Exposure to non-steroidal anti-inflammatory drugs during pregnancy and risk of miscarriage: population-based cohort study. *BMJ* 2003; **327**: 368–70.

43. Habel LA, Zhao W, Stanford JL. Daily aspirin use and prostate cancer risk in a large, multiracial cohort in the US. *Cancer Causes Control* 2002; **13**: 427–34.

44. Karter AJ, Thom DH, Liu J, Moffet HH, Ferrara A, Selby JV. Use of antibiotics is not associated with decreased risk of myocardial infarction among patients with diabetes. *Diabetes Care* 2003; **26**: 2100–6.

45. Sidney S, Petitti DB, Soff GA, Cundiff DL, Tolan KK, Quesenberry CP Jr. Venous thromboembolic disease in users of low-estrogen combined estrogen–progestin oral contraceptives. *Contraception* 2004; **70**: 3–10.

46. Brown JB, Nichols GA, Perry A. The burden of treatment failure in type 2 diabetes. *Diabetes Care* 2004; **27**: 1535–40.

47. Mullooly JP, Maher JE, Drew L, Schuler R, Hu W. Evaluation of the impact of an HMO's varicella vaccination program on incidence of varicella. *Vaccine* 2004; **22**: 1480–5.

48. Brown JB, Pedula K, Barzilay J, Herson MK, Latare P. Lactic acidosis rates in type 2 diabetes. *Diabetes Care* 1998; **21**: 1659–63.

49. Johnson RE, McFarland BH. Lithium use and discontinuation in a health maintenance organization. *Am J Psychiatry* 1996; **153**: 993–1000.

50. Weiss SR, McFarland BH, Burkhart GA, Ho PT. Cancer recurrence and secondary primary cancers after use of antihistamines or antidepressants. *Clin Pharmacol Ther* 1998; **63**: 594–9.

51. Chan KA, Truman A, Gurwitz JH, Hurley JS, Martinson B, Platt R *et al.* A cohort study of the incidence of serious acute liver injury in diabetic patients treated with hypoglycemic agents. *Arch Intern Med* 2003; **163**: 728–34.

52. Graham DJ, Green L. *Final Report: Liver Failure Risk with Troglitazone.* Rockville, MD: Office of Postmarketing Drug Risk Assessment, Center for Drug Evaluation and Research, Food and Drug Administration, 2000.

53. Delea TE, Edelsberg JS, Hagiwara M, Oster G, Phillips LS. Use of thiazolidinediones and risk of heart failure in people with type 2 diabetes: a retrospective cohort study. *Diabetes Care* 2003; **26**: 2983–9.

54. Alexander M, Grumbach K, Selby J, Brown AF, Washington E. Hospitalization for congestive heart failure: explaining racial differences. *JAMA* 1995; **274**: 1037–42.

55. Iribarren C, Karter AJ, Go AS, Ferrara A, Liu JY, Sidney S *et al.* Glycemic control and heart failure among adult patients with diabetes. *Circulation* 2001; **103**: 2668–73.

56. Rosenbaum PR, Rubin DB. The central role of the propensity score in observational studies of causal effects. *Biometrika* 1983; **70**: 41–5.

57. Goodwin FK, Fireman B, Simon GE, Hunkeler EM, Lee J, Revicki D. Suicide risk in bipolar disorder during treatment with lithium and divalproex. *JAMA* 2003; **290**: 1467–73.

58. Farber HJ, Chi FW, Capra A, Jensvold NG, Finkelstein JA, Lozano P *et al.* Use of asthma medication dispensing patterns to predict risk of adverse health outcomes: a study of Medicaid-insured children in managed care programs. *Ann Allergy Asthma Immunol* 2004; **92**: 319–28.

59. Farber HJ, Capra AM, Lozano P, Finkelstein JA, Quesenberry C, Jensvold N *et al.* Misunderstanding of asthma medications: effects on adherence. *J Asthma* 2003; **40**: 17–25.

60. Levin TR, Schmittdiel JA, Henning JM, Kunz K, Henke CJ, Colby CJ *et al.* A cost analysis of a *Helicobacter pylori* eradication strategy in a large health maintenance organization. *Am J Gastroenterol* 1998; **93**: 743–7.

61. Ray GT, Butler JC, Lieu TA, Black SB, Shinefield HR, Fireman BH *et al.* Observed costs and health care use of children in a randomized controlled trial of pneumococcal conjugate vaccine. *Pediatr Inf Dis J* 2002; **21**: 361–5.

62. Johnson RE, McFarland BH. Anti-psychotic drug exposure in a Health Maintenance Organization. *Medical Care* 1993; **31**: 432–44.

63. Johnson RE, McFarland BH, Nichols G. Changing patterns of antidepressant use in an HMO. *Pharmacoeconomics* 1997; **11**: 274–86.

64. Johnson RE, McFarland BH. Lithium use and discontinuation in an HMO. *Am J Psychiatry* 1996; **153**: 993–1000.

65. Johnson RE, McFarland BH, Corelle CA, Woodson GT. Estimating daily dose for pharmacoepidemiologic studies: alprazolam as an example. *Pharmacoepidemiol Drug Saf* 1994; **3**: 139–45.

66. Johnson RE, McFarland BH, Woodson G. Whither triazolam? *Medical Care* 1997; **35**: 303–10.

67. McFarland BH. Comparing period prevalences. *J Clin Epidemiol* 1996; **49**: 473–82.

68. Feldstein A, Simon SR, Schneider J, Krall M, Laferriere D, Smith DH *et al.* Using in-depth interviews to design computerized alerts to enhance outpatient prescribing safety. *Jt Comm J Qual Saf* in press.

69. Butler J, Arbogast PG, BeLue R, Daugherty J, Jain MK, Ray WA *et al.* Outpatient adherence to beta-blocker therapy after acute myocardial infarction. *J Am Coll Cardiol* 2002; **40**: 1589–95.

70. Brown JB, Delea TE, Nichols GA, Edelsberg J, Elmer PJ, Oster G. Use of oral antithrombotic agents among health maintenance organization members with atherosclerotic cardiovascular disease. *Arch Intern Med* 2002; **162**: 193–9.

71. Keith DS, Nichols GA, Gullion CM, Brown JB, Smith DH. Longitudinal follow-up and outcomes among a population with chronic kidney disease in a large managed care organization. *Arch Intern Med* 2004; **164**: 659–63.

72. Smith DH, Gullion CM, Nichols G, Keith DS, Brown JB. Cost of medical care for chronic kidney disease and comorbidity among enrollees in a large HMO population. *J Am Soc Nephrol* 2004; **15**: 1300–6.

73. Ritzwoller D, Shetterly S, Yamasaki K, France E, Gershman K, Shupe A *et al*. Assessment of the effectiveness of the 2003–04 influenza vaccine among children and adults—Colorado, 2003. *Morbidity Mortality Weekly Report* 2004; **53**: 707–10.

74. Raebel MA, Lyons EE, Andrade SE, Chan KA, Chester EA, Davis RL *et al*. Laboratory monitoring of high risk drugs at initiation of therapy in ambulatory care. HMO Research Network 10th Annual Conference, May 5, 2004, Detroit, MI.

16

The HMO Research Network

K. ARNOLD CHAN[1], ROBERT L. DAVIS[2], MARGARET J. GUNTER[3], JERRY H. GURWITZ[4], LISA J. HERRINTON[5], WINNIE W. NELSON[6], MARSHA A. RAEBEL[7], DOUGLAS W. ROBLIN[8], DAVID H. SMITH[9] and RICHARD PLATT[1]

[1] Harvard Medical School, Boston, Massachusetts, USA; [2] University of Washington, Seattle, Washington, USA; [3] Lovelace Clinic Foundation, Albuquerque, New Mexico, USA; [4] University of Massachusetts Medical School, Worcester, Massachusetts, USA; [5] Division of Research, Kaiser Permanente Northern California, Oakland, California, USA; [6] Health Partners Research Foundation, Minneapolis, Minnesota, USA; [7] Kaiser Permanente Colorado, Denver, Colorado, USA; [8] Department of Research, Kaiser Permanente Georgia, Atlanta, Georgia, USA; [9] Center for Health Research, Kaiser Permanente Northwest, Portland, Oregon, USA.

INTRODUCTION

The HMO Research Network (http://www.hmoresearchnetwork. org) is a consortium of 14 health plans. It advances population-based health and health care research in the public domain by using health plans' defined populations, their clinical systems, and their data resources to address important medical care and public health questions.[1] Each of the health plans is home to a research unit that develops and implements its own research portfolio. In addition, these research groups work together through a variety of formal and informal collaborations. The HMO Research Network Center for Education and Research on Therapeutics (CERT) is one of several research collaborations that involve network members; others include the Cancer Research Network funded by the National Cancer Institute,[2] an Integrated Delivery Systems Research Network[3] funded by the Agency for Healthcare Research and Quality (AHRQ), and a Collaborative Clinical Studies Network funded by the National Institute of Health (NIH). The Vaccine Safety Datalink of the National Immunization Program[4] is also comprised largely of members of the HMO Research Network.

Several of the HMO Research Network members have vigorous research programs in pharmacoepidemiology, some of which are described elsewhere (see Chapters 14, 15, and 17). We focus in this chapter on multicenter pharmacoepidemiology studies within the Network. A large proportion of these studies are conducted as part of the HMO Research Network CERT, which includes 10 of the Network's 14 member organizations. We therefore concentrate here on describing the ways in which HMO Research Network members collaborate in this research through their participation in the CERT. This CERT is one of seven centers

Pharmacoepidemiology, Fourth Edition   Edited by B.L. Strom
© 2005 John Wiley & Sons, Ltd

created in response to a congressional mandate in 1999 (see also Chapters 6, 17, and 18).[5] The mission of the CERTs includes research and education to advance the optimal use of drugs, medical devices, and biological products (http://www.certs.hhs.gov).[6] Sponsors for research include AHRQ, NIH, Centers for Disease Control and Prevention, nonprofit foundations, and private organizations. We describe here our data capacity, operational principles, data development process, and the types of studies the HMO Research Network conducts.

DESCRIPTION

MEMBER HEALTH PLANS

There are 14 members in the HMO Research Network: they are Group Health Cooperative in Washington State and Northern Idaho, Harvard Pilgrim Health Care in Eastern Massachusetts, HealthPartners Research Foundation in Minnesota, Henry Ford Health System—Health Alliance Plan in Michigan, Kaiser Permanente Colorado, Kaiser Permanente Georgia Region, Kaiser Permanente Hawaii Region, Kaiser Permanente Northern California, Kaiser Permanente Northwest in Oregon, Kaiser Permanente Southern California, Lovelace Health System in New Mexico, Meyers Primary Care Institute/Fallon Healthcare in central Massachusetts, Scott and White Memorial Hospital in Texas, and UnitedHealthcare (which brings together commercial health plans in several states).

The 10 members of the HMO Research Network CERT are described in Table 16.1. They serve geographically and ethnically diverse populations with a broad age range and relatively low turnover rate; together, the health plans have nearly 11 million members, representing approximately 4% of the US population, enough to address many topics that are beyond the power of their individual populations. A wide array of medical care delivery models is represented, including staff model, group and network model, and independent physicians associations (IPA). Each health plan has an internal research center staffed by full-time investigators with expertise in the requisite research domains and who are also skilled in working with the health plans' providers, their members, and their data to perform research in a wide array of public health areas.

LEADERSHIP AND ORGANIZATION OF THE HMO RESEARCH NETWORK CERT

The HMO Research Network CERT functions through a leadership team comprised of the Principal Investigator (Dr Richard Platt of Harvard Pilgrim Health Care and Harvard Medical School), site-Principal Investigators at each health plan, and investigators at the Coordinating Center located at the Channing Laboratory, a Harvard Medical School research laboratory at the Brigham and Women's Hospital. Individual projects may involve some or all of the HMO Research Network's members, depending on the needs of the specific project and each HMO's willingness and ability to participate. Each health plan decides individually whether or not to participate in any collaborative activity.

DATA DEVELOPMENT ACROSS HEALTH PLANS

The general strategy for accomplishing research goals is for each health plan-based research group to work with its own data through the creation of either extracts (i.e., subsets of the raw data files) or summaries (i.e., analytic data files with summary variables), whichever is appropriate for a specific question. The initial phase of each investigation is devoted to creating a common study protocol and to achieving common definitions for requisite data elements. Investigators, programmers, and data managers at each site confer to ensure uniform application and integrity of a study's protocol and design. Thus, the local investigative teams, with expert knowledge of each health plan's population, practices, and records, expedite data access and ensure that data are used and interpreted properly.

To ensure consistent implementation of study protocols across multiple sites, respect for the proprietary nature of health plans' data, and compliance with Health Insurance Portability and Accountability Act (HIPAA) regulations, we have developed data management and analysis strategies that substantially reduce the amount of data that must be transferred between collaborating organizations. Source data are retained at each health plan, and often no person-level data leave the health plans. When person-level data are moved across sites, only data elements needed to support predefined analyses are transferred after appropriate de-identification. In many cases, person-level data is fully de-identified by HIPAA standards.

DATA ELEMENTS IN AUTOMATED DATABASES

Demographic Data

Date of birth and gender are routinely available. In addition, we impute race and socioeconomic status using Census data by geocoding the addresses of health plan members and linking to 2000 US Census data, using the methods of Krieger and colleagues.[7]

Table 16.1. Characteristics of the HMOs as of 2002

	Group Health Cooperative	Harvard Pilgrim	HealthPartners	Fallon	Kaiser Permanente Northern California	Kaiser Permanente Northwest	Kaiser Permanente Colorado	Kaiser Permanente Georgia	Lovelace Health System	United Healthcare
Year established	1947	1969	1957	1977	1945	1942	1969	1985	1973	1988
Structure (%)										
Staff/group	76	30	35/65	64	100	100	100	90	9	0
Independent physicians association		70		36		0	0	10	91	0
Preferred provider	24	0	0	0		0	0		0	100
Clinic sites	35	14[a]	681	22	151	26	18	11	10	N/A
Hospitals	2	21[a]	161	1	17	1	3	3	1	N/A
Staff physicians	640	802[a]	570	246	4400	725	576	230	258	0
Contracted physicians	6633	116[a]	3355	2300			1855	2366	4174	497 906
Primary care providers	420	196[a]	4411	960		326	270	807	83	249 799
Total enrollment (000s)	582	804	650	207	3200	450	368	272	239	4042
Age, years (%)										
<24	33	32	36	30	34	32	30	35	41	36
25–64	55	60	55	53	56	56	55	59	49	46
65+	12	7	9	17	9	12	15	6	10	18
Gender, Female (%)	53	52	53	51	51	52	52	52	52	49
Race (%)										
White	89	77	66	87	67	88	70	59	56	—
African American	4	17	15	2	6	2	4	33	1	—
Asian American	5	2	9	3	13	2	3	2	1	—
Native American	1	<1	2	<1	1	1	1	1	2	—
Hispanic	1	4	8	8	10	4	15	4	39	—
Other	0	0	4	0	<1	3	7	1	1	—
Retention of members (1990) (% at one year)	88	86	84	86	84	84	90	87	86	80

[a] Staff-group component only.

Membership Status

Each health plan maintains detailed information on dates of enrollment, termination of membership, and change in benefit plans for each health plan member for billing purposes. This information is usually used to qualify and identify subjects with incident drug use in inception cohorts.[8] Annual membership turnover rates are between 10% and 15% for general health plan membership in most plans. Membership retention is much higher among patients with chronic diseases. For example, Field and colleagues demonstrated that after diagnosis of cancer, retention rates for survivors were 96% at one year and 84% at five years.[9]

Drug Exposure

Approximately 90% of members have a pharmacy benefit that provides a strong financial incentive for them to receive their drugs through a mechanism that results in a claim for reimbursement. Each drug dispensing record contains a unique National Drug Code (NDC) that identifies the active ingredient(s), dose, formulation, and route of administration. Amount dispensed, days of supply, and prescribing physicians are also included in the dispensing records. Based on the NDC dictionary published by the FDA and commercial data sources, a comprehensive drug dictionary has been built and is updated regularly at the Coordinating Center. Drugs that are administered intravenously in special clinics or office visits can be identified by either the dispensing record or a special designation, such as the Health Care Financing Agency Common Procedure Coding System codes, for the particular office visit during which the drug was administered. However, ascertainment of drug exposure using these automated dispensing records may not provide a complete picture. Information on drugs that are used during hospitalizations is usually not available. Some benefit plans, for instance Medicare+choice plans, have an annual drug expenditure limit, beyond which medications have to be paid out-of-pocket by the member. The health plans typically have no record of dispensings for drugs after the limit has been reached, and do not have information on the use of over-the-counter medications.

Diagnoses

Diagnoses associated with hospitalizations or ambulatory visits can be identified from automated claims or health plans' electronic ambulatory medical records. Most diagnoses are recorded in standard ICD-9-CM codes. Plan-specific ambulatory diagnosis codes have been translated into ICD-9-CM codes for research purposes.

Procedures/Special Examinations

Hospital and ambulatory procedures (laboratory tests, radiology examinations, endoscopy examinations, surgeries, or others) are coded according to the ICD-9-CM, Current Procedural Terminology (CPT), or plan-specific systems. The Coordinating Center works with investigators to compile a comprehensive list of procedure codes for each specific study on an as-needed basis.

Electronic Medical Records

In addition to claims data, medical records for ambulatory visits are currently available electronically in six plans. Most of the remainder are adopting electronic medical records. These automated records allow efficient access to vital signs, laboratory test results, prescribing data (versus dispensing data from claims), and full-text clinician notes. Text search for symptoms and signs that are not coded in the systems described above can be conducted to identify clinical conditions that are markers for underlying diseases. One example is to search for the term "syncope," which may be a result of arrhythmia.[10]

LINKAGE TO EXTERNAL REGISTRIES AND DATA SOURCES

Health plan data can be linked with external data for research purposes. For example, linkage to cancer registries and the National Death Index have been performed to ascertain cancer and mortality outcomes.

FULL-TEXT MEDICAL RECORDS

In addition to automated data, review of medical records is warranted in certain types of research. Full-text medical records are either available within the health plan or are requested from hospitals and other medical care providers. We typically receive more than 80% of records requested for these purposes.

DATA DEVELOPMENT PROCEDURES

At the beginning of each research project, the Coordinating Center works with the lead investigator to prepare a Data Development Plan. Detailed instructions are then provided to investigators at each health plan to prepare the source data described above in standard format. SAS programs are developed at the Coordinating Center and executed at each site to qualify study subjects and generate study-specific data elements. The centrally developed SAS programs ensure consistent implementation of the study protocols across multiple sites and decrease the programming costs. For descriptive studies in which the reportable results are aggregate data,[11] site-specific tables are generated by standard SAS programs from source data at each site and are combined at the Coordinating Center to support the final analyses; there is no need to transfer person-level data.

When there is a compelling need to generate a combined data set with person-level data for complex statistical analyses, we share the minimum data necessary. Typically, none of the 18 personally identifiable HIPAA data elements is included in a person-level data set. The following processes are used to minimize the amount of detailed information that leaves the originating health plan:

- Age: date of birth is not shared. Age as of an index event, e.g. hospital discharge with a diagnosis of acute myocardial infarction, is calculated in study-appropriate groups, e.g., 5-year intervals for adults.
- Dates: occurrences of all other events of interest are specified relative to the index event, such as the dispensing of a β-blocker 35 days after a hospitalization for acute myocardial infarction or the dispensing of an anti-epileptic drug 150 days before delivery of a baby. While preserving the temporal sequence of events of interest, data prepared in this fashion have no date at the person level that is shared outside of the HMO.

Specific diagnosis and procedure codes are grouped into clinically meaningful entities.

- Drugs of interest are grouped into therapeutic classes or individual drugs.
- Composite scores, such as the Chronic Disease Score[12] or the Charlson comorbidity index,[13] are computed at the sites, and the scores (or, if necessary, their components) are transmitted. The individual data elements, such as specific drug dispensings that contribute to the score, are not shared.
- A randomly generated Study Identifier (ID) replaces the unique health plan identifier for each study subject. The crosswalks between the HMO identifier and the Study ID are securely stored at each site. The Study IDs are not reused, such that the same person identified in different studies would not carry the same Study ID. In some cases, more than one Study ID is used for a person in a single study, if the unit of analysis is a specific

clinical event. For instance, an analysis of patterns of laboratory testing associated with drug prescribing might assign different Study IDs to the same person for each of two target drugs.

- These analysis data sets are transferred from each site to the Data Coordination Center for quality check and concatenation. The combined data set, with identities of health plans disguised, is then provided to the lead investigator for final analysis. In some circumstances, for instance in some studies of quality of care, the link to individual health plans is destroyed after data quality checking.

Collectively these processes ensure valid collection and transformation of data and maximal protection of patients' privacy and of the health plans' proprietary information.

STRENGTHS

The large and diverse defined populations, the varied delivery models and practice patterns, together with automated claims data, access in many plans to full-text medical records, access to providers, and ability to work with the health plans' members are valuable assets for research requiring large, diverse populations and delivery systems. Large cohorts can be identified to evaluate incidence of rare events and to study these events among sufficiently large numbers of patients with certain comorbidities, such as hypertension, diabetes, and congestive heart failure. The diverse ethnic composition of the health plans (Table 16.1) allows for studies that are more likely to be generalizable in the US than may be the case in single health plans. While even larger populations are available from other data sources in the US, including pharmacy benefit managers and proprietary databases based on insurance claims, the health plans' access to medical records (in written or electronic format) for confirmation of clinical events is essential for certain studies.

Coordination and data development infrastructure enables both observational and intervention studies efficiently across HMOs. Human subjects committees of the health plans have approved the data development processes that have been developed to protect health plan members' privacy and confidentiality. Since its establishment in 2000, this network has demonstrated its ability to assess therapeutics for adults and children, to test interventions to improve care, and to disseminate proven care improvement methods to clinicians and to patients.

WEAKNESSES

The general limitations of health plan-based data sources apply to the HMO Research Network. The most important of these are absence of population groups that are uninsured, underrepresentation in some HMOs of the elderly, turnover of the population, carveouts of some services, caps on certain services, some constraints on formularies, and lack of information on potential confounders that are not captured in automated data or written medical records. Some of these limitations have been discussed in the sections describing the membership, diagnosis, drug dispensings, and procedures data. While the data are rich in elements related to health care, race and ethnicity and lifestyle factors such as smoking and alcohol consumption are not yet readily available. Even if medical records are available for review, certain lifestyle factors may not be validly recorded and abstraction of this information would be time consuming and labor intensive. At present, the need for study-by-study approval from each health plan's human subjects protection committee adds to the administrative requirements; the Network is working to develop simpler systems for human subjects oversight.

PARTICULAR APPLICATIONS

OBSERVATIONAL STUDIES

Study designs commonly used in pharmacoepidemiologic studies based on automated data can be readily implemented in the HMO Research Network data environment. Many studies use a retrospective cohort of health plan members with common attributes, as the high costs normally associated with obtaining exposure information for all subjects in a population are greatly reduced by availability of computerized pharmacy and clinical data. Exposure cohorts may be identified on the basis of personal characteristics, (e.g., children), drug dispensing (e.g. medications for asthma), diagnoses (e.g., diabetes), delivery of care (e.g., survivors of hospitalization for congestive heart failure), or type of care (e.g., network versus IPA, internist versus family practitioner).

This Network is also an efficient environment for nested case–control studies. This approach is often preferred when it is necessary to review medical records, for instance to ascertain exposure status. To perform these studies, investigators typically first identify HMO members with specific diagnosis, test, or procedure codes in the automated outpatient or inpatient records representing incident disease from a specified cohort. A sample of the cohort members, matched to the cases by gender, age, and other clinical attributes, can be selected as the control group. With the patient identifier as the link, information on outpatient drug exposures is obtained from the pharmacy database. One such example is a study on the use of statins and reduced risk of fracture.[14]

Underlying illness is an important confounder in many studies. We have implemented methods to calculate two comorbidity indices for study subjects: the Chronic Disease Score and the Deyo version of the Charlson Index. Either of these indices may be controlled for in statistical analyses. The Chronic Disease Score is a metric based on outpatient utilization of drugs for chronic diseases to represent a study subject's general health status, and was developed in one HMO[15] and validated in multiple HMOs in predicting subsequent hospitalizations.[11] The Charlson Index was originally developed with information based on manual abstraction of medical records[16] and then implemented with automated claims data.[13]

INTERVENTION STUDIES

Health plans are often ideal environments in which to test interventions to evaluate the efficacy and effectiveness of new therapies and to assess new methods, technologies and policies to support prescribing, to improve therapeutic monitoring, and to improve compliance with prescribed therapy. Advantages of interventions in these settings include the ability to use health plans' data systems to identify potential study subjects and to perform important parts of follow-up, the ability to study interventions under "real-life" conditions, the prospect of good generalizability because the populations are relatively unselected, and the fact that feasible and effective interventions are likely to be adopted in conventional practice settings.

Depending on the question under study, the units of intervention can be practices, physicians, pharmacists, or health plan members. In addition to conventional randomized trials, quasi-randomized designs may be efficient ways to achieve comparability. An example of a quasi-randomized study would be the phased introduction of reminder letters to patients who fail to renew prescriptions for medications intended for chronic use, with the order of the mailings being chosen in a way that is unrelated to the individuals' known medical status. Cluster randomization, in which entire practices are assigned to one or another intervention, is also well suited to the health plan environment. Cluster randomization may be particularly informative and efficient for assessing two different treatments that are indicated for the same condition.

TYPES OF PHARMACOEPIDEMIOLOGIC STUDIES

Assessment of Prescribing Practices

Description of the use of most drugs in large, defined, ambulatory populations can be achieved with large automated record linkage systems, and these data sources allow understanding of the frequency of exposure to individual drugs, drug combinations, and the indications for their use. This information can also be developed to understand drug exposure in special population groups, such as the very young,[11,17,18] pregnant women,[19] or the elderly.[20] Finkelstein and colleagues assessed information on dispensing of antibiotics for 225 000 children younger than 18 (25 000 from each of nine HMOs) from 1995 through 2000 and linked ambulatory diagnoses in close temporal proximity to these dispensings to describe secular trends in antibiotic utilization.[11] Evaluating drug use before and during pregnancy, Andrade and colleagues identified 152 531 deliveries from 1996 through 2000 and found that about 65% of the mothers received a prescription drug other than a vitamin or mineral supplement during the 270 days before delivery, and nearly half of pregnant women were prescribed drugs from category C (no evidence supporting safety) of the FDA risk classification system.[19] Two other examples are the undertreatment of osteoporosis among postmenopausal women following a fracture[21] and the evaluation of the change in utilization patterns of postmenopausal hormone replacement therapy after the publication of the results of the Women's Health Initiatives that demonstrated an increased risk of adverse cardiovascular outcomes among women receiving hormone replacement therapy.[22]

Studies of Drug Safety

Large health care delivery systems are major resources for identifying and quantifying adverse drug reactions. This Network has used its data resources to address postmarketing drug safety issues, for instance the incidence of serious acute liver injury among patients using hypoglycemic agents[23] and the association between alendronate and gastroduodenal perforation, ulcer, and bleeding.[24]

Safe Use of Drugs and Therapeutic Agents

Delivery systems are important settings in which to assess the appropriateness of drug therapy, including failure to provide or adhere to indicated therapy. With empirical data at hand, investigators can design interventions involving prescribers, pharmacists, and patients to improve safe use of medications. HMO Research Network investigators have assessed the prevalence of baseline laboratory testing recommended in the package insert of medications when patients started to use these drugs[25] and intervention studies are carried out at selected health plans to improve the adherence to these laboratory monitoring guidelines. In addition, Network investigators are working with physicians to develop and test high-impact alerts to prevent inappropriate prescribing in environments that use computerized physician order entry. An example is an alert that signals a clinician when an order is entered for a long-acting benzodiazepine and the patient is over 65, guiding the clinician to alternatives. A separate pharmacy-level intervention provides alerts to pharmacists when patients present a prescription for a drug that requires laboratory monitoring.[26] We are also testing group academic detailing methods in the practice setting to support improved prescribing in environments without extensive office automation systems. Finally, the HMO Research Network conducts interventions that target patients, for instance to enhance adherence to β-blockers after myocardial infarction.

Very Rare Diseases

The HMO Research Network large population allows assessment of certain rare conditions and/or rare exposures that would otherwise be extremely difficult to study. Churg–Strauss syndrome is a condition of vasculitis and pulmonary eosinophilia that has been increasingly reported as a potential complication of asthma treatment. Because this disease occurs in only a few persons per million each year, only resources with extraordinarily wide coverage can address quantitative questions such as the relation of Churg–Strauss syndrome to asthma therapies. This represents ongoing research.[27]

Effectiveness Studies

A related use of record linkage systems is in the evaluation of drug effectiveness, i.e., their effect under conditions of actual use, rather than under clinical trial conditions. For example, a current HMO Research Network CERT project addresses the relationship between dosing appropriateness of angiotensin-converting enzyme inhibitors and the rate of re-hospitalization for congestive heart failure.

Economic and Cost-Effectiveness Studies

Cost-effectiveness studies depend on information derived from large linked databases to estimate prevalence of conditions of interest, and specific outcomes following different treatment strategies. Such information can often be obtained from the automated databases at the HMOs and entered into complex simulation models to support cost-effectiveness studies.

DRUG POLICY STUDIES

Formulary restrictions, copayments, and other controls on prescribing or access are common features of health care coverage whose impact on overall costs and health outcomes are not well understood. For example, it is clear that in some cases caps on drug benefits result in both worse health outcomes and increased costs.[28] These restrictions have their greatest impact on the most vulnerable sections of our population.[29] An HMO Research Network CERT study demonstrated a 19% decrease in adherence to oral hypoglycemic therapy following increase in copayments by more than $10 per month.[30]

STUDIES INVOLVING HEALTH PLAN MEMBERS

The HMO Research Network conducts a variety of studies that involve direct contact with health plan members. Some of these focus on individuals with specific conditions, such as the intervention described above to increase adherence to β-blockers after myocardial infarction. Others utilize data on health plan members without specific diseases. For example, a recent study assessed health plan members' preferences about notification of medical error[31] or of the effectiveness of educational literature regarding judicious antibiotic use.[32]

THE FUTURE

We intend to continue the types of studies described above. We also anticipate placing additional emphasis on understanding comparative effectiveness of different therapies with similar indications, and improving the safe and effective use of therapies through better decision support systems both for clinicians and patients. The latter will be directed at reducing inappropriate or unsafe use, but also at encouraging appropriate therapy, particularly of therapies used for chronic conditions. These efforts are likely to rely increasingly on direct interactions, including intervention studies that involve clinicians, pharmacists, and health plan members.

ACKNOWLEDGMENT

All the authors are affiliated with the Centers for Education and Research on Therapeutics (CERTs) program funded by the Agency for Health care Research and Quality (grant number U18HS010391).

REFERENCES

1. Vogt TM, Elston-Lafata J, Tolsma D, Greene SM. The role of research in integrated healthcare systems: the HMO Research Network. *Am J Manag Care* 2004; **10**: 643–8.

2. Wagner EH, Brown M, Field TS, Fletcher S, Geiger AM, Herrinton LJ *et al*. Collaborative cancer research across multiple HMOs: the Cancer Research Network. Abstract presented at the HMO Research Network CERTs Annual Meeting, Denver, CO, April, 2003. Available at: http:/ /www.hmoresearchnetwork.org/ archives/2003abst/03_pa_50.pdf. Accessed: December 5, 2004.

3. Selby J, Fraser I, Gunter M, Peterson E, Martinson B. Results from IDSRN rapid cycle research projects. Abstract presented at the 9th Annual HMO Research Network Conference, April 2, 2003. Available at: http://www.hmoresearchnetwork.org/archives/ 2003abst/03_ca_a4.pdf. Accessed: December 5, 2004.

4. Chen RT, DeStefano F, Davis RL, Jackson LA, Thompson RS, Mullooly JP *et al*. The Vaccine Safety Datalink: immunization research in health maintenance organizations in the USA. *Bull World Health Organ* 2000; **78**: 186–94.

5. Platt R, Davis R, Finkelstein J, Go AS, Gurwitz JH, Roblin D *et al*. Multicenter epidemiologic and health services research on therapeutics in the HMO Research Network Center for Education and Research in Therapeutics. *Pharmacoepidemiol Drug Saf* 2001; **10**: 373–7.

6. Califf R. The Centers for Education and Research on Therapeutics. The need for a national infrastructure to improve the rational use of therapeutics. *Pharmacoepidemiol Drug Saf* 2002; **11**: 319–27.

7. Krieger N, Chen JT, Waterman PD, Soobader M-J, Subramanian SV, Carson R. Geocoding and monitoring US socioeconomic inequalities in mortality and cancer incidence: does choice of area-based measure and geographic level matter? The Public Health Disparities Geocoding Project. *Am J Epidemiol* 2002; **156**: 471–82.

8. Ray WA, Maclure M, Guess HA, Rothman KJ. Inception cohorts in pharmacoepidemiology. *Pharmacoepidemiol Drug Saf* 2001; **10** (suppl 1): 64–5.

9. Field TS, Cernieux J, Buist D, Geiger A, Lamerato L, Hart G *et al*. Retention of enrollees following a cancer diagnosis within health maintenance organizations in the Cancer Research Network. *J Natl Cancer Inst* 2004; **96**: 148–52.

10. Hanrahan JP, Choo PW, Carlson W, Greineder D, Faich GA, Platt R. Terfenadine-associated ventricular arrhythmias and QTc interval prolongation—a retrospective cohort comparison with other antihistamines among members of a health maintenance organization. *Ann Epidemiol* 1995; **5**: 201–9.

11. Finkelstein JA, Stille C, Nordin J, Davis R, Raebel MA, Roblin D *et al*. Decreasing antibiotic use among US children: the impact of changing diagnosis patterns. *Pediatrics* 2003; **112**: 620–7.

12. Putnam KG, Buist DSM, Fishman P, Andrade SE, Boles M, Chase GA *et al*. Chronic disease score as a predictor of subsequent hospitalization: a multiple HMO study. *Epidemiology* 2002; **13**: 340–6.

13. Deyo RA, Cherkin DC, Ciol MA. Adapting a clinical comorbidity index for use with ICD-9-CM administrative databases. *J Clin Epidemiol* 1992; **45**: 613–19.

14. Chan KA, Andrade SE, Boles M, Buist DSM, Chase GA, Dohanue JG *et al*. Inhibitors of hydroxymethylglutaryl-coenzyme A reductase and risk of fracture among older women. *Lancet* 2000; **355**: 2185–8.

15. Von Korff M, Wagner EH, Saunders K. A chronic disease score from automated pharmacy data. *J Clin Epidemiol* 1992; **45**: 197–203.

16. Charlson ME, Pompei P, Ales KL, MacKenzie CR. A new method of classifying prognostic comorbidity in longitudinal studies: development and validation. *J Chron Dis* 1987; **40**: 373–83.

17. McPhillips H, Davis RL, Hecht JA, Stille CJ. Off-label prescription drug use in children. Abstract presented at the 9th Annual HMO Research Network Conference, April 2, 2003. Available at: http://www.hmoresearchnetwork.org/archives/2003abst/03_pa_32.pdf. Accessed: December 5, 2004.

18. Stille CJ, Andrade SE, Huang SS, Nordin J, Raebel MA, Go AS *et al*. Increased use of second-generation macrolide antibiotics for children in nine health plans in the United States. *Pediatrics* 2004; **114**: 1206–11.

19. Andrade SE, Gurwitz JH, Davis RL, Chan KA, Finkelstein JA, Fortman K *et al*. Prescription drug use in pregnancy. *Am J Obstet Gynecol* 2004; **191**: 398–407.

20. Simon SR, Chan KA, Soumerai SB, Wagner AK, Andrade SE, Feldstein AC *et al*. Potentially inappropriate medication use by elderly persons in US Health Maintenance Organizations, 2000–2001. *J Am Geriatr Soc* 2005; **53**: 227–32.

21. Andrade SE, Majumdar SR, Chan KA, Buist DSM, Go AS, Goodman MJ *et al*. Low frequency of treatment of osteoporosis among postmenopausal women following a fracture. *Arch Intern Med* 2003; **163**: 2052–7.

22. Buist DSM, Newton KM, Miglioretti DL, Beverly K, Connelly MT, Andrade SE *et al*. Hormone therapy prescribing patterns in the United States. *Obstet Gynecol* 2004; **104**: 1042–50.

23. Chan KA, Truman A, Gurwitz J, Hurley JS, Martinson B, Platt R *et al*. A cohort study of the incidence of serious acute liver injury in diabetic patients treated with hypoglycemic agents. *Arch Intern Med* 2003; **163**: 728–34.

24. Donahue JG, Chan KA, Andrade SE, Beck A, Boles M, Buist DS *et al*. Gastric and duodenal safety of daily alendronate. *Arch Intern Med* 2002; **162**: 936–42.

25. Raebel MA, Lyons EE, Ellis JL, Long CL, Andrade S, Simon SR *et al*. Laboratory monitoring of high risk drugs at initiation of therapy in ambulatory care. Abstract presented at the 10th Annual HMO Research Network Conference, May 2004. Available at: http://www.hmoresearchnetwork.org/archives/2004abst/04_pa_24.pdf. Accessed: December 5, 2004.

26. Raebel MA, Magid DJ, Lyons EE, Miller C, Chester EA, Bodily MA. Improving laboratory monitoring at initiation of high risk drug therapy: a randomized practical clinical trial. Abstract presented at the 10th Annual HMO Research Network Conference, May 2004. Available at: http://www.hmoresearchnetwork.org/archives/2004abst/04_pa_25.pdf. Accessed: December 5, 2004.

27. Harrold LR, Andrade SE, Eisner M, Buist AS, Go A, Vollmer WM *et al*. Identification of patients with Churg–Strauss syndrome (CSS) using automated data. *Pharmacoepidemiol Drug Saf* 2004; **13**: 661–7.

28. Soumerai SB, McLaughlin T, Ross-Degnan D, Casteris CS, Bollini P. Impact of a Medicaid drug limit on use of psychotropics and acute mental health care among schizophrenic patients. *N Engl J Med* 1994; **331**: 650–5.

29. Soumerai SB, Ross-Degnan D. Inadequate prescription drug coverage for Medicare enrollees—a call to action. *N Engl J Med* 1999; **340**: 722–8.

30. Roblin DW, Platt R, Goodman MJ, Hsu JT, Nelson WW, Smith DH *et al*. Effect of changes in medication cost-sharing on oral hypoglycemic use among diabetes patients. Abstract presented at the 10th Annual HMO Research Network Conference, May 4, 2004. Available at: http://www.academyhealth.org/2004/abstracts/medicare.pdf. Accessed: December 5, 2004.

31. Mazor KM, Simon SR, Yood RA, Martinson BC, Gunter MJ, Reed GW *et al*. Health plan members' views about disclosure of medical errors. *Ann Intern Med* 2004; **140**: 409–16.

32. Finkelstein J, Rifas S, Kleinman K, Stille C. Parental knowledge and attitudes on antibiotic use: results of a 16-community trial. Presented at the Pediatric Academic Societies: San Francisco, CA, May 1–4, 2004.

17

UnitedHealth Group

DEBORAH SHATIN[1], NIGEL S.B. RAWSON[1] and ANDY STERGACHIS[2]

[1] Center for Health Care Policy and Evaluation, UnitedHealth Group, Minneapolis, Minnesota, USA;
[2] Department of Epidemiology, Department of Pharmacy, University of Washington, Northwest Center for Public Health Practice, Seattle, Washington, USA.

INTRODUCTION

UnitedHealth Group is a diversified company providing health and well-being services to more than 50 million members throughout the United States. The company established the Center for Health Care Policy and Evaluation in 1989 as a private sector research institute with an independent research agenda. The Center was created to foster objective public health research for UnitedHealth Group-affiliated health plans and specialty companies (such as Uniprise, which provides benefits programs to leading businesses in the United States, and AmeriChoice, which provides public sector health care programs) as well as Federal, state, and private sector clients.

UnitedHealth Group provides a link to affiliated health care plans and their electronic administrative claims data. Typically, each affiliated health plan contracts with a large network of physicians and hospitals to provide health care services. These arrangements result in access to medical management information data reflecting a broad cross-section of the population, which provides UnitedHealth Group researchers and their collaborators with unique research opportunities. The Center for Health Care Policy and Evaluation uses a subset of the electronic claims data, the research databases, to conduct a variety of customized studies, including pharmacoepidemiologic research, analyses of health care quality, performance and outcomes, and economic evaluations, often in collaboration with academicians and/or government agencies.

This chapter describes UnitedHealth Group and the research databases that link various health care services data files, and the advantages and disadvantages of utilizing these databases for pharmacoepidemiologic research, including studies of adverse events and the effectiveness of strategies for risk communication. The chapter also includes examples of such studies performed by the Center for Health Care Policy and Evaluation, and future directions for postmarketing surveillance and pharmacoepidemiologic research in this setting. Although the focus of this chapter is public health research,[1] UnitedHealth Group data are accessible for commercial uses through other areas of the company.[2,3] However, the Center works independently of these groups to maintain the confidential nature of its government-funded pharmacoepidemiologic research.

Pharmacoepidemiology, Fourth Edition   Edited by B.L. Strom
© 2005 John Wiley & Sons, Ltd

DESCRIPTION

OVERVIEW OF UNITEDHEALTH GROUP

UnitedHealth Group (www.unitedhealthgroup.com) is a national health care company serving consumers, managers, and health care professionals. Founded in 1974, the company serves more than 50 million persons through a continuum of health care and specialty services. These services include point of service arrangements, preferred provider organizations, managed indemnity programs, Medicaid and Medicare managed care programs, and senior and retiree insurance programs. Other services include managed mental health and substance abuse services, care coordination, specialized provider networks, third-party administration services, employee assistance services, evidence-based medicine services, and information systems.

UnitedHealth Group-affiliated health plans presently reach over 16 million people across the United States.[4] The health plans are located in all geographic regions and include both urban and rural representation. The members of the plans are predominantly employer-based groups but also include individuals from the Medicaid and Medicare populations. To serve these customers, the company arranges access to care with more than 400 000 physicians and 3300 hospitals. Over 50% of all hospitals in the United States are part of the network.

Although managed care is often viewed as a unitary concept and was the initial health maintenance organization (HMO) model,[5,6] plan structures vary and range from staff or group models to independent practice associations. UnitedHealth Group-affiliated health plans are typically independent practice association models, with open access to a wide network of health professionals, although some have offered gatekeeper or capitated models. Nevertheless, the emphasis remains primarily open access and discounted fee-for-service payment models.

RESEARCH DATABASES

The research databases typically used for public health research presently consist of current and historical medical and pharmacy administrative claims data submitted by 11 UnitedHealth Group-affiliated health plans that are geographically diverse, being situated in the northeastern, southeastern, midwestern, and western regions of the United States. The administrative claims research databases are large longitudinal databases, containing more than 10 years of data from 1993 to the present. In 2002, there were a total of approximately 3.8 million members and 2.8 million member-years,

representing commercial, Medicaid, and Medicare populations. For the purpose of pharmacoepidemiologic evaluations for postmarketing drug surveillance, analyses typically are restricted to those members having a drug benefit. More than 90% of commercial members and most Medicaid members in the research databases have a prescription drug benefit. Since Medicare drug benefits vary depending on the plan, pharmacy files may not capture all prescribed drugs if Medicare beneficiaries reach their drug benefit limits. The number of members in the research databases varies from year to year but is expected to continue to increase.

The research databases are used to link files longitudinally at the individual level and are organized from the following components (Table 17.1):

- *Membership data.* A member enrollment file stores demographic information on all health plan members, including dependents. Data elements include date of birth, gender, place and type of employment, and benefit package as well as linkage to dates of enrollment and disenrollment. A unique identifier is assigned to each member at the time of enrollment and is retained if a member disenrolls and later re-enrolls. Precautions are taken to safeguard the confidentiality of individually identifiable information and Protected Health Information as required by state and Federal regulations.

- *Medical claims.* A claim form must be submitted by a health care professional in order to receive payment for any covered service. Medical claims are collected from all health care sites (e.g., inpatient, hospital outpatient, emergency room, surgery center, physician's office) for virtually all types of covered services, including specialty, preventive, and office-based injections and other treatment. Claims are submitted electronically or by mail.

- *Pharmacy claims.* Claims for covered pharmacy services typically are submitted electronically by the pharmacy at the time a prescription is filled. The claims history is a profile of all prescription drugs covered by the health plan and filled by the member. Each claim specifies the pharmacy code, drug name, date dispensed, dosage of medication dispensed, duration of the prescription in days, and quantity dispensed.

- *Health professional data.* A separate file contains data on the health plan's participating physicians and other health professionals, including type and location, as well as physician specialty or subspecialty. A unique identification number is assigned to each health professional and institution. Precautions are taken to protect the identity of health professionals.

Table 17.1. Data elements included in the UnitedHealth Group research databases

Type of data	Selected administrative data elements
Membership	Health plan identifier Member identifier Date of birth Gender Date of enrollment Date of disenrollment
Medical claims: ambulatory	Health plan identifier Member identifier Physician specialty Physician identifier Date service provided ICD-9-CM diagnosis code CPT-4 procedure code Place of service Amount claimed
Medical claims: institutional	Health plan identifier Member identifier Facility identifier Beginning date of service Ending date of service Principal ICD-9-CM diagnosis code Other ICD-9-CM diagnosis codes CPT-4 procedure codes Revenue code Amount claimed
Pharmacy claims	Health plan identifier Member identifier Prescribing physician identifier Pharmacy identifier National Drug Code (NDC) Generic code Drug name Drug strength Dosage form Quantity of drug dispensed Days supply Date filled Amount claimed
Physician	Health plan identifier Physician specialty Physician or facility identifier Prescribing physician identifier Physician or facility name Physician or facility mailing address

The components of these databases are directly applicable to addressing pharmacoepidemiologic research questions regarding drug exposures and adverse events, as well as the effectiveness of risk communications. The various files described above are incorporated into internal software designed to facilitate the investigation of pharmacoepidemiologic research issues. Research capabilities include:

- *Performing record and file linkages.* Enrollment, medical claims, pharmacy claims, and physician claims can be integrated by linking members' discrete records, inpatient claims, outpatient claims and pharmacy claims to member and health professional data. These linkages allow for the analyses of episodes of care and the investigation of procedures and treatments regardless of the location of care.
- *Constructing longitudinal histories.* Information on diagnosis, treatments, and the occurrence of adverse clinical events, as coded on claims, can be tracked across time. In addition, adherence to recommended patient laboratory and other testing and persistency of use for specific medications can be evaluated. To facilitate these processes, more complete longitudinal histories are constructed by tracking members who have had multiple enrollment periods and identification numbers within and across plans. Similarly, programs have been written to combine data from physicians with multiple identification numbers.
- *Identifying denominators to calculate rates.* The research databases can be used to calculate population-based rates, and to adjust resource use rates for the effects of partial-year enrollment. Through the member enrollment file, all individuals eligible to receive medical services or outpatient pharmacy services are identified. These populations can be defined by age, gender, benefit status, period and duration of enrollment, or geography. Through the medical and pharmacy claims, subgroups of the membership can be identified for calculating the prevalence and incidence of specific diseases and conditions or utilization of particular treatments.
- *Identifying treatment at a particular point in time.* The ability to identify and track treatment is a critical function in pharmacoepidemiologic research. For instance, specific treatments can be identified using pharmacy and procedure codes.
- *Identifying cases and controls for study.* Programs have been developed and tested to identify and select cases and controls for study based on eligibility criteria such as insurance benefit status, age, current and/or continuous enrollment during a specific period of time, disease diagnosis, and covered medical procedures or drug therapies.
- *Identifying the treating physician.* For many studies, it is essential to attribute members' health care to a particular

physician or other health professional. For example, researchers may want to locate a medical record for the collection of detailed clinical information not captured in the claims data. Because members receive care from multiple physicians, logic algorithms have been developed to identify the physician who provided the majority of care or key treatments for a particular medical condition during the study period of interest.

- *Calculating person-time at risk and time of event occurrence.* The databases contain the data elements necessary to calculate person-time at risk, i.e., the date on which the prescription was filled, the amount dispensed, the duration of the prescription (days' supply), and the period and duration of enrollment for each member. The drug strength, amount dispensed, and days' supply fields can be used to estimate the total dose per prescription, the cumulative dose, or the time-at-risk above a recommended dose. Software has also been developed to calculate the number of days that members have been enrolled in the plan. Disenrollment from the health plan is a factor in establishing person-time at risk for drug exposures or drug therapy.

- *Obtaining medical record abstractions for validation purposes.* The current process to abstract medical records has been developed in collaboration with UnitedHealth Group-affiliated health plans, and has been successfully used for a number of studies. Although time consuming, the process is designed to ensure efficiency and data integrity, to protect data confidentiality, to maintain the health plans' relationship with its providers, and to minimize provider burden. The abstractors typically are registered nurses with substantial experience in abstracting medical records (they may be employed by the health plan or hired as independent contractors after signing a confidentiality agreement). Staff and their research collaborators design the abstract tool and detailed abstracting instructions, and train the abstractors. Study staff answer physician or facility questions, as well as any research-related concerns. After the removal of the patient's personal identifiers, completed abstract forms are sent for review, data entry, and linkage to the administrative data.

- *Evaluating the impact of risk communication efforts.* Successful government management of drug safety risks requires effective communication with health care providers and the public. The evaluation of the effectiveness of risk communication efforts requires data on real-world medical practice. The research databases provide nationally representative information on actual clinical practice for these evaluations, for example whether testing recommended by the Food and Drug

Administration (FDA) labeling is completed prior to exposure to a new drug.

CONFIDENTIALITY AND PATIENT PRIVACY

Confidentiality and patient privacy have always been of paramount importance at UnitedHealth Group. With the implementation of the Health Insurance Portability and Accountability Act (HIPAA) regulations, all research is required to use the minimum necessary personal health information, full documentation of such use, institutional review board approval with informed consent or waiver, and HIPAA authorization (or waiver or exempt status, if applicable) for all Federally funded research.

Prior to the introduction of HIPAA, there was concern that the new regulations would compromise health care research that required access to medical records. In a study conducted in 1998 in Minnesota, which at that time had its own stringent regulations necessitating study-specific informed consent, the ability to successfully perform medical record abstractions was reduced to a rate of approximately 20%.[7] Moreover, as part of a multi-organization study of the relationship between rotavirus vaccination and intussusception,[8] in which medical record abstraction for case validation took place at two points in time shortly before and after the passage of HIPAA, the medical records abstraction completion rate for UnitedHealth Group's network of hospitals and physicians' offices dropped from 100% to 73%.[9] However, in a recent investigation conducted post-HIPAA implementation, 90% of the hospital medical record abstractions were successfully completed. This may reflect the reliance on institutional procedures and processes as part of HIPAA implementation so that, with less uncertainty, participation increased. However, participation is likely to vary by specific hospital or physician office in each study, thereby affecting abstraction completion rates.

STRENGTHS

The research databases provide an efficient and unobtrusive method to identify and study exposures to prescription drugs and biologics. Further, drug or biologic utilization and potential adverse events identified within United-Health Group-affiliated plans reflect usual practice within the general medical community. Whereas clinical trials for new drugs are typically conducted in university or other unique settings to determine efficacy, postmarketing surveillance enables researchers to determine the effectiveness when usage has diffused to the broader medical community.[10]

The varied types of plan locations and differences in characteristics of populations, in combination with the large size of the databases, provide unique advantages to conduct pharmacoepidemiologic research studies. The diverse demographic characteristics of members increase the utility of these databases when conducting this type of research. Specifically, populations of children (almost 1 million in 2000), pregnant women (approximately 32 000 deliveries in 2000), and the elderly (over 210 000 were 65 years of age or older in 2000) in the research databases are sufficient for most analyses. In addition, the use of these standardized databases provides both numerators and denominators for exposures to drugs and allows the estimation of incidence and prevalence. Further, rare exposures and rare outcomes (such as birth defects) can be detected given the size of the databases. Table 17.2 provides a listing of the top 25 drug exposures for health plan members in 2002, ranked by the number of members available for analysis.

The databases also provide the ability to link various types of files longitudinally for individual members regardless of the site of service, as described above. Thus, adverse events and outcomes may be analyzed considering temporality in relation to drug exposure through pharmacy claims and linking such varied health services as hospitalization, emergency department use, physician visits, and any other site of health care service. Further, with respect to pharmacy claims, the prescribing physicians can be determined as well as their specialty and location. Claims submissions are generally complete, since claims must be submitted by health professionals for payment in most of the UnitedHealth Group-affiliated health plans.

Several studies that utilize other data sources in addition to administrative data have been conducted, including medical records information and surveys. As Iezzoni[11] suggests, administrative claims data are useful for quality assessment and as a screening tool to identify quality problems. Similarly, the databases can be used to identify cases and controls or cohorts for study[5] and additional information then can be obtained from medical records. This supplemental information can be crucial in pharmacoepidemiologic research studies. For example, through the abstraction of medical records, one can confirm a diagnosis and obtain additional information on risk factors and outcomes. Building on the above strengths of the administrative claims data, supplemented by other data sources, UnitedHealth Group has had experience conducting both cohort and case–control studies.

Table 17.2. Top 25 outpatient prescription drugs from 11 UnitedHealth Group health plans in 2002

Drug name	No. of members	No. of prescriptions
Amoxicillin	384 174	516 073
Azithromycin	300 852	387 059
Acetaminophen w/hydrocodone	264 633	597 764
Amoxicillin w/potassium clavulanate	179 555	230 678
Cephalexin	157 596	194 055
Albuterol	111 953	235 995
Ibuprofen	111 034	169 961
Atorvastatin	109 174	603 764
Acetaminophen w/ propoxyphene	109 104	216 560
Acetaminophen w/ oxycodone	102 615	172 863
Prednisone	101 006	174 887
Levothyroxine	97 721	654 086
Cetirizine	87 474	231 652
Loratadine	86 503	225 331
Fexofenadine	84 403	226 063
Ciprofloxacin	84 333	109 604
Sulfamethoxazole w/trimethoprim	83 525	115 602
Acetaminophen w/codeine	82 162	121 055
Naproxen	81 921	133 290
Levofloxacin	81 802	107 206
Alprazolam	77 943	287 092
Methylprednisolone	75 896	90 603
Clarithromycin	75 088	90 230
Penicillin V	68 814	82 523
Fluconazole	66 443	109 930

WEAKNESSES

Large databases must be used "judiciously"[12] and require recognition of limitations as well as advantages.[13] The constraints of a database must be recognized in order to fully understand and utilize data appropriately.[6,14–16]

For the research databases described above, there are certain structural constraints that limit access to obtaining all possible prescription drug claims. Like many other resources for pharmacy management services, data on the use of inpatient drugs are not available. In addition, given the pharmacy benefit structure, if the cost of a prescription drug is lower than the copayment amount, the prescription may not be included in the database since no prescription claim may be submitted. Overall, if a drug is not covered on the preferred drug list, exposures to that specific drug may be limited since the copayment is higher. As the list of exposures for the top 25 drugs suggests (Table 17.2), drug exposure is sizable. However, these omissions have implications both to sample size, and to controlling for confounding by the omitted drugs.

A limitation of claims data with respect to characterizing exposure to drugs is a lack of information on patient adherence with the therapeutic regimen. A number of fields related to filling a prescription are provided in the pharmacy claim, such as dates filled, amount dispensed, and days' supply that allow for proxy measures of adherence and persistency.

With respect to the completeness of the databases, some plans that have different financial incentives from the typical discounted fee-for-service mechanism may not have complete data. If reimbursement to a specialist is capitated and there is no requirement to submit a bill for payment, that service may not be included as part of the databases. This disadvantage may be addressed by excluding this small number of plans from data extraction for research studies. Another disadvantage is that certain variables that would be of interest are not available in the electronic claims databases, e.g., race/ethnicity and cigarette smoking history. If necessary for a specific study, this information may be determined through a review of the medical record. However, since medical records are not standardized, it is possible that this information still may not be available.

Another limitation is the claims lag or the length of time required to obtain all claims for a given time frame. The claims lag is short for pharmacy claims (1 month) but is longer for physician and facility claims (7–8 months). The claims lag may be variable across study years and should be taken into account in the design of a study.

Since approximately 90% of the members are enrolled in employment-based plans, the elderly are under-represented in the research databases. To some extent, this is reflected in the order of the medications in Table 17.2. Thus, the data cannot be used to estimate total population-based health care utilization, but they can provide reliable estimates for persons under the age of 65 years.

In summary, certain disadvantages of using the administrative claims databases may be taken into account or minimized through study design or the use of proxy measures. Others must be noted in the study findings. The following examples provide empirical information on both the strengths and limitations of the data and present specific applications of the utilization of the databases to address pharmacoepidemiologic research questions.

PARTICULAR APPLICATIONS

DRUG UTILIZATION

There is a lack of systematic evaluation of the pediatric use of psychotropic medications in the United States, despite widespread interest and concern. This situation led to a retrospective observational study being carried out to describe the ambulatory use of psychotropic drugs by children and adolescents in a large, geographically diverse population.[17] Administrative claims data for 1995–1999 for members under the age of 20 years in six affiliated health plans were used to calculate the prevalence of use of four major therapeutic drug classes relevant to the treatment of attention-deficit hyperactivity disorder or depression: central nervous system stimulants (CNSSs), selective serotonin reuptake inhibitors (SSRIs), tricyclic antidepressants (TCAs), and other antidepressants. Changes over time by age, gender, geographic region, and prescriber specialty were analyzed in each drug group.

The prevalence of CNSS, SSRI, and other antidepressant use increased steadily over the 5-year study period (23.8 to 30.0 per 1000, 7.9 to 12.8 per 1000, and 1.9 to 5.6 per 1000, respectively), whereas TCA use fell from 5.2 to 4.1 per 1000. Use of CNSSs and TCAs was consistently higher among males and use of SSRIs was consistently higher among females. The prevalence of CNSS and SSRI use varied across the six health plans and, interestingly, the plan with the lowest prevalence of CNSS use had the highest prevalence of SSRI use. Pediatricians were the most frequent prescribers of CNSSs, while psychiatrists were most likely to prescribe SSRIs.

Another drug utilization study evaluated the use of ticlopidine and clopidogrel in association with percutaneous coronary revascularization procedures in 12 affiliated health plans over the three-year period 1996–1998.[18] At the time, such use was considered "off-label" and common, especially in individuals aged less than 60 years. More than three-quarters of coronary stent patients in 1998 filled a prescription for either drug within two weeks of implantation. Subsequently, ticlopidine and clopidogrel were labeled for this indication.

ADVERSE EVENT EVALUATION

Troglitazone was the first thiazolidinedione approved in the United States for the treatment of type 2 diabetes. Its mechanism of action differed from other oral antidiabetic agents by increasing the response of muscle and adipose tissue to circulating insulin.[19] During the clinical trial phase, serum liver transaminase levels greater than three times the upper limit of the normal range were found in 1.9% of the troglitazone treated patients and three patients developed jaundice.

Soon after marketing began in March 1997, cases of acute liver failure (ALF) in patients taking troglitazone were reported to the FDA. Letters were sent to physicians warning of the risk of ALF and recommending regular liver enzyme monitoring,[20] but cases continued to be reported to the FDA and elsewhere.[21–26] The FDA convened an advisory committee in March 1999 to review data on 43 US cases of ALF and to decide whether troglitazone should be discontinued. However, the drug remained on the market for another year, by which time 94 cases of ALF had been reported. A study was performed in collaboration with the CDER to estimate the incidence rates of idiopathic ALF and hospitalized acute liver injury in a large, inception cohort of troglitazone users.[27]

The administrative claims data were used to identify members from 12 health plans with at least one troglitazone prescription between April 1, 1997 and December 31, 1998, who had a minimum of 90 days of continuous enrollment before their index (first) troglitazone prescription during the study period. Person-years of exposure to troglitazone were calculated for each patient based on the cumulative days' supply of all prescriptions filled during the observation time period.

The hospital claims data were searched for International Classification of Diseases (ICD-9-CM) and current procedural terminology (CPT-4) codes to identify hospitalizations indicating a discharge diagnosis of liver disease or procedures suggesting possible liver disease, e.g., liver biopsy or transplantation, occurring after the date of the index prescription. Claims data for the patients identified were examined for evidence of other conditions, such as viral hepatitis, metastatic cancer, or chronic liver disease, which might explain the liver disorder. For those patients whose administrative claims data were suggestive of ALF or inconclusive, hospital medical records were reviewed. For a diagnosis of ALF, hepatic encephalopathy, liver transplantation, or death in the setting of acute, severe liver injury was required.

A total of 7568 patients with 4020 person-years of exposure to troglitazone were identified for the inception cohort. Of 19 patients who had a liver-related hospitalization after their index prescription, 10 were excluded on the basis of the review of their claims data. Medical records were sought for the other nine patients. The record for one patient could not be obtained because it was a psychiatric admission and another was found to be a claims error. Of the remaining seven, one patient had hemachromatosis with cirrhosis and another had hepatitis C. For the other five patients, acute liver injury was documented in the hospital records for which alternative explanations were not apparent (Table 17.3).

Table 17.3. Summary of five patients hospitalized with troglitazone-induced acute liver failure[a]

Age (years)	Sex	Outcome	Duration of troglitazone use (months)	Other diabetes therapy	Alanine aminotransferase[b] (IU/L)	Aspartate aminotransferase[b] (IU/L)	Total bilirubin[b] (mg/dl)	Alkaline phosphatase[b] (IU/L)	Medical procedures[c]
55[de]	F	Discharged with jaundice	1	Insulin	167 (≤40)	171 (5–40)	10.4 (≤1.5)	315 (4–120)	ERCP: normal Liver ultrasound: normal
57	M	Recovered	9	Insulin Metformin	978 (10–60)	1266 (10–43)	12.5 (≤1.0)	217 (42–121)	CT of abdomen: no liver abnormality noted
67[d]	F	Recovered	5	Insulin	62 (4–40)	97 (15–45)	3.1 (<1.5)	63 (37–117)	CT of abdomen: normal
77[f]	M	Recovered	0.5	Insulin	97	338 (5–45)			
85[d]	M	Died	5	Insulin	608 (10–45)	416 (10–45)	15.6 (≤1.0)	144 (50–136)	ERCP: normal Liver ultrasound: normal

[a] Patients were initially identified from claims data and additional clinical data were obtained from medical record abstractions.
[b] Relevant normal ranges in parentheses.
[c] ERCP, endoscopic retrograde cholangiopancreatography; CT, computerized tomography.
[d] Patients had documented normal serum transaminase levels before onset of liver injury.
[e] Patient enrollment ended shortly after hospital discharge and eventual outcome unknown.
[f] Patient had "normal laboratory evaluation" before onset of liver injury.
Reproduced by permission of the American Journal of Gastroenterology.[27]

In four of these, hospitalization was judged to be the direct result of troglitazone-induced hepatotoxicity, while in the fifth patient, elevated serum transaminase and creatinine kinase levels were noted after admission for a urinary tract infection and were diagnosed as troglitazone-related. The estimated incidence rates of acute idiopathic liver injury per million person-years, with 95% confidence intervals, were 1244 (404, 2900) for hospitalization ($n=5$), 995 (271, 2546) for hospitalized jaundice ($n=4$), and 240 (6, 1385) for ALF ($n=1$).

IMPACT OF RISK COMMUNICATION

As the number of cases of ALF in patients taking troglitazone reported to the FDA increased, four separate "Dear Healthcare Professional" letters were sent by the manufacturer to physicians nationwide, each successively recommending an increase in liver enzyme monitoring, and associated changes were made to the drug's labeling. These risk management efforts provided an opportunity to study their impact on behavior and to assess their effectiveness.[20]

Claims data from UnitedHealth Group-affiliated health plans were used to establish four cohorts of troglitazone patients with at least 90 days of enrollment before their first prescription for this drug during four consecutive time periods representing four progressively stringent liver monitoring recommendations (Table 17.4). The proportion of eligible patients in each cohort that received baseline, monthly (for up to six months of continuous use) and complete (baseline and monthly) enzyme monitoring, based on computerized laboratory claim records, was evaluated.

Baseline testing increased from 15% before any FDA liver enzyme monitoring recommendations (cohort 1) to 45% following four separate FDA interventions (cohort 4). In cohort 4, 33% of the patients had follow-up testing after one month of troglitazone treatment, which fell to 13% after five months of continuous use. In all four cohorts, less than 5% received all the recommended enzyme tests by the third month of continuous use, indicating that the risk management efforts did not achieve meaningful or sustained improvement. The study concluded that further evaluation of the impact of FDA regulatory actions and risk communication is required.

More recently, the effect of risk communications concerning the need for tuberculin skin testing before commencing therapy with infliximab, a tumor necrosis factor α antagonist biologic product used to treat serious inflammatory diseases, has been assessed.[28] Infliximab was first marketed in late 1998 and, by May 2001, 70 patients were reported to the FDA to have tuberculosis following infliximab therapy.[29] Subsequently, a range of increasingly stringent risk communications and labeling changes occurred, including the recommendation for tuberculin skin testing. The communications included "Dear Healthcare Professional" letters sent to rheumatologists and gastroenterologists, pharmaceutical company education efforts, presented and published scientific reports of tuberculosis cases, and FDA advisory committee meetings. Preliminary results from the evaluation of the effect of these communications[28] suggest that recommended tuberculin skin testing prior to infliximab therapy increased two-fold but remains much less than optimal. Moreover, over time the testing was increasingly completed prior to exposure to infliximab, as recommended in the labeling.

THE FUTURE

Postmarketing surveillance and pharmacoepidemiologic research studies are, by necessity, conducted in the context of a rapidly changing health care environment. Looking to the future, this dynamic environment has implications

Table 17.4. The four cohorts used to investigate the impact of progressively stringent liver monitoring recommendations for troglitazone

Study cohort	Inclusive dates	Liver enzyme monitoring recommendations	Cohort size
1	Apr. 1, 1997–Oct. 27, 1997	None	2307
2	Dec. 1, 1997–Jun. 30, 1998	Baseline, monthly, 6 times	2823
3	Jul. 28, 1998–Jan. 26, 1999	Baseline, monthly, 8 times	1673
4	Mar. 26, 1999–Sep. 24, 1999	After advisory meeting, baseline, monthly, 12 times from mid-June to end of period	800

Reproduced by permission of the *Journal of the American Medical Association*.[20]

for the nature of the data obtained, the ability to obtain information, and the characteristics of the general and specific populations that form the basis of these types of studies. Changes in the health care system, given the concern with the rising cost of health care, will continue to impact the health benefits structure, including pharmacy benefits coverage. As the pharmacy benefit structure is broadened to include coverage across a larger number of defined tiers (e.g., brand, generic, and not on the preferred drug list), certain transactions may not be captured in the pharmacy files if the cost is lower than the copayment. This may, however, be balanced by the increasing cost of prescription drugs.

With respect to the ability to obtain data, additional automation will be available in the future for health care companies such as UnitedHealth Group. Laboratory test results and medical records are becoming available electronically. However, this process is being limited both by a lack of standards and by the potential high cost to implement electronic medical records across a diverse network of independent practitioners. Concern about the confidentiality of medical information also may be a factor. The size of the research databases will increase in the future as other affiliated health plans are added to the research databases using commonly defined data elements.

The importance of pharmacoepidemiology and the ability to conduct postmarketing studies will become increasingly critical in the future due to a number of factors relating to changing characteristics of the American population. First, changes attributable to the aging of the population will augment the need for a better understanding of the use of prescribed medications in the older population, including variations in metabolism and appropriate dosages. Second, as the population ages, more Americans are likely to receive a larger number of medications due to the prevalence of chronic disease in this group, raising polypharmacy questions. Increased use of over-the-counter drugs, alternative medications, and devices also will need to be explored. Third, developments in the biotechnology field are resulting in new and expensive, but potentially more effective products, whose adverse effects need to be addressed. Finally, the commercial incorporation of pharmacogenomic data to target appropriate patients should increase both the effectiveness and safety profiles of new therapies.

With the acceleration of innovation, postmarketing evaluations will become more crucial as society attempts to balance public health concerns, individual access to new therapies, and increasing costs. The challenge for the future will be in balancing these competing demands

and values. The information gained from the results of pharmacoepidemiologic research using data from nationally representative health care settings will help to meet this challenge.

REFERENCES

1. Shatin D, Drinkard C, Stergachis A. UnitedHealth Group. In: Strom BL, ed., *Pharmacoepidemiology*, 3rd edn. Chichester: John Wiley & Sons, 2000; pp. 295–305.
2. Enger C, Cali C, Walker AM. Serious ventricular arrhythmias among users of cisapride and other QT-prolonging agents in the United States. *Pharmacoepidemiol Drug Saf* 2002, **11**: 477–86.
3. Cole JA, Loughlin JE, Ajene AN, Rosenberg DM, Cook SE, Walker AM. The effect of zanamivir treatment on influenza complications: a retrospective cohort study. *Clin Ther* 2002; **24**: 1824–39.
4. Tuckson R. Costs of health care administration in the United States and Canada. *N Engl J Med* 2003; **349**: 2462–3.
5. Selby JV. Linking automated databases for research in managed care settings. *Ann Intern Med* 1997; **127**: 719–24.
6. Shatin D. Organizational context and taxonomy of health care databases. *Pharmacoepidemiol Drug Saf* 2001; **10**: 367–71.
7. McCarthy DB, Shatin D, Drinkard CR, Kleinman JH, Gardner JS. Medical records and privacy: empirical effects of legislation. *Health Serv Res* 1999; **34**: 417–25.
8. Kramarz P, France EK, DeStefano F, Black SB, Shinefield H, Ward JI *et al*. Population-based study of rotavirus vaccination and intussusception. *Pediatr Infect Dis J* 2001; **20**: 410–16.
9. Shatin D, Manda B. Vaccine safety: a case study of the impact of privacy concerns on public health research. Presentation at the Office of Research Integrity Conference, Potomac, MD, November 2002.
10. Brook RH, Lohr KN. Efficacy, effectiveness, variations, and quality: boundary-crossing research. *Med Care* 1985; **23**: 710–22.
11. Iezzoni LI. Assessing quality using administrative data. *Ann Intern Med* 1997; **127**: 666–74.
12. Hui SL. Measuring quality, outcomes, and cost of care using large databases. *Ann Intern Med* 1997; **127**: 665.
13. Rawson NSB, D'Arcy C. "Validity" and reliability: idealism and reality in the use of computerized health care databases for pharmacoepidemiological research. *Post Market Surveill* 1991; **5**: 31–55.
14. Wray NP, Ashton CM, Kuykendall DH, Hollingsworth JC. Using administrative databases to evaluate the quality of medical care: a conceptual framework. *Soc Sci Med* 1995; **40**: 1707–15.
15. Rawson NSB, D'Arcy C. Assessing the validity of diagnostic information in administrative health care utilization data: experience in Saskatchewan. *Pharmacoepidemiol Drug Saf* 1998; **7**: 389–98.
16. Rawson NSB. Health care utilization databases [editorial]. *Can J Clin Pharmacol* 1998; **5**: 203–4.

17. Shatin D, Drinkard CR. Ambulatory use of psychotropics by employer-insured children and adolescents in a national managed care organization. *Ambul Pediatr* 2002; **2**: 111–19.

18. Shatin D, Schech SD, Brinker A. Ambulatory use of ticlopidine and clopidogrel in association with percutaneous coronary revascularization procedures in a national managed care organization. *J Interven Cardiol* 2002; **15**: 181–6.

19. Imura H. A novel antidiabetic drug, troglitazone: reason for hope and concern [editorial]. *N Engl J Med* 1998; **338**: 908–9.

20. Graham DJ, Drinkard CR, Shatin D, Tsong Y, Burgess MJ. Liver enzyme monitoring in patients treated with troglitazone. *JAMA* 2001; **286**: 831–3.

21. Gitlin N, Julie NL, Spurr CL, Lim KN, Juarbe HM. Two cases of severe clinical and histologic hepatotoxicity associated with troglitazone. *Ann Intern Med* 1998; **129**: 36–8.

22. Neuschwander-Tetri BA, Isley WL, Oki JC, Ramrakhiani S, Quiason SG, Phillips NJ *et al*. Troglitazone-induced hepatic failure leading to liver transplantation: a case report. *Ann Intern Med* 1998; **129**: 38–41.

23. Shibuya A, Watanabe M, Fujita Y, Saigenji K, Kuwao S, Takahashi H *et al*. An autopsy case of troglitazone-induced fulminant hepatitis. *Diabetes Care* 1998; **21**: 2140–3.

24. Herrine SK, Choudhary C. Severe hepatotoxicity associated with troglitazone [letter]. *Ann Intern Med* 1999; **130**: 163–4.

25. Murphy EJ, Davern TJ, Shakil AO, Shick L, Masharani U, Chow C *et al*. Troglitazone-induced fulminant hepatic failure. *Dig Dis Sci* 2000; **45**: 549–53.

26. Jagannath S, Rai R. Rapid-onset subfulminant liver failure associated with troglitazone [letter]. *Ann Intern Med* 2000; **132**: 677.

27. Graham DJ, Drinkard CR, Shatin D. Incidence of idiopathic acute liver failure and hospitalized liver injury in patients treated with troglitazone. *Am J Gastroenterol* 2003; **98**: 175–9.

28. Shatin D, Rawson NSB, Braun MM, Manda B, Curtis J, Moreland LW *et al*. Impact of risk communication on tuberculosis testing for infliximab users [abstract]. *Pharmacoepidemiol Drug Saf* 2003; **12** (suppl 1): S129–30.

29. Keane J, Gershon S, Wise RP, Mirabile-Levens E, Kasznica J, Schwieterman WD *et al*. Tuberculosis associated with infliximab, a tumor necrosis factor α-neutralizing agent. *N Engl J Med* 2001; **345**: 1098–104.

18

Medicaid Databases

SEAN HENNESSY[1], JEFFREY L. CARSON[2], WAYNE A. RAY[3] and BRIAN L. STROM[1]

[1]University of Pennsylvania School of Medicine, Philadelphia, Pennsylvania, USA; [2]University of Medicine and Dentistry of New Jersey—Robert Wood Johnson Medical School, New Brunswick, New Jersey, USA; [3]Vanderbilt University School of Medicine, Nashville, Tennessee, USA.

INTRODUCTION

Medicaid is currently the largest US government-funded program that pays for both outpatient prescription drugs and medical care. Medicaid data have been used for pharmacoepidemiologic research since the early 1980s, and continue to be used actively today. This chapter reviews the current status of Medicaid data, including its advantages, disadvantages, and appropriate uses within pharmacoepidemiology.

DESCRIPTION

DESCRIPTION OF THE MEDICAID PROGRAM

Medicaid was established by the Social Security Amendment of 1965, which also established Medicare.[1] Although this chapter focuses on *Medicaid*, a brief discussion of *Medicare* is provided to distinguish the two programs.

Medicare is funded solely by the US Federal government, and administered by the Centers for Medicare and Medicaid Services (CMS), a Federal agency within the Department of Health and Human Services. Medicare provides health care coverage for virtually all individuals aged 65 years and older, some disabled people younger than 65, and persons with end-stage renal disease. While Medicare has not historically paid for outpatient drugs, the Medicare Prescription Drug, Improvement, and Modernization Act of 2003 provides for limited pharmaceutical coverage beginning in 2006. If, as is hoped, this pharmaceutical benefit is structured in such a way that all drug data are readily available and linkable to other Medicare data, then the resulting information resource will be enormously valuable for researchers seeking to improve public health.

In contrast to Medicare, *Medicaid* is funded jointly by the Federal government and by individual state governments, and is administered by states with Federal oversight. Medicaid provides benefits to US citizens and lawfully admitted immigrants, if they belong to one of three general groups: (i) low-income pregnant women and families with children, (ii) persons with chronic disabilities, and (iii) low-income seniors, including those receiving Medicare benefits.

Pharmacoepidemiology, Fourth Edition   Edited by B.L. Strom

Table 18.1. Mandatory and optional Medicaid services under US Federal law[1]

Mandatory services	Optional services
Inpatient hospital services	Podiatrists' services
Outpatient hospital services	Optometrists' services
Rural health clinic and Federally qualified health center services	Chiropractors' services
Laboratory and X-ray services	Psychologists' services
Nurse practitioners' services	Medical social worker services
Nursing facility services and home health services for individuals aged 21+	Nurse anesthetists' services
Early and periodic screening, diagnosis, and treatment for individuals under age 21	Private duty nursing
	Clinic services
Family planning services and supplies	Dental services
Physicians' services	Physical therapy
Medical and surgical services of a dentist	Occupational therapy
Nurse-midwife services	Speech, hearing, and language disorders
	Prescribed drugs
	Dentures
	Prosthetic device
	Eyeglasses
	Diagnostic service
	Screening services
	Preventative services
	Rehabilitative services
	Intermediate care facilities/mentally-retarded services
	Inpatient psychiatric services for under age 21
	Christian Science nurses
	Christian Science sanatoriums
	Nursing facility services for under age 21
	Emergency hospital services
	Personal care services
	Transportation services
	Case management services
	Tuberculosis-related services
	Inpatient and nursing facility services for 65+ in institutions for mental diseases

Medicaid does *not* provide coverage for even the poorest individuals unless they belong to one of these specifically designated groups. Each state establishes its own Medicaid eligibility rules within general Federal guidelines. Most states also have "state-only" programs that pay for medical services for specific categories of persons who do not qualify under any Federally specified category. However, states cannot use Federal Medicaid funds to pay for state-only programs unless they obtain a special waiver.

The types of services provided under Medicaid also vary by state within Federal guidelines. Table 18.1 lists services that all states are required to provide, as well as optional services for which states may use Federal Medicaid funds. Mandatory services include inpatient hospital services, outpatient hospital services, and physician services. Although states are not required to cover outpatient prescription drugs, all 50 states and the District of Columbia provide such coverage for at least some categories of enrollees.[2]

However, not all states provide prescription drug coverage for all categories of enrollees. For example, some states

exclude "medically needy" individuals (who have income or resources exceeding the criteria for "categorically needy") from prescription drug benefits.

Medicaid programs function as a payer rather than as a direct provider of health care services. Most Medicaid programs include some beneficiaries who receive services on a fee-for-service basis and others enrolled in capitated plans. In fee-for-service plans, health care providers such as physicians, hospitals, and pharmacies bill Medicaid for specific goods and services provided, such as physician visits, hospitalizations, and prescription drugs. In capitated plans, an insurance company is paid a certain amount per person per time period (e.g., month) to cover all or specific aspects of that enrollee's health care. Importantly for researchers, the degree of completeness of encounter information for patients in capitated plans depends on the specific plan.

Health care providers participating in Medicaid must accept Medicaid payment as payment in full, although states may impose nominal deductibles, co-insurance, or copayments on some Medicaid beneficiaries for certain

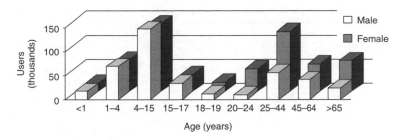

Figure 18.1. Age and sex distribution of Missouri Medicaid users, December 2003. Available at: www.health.state.mo.us/MedicaidMICA/medicaid.html. Accessed: April 9, 2004.

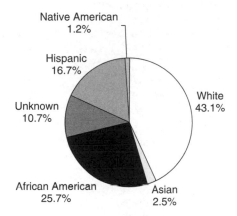

Figure 18.2. Race distribution of US Medicaid users, fiscal year 1998.[1]

services. For example, most state Medicaid programs allow pharmacies to charge patients a fee ranging from $0.50 to $5.00 for each outpatient prescription.[2]

CHARACTERISTICS OF MEDICAID RECIPIENTS

In 2002, 51 million persons, or 16% of the US population, received health care services through Medicaid.[3] The age and sex distribution of recipients in Missouri is presented in Figure 18.1, as an example, and the race distribution nationally is presented in Figure 18.2. As is apparent, children, females, and nonwhites are overrepresented.

Tables 18.2–18.4 present the most frequently dispensed outpatient drugs, most frequent outpatient diagnoses, and most frequent principal inpatient diagnoses in Medicaid recipients.

SOURCES OF MEDICAID DATA FOR RESEARCH

CMS is a major source of Medicaid data for researchers. CMS receives data from individual state Medicaid programs, and performs extensive editing, range checks, and comparisons with previous data from that state when preparing Medicaid Analytic Extract (MAX) files. Anomalies identified by CMS are resolved whenever possible through contact with the state. When anomalies cannot be resolved, they are documented for data users. Crude data from the Medicaid Statistical Information System (MSIS) are also available, but do not undergo the same quality assurance procedures that MAX data undergo. There is currently a lag of approximately four years between the end of a calendar year and when MAX data from that year become available from CMS. Since 1997, the University of Minnesota School of Public Health's Research Data Assistance Center (ResDAC) has, through a contract with CMS, provided free assistance to academic, government, and nonprofit researchers interested in using Medicaid and Medicare data for research. The data are obtained from CMS. However, ResDAC maintains a website of information on Medicaid and Medicare data, conducts workshops and seminars, and provides individual technical assistance to researchers, including obtaining prices for data from CMS, assisting in preparation of data requests, and providing technical assistance in the use of the data once they have been provided by CMS. The address of the ResDAC website is www.resdac.umn.edu.

Pharmacoepidemiologic research has also been conducted using data obtained directly from individual states, including California,[4] New Jersey,[5] New York,[6] and Tennessee.[7]

Commercial data vendors used to be a common source of Medicaid data, but few currently provide such data now that they are available from CMS. One exception is Jen Associates, Inc., which can provide data derived from the MSIS system for requests that have been approved by CMS.

DATA STRUCTURE

CMS provides Medicaid data in five distinct types of MAX files: Personal Summary file, Inpatient file, Prescription Drug file, Long Term Care file, and Other Therapy file.

Table 18.2. Top 50 prescription medications dispensed in the US Medicaid program, 2001

Medication	Total Medicaid prescriptions, 2001
Albuterol	9 308 721
Furosemide	8 663 918
Amoxicillin	7 692 866
Hydrocodone bitartrate/acetaminophen	7 183 995
Levothyroxine	6 570 946
Potassium chloride	6 094 356
Ibuprofen	5 489 219
Risperidone	5 441 273
Atorvastatin	4 891 752
Amlodipine	4 885 734
Sertraline	4 760 490
Olanzapine	4 743 997
Lansoprazole	4 734 329
Celecoxib	4 698 648
Paroxetine	4 665 186
Divalproex	4 527 513
Omeprazole	4 337 952
Metformin	4 060 659
Azithromycin	4 056 493
Codeine phosphate/acetaminophen	3 988 544
Lisinopril	3 937 950
Warfarin	3 908 460
Lorazepam	3 854 789
Ranitidine	3 818 499
Atenolol	3 655 953
Acetaminophen	3 635 473
Gabapentin	3 579 417
Loratadine	3 529 864
Alprazolam	3 458 869
Rofecoxib	3 371 884
Propoxyphene/acetaminophen	3 310 518
Trazodone	3 206 663
Conjugated estrogens	3 058 703
Clonazepam	3 054 568
Diltiazem	2 904 396
Amoxicillin/clavulanate	2 867 826
Hydrochlorothiazide	2 863 837
Aspirin	2 862 846
Fluoxetine	2 816 519
Nitroglycerin	2 733 739
Cephalexin	2 727 789
Glipizide	2 685 459
Amitriptyline	2 658 852
Zolpidem	2 588 363
Clonidine	2 557 638
Carbamazepine	2 553 587
Methylphenidate	2 522 252
Metoprolol	2 507 163
Phenytoin	2 484 911
Trimethoprim/sulfamethoxazole	2 424 212

Source: http//www.cms.hhs.gov/medicaid/drugs/drug5.asp. Accessed: April 8, 2004.

Table 18.3. Top 50 primary diagnoses from outpatient physician visits by Medicaid recipients

ICD-9 code	Diagnosis text	Outpatient physician visits in 2001
V20.2	Routine infant or child health check	5 260 582
V22.1	Supervision of other normal pregnancy	3 607 492
382.9	Unspecified otitis media	2 167 722
465.9	Acute upper respiratory infections of unspecified site	2 132 450
462	Acute pharyngitis	1 579 287
490	Bronchitis, not specified as acute or chronic	1 501 395
314.01	Attention deficit disorder of childhood with hyperactivity	1 260 376
250.00	Type two diabetes mellitus without mention of complication, not stated as uncontrolled	1 139 414
493.90	Asthma, unspecified type	851 464
401.9	Unspecified essential hypertension	784 803
463	Acute tonsillitis	776 259
789.00	Abdominal pain, unspecified site	634 916
558.9	Other and unspecified noninfectious gastroenteritis and colitis	585 861
034.0	Streptococcal sore throat	542 718
V24.2	Routine postpartum follow-up	496 825
311	Depressive disorder, NEC	460 767
530.81	Esophageal reflux	414 958
599.0	Urinary tract infection, site not specified	402 427
466.0	Acute bronchitis	396 628
V70.0	Routine general medical examination at a health care facility	382 312
692.9	Contact dermatitis and other eczema, unspecified cause	353 717
414.00	Coronary atherosclerosis of unspecified type of vessel, native or graft	352 986
473.9	Unspecified sinusitis (chronic)	351 115
079.99	Unspecified viral infection	338 975
486	Pneumonia, organism unspecified	324 195
487.1	Influenza with other respiratory manifestations	322 596
714.0	Rheumatoid arthritis	313 263
706.1	Other acne	304 847
296.20	Major depressive affective disorder, single episode, unspecified degree	302 378
496	Chronic airway obstruction, NEC	274 114
564.0	Constipation	271 373
626.0	Absence of menstruation	261 754
722.10	Displacement of lumbar intervertebral disc without myelopathy	256 698
242.00	Toxic diffuse goiter without mention of thyrotoxic crisis or storm	252 836
784.0	Headache	252 689
V72.3	Gynecologic examination	245 179
786.50	Unspecified chest pain	243 959
346.90	Migraine, unspecified without mention of intractable migraine	242 375
V23.9	Supervision of unspecified high-risk pregnancy	234 648
250.01	Type one diabetes mellitus without mention of complication, not stated as uncontrolled	233 052
428.0	Congestive heart failure, unspecified	232 102
278.00	Obesity, unspecified	229 727
250.02	Type two diabetes mellitus without mention of complication, uncontrolled	227 833
244.9	Unspecified acquired hypothyroidism	223 702
691.0	Diaper or napkin rash	219 288
296.7	Bipolar affective disorder, unspecified	213 080
796.2	Elevated blood pressure reading without diagnosis of hypertension	204 225
295.90	Unspecified type schizophrenia, unspecified state	199 831
682.9	Cellulitis and abscess of unspecified sites	199 340
845.00	Unspecified site of ankle sprain	198 632

Source: 2001 National Ambulatory Medical Care Survey.

Table 18.4. Top 50 principal diagnoses from 2001 admissions to acute care hospitals by Medicaid enrollees

ICD-9 code	Diagnosis text	Discharges
V27.0	Outcome of delivery—single liveborn	1 222 689
V30.00	Single liveborn born in hospital without mention of cesarean delivery	911 798
V30.01	Single liveborn born in hospital delivered by cesarean delivery	276 378
486	Pneumonia, organism unspecified	126 714
276.5	Volume depletion disorder	72 415
466.11	Acute bronchiolitis due to respiratory syncytial virus (RSV)	57 385
428.0	Congestive heart failure, unspecified	55 780
466.19	Acute bronchiolitis due to other infectious organisms	47 180
V27.9	Unspecified outcome of delivery	42 848
493.92	Asthma, unspecified type, with (acute) exacerbation	41 131
558.9	Other and unspecified noninfectious gastroenteritis and colitis	38 451
311	Depressive disorder, NEC	37 985
414.01	Coronary atherosclerosis of native coronary vessel	37 295
282.62	Hb-SS disease with crisis	35 927
577.0	Acute pancreatitis	35 627
644.03	Threatened premature labor, antepartum	34 301
295.70	Schizo-affective type schizophrenia, unspecified state	33 096
491.21	Obstructive chronic bronchitis, with (acute) exacerbation	33 087
599.0	Urinary tract infection, site not specified	30 619
042	Human immunodeficiency virus (HIV) disease	29 692
V57.89	Other specified rehabilitation procedure, NEC	28 490
646.63	Antepartum infections of genitourinary tract	26 267
540.9	Acute appendicitis without mention of peritonitis	23 902
296.33	Major depressive affective disorder, recurrent episode, severe degree, without mention of psychotic behavior	23 187
298.9	Unspecified psychosis	22 158
401.9	Unspecified essential hypertension	21 718
493.91	Asthma, unspecified type, with status asthmaticus	21 425
682.6	Cellulitis and abscess of leg, except foot	21 211
V58.1	Chemotherapy encounter	20 253
648.93	Other current conditions classifiable elsewhere of mother, antepartum	20 233
V31.01	Twin, mate liveborn, born in hospital delivered by cesarean delivery	20 169
493.90	Asthma, unspecified type, unspecified	19 744
296.20	Major depressive affective disorder, single episode, unspecified degree	19 693
079.99	Unspecified viral infection	18 731
291.81	Alcohol withdrawal	18 346
295.34	Paranoid type schizophrenia, chronic state with acute exacerbation	18 125
296.34	Major depressive affective disorder, recurrent episode, severe degree, specified as with psychotic behavior	17 851
530.81	Esophageal reflux	17 400
574.10	Calculus of gallbladder with other cholecystitis, without mention of obstruction	17 139
518.81	Acute respiratory failure	16 908
292.0	Drug withdrawal syndrome	16 741
410.71	Subendocardial infarction, initial episode of care	15 366
296.7	Bipolar affective disorder, unspecified	14 333
295.74	Schizo-affective type schizophrenia, chronic state with acute exacerbation	14 287
296.30	Major depressive affective disorder, recurrent episode, unspecified degree	14 268
465.9	Acute upper respiratory infections of unspecified site	14 234
571.2	Alcoholic cirrhosis of liver	13 567
998.59	Other postoperative infection	13 168
V27.2	Outcome of delivery—twins both liveborn	12 422
303.91	Other and unspecified alcohol dependence, continuous drinking behavior	12 400

Source: 2001 National Hospital Discharge Survey.

There is one of each of these types of file for each state for each calendar year. Each file type will be described briefly.

The Personal Summary file contains one record per individual enrolled in that state's Medicaid program for at least one day during the relevant year. This file includes demographic data (including date of birth, sex, race, and zip code), identifies which months the person was enrolled in Medicaid, and which months (if any) the person participated in a managed care plan. Dates of death are included, although they appear to be incomplete in at least some states. More complete death information can be obtained by linking Medicaid data to external data such as the Death Master File available from the Social Security Administration, from the National Death Index maintained by the Centers for Disease Control and Prevention, or from individual state vital statistics registries.

The Inpatient file contains information on hospitalizations. Available information includes a code identifying the hospital, admission date, discharge date, discharge status, up to nine diagnoses (coded in the International Classification of Diseases, 9th edition, Clinical Modification; ICD-9-CM), up to six procedures (coded in Current Procedural Terminology CPT-4 or ICD-9-CM, or other coding systems), and payment information. The Inpatient file does not contain information on drugs received in the hospital. Therefore Medicaid data are not useful for studying inpatient drug exposures.

The Prescription Drug file contains one record for each reimbursed outpatient or nursing home prescription. Drugs are coded in a nonhierarchical system known as the National Drug Code (NDC). The first five digits of the NDC indicate the drug's manufacturer. The next four digits are assigned by the manufacturer, and indicate the product, including drug, strength, and dosage form. Unfortunately, product codes for the same drug are not standard across manufacturers. The last two digits of the NDC indicate the package size that was purchased by the pharmacy. Researchers wishing to use the Medicaid Prescription Drug file must obtain a drug database to translate from NDC to drug, strength, dosage form, etc. NDC databases are available for license from private-sector firms such as First DataBank and Medi-Span. In addition to NDC, records in the Prescription Drug file also include the date the drug was dispensed, the identification number of the prescriber (although this field is often missing), the quantity dispensed (e.g., number of tablets), whether the prescription was new or a refill, cost information, and the intended duration of the prescription as estimated by the pharmacy ("days supply"). However, in about 18% of physician prescriptions, the days supply is ambiguous because the amount used depends on administration technique (e.g., creams and eye drops), or because the dosage directions allow for variation in dose (e.g., "take as needed").[8] Even when the days supply can be determined unambiguously from the written prescription, it may not always be accurately recorded by the pharmacy. For example, one study found that 36% of prescriptions for chronically administered medications had a recorded days supply that differed by more than five days from the true value as determined by investigators.[8] Therefore, the days supply field must be interpreted cautiously. Most states limit reimbursement to a maximum of a 30-, 31-, or 34-day supply, although some states will pay for a larger supply (e.g., 90 days) for chronically administered drugs.[2] Some states also limit the number of prescriptions reimbursed per month.[2] Most states also have lists of drugs that will be reimbursed only if prior authorization is obtained. Most states cover certain categories of non-prescription drug if a prescription is written.

The Long Term Care file contains encounter records for long term care services provided by skilled nursing facilities, intermediate care facilities, and independent psychiatric facilities. Fields include facility type, dates of service, diagnosis, and discharge status.

The Other Therapy file contains encounter records for all non-institutional Medicaid services, including physician services, laboratory, radiology, and clinic services. Capitation payments for persons in capitated managed care plans are also included. For laboratory and radiology encounter records, the type of test, but not its results, is reported. Date of service, type of service, and, if applicable, diagnosis or procedure code are reported.

Other types of data have been linked to Medicaid data to enhance its utility. For example, Medicare data have been linked to increase the proportion of medical care encounters identified among individuals who are eligible for both Medicare and Medicaid.[9] Such a link can be very important, since Medicaid encounter records can fail to document a considerable proportion of care provided to individuals who are simultaneously eligible for both Medicare and Medicaid.[10] Medicaid data have also been linked to mortality data such as the Social Security Administration Death Master File,[11] National Death Index,[12] and state vital statistics registries.[13] Linkage to birth certificate data is needed for studies of the effects of fetal exposure to medications and for evaluations of the effects on newborns of policies that affect prenatal care.[14] Drivers license data and police reports of injurious crashes have also been linked to Medicaid data.[15] Finally, cancer registries have been linked to Medicaid data to study possible carcinogenic effects of medications.[16] The accuracy and completeness of such linkages cannot be assumed, but rather need to be evaluated by researchers relying on them.

STRENGTHS

An important strength of Medicaid databases is their large size, which permits the study of infrequently used drugs and rare outcomes. More than ten states (e.g., California, New York) have over a million Medicaid recipients each. A related strength is that studies using existing sources such as Medicaid data are much less expensive than similarly sized studies in which data are collected *de novo*.

Another strength of Medicaid data is that the outpatient prescription encounter records accurately record the date, NDC, and quantity dispensed by the pharmacy for each Medicaid beneficiary. Because this information determines the payment provided by the Medicaid program to the pharmacy, it is subject to regulatory audit and has been shown to be highly accurate in a validation study conducted in the early 1980s.[17] Medicaid prescription data reflect what was dispensed by the pharmacy, which is one step closer to biologic ingestion than what was prescribed, which is recorded in medical record databases such as the General Practice Research Database (see Chapter 22). Of course, patients may not take all of the medicine dispensed as directed. However, for chronically administered drugs, dispensing records have been found to accurately reflect cumulative exposure and gaps in medication supply when compared with electronic medication containers,[18] which are currently considered the best available means of measuring medication ingestion in community-dwelling patients. Because patients have a financial incentive to use Medicaid to purchase their drugs instead of paying for them out-of-pocket, it seems reasonable to expect that pharmacy encounter records capture the vast majority of prescription drug use, particularly in the low-income populations that are served by Medicaid.

Like prescription records, encounter records that code for clinical procedures determine the amount of money paid to the health care provider. Therefore, procedure records are audited to detect fraud, and would thus be expected to be highly accurate with regard to performance of that procedure. Wysowski and Baum performed medical record validation in a Medicaid study that used presence of a surgical procedure code as part of an algorithm to identify cases of hip fracture.[19] They found that, while all of the procedures billed for were actually performed, some of the procedures were used to correct orthopedic conditions other than hip fracture.

Another potential strength of Medicaid is overrepresentation of certain populations. Medicaid has substantially greater proportions of pregnant women, young children, and African Americans than other data sets. Approximately 11% of Medicaid beneficiaries are 65 years of age or older.[1] Because populations that are overrepresented in Medicaid are often underrepresented in randomized trials, the opportunity to study them in Medicaid is particularly valuable. Two examples of traditionally underrepresented populations that were studied with Medicaid data include studies of fetal metronidazole exposure and childhood cancer,[20] and of angiotensin converting enzyme inhibitors and angioedema in African Americans.[21]

WEAKNESSES

GENERALIZABILITY

Medicaid recipients are not representative of the general population with respect to factors such as age, race, income, and disability status. Therefore, some results may not generalize well to the broader population. This is particularly true of descriptive studies of health care utilization. For example, newborn deliveries account for 40% of hospital admissions within Medicaid beneficiaries, but only 16% of admissions in the non-Medicaid US population.[22] However, the generalizability of etiologic studies is compromised only for biologic relationships that vary based on factors that differ between Medicaid and non-Medicaid populations. Thus, the results of etiologic studies have generally been consistent between Medicaid and non-Medicaid populations. For example, Medicaid studies evaluating the gastrointestinal side effects of nonsteroidal anti-inflammatory drugs have produced similar results to those performed in other populations.[23]

DIAGNOSTIC TERMINOLOGY

Diagnoses in Medicaid are coded using the ICD-9-CM coding scheme. While this coding system is the most common scheme used for administrative purposes, its use can be problematic for researchers for several reasons. First, there are often many ICD-9-CM codes compatible with a single clinical condition. For example, upper gastrointestinal bleeding from a duodenal ulcer can be coded as upper gastrointestinal bleeding not otherwise specified (ICD-9-CM code 578.9), hematemesis (578.0), melena (578.1), acute duodenal ulcer with bleeding (532.0), peptic ulcer with bleeding (533.0), etc. Therefore, it is usually necessary to include many different ICD-9-CM codes to identify an outcome of interest.

Second, there is no incentive for providers to use the most specific code available, such as duodenal ulcer with bleeding rather than peptic ulcer with bleeding or upper gastrointestinal bleeding, not otherwise specified. Thus, one must be careful not to over-interpret such distinctions within claims data. In general, researchers using claims data should be "lumpers" rather than "splitters."

Third, ICD-9-CM codes do not always precisely fit the clinical condition of interest. Therefore, several sets of codes are often needed to define the same disease. For example, in a study of zomepirac and hypersensitivity reactions[24] investigators used six different definitions of hypersensitivity reactions: (i) bronchospasm and laryngospasm, (ii) shock, other than septic and cardiogenic shock, (iii) allergy unspecified, (iv) allergic skin reactions such as urticaria, (v) adverse effects of medicinal and biological substances, and (vi) the subset of each of the first five code groups that was felt to best approximate the syndrome of anaphylaxis without including too much non-anaphylactic disease.

Fourth, the ICD-9-CM coding scheme is often too non-specific for research purposes. For example, the code for erythema multiforme (695.1) includes erythema multiforme major, erythema multiforme minor, Stevens–Johnson syndrome, toxic epidermal necrolysis, staphylococcal scalded skin syndrome, and other conditions. Some of these conditions may share common etiologies, while others clearly do not. When coded encounter diagnoses are not specific enough, researchers must use primary medical records to distinguish among clinical conditions.

Finally, outcomes that do not reliably result in encounters with health care providers may be under-ascertained. This can introduce bias into the findings of analytic studies if the likelihood that a given clinical condition leads to medical care is related to use of a particular medication.

LIMITATIONS IN PRESCRIPTION COVERAGE

Only drugs covered by Medicaid can be studied using Medicaid encounter data. A number of drug categories are generally not covered by Medicaid, such as agents for fertility, weight loss, hair growth, cosmetic effect, and smoking cessation. Therefore, these agents cannot be studied using Medicaid data. Many states also require prior approval before reimbursing for certain drugs, such as human growth hormone, nonsedating antihistamines, and more expensive nonsteroidal anti-inflammatory agents. The coverage of injectable drugs and adult vaccines also varies by state, although coverage for many childhood vaccines is required by Federal law. Whether injectable drugs are recorded as prescription encounters or other types of encounters also varies by state. Finally, states vary in their coverage of non-prescription drugs.

CONFOUNDING

A concern of most pharmacoepidemiology studies is the potential for confounding by factors such as age, sex,

indications and contraindications for drug therapy, concomitant drug therapy, and underlying diagnoses. When information on these factors is available, it can be controlled for by using one or more standard epidemiological approaches such as exclusion, matching, stratification, or mathematical modeling. Each of these approaches requires that the confounding variable (or a sufficiently correlated variable) be recorded. However, Medicaid lacks information on many potentially important confounding factors, including smoking, exercise, diet, environmental exposures, illicit drug use, alcohol use, occupation, family history, and use of many over-the-counter drugs.

Measured variables can sometimes be used as proxies for unmeasured variables. For example, presence of alcohol-related illnesses such as alcoholic cirrhosis, alcoholic hepatitis, delirium tremens, etc., can be used as a surrogate for alcohol abuse.[25] However, while the positive predictive value of these proxies is probably quite high, reliance on them almost certainly results in under-ascertainment of alcohol abuse. Other factors, such as occupational exposures, diet, and exercise, cannot be controlled for at all without supplemental data.

To address this weakness, researchers using Medicaid data have used primary medical records to obtain information on potential confounding factors in a subset of subjects. For example, in a study of drug-induced liver disease, investigators excluded cases with a history of significant alcohol use recorded in their medical record.[26] This approach can only be successful for variables for which the information is reliably recorded in the medical record. For example, in a study of liver disease, alcohol use would be expected to be reliably recorded in the clinical record, since alcohol is one of the most common causes of liver disease. In contrast, smoking may not be reliably recorded in the clinical records of patients with liver disease, since smoking is not believed to be related to liver disease. In contrast, smoking would be expected to be recorded reliably in the medical records of patients with lung cancer, since smoking is a widely recognized risk factor for lung cancer.

Another approach to handling confounding by factors not recorded in encounter data is to perform medical record review within the cases to assess the relationship between the confounding factor and the exposure of interest (see also Chapter 48). As above, this approach can be useful only for potential confounders that are reliably recorded in the clinical records of subjects with the outcome. It is based upon the fact that, in the absence of effect modification, a true confounder will have a different prevalence in exposed and unexposed cases.[27] This approach was used in a study of nonsteroidal anti-inflammatory drugs and peptic ulcer disease, which found that among cases of peptic ulcer disease, current NSAID was unrelated to smoking status.[28] Therefore, provided that NSAIDs have the same effect on risk of peptic ulcer disease among smokers and nonsmokers, smoking could not confound the relationship between NSAIDs and peptic ulcer disease.

One approach to reduce the potential for confounding by measured and unmeasured factors in Medicaid-based studies is to use a reference group that is similar to users of the drug of interest. This can be accomplished by comparing users of drugs from the same therapeutic class,[11] or comparing rates of outcomes in the same subjects between their time on versus time off the drug,[15,29] or through use of a case-crossover design,[30] as described in Chapter 48. However, because the risk of an event of interest may be positively or negatively associated with choice of a particular agent within a class (e.g., avoidance of long-acting benzodiazepines in frail patients) or with reasons for starting or stopping a drug (e.g., a prodromal symptom of the disease under study), such approaches may reduce, but do not eliminate, the potential for confounding.

Despite the availability of a variety of approaches to reduce confounding, the potential for confounding by unmeasured factors may be so great as to render a Medicaid study of a given relationship inadvisable. For example, comparisons of rates of suicide among users of different antidepressants could be substantially confounded by baseline differences in severity of depression among recipients of different antidepressants, a factor that is not readily obtainable from encounter records.

DATA VALIDITY

Probably the most important concern with using administrative data for research is its validity, which is also discussed in Chapter 45. A study funded by the US Food and Drug Administration and performed by the Research Triangle Institute (RTI) in the early 1980s compared Medicaid encounter data from Michigan and Minnesota to its primary sources, i.e., clinical records in hospitals, physician offices, pharmacies, etc.[17] The results of this study suggested that the demographic and drug data appeared to be of extremely high quality. For example, within pre-established limits, year of birth agreed in 94% of sampled patients, and could not be determined from the medical records in another 2.5%. Sex agreed in 95% of patients, yet was missing from some states for 10% of subjects, and could not be determined from the medical records in another 4%. Date of dispensing of prescriptions agreed in 97% of prescriptions. Regarding medical services, of those records that could be evaluated,

93% of the services in Medicaid encounter data could be found in the provider records within one week of the Medicaid encounter date. However, in 17% of those, the provider record included a previous or subsequent visit that was not included in the Medicaid encounter data. Diagnostic agreement to at least three digits of the ICD-9-CM code occurred in 41% of records, while agreement within a broad diagnostic category in another 16% (i.e., same body system and/or type of illness). These results suggest that the validity of diagnostic data must be considered in the context of each individual study outcome.

Several levels of validity of diagnosis data need to be considered when using Medicaid encounter data. The first is whether the encounter diagnosis accurately reflects the clinical diagnosis listed on the medical record. The second level is whether the clinical diagnosis made and recorded by the physician is correct. For example, a physician may diagnose a skin rash as erythema multiforme, when it is actually some other skin disorder. Specific clinical criteria need to be developed to validate diagnoses in this way. However, primary medical records do not always include enough detail to permit this second level of validation.

The validity of a number of specific Medicaid encounter diagnoses have been examined using primary medical records, with each study illustrating strengths and weaknesses of Medicaid data. In a study of the validity of neutropenia diagnoses in Medicaid, the encounter diagnosis was verified by laboratory information in 192 of 198 clinical records available, yielding a positive predictive value of 97%.[31] However, the purpose of the study was to investigate incident cases of neutropenia, yet 13.5% of the cases had recurrent neutropenia, and 9.9% had cyclic neutropenia. Thus, even when the encounter diagnosis was highly accurate, other information from the medical record was needed to characterize cases accurately.

For a Medicaid study of Stevens–Johnson syndrome, the hospital records of 249 cases with an inpatient diagnosis of "erythema multiforme" (ICD-9-CM code 695.1) were sought from three states.[32] Of these, 128 (51.4%) medical records were available. Of these, 121 (94.5%) subjects had received a clinical diagnosis that was potentially compatible with the encounter diagnosis. However, upon review by a study dermatologist, a diagnosis of erythema multiforme minor or major was confirmed in only 42% of those with the relevant encounter diagnosis. This study confirmed that this ICD-9-CM diagnosis code includes several unrelated conditions, and that the clinical diagnoses are not always accurate.

For a Medicaid study of drug-induced acute liver disease, the medical records of 414 subjects with an encounter diagnosis of liver disease were reviewed.[26] One of the goals of this review was to exclude patients with identifiable non-drug causes of liver disease. Of the records reviewed, 15.9% were alcoholics, 31.9% had acute hepatitis A or B, 13.5% were injecting drug users, 8.2% had acute cholecystitis or choledocholithiasis, and 4.1% had received a transfusion within 6 months. No liver diagnosis was found in 10.6%, and 5.7% had chronic liver disease. Of the 169 cases of acute idiopathic liver disease, many were hospitalized for reasons other than liver disease, and had very mild liver disease. Thus, this study found that Medicaid encounter data has a high positive predictive value for the diagnosis of acute liver disease. However, the results suggest that primary medical records are essential for studying drug-induced hepatitis, to exclude non-drug causes of liver disease, and to obtain other information not included in the encounter data.

Our experience suggests that in each study, with few exceptions, investigators should obtain medical records in at least a sample of outcomes to confirm the validity of the encounter diagnoses, characterize the severity of the disease, and obtain information on potential confounding variables not found in the encounter data. One potential exception is studies of outcomes for which encounter diagnoses have previously been found to be sufficiently valid. Another potential exception is studies using a procedure or a prescription for a drug as the outcome of interest. For example, a study investigating metoclopramide-induced parkinsonism found an association between a new prescription for levodopa and prior exposure to metoclopramide.[33] This seems like a reasonably specific (although perhaps insensitive) way to identify drug-induced parkinsonism, since Medicaid prescription claims accurately reflect what was dispensed, and the vast majority of levodopa use is for parkinsonism.

Examining the validity of diagnosis codes requires review of clinical records, which must frequently be done without subject contact, since contacting Medicaid beneficiaries who experienced specific outcomes years ago may be impossible or impracticable. Under the Privacy Rule of the Health Insurance Portability and Accountability Act (HIPAA), researchers with necessary documentation can legally request the hospital records of specific patients even without patient contact (see also Chapter 38). Necessary documentation includes waivers of informed consent and of HIPAA authorization granted by an institutional review board, and a data use agreement with the agency providing the encounter data (e.g., CMS or the individual Medicaid agency). In most circumstances, hospitals would be required to record (in HIPAA parlance, "account for") such disclosures of protected health information, and report those disclosures to any of their patients who were subjects in the study and who request this information. At present, there is little experience upon which to gauge the willingness of hospitals to provide researchers with access to medical records data using this mechanism. Unfortunately, if investigators are unable to obtain clinical records because of regulatory impediments, the utility of Medicaid encounter data to improve public health will be compromised.

IDENTIFYING ENROLLED PERSON-TIME

Studies using Medicaid data can validly include only person-time during which subjects would have had health care services reimbursed by Medicaid if they had occurred. Thus, the need to identify *enrolled person-time* is crucial, as investigators need to distinguish periods of health from periods of ineligibility. In studies that follow each subject for the expected duration of a given prescription, only a small proportion of subjects would be expected to become ineligible during the short follow-up period following the prescription. Thus, this issue may be relatively unimportant in this context. In contrast, this issue may be more important in case–control studies, in which a necessary step is to identify a representative sample of person-time in the source population that gave rise to the cases,[34] and in cohort studies with unexposed comparison groups.

One way to identify enrolled person-time is to use the information from the Personal Summary (i.e., enrollment) file, which lists the Medicaid enrollment dates for each subject enrolled in the program for each month during that year. This approach has been used in prior studies.[7,13,15,29,35] There are two potential problems with relying on this information. The first is that, for subjects enrolled in capitated plans, it is uncertain whether encounter-level information such as hospitalizations and physician visits will be recorded in the encounter files. Since 1999, states have been required to provide CMS with encounter data for individuals enrolled in capitated plans. However, despite this requirement, encounter data for those enrolled in capitated plans appears to be incomplete in at least some states. The problem of missing encounter data for persons enrolled in capitated plans can be avoided by excluding person-time during which the individual was enrolled in a capitated plan. The second potential problem is that anecdotal experience has suggested that enrollment information from some states may be inaccurate. In particular, the experience has been that individuals are sometimes retroactively enrolled, e.g., when they become medically eligible, and encounters from retroactively enrolled periods may be incomplete.

Another approach to reducing this potential problem is to restrict consideration to time periods in which Medicaid encounters are present within some specified period (e.g., six months) both before and after the person-time under study.[24,25,32,36–39] Naturally, this approach will miss fatal outcomes. It also is unable to differentiate periods of ineligibility from periods of health.

PARTICULAR APPLICATIONS

METHODOLOGIC STUDIES

Hennessy and colleagues performed descriptive analyses to assess the integrity of data that were provided by a commercial vendor for six Medicaid programs.[10] They found that prescription encounter records appeared to be intermittently missing in some states, and that there was no valid marker for inpatient hospitalizations for some states. In addition, hospitalizations in those aged 65 years and above appeared to be missing to varying degrees in all states, presumably because Medicare was the primary payer for such hospitalizations. Mismatches between diagnostic and demographic information (e.g., female disorders in males) were rare. The authors recommended that whenever possible, descriptive analyses of the underlying administrative data be used to identify potentially important data anomalies.[10]

McKenzie and colleagues examined the validity of Medicaid pharmacy encounter records to estimate drug use in elderly nursing home residents.[40] They found good agreement between Medicaid encounter records and nursing home records for presence or absence of drug ingestion (positive and negative predictive values >85%), and that doses recorded using the two databases correlated well (correlation coefficients from 0.66 to 0.97).[40]

Another example of a methodologic study performed in Medicaid is the study of data validity performed by the Research Triangle Institute, described above.[17]

CONTENT AREA STUDIES

Medicaid data are used for descriptive drug utilization studies, which are described in Chapter 27. For example, dosReis and colleagues used Medicaid data to examine doses of different antipsychotic agents used in persons with schizophrenia. They found that the average dose (in chlorpromazine equivalents) was 729 mg/d for high-potency agents, and 304 mg/d for low-potency agents.[41]

Medicaid data are also commonly used for etiologic studies. For example, Ray and colleagues used Tennessee Medicaid data to examine the association between antipsychotic drugs and risk of sudden cardiac death.[13] They found that at doses of greater than 100 mg/d of chlorpromazine equivalents, the rate ratio for use of any antipsychotic drug was 2.39 (95% confidence interval (CI), 1.77–3.22).[13] Hennessy and colleagues used Medicaid data from three states to study the risk of a composite outcome of sudden death or ventricular arrhythmia in persons with schizophrenia who received antipsychotics.[11] The primary comparison was thioridazine versus haloperidol. They found no overall difference in the rate of the composite outcome, although thioridazine had a higher risk of the composite outcome at doses of 600 mg/d or greater in chlorpromazine equivalents (rate ratio 2.6, 95% CI 1.0–6.6). A dose–response relationship was evident for thioridazine but not for haloperidol.[11]

Medicaid data are also used for studies that evaluate the effects of public policies. For example, McCombs and colleagues used California Medicaid data to examine the effect of initial addition of selective serotonin reuptake inhibitors to the California Medicaid formulary. They found that formulary addition resulted in an immediate and sustained increase in the proportion of depressed patients initiating antidepressant therapy.[42] As another example, Soumerai and colleagues used Medicaid data from New Hampshire and New Jersey to examine the effect of a three-prescription monthly limit (cap) on the use of psychotropic drugs and acute mental health care by persons with schizophrenia. They found that the cap resulted in immediate reductions in the use of psychotropic agents, including antipsychotic drugs, and a sharp increase in the use of acute mental health services. Removal of the cap led to reversion to baseline levels. The cost of the cap exceeded its drug cost savings by a factor of 17.[43]

APPROPRIATE ROLE OF MEDICAID DATA IN PHARMACOEPIDEMIOLOGY

Medicaid data are especially useful for research in several circumstances. Many pharmacoepidemiology studies require very large sample sizes, since they examine rare exposures, outcomes, or both. If a rapid answer is required because of public health concerns, then using pre-existing databases is often preferable. Similarly, if financial resources are limited, then studies using existing databases can generally be performed at significantly lower cost compared to studies using *de novo* data collection. Finally, administrative databases are preferable when studies are especially prone to information bias, such as a study of drug-induced birth defects that relies on maternal recall of drugs taken during pregnancy.

There are also several situations when Medicaid data should not be used for pharmacoepidemiology studies. First, Medicaid data cannot be used to study in-hospital drug use, since information on inpatient medication use is unavailable. Second, Medicaid data may capture only a small and variable proportion of non-prescription drug use. Third, Medicaid data should not be used to study outcomes that will not reliably come to medical attention, such as minor nausea and mild skin rashes. In addition, if researchers are unable to gain access to clinical records to verify at least a subset of outcomes identified by encounter diagnoses, and the encounter diagnoses of interest have not previously been shown to be valid, then Medicaid data should generally not be used. Fourth, Medicaid data should not be used for studies in which there is likely to be important confounding by factors not recorded in Medicaid data. For example, it usually would not be appropriate to use Medicaid data for a study of lung cancer in which smoking may be an important confounder, since smoking history is unavailable. Fifth, Medicaid data should not be used if the ICD-9-CM coding system does not adequately describe the outcome of interest. An example would be a study of warfarin-induced skin necrosis. There also are times when this coding system is too nonspecific, so that related diseases are grouped together. An example would be a study of drug-induced retroperitoneal fibrosis, since retroperitoneal fibrosis is grouped into the code for urethral obstruction. Sixth, Medicaid data may not be suitable to study long-term effects of drugs if frequent eligibility changes result in many subjects losing benefits. Finally, Medicaid (or other automated databases) should not be used if crucial study variables need to be determined via patient contact, such as depression, blood pressure, serum cholesterol, or genetic factors (see Chapter 37).

THE FUTURE

Very large studies can be performed with Medicaid databases in a relatively quick and inexpensive way. These databases permit studies of both inpatient and outpatient diseases, and sometimes permit calculation of incidence rates.

A major concern in using this type of database is the validity of the diagnosis data. Thus, the ability to obtain clinical records to validate encounter diagnoses is crucial. Provided that appropriate steps are taken, health care providers are permitted under HIPAA to provide investigators with access to clinical records even without patient contact. However, current experience does not allow us to gauge the willingness of providers to do so. This is a problem that must be resolved if these resources are to continue to demonstrate maximum utility.

ACKNOWLEDGMENTS

We thank Charles E. Leonard, PharmD for generating several of the tables and figures in this chapter. We also thank Gerrie Barosso, RD, MPH, MS for commenting on a draft of this chapter. Ms Barosso's work is supported by CMS contract 500–01–0043 to the University of Minnesota School of Public Health.

REFERENCES

1. *A Profile of Medicaid*. Washington, DC: US Department of Health and Human Services, 2000.
2. *Pharmaceutical Benefits under State Medical Assistance Programs*. Reston, VA: National Pharmaceutical Council, 2003.
3. Iglehart JK. The dilemma of Medicaid. *N Engl J Med* 2003; **348**: 2140–8.
4. Menzin J, Boulanger L, Friedman M, Mackell J, Lloyd JR. Treatment adherence associated with conventional and atypical antipsychotics in a large state Medicaid program. *Psychiatr Serv* 2003; **54**: 719–23.
5. Wang PS, Walker AM, Tsuang MT, Orav EJ, Glynn RJ, Levin R *et al*. Dopamine antagonists and the development of breast cancer. *Arch Gen Psychiatry* 2002; **59**:1147–54.
6. Laine C, Zhang D, Hauck WW, Turner BJ. HIV-1 RNA viral load monitoring in HIV-infected drug users on antiretroviral therapy: relationship with outpatient care patterns. *J Acquir Immune Defic Syndr* 2002; **29**: 270–4.
7. Ray WA, Meredith S, Thapa PB, Hall K, Murray KT. Cyclic antidepressants and the risk of sudden cardiac death. *Clin Pharmacol Ther* 2004; **75**: 234–41.
8. Farris KB, Kaplan B, Kirking DM. Examination of days supply in computerized prescription claims. *J Pharmacoepidemiol* 1994; **3**: 63–76.
9. Wang PS, Levin R, Zhao SZ, Avorn J. Urinary antispasmodic use and the risks of ventricular arrhythmia and sudden death in older patients. *J Am Geriatr Soc* 2002; **50**: 117–24.
10. Hennessy S, Bilker WB, Weber A, Strom BL. Descriptive analyses of the integrity of a US Medicaid claims database. *Pharmacoepidemiol Drug Saf* 2003; **12**: 103–11.
11. Hennessy S, Bilker WB, Knauss JS, Margolis DJ, Kimmel SE, Reynolds RF *et al*. Cardiac arrest and ventricular arrhythmia in patients taking antipsychotic drugs: cohort study using administrative data. *BMJ* 2002; **325**: 1070.
12. Staffa JA, Jones JK, Gable CB, Verspeelt JP, Amery WK. Risk of selected serious cardiac events among new users of antihistamines. *Clin Ther* 1995; **17**: 1062–77.
13. Ray WA, Meredith S, Thapa PB, Meador KG, Hall K, Murray KT. Antipsychotics and the risk of sudden cardiac death. *Arch Gen Psychiatry* 2001; **58**: 1161–7.

14. Ray WA, Gigante J, Mitchel EF Jr, Hickson GB. Perinatal outcomes following implementation of TennCare. *JAMA* 1998; **279**: 314–16.

15. Ray WA, Fought RL, Decker MD. Psychoactive drugs and the risk of injurious motor vehicle crashes in elderly drivers. *Am J Epidemiol* 1992; **136**: 873–83.

16. Wang PS, Walker AM, Tsuang MT, Orav EJ, Glynn RJ, Levin R *et al.* Dopamine antagonists and the development of breast cancer. *Arch Gen Psychiatry* 2002; **59**: 1147–54.

17. Lessler JT, Harris BSH. *Medicaid Data as a Source for Postmarketing Surveillance Information.* Research Triangle Park, NC: Research Triangle Institute, 1984.

18. Choo PW, Rand CS, Inui TS, Lee ML, Cain E, Cordeiro-Breault M *et al.* Validation of patient reports, automated pharmacy records, and pill counts with electronic monitoring of adherence to antihypertensive therapy. *Med Care* 1999;**37**: 846–57.

19. Wysowski DK, Baum C. The validity of Medicaid diagnoses of hip fracture. *Am J Public Health* 1993; **83**: 770.

20. Thapa PB, Whitlock JA, Brockman Worrell KG, Gideon P, Mitchel EF, Jr., Roberson P *et al.* Prenatal exposure to metronidazole and risk of childhood cancer: a retrospective cohort study of children younger than 5 years. *Cancer* 1998; **83**: 1461–8.

21. Brown NJ, Ray WA, Snowden M, Griffin MR. Black Americans have an increased rate of angiotensin converting enzyme inhibitor-associated angioedema. *Clin Pharmacol Ther* 1996; **60**: 8–13.

22. *National Hospital Discharge Survey 2001.* Hyattsville, MD: National Center for Health Statistics, 2003.

23. Henry D, Lim LL, Garcia Rodriguez LA, Perez GS, Carson JL, Griffin M *et al.* Variability in risk of gastrointestinal complications with individual non-steroidal anti-inflammatory drugs: results of a collaborative meta-analysis. *BMJ* 1996; **312**: 1563–6.

24. Strom BL, Carson JL, Morse ML, West SL, Soper KA. The effect of indication on hypersensitivity reactions associated with zomepirac sodium and other nonsteroidal antiinflammatory drugs. *Arthritis Rheum* 1987; **30**: 1142–8.

25. Carson JL, Strom BL, Duff A, Gupta A, Das K. Safety of nonsteroidal anti-inflammatory drugs with respect to acute liver disease. *Arch Intern Med* 1993; **153**: 1331–6.

26. Carson JL, Strom BL, Duff A, Gupta A, Shaw M, Das K. The feasibility of studying drug-induced acute hepatitis with use of Medicaid data. *Clin Pharmacol Ther* 1992; **52**: 214–19.

27. Ray WA, Griffin MR. Use of Medicaid data for pharmacoepidemiology. *Am J Epidemiol* 1989; **129**: 837–49.

28. Griffin MR, Ray WA, Schaffner W. Nonsteroidal anti-inflammatory drug use and death from peptic ulcer in elderly persons. *Ann Intern Med* 1988; **109**: 359–63.

29. Ray WA, Griffin MR, Downey W. Benzodiazepines of long and short elimination half-life and the risk of hip fracture. *JAMA* 1989; **262**: 3303–7.

30. Maclure M. The case-crossover design: a method for studying transient effects on the risk of acute events. *Am J Epidemiol* 1991; **133**: 144–53.

31. Strom BL, Carson JL, Schinnar R, Snyder ES, Shaw M. Descriptive epidemiology of agranulocytosis. *Arch Intern Med* 1992; **152**: 1475–80.

32. Strom BL, Carson JL, Halpern AC, Schinnar R, Snyder ES, Shaw M *et al.* A population-based study of Stevens–Johnson syndrome. Incidence and antecedent drug exposures. *Arch Dermatol* 1991; **127**: 831–8.

33. Avorn J, Gurwitz JH, Bohn RL, Mogun H, Monane M, Walker A. Increased incidence of levodopa therapy following metoclopramide use. *JAMA* 1995; **274**: 1780–2.

34. Rothman KJ, Greenland S. *Modern Epidemiology*, 2nd edn. Philadelphia, PA: Lippincott-Raven, 1998.

35. Ray WA, Griffin MR, Downey W, Melton LJ3d. Long-term use of thiazide diuretics and risk of hip fracture. *Lancet* 1989; **1**: 687–90.

36. Carson JL, Strom BL, Soper KA, West SL, Morse ML. The association of nonsteroidal anti-inflammatory drugs with upper gastrointestinal tract bleeding. *Arch Intern Med* 1987; **147**: 85–8.

37. Carson JL, Strom BL, Schinnar R, Duff A, Sim E. The low risk of upper gastrointestinal bleeding in patients dispensed corticosteroids. *Am J Med* 1991; **91**: 223–8.

38. Carson JL, Strom BL, Duff A, Gupta A, Shaw M, Lundin FE *et al.* Acute liver disease associated with erythromycins, sulfonamides, and tetracyclines. *Ann Intern Med* 1993; **119**: 576–83.

39. Strom BL, Carson JL, Schinnar R, Snyder ES, Shaw M, Lundin FE Jr. Nonsteroidal anti-inflammatory drugs and neutropenia. *Arch Intern Med* 1993; **153**: 2119–24.

40. McKenzie DA, Semradek J, McFarland BH, Mullooly JP, McCamant LE. The validity of Medicaid pharmacy claims for estimating drug use among elderly nursing home residents: the Oregon experience. *J Clin Epidemiol* 2000; **53**: 1248–57.

41. dosReis S, Zito JM, Buchanan RW, Lehman AF. Antipsychotic dosing and concurrent psychotropic treatments for Medicaid-insured individuals with schizophrenia. *Schizophr Bull* 2002; **28**: 607–17.

42. McCombs JS, Shi L, Croghan TW, Stimmel GL. Access to drug therapy and substitution between alternative antidepressants following an expansion of the California Medicaid formulary. *Health Policy* 2003; **65**: 301–11.

43. Soumerai SB, McLaughlin TJ, Ross-Degnan D, Casteris CS, Bollini P. Effects of a limit on Medicaid drug-reimbursement benefits on the use of psychotropic agents and acute mental health services by patients with schizophrenia. *N Engl J Med* 1994; **331**: 650–5.

19

Health Services Databases in Saskatchewan

WINANNE DOWNEY, MARYROSE STANG, PATRICIA BECK, WILLIAM OSEI
and JAMES L. NICHOL

Population Health Branch, Saskatchewan Health, Regina, Saskatchewan, Canada.

INTRODUCTION

Saskatchewan is one of ten provinces and three territories in Canada. It is located in western Canada and has a relatively stable population of about one million people, or about 3.2% of the population of Canada.

Saskatchewan has a publicly funded health system. Within this system, Saskatchewan Health, a provincial government department, and 13 health authorities provide health services to the citizens of Saskatchewan. With funding from Saskatchewan Health, the health authorities plan and deliver most services to people within their geographic jurisdictions based on the needs of their residents. Saskatchewan Health coordinates province-wide programs such as the Prescription Drug and Medical Care Insurance Plans.

In almost all of the provincially funded programs, residents of the province enjoy universal health insurance. There is no eligibility distinction based on socioeconomic status. As a by-product of these universal health care programs, Saskatchewan Health has been accumulating a large amount of health care information in computerized databases over a number of years. These databases have been recognized as a resource for pharmacoepidemiologic, drug utilization review, health economics, and other health services research. Publications of studies based on the data reflect the value of the databases for this research.[1-98]

DESCRIPTION

The major databases include the registry of the eligible population, prescription drug data, hospital services data, physician services data, the cancer registry, and vital statistics data. These are described in more detail below.

ELIGIBLE POPULATION

Saskatchewan residents are entitled to receive benefits through the health care system once they have established residence and have registered with Saskatchewan Health. A Health Services Number (HSN), assigned at registration, is a lifetime number that uniquely identifies each beneficiary. The HSN is captured in records of health service utilization and enables linkage of the computer databases.

Pharmacoepidemiology, Fourth Edition   Edited by B.L. Strom
© 2005 John Wiley & Sons, Ltd

Saskatchewan Health maintains an accurate, comprehensive, and current population registry that includes all residents eligible for health coverage (the "covered population"). As of June 30, 2003, more than one million people were eligible for health benefits (Table 19.1).[99] Excluded from eligibility, and therefore from the population registry, are people whose health care is fully funded Federally. This category, which includes members of the Royal Canadian Mounted Police, members of the Canadian Forces, and inmates of Federal penitentiaries, accounts for less than 1% of the total population. Consequently, the population registry (together with specific health services information) enables study of all segments of the population, including children, women of childbearing age, and the elderly.

The population registry captures demographic and coverage data on every member of the eligible population (Table 19.2). It is updated daily for name or address changes, births, deaths, new residents, departing residents, and those qualifying for extended health benefits. The registry is verified and updated through a variety of mechanisms which signal changes in eligibility, identification, or demographic data. Transactions for an insured health service are checked against the population registry for eligibility of the claimant and for accuracy of identification and demographic information; inconsistencies are manually checked.

PRESCRIPTION DRUG DATA

All Saskatchewan residents are eligible for benefits under the Prescription Drug Plan (the "Drug Plan"), with the exception of approximately 9% of the population (primarily registered Indians) who have their prescription costs paid for by another government agency. (Those ineligible for prescription coverage can be excluded from studies.)

Drugs covered by the Drug Plan are listed in the Saskatchewan Formulary. Some drugs are listed with restricted status and covered only when certain criteria are met. Criteria for coverage for drugs under restricted status are different for each drug and include considerations such as:

- the drug is used infrequently because therapeutic alternatives covered without restriction are usually effective, but are contraindicated or ineffective because of the clinical condition of the individual patient;
- the drug has the potential for the development of widespread inappropriate use;
- the drug is more expensive than drugs covered without restriction and offers an advantage in only a limited number of indications.

Coverage for some antibiotics, for example, is restricted to use as second line therapy in cases where the infection is resistant or not responding to alternatives or the patient is allergic to alternatives. All drugs listed in the Saskatchewan Formulary are intended for outpatients, including residents of long-term care facilities. The Formulary is published annually and updated quarterly; as of July 2003, it included over 3500 drug products.[100] Listed drugs are under continuous review; new drug products are evaluated as applications are made and are added if they meet the standards of professional expert committees that aid the provincial government. With the exception of insulin and diabetes testing supplies, drugs must be prescribed by a licensed practitioner in order to be covered.

The Drug Plan began providing benefits to residents on September 1, 1975. When the program began, consumers paid a portion of the professional fee, and Saskatchewan Health paid the pharmacy for the remainder of the prescription cost; those individuals who could not afford to pay even a portion of the prescription fee were entitled to benefits without any payment. Since then the program's cost-sharing structure has undergone several changes and it currently operates as an income-based support program. Data are collected on an individual basis. Data are captured on

Table 19.1. Eligible population by age and sex: June 30, 2003

Age (years)	Females	Males	Total
Under 1	5 651	5 945	11 596
1–9	56 787	59 167	115 954
10–19	75 829	79 873	155 702
20–29	67 645	70 059	137 704
30–39	64 563	63 858	128 421
40–49	77 508	78 390	155 898
50–59	56 199	57 951	114 150
60–69	39 334	37 797	77 131
70–79	35 394	29 891	65 285
80–89	23 766	14 232	37 998
90+	5 601	2 313	7 914
Total	508 277	499 476	1 007 753

Table 19.2. Information contained in the population registry

Name
Health Services Number
Sex
Marital status
Date of birth
Residence information
Indicator for registered Indian status
Dates of coverage initiation and termination
Reason for coverage termination (e.g., died, left the province)

all prescriptions for drugs listed in the Formulary and dispensed to eligible beneficiaries, regardless of the level of benefit provided.

There are a number of validation checks made on the data. The computerized claims processing system checks each transaction for identification and demographic accuracy, claimant eligibility, and drug coverage under the Drug Plan. The immediate visual feedback incorporated in the point-of-service (POS) computer–telecommunication claims processing system provides an additional verification check at the pharmacy level during data entry. In addition, drug utilization review and program evaluations using the drug data are ongoing within the Drug Plan; to some extent, this data usage affords validation.

The database contains information from September 1975 to June 1987 and from January 1989 to date. Drug data are incomplete from July 1987 to December 1988. (During that 18-month period, data were collected from consumer-submitted claims rather than pharmacy claims and data were recorded by family unit rather than by individual.) Data include patient, drug, prescriber, pharmacy, and cost information (Table 19.3). The drug

classification schemes used enable analysis of drugs at a brand, generic, or class level; customized programs facilitate categorization into various therapeutic and/or pharmacologic groups. Because the patient is identified by the HSN, the drug data can be linked to the population registry to compile information on the age, sex, and residence of users of a product. The prescriber number can be linked with a physician registry for additional information, such as prescriber specialty. The pharmacy number enables classification by location, type of pharmacy (chain or independent), and prescription volume. The drug database does not include information on most nonformulary prescription drug use, most over-the-counter drug use, use of professional samples, or in-hospital medications. In addition, it does not include information about the dosage regimen prescribed, the reason the drug was prescribed, days supply or patient compliance.

In the fiscal year 2002–03, approximately 8.4 million prescription claims were processed by the Drug Plan (Table 19.4). Of those eligible, 68% received prescriptions;

Table 19.3. Information contained in the prescription drug database

Patient information
  Health Services Number
  Sex
  Year of birth; age
  Designation of program (e.g., social assistance, palliative care)
Drug information
  Pharmacologic–therapeutic classification[a]
  Drug identification number (DIN)[b]
  Drug active ingredient number (AIN)[b]
  Generic and brand names
  Strength and dosage form
  Manufacturer of drug
  Date dispensed
  Quantity dispensed
Prescriber information
  Prescriber identification number
Dispensing pharmacy information
  Pharmacy identification number
Cost information
  Unit cost of drug materials
  Dispensing fee
  Mark-up
  Drug Plan share of total cost
  Total cost

[a] The American Hospital Formulary Service classification system is used.
[b] Assigned by the Therapeutics Product Directorate of Health Canada.

Table 19.4. Prescriptions covered by the Drug Plan by pharmacologic–therapeutic classification, 2002–03

Pharmacologic–therapeutic classification[a]	Number of prescriptions
8: 00 Anti-infectives	639 048
10: 00 Antineoplastic drugs	1 043
12: 00 Autonomic drugs	266 165
20: 00 Blood formation and coagulation	168 285
24: 00 Cardiovascular drugs	2 271 413
28: 00 Central nervous system drugs	1 714 968
36: 00 Diagnostic agents	106 611
40: 00 Electrolytic, caloric, and water balance	582 745
48: 00 Cough preparations	867
52: 00 Eye, ear, nose, and throat preparations	270 729
56: 00 Gastrointestinal drugs	421 519
60: 00 Gold compounds	294
64: 00 Metal antagonists	357
68: 00 Hormones and substitutes	1 155 371
84: 00 Skin and mucous membrane preparations	269 634
86: 00 Spasmolytics	42 820
88: 00 Vitamins	73 117
92: 00 Unclassified	365 869
Total	8 350 855

[a] The American Hospital Formulary Service classification system is used.
Provided by: Drug Plan and Extended Benefits Branch, Saskatchewan Health, Regina, Saskatchewan.

21% of individuals receiving prescriptions were 65 years or older and they received over 47% of all prescriptions processed under the Drug Plan.

HOSPITAL SERVICES DATA

Under the hospital care insurance program, hospitals provide medically necessary services without charge to beneficiaries. All members of the covered population are eligible to receive benefits. Data are collected on every hospital separation and day surgery case, thus creating a central data bank of diagnostic and other health information on a defined population. (In Saskatchewan, a separation is defined as the discharge, transfer, or death of an inpatient.)

Five large provincial hospitals provide a full range of hospital services to the populace in their immediate areas, serve as the tertiary referral centers for specialized services, and play a major role in research and education. Six regional hospitals serve as referral centers for the people from outside their immediate vicinity, provide basic hospital care to residents in their immediate locale, and assume a limited role in education. Most acute care hospitals are classified as district, northern, or community hospitals that serve the local populace and offer a more limited range of services than the provincial or regional hospitals.

Data are collected from all hospitals in the province. Included in the database are all acute care inpatient separations, day surgeries, long-term care separations on patients who occupy a bed in a general hospital, inpatient psychiatric separations on patients treated in general hospitals, active rehabilitation therapy in general hospitals, and out-of-province hospital separations involving a member of the covered population.

All health service transactions are cross-checked with the population registry for patient eligibility and for identification and demographic accuracy. There are computer programs designed to detect illogical entries. Beginning in 1984–85, diagnostic data for over one half of the separations were processed by a national body, now known as the Canadian Institute for Health Information (CIHI); since 1998–99, all separations have been processed by CIHI. CIHI assigns additional fields to each record such as the Case Mix Group (CMG) and Resource Intensity Weight (RIW) based on the discharge diagnoses and procedures performed in hospital. The CMG and RIW values enable estimation of costs associated with a given hospitalization.

The hospital separation database includes patient, diagnostic, treatment, and other information (Table 19.5).

Table 19.5. Information contained in the hospital separation database

Patient information
  Health Services Number
  Sex
  Date of birth
Diagnostic and treatment information
  Most responsible diagnosis
  Other diagnoses (number potentially available varies
    depending on the time period)
  Principal procedure
  Other procedures (number potentially available varies
    depending on the time period)
  Accident code (external cause code)
Other
  Admission and discharge dates
  Length of stay
  Admission and separation types
  Case mix group
  Resource intensity weight
  Attending physician
  Attending surgeon (if applicable)
  Hospital identification number

Standard diagnostic and procedure classification systems are used. In data collected up to March 31, 2002, diagnoses are recorded using four-digit codes based on the International Classification of Diseases, Ninth Revision (ICD-9)[101] and procedures are recorded using four-digit codes based on the Canadian Classification of Diagnostic, Therapeutic, and Surgical Procedures (CCP).[102] Effective April 2002, diagnoses and procedures are recorded using the International Statistical Classification of Diseases and Related Health Problems, Tenth Revision, Canada (ICD-10-CA)[103] and the Canadian Classification of Health Interventions (CCI).[104] Diagnostic coding for the majority of hospital discharges is undertaken at the hospital level, usually by health records administrators. Limited routine validation of the accuracy of this coding procedure is undertaken centrally by CIHI. The data are accessible electronically from 1970 to the present.

In 2001–02, there were 140 791 inpatient separations for adults and children. Table 19.6 provides a breakdown of the inpatient separations by the ICD-9 diagnostic chapter of the most responsible diagnosis.

PHYSICIAN SERVICES DATA

In Saskatchewan, most physician services are an insured benefit. All members of the covered population are eligible to receive benefits. Medical, surgical, obstetric,

Table 19.6. Inpatient hospitalizations by ICD-9 diagnostic chapter for most responsible diagnosis, 2001–02

ICD-9 chapter		ICD-9 codes	Number of separations
I.	Infectious and parasitic diseases	001–139	2 286
II.	Neoplasms	140–239	7 617
III.	Endocrine, nutritional and metabolic diseases, and immunity disorders	240–279	3 261
IV.	Diseases of the blood and blood-forming organs	280–289	1 288
V.	Mental disorders	290–319	6 285
VI.	Diseases of the nervous system and sense organs	320–389	2 786
VII.	Diseases of the circulatory system	390–459	18 394
VIII.	Diseases of the respiratory system	460–519	13 159
IX.	Diseases of the digestive system	520–579	15 757
X.	Diseases of the genitourinary system	580–629	7 441
XI.	Complications of pregnancy, childbirth, and the puerperium	630–676	14 157
XII.	Diseases of the skin and subcutaneous tissue	680–709	1 733
XIII.	Diseases of the musculoskeletal system and connective tissue	710–739	6 363
XIV.	Congenital anomalies	740–759	840
XV.	Conditions originating in the perinatal period	760–779	3 090
XVI.	Symptoms, signs, and ill-defined conditions	780–799	8 391
XVII.	Injury and poisoning	800–999	11 458
Supplementary classification of factors influencing health status and contacts with health services		V01–V80	16 485
Total			140 791

Provided by: Health Information Solutions Centre, Saskatchewan Health, Regina, Saskatchewan.

anesthesia, and diagnostic services are included. A small number of physician services are not insured (e.g., cosmetic surgery, examinations for employment or insurance). A beneficiary may seek services from any general practitioner desired, while physicians retain the ability to accept or decline any patient.

Data collected are based primarily on physicians' claims for payment on a fee-for-service basis. There are also a number of other physicians on alternative payment arrangements (e.g., salary, contract). Under these arrangements, physicians may submit shadow or dummy claims. However, not all services provided may be captured consistently. In 2002–03, these non-fee-for-service funding arrangements accounted for about 26% of expenditure or physician-delivered services.[105]

Claims received from physicians contain patient identifiers, details regarding the service provided, and a diagnosis. Submitted claims are subjected to a series of computer checks to determine the validity of the claim data. Transactions are cross-checked with the population registry for patient eligibility and identification. Other internal computer checks are in place to check accuracy and to detect illogical entries. Claims rejected during the computer processing are reviewed manually.

Considerable patient, physician, diagnostic, and service information is available by using the claims file and the

physician registry file (Table 19.7). Diagnoses are recorded using three-digit ICD-9 codes (ICD-8 coding was used in data prior to 1979) and about 40 diagnostic codes assigned by the Medical Services Branch in Saskatchewan Health to

Table 19.7. Information available on physicians and physician services

Patient information
  Heath Services Number
  Age
  Sex
  Location of residence
  Indicator for registered Indian status
Physician information
  Physician specialty
  Referring physician
  Clinic
  Age
  Sex
  Place and year of graduation
Diagnostic and service information
  Date of service
  Service code
  Type of service
  Diagnosis (3-digit ICD-9 code)
  Location of service (e.g., office, inpatient, outpatient, home, other)
  Billing information (amount paid, date of payment)

facilitate coding of routine diagnostic tests and select conditions. Procedures are coded using fee-for-service codes from a payment schedule.[106] Fee-for-service codes are established through consultation between Saskatchewan Health and the Saskatchewan Medical Association. Because diagnostic data are given only to support the claim for payment and because only one three-digit ICD-9 code is recorded per visit, health outcome studies should not be done with unvalidated physician services data alone. When used in conjunction with the other databases, however, the outpatient physician services data can play a useful role in data linkage projects. Claims data are accessible electronically from 1971 to the present; however, for practical purposes, data are typically used from 1975 forward.

In 2002–03, more than 10 million services were provided by physicians. Table 19.8 shows the distribution of these services by ICD-9 diagnostic chapter.

CANCER SERVICES DATA

The Saskatchewan Cancer Program encompasses prevention, early detection, diagnosis, treatment, and follow-up of patients as well as research and education for malignant or pre-malignant disease. Provincial legislation mandates that

information from medical professionals and hospital records required to complete the cancer registration must be provided to the Saskatchewan Cancer Agency. Thus, the cancer registry has a record of all people in the province diagnosed with cancer. Approximately 95% of cancer notifications are from specialist referral or a pathology report, 5% are from death registrations or autopsy (singly or combined), and a small number are through physician claims. In situ cancers and some neoplasms of uncertain behavior are also registered and followed. Within Canada, patients who move out of the province receive continued surveillance through the appropriate provincial cancer clinic. All cases of invasive cancer are maintained in a follow-up program for a minimum of 10 years. The rate of loss-to-follow-up is approximately 3%.

This population-based registry was established in 1932.[107] Complete computerized data for all cancer sites are available since 1967. For research purposes, data are usually only used from 1970 forward because these data have been used more and are considered more stable than the 1967–1969 data. The cancer registry contains identification, case, death, and review information (Table 19.9) and can be related to radiotherapy and in-clinic chemotherapy treatment data. Both confirmed and suspected cases of cancer are registered.

Table 19.8. Physician services by ICD-9 diagnostic chapter, 2002–03

ICD-9 chapter		ICD-9	Number of services	Number of patients
I.	Infectious and parasitic diseases	001–139	326 496	132 023
II.	Neoplasms	140 239	222 182	60 184
III.	Endocrine, nutritional and metabolic diseases, and immunity disorders	240–279	368 355	120 234
IV.	Diseases of the blood and blood-forming organs	280–289	104 228	29 641
V.	Mental disorders	290–319	569 255	122 438
VI.	Diseases of the nervous system and sense organs	320–389	809 452	226 858
VII.	Diseases of the circulatory system	390–459	975 200	173 495
VIII.	Diseases of the respiratory system	460–519	1 072 011	338 163
IX.	Diseases of the digestive system	520–579	362 913	127 264
X.	Diseases of the genitourinary system	580–629	604 282	170 470
XI.	Complications of pregnancy, childbirth, and the puerperium	630–676	79 206	17 507
XII.	Diseases of the skin and subcutaneous tissue	680–709	429 972	171 472
XIII.	Diseases of the musculoskeletal system and connective tissue	710–739	581 357	211 469
XIV.	Congenital anomalies	740–759	15 633	6 264
XV.	Conditions originating in the perinatal period	760–779	9 770	3 780
XVI.	Symptoms, signs, and ill-defined conditions	780–799	734 635	247 390
XVII.	Injury and poisoning	800–999	666 485	225 046
Supplementary classification of factors influencing health status and contacts with health services		V01–V80	2 514 516	473 520
All other diagnoses			7 726	4 324
Total			10 453 674	850 356[a]

[a] Does not equal column total; some patients are counted in more than one chapter.
Provided by: Medical Services Branch, Saskatchewan Health, Regina, Saskatchewan.

Table 19.9. Basic information contained in the cancer registry

Patient information
　　Health Services Number
　　Name
　　Sex
　　Date and place of birth
　　Address
　　Marital status
Case information
　　Registration information (including tentative diagnosis, height, and weight)
　　Final diagnostic information (ICD-O, behavior, grade)
　　Staging information (as reported but most complete for breast and colorectal)
　　Metastases at diagnosis
　　Date of diagnosis
　　Method of diagnosis
　　Pathology report and hospital record numbers
　　Type of surgery, chemotherapy, and radiotherapy treatment indicators at diagnosis (within four months)
　　Disease status (with or without evidence of disease at end of treatment)
　　Follow-up type
Review information
　　Review date
　　Physician identifier
　　Type of review
　　Recurrence, metastases, and treatment information (surgery, chemotherapy, radiotherapy)
　　Performance status
　　Disease status
　　Weight
Death information
　　Date and place of death
　　Primary and secondary cause of death
　　Disease status at death
　　Autopsy status

In 2002, the overall cancer incidence rates were 476.6 per 100 000 for males and 414.6 for females. Incidence rates by cancer site are shown in Table 19.10.

VITAL STATISTICS

All birth, death, stillbirth, and marriage data are collected by Saskatchewan Health. Electronic data are readily accessible from 1979 to the present. Cause of death is recorded by a physician or coroner on a Medical Certificate of Death form. The causes of death recorded on this form are keyed electronically and an algorithm is applied to determine the underlying cause of death in accordance with World Health Organization criteria. If updated information such as an autopsy diagnosis is received, it takes priority over the previously submitted Medical Certificate of Death information. For events occurring up to and including 1999, four-digit ICD-9 codes are used to report cause(s) of death; since January 2000, coding is based on the International Statistical Classification of Diseases and Related Health Problems, Tenth Revision (ICD-10).[108]

Live birth registrations record obstetrical information and infant information. Completion of the Live Birth Registration Form is the responsibility of the family. Although health information regarding the infant is not captured on the birth registration form, some information regarding the health of the infant, especially major congenital anomalies, may be found in the hospital services database because most births (over 99%) occur in a hospital. Stillbirth registrations include a "medical certificate" section, which is completed and signed by a physician or coroner.

Although vital statistics data prior to 1992 do not include the HSN, those records can be searched by name or by the vital statistics registration number for linkage with other databases.

Table 19.10. Incidence rates per 100 000 by cancer site, 2002

Cancer site	Incidence rate per 100 000	
	Males	Females
Lip	4.5	1.6
Oral cavity	3.5	3.7
Head and neck	4.3	1.7
Esophagus	7.5	2.3
Stomach	11.6	5.8
Colon	40.4	41.0
Rectum	26.3	17.3
Liver	3.1	1.0
Gall bladder and biliary tract	2.6	5.2
Pancreas	10.6	7.4
Digestive tract	1.8	2.7
Larynx	4.5	0.8
Trachea, bronchus, lung	63.2	49.1
Respiratory system	2.6	1.7
Bone and connective tissue	3.1	4.5
Malignant melanoma of skin	10.6	12.6
Breast	1.0	125.0
Cervix: invasive	—	5.8
Uterus	—	23.7
Ovary	—	13.6
Female genital organs	—	2.7
Prostate	151.3	—
Male genital organs	8.0	—
Kidney	14.9	7.6
Bladder	19.8	5.0
Other urinary tract	2.9	1.4
Brain and central nervous system	6.7	4.7
Thyroid	3.1	9.1
Other endocrine glands	0.4	0.2
Lymphoma	21.0	15.5
Hodgkin's disease	3.1	2.9
Multiple myeloma	5.3	4.7
Leukemia	18.1	10.3
Primary site unknown	10.6	11.6
Other primary sites	10.2	12.4
Total	476.6	414.6

Provided by: Saskatchewan Cancer Agency, Regina, Saskatchewan.

OTHER SASKATCHEWAN HEALTH INFORMATION

A variety of health services data are available and can be either linked with the HSN or manually reviewed to provide additional information on study populations. Examples of these data include supportive care services (e.g., long-term care and home care services), some publicly funded mental health services, and laboratory services provided by the Saskatchewan Health Provincial Laboratory. The tenure and completeness of the information in these databases are variable, and the suitability of these data for research would be dependent on the particular project.

MEDICAL RECORDS

Hospital record abstraction has been used for a number of studies to collect additional information to complement or validate information derived from the administrative databases.[9–12,17–21,26–31,33–38,45–53,59,60,65,66,71,83] Medical records in hospitals are accessible upon approval from individual health authorities and affiliated facilities. To date, all those approached have permitted use of their records. Records are accessed by Saskatchewan Health personnel. Personal identifiers are available to the abstractor but are removed before information leaves the facility. The final records are coded with a pseudo-identifier. Record retrieval rates have been excellent and typically exceed 95%.

Primary health records held by physicians have been accessed for research on several occasions.[71,74,83] The process has been varied and has included both Saskatchewan Health abstractors visiting physician clinics and physician self-reporting. To date, physician participation and record retrieval rates are much lower than the rates achieved with institution-held records.[83]

STRENGTHS

SUBJECT IDENTIFICATION

One of the greatest advantages of Saskatchewan's health databases is the use of the unique HSN to identify individuals. This number is used to code all health care services and hence can be used to link data from any of the computerized databases electronically.

POPULATION-BASED DATA

Saskatchewan is a geopolitical entity composed of over 1 million people. The registry is dynamic and updated daily; therefore, it is very useful for providing current, valid denominator data. Health services data are recorded for nearly the entire population.

ELECTRONICALLY LINKABLE DATA

Data housed within Saskatchewan Health are electronically linkable. This means that information can be compiled across the databases and over time. It also means that data can be merged and sorted on the basis of age, sex, geographic location, diagnosis, and a variety of other parameters.

CROSS-SECTIONAL AND LONGITUDINAL STUDIES

It is possible to carry out both cross-sectional and longitudinal outcome studies by linking data from two or more databases. Given the long tenure of the databases, it is possible to compile information about prior drug use and previous disease experience for study populations.

OUTPATIENT PRESCRIPTION DRUG DATA

The Saskatchewan Formulary is extensive and lists over 3500 drug products (as of 2003). The database captures the majority of prescription drug use in the province.

DIAGNOSTIC CODING WITH THE INTERNATIONAL CLASSIFICATION OF DISEASES

Both the hospital separation and the physician services data use the ICD-9 coding system for diagnoses and, for more recent hospital data, the ICD-10-CA. Depending on the time period, hospital data include a varying number of discharge diagnoses, currently up to 25. The physician services data include one three-digit code per visit. The advantage of using the standard international coding system is that other agencies and other researchers can compare information from Saskatchewan with that from other jurisdictions.

MEDICAL RECORD ACCESSIBILITY

Medical records in hospitals are accessible upon approval from individual health authorities and affiliated facilities. Cooperation by individual health authorities and affiliated facilities to allow access to records has been excellent. Availability of records in the institutions has ranged from 95% to 100%, depending on the age of the record.

DATA VERIFIED AND VALIDATED

For pharmacoepidemiologic studies, it is important that data validity and reliability be evaluated. Data integrity is the responsibility of the respective administrative programs within Saskatchewan Health. The various claims processing systems have built-in audit and eligibility checks.

For research purposes, further validation is necessary. Validation, mostly by hospital chart review, has been built into a number of studies using Saskatchewan data. A wide range of conditions have been validated in this way, including rheumatoid arthritis,[28,29] hip fractures,[10,11,17,34] gastrointestinal bleeding,[9,47,51] asthma-related conditions,[18,21,26,30,31,33,35,36,45,46,50] puerperal seizures,[12] stroke,[66] liver injury,[20,27] and acute renal failure.[53] The validity of the diagnostic data is generally very good, but is dependent upon the ability of a diagnostic code to properly represent the condition in question and therefore varies with the condition. For example, for hip fracture diagnoses the sensitivity was over 99%,[10] whereas for gastrointestinal bleeding and/or perforation it was 77%[9] based on the particular case definition used in the study. Therefore, validity should be quantified for each condition studied.

Rawson and colleagues conducted a comprehensive validation study on several diagnoses and procedures in the database. The agreement between hospital data and clinical charts was excellent for hysterectomy,[49] ischemic heart disease,[38] and chronic obstructive pulmonary disease.[38]

Rawson and Robson also studied the concordance of the recording of neoplasms in the Saskatchewan cancer registry with that in hospital charts and death registrations for 368 patients.[76] The results suggested a high degree of consistency among the three data sources.

WEAKNESSES

The health databases have been constructed by the Saskatchewan government primarily for program management purposes. Research, therefore, is a secondary use, and the databases may not be well suited to some types of studies. As well, being administrative in nature, changes in policy and/or program features may influence the data collected. The gap in the drug database from July 1987 to December 1988 is an example of how a program change affected the completeness of the data collected.

The current population of Saskatchewan is relatively small for the evaluation of rare risks. To some extent, this limitation is mitigated by the fact that over 25 years of drug exposure data and almost 30 years of outcome/diagnostic data are available. Nevertheless, the databases still may be too small to evaluate low prevalence exposures or rare outcomes.

There are some limitations regarding exposure data. The Drug Plan operates on a formulary system. While the Saskatchewan Formulary is extensive (over 3500 drug products in 2003), the drug must be covered by the Drug Plan in order for records of its use to be included in the drug database. Consequently, it is not always possible to study exposure to prescription drugs as soon as they are available on the Canadian market. As well, there is no centralized computer database on inpatient drug use, over-the-counter drug use, or use of alternative therapies.

Diagnostic information is derived primarily from hospital separation or physician billing data. If the outcome does not result in any medical attention, it cannot be identified. Also, if the outcome does not result in hospitalization, the diagnostic information is weaker because it is based on physician billing data, which have less complete and less specific diagnostic coding. The lack of a complete, centralized laboratory information database limits the ability to detect outcomes that must be identified and/or confirmed by specific test results.

In any epidemiologic analyses, information on confounding is important. The databases do not contain information on some potentially important confounding variables (e.g., smoking, alcohol use, occupation, and family history). Study designs must consider alternative methods of obtaining the necessary information on confounding factors, for example use of medical records, as discussed above, or patient surveys.[72]

Some of these limitations may be offset by the ability to access individual patient records to obtain information not included in the computer databases. This is a manual process, however, and is therefore more time consuming and expensive.

PARTICULAR APPLICATIONS

LOGISTICS OF ACCESSING DATA

Researchers interested in using the data may submit proposals to Saskatchewan Health. Policies and procedures are in place that enable the data to be used for research while maintaining beneficiary and provider confidentiality and database integrity. Researchers using the data have included those from academia, other governments, the pharmaceutical industry, other private companies, and practitioners.

The prime consideration for use of the databases is confidentiality of both recipients and providers of services. Identifiable information including, for example, the identity of the patient, physician, pharmacy, or hospital will not be released without consent. Furthermore, Saskatchewan Health will not allow source files, even if pseudo-identified, to be released; only aggregated information or limited fields of non-identifiable information at a person-level may be released. Further, information collected directly from study subjects will not be linked with the administrative data without the explicit consent of the study subjects. Any data use and release must be consistent with the terms and conditions of *The Health Information Protection Act* (HIPA) of Saskatchewan, which became effective September 1, 2003.[109] Research which requires use and disclosure of identifiable personal health information must be approved by a research ethics committee which has been designated under the HIPA.

The Research Services Unit of the Population Health Branch has responsibility for conducting and/or facilitating pharmacoepidemiologic and other outcomes research, and is the point of contact for investigators who are interested in using the data for research. Personnel in the Unit have combined expertise in project management, research methodology, and analyses as well as extensive experience in using the large computerized databases for pharmacoepidemiologic and epidemiologic research.

The Saskatchewan databases have been used for a variety of studies. To illustrate the types of pharmacoepidemiologic studies that have been conducted, synopses of several projects are outlined below.

EXAMPLES OF USES

Drug Use Reviews and Patterns of Drug Utilization

1. The outpatient prescription drug database was used by Joffe *et al.* to examine the use of fluoxetine in Saskatchewan between January 1992 and June 1996.[79] Fluoxetine users during this time period were 68.2% female and 17.4% were 65 years of age or older. The average length of treatment was 88.1 days; only 18.9% of users filled prescriptions for six months. Switching to another antidepressant occurred in 13.6% of subjects. The authors concluded that further research was warranted to investigate potential underutilization of fluoxetine.

2. Bourgault *et al.* conducted a cohort study of 35 631 subjects who started therapy with angiotensin-converting enzyme (ACE) inhibitors, β-blockers, or calcium antagonists (CAs) between January 1, 1990 and December 31, 1993 according to data in the outpatient prescription drug database.[77] Follow-up data for up to seven years were compiled for this cohort from the population registry and the drug, physician services, and hospital separation databases. Patterns and determinants of use of major antihypertensive drug classes were examined, including both initial treatment and subsequent modifications to therapy. They analyzed a subset of 19 501 subjects who were between 40 and 79 years of age and had no recognized cardiac disease, and found that ACE inhibitors and CAs were increasingly used as initial therapy and that only 11.5% of study subjects continuously used the agent with

which treatment was initiated. A high number of patients, particularly among the β-blocker users, discontinued therapy early after treatment initiation. Patients initiating therapy with combination drugs were less likely to modify their treatment regimen. Patient characteristics such as age, sex, and the presence of risk factors appeared to be correlated with initial drug choice but none emerged as predictors of the rates of treatment modification. The study confirmed patterns of use of antihypertensive agents were highly variable, with a high frequency of treatment interruptions and modifications.

Studies of Drug Exposure and Health Outcomes

1. Beck *et al.* conducted a historical cohort study to investigate a possible association between 3-hydroxy3-methylglutaryl coenzyme A reductase inhibitor ("statin") cholesterol-lowering drugs and the risk of breast cancer.[92] Subject selection was based on information in the outpatient prescription drug database, the population registry, and the Saskatchewan Cancer Agency (SCA) registry.

The study cohort included 13 592 statin users and 53 880 nonexposed subjects. Subjects were followed for up to 8.5 years (mean 4.2 years). Among women aged 55 years or younger, statin use was not associated with breast cancer incidence. In women older than 55 years, the relative rate of breast cancer was 1.15 (95% CI 0.97–1.37). Rate ratios were also stratified by length of exposure to statins and prior use of hormone replacement therapy (HRT) and oral contraceptives. Among women over 55 years, these stratified analyses revealed an increase in breast cancer risk in short-term statin users, which may possibly be explained by surveillance bias. An increase in breast cancer risk was also seen in statin users with long-term (>6 years) HRT use (RR 2.04; 95% CI 1.20, 3.46).

The investigators concluded that the risk of breast cancer associated with statin use in postmenopausal women appears to be small if such a risk exists at all. Further studies are necessary to determine if short-term statin use and statin use with long-term HRT are associated with breast cancer.

2. A large population-based nested case–control study was conducted by Csizmadi *et al.* to investigate the association between colorectal cancer and HRT in post-menopausal women.[98] Cases were identified from the SCA cancer registry. Age-matched controls were selected from the population registry. HRT history was compiled from the outpatient prescription drug database. A subset of these compiled data was analyzed to investigate the effects on risk of colorectal cancer of two different HRT formulations: oral estrogen (OE) and transdermal estrogen (TDE). Rates of use of OE and TDE were 22.7% and 2.7%, respectively, among cases and 25.3% and 4.1%, respectively, among controls. The odds ratios (ORs) for less than three years and for three years and more of TDE use and colorectal cancer compared to women who had never used HRT were 0.69 and 0.33, respectively. The ORs for OE use were 0.9 and 0.75, respectively. The findings suggest that there may be a differential risk reduction of colorectal cancer between the HRT formulations.

Studies of Drug Use in Infants and Children

Wang *et al.* used the Saskatchewan health databases to assess the level of antibiotic overprescribing for upper respiratory infections (URIs) for young children less than five years of age in 1995.[67]

Respiratory diagnoses (ICD-9 codes 381, 460–466, 480–487) were identified from the physician claims database and linked to antibiotic prescriptions dispensed within seven days of the date of diagnosis. There were 140 892 visits for URIs by 38 848 children during 1995. Antibiotics are not indicated for acute URI, acute bronchitis and bronchiolitis, the common cold, serous otitis media, acute laryngitis, and influenza. Percentages of visits for these conditions resulting in an antibiotic prescription were 36%, 50%, 16%, 21%, 34%, and 22%, respectively.

Pharmacoeconomic Studies

A research project was undertaken by Simpson *et al.* to estimate health care expenditures for diabetes and its major complications.[93]

The study population consisted of 38 124 people who were assumed to have diabetes in 1996 based on the presence of one or more records for insulin or an oral antidiabetic agent in the drug database, two or more physician service claims for diabetes (ICD-9 code 250) within a two-year period, or one or more hospitalizations with a diagnostic code for diabetes as the primary, secondary, or tertiary diagnosis from 1991 to 1996 inclusive. For this diabetic cohort, information on prescription drug use, hospitalizations, and physician services in 1996 was abstracted from the respective databases. Expenditures for prescription drugs and physician services were taken directly from the corresponding database records. Hospitalization expenditures were estimated using the resource intensity weight (RIW) variable on the hospital record and multiplying it by a cost per RIW.

The study found that the 38 124 study population assumed to have diabetes in 1996 represented about 3.6% of the Saskatchewan population, whereas the estimated health care expenditures of $134.3 million for that population were approximately 15% of estimated expenditures for hospitalization, physician services, and prescription drugs in that year. There was a large variation in cost among individuals with diabetes. Patients with no complications had the lowest cost and those with renal complications had the highest cost. Also, as the number of complications increased in a diabetic patient, so did the expenditures. The study concluded that actions to prevent or control comorbidity in diabetes would yield significant cost savings.

Although this was a broad economic analysis as opposed to a pharmacoeconomic study per se, it illustrates the capabilities of the databases for cost analyses.

THE FUTURE

One of the areas of focus of the blueprint for Saskatchewan's health system is an emphasis on quality, efficiency, and accountability.[110] A Health Information Solutions Centre, a new branch within Saskatchewan Health, is working closely with regional health authorities and others to invest in information technologies to support better access to information in order to enhance initiatives in these areas.[111] As these information systems are developed, the scope and quality of data available for research may be enhanced.

One initiative under development is the collection of data by Saskatchewan Health on all prescription drug use by all residents of Saskatchewan. As with the outpatient prescription drug data currently collected on drugs listed in the Saskatchewan Formulary, pharmacies will submit the prescription information; however, it will now include all prescription drugs dispensed to any resident eligible for Saskatchewan Health coverage. This will mean complete capture of information on all outpatient prescription drugs used, regardless of who pays for the prescription. It is expected this new system will be functioning fully by July 2005. When operational, this may enable research on drug use by Saskatchewan residents as soon as the drugs are first marketed in Canada. This would be a valuable resource to enhance the capability of pharmacoepidemiologic studies that would not be limited by program coverage criteria.

Preservation of confidentiality of personal health information will continue to be of paramount importance. HIPA, which became effective September 1, 2003, establishes a common set of rules for everyone in the health system. It emphasizes protection of privacy of personal health information while ensuring that, with proper precautions, information is available to provide efficient health services. Research under specific conditions continues to be a permitted use of health services information.

The value of the Saskatchewan health databases as a resource for pharmacoepidemiologic research has been demonstrated. As enhancements of the databases continue and as the information is used in a responsible manner, the databases will continue to contribute to providing valuable information on public health issues related to drug use.

ACKNOWLEDGMENTS

We gratefully acknowledge our colleagues in both Saskatchewan Health, in particular, Andrea Laturnas, Sheena McRae, Duane Mombourquette, Carmelle Mondor, and Ronn Wallace, and the Saskatchewan Cancer Agency, in particular, Bill Morton and Jon Tonita, for their critical review of the respective program descriptions and data provision. We also gratefully acknowledge Maureen Jackson for her constructive comments on the manuscript overall and Lyn Yeo for her layout and editorial assistance.

REFERENCES

1. Skoll EL, August RJ, Johnson GE. Drug prescribing for the elderly in Saskatchewan during 1976. *Can Med Assoc J* 1979; **121**: 1074–81.
2. Schnell BR. A review of the use of prescription drugs in Saskatchewan. *Can Pharm J* 1981; **7**: 267–70.
3. Power B, Downey W, Schnell BR. Utilization of psychotropic drugs in Saskatchewan. *Can J Psychiatry* 1983; **28**: 547–51.
4. West R, Sherman GJ, Downey W. A record linkage study of valproate and malformations in Saskatchewan. *Can J Public Health* 1985; **76**: 226–8.
5. Quinn DMP. Prevalence of psychoactive medication in children and adolescents. *Can J Psychiatry* 1986; **31**: 575–80.
6. Guess HA, West R, Strand LM, Helston D, Lydick E, Bergman U *et al.* Hospitalization for renal impairment among users and non-users of nonsteroidal anti-inflammatory drugs in Saskatchewan, Canada, 1983. In: Rainsford KD, Velo GP, eds, *Side-Effects of Anti-Inflammatory Drugs, Part 2: Studies in Major Organ Systems.* Lancaster, PA: MTP Press, 1987; pp. 367–74.
7. Babiker IE. Comparative efficacy of long-acting depot and oral neuroleptic medications in preventing schizophrenic recidivism. *J Clin Psychiatry* 1987; **48**: 94–7.
8. Hogan DJ, Strand LM, Lane PR. Isotretinoin therapy for acne: a population-based study. *Can Med Assoc J* 1988; **138**: 47–50.
9. Guess HA, West R, Strand LM, Helston D, Lydick EG, Bergman U, Wolski K. Fatal upper gastrointestinal hemorrhage

or perforation among users and nonusers of nonsteroidal anti-inflammatory drugs in Saskatchewan, Canada 1983. *J Clin Epidemiol* 1988; **41**: 35–45.

10. Ray WA, Griffin MR, Downey W, Melton LJ. Long-term use of thiazide diuretics and risk of hip fracture. *Lancet* 1989; **i**: 687–90.

11. Ray WA, Griffin MR, Downey W. Benzodiazepines of long and short elimination half-life and the risk of hip fracture. *JAMA* 1989; **262**: 3303–7.

12. Rothman KJ, Funch DP, Dreyer NA. Bromocriptine and puerperal seizures. *Epidemiology* 1990; **1**: 232–8.

13. Blackburn JL, Downey FW, Quinn TJ. The Saskatchewan program for rational drug therapy: effects on utilization of mood-modifying drugs. *Drug Intell Clin Pharm* 1990; **24**: 878–82.

14. Thiessen BQ, Wallace SM, Blackburn JL, Wilson T, Bergman U. Increased prescribing of antidepressants subsequent to beta-blocker therapy. *Arch Intern Med* 1990; **150**: 2286–90.

15. O'Reilly R. Are the monoamine oxidase inhibitors facing extinction? *Can J Psychiatry* 1991; **36**: 186–9.

16. Horwitz RI, Spitzer W, Buist S, Cockcroft D, Ernst P, Habbick B *et al.* Clinical complexity and epidemiologic uncertainty in case–control research: fenoterol and asthma management. *Chest* 1991; **100**: 1586–91.

17. Ray WA, Griffin MR, Malcolm E. Cyclic antidepressants and the risk of hip fracture. *Arch Intern Med* 1991; **151**: 754–6.

18. Spitzer WO, Suissa S, Ernst P, Horwitz RI, Habbick B, Cockcroft D *et al.* The use of β-agonists and the risk of death and near death from asthma. *N Engl J Med* 1992; **326**: 501–6.

19. Garcia Rodriguez LA, Walker AM, Perez Gutthann S. Nonsteroidal anti-inflammatory drugs and gastrointestinal hospitalizations in Saskatchewan: a cohort study. *Epidemiology* 1992; **3**: 337–42.

20. Garcia Rodriguez LA, Perez Gutthann S, Walker AM, Lueck L. The role of nonsteroidal anti-inflammatory drugs in acute liver injury. *BMJ* 1992; **305**: 865–8.

21. Ernst P, Spitzer WO, Suissa S, Cockcroft D, Habbick B, Horwitz RI *et al.* Risk of fatal and near-fatal asthma in relation to inhaled corticosteroid use. *JAMA* 1992; **268**: 3462–4.

22. Suissa S, Spitzer WO, Abenhaim L, Downey W, Gardiner RJ, Fitzgerald D. Risk of death from human insulin. *Pharmacoepidemiol Drug Saf* 1992; **1**: 169–75.

23. Quinn K, Baker M, Evans B. A population-wide profile of prescription drug use in Saskatchewan, 1989. *Can Med Assoc J* 1992; **146**: 2177–86.

24. Suissa S, Hemmelgarn B, Spitzer WO, Brophy J, Collet JP, Cote R *et al.* The Saskatchewan oral contraceptive cohort study of oral contraceptive use and cardiovascular risks. *Pharmacoepidemiol Drug Saf* 1993; **2**: 33–49.

25. Rawson NSB. An acute adverse drug reaction alerting scheme using the Saskatchewan Health datafiles. *Drug Invest* 1993; **6**: 245–56.

26. Habbick BF, for the Saskatchewan Asthma Epidemiology Project Team. The Saskatchewan Asthma Epidemiology Project. *Sask Med J* 1993; **4**: 4–7.

27. Perez Gutthann S, Garcia Rodriguez LA. Increased risk of hospitalizations for acute liver injury in a population with exposure to multiple drugs. *Epidemiology* 1993; **4**: 497–501.

28. Tennis P, Bombardier C, Malcolm E, Downey W. Validity of rheumatoid arthritis diagnoses listed in the Saskatchewan hospital separations database. *J Clin Epidemiol* 1993; **46**: 675–83.

29. Tennis P, Andrews E, Bombardier C, Wang Y, Strand L, West R *et al.* Record linkage to conduct an epidemiologic study on the association of rheumatoid arthritis and lymphoma in the province of Saskatchewan, *Can. J Clin Epidemiol* 1993; **46**: 685–95.

30. Ernst P, Habbick B, Suissa S, Hemmelgarn B, Cockcroft D, Buist AS *et al.* Is the association between inhaled beta-agonist use and life-threatening asthma because of confounding by severity? *Am Rev Respir Dis* 1993; **148**: 75–9.

31. Suissa S, Ernst P, Boivin JF, Horwitz R, Habbick B, Cockcroft D *et al.* A cohort analysis of excess mortality in asthma and the use of inhaled beta-agonists. *Am J Respir Crit Care Med* 1994; **249**: 604–10.

32. Risch HA, Howe GR. Menopausal hormone usage and breast cancer in Saskatchewan: a record-linkage cohort study. *Am J Epidemiol* 1994; **139**: 670–83.

33. Hemmelgarn B, Blais L, Collet, JP, Ernst P, Suissa S. Automated databases and the need for fieldwork in pharmacoepidemiology. *Pharmacoepidemiol Drug Saf* 1994; **3**: 275–82.

34. Lichtenstein MJ, Griffin MR, Cornell JE, Malcolm E, Ray WA. Risk factors for hip fractures occurring in the hospital. *Am J Epidemiol* 1994; **140**: 830–8.

35. Suissa S, Blais L, Ernst P. Patterns of increasing β-agonist use and the risk of fatal or near-fatal asthma. *Eur Respir J* 1994; **7**: 1602–9.

36. Ernst P, Hemmelgarn B, Cockcroft DW, Suissa S. Overreliance on bronchodilators as a risk factor for life-threatening asthma. *Can Respir J* 1995; **2**: 34–9.

37. Tennis P, Cole TB, Annegers JF, Leestma JE, McNutt M, Rajput A. Cohort study of incidence of sudden unexplained death in persons with seizure disorder treated with antiepileptic drugs in Saskatchewan, Canada. *Epilepsia* 1995; **36**: 29–36.

38. Rawson NSB, Malcolm E. Validity of the recording of ischaemic heart disease and chronic obstructive pulmonary disease in the Saskatchewan health care datafiles. *Stat Med* 1995; **14**: 2627–43.

39. Neutel I, Downey W, Senft D. Medical events after a prescription for a benzodiazepine. *Pharmacoepidemiol Drug Saf* 1995; **4**: 63–73.

40. Habbick B, Baker MJ, McNutt M, Cockcroft DW. Recent trends in the use of inhaled β_2-adrenergic agonists and inhaled corticosteroids in Saskatchewan. *Can Med Assoc J* 1995; **153**: 1437–43.

41. Neutel CI. Risk of traffic accident injury after a prescription for a benzodiazepine. *Ann Epidemiol* 1995; **5**: 239–44.

42. Neutel CI, Maxwell CJ. The benzodiazepine treadmill—does one prescription lead to more? *Pharmacoepidemiol Drug Saf* 1996; **5**: 39–42.

43. Remillard AJ. A pharmacoepidemiological evaluation of anti-cholinergic prescribing patterns in the elderly. *Pharmacoepidemiol Drug Saf* 1996; **5**: 155–64.

44. Albright PS, Livingstone S, Keegan DL, Ingham M, Shrikhande S, LeLorier J. Reduction in healthcare resource utilisation and costs following the use of risperidone for patients with schizophrenia previously treated with standard antipsychotic therapy. A retrospective analysis using the Saskatchewan Health linkable databases. *Clin Drug Invest* 1996; **11**: 289–99.

45. Joseph KS, Blais L, Ernst P, Suissa S. Increased morbidity and mortality related to asthma among asthmatic patients who use major tranquillisers. *BMJ* 1996; **312**: 79–83.

46. Suissa S. The case–time–control design. *Epidemiology* 1996; **6**: 248–53.

47. Raiford DS, Perez Gutthann S, Garcia Rodriguez LA. Positive predictive value of ICD-9 codes in the identification of cases of complicated peptic ulcer disease in the Saskatchewan hospital automated database. *Epidemiology* 1996; **7**: 101–4.

48. Suissa S, Hemmelgarn B, Blais L, Ernst P. Bronchodilators and acute cardiac death. *Am J Respir Crit Care Med* 1996; **154**: 1598–1602.

49. Edouard L, Rawson NSB. Reliability of the recording of hysterectomy in the Saskatchewan health care system. *Br J Obstet Gynaecol* 1996; **103**: 891–7.

50. Blais L, Ernst P, Suissa S. Confounding by indication and channeling over time: the risks of β$_2$-agonists. *Am J Epidemiol* 1996; **144**: 1161–9.

51. Perez Gutthann S, Garcia Rodriguez LA, Raiford DS. Individual nonsteroidal anti-inflammatory drugs and other risk factors for upper gastrointestinal bleeding and perforation. *Epidemiology* 1996; **8**: 18–24.

52. Rawson NSB, Malcolm E, D'Arcy C. Reliability of the recording of schizophrenia and depressive disorder in the Saskatchewan health care datafiles. *Soc Psychiatry Psychiatr Epidemiol* 1997; **32**: 191–9.

53. Perez Gutthann S, Garcia Rodriguez LA, Raiford DS, Duque Oliart A, Ris Romeu J. Nonsteroidal anti-inflammatory drugs and the risk of hospitalization for acute renal failure. *Arch Intern Med* 1996; **156**: 2433–9.

54. Johnson JA, Wallace SM. Investigating the relationship between β-blocker and antidepressant use through linkage of the administrative databases of Saskatchewan Health. *Pharmacoepidemiol Drug Saf* 1997; **6**: 1–11.

55. Maxwell CJ, Neutel CI, Hirdes JP. A prospective study of falls after benzodiazepine use: a comparison of new and repeat use. *Pharmacoepidemiol Drug Saf* 1997; **6**: 27–35.

56. Senthilselvan A. Prevalence of physician-diagnosed asthma in Saskatchewan 1981 to 1990. *Chest* 1998; **114**: 388–92.

57. Blais L, Suissa S, Boivin J-F, Ernst P. First treatment with inhaled corticosteroids and the risk of admissions to hospital for asthma. *Thorax* 1998; **53**: 1025–9.

58. Blais L, Ernst P, Boivin J-F, Suissa S. Inhaled corticosteroids and the prevention of readmission to hospital for asthma. *Am J Respir Crit Care Med* 1998; **158**: 126–32.

59. Rawson NSB, Rutledge Harding S, Malcolm E, Lueck L. Hospitalizations for aplastic anemia and agranulocytosis in Saskatchewan: incidence and associations with antecedent prescription drug use. *J Clin Epidemiol* 1998; **51**: 1343–55.

60. Rawson NSB, D'Arcy C. Assessing the validity of diagnostic information in administrative health care utilization data: experience in Saskatchewan. *Pharmacoepidemiol Drug Saf* 1998; **7**: 389–98.

61. Rawson NSB, Blackburn JL, Baker MJ. Prescription-episodes to study drug utilization with the Saskatchewan Drug Plan datafile. *J Soc Adm Pharm* 1998; **15**: 241–51.

62. Suissa S, Bourgault C, Barkun A, Sheehy O, Ernst P. Antihypertensive drugs and the risk of gastrointestinal bleeding. *Am J Med* 1998; **105**: 230–5.

63. Caro JJ, Salas M, Speckman JL, Raggio G, Jackson JD. Persistence with treatment for hypertension in actual practice. *Can Med Assoc J* 1999; **160**: 31–7.

64. Caro JJ, Salas M, Speckman JL, Raggio G, Jackson JD. Effect of initial drug choice on persistence with antihypertensive therapy: the importance of actual practice data. *Can Med Assoc J* 1999; **160**: 41–6.

65. Stang MR, Wysowski DK, Butler-Jones D. Incidence of lactic acidosis in metformin users. *Diabetes Care* 1999; **22**: 925–7.

66. Liu L, Reeder B, Shuaib A, Mazagri R. Validity of stroke diagnosis on hospital discharge records in Saskatchewan, Canada: implications for stroke surveillance. *Cerebrovasc Dis* 1999; **9**: 224–30.

67. Wang EEL, Einarson TR, Kellner JD, Conly JM. Antibiotic prescribing for Canadian preschool children: evidence of overprescribing for viral respiratory infections. *Clin Infect Dis* 1999; **29**: 155–60.

68. Bourgault C, Elstein E, LeLorier J, Suissa S. Reference-based pricing of prescription drugs: exploring the equivalence of angiotensin-converting-enzyme inhibitors. *Can Med Assoc J* 1999; **160**: 255–60.

69. Caro JJ, Migliaccio-Walle K, for CAPRA. Generalizing the results of clinical trials to actual practice: the example of clopidogrel therapy for the prevention of vascular events. *Am J Med* 1999; **107**: 568–72.

70. Rawson NSB, Rawson MJ. Acute adverse event signalling scheme using the Saskatchewan administrative health care utilization datafiles: results for two benzodiazepines. *Can J Clin Pharmacol* 1999; **6**: 159–66.

71. Walker AM, Szneke P, Weatherby LB, Dicker LW, Lanza LL, Loughlin JE *et al*. The risk of serious cardiac arrhythmias among cisapride users in the United Kingdom and Canada. *Am J Med* 1999; **107**: 356–62.

72. Sharpe CR, Collet JP, McNutt M, Belzile E, Boivin JF, Hanley JA. Nested case–control study of the effects of non-steroidal anti-inflammatory drugs on breast cancer and stage. *Br J Cancer* 2000; **83**: 112–20.

73. Suissa S, Ernst P, Benayoun S, Baltzan M, Cai B. Low-dose inhaled corticosteroids in the prevention of death from asthma. *N Engl J Med* 2000; **343**: 332–6.

74. West S, Richter A, Melfi C, McNutt M, Nennstiel M, Mauskopf J. Assessing the Saskatchewan databases for

outcomes research studies of depression and its treatment. *J Clin Epidemiol* 2000; **53**: 823–31.

75. Jick SS, Kremers HM, Vasilakies-Scaramozza C. Isotretinoin use and risk of depression, psychotic symptoms, suicide, and attempted suicide. *Arch Dermatol* 2000; **136**: 1231–6.

76. Rawson NSB, Robson DL. Concordance on the recording of cancer in the Saskatchewan Cancer Agency registry, hospital charts, and death registrations. *Can J Public Health* 2000; **5**: 390–3.

77. Bourgault C, Rainville B, Suissa S. Antihypertensive drug therapy in Saskatchewan: patterns of use and determinants in hypertension. *Arch Intern Med* 2001; **161**: 1873–9.

78. Benayouan S, Ernst P, Suissa S. The impact of combined inhaled bronchodilator therapy in the treatment of COPD. *Chest* 2001; **119**: 85–92.

79. Joffe RT, Iskedjian M, Einarson TR, O'Brien BJ, Stang MR. Examining the Saskatchewan health drug database for antidepressant use: the case of fluoxetine. *Can J Clin Pharmacol* 2001; **8**: 146–52.

80. Dyck RF, Klomp H, Tan L. From "thrifty genotype" to "hefty fetal phenotype": the relationship between high birthweight and diabetes in Saskatchewan registered Indians. *Can J Public Health* 2001; **92**: 340–4.

81. Bourgault C, Elstein E, Baltzan MA, Le Lorier J, Suissa S. Antihypertensives and myocardial infarction risk: the modifying effect of history of drug use. *Pharmacoepidemiol Drug Saf* 2001; **10**: 287–94.

82. Sharpe CR, Collet JP, Belzile E, Hanley JA, Boivin JF. The effects of tricyclic antidepressants on breast cancer risk. *Br J Cancer* 2002; **86**: 92–7.

83. Rawson N, Cox J, Stang MR, Rawson M. New use of antiarrhythmia drugs in Saskatchewan. *Can J Cardiol* 2002; **18**: 43–50.

84. Rawson N. Ethical issues in pharmacoepidemiologic research using Saskatchewan administrative health care utilization data. *Pharmacoepidemiol Drug Saf* 2001; **10**: 607–12.

85. Csizmadi I, Benedetti A, Boivin JF, Hanley, JA, Collet JP. Use of postmenopausal estrogen replacement therapy from 1981 to 1997. *Can Med Assoc J* 2002; **166**: 187–8.

86. Marentette MA, Gerth WC, Billings DK, Zarnke KB. Antihypertensive persistence and drug class. *Can J Cardiol* 2002; **18**: 649–56.

87. Ernst P, Cai B, Blais L, Suissa S. The early course of newly diagnosed asthma. *Am J Med* 2002; **112**: 44–8.

88. Suissa S, Ernst P, Kezouh A. Regular use of inhaled corticosteroids and the long term prevention of hospitalization for asthma. *Thorax* 2002; **57**: 880–4.

89. Benayoun S, Ernst P, Suissa S. The impact of combined inhaled bronchodilator therapy in the treatment of COPD. *Chest* 2001; **119**: 85–92.

90. Collet JP, Sharpe C, Belzile E, Boivin JF, Hanley J, Abenhaim L. Colorectal cancer prevention by non-steroidal anti-inflammatory drugs: effects of dosage and timing. *Br J Cancer* 1999; **81**: 62–8.

91. Johnson J, Majumdar S, Simpson S, Toth E. Decreased mortality associated with the use of metformin compared with sulfonylurea monotherapy in type 2 diabetes. *Diabetes Care* 2002; **25**: 2244–8.

92. Beck P, Wysowski D, Downey W, Butler-Jones D. Statin use and the risk of breast cancer. *J Clin Epidemiol* 2003; **56**: 280–5.

93. Simpson S, Corabian P, Jacobs P, Johnson J. The cost of major comorbidity in people with diabetes mellitus. *Can Med Assoc J* 2003; **168**: 1661–7.

94. Senthilselvan A, Lawson J, Rennie D, Dosman J. Stabilization of an increasing trend in physician-diagnosed asthma prevalence in Saskatchewan, 1991 to 1998. *Chest* 2003; **124**: 438–48.

95. Mitchell C, Simpson S, Johnson J. The cost of blood glucose test strips in Saskatchewan, 1996: a retrospective database analysis. *Can J Diabetes* 2003; **27**: 149–53.

96. Dyck R, Klomp H, Tan L, Stang MR. An association of maternal age and birth weight with end-stage renal disease in Saskatchewan: sub-analysis of registered Indians and those with diabetes. *Am J Nephrol* 2003; **23**: 395–402.

97. Suissa S, Assimes T, Brassard P, Ernst P. Inhaled corticosteroid use in asthma and the prevention of myocardial infarction. *Am J Med* 2003; **115**: 377–81.

98. Csizmadi I, Collet J-P, Benedetti A, Boivin J-F, Hanley JA. The effects of transdermal and oral oestrogen replacement therapy on colorectal cancer risk in postmenopausal women. *Br J Cancer* 2004; **90**: 76–81.

99. Health Information Solutions Centre. *Covered Population 2003*. Regina, SK: Saskatchewan Health, 2003.

100. Drug Plan and Extended Benefits Branch, Saskatchewan Health. *Formulary*, 53rd edn. Regina, SK: Saskatchewan Health, 2003.

101. World Health Organization. *Manual of the International Statistical Classification of Diseases, Injuries, and Causes of Death*, 9th revision. Geneva: WHO, 1977.

102. Statistics Canada. *Canadian Classification of Diagnostic, Therapeutic, and Surgical Procedures*. Ottawa: Minister of Supply and Services, 1986.

103. *International Statistical Classification of Diseases and Related Health Problems* (ICD-10-CA) [monograph on CD-ROM], 10th revision. Ottawa: Canadian Institute for Health Information, 2003.

104. *Canadian Classification of Health Interventions* (CCI) [monograph on CD-ROM]. Ottawa: Canadian Institute for Health Information, 2003.

105. Medical Services Branch, Saskatchewan Health. *Annual Statistical Report 2002–2003*. Regina, SK: Saskatchewan Health, 2003.

106. Medical Services Branch, Saskatchewan Health. *Payment Schedule for Insured Services Provided by a Physician October 2003*. Regina, SK: Saskatchewan Health, 2003.

107. Tonita J, Alvi R, Watson F, Robson D. *Saskatchewan Cancer Control Report: Profiling Trends in Cancer, 1970–2001*. Regina, SK: Saskatchewan Cancer Agency, 2003.

108. World Health Organization. *International Statistical Classification of Diseases and Related Health Problems* (ICD-10), 10th revision. Geneva: WHO, 1992.

109. *The Health Information Protection Act*, Chapter H-0.021, Statutes of Saskatchewan (1999).

110. Saskatchewan Health. *The Action Plan for Saskatchewan Health Care*. Regina, SK: Saskatchewan Health, 2001.

111. Saskatchewan Health. *The Action Plan for Saskatchewan Health Care: Progress Report*. Regina, SK: Saskatchewan Health, 2003.

20

Automated Pharmacy Record Linkage in The Netherlands

HUBERT G. LEUFKENS[1] and JOHN URQUHART[2]

[1] Department of Pharmacoepidemiology and Pharmacotherapy, Utrecht Institute for Pharmaceutical Sciences (UIPS), The Netherlands; [2] Department of Epidemiology, Maastricht University, Maastricht, The Netherlands, and AARDEX Ltd, Zug, Switzerland and Palo Alto, California, USA.

INTRODUCTION

Pharmacoepidemiology, as a scientific and clinical discipline, has shown remarkable growth and advancement during the past decade in The Netherlands and, as in other countries, it has many antecedents, each with some decades of history. The traditions of academic medicine in The Netherlands are long and strong. Bedside teaching as a basic pedagogic device was pioneered by Herman Boerhaave in Leiden in the early 18th century, attracting students from as far as Japan. Around the turn of the last century, van't Hoff's discovery of osmosis and Einthoven's discovery and development of electrocardiography laid important scientific foundations for modern medicine; both were early Nobel Laureates. Clinical research developed in The Netherlands in parallel with other Western countries, with increasing use of randomized clinical trials after the Second World War.

In the late 1980s, a number of Dutch clinical pharmacologists began shifting towards observational studies, bridging the gap between clinical pharmacology and epidemiology. Notable findings in this work have been, for example, the role of dietary potassium intake in prevention of cardiovascular disease,[1] information about the risks of stroke in patients on antihypertensive treatment,[2] and the adverse effects on the cardiovascular system of the use of nonsteroidal anti-inflammatory drugs (NSAIDs).[3] The latter study has stimulated further pharmacoepidemiologic research with the PHARMO system (more about this later) on the association between exposure to NSAIDs and adverse cardiovascular effects. Heerdink et al. found a twofold-increased risk of hospitalization for congestive heart failure (CHF) during periods of concomitant use of diuretics and NSAIDs compared with use of diuretics only.[4] A few years later, Feenstra et al. were able to differentiate NSAID-induced risk between patients with incident and prevalent CHF.[5] Using data from the Rotterdam Study (more about this later) an NSAID-induced relative risk of incident CHF of 1.1 (95% CI=0.7–1.7) was found. In patients with prevalent

Pharmacoepidemiology, Fourth Edition   Edited by B.L. Strom

CHF the relative risk of a relapse of disease was 9.9 (95% CI = 1.7–57.0). As elsewhere, the long-term consequences of oral contraceptive use became a focus of what we would today call pharmacoepidemiologic research, with a series of studies investigating the preventive effect of oral contraceptives on the risk of rheumatoid arthritis,[6,7] followed during the mid- and late 1990s by a surge of Dutch studies on the mechanisms and magnitude of venous and arterial risk with so-called third-generation oral contraceptives.[8–10]

Two notable antecedents of Dutch pharmacoepidemiology are pharmacovigilance and drug utilization research. The Dutch pharmacovigilance system began in the 1960s, and has generated a succession of signals of suspected adverse effects, pharmacoepidemiology studies to test them, and the finding of new signaling methods for drug risks.[11,12] Nowadays, The Netherlands Pharmacovigilance Foundation, called LAREB, plays an innovative role in signal detection, strengthening, and evaluation. The system is strongly based on liaison between pharmacists and physicians, and plays a key role in assuring patient safety, in close collaboration with national regulatory agencies and academic centers.[13,14] Drug utilization research dates back to the early 1970s under the WHO Drug Utilization Research Group, recently renamed EuroDURG, strengthening methods for ascertaining drug exposure[15,16] (see also Chapter 27).

Progress in pharmacoepidemiology in The Netherlands has, as elsewhere, been closely related to specific features of the systems for health care delivery and its reimbursement. The discipline could flourish in environments where there is good access to data on the variability of drug exposure, diagnoses, reasons for hospitalization, clinical status, and outcomes.[17] Yet there is no Valhalla where all these sources of information freely come together, so the possibilities for pharmacoepidemiologic research vary greatly from one country to another, and within countries, as the different chapters in this section of this book demonstrate. Indeed, differences in the organization and reimbursement of health care that are trivial from an administrative perspective can have major impacts on the possibilities for epidemiologic research—a point that epidemiologists have traditionally found difficult to communicate to administrators. It was not long ago that Ellwood underscored the value of administrative and reimbursement arrangements that facilitate the collection of data on the vast array of natural experiments that comprise routine health care for outcomes research.[18] Building a bridge between (clinical) epidemiology and outcomes research based on such data from routine health care remains a major challenge. As we shall see later in this chapter, there has been for decades a very productive "loyalty culture" in Dutch health care of patients seeking cure and medical assistance through a single GP practice for their primary care and through a single designated pharmacy for their outpatient prescription drugs.

DESCRIPTION

DUTCH MEDICINE

Pharmacoepidemiology in The Netherlands is naturally imbedded in the principles of medicine as practiced in this country of approximately 16.5 million people.[19] Demographically, The Netherlands is similar to the other Western countries—very low mortality rates until past age 60, with an increasing population of elderly, in which females outnumber males. The three main causes of death are, as in other technologically advanced countries, coronary heart disease and other cardiovascular diseases, the various cancers, and accidents. Per capita expenditures on health care are in line with other western European countries, and about half of those in the United States. One searches in vain, however, for substantive differences in public health indices between The Netherlands and the United States.

The drug regulatory system in The Netherlands has been widely acknowledged as one of the most influential and proactive in Europe, and plays an important role in European regulatory affairs within the framework of the European Medicines Agency (EMEA) in London. Dutch regulators and assessors belong to the most frequently involved authorities in bringing new drugs to European patients and in keeping track of the course of events connected to the new drug after marketing authorization is granted. By tradition, governmental and reimbursement policies, as well as the leadership in the medical profession, show a certain reluctance towards new pharmaceutical products. Rising health care costs, but also a culture of skepticism among prescribers and other decision makers regarding medical technology, reinforce this policy.[20]

The Dutch system of medicine is based on primary care physicians—general practitioners (GPs) called "house doctors" (*huisarts*)—who practice in the community but not in hospitals, referring ambulatory patients to specialists for out- or inpatient care, as circumstances require. Hospital care, as in other continental countries, is provided by full-time staff physicians who are specialists of various kinds. Medical care, including prescription drugs, is essentially fully paid for by public or private insurers. Health care of essentially uniform quality is provided to all citizens. Hospitals are organized regionally, with well-defined catchment areas. It is, in principle, possible to link data from the community and hospitals, although with strict attention to anonymization, as discussed later. So far, neither Dutch medicine nor the Dutch pharmaceutical industry is much influenced by the tort system of medical malpractice and product liability that is so prominent in the United States, and increasing in the United Kingdom.

The public insurers are in most cases regional agencies, in the past collectively called *Ziekenfonds* ("Sickfunds"), but nowadays are parts of conglomerates of health insurance companies, which represent a typical Dutch blend of both nonprofit and commercial, stockmarket-driven insurers. They provide essentially complete insurance coverage for approximately two-thirds of the population whose incomes fall below a defined annual level. Patients covered by these public insurance schemes are required to designate a general practitioner for primary care and a community pharmacy for all reimbursed prescription drugs. The remaining third of the population are covered by private insurers, usually organized through their employer.

All insurers are nominally in competition with one another, but it is a muted form of competition that has, thus far, avoided serious poaching on each other's actuarial bases. In this economic context, contemporary health care policies are increasingly driven by cost-containment and efficiency factors, thereby challenging the sustainability of a collective, solidarity based, health care system as it has existed for the past four to five decades.[19] This interplay between economic, demographic (e.g., extension of the European Union and globalization), and socioeconomic factors, technological change, and other forces in the health care market, may result in very different scenarios for the future.[21]

GENERAL PRACTICE SYSTEM

Computerization of general practices began in the late 1980s. Debate and confusion about taxonomy and software have impeded its development, as has the lack of any distinct economic incentive for physicians to abandon paper-based records. This situation contrasts sharply with the almost complete computerization of community pharmacies during the 1980s, facilitated by distinct economic incentives, a well-developed taxonomy for products, and major investment in the development and marketing of several competing systems of software.

Since the late 1970s, a large number of (mainly) academically-driven research networks of "sentinels" in general practice have been established among primary care physicians, doing population-based pharmacoepidemiology studies. For example, Hoes conducted a case–control study among hypertensive patients, demonstrating an association

between the use of potassium-wasting diuretics and an increased risk of sudden cardiac death, based on data collected through a network of GPs in Rotterdam.[22] Pharmacy data were used to validate the drug exposure data provided by the GPs. No significant discrepancies between the two sets of data were found, which is noteworthy, in view of numerous examples of incomplete prescribing information from paper-based GP records.

A very powerful development in making use of the GP as a resource for pharmacoepidemiology has been the establishment of the Integrated Primary Care Information (IPCI) system, which is a research-oriented database with information from computerized patient records of GPs throughout The Netherlands. The system has been developed by the Department of Medical Informatics in collaboration with the Pharmacoepidemiology Unit of the Erasmus University Medical School.[23] The database includes all demographic information, patient complaints, symptoms and diagnosis (International Classification of Primary Care; ICPC), laboratory tests, discharge and consultant letters, and detailed prescription information (drug name, ATC code, dosing information and indication). The system maintains a network of 150 general practitioners, covers over 500 000 people, is population-based, and provides a powerful tagging system enabling prospective follow-up of clinically well-defined target groups. As the system is close to general practice, it is a very suitable resource to evaluate doctor-specific prescribing behavior in the context of information about the indication of prescribing. This aspect is exemplified by a follow-up study of prescribing behavior in the aftermath of a controversial press campaign in 2002 by the pharmaceutical industry to promote more attention for onychomycosis, thereby anticipating more prescriptions for a new drug product for that indication (i.e., terbinafine).[24] Direct-to-consumer marketing is illegal in the EU. IPCI data showed that the consultation rate for onychomycosis increased, that the prescription rates for one of the older, and cheaper, antimycotic drugs (i.e., itraconazole) decreased, and that prescription volume of terbinafine more than doubled. After the campaign was stopped, rates of consultations and prescriptions dropped again.

The database has also shown its strengths for conducting population-based case–control studies, for instance in relation to the question of whether antipsychotics are associated with prolongation of QT interval and sudden cardiac death.[25] A total of 554 cases of sudden cardiac death were evaluated with data retrieved from IPCI. Current use of antipsychotics was found to be associated with a threefold increased risk of sudden cardiac death, even at a low dose and for indications other than schizophrenia.

THE DUTCH COMMUNITY PHARMACY SYSTEM

Dutch community pharmacies are typically three to four times larger than their counterparts in other western European countries or North America, having 8000–10 000 patients per pharmacy. Dutch pharmacies essentially limit themselves to prescription drugs, and have virtually none of the long shelves of consumer products that one finds in pharmacies in the United States, Canada, and the United Kingdom. Dutch pharmacies do carry over-the-counter products, but keep them behind the counter. In the past decades, the government has acted in various ways to restrict pharmacists' incomes, but most Dutch community pharmacies continue to be economically strong. Computerization of pharmacy records, and thus the compilation of prescription drug histories, is almost universal. Although recent public policies on pharmaceutical services aim to encourage patients to seek the most cost-effective pharmaceutical care available, and if necessary to switch from one pharmacy to another, practice and research show that mobility between pharmacies, which would hamper continuity and completeness of prescription drug histories, is virtually nonexistent so far. As most patients are fully reimbursed for their prescription drugs, economic incentives for between-pharmacy shopping are practically absent. Personal service and the provision of pharmaceutical care remain the main basis for competition among pharmacies.

Grouping patients as recipients of a particular pharmaceutical is thus possible by linking medication files, creating a pharmacy-based cohort, as first defined by Borden and Lee at Upjohn in the 1970s.[26] Their method consisted of the identification and follow-up of patients whose treatment with a certain pharmaceutical was defined by pharmacy records showing that the product in question had been dispensed to them. This approach has now been widely adopted. For example, recipients of acitretine in The Netherlands were traced nationally through pharmacies and dispensing physicians, after it became known that the teratogen etretinate was a metabolite of acitretine. A written survey to all pharmacies and dispensing physicians was responded to by 87% of all dispensers, representing the same proportion of recipients of etretinate.[27]

The same approach has been applied by Souverein et al. in building a cohort of early users of sildenafil, in order to monitor prospectively the occurrence of any adverse events in patients exposed to this drug.[28] Most of the cohort participants ($N=3477$) were untreated for erectile dysfunction before sildenafil came on the market and showed high prevalence of cardiovascular morbidity and/or diabetes.

Using this unique source of drug exposure information, several networks of so-called "sentinel" pharmacies have been developed for pharmacoepidemiologic research.[29] More on this will follow.

MEDICAL RECORD LINKAGE

There is widespread, deep-seated resistance in The Netherlands to the use of a unique personal identification number. Identification for insurance purposes is done by an anonymized family number, with substring codes used to distinguish individuals within the family, to enable linkage of individual patients' records. To address the occasional need to ascertain specific information from an individual patient's medical records, in several studies community pharmacists have acted as an intermediary between the epidemiology researcher and the responsible physician. Coded and sealed envelopes were used for the exchange of information, maintaining the patients' anonymity but allowing correlation of drug exposure information with the corresponding patients' medical data. In one of these studies, however, the response rate of the GPs was only 81%, which could be a substantial obstacle to certain study designs.[30] Moreover, the procedure was time consuming and costly. The same sealed envelope scheme was used by Petri et al. to search for clinical signs of Parkinson's disease in recipients of flunarizine.[31]

In the early 1990s, a formal system of record linkage was developed, called PHARMO. Developed by Herings and Stricker, it links community pharmacy and hospital data within established hospital catchment regions, on the basis of patients' birth date, gender, and GP code, preserving anonymity. While there are certain probabilistic aspects of the linkage, the combination of these three data items yields a sensitivity and specificity of over 95%.[32] The PHARMO system has been expanded to a population of over 500 000, is population based, links all prescription drug data to hospital data, and has been used to study a large number of drug effects severe enough to require hospitalization.[4,9,33] Nowadays, PHARMO has linked also to primary care data, population surveys, laboratory and genetic data, cancer and accident registries, mortality data, and economic outcomes. Even in the absence of a unique patient identifier—which remains missing in The Netherlands—the PHARMO system provides a powerful approach for conducting follow-up studies, case–control studies, and other analytical epidemiologic studies for evaluating drug-induced effects. The data collection is longitudinal and goes back to 1987. The system has well-defined denominator information, allowing incidence and prevalence estimates, and is relatively cheap because existing databases are used and linked. Recently, the spin-out of PHARMO from the Department of Pharmacoepidemiology and Therapeutics at Utrecht University into an economically independent venture has ratified the scientific, clinical, and commercial value of Dutch pharmacy records for pharmacoepidemiology. PHARMO figures in a large number of applications discussed elsewhere in this chapter.

Two more recent developments in Dutch pharmacy record linkage are the Rotterdam Study and the PREVEND study, both very potent resources for pharmacoepidemiologic research. The Rotterdam Study started in 1990 as a population-based prospective follow-up study.[34] All 10 275 residents of the Ommoord suburb in Rotterdam aged 55 years or over were invited to participate. In total, 7983 (78%) subjects gave written informed consent and for 86% of these blood samples are available. The baseline measurements include a physical examination, demographic data, medical history, family history of diseases, and lifestyle factors. Moreover, blood samples are drawn for DNA extraction. Pharmacy records have been linked to this cohort since 1991. Several examples bring to light the potential of the Rotterdam study in evaluating drug–effect associations. Van Leeuwen et al. studied the possible role of cumulative exposure of cholesterol lowering drugs in protecting against age-related maculopathy,[35] and in the same cohort the use of the calcium channel blocker verapamil was found to be associated with increased cancer risk.[36] The strengths of pharmacy record linkage, providing detailed and valid exposure information, have been shown particularly in a study on the use of diuretics and hip fractures ($N = 281$ cases).[37] Relative to nonuse, current use of thiazides for more than 365 days was statistically significantly associated with a lower risk for hip fracture (hazard ratio, 0.46; 95% CI 0.21–0.96). There was no clear dose dependency and after thiazide use was discontinued, the lower risk disappeared.

The PREVEND (Prevention of Renal and Vascular End-stage Disease) study has been initiated by Groningen University and is based on a cohort of patients with microalbuminuria identified in the general population. This group and an equally sized sample of non-microalbuminuria subjects (total group $N = 8592$) are being followed for various outcomes, and linkage to pharmacy records has been achieved in order to conduct pharmacoepidemiologic research.[38,39]

STRENGTHS

The most important advantage of the Dutch system lies in its virtually complete coverage of a relatively homogeneous population of reasonable size. We believe that the quality of data on drug exposure in The Netherlands is second to none, because of three factors:

1. computerized dispensing records are subject to financial audit because they are the basis for reimbursement;
2. a long tradition that patients frequent a single GP and pharmacy;
3. the practical lack of economic incentives for between-pharmacy shopping (although, as said before, governmental policies strive to mobilize patients).

It is one of those more or less dreadful paradoxes in Dutch health care that one governmental stakeholder (e.g., department of economic affairs) pushes for more competition and efficiency in the health care sector, while another department with a formal task of preventing drug-related risk and increasing patient safety relies heavily on the availability of high quality data on drug exposure and (possibly) related outcomes. Nonetheless, data on drug exposure can be linked extensively to various outcomes and to data on possible confounders or effect modifiers. With respect to the latter, the strong increase in possibilities of linking genetic information to studies evaluating drug exposure–outcomes associations is an important development.[40]

Yet, it is not only genetics that drives more focus on molecular pharmacoepidemiology in The Netherlands. Researchers in the field of understanding the nature and extent of drug effects have found their way to laboratory medicine and other resources where biochemical and other clinical "signatures" of patient outcomes can be ascertained. The series of studies on drug-induced deep vein thrombosis and embolism (VTE) including laboratory data on a plethora of various thrombotic factors has already been mentioned. In the context of the well-developed tradition of Dutch research on thrombotic events and their correlates, Schalekamp et al. used data from a network of anticoagulation clinics in order to evaluate the role of CYP2C9 genotypes in causing problems with acenocoumarol anticoagulation.[41] A similar approach of linking such data to drug exposure data has been applied by Visser et al.[42] These studies show very nicely the complex interplay between genetics, adjusted prescribing behavior, and feedback information based on phenotypic assessment of the coagulation status. Movig et al. have linked pharmacy-based drug exposure data on the use of serotonergic antidepressants to both clinical laboratory and hospitalization data for the identification of cases of possible drug-induced hyponatremia.[43] With such work leading the way, we anticipate a surge in the application of laboratory biomarkers in Dutch pharmacoepidemiologic research, on both intended and adverse drug effects (see also Chapter 37).

WEAKNESSES

The Dutch system is not immune from problems, such as unreliable or outdated information in the patient file undermining the quality of pharmacy records. Patient files in pharmacies are maintained mostly by pharmacists, on the basis of information provided by patients, relatives of patients, or local administrative sources. This eclectic sourcing of information limits the value of demographic information contained in pharmacy computers.

There is an ongoing need for quality assessment of data for epidemiology research that are derived from medical information systems. As in many countries, the patient's medical record, being in the past a personal registry compiled by the individual health professional, has become a target for numerous interest groups, e.g., insurance companies, regulators, consumer organizations, lawyers involved in liability actions, and epidemiologists. There is thus a need for careful monitoring of the quality of medical registries, including the process of data recording, its completeness, and its validity. For reasons already discussed, pharmacy dispensing data are of generally high quality. However, proper evaluation of the quality and validity of data is always needed.[44,45]

A second weakness is the size of the country, and thus the population exposed to certain drugs, together with the general reluctance within the medical community, especially within general practice, to adopt new drugs after marketing approval. Rare events, in particular when exposure is small, are difficult to study. We have experienced this limitation when several case reports of the occurrence of Achilles tendon rupture were attributed to the use of quinolones, but the epidemiologic evidence for this association was still scanty. Van der Linden *et al.* had to study this association in available UK databases as Dutch data on both exposure to quinolones and the outcome of interest (e.g., Achilles tendon rupture) were too limited to achieve a reasonable sample size.[46]

Probably the biggest potential risks to the future of the Dutch pharmacy database are the consequences of politically motivated tinkering with a health care system that has worked very effectively and, relative to other countries, economically. Yet there is, as stated before, a strong sense that health care costs must be reduced, which has led to a series of recent changes that, from the perspective of the situations in health care in other countries, suggest failure to heed the warning: 'if it ain't broke, don't fix it.' In a certain sense, we suffer the consequences of having a system of health care that evolved before extensive, effective regulatory (e.g., negative lists, patient copayment, reimbursement restrictions) interventions were possible.

Effective interventions are the dividends of the large investment in biomedical research that all advanced nations have made since the end of the Second World War. So, interventions that "work" have grown in number, complexity, and cost, with steeply accelerating growth during the past two decades. But they have arrived piecemeal, changing the face of medicine in the fashion of a complex picture-puzzle only gradually coming together, unguided by a view of the complete picture. The political and economic reactions have been similarly piecemeal, naturally lagging behind the technological changes, as the political and economic reactions develop in response to, never in anticipation of, accumulating problems created by growing costs, ethical dilemmas, and—the ultimate dividend—demographic changes.

PARTICULAR APPLICATIONS

THE DIMENSION OF TIME IN DRUG EXPOSURE

The ascertainment of drug exposure is determined by various factors. Time is a crucial variable that has the power to reject hypotheses about causality, e.g., when the putative adverse reaction precedes the first record of dispensing of the suspected drug. Thus, in assessing causal relationships between drug use and suspected events, it is essential to verify the temporal sequence of events in relation to exposure to the drug.[29] This very basic point is not an easy one to apply, because of the prevalence of timing errors in casual reporting: an ostensibly minor error in data entry can transpose the onset of drug exposure, or the onset of disease, negating or supporting a hypothesis about causality.

A time-oriented database consists essentially of three distinct types of variables: headers (e.g., referring to patient characteristics like birth date and gender), point events (referring to a certain event in time, e.g., hospitalization, onset of adverse drug effect), and interval events (referring to the calculated duration between point events, e.g., duration of drug therapy, length of stay in hospital). Interest focuses not only on the interval between the beginning and end of drug exposure, termed the "risk window", but on periods prior to, and after, the risk window, for these provide information on events in the patient's life at times proximate to, but outside, the risk window.[47] When the date of the first dispensing of drug is known, one can calculate, from the amount dispensed and the prescribed daily dose, the expected, or "legend," period of treatment. Thus, Dutch pharmacy records provide a sound basis for estimating the duration of drug exposure.

There are practical problems, however. The onset of drug exposure is putatively defined by the date of drug dispensing to the patient, but is subject to uncertainties about when the patient actually began taking the medicine, which is not necessarily coincident with the dispensing date. Greater uncertainty attends definition of the cessation of exposure. When there have been one or more refills of the same prescription, one can examine the intervals between refills for evidence of delay due to omitted doses, or to be more sophisticated, one can measure continuity of compliance with prescribed drug regimens with electronic medication event monitors.[48,49] When the last refill has been dispensed, one faces the question of defining when the last dose is likely to have been taken, and how long the effects of treatment may linger after the last dose was taken. An unfortunate lacuna in clinical pharmacology is its one-sided focus on studying, with great care and diligence, the temporal details of the onset of drug action, while almost totally ignoring the variability in drug action due to variable patient compliance[50] (see also Chapter 46).

Petri *et al.* used the risk window approach to assess a postulated association between the antimigraine/antivertigo drug flunarizine and mental depression.[31] That study, which pioneered the use of computerized Dutch pharmacy records, identified 1284 ever-recipients of flunarizine, 180 (14%) of whom had, at one time or another during the study interval, been prescribed also an antidepressant. If, as postulated, flunarizine did trigger mental depression, one would have expected to see a flurry of antidepressant prescribing in the wake of flunarizine prescribing. Of course, in an ideal world, the appearance of signs of depression would lead physicians to terminate the prescription for flunarizine rather than add a prescription for an antidepressant, but the reality is that physicians are, on the whole, much more likely to start new prescriptions rather than to stop old ones, unless there is a very well characterized adverse effect of a previously prescribed drug.

DIMENSIONS OF DRUG EXPOSURE AND ITS CORRELATES

Important dimensions in interpreting the correlates of drug exposure are the patient's profile and health status.[17] The profile includes age, gender, education, socioeconomic status, and estimated compliance with prescribed pharmacotherapy. Health status is judged on the basis of information about disease severity and comorbidity—simple words that stand

for considerable complexity. An often-overlooked factor whose importance cannot be overemphasized in judging health status is the patient's prescription drug history within the past several years.

Use of the prescription drug history alone as an indicator of health status and prognosis remains an under-explored topic. On its face, several things are evident. First, the writing of a prescription represents a summary medical judgment that the prescribed agent's indications are appropriate for the patient's present situation, as perceived and interpreted by the prescribing physician. Those perceptions and interpretations may be irrational or otherwise wrong, which one cannot, of course, judge from the prescription—though a clear clash between the indications and contraindications of concomitantly prescribed agents may signal irrational prescribing. More information can, of course, be gained from the physician's notes written around the same time, but at considerably greater cost. Whether the added information to be gleaned from physicians' notes justifies the gleaning costs depends on the importance of the question at issue.

A second consideration is that drugs differ widely in the specificity of their indications, so the clinical information implicit in a first prescription will depend on the drug, its indications, and the other agents with which it is co-prescribed.[17,50] Whether or not a first prescription is refilled, and for how long, gives an indication of whether it has struck enough of a perceived balance of good and ill to warrant its continuation.

A third point is that many physicians prescribe certain drugs as a way of buying time, to see after some days or weeks how a patient's complaints either resolve or become more indicative of a specific medical problem.

Obviously, the prescription drug history is far from a complete medical record, but can nevertheless tell a great deal. It has been this very principle that has driven Dutch pharmacy record linkage to successful and challenging avenues for pharmacoepidemiologic research.

CHANNELING

Comparisons are the sinew of observational epidemiologic studies, but they depend on comparing like with like. One source for misclassification occurs when drugs with more or less identical pharmacology and indications are assumed to be used by patients with more or less identical profiles and health status.[17] Figure 20.1(a), however, shows a prototypical description of the distribution of several patient populations along the dimension of disease severity. Patients included in randomized clinical trials (RCTs) often are positioned at the right side of the figure in order to get enough impact versus

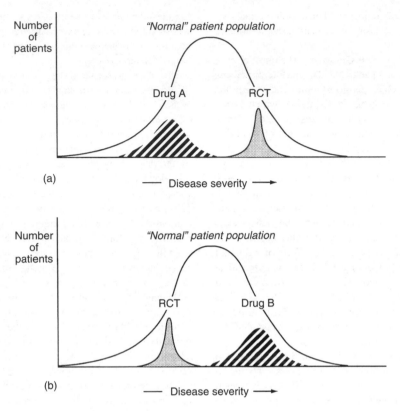

Figure 20.1. Two theoretical distributions of dosage severity in a "normal" patient population, in a randomized clinical trial population, and in patients receiving drugs in normal medical practice.

placebo to show efficacy. In the example of Figure 20.1(a), usual recipients of Drug A in everyday medical practice are positioned in the mild–moderate region.

Figure 20.1(b) shows rather an opposite picture of the RCT population, in the mild–moderate region of the population distribution of severity. This situation probably prevails in most RCTs, which exclude patients who have complex health problems associated with multiple diseases: the RCT population tends to be recruited from the low end of severity, in the interest of simplicity of analysis. Consequently, the profile and health status of patients prescribed Drug B in routine practice may differ considerably from patients in the RCTs. Inman reported data supporting this situation in his PEM study of the osmotic pump formulation of indomethacin (Osmosin®, Indosmos®) and other NSAIDs[51] (see also Chapter 12). The new formulation of indomethacin had been promoted as a form of the drug less likely than the conventional capsule form to produce gastrointestinal side effects, thereby prompting many physicians to choose

the osmotic pump formulation for patients with a history of gastrointestinal problems. One of us has termed this phenomenon "channeling".[52] It highlights one of the basic, often difficult to answer questions in pharmacoepidemiology: "did the drug bring the problems to the patient, or did the patient bring the problems to the drug?"[17] One way to judge this matter is to compare the frequencies with which recipients of ostensibly identical agents are co-prescribed other agents that indicate more severe disease. Some examples will be used to illustrate this point.

Channeling may explain the flow of adverse reaction reports from an NSAID that was formulated and promoted in a manner very similar to that of Osmosin®.[51,53] In January 1989, SmithKline Beecham introduced into the Dutch market a controlled-release formulation (Oscorel®, Oruvail®) of the established NSAID ketoprofen. The product was heavily promoted with claims of safety with respect to gastrointestinal toxicity. In the first year after introduction of this product, the national authorities received a surge of case reports of gastrointestinal bleeding and/or perforation in recipients of Oscorel®. This observation led to a pharmacy-based study in which 837 patients receiving first prescriptions for Oscorel® were identified. The drug use histories of these patients over the period 1987–88 were searched for prescribing of agents indicated for the treatment of peptic ulcer disease. It was found that 24.1% of Oscorel® recipients had received anti-ulcer drugs, versus 15.7% in a reference population (RR = 1.54; 95% CI = 1.36–1.74). This pattern of channeling of Oscorel® toward patients with a history of gastrointestinal disease was recognized in time to help interpret the adverse reaction reports, and to prevent an incorrect conclusion, simply on the basis of adverse reaction reports, that the product was more prone than the conventional form of ketoprofen or other NSAIDs to cause gastrointestinal problems.

Another example where channeling has occurred is in the prescribing of the several inhalational beta-2 agonists salbutamol, terbutaline, and fenoterol. To evaluate the role of channeling in the controversy over the mortality risk attributed to fenoterol, Petri et al. examined the extent to which fenoterol is channeled into use by high-risk asthma patients, by studying the co-prescribing of beta-2 agonists marketed in The Netherlands with systemic corticosteroids, as an indicator of asthma severity.[54] Compared to patients prescribed inhalational salbutamol, approximately twice the proportion of patients prescribed inhalational fenoterol were concomitantly prescribed systemic steroids; patients prescribed inhalational terbutaline were intermediate in respect to the prescribing of systemic steroids. These data indicate that, in The Netherlands, fenoterol was channeled into use in patients with severe asthma. These different usage patterns appear to relate to the sequence with which the products were introduced into the market, with the later entering products having been promoted mainly to specialists for patients with more severe disease.

Since the first channeling studies, other examples of substantial channeling have been found. Egberts et al. observed that patients receiving newly introduced antidepressants during the first year after their introduction were not comparable to patients who were receiving longer-available antidepressants of the tricyclic class.[55] The recipients of the newly introduced agents tended to be patients who had failed to respond satisfactorily to older agents. Of course, failure to respond has a dual origin: pharmacological non-response and clinically unrecognized noncompliance, so when the latter problem is the true reason for failed treatment, there is a high likelihood that the new treatment will similarly fail, unless the patient chooses that moment to commence proper dosing. It is important to recognize channeling, because it

signifies the role of confounding by indication (see also Chapter 40), demonstrating that drugs which may be scarcely distinguishable on clinical pharmacological grounds nevertheless end up being used by patients with quite different health status and prognosis.[56]

Drug effects may also differ in treated and untreated patients because channeling or confounding by indication is driven by a factor making doctors reluctant to prescribe the drug for a particular patient. Feenstra et al. have evaluated the effects of confounding by contraindication on risk factors for death in patients taking ibopamine after its use was restricted in early September 1995.[57] In a cohort of 1146 patients with congestive heart failure and exposed to ibopamine, they found an adjusted risk for death associated with current use of ibopamine of 2.62 (95% CI, 1.76–3.90) before September 1995 and 0.93 (95% CI, 0.84–1.02), after that date. This marked inversion of the relative risk was interpreted as the result of confounding by contraindication. In other words, the drug in question was prescribed significantly less to susceptible patients after regulatory action was taken in September 1995.

UNDERTREATMENT

There has been growing attention in Dutch pharmacoepidemiology to answering the question: do patients use available efficacious and safe medicines in such a fashion that maximum clinical benefit can be achieved? Undertreatment may be the result of premature discontinuation of chronic therapy and various studies have shown shocking data on patients interrupting therapy while clinical evidence would urge them to stay on the prescribed treatment regimens, particularly in the field of psychotropics, cardiovascular therapy, and others.[48,58,59] Automated pharmacy record linkage stratifying patients into "to be treated" and "not to be treated" has produced evidence that many patients with risk factors for preventable negative outcomes are undertreated. Schelleman and colleagues evaluated the undertreatment of hypertension in a Dutch population.[59] Only about one out of five men and two out of five females with hypertension were treated according to existing evidence-based guidelines. This finding of a considerable proportion of hypertensives being untreated and uncontrolled has previously been linked by Klungel et al. to significant proportions of attributable cases of stroke.[60] For untreated hypertensive men and women who should have been treated, he found proportions of preventable strokes being 22.8% and 25.4%, respectively.

Discontinuation of chronic drug therapy has been found to be associated with various factors, among them pill scares driving patients away from their therapy, as was found in the case of patients using ceruvistatin (Baycol®, Lipobay®). After this drug was withdrawn from the market for safety reasons, a significantly higher proportion of patients stopped statin therapy in contrast to patients using other lipid-lowering drugs.[61]

THE FUTURE

As said before, the Dutch health care system is moving ahead in the direction of more market forces, freedom of choice by patients, and more emphasis on cost containment and efficiency.[19] The full implications for pharmacoepidemiologic research are not clear yet, but the strong actuarial basis of the GP and pharmacy system will most likely continue as the solid basis for primary patient care and medical record keeping. Record linkage has been adopted nowadays not only by epidemiologists but also by policy analysts and health care managers in order to facilitate continuity of care, transparency, and accountability. The development of a national electronic patient dossier (EPD) has been embraced as a national priority in health policy. This flow of common interests will drive automated pharmacy record linkage along new avenues. Therefore, the future will see more work on record linkage, to be sure, but also work to help define the contributions that the prescription drug history can make in the evaluation of health status, and the uses of objective, quantitative information on drug exposure and patient compliance to improve the quality and efficiency of ambulatory health care.

While the small size of The Netherlands has certain inherent disadvantages, it has a number of advantages, too. It is, for example, possible to have personal contact with all the leading experts in a given field, which creates the possibility of extensive "learning" before starting with "confirming".[62] There is the large number of communities in which a single pharmacy and five or six primary care physicians together constitute the core of pharmacotherapy in their area. These communities provide powerful environments for identification of susceptible patients for adverse drug effects, interaction risks, undertreatment, and noncompliance. This strategy of "patient typing," starting from the scope of epidemiology towards clinical and molecular sciences, will be key to solving society's needs in the field of patient safety and pharmacovigilance. This approach requires the availability of extensive and longitudinal data on drug exposure, advanced medical record linkage systems, and an integrative knowledge base of pharmacoepidemiology, clinical epidemiology, and relevant fields in molecular epidemiology, e.g., laboratory medicine and genetics. There is increasing evidence that both the efficacy of drugs (e.g.,

antihypertensives, asthma drugs) and their safety (e.g., slow metabolizers and risky dosing) have their genetic correlates.[40] These findings argue for innovative approaches to integrate research on drug exposure, patient characteristics of various types, and outcomes. There is increasing evidence that bad response to drug therapy is correlated with both patient factors (disease severity, comorbidity, metabolism, genetics) and utilization factors (quality of diagnosis, inappropriate prescribing, concomitant use of other drugs, noncompliance and other patterns of interrupted drug usage).

Moreover, there is an ongoing trend to develop proactively for all (future) drug products, risk management activities including the preparation of pharmacovigilance specification during the medicinal product development program (see Chapter 33). Regulators, the medical–pharmaceutical profession, industry, and academia are joining forces to get the most out of the Dutch system of automated pharmacy record linkage to solve today's and tomorrow's questions regarding comparative risk/benefit evaluation after the drug has been used widely in daily practice. Risk/benefit comparisons of different drug therapies are subjects for observational epidemiologic studies, a logical next step after the conduct of randomized clinical trials designed to provide evidence for efficacy.[63]

The future will require more work on better methods. Observational studies on drug risks are often subject to scientific debate because factors like confounding by indication, channeling bias, and other types of misclassification may cause flaws in the interpretation of the results of such studies.[52,58] Because of commercial interests being an important feature of today's pharmaceutical marketplace, these questions need careful and independent scientific consideration and advancement of better methodologies. Identifying individual patient characteristics is considered an important strategy to improve like-with-like, and automated pharmacy records are nowadays a recognized mainstay in that process.

REFERENCES

1. Kok FJ, Vandenbroucke JP, Van der Heide-Wessel C, Van der Heide RM. Dietary sodium, calcium, and potassium and blood pressure. *Am J Epidemiol* 1986; **123**: 134–8.
2. Jansen PAF, Schulte BPM, Meyboom RHB, Gribnau FWJ. Antihypertensive treatment as a possible cause of stroke in the elderly. *Age Ageing* 1986; **15**: 129–38.
3. Ouweland FA van, Gribnau FWJ. Nonsteroidal anti-inflammatory drugs as a prognostic factor in acute pulmonary edema. *Arch Intern Med* 1987; **147**: 176–9.
4. Heerdink ER, Leufkens HG, Herings RM, Ottervanger JP, Stricker BH, Bakker A. NSAIDs associated with increased risk

of congestive heart failure in elderly patients taking diuretics. *Arch Intern Med* 1998; **158**: 1108–12.

5. Feenstra J, Heerdink ER, Grobbee DE, Stricker BH. Association of nonsteroidal anti-inflammatory drugs with first occurrence of heart failure and with relapsing heart failure: the Rotterdam Study. *Arch Intern Med* 2002; **162**: 265–70.

6. Vandenbroucke JP, Valkenburg HA, Boersma JW, Cats A, Festen JJM, Huber-Bruning O *et al*. Oral contraceptives and rheumatoid arthritis: further evidence for a preventive effect. *Lancet* 1982; **ii**: 839–42.

7. Hazes JMW, Dijkmans BAC, Vandenbroucke JP, Vries RPR, Cats A. Reduction of the risk of rheumatoid arthritis among women who take oral contraceptives. *Arthritis Rheum* 1990; **33**: 173–9.

8. Bloemenkamp KW, Rosendaal FR, Helmerhorst FM, Buller HR, Vandenbroucke JP. Enhancement by factor V Leiden mutation of risk of deep-vein thrombosis associated with oral contraceptives containing a third-generation progestagen. *Lancet* 1995; **346**: 1593–6.

9. Herings RM, Urquhart J, Leufkens HG. Venous thromboembolism among new users of different oral contraceptives. *Lancet* 1999; **354**: 127–8.

10. Tanis BC, van den Bosch MA, Kemmeren JM, Cats VM, Helmerhorst FM, Algra A *et al*. Oral contraceptives and the risk of myocardial infarction. *N Engl J Med* 2001; **345**: 1787–93.

11. van der Klauw MM, Stricker BH, Herings RM, Cost WS, Valkenburg HA, Wilson JH. A population based case–cohort study of drug-induced anaphylaxis. *Br J Clin Pharmacol* 1993; **35**: 400–8.

12. Egberts TC, Smulders M, de Koning FH, Meyboom RH, Leufkens HG. Can adverse drug reactions be detected earlier? A comparison of reports by patients and professionals. *BMJ* 1996; **313**: 530–1.

13. De Bruin ML, van Puijenbroek EP, Egberts AC, Hoes AW, Leufkens HG. Non-sedating antihistamine drugs and cardiac arrhythmias—biased risk estimates from spontaneous reporting systems? *Br J Clin Pharmacol* 2002; **53**: 370–4.

14. van Puijenbroek E, Diemont W, van Grootheest K. Application of quantitative signal detection in the Dutch spontaneous reporting system for adverse drug reactions. *Drug Saf* 2003; **26**: 293–301.

15. Haayer-Ruskamp FM. Drug utilization studies in The Netherlands. *Pharm Weekbl Sci* 1990; **12**: 91–6.

16. Hekster YA, Vree TB. Drug utilization research in clinical practice. *Drug Intell Clin Pharm* 1986; **20**: 679–82.

17. Leufkens HG, Urquhart J. Variability in patterns of drug usage. *J Pharm Pharmacol* 1994; **46**: 433–7.

18. Ellwood P. Shattuck lecture: outcomes management. *N Engl J Med* 1988; **318**: 1549–56.

19. Schrijvers AJP, ed., *Health and Health Care in The Netherlands. A Critical Self-Assessment by Dutch Experts in the Medical and Health Sciences.* Utrecht: De Tijdstroom, 1998.

20. Zwart-van Rijkom JE, Leufkens HG, Busschbach JJ, Broekmans AW, Rutten FF. Differences in attitudes, knowledge and use of economic evaluations in decision making in The Netherlands.

The Dutch results from the EUROMET Project *Pharmacoeconomics* 2000; **18**: 149–60.

21. Leufkens HG, Haaijer-Ruskamp F, Bakker A, Dukes G. Scenario analysis of the future of medicines. *BMJ* 1994; **309**: 1137–40.

22. Hoes AW, Grobbee DE, Lubsen J, Man in't Veld AJ, van der Does E, Hofman A. Diuretics, beta-blockers, and the risk for sudden cardiac death in hypertensive patients. *Ann Intern Med* 1995; **123**: 481–7.

23. Van der Lei J, Duisterhout JS, Westerhof HP *et al*. The introduction of computer-based patient records in The Netherlands. *Ann Intern Med* 1993; **119**: 1036–41.

24. Jong GW 't, Stricker BH, Sturkenboom MC. Marketing in the lay media and prescriptions of terbinafine in primary care: Dutch cohort study. *BMJ* 2004; **328**: 931.

25. Straus SM, Bleumink GS, Dieleman JP, van der Lei J, 't Jong GW, Kingma JH *et al*. Antipsychotics and the risk of sudden cardiac death. *Arch Intern Med* 2004; **164**: 1293–7.

26. Borden EK, Lee JG. A methodologic study of postmarketing drug evaluation using a pharmacy-based approach. *J Chron Dis* 1982; **35**: 803.

27. Stricker BHCh, Barendregt M, Herings RMC, De Jong-van den Berg LTW, Cornel MC, De Smet PAGM. Ad hoc tracing of a cohort of patients exposed to acitretine (Neotigason) on a nation wide scale. *Eur J Clin Pharmacol* 1992; **42**: 555–7.

28. Souverein PC, Egberts AC, Sturkenboom MC, Meuleman EJ, Leufkens HG, Urquhart J. The Dutch cohort of sildenafil users: baseline characteristics. *Br J Urology* 2001; **87**: 648–53.

29. Urquhart J. Time to take our medicines, seriously (inaugural professorial lecture, University of Limburg, April 3, 1992). *Pharm Weekbl* 1992; **127**: 769–76.

30. Leufkens HG, Ruter EM, Ameling CB, Hekster YA, Bakker A. Linkage of pharmacy data on heavy users of nonsteroidal anti-inflammatory drugs to information from general practitioners. *J Pharmacoepidemiol* 1991; **2**: 67–77.

31. Petri H, Leufkens H, Naus J, Silkens R, Hessen P van, Urquhart J. Rapid method for estimating the risk of acutely controversial side effects of prescription drugs. *J Clin Epidemiol* 1990; **43**: 433–9.

32. Herings RMC, Stricker BHC, Nap G, Bakker A. Pharmaco-morbidity linkage: a feasibility study comparing morbidity in two pharmacy-based exposure cohorts. *J Epidemiol Community Health* 1992; **46**: 136–40.

33. Herings RM, de Boer A, Stricker BH, Leufkens HG, Porsius A. Hypoglycaemia associated with use of inhibitors of angiotensin converting enzyme. *Lancet* 1995; **345**: 1195–8.

34. Hofman A, Grobbee DE, de Jong PT, van den Ouweland FA. Determinants of disease and disability in the elderly: the Rotterdam Elderly Study. *Eur J Epidemiol* 1991; **7**: 403–22.

35. van Leeuwen R, Vingerling JR, Hofman A, de Jong PT, Stricker BH. Cholesterol lowering drugs and risk of age related maculopathy: prospective cohort study with cumulative exposure measurement. *BMJ* 2003; **326**: 255–6.

36. Beiderbeck-Noll AB, Sturkenboom MC, van der Linden PD, Herings RM, Hofman A, Coebergh JW *et al*. Verapamil is

associated with an increased risk of cancer in the elderly: the Rotterdam study. *Eur J Cancer* 2003; **39**: 98–105.

37. Schoofs MW, van der Klift M, Hofman A, de Laet CE, Herings RM, Stijnen T *et al*. Thiazide diuretics and the risk for hip fracture. *Ann Intern Med* 2003; **139**: 476–82.

38. Monster TB, Janssen WM, de Jong PE, de Jong-van den Berg LT. PREVEND Study Group. The impact of antihypertensive drug groups on urinary albumin excretion in a non-diabetic population. *Br J Clin Pharmacol* 2002; **53**: 31–6.

39. Atthobari J, Monster TB, de Jong PE, de Jong-van den Berg LT. PREVEND Study Group. The effect of hypertension and hypercholesterolemia screening with subsequent intervention letter on the use of blood pressure and lipid lowering drugs. *Br J Clin Pharmacol* 2004; **57**: 328–36.

40. Maitland-van der Zee AH, de Boer A, Leufkens HG. The interface between pharmacoepidemiology and pharmacogenetics. *Eur J Pharmacol* 2000; **410**: 121–30.

41. Schalekamp T, van Geest-Daalderop JH, de Vries-Goldschmeding H, Conemans J, Bernsen Mj M, de Boer A. Acenocoumarol stabilization is delayed in CYP2C93 carriers. *Clin Pharmacol Ther* 2004; **75**: 394–402.

42. Visser LE, Schaik RH, Vliet Mv M, Trienekens PH, De Smet PA, Vulto AG *et al*. The risk of bleeding complications in patients with cytochrome P450 CYP2C9*2 or CYP2C9*3 alleles on acenocoumarol or phenprocoumon. *Thromb Haemost* 2004; **92**: 61–6.

43. Movig KL, Leufkens HG, Lenderink AW, Egberts AC. Validity of hospital discharge International Classification of Diseases (ICD) codes for identifying patients with hyponatremia. *J Clin Epidemiol* 2003; **56**: 530–5.

44. De Jong van den Berg LTW, van den Berg PB, Haayer-Ruskamp FM, Dukes MNG, Wesseling H. Investigating drug use in pregnancy. Methodological problems and perspectives. *Pharm Weekbl Sci* 1991; **13**: 32–8.

45. Lau HS, Boer de A, Beuning KS, Porsius A. Validation of pharmacy records in drug exposure assessment. *J Clin Epidemiol* 1997; **50**: 619–25.

46. Linden PD van der, Sturkenboom MC, Herings RM, Leufkens HM, Rowlands S, Stricker BH. Increased risk of achilles tendon rupture with quinolone antibacterial use, especially in elderly patients taking oral corticosteroids. *Arch Intern Med* 2003; **163**: 1801–7.

47. Staa TP van, Abenhaim L, Leufkens HG. A study of the effects of exposure misclassification due to the time-window design in pharmacoepidemiologic studies. *J Clin Epidemiol* 1994; **47**: 183–9.

48. Meijer WE, Bouvy ML, Heerdink ER, Urquhart J, Leufkens HG. Spontaneous lapses in dosing during chronic treatment with selective serotonin reuptake inhibitors. *Br J Psychiatry* 2001; **179**: 519–22.

49. Klerk E de, van der Heijde D, Landewe R, van der Tempel H, Urquhart J, van der Linden S. Compliance in rheumatoid arthritis, polymyalgia rheumatica, and gout. *J Rheumatol* 2003; **30**: 44–54.

50. Urquhart J. Pharmacodynamics of variable patient compliance: implications for pharmaceutical value. *Adv Drug Delivery Rev* 1998; **33**: 207–19.

51. Inman B. Comparative study of five NSAIDs. *PEM News* 1985; **3**: 3–134.

52. Petri H, Urquhart J. Channeling bias in the interpretation of drug effects. *Stat Med* 1991; **10**: 577–81.

53. Leufkens HG, Urquhart J, Stricker BHCh, Bakker A, Petri H. Channeling of controlled release formulation of ketoprofen (OSCOREL) in patients with history of gastrointestinal problems. *J Epidemiol Community Health* 1992; **46**: 428–32.

54. Petri H, Urquhart J, Herings R, Bakker A. Characteristics of patients prescribed three different inhalational beta-2 agonists: an example of the channeling phenomenon. *Postmarket Surveill* 1991; **5**: 57–65.

55. Egberts ACG, Lenderink AW, Koning de FHP, Leufkens HGM. Channeling of three newly introduced antidepressants to patients not responding satisfactorily of previous treatment. *J Clin Psychopharmacol* 1997; **17**: 149–55.

56. Grobbee DE, Hoes AW. Confounding and indication for treatment in evaluation of drug treatment for hypertension. *BMJ* 1997; **315**: 1151–4.

57. Feenstra J, Grobbee DE, in 't Veld BA, Stricker BHCh. Confounding by contraindication in a nationwide cohort study of risk for death in patients taking ibopamine. *Ann Intern Med* 2001; **134**: 569–72.

58. Herings RM, Erkens JA. Increased suicide attempt rate among patients interrupting use of atypical antipsychotics. *Pharmacoepidemiol Drug Saf* 2003; **12**: 423–4.

59. Schelleman H, Klungel OH, Kromhout D, de Boer A, Stricker BH, Verschuren WM. Prevalence and determinants of under-treatment of hypertension in the Netherlands. *J Hum Hypertens* 2004; **18**: 317–24.

60. Klungel OH, Stricker BH, Paes AH, Seidell JC, Bakker A, Vok Z *et al*. Excess stroke among hypertensive men and women attributable to undertreatment of hypertension. *Stroke* 1999; **30**: 1312–18.

61. Mantel-Teeuwisse AK, Klungel OH, Egberts TC, Verschuren WM, Porsius AJ, de Boer A. Failure to continue lipid-lowering drug use following the withdrawal of cerivastatin. *Drug Saf* 2004; **27**: 63–70.

62. Sheiner LB. Learning versus confirming in clinical drug development. *Clin Pharmacol Ther* 1997; **61**: 275–91.

63. Stricker BHCh, Psaty BM. Detection, verification, and quantification of adverse drug reactions. *BMJ* 2004; **329**: 44–7.

21

The Tayside Medicines Monitoring Unit (MEMO)

LI WEI, JOHN PARKINSON and THOMAS M. MACDONALD

Medicines Monitoring Unit, University of Dundee, Ninewells Hospital & Medical School, Dundee, UK.

INTRODUCTION

The National Health Service in Scotland (NHSiS) is a tax funded, free at the point of consumption, cradle to grave service. In Scotland there is very little private health care and as there are no socioeconomic eligibility distinctions, the level of health care given to an individual is based on need alone.

The Medicines Monitoring Unit (MEMO) is a university-based organization that works closely with the NHSiS to record-link health care data sets for the purposes of carrying out research. MEMO was founded in the late 1980s to perform in-hospital studies of adverse reactions. However, because most prescribing occurs in the community, in the 1990s the research direction changed towards community-based studies. Since then the MEMO has done many studies to detect and quantify serious drug toxicity in the community, using record linkage techniques. However, MEMO has also diversified its activities to undertake outcomes research, economic, genetic, drug utilization, and disease epidemiologic studies. The potential of the MEMO system to undertake most, if

not all, aspects of pharmacoepidemiology addressed in this book was described in 1994.[1]

MEMO has traditionally used data from the Tayside region of Scotland, which is geographically compact and serves over 400 000 patients. It has a low rate of patient migration with, for example, only 5% of nearly 4000 cimetidine users lost to follow-up in a five-year period.[2] Health care for the region is coordinated by NHS Tayside (www.nhstayside.scot.nhs.uk), part of the NHSiS. NHS Tayside maintains a computerized record of all patients registered with general practitioners. Additionally, Tayside has been at the forefront of generating managed clinical networks for chronic diseases such as diabetes (www.diabetes-healthnet.ac.uk), heart disease (www. hearts.org.uk) and endocrine disorders (www.tayendoweb. co.uk). More such managed clinical networks are in development in the newly-opened Clinical Technology Centre, a collaborative venture between MEMO (the University of Dundee) and the NHSiS. The engines that drive these chronic disease management systems are based around a large regional database that stores health care and related data for the

Pharmacoepidemiology, Fourth Edition   Edited by B.L. Strom
© 2005 John Wiley & Sons, Ltd

purpose of day to day clinical care. This database is called the Scottish Care Information (SCI) system (www. show.scot.nhs.uk/nhsstaff/indexstaff.htm). Data from this system are available to MEMO, as well as other data that may be stored in computer systems not yet attached to the regional database or that can be obtained from paper case records.

At the heart of the MEMO record linkage system is the dispensed prescribing data set, which is unique to the UK. In the absence of data on whether patients actually take their medications as directed, this is the acknowledged prime

data set in which to establish exposure and drug utilization patterns. There are other key electronic data sets regularly used by MEMO. The most important of these are the national Scottish Morbidity Record (SMR) databases (www.statistics. gov.uk/STATBASE/Source.asp?vlnk=1106&more=Y) that make up the electronic health records for Scotland (see Table 21.1). A manual for these SMR databases is also available.[3] As well as the databases in the table there are also SMR06 (cancer registration), SMR13 (community dental services), SMR20 (cardiac surgery), and SMR22

Table 21.1. Scottish Morbidity Record details

From 1996	Date began	Information collected	Content of data
SMR00	1991	First (mandatory) and return (optional) attendances at outpatient clinics in all specialties (except Accident and Emergency); includes procedural information	Individual patient records, each based on a single episode of care. Three basic areas of information are captured: patient's identification and demographic details, episode management details (includes contract data), and clinical information (optional)
SMR01	1961	Hospital inpatient and day case episodes in general and acute specialties. In 1978, SMR01 also collected previously unrecorded data on day cases	Individual patient records, each based on a single episode of care. Three basic areas of information are captured: patient's identification and demographic details, episode management details (includes contract data), and clinical information
SMR02	1969	Maternity inpatient and day case episodes	Individual patient records, each based on a single episode of care, including domiciliary deliveries. Four basic areas of information are captured: as above including clinical information, obstetric specific details, and in delivery cases, details about babies
SMR02D	1996	Home births, planned or unexpected, with no hospital admission	Individual patient records as for SMR02, except that date of admission and discharge are not completed. Some fields in the episode management section are preprinted with hard codes such as location code which is always D201N
SMR04	1963	Inpatient and day case episodes for mental health specialties	Individual patient records consisting of two parts: part 1 completed on admission and part 2 completed on discharge. Three basic areas of information are captured: patient's identification and demographic details, episode management details (includes contract data), and clinical information at the time of admission and discharge
SMR11	1975	Sick baby inpatient episodes	Individual patient records, each based on a single episode of care. Four basic areas of information are captured: patient's identification and demographic details, episode management details (includes contract data), clinical information, and specific details about sick babies
SMR50	1996	Inpatient episodes in hospitals and units providing continuing care for the elderly (geriatric long stay)	Individual patient records consisting of two parts: part 1 completed on admission and part 2 completed on discharge. Three basic areas of information are captured: patient's identification and demographic details, episode management details (includes contract data), and clinical information at the time of admission and discharge

Source: www.show.scot.nhs.uk/indicators/SMR/main.htm.

(drug misuse) databases. In addition there is the Scottish Immunisation Recall System (SIRS), which tracks all childhood immunization in Scotland (www.isdscotland. org/isd/info3.jsp?pContentID = 1882&p_applic= CCC&p_ service = Content.show&).

MEMO also makes use of Tayside regional biochemistry, pathology, hematology, microbiology, and hospital clinic data as well as data sets imported or created specifically for research projects. These databases are discussed in greater detail below.

MEMO also now uses Scotland-wide data. Record linkage of Scotland-wide data using patients' names, dates of birth, and addresses has been pioneered by the NHSiS Information and Statistics Division (ISD). It has mainly been used for evaluation of health care activity and outcomes research. In conjunction with MEMO, the ability to link dispensed prescribing data to hospitalizations for the total 5 million population of Scotland has been demonstrated. This allows the evaluation of drug safety and accurate quantification of risk of adverse drug reactions with less commonly prescribed drugs. Such work has shown the utility of the record-linkable Scottish unique identifier, and as a result about 85% of all prescriptions now contain this identifier. This now enables large-scale cost-efficient database tracking studies that we believe will become the norm in future pharmacovigilance and outcomes research. Additionally, the managed care networks already operating in Tayside are now being rolled out over all of Scotland.

Importantly, whether working with Tayside or Scottish data, MEMO has been at the forefront of ensuring compliance with the principles of good epidemiologic practice (GEP) with regard to the use of observational data.[4] A recent *British Medical Journal* commentary[5] praised MEMO researchers for paying careful attention to the protection of patient confidentiality by using modern anonymization technologies.

DESCRIPTION

PATIENT IDENTIFICATION

Every person who is registered with a general medical practitioner (GP) in Scotland is allocated a unique identifying number known as the Community Health Index number (CHI number). This is a ten-digit integer, the first six digits indicating the date of birth, digits seven and eight giving region of residence information, the ninth digit indicating sex, and the tenth digit incorporating a checksum to ensure the validity of the number. The CHI number maps to a data set (Table 21.2) that forms an extremely useful resource to the NHS and also serves as a useful roster file in epidemiologic studies.

For practical purposes, the entire Tayside population is registered with a GP and thus appears in the central computerized records held by the Health Board, the Community Health Master Patient Index (Table 21.2). This file also contains GP and address details, and a log of deceased persons along with the dates of death. The demographic composition of the Tayside population can therefore be readily obtained.

The CHI number is used as the patient identifier for most health care activity in Tayside, be this primary care or hospital inpatient care. For any data with just a name and address, MEMO has powerful software that enables the CHI to be added.

DISPENSED PRESCRIPTION DRUG DATA

In Scotland, all community prescribing is performed by GPs, sometimes on the advice of hospital physicians. Only hospital inpatients receive drugs by a different mechanism. MEMO has devised a method of capturing all GP prescribing. When a patient receives a prescription from a doctor, he/she takes it to any of the community pharmacies where the prescription is dispensed. The pharmacist then

Table 21.2. Community Health Number (CHI) core demographic database (Community Health Master Patient Index)

CHI number
NHS number
Date of birth
Surname
Birth surname
First forename
Second forename
Sex
Marital status
Previous surname
Date surname changed
Address
Postcode
Alternative forename
Area of residence
Reason for transfer
Previous address
Previous postcode
GP code
GP GMC number
Date accepted onto GP list
GP name
Practice code
Contact date
List of other hospital contacts
Various local codes

sends the original prescription form to the Practitioner Services Division (PSD) part of the ISD of the NHSiS in Edinburgh to obtain reimbursement.

After paying the pharmacists and dealing with any appeals, the PSD sends the cashed prescription forms to MEMO, where they are stored on a database linked to the CHI number. The following section describes the system that has been developed to perform this task.

ASCRIBING THE UNIQUE IDENTIFIER NUMBER TO PRESCRIPTIONS

All prescriptions are electronically scanned and read by powerful optical character recognition (OCR) software that runs multiple algorithms to obtain the best recognition for differing type faces and font sizes. Each area of the prescription is read against a dictionary of the text that might be expected (name, address, drug name, dose instruction, doctor name, date, pharmacy name) to generate an OCR best recognition. Both the actual text scanned and the OCR recognition are stored in the database. The objective at this stage is to "sort" all prescriptions by drug items so that data entry can then concentrate on prescriptions by name of drug or by BNF code, making the data entry more time efficient.

The next stage involves the reconciliation of all data that have not been picked up accurately by the OCR system. At this stage, all prescriptions are viewed electronically on screen by a data entry clerk, who validates data and enters handwritten prescriptions that the OCR has failed to read. Another data entry operation then adds the CHI number to the prescriptions where this is missing (about 15% of prescriptions), as well as verifying the dosing instructions.

This system ascribes in excess of 98% of CHI numbers to prescriptions on the first pass. The remaining 2% consist of persons who have recently changed address within Tayside or moved into Tayside from outside, and those visitors that are not registered with GPs. The Community Health Master Patient Index is continually updated by NHS Tayside but nevertheless the copy held in MEMO is always a little out of date. Consequently, data on those patients not identified on the first pass are entered manually and reconciled when the CHI number update data are available.

In January 2005, MEMO radically altered the way it captures dispensed prescribing information to make the process more efficient. In brief, MEMO receives all prescriptions electronically as scanned images. Accompanying these image files is a text file that consists of details of the prescription drug, the cost, the prescribing doctor code, the practice code and (in 75–80%) the CHI number. MEMO uses these data sources to create a dispensed drug file that has complete CHI ascribed and also has dose and duration of treatment added. This solution is scaleable to Scotland.

PRESCRIBER DATA

The code number of the GP with whom the patient is registered is known and the code number of the GP issuing the script is held with each prescription record. Repeat prescriptions may be written by GP partners in rotation. This method of data collection allows the identification of the prescriber who initiated a course of treatment.

HOSPITAL DATA

Since 1961, all hospitals in Scotland have been required to compile and return coded information on all acute inpatient admissions, forming the basis of the Scottish Morbidity Record 1 (SMR1), which contains administrative, demographic, and diagnostic information. In Tayside this is coded by medical clerks before being entered onto computer and subjected to quality control. The data are then sent to the ISD. Each SMR1 record has one principal and five other diagnostic fields coded according to the International Classification of Diseases, 9th revision (ICD-9).[6] There is also one main operation or procedure field and three others coded according to the Office of Population and Census Surveys, 4th revision (OPCS4) classification.[7] In 1996, the NHS introduced the 10th Revision of the ICD codes.[8] In Tayside there are approximately 63 000 hospital discharges per year. MEMO has in-house historical SMR1 data going back to 1980. These data allow for a past medical history of hospitalization for a condition to be controlled.

The SMR1 database contains details of deaths certified in hospital, which may be up to 85% of the total mortality. The Community Health Master Patient Index records the date of death of subjects in the Tayside population, while information on the certified cause of death of patients is provided to MEMO by the Registrar General. Population-based morbidity and mortality studies are thus feasible.

OTHER IN-HOSPITAL DATA

Any health care data set that is indexed by the CHI number can be linked into MEMO's record-linkage database, including other Scottish Morbidity Record returns supplied by ISD. In MEMO, commonly used data sets are the cancer registration database (SMR06), child development records, maternity records (SMR02), psychiatric records (SMR04), and neonatal discharges (SMR11).

CLINICAL LABORATORY DATA

Clinical laboratory data for the Tayside region since 1989 are held on a computerized archive in the Department of Biochemical Medicine in Ninewells Hospital. The database has CHI-specific biochemical, hematology, microbiology, virology, and serology laboratory results and reports. CHI-specific results from all pathology investigations since 1990 for Tayside are stored electronically in MEMO. Those data can be record-linked to the MEMO database to complete the clinical characteristics of disease or hospital admission. It also allows investigators to study the effectiveness of drug treatments such as lipid-lowering drugs and antidiabetic drugs by monitoring serum lipid profile, serum glucose level, glycosylated hemoglobin levels, etc.

PRIMARY CARE DATA

Health care data stored on GP computer systems are increasingly available. At present such linkages are done *ad hoc* for each study, but this is becoming increasingly integrated using new purpose-built data extraction software. In particular, access to data such as smoking, alcohol use, body mass index, blood pressure, visits to GP and nurses, as well as access to symptoms and diagnoses are possible. MEMO also has a bank of research nurses who extract data written in paper case records, providing a methodology for accessing all GP data held in a patient's record since birth.[9]

GEOGRAPHIC DATA

All patients and their addresses are known, including post code, and information is available from the decennial census regarding the relative deprivation levels of small area post code areas in the form of the Carstairs deprivation score.[10] This is a z-score using the following census variables: unemployment, overcrowding, male car ownership, and low social class. The Carstairs deprivation score can be used as an indicator of the socioeconomic status of patients.[11]

Studies of geographic variation in prescribing and outcome are also feasible. Post code data also allow the merging of other types of environmental data into the data set. As examples of the breadth of types of research that can be done, it is possible to merge climatic and meteorological data. These are available for small areas of Tayside, with automated stations providing readouts as granular as every few minutes. It is thus possible to study the effect of climatic conditions on health, or surrogates of health such as prescribing. As another example, the dates and locations of flowering of crops, such as rapeseed oil, can be accurately determined. It is thus possible to study the relationship between flowering and the prescribing of anti-allergy drugs. Finally, the distance between any two post code areas can be determined accurately and this provides the opportunity to study the effect on health outcome of distance from heath care facilities.

DARTS AND HEARTS MANAGED CLINICAL NETWORK DATABASES

MEMO has facilitated the development of clinical systems to promote seamless care of patients across all parts of the health care system; as such all health care professionals use just one information technology (IT) system. The Diabetes Audit and Research in Tayside Scotland (DARTS) database is the most developed of these resources and essentially is record-linkage, at source, in real time at the point of care delivery.[9] These databases provide rich and detailed data on the disease phenotype, severity, complications, associated comorbidities, non-drug treatments, demographics, etc. The DARTS system has now been adopted nationally in Scotland and is known as SCI-DC (www.show.scot.nhs.uk/crag).

BIRTH COHORT 1952–1967 (WALKER DATA SET)

This birth cohort, named after the professor of obstetrics who created it, is a database of more than 48 000 birth records that contain meticulously recorded details of pregnancy, labor, birth, and care before discharge for babies born in the Dundee area in the 1950s. MEMO has been able to add the CHI to over 21 000 children, presently alive and living in Tayside (now aged 37–51), and additionally over 15 000 mothers and fathers. Linkage across siblings and over two and three generations is now possible. This data set forms a powerful resource for familial genetic studies by linking with the phenotypic data available within the other data sets, with intermediate phenotypic data obtained at the time of sample collection as well as future database tracking.[12]

AMBULANCE AND EMERGENCY DEPARTMENT DATA

MEMO has the ability to obtain data on ambulance use and emergency visits to the Accident and Emergency departments. Such data have enabled MEMO to provide a complete picture of all resources used by diabetic patients who have hypoglycemic attacks that require NHS hospital treatment but who do not require hospitalization.[13]

OTHER OUTCOME DATA SETS

Other health care data sets are available in Tayside that are not indexed by CHI number. However, provided that some patient demographic details are present, such as name, date of birth, and post code, MEMO can usually identify the correct CHI number in the same way that CHI numbers are identified for prescriptions. Thus, biochemical laboratory reports filed on computer tape back to 1977 and computerized records of histopathology reports have been used. MEMO has also constructed a database of 100 000 endoscopy and colonoscopy procedures,[14] and, in collaboration with Tayside Police, a database of subjects involved in 22 000 road traffic accidents in Tayside.[15]

PATIENT-REPORTED OUTCOMES

Over the past three years MEMO has conducted a number of studies involving direct contact with patients in order to obtain quality-of-life information, patient-reported outcomes such as diabetes-related hypoglycemic attacks managed at home, or the effects of asthma on day- and night-time activities (see also Chapter 42). More recent work is aimed at understanding factors that lead to non-adherence to medications (see also Chapter 46).

GENETIC DATA–PHENOTYPIC LINKAGE

The linkage of genetic information with phenotypic data is a task being undertaken in many parts of the world (see Chapter 37). The molecular biology techniques used to detect and analyze genetic information are now fairly routine, having been enabled by increasingly powerful and rapid technological advances. However, the phenotypic component is the area that deserves most care as linkage of genetic data to phenotypic data of unknown, poor, or mediocre quality is at best poor science and at worst likely to miss important associations. The quality of Tayside data as recorded in the various data sets, the coverage of the data sets, the cradle to grave single data collection point nature, as well as the new managed care clinical networks produce phenotypic data of high quality that enable pharmacogenetics and pharmacogenomic research.[16]

CONFIDENTIALITY, ETHICS, AND GOOD EPIDEMIOLOGIC PRACTICE

European and UK data protection law,[17] NHS guidelines, and research governance requirements (www.show.scot. nhs.uk/cso/ResGov/ResGov.htm), as well as published codes of GEP, clearly dictate what can and cannot be done with UK health care data as well as defining how such data should be managed in observational studies (see also Chapter 38). The tight geographic nature of data used by MEMO as well as the fact that the data come from one NHSiS region, along with the climate of "nervousness" that surrounds data linkage, particularly for genetic purposes, have meant that MEMO has had to undergo a radical evolution to allow it to continue doing pharmacoepidemiology and other research. We suspect that all other European and UK data sets will also be forced to follow this route. This evolution has seen MEMO split into three separate organizations over three physical locations in order to separate subject identifiable data from researchers. MEMO has also developed powerful in-house built software for anonymization and project management. In addition, MEMO now undergoes external audit of all activities, the project management and external audit having as their main focus adherence to GEP.

The three separate organizations are:

1. The NHS Clinical Technology Centre. This center stores and processes all of the NHS subject-specific data. It also runs the IT systems for clinical care. No research is undertaken by this group.
2. The MEMO/HIC/NHS Clinical Interface Unit. This unit acts as a research "bureau service" in that it provides anonymous record-linked data for research. The unit takes in data with patients' names and addresses and exchanges these for the CHI number and then, because the CHI is a personal identifier (containing sex and date of birth identifiers), exchanges the CHI for an anonymized number (ANO-CHI). The conversion to ANO-CHI is done using custom-written software called CLAM (CLeaning and Anonymization by Mapping) that also cleans data, so ensuring that codes and dates are in the correct format. A further anonymization is then undertaken prior to release of data for a research project. This final anonymization ensures that data from separate studies cannot be linked without referral back to the ANO-CHI level, and this can only be done against strictly controlled approved protocols under the control of the Tayside Caldicott Guardians (the government-appointed guardians of subject identifiable health data).
3. The Health Informatics Centre (HIC). This is the new custom-built center that now houses the research and biostatistics part of MEMO. The HIC also brings together the Dental Health Services Research Unit, the researchers within the Tayside Centre for General Practice, the Departments of Public Health, Economics, and Geography, and other partners in the Social Dimensions

of Health Institute, to create a powerful collaborative research grouping capable of ensuring that maximum utility is gained from all the available health, dental, and well-being data in both Tayside and Scotland.

A further benefit of HIC that has been enabled by the standard operating procedures (SOPs) and project management systems now in place means that research on Tayside data can now be undertaken by researchers external to Tayside, provided they agree to adhere to our published SOPs.

Of equal importance is the way the project management system "forces" GEP. Thus the system ensures that protocols, ethics, original data files, transformed data files, programs used to transform and analyze the data, results of analyses, reports, publications, funding sources, and spending are tracked, locked (in an auditable form), and archived for 15 years. It also provides a data compliance tool that prevents access to person-level anonymous data without ethical committee approval and other governance approvals. In addition, an approved protocol must list the data required as well as the analyses that will be undertaken, both requirements of GEP. Deviations from the protocol or protocol amendments must go through a similar process as protocol amendments in clinical trial research. However, the system does not prevent the access to aggregate data within the individual data sets that is required in order to undertake power calculations or to assess study feasibility. Power calculations are a further requirement within GEP and an absolute requirement for our local research ethics committee before the granting of an approval for a hypothesis testing study.

STRENGTHS

PATIENT IDENTIFICATION

One of the greatest advantages of using data from Tayside is the unique patient identifier. This allows for relative ease of record linkage and, since this number is also age- and sex-specific, it is relatively easy to choose age-, sex-, GP-, or practice-matched comparator groups from the population. Selection of patients for both cohort and case–control studies is thus efficient.

POPULATION-BASED DATA

MEMO is regularly supplied with updated copies of the Community Health Master Patient Index from NHS Tayside, and uses this to track the population of patients alive and resident in Tayside on a daily basis to define study populations

for drug safety studies. Unlike clinical trials, which focus on highly selected patients, this observational approach allows "real-world" populations to be studied representing all socioeconomic groups and within a universal health care coverage scheme. Such population-based data allow the calculation of incidence rates, excess risk, and attributable risk.[18]

DRUG EXPOSURE DATA

The data captured at MEMO represent prescriptions that have been dispensed at a pharmacy and so primary noncompliance is eliminated. In a study carried out to assess the extent of primary noncompliance in Tayside, a large family practice (11 500 patients) wrote all prescriptions in duplicate (carbon copy) forms over a three-month period.[19] The copies were sent to MEMO. The original top-copy forms that were redeemed by patients at community pharmacies were also returned to MEMO after the pharmacists had been reimbursed by the NHS. Duplicate forms for which no original was present represented the prescriptions that were not redeemed. Figure 21.1 shows the rate of primary noncompliance by age and sex, and it is clear that in some age groups this is a significant problem.

ACCESSIBILITY TO MEDICAL RECORDS

A major strength of MEMO is the ability to examine original hospital case records where necessary. This allows for quality control of the computerized data and can also deal with some elements of confounding. For example, persons admitted with gastrointestinal bleeding are nearly always asked about their previous ingestion of aspirin and nonsteroidal anti-inflammatory drugs. Over-the-counter (OTC) preparations are not recorded in the MEMO drug exposure database

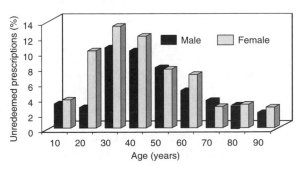

Figure 21.1. Primary noncompliance with prescribed medication.[19]

and this confounding can be partly controlled by such data. Similarly, information may be available on potential confounding factors such as smoking and alcohol consumption.[20]

Several studies validating the computerized diagnostic data with the case medical records have been carried out. Within the NHS, such case record searching for the purposes of drug safety evaluation is ethically permissible.[21]

HIGH DIAGNOSTIC ACCURACY

Record linkage of data sets using a diagnostic algorithm rather than the use of a single diagnosis code from one data set improves the specificity and sensitivity of diagnoses. In addition, the access to case medical records further improves accuracy.

LOW/NO MISSING DATA

By using data from computer systems, MEMO data are not subject to missing data on hospitalizations or data that may have transcription errors. Historically, this has been a known problem for primary care data sets.

COLLABORATIVE CULTURE

MEMO could not have achieved what it has over the past 14 years without a strong and collaborative relationship with the NHSiS in Tayside and the ISD of the NHSiS. This collaboration has been two-way, in enabling a wide range of research and, in return, influencing and building the IT systems that improve the delivery of patient care. The new collaborative HIC will further maximize the research output from the MEMO data set.

PATIENT ACCESS

MEMO is able to use its data sets to generate lists of subjects who meet set criteria for entry to certain types of prospective studies. Such work is done under a detailed SOP ensuring patient confidentiality and in conjunction with the subject's primary care doctor, who is the point of contact with the patient. It is hoped that this new initiative will assist with the identification of subjects as possible subjects for inclusion in clinical trials.

RANDOMIZED SIMPLIFIED TRIALS AND RANDOMIZED EPIDEMIOLOGY

Access to patients, collaboration with primary care, and the MEMO data sets enable cost-efficient randomized Phase IV real-world studies of safety and/or effectiveness to be done at low cost (see also Chapter 39). These studies can contribute significantly to risk management plans after licensing (see also Chapter 33). They can also be used to produce the data on effectiveness that are increasingly demanded by health service providers. In such studies, patients are recruited according to good clinical practice by their primary care physician. They are then randomized by MEMO to receive a study drug prescription or a comparator drug prescription, prescribed in the normal manner within the NHS. The relevant data sets are then tracked for exposure and outcomes. Once randomized, subjects are treated in the same way as other subjects. These trials are open but the endpoints can be assessed by a committee blinded to treatment allocation—the so-called PROBE (Prospective, Randomized, Open, Blinded Endpoint) design. Importantly, those randomized into such studies can be compared with those who are not randomized to determine if those randomized are representative of the real-world population who get such drug treatment.

A recent UK government initiative, called the Pharmaceutical Industry Competitive Task Force (www.advisory bodies.doh.gov.uk/pictf), means that industry bears only the incremental cost to the NHS of carrying out such trials.

Philosophically, there are two types of large randomized study that can be carried out using this methodology. Where a hypothesis is being tested, then this is a simplified clinical trial and the power calculation is done on the endpoint of interest. However, it is also possible to randomize subjects without an *a priori* hypothesis. In such cases these trials can be regarded as randomized epidemiologic studies without a prior hypothesis. These trials might be conservatively powered for mortality equivalence between treatments. However, the database can also be used for one or perhaps more hypothesis testing studies on signals that arise following marketing. Since follow-up of these cohorts is inexpensive, such trials can continue for as long as is deemed appropriate. The follow-up of trial cohorts using such record linkage in Scotland has previously been shown to be useful and comparable to traditional methods.[22] The great advantage of these trials over traditional observational studies is that the play of chance minimizes the differences between the treatment groups at baseline (see Chapter 39). This avoids the issues of channeling bias and confounding by indication or contraindication[23] (see also Chapters 40 and 47). While methodologies have been developed to cope with these issues[24] (see also Chapter 40), there remains the lingering problem of residual confounding. A criticism of such studies is that because there is no experimental control following randomization then with the passage of time they become more observational in nature. However, it is our belief that the benefits of baseline randomization far outweigh any subsequent arguments of this nature.

WEAKNESSES

POPULATION SIZE AND DRUG USE

The current population of Tayside is approximately 400 000, which is comparatively small for many pharmacovigilance studies. However, 400 000 is an adequate size for many other types of pharmacoepidemiology studies.

Drug exposure data in Tayside are only available from 1989 and cover only a limited set of drugs until January 1993 (from when all dispensed prescriptions have been collected).

OTC AND HOSPITAL-DISPENSED MEDICATIONS

Another weakness is the inability to capture directly exposure to OTC drugs or drugs prescribed in hospital. People use OTC medications such as aspirin, ibuprofen, paracetamol (acetaminophen), and others for their symptoms.

INDICATION FOR USE

Given that confounding by indication is arguably one of the most difficult potential sources of error in pharmacoepidemiologic research (see Chapter 40), one of MEMO's biggest weaknesses is that the diagnostic indication for prescribing is not available. Where the indication for a drug is wide (e.g., beta adrenoceptor blocking drugs can be given for indications varying from anxiety to hypertrophic cardiomyopathy), this can lead to difficulties. In addition, there is a certain amount of "over-coding" that happens in primary care data sets where the coded diagnosis given at the time of prescription is assigned for convenience and may be incorrect.

INACCURATE DIAGNOSIS

One of the criticisms leveled at record linkage studies is the inaccuracy of computerized medical diagnoses (see Chapter 45). In MEMO, the discharge diagnoses for SMR1 are abstracted from the clinical discharge summaries by specially trained coding clerks. These clerks on occasions have to interpret "soft diagnoses," such as symptoms for which no cause can be found. In addition, nonstandard terminology may be employed to describe an illness, for example eponymous terms, and so the coding of diagnoses may be imprecise. Computerized algorithms exist to detect and reject the most glaring errors, but errors of interpretation persist within the database. In addition, these SMR databases are continuously audited by the ISD of the NHSiS (www.isdscotland.org/isd/collect2.jsp?pContentID=1607&p_applic=CCC&p_service=Content.show&) and the quality and accuracy of the data they contain is consistently high.[25] These data demonstrate the continuous improvements in data quality that are being achieved and allow for increasing confidence in the results of purely electronic studies. Several validation studies of the accuracy of hospital discharge data in Scotland have also been performed, comparing the coded diagnoses with diagnoses inferred by one or more senior doctors who have reviewed the original case records.[26–28] These studies have largely confirmed the accuracy of computerized data. However, ultimately, access to primary medical records is critical here.

EPISODES AND ADMISSION

Another issue that must be appreciated with computerized SMR data is that the currency is the "consultant episode of care." In other words, a patient who is hospitalized with a gastrointestinal hemorrhage under the care of an internist and who then gets transferred to the care of a surgeon, gets transferred to an intensive care specialist postoperatively, and then back to an internist prior to discharge will have four computerized admission and discharge records, each containing diagnostic terms and procedure terms. Government statistics on health care activity, often used in determining power calculations for drug safety studies, list these consultant episodes and not hospital admission events. Typically, 100 consultant episodes would translate into about 70 admission and discharge events. The weakness of this system is that consultant episodes must be reconciled into admission and discharge events. The strength is that more diagnostic terms are used and the likelihood of incorrect coding is minimized. In addition, a major benefit of these episodes of care data is the ability to "cost" hospitalizations. Each facility the patient is treated in carries a different NHS tariff cost. The economic evaluation of health care interventions is assuming increasing importance within any health care system so these data are of increasing importance.

PARTICULAR APPLICATIONS

DRUG UTILIZATION RESEARCH

MEMO is able to produce very detailed drug utilization data, broken down by age, sex, date, day of the week prescribed, prescriber, generic or proprietary dispensing, co-prescribing, acute prescribing, and/or repeat prescribing, dose, and duration. Specific studies can then be carried out to examine in more detail how drugs are prescribed and used in Tayside, from the standpoint of either the prescriber or the patient. This is important as the safety and efficacy of drugs may depend on whether they are used properly (see also Chapters 27, 28, and 29).

One important dimension is the audit of GP prescribing in the population, although GP-specific data are analyzed anonymously and individual GPs are never identified. For example, one study identified rare instances of potentially hazardous co-prescribing of β-antagonists and β-agonists to patients in Tayside likely to have asthma or chronic obstructive airways disease, by linking the dispensed prescribing database to hospital admission records.[29] Another study exploited the detailed data on dose and duration (inferred from the total amount dispensed and the dosage instructions) and showed that various antidepressants are often prescribed at ineffective doses for insufficient durations.[30] The processing of prescribing data according to the demographic characteristics of prescribing GPs has also yielded some useful insights into the characteristics of "good" prescribers. For example, differences in the prescribing of antibiotics and psychotropic medication have been seen between GP registrar training and non-training practices.[31] Prescribing might also vary by patient factors, independent of need or disease severity, an example being the variation in the use of statin therapy by socioeconomic status.[11]

A related issue is patient adherence with medication. By assessing how medication is collected by patients, in terms of numbers of prescriptions dispensed and intervals between them, and linking this to outcome data sets, it is possible to assess the effects of adherence. For example, about 64% of patients adhere to statin treatment after a myocardial infarction. Those who adhere have considerably better outcomes than those who do not.[32] Other studies of patient adherence have been done in diabetes,[33,34] heart failure,[35] and asthma[36] (see also Chapter 46).

COHORT STUDIES

A number of cohort studies have been conducted in recent years using the MEMO record-linkage database. For example, cohort study designs have been used to evaluate the risk profile of nonsteroidal anti-inflammatory drugs (NSAIDs).[14,23,37] A recent study has examined the effect of channeling bias with newer NSAIDs.[23] We also used a cohort design to examine the interaction between aspirin and ibuprofen,[38] to calculate the resource costs of prescribing low dose aspirin in the setting of the NHS,[39] to study the pharmacoeconomics of different NSAID treatment strategies,[40] and to investigate hypersensitivity reactions to NSAIDs.[41]

We have also used the cohort design to study the drug treatment of Parkinson's disease,[42] to study the associations between exposure to allopurinol[43] and social deprivation[44] and hospitalization for heart failure, to study the effects of β-blockers on the secondary prevention of coronary disease,[45] and to study the association between glucocorticoids and cardiovascular disease.[18]

CASE–CONTROL STUDIES

The case–control design has been used in a range of MEMO studies. Cases are identified from one of the SMR databases, and matched sets of either "community" controls (from the study population) or "hospital" controls (from patients admitted to the same hospital as the case but with a diagnosis unrelated to exposure) can be generated efficiently. Exposure frequencies can be calculated for cases and controls using data from the dispensed prescribing database, and exposure odds ratios calculated. It is also possible to adjust for confounding from other drug use and for other covariates assembled from other MEMO databases. For example, we have studied the associations between topical NSAIDs and hospitalization for upper gastrointestinal hemorrhage and perforation,[46] NSAIDS and acute renal failure,[47] acute appendicitis,[48] and acute colitis.[49] More recent case-control studies have examined the role of prior exposure to antibiotics in the etiology of trimethoprim resistant bacteriuria.[50,51]

CASE-CROSSOVER STUDIES

The case-crossover design was employed in a study examining the risks of road traffic accidents associated with benzodiazepine use.[15] In this design, only cases who had experienced a road traffic accident were considered. The "controls" were the same cases at earlier times, hence the name case-crossover design. There were 19 386 subjects in this study and a dose–response relation was found between benzodiazepine use and road traffic accident. The case-crossover design is suitable for the evaluation of transient risks, and because cases are used as their own controls, some problems of confounding can be dealt with neatly (see Chapter 48).

OTHER STUDIES

MEMO has made contributions to research on compliance with glucose monitoring in diabetes,[52] drug use during pregnancy,[53] pharmacoeconomics and disease management,[54–56] disease epidemiology,[57–61] and drug overdose studies.[62–64]

METHODOLOGICAL STUDIES

MEMO has also provided the setting for some methodological work in pharmacoepidemiology. Work on the cohort method has focused on the selection of comparator groups and whether the length of "risk windows" influences the estimate of effect.[65] This is the length of time after a drug has been prescribed during which a potential side effect might be identified. Other examples include studies on propensity score methodology,[66-68] design issues for drug epidemiology,[69] sample size for cohort studies,[70] adjusting for missing data,[71] Bayesian risk-analysis,[72] and case-crossover and case-time-control designs.[73]

OTHER RESEARCH APPLICATIONS

An interesting application of record-linkage in MEMO is the compilation of patient-specific disease registers using information from different sources. For example, a validated diabetic register of all patients (treated or nontreated) with type 1 and type 2 diabetes has been constructed.[9] This is known as the DARTS initiative, a collaboration among MEMO, all GP practices in Tayside, and the Diabetes Units in three health care trusts. The register is compiled by record-linking data from eight independent data sources: SMR01, four diabetes clinics in three health care trusts, and a mobile eye van that has been operating in Tayside since 1990 performing community retinopathy screening, all of which use the CHI number routinely as a patient identifier. Data from MEMO's dispensed prescribing database (which includes glucose monitoring equipment) and the results of biochemistry tests in hospitals are also used. An example of the use of this database in pharmacoepidemiology was the association between angiotensin converting enzyme inhibitor use and hypoglycemia in diabetes,[74] but it has also been used for other epidemiological research.[75] The register has recently been used to link pharmacoepidemiology to genetics research. For example, we have recently shown that the ARE2 allele of PPP1R3A was associated with a male preponderance to early type 2 diabetes.[76] Other such registers are becoming available and are increasingly being used for research.[59-61]

The incorporation of cost into the MEMO dispensed prescribing database also makes this an important resource for pharmacoeconomic research, particularly that which recognizes the cost of adverse reactions to drugs that occur in the community,[39,40,54-56,60,77,78] an aspect which is often overlooked (see also Chapter 41).

THE FUTURE

The establishment of the HIC will see an increase in the range and volume of research undertaken using Tayside and Scottish data. Scotland now has its own Centre for Adverse Reactions to Drugs (www.show.scot.nhs.uk/CSMScotland) and this is a further driver for the development of Scotland-wide adverse drug reaction data. The uptake of managed care networks across Scotland will enable access to large data sets that are rich in detail. The inclusion of the unique identifier on all prescriptions will see a further change in the methods used by MEMO to create the prescription data set. New electronic links are being established to speed the flow of prescription data into MEMO, to make the dispensed prescribing data set larger and current. Confidentiality issues and GEP will remain key issues, particularly as more genetic research is undertaken that links phenotype to genotype. MEMO/HIC will also be increasing the number of patient representatives who sit on key advisory committees.

In conclusion, MEMO has realized its potential as a comprehensive record linkage system that not only can be used for the detection and quantification of serious drug toxicity, but also can be used for a wide range of research in health care. We are confident that along with randomized clinical trials, record-linkage studies will continue to add great value to health care research.

REFERENCES

1. MacDonald TM, McDevitt DG. The Tayside Medicines Monitoring Unit (MEMO). In: Strom BL, ed., *Pharmacoepidemiology*, 2nd edn. Chichester: John Wiley & Sons, 1994; pp. 245–55.
2. Beardon PHG, Brown SV, McDevitt DG. Four-year mortality among cimetodine takers in Tayside: results of a controlled study using record linkage. *Pharm Med* 1988; **3**: 333–9.
3. NHS in Scotland, Information and Statistics Division. *SMR Data Manual*, version 1.3. Edinburgh: NHSiS, 2000. Available at: http://www.isdscotland.org/isd/files/SMRDM_intro.pdf.
4. International Society for Pharmacoepidemiology. Guidelines for Good Pharmacoepidemiology Practices (GPP). Available at: http://www.pharmacoepi.org/resources/guidelines_08027.cfm.
5. Wilson P. Commentary: legal issues of data anonymisation in research. *BMJ* 2004; **328**: 1300–1.
6. World Health Organization. *Manual of the International Statistical Classification of Diseases, Injuries and Causes of Death*, 9th revision, vol. 1. Geneva: World Health Organization, 1977.
7. Office of Population Censuses and Surveys. *Tabular List of the Classification of Surgical Operations and Procedures*, 4th revision. London: HMSO, 1990.

8. World Health Organization. *International Statistical Classification of Diseases and Related Health Problems*, 10th revision. Geneva: World Health Organization, 1992.

9. Morris AD, Boyle DI, MacAlpine R, Emslie-Smith A, Jung RT, Newton RW *et al*. The diabetes audit and research in Tayside Scotland (DARTS) study: electronic record linkage to create a diabetes register. DARTS/MEMO Collaboration. *BMJ*. 1997; **315**: 524–8.

10. Carstairs V. Deprivation and health in Scotland. *Health Bull* (Edinb) 1990; **48**: 162–75.

11. Wei L, MacDonald TM, Davey PG. Relation between socio-economic deprivation and statin prescribing in post myocardial infarction patients: a population based study. *Pharmacoepidemiol Drug Saf* 2002; **11** (suppl): S151.

12. Libby G, Smith A, McEwan NF, Chien PFW, Greene SA, Forsyth JS *et al*. The Walker Project: a longitudinal study of 48,000 children born 1952–66 (aged 36–50 years in 2002) and their families. Study methodology. *Paediatr Perinat Epidemiol* 2004; **18**: 302–12.

13. Leese GP, Wang J, Broomhall J, Kelly P, Marsden A, Morrison W *et al*. Frequency of severe hypoglycemia requiring emergency treatment in type 1 and type 2 diabetes: a population-based study of health service resource use. *Diabetes Care* 2003; **26**: 1176–80.

14. MacDonald TM, Morant SV, Robinson GC, Shield MJ, McGilchrist MM, Murray FE *et al*. Association of upper gastrointestinal toxicity of non-steroidal anti-inflammatory drugs with continued exposure: cohort study. *BMJ* 1997; **315**: 1333–7.

15. Barbone F, McMahon AD, Davey PG, Morris AD, Reid IC, McDevitt DG *et al*. Association of road-traffic accidents with benzodiazepine use. *Lancet* 1998; **352**: 1331–6.

16. Doney AS, Fischer B, Cecil JE, Boylan K, McGuigan FE, Ralston SH *et al*. Association of the Pro12Ala and C1431T variants of PPARG and their haplotypes with susceptibility to Type 2 diabetes. *Diabetologia* 2004; **47**: 555–8.

17. Data Protection Act, Chapter 29. London: The Stationery Office, 1998.

18. Wei L, MacDonald TM, Walker BR. Taking glucocorticoids by prescription is associated with subsequent cardiovascular disease. *Ann Intern Med* 2004; **141**: 764–70.

19. Beardon PH, McGilchrist MM, McKendrick AD, McDevitt DG, MacDonald TM. Primary non-compliance with prescribed medication in primary care. *BMJ* 1993; **307**: 846–8.

20. Evans JM, McMahon AD, Steinke DT, McAlpine RR, MacDonald TM. Do H_2-receptor antagonists cause acute pancreatitis? *Pharmacoepidemiol Drug Saf* 1998; **7**: 383–8.

21. The Scottish Office, Home and Health Department. Local Research Ethical Committees. Edinburgh: HMSO, 1992; p. 9.

22. The West of Scotland Coronary Prevention Study Group. Computerised record linkage: compared with traditional patient follow-up methods in clinical trials and illustrated in a prospective epidemiological study. *J Clin Epidemiol* 1995; **48**: 1441–52.

23. MacDonald TM, Morant SV, Goldstein JL, Burke TA, Pettitt D. Channelling bias and the incidence of gastrointestinal haemorrhage in users of meloxicam, coxibs, and older, non-specific nonsteroidal anti-inflammatory drugs. *Gut* 2003; **52**: 1–6.

24. Morant SV, Pettitt D, MacDonald TM, Burke TA, Goldstein JL. Application of a propensity score to adjust for channelling bias with NSAIDs. *Pharmacoepidemiol Drug Saf* 2004; **13**: 345–53.

25. Scottish Health Statistics. Appendixes. Available at: http://www.show.scot.nhs.uk/isdonline/Scottish_Health_Statistics/SHS98/Appendix.pdf.

26. Pears J, Alexander V, Alexander GF, Waugh NR. Audit of the quality of hospital discharge data. *Health Bull* 1992; **50**: 356–61.

27. Kohli HS, Knill-Jones RP. How accurate are SMR1 (Scottish Morbidity Record 1) data? *Health Bull* 1992; **50**: 14–23.

28. Park RH, McCabe P, Russell RI. Who should log SHIPS? The accuracy of Scottish Hospital Morbidity Data for Wilson's disease. *Health Bull* 1992; **50**: 24–8.

29. Evans JM, Hayes JL, Lipworth BJ, MacDonald TM. Potentially hazardous co-prescribing of beta-adrenoceptor antagonists and agonists in the community. *Br J Gen Pract* 1996; **46**: 423–5.

30. MacDonald TM, McMahon AD, Reid IC, Fenton GW, McDevitt DG. Antidepressant drug use in primary care: a record linkage study in Tayside, Scotland. *BMJ* 1996; **313**: 860–1.

31. Steinke DT, Bain DJ, MacDonald TM, Davey PG. Practice factors that influence antibiotic prescribing in general practice in Tayside. *J Antimicrob Chemother* 2000; **46**: 509–12.

32. Wei L, Wang J, Thompson P, Wong S, Struthers AD, MacDonald TM. Adherence to statin treatment and readmission of patients after myocardial infarction: a six year follow up study. *Heart* 2002; **88**: 229–33.

33. Morris AD, Boyle DIR, McMahon AD, Pearce H, Evans JMM, Newton RW, *et al*. ACE inhibitor use is associated with hospitalisation for severe hypoglycaemia in patients with diabetes. *Diabetes Care* 1997; **20**: 1363–7.

34. Donnan PT, MacDonald TM, Morris AD. Adherence to prescribed oral hypoglycaemic medication in a population of patients with type 2 diabetes: a retrospective cohort study. *Diabet Med* 2002; **19**: 279–84.

35. Struthers AD, Anderson G, MacFadyen RJ, Fraser C, MacDonald TM. Nonadherence with ACE inhibitors is common and can be detected in clinical practice by routine serum ACE activity. *Congest Heart Fail* 2001; **7**: 43–46, 50.

36. McMahon AD, Lipworth BJ, Davey PG, Morris AD, MacDonald TM. Compliance with inhaled corticosteroids and control of asthma. *Pharmacoepidemiol Drug Saf* 2000; **9**: 293–303.

37. McMahon AD, Evans JM, White G, Murray FE, McGilchrist MM, McDevitt DG *et al*. A cohort study (with re-sampled comparator groups) to measure the association between new NSAID prescribing and upper gastrointestinal hemorrhage and perforation. *J Clin Epidemiol* 1997; **50**: 351–6.

38. MacDonald TM, Wei Li. Effect of ibuprofen on cardioprotective effect of aspirin. *Lancet* 2003; **361**: 573–4.

39. Morant SV, McMahon AD, Cleland JG, Davey PG, MacDonald TM. Cardiovascular prophylaxis with aspirin: costs of supply and management of upper gastrointestinal and renal toxicity. *Br J Clin Pharmacol* 2004; **57**: 188–98.

40. Morant SV, Shield MJ, Davey PG, MacDonald TM. A pharma-coeconomic comparison of misoprostol/diclofenac with diclofenac. *Pharmacoepidemiol Drug Saf* 2002; **11**: 393–400.

41. McMahon AD, Evans JMM, MacDonald TM. Hypersensitivity reactions associated with exposure to naproxen and ibuprofen: a cohort study. *J Clin Epidemiol* 2001: **54**: 1271–4.

42. Donnan PT, Steinke DT, Stubbings C, Davey PG, MacDonald TM. Selegiline and mortality in subjects with Parkinson's disease: a longitudinal community study. *Neurology* 2000; **55**: 1785–9.

43. Struthers AD, Donnan PT, Lindsay P, McNaughton D, Broomhall J, MacDonald TM. The effects of allopurinol on mortality and hospitalisations in chronic heart failure: a retrospective cohort study. *Heart* 2002; **87**: 229–34.

44. Struthers AD, Anderson G, Donnan PT, MacDonald TM. Social deprivation increases cardiac hospitalisations in chronic heart failure independently of disease severity and of diuretic non-adherence. *Heart* 2000; **83**: 12–16.

45. Wei L, Flynn R, Murray GD, MacDonald TM. Use and adherence to beta-blockers for secondary prevention of myocardial infarction: who is not getting treatment? *Pharmacoepidemiol Drug Saf* 2004; **13**: 761–6.

46. Evans JM, McMahon AD, McGilchrist MM, White G, Murray FE, McDevitt DG *et al*. Topical non-steroidal anti-inflammatory drugs and admission to hospital for upper gastrointestinal bleeding and perforation: a record linkage case–control study. *BMJ* 1995; **311**: 22–6.

47. Evans JM, McGregor E, McMahon AD, McGilchrist MM, Jones MC, White G *et al*. Non-steroidal anti-inflammatory drugs and hospitalization for acute renal failure. *Q J Med* 1995; **88**: 551–7.

48. Evans JM, Macgregor AM, Murray FE, Vaidya K, Morris AD, MacDonald TM. No association between non-steroidal anti-inflammatory drugs and acute appendicitis in a case–control study. *Br J Surg* 1997; **84**: 372–4.

49. Evans JM, McMahon AD, Murray FE, McDevitt DG, MacDonald TM. Non-steroidal anti-inflammatory drugs are associated with emergency admission to hospital for colitis due to inflammatory bowel disease. *Gut* 1997; **40**: 619–22.

50. Donnan PT, Wei L, Steinke DT, Phillips G, Clarke R, Noone A *et al*. Presence of bacteriuria caused by trimethoprim resistant bacteria in patients prescribed antibiotics: multilevel model with practice and individual patient data. *BMJ* 2004; **328**: 1297–301.

51. Steinke DT, Seaton RA, Phillips G, MacDonald TM, Davey PG. Prior trimethoprim use and trimethoprim-resistant urinary tract infection: a nested case–control study with multivariate analysis for other risk factors. *J Antimicrob Chemother* 2001; **47**: 781–7.

52. Evans JMM, Newton RW, Ruta DA, MacDonald TM, Stevenson R, Morris AD. Frequency of blood glucose monitoring in relation to glycaemic control: observational study with diabetes database. *BMJ* 1999; **319**: 83–6.

53. Olesen C, de Vries CS, Thrane N, MacDonald TM, Larsen H, Sorensen HT. The EuroMAP Group. Effect of diuretics on fetal growth: a drug effect or confounding by indication? Pooled Danish and Scottish cohort data. *Br J Clin Pharmacol* 2001; **51**: 153–7.

54. Davey PG, McMahon AD, Barbone F, Gillespie WG, Rizvi KA, MacDonald TM. The effect of hip replacement on prescribing of NSAIDs, ulcer healing drugs and hospitalization—a matched cohort study. *Pharmacoepidemiol Drug Saf* 1999; **8**: 423–31.

55. Davey PG, Clarkson P, MaMahon A, MacDonald TM. Costs associated with symptomatic systolic heart failure. *Pharmacoeconomics* 1999; **16**: 399–407.

56. Davey PG, McMahon AD, Irwin D, Anderson P, Morris AD, MacDonald TM. The influence of case mix, site selection and methods biases on costs of hospitalization for acute exacerbations of chronic obstructive airway disease and lower respiratory tract infections. *Value Health* 1999; **2**: 333–41.

57. Donnan PT, Boyle DI, Broomhall J, Hunter K, MacDonald TM, Newton RW *et al*. Prognosis following first acute myocardial infarction in type 2 diabetes: a comparative population study. *Diabet Med* 2002; **19**: 448–55.

58. Evans JM, Wang J, Morris AD. Comparison of cardiovascular risk between patients with type 2 diabetes and those who had had a myocardial infarction: cross sectional and cohort studies. *BMJ* 2002; **324**: 939–42.

59. Steinke DT, Weston TL, Morris AD, MacDonald TM, Dillon JF. The epidemiology of liver disease in Tayside database: a population-based record-linkage study. *J Biomed Inform* 2002; **35**: 186–93.

60. Steinke DT, Weston TL, Morris AD, MacDonald TM, Dillon JF. Epidemiology and economic burden of viral hepatitis: an observational population based study. *Gut* 2002; **50**: 100–5.

61. Flynn RWV, MacDonald TM, Morris AD, Jung RT, Leese GP. The thyroid epidemiology and research study (TEARS): thyroid dysfunction in the general population. *J Clin Endocrinol Metab* 2004; **89**: 3879–84.

62. Sheen CL, Dillon JF, Bateman DN, Simpson KJ, MacDonald TM. Paracetamol-related deaths in Scotland, 1994–2000. *Br J Clin Pharmacol* 2002; **54**: 430–2.

63. Sheen CL, Dillon JF, Bateman DN, Simpson KJ, MacDonald TM. Paracetamol toxicity: epidemiology, prevention and costs to the health care system. *Q J Med* 2003; **95**: 609–19.

64. Sheen CL, Dillon JF, Bateman DN, Simpson K, MacDonald TM. Paracetamol pack size restriction: the impact on paracetamol poisoning and over-the-counter supply of paracetamol, aspirin and ibuprofen. *Pharmacoepidemiol Drug Saf* 2002; **11**: 329–31.

65. McMahon AD, Evans JMM, McGilchrist MM, McDevitt DG, Macdonald TM. Drug exposure risk windows and unexposed comparator groups for cohort studies in pharmacoepidemiology. *Pharmacoepidemiol Drug Saf* 1998; **7**: 275–80.

66. Wang J, Donnan PT, Steinke D, MacDonald TM. The multiple propensity score for analysis of dose–response relationships in drug safety studies. *Pharmacoepidemiol Drug Saf* 2001; **10**: 105–11.

67. Wang J, Donnan PT. Propensity score methods in drug safety studies: practice, strengths and limitations. *Pharmacoepidemiol Drug Saf* 2001; **10**: 341–4.

68. Wang J, Wei L, MacDonald TM. Adjustment using the propensity of adherence: theory, simulation and practical application. *Pharmacoepidemiol Drug Saf* 2002; **11** (suppl): S207.

69. McMahon AD, MacDonald TM. Design issues for drug epidemiology. *Br J Clin Pharmacol* 2000; **50**: 419–25.

70. McMahon AD, MacDonald TM. Sample size for cohort studies in pharmacoepidemiology. Design issues for drug epidemiology. *Pharmacoepidemiol Drug Saf* 1997; **6**: 331–5.

71. Wang J, Donnan PT. Adjusting for missing data in record linkage outcome studies. *J Appl Stat* 2002; **29**: 873–84.

72. Wang J, Donnan PT, MacDonald TM. An approximate Bayesian risk-analysis for the gastro-intestinal safety of ibuprofen. *Pharmacoepidemiol Drug Saf* 2002; **11**: 695–701.

73. Donnan PT, Wang J. The case-crossover and case–time–control designs in pharmacoepidemiology. *Pharmacoepidemiol Drug Saf* 2001; **10**: 259–62.

74. Morris AD, Boyle DI, McMahon AD, Pearce H, Evans JM, Newton RW, Jung RT, MacDonald TM. ACE inhibitor use is associated with hospitalization for severe hypoglycemia in patients with diabetes. DARTS/MEMO Collaboration. Diabetes Audit and Research in Tayside, Scotland. Medicines Monitoring Unit. *Diabetes Care* 1997; **20**: 1363–7.

75. Ellis JD, Evans JM, Ruta DA, Baines PS, Leese G, MacDonald TM, Morris AD. Glaucoma incidence in an unselected cohort of diabetic patients: is diabetes mellitus a risk factor for glaucoma? DARTS/MEMO collaboration. Diabetes Audit and Research in Tayside Study. Medicines Monitoring Unit. *Br J Ophthalmol* 2000; **84**: 1218–24.

76. Doney AS, Fischer B, Cecil JE, Cohen PT, Boyle DI, Leese G *et al*. Male preponderance in early diagnosed type 2 diabetes is associated with the ARE insertion/deletion polymorphism in the PPP1R3A locus. *BMC Genet* 2003; **4**: 11.

77. MacDonald TM. The economic evaluation of antibiotic therapy: relevance to urinary tract infection. *J Antimicrob Chemother* 1994; **33** (suppl A): 137–45.

78. MacDonald TM, Collins D, McGilchrist MM, Stevens J, McKendrick AD, McDevitt DG, Davey PG. The utilisation and economic evaluation of antibiotics prescribed in primary care. *J Antimicrob Chemother* 1995; **35**: 191–204.

22

The UK General Practice Research Database

JOEL M. GELFAND[1], DAVID J. MARGOLIS[1] and HASSY DATTANI[2]

[1] Department of Dermatology and Center for Clinical Epidemiology and Biostatistics, University of Pennsylvania, Philadelphia, Pennsylvania, USA; [2] Epidemiology and Pharmacology Information Core, London, UK.

INTRODUCTION

The study of the distribution and determinants of disease is often challenged by the substantial costs of collecting health information from individuals and logistical difficulties of using this information to answer epidemiologic questions. The challenge of efficiently obtaining health data is magnified when researchers are studying rare but medically important diseases (e.g., most cancers occur with a frequency of less than 1 per 10 000 person-years), diseases that persist for or evolve over many years, or when examining relatively modest associations that are of public health significance. One potential method for studying rare outcomes is a case–control study, but a major challenge of this epidemiologic design is to study samples of patients that are representative of their source population. As a result, studies of well-defined populations for which data have been collected in a reliable and routine fashion offer a significant advantage to the epidemiologic researcher in that they improve the internal and external validity of a study.

The use of existing databases that capture information on large numbers of patients offers tremendous scientific opportunity to study epidemiologic aspects of disease. For example, databases that capture longitudinal health information on patients offer the opportunity to perform retrospective cohort studies in large numbers of patients in a timely and cost efficient manner. Databases that collect health information can be divided into two broad categories: those that collect information for administrative purposes such as filing claims for payment, and those that serve as the patient's medical record and therefore are a primary means by which physicians track health information on their patients. Several other chapters in this textbook describe many of the administrative databases used for epidemiologic research (see Chapters 13–21). Administrative databases are often inferior to medical records databases when studying the presence or absence of a disease because their intended purpose is often for billing. As a result, they often fail to capture important health data (e.g., family history, lifestyle practices) and the health care data that are captured may suffer from significant validity limitations in that their purpose was for the generation of a bill or payment and not patient care. In contrast, the purpose of a medical record database is to provide a health care provider with information needed to care for a patient. While on face value this information may seem to be of superior quality for epidemiologic studies,

Pharmacoepidemiology, Fourth Edition   Edited by B.L. Strom
© 2005 John Wiley & Sons, Ltd

medical record databases can also have limitations in that the collection of data is for patient care and not necessarily for scientific studies. Therefore, the information recorded or even the way that data is quantified by the health care provider in the database may not reflect the interests of the epidemiologic investigator. This chapter will focus on the General Practice Research Database (GPRD), which is generally considered to be the largest medical records database that is in routine use for epidemiologic investigation, and the one which has been used most extensively for published pharmacoepidemiologic research.

DESCRIPTION

HISTORY AND EVOLUTION OF THE GPRD

The GPRD was started in June 1987 as a tool for conducting public health research. The system of health care delivery in the UK allows a unique opportunity for researchers to study data on a well-defined population. In the UK, virtually all of the patient's care is coordinated by the general practitioner (GP) through the National Health Service (NHS). When patients are referred for specialty care, a treatment plan is initiated by the consultant but ultimately chronic therapies are prescribed and monitored by the GP. When patients are seen by specialists or in the hospital, future treatment is directed through the GP, ultimately allowing for capture of this information as well.

The GPRD was established for the purpose of allowing researchers to conduct high quality epidemiologic studies based on data that are routinely recorded by the GP. The database contains information on both medical diagnoses and prescription medications, which are recorded by the GP as part of the patient's medical record. The GPRD initially was called the Value Added Medical Products (VAMP) Research Databank. VAMP provided general practitioners with computerized software that enabled them to contribute anonymized data to a central database. The computerized software was designed so that it would ultimately replace the written medical record. The software was developed by Dr Alan Dean, a practicing GP in the UK[1] and a VAMP director. VAMP initially signed an agreement with approximately 1000 practices representing about 3000 general practitioners nationally and represent-ative of general practices in the UK whereby the GPs agreed to (i) receive training in standardized data entry, (ii) provide a copy of the entire medical record data to VAMP (stripped of identifiers), and (iii) provide anonymized photocopied referral letters to hospitals and specialists, for use in specific research studies. VAMP also entered into an agreement with the Boston Collaborative Drug Surveillance Program (BCDSP), whereby BCDSP reorganized the raw data into an analyzable format. BCDSP then performed a series of studies to evaluate the completeness and accuracy of the recorded data in collaboration with VAMP.

The administration of the GPRD has undergone several changes since it was initiated by VAMP in 1987. VAMP was acquired by Reuters Health Information in 1993, which in turn donated the research database to the UK Department of Health in 1994, with the stipulation that the database be used for research, on a nonprofit basis. From 1994 until 1999 the database was operated by the Office for National Statistics (ONS). In 1995, Vision, a Windows-based software system created by Reuters for managing patient information, was introduced and subsequently became the dominant data entry system used by GPs in the GPRD. Management of the GPRD was transferred to the UK Medicines Control Agency in April 1999 and this agency became part of the newly created Medicines and Healthcare products Regulatory Agency (MHRA) in April 2003.

Despite the changes in the administration of the GPRD during this time period, high-quality data collection and validation have been maintained.[2] However, since the inception of data collection the overall participation of practices has decreased.[3] In 1987 there were over 700 practices participating. The number of practices declined to 520 in 1995 and declined further to 365 in 2000. Further diminishing the overall size of the GPRD, the Epidemiology and Pharmacology Information Core (EPIC), a vendor of the GPRD, which grew out of VAMP, has recommended not using data from practices that have not met quality assurance criteria allowing them to receive the "up to standard" desig-nation (see "Data collection and structure"). Additionally, the BCDSP, in its licensed copy of the GPRD, has dropped almost half of all original VAMP practices due to lapses in data entry, unwillingness to provide clinical records, a change in computer systems of the practices, or based on requests of the practices that their data be removed.[4]

The GPRD has been used internationally by researchers from academia, regulatory authorities, and industry. A recent review of protocols using GPRD data showed that the database is used for pharmacoepidemiology (56%), disease epidemiology (30%), drug utilization (10%), pharma-coeconomics (4%), and environmental hazards (1%).[2] There have been over 250 publications in peer-reviewed journals using GPRD. Existing data sets from the GPRD have been studied extensively by EPIC, BCDSP, members of the pharmaceutical industry, and several independent academic centers. Details on use and applications of the GPRD can be found in the section on "Particular applications."

DATA COLLECTION AND STRUCTURE

In any given year, GPs who are members of the GPRD collect data on about 3 million patients, which translates into about 37 million person-years of follow-up between 1987 and 2002.[1–3,5] Continuous information has been collected for 6 years or more in most of the practices.[3] About 5% of the UK population is included in the GPRD, which is broadly representative of the general UK population in terms of age, sex, and geographic distributions. The database covers approximately 6.4% of the population in England, 5.1% in Wales, 2.8% in Scotland, and 5.8% in Northern Ireland.[5] There is a slight underrepresentation of smaller practices and of practices in northern England. Since 1994 data have been collected by approximately 1500 general practitioners who work in 500 practices across the UK.[1]

GPs use their software primarily to create electronic medical records and for the purpose of managing their patients. Since it is the patient's medical record, the GPRD offers a significant advantage over administrative databases. GPs were initially trained in data entry by VAMP and their data were reviewed to ensure that they were of sufficient quality for research studies. For example, practices were required to record a minimum 95% of prescribing and relevant patient encounters. Also, practitioners were required to record medical events for each acute prescription issued, and all events leading to hospitalization or referral. VAMP initially identified practices meeting these quality criteria and coded them as "up to standard." The first "up to standard date" was assigned to a practice in 1987, but most practices did not become up to standard until 1990–91. Data quality assurance was performed by VAMP until 1994 when the database was donated to the UK Department of Health. The UK ONS was responsible for quality assurance from 1995 to 1999, followed by the Medicines Control Agency. GPs receive nominal financial inducements for their participation in this program, and many participate because they believe they are providing a valuable research service and because the computerized system improves their practice.[2,5]

GPs use the computer software to enter data into different files (see Table 22.1). Data collected electronically by general practitioners include demographics (age and sex); medical diagnoses that are part of routine care or resulting from hospitalizations, consultations, or emergency care, along with the date and location (e.g., GP's office, hospital, consultant) of the event and an option for adding free text; referrals to hospitals and

Table 22.1. Data collected by general practitioners using Vision software, organized by file name

File name	Description
Patient	Patient details, demographic, and registration information
Clinical	Clinical data, contains medical coded information related to office visits, including blood pressure measurements
Consultation	Details of consultations, links items related to specific visits
Test	Test results, for some practices downloaded electronically from pathology laboratory
Immunization	Immunization details
Referral	Information on referral for specialist consultation
Therapy	Issued acute and repeat prescriptions and all associated details

specialists; all prescriptions, including date of prescription, formulation, strength, quantity, and dosing instructions, indication for treatment for all new prescriptions (cross-referenced to medical events on the same date), and events leading to withdrawal of a drug or treatment; vaccinations and prescription contraceptives; and miscellaneous information such as smoking, height, weight, immunizations, pregnancy, birth, death, date entering the practice, date leaving the practice, and laboratory results.

Diagnoses were recorded using Oxford Medical Information System (OXMIS) codes until newer versions of the GP system were made available in 1995 when the Read coding system was introduced. OXMIS codes are similar to ICD-9 codes; however OXMIS codes allow for more detailed diagnostic coding. Currently all GPRD data are coded in Read codes, which are alphanumeric codes that group and define illnesses using a hierarchical nosologic system. The Read codes are a very comprehensive coded clinical language developed in the UK and funded by the NHS. The codes include terms relating to observations (signs and symptoms), diagnoses, procedures, and laboratory and radiologic tests.

Prescriptions were originally entered using Prescription Pricing Authority (PPA) codes and are currently entered using Multilex codes issued by First Databank. Drug codes provide detailed information on the drug, dose, and route of administration. Patients in the GPRD are also issued a number that identifies people residing at the same address or not at the same address but who are family members. This data field, in combination with the date of birth of children and the delivery code in the mother's record, can be linked to identify mothers and their children.[6]

ACCURACY AND COMPLETENESS OF THE GPRD

Extensive studies have been performed to evaluate the accuracy of the GPRD. The validity of specialists' information and its capture by GPs in the GPRD have been well documented with studies demonstrating that 87% of diagnoses from specialist letters were documented electronically.[7] There is also good agreement between GPRD prescribing data and national data from the PPA.[8] Due to the UK's requirement for printed prescriptions and because the GP computer system provides this service for the GP, pharmacy information is very well documented in the GPRD.

The validity of using the GPRD to study a wide range of medical conditions, including atrial fibrillation,[9] cancer,[10] cataract,[11] chronic obstructive pulmonary disease,[12] inflammatory bowel disease,[13] lymphoma,[14] myocardial infarction,[15] Paget's disease,[16] pregnancy outcomes,[17] pressure ulcers,[18] psychosis,[19] suicide,[20] and venous thromboembolism,[21] has been demonstrated by comparing the computer record to direct queries of the general practitioners.[3,5,13,14] The rates of breast cancer, influenza, intussusception in children, autism, colorectal cancer, cataracts, and psoriasis have been similar to external measures of disease frequency in the UK.[4,22]

The database may not contain data on every patient characteristic or disease characteristic that may be required for a study. For example, information on occupation, employment, and socioeconomic status is not available electronically. Furthermore, as per GPRD data recording instructions, general practitioners do not routinely collect information on all encounters. Only consultations for significant events, both current and from the past, and those which require a new diagnosis or a change in therapy are routinely recorded and therefore collected. As a result, visits for acute conditions are more likely to be represented, while the frequency of visits for chronic conditions such as asthma and diabetes may be underreported, although the presence of such conditions will be well recorded in the database.[8] For example, studies have shown good agreement between GPRD rates of acute conditions such as chicken pox and hayfever, and rates of these conditions observed in the 4th National Morbidity Survey in General Practice. However, in chronic conditions, such as asthma and diabetes, GPRD consultation rates are 10–20% lower than those observed in the National Morbidity Survey.[8] However, as noted above, the presence of a chronic disease is well reported. For example, patient treatment of asthma (e.g., prescription records) has shown good agreement with external surveys,[8] suggesting that GPRD can be used to track chronic diseases by utilizing algorithms that include diagnostic codes and treatment records. Finally, it should be noted that many of the validation studies performed have been in subsets of the full GPRD from the BCDSP or EPIC. Therefore, studies using the full GPRD or versions different from those studied by EPIC or BCDSP may not have the same degree of completeness or accuracy.[4]

STRENGTHS

POPULATION-BASED DATA

As a data source GPRD provides researchers the opportunity to design studies using population-based methods, which minimizes selection bias and improves the validity of epidemiologic studies. Population-based studies are defined as those in which the cases (e.g., individuals with disease) are a representative sample of all cases in a precisely defined population and the controls are directly sampled randomly from this population.[23] The GPRD represents a defined population, which allows investigators to study all patients with a given disease and gives them the ability to study control patients from the same source population from which those with the disease of interest are derived. Therefore, even in conducting case–control studies, the GPRD offers a significant advantage for epidemiologic studies over traditional hospital-based designs. Furthermore, the GPRD is broadly representative of the UK population in general, suggesting that findings from the GPRD should generalize to the broader UK population.

The well-defined population of the GPRD also allows investigators to study families and to link health events in mothers to outcomes in their children. Finally, all individuals in the GPRD are assigned a practice number as well, allowing researchers to measure individual practice effects on health outcomes.

SIZE OF THE DATABASE

On average in any particular year between 1991 and 1996 there are about 3.4 million active patients represented in the GPRD. The cumulative experience of the GPRD yields about 9.8 million patients followed for over 37 million person-years. As a result, the GPRD can be used by researchers to study rare outcomes using cohort designs for medical conditions with incidence rates of less than $1/10\,000$ with sufficient statistical power. The number of practices, and therefore GPs, participating in the GPRD has been decreasing for the past 5 years. As a result, the total number of active patients represented in a year in the GPRD from 1997 onward has decreased to an average of 2.2 million.

VALIDITY OF INFORMATION

As described above ("Accuracy and completeness of the GPRD"), the validity of the GPRD has been extensively studied. Studies have demonstrated good agreement between the electronic medical record and capture of information from specialists.[7] A variety of individual diagnoses have been validated by direct query of the general practitioners, and the accuracy of information on prescription medications has also been demonstrated.[8] Additionally, the quality of data submitted by GPs is also under ongoing internal scrutiny by administrators of the GPRD. As a result, the GPRD is one of the best-studied sources of health data available for epidemiologic investigations.

ACCESS TO ORIGINAL MEDICAL RECORDS

At least one vendor of the GPRD and the MHRA has the capacity to allow investigators the opportunity, through an intermediate, to obtain anonymized copies of the patient's (non-electronic) medical record and a more detailed review of the patient's health history. This capacity allows researchers to verify information captured on death certificates and letters from specialists. Studies in which medical records have been requested have resulted in response rates of over 80% and in many cases over 90%, with the majority of requests being met within 3 months.[1]

This service also allows investigators to send questionnaires to the general practitioners about individual patients. In some instances, researchers can have questionnaires completed by individual patients by working through the general practitioner. All data from questionnaires or paper-based medical records are stripped of personally identifying information prior to being sent to the researcher.

WEAKNESSES

COMPLETENESS OF DATA

The GPRD is in most cases used by the GP as the patient's medical record, and therefore information generated by the GP is expected to be complete. However, information from specialists as well as events that occur in the hospital may not be fully captured in the electronic medical record. Communication from specialists, discharge summaries from hospitals, and test results from pathology laboratories are often received in hard copy and must be manually entered into the computer. Since this can be a time-consuming process, some practices will only enter information that will affect the care of the patient in the future. Therefore, with

test results it is likely that only the abnormal results are entered onto the computer for collection and inclusion in the GPRD. Agreement between the GPRD and data from specialists and hospitalizations has generally been quite good (about 90%).[1] However, this indicates that about 10% of the time, data from hospitalizations or specialists may be missing. In particular, minor medical events are more likely to be missed than medically significant diagnoses or events. Information on treatments that are restricted by the NHS to specialist care (e.g., psoralen plus ultraviolet A therapy, cytotoxic/chemotherapy) may be particularly problematic. Data on non-prescription medications and treatments given in the hospital are not readily available. Data on nonsignificant medical events and exposures to medications that occurred prior to enrollment in the GPRD and are no longer active clinical issues may also not be documented in the electronic medical record. Furthermore, data on important confounding variables such as smoking, alcohol use, and body weight and height are only available for about 70% of patients.[1] One study demonstrated that the positive predictive value for having ever smoked was 86%, current smoking was 70%, and former smoking 60%.[24] The prevalence of former smoking as recorded in the GPRD is lower than would be expected based on external survey data.[25] Use of the GPRD for more detailed diagnostic studies may be problematic. For example, investigators have determined that a diagnostic coding algorithm cannot reliably identify patients with pneumococcal pneumonia based on query of the GP, although investigators can reliably determine that a patient had pneumonia.[26]

COMPLEXITY AND COSTS OF COMPUTER HARDWARE/SOFTWARE NEEDED TO WORK WITH GPRD

The size and complexity of the GPRD database requires that individuals or institutions working with it have adequate computer software and hardware, as well as experienced data managers. Technical requirements for working with the GPRD will vary according to the vendor. The UK MHRA offers GPRD through a web-enabled link, which requires knowledge of the particular application into which the data are loaded and stable telecommunications links. EPIC supplies GPRD as a set of flat text files which can be imported into any application but requires hardware and data storage facilities. Actual use of the GPRD may vary from user to user with respect to the size of the database, the fields of the database available for review, and whether data are available as individual records or tables. For example, our academic institution recently received a full GPRD data set from EPIC. This version of the GPRD contains all information in the GPRD from 1988 to 2002. The full size of the GPRD was approximately 54 gigabytes. It is currently residing on a Sun Microsystems Enterprise™ server running the Solaris operating system in a Unix environment. The unit requires 170 gigabytes of disk storage. The database is implemented using Oracle's® relational database. The database tools include Oracle's Internet developer's suite of tools, such that clients within our server environment can access the GPRD in real time using Oracle Discover®, as well as by using an SAS©-based interface. With these tools it has been possible for clients, using Ethernet-connected PCs, to download data and convert the data into several different database programs, including Microsoft Access© and Visual Dbase© and statistical packages such as Stata®, SAS©, and SPSS®.

PARTICULAR APPLICATIONS

Access to the latest version of GPRD (as of January 2004), can be purchased through the MHRA (available at www.gprd.com). Additionally, a static version of GPRD updated through March 2002 is available from EPIC (www.epic-uk.org). All studies using GPRD data must be approved by the Scientific and Ethical Advisory Board (SEAG). SEAG's primary role is to ensure that scientific and ethical standards for use of the GPRD are maintained.

The GPRD has been used for a variety of studies that examine pharmacoepidemiology, disease epidemiology, and pharmacoeconomics. The GPRD is particularly useful for cohort and case–control study designs. As with any study utilizing a pre-existing database, the investigators must fully understand how well the database captures information on the diseases and exposures the investigator wishes to examine. In some circumstances, the investigators may need to perform additional validation studies when using the GPRD to ensure the accuracy of their findings. A common limitation of using existing databases for pharmacoepidemiology studies is that the presence of a prescription does not guarantee that the patient actually took the medication. Furthermore, for some studies the GPRD may not be an appropriate data source. For example, the GPRD would not have information on medication exposures that occurred prior to the patient enrolling in the GPRD. Additionally, the GPRD on average has about 6 years of observation time. Therefore, outcomes with long latency periods may not be appropriate for studies using the GPRD.

Investigators have frequently used case–control, cohort, and nested case–control designs to address scientific hypotheses in the GPRD. Nested case–control studies have taken advantage of the ability to contact the GP for additional health information or supportive documentation through a third party vendor. Since the GPRD collects data longitudinally, investigators are able to perform incidence studies and can model outcomes using time to event analyses. A comprehensive listing of published papers using GPRD data is available at www.gprd.com. Here, we briefly review some of the major health outcomes that have been studied using the GPRD.

The GPRD has been a very useful tool to study patients with diabetes. Investigators have studied outcomes associated with diabetes, such as erectile dysfunction,[27] stillbirth,[28] and rates of acute liver injury.[29] Pharmacoepidemiology studies have examined the risk of incident diabetes associated with antipsychotic medications,[30] and have examined rates of hypoglycemia associated with different forms of insulin[31] and sulfonylureas.[32] Gastrointestinal disorders have also been studied using GPRD data. Investigators have examined the risk of lymphoma associated with inflammatory bowel disease,[14] the association of obesity and liver disease,[33] and the natural history of irritable bowel syndrome.[34] Cardiovascular studies have examined the incidence of newly diagnosed heart failure in general practice,[35] the effect of aspirin and non-aspirin anti-inflammatory drugs in the primary prevention of myocardial infarction in postmenopausal women,[36] and the risk of first myocardial infarction in users of antibiotics[37] and patients with acute respiratory tract infections.[38] Neurological diseases such as multiple sclerosis,[39] Parkinson's disease,[40] and seizure disorders[41] have been studied in the GPRD, as have psychiatric outcomes such as depression,[42] schizophrenia,[43] and suicide.[44,45] Dermatologic disorders studied include acne,[46] psoriasis,[22] eczema,[47] pressure ulcers,[48] venous leg ulcers,[18] and serious skin reactions to medications.[49] The GPRD has been also used to study cancer of the ovary,[50] breast,[51] colon, kidney, bladder, esophagus, pancreas, lung, prostate, and lymph glands.[14,52,53]

The GPRD has been used as an abundant source of scientific data for pharmacoepidemiologic investigations. For example, vaccine studies have explored the relationship between oral polio vaccine and intussusception,[55] measles, mumps, and rubella (MMR) vaccine and idiopathic thrombocytopenic purpura,[55] MMR and autism,[56] and the safety of influenza vaccination in patients with asthma or chronic obstructive pulmonary disease.[57] Patterns of hormone replacement therapy (HRT) use have been examined.[58] The relationship of HRT and a variety of outcomes, including acute myocardial infarction,[59] venous thromboembolism,[60] chronic wounds such as pressure ulcers and venous leg ulcers,[18] Alzheimer's disease,[61] irritable bowel syndrome,[62] and systemic or discoid lupus,[63] has been studied in the GPRD. The GPRD has also been used to study a variety of outcomes associated with nonsteroidal anti-inflammatory drugs (NSAIDs). Investigators have examined the relationship of these commonly prescribed medications and myocardial infarction,[64] thromboembolic events in rheumatoid arthritis patients,[65] chemoprevention of cancer,[66] upper gastrointestinal bleeding,[67] and heart failure.[68] Additional examples of pharmacoepidemiologic studies include investigations of the incidence of serious skin reactions and acute liver toxicity associated with oral anti-fungal medication,[49,69] the relationship between the treatment of acne vulgaris and depression[70] and acute liver disease,[71] the effect of inhaled corticosteroids on a variety of outcomes such as survival in patients with chronic obstructive pulmonary disease,[72] the risk of cataract development[73] and hip fracture,[74] and adverse events associated with anticonvulsant medications such as congenital abnormalities,[17] sudden death[75,76] and fertility.[75]

THE FUTURE

Recent changes within the UK NHS, such as a move towards "fee for service" payments for items such as general health screens for newly registered patients, have led to a greater emphasis on the quality of data recorded in GP computer systems. Information extracted from these systems will be used by GP practices to secure additional payments related to the standard of clinical care they provide. These initiatives present GPs with an incentive to ensure that the data entered into their systems is accurate and complete. Consequently, data extracted from UK GP systems in the future are likely to be of a much higher quality than they have been in the past and will, therefore, continue to be an important resource for epidemiologic investigations.

GPRD data have always been collected from VAMP systems and are, at present, collected from the latest version, called Vision. Although the Vision system is used by more than 1500 GP practices in the UK, only about 370 of these currently supply data for inclusion into GPRD. The MHRA has ongoing efforts to recruit more practices into the GPRD. The major obstacle to recruitment is that they are limited only to the practices that use the Vision software.

Since the complexity of the GP system has increased, doctors can use it for a wider range of purposes. While this results in the collected data being more complex, it also means that the data are more comprehensive. The system incorporates a number of structured data areas so that the system prompts the doctor to enter a whole series of items related to a specific problem. Also, the system now enables referral letters to be written directly from the consultation record, which automatically records the referral. Referral information is extracted as a separate file now as opposed to a manually entered flag in the medical record in the older versions of the GP system. In order to overcome the difficulties associated with the more complicated data structures of the Vision system, the managers of GPRD have loaded the data into an object-oriented database known as Full Feature GPRD (FFGPRD). In addition to the historically available variables described above ("Data collection and structure"), FFGPRD includes the functionality to perform queries within the system.

Currently, an updated version of GPRD is available via the Internet (www.gprd.com) from a single vendor, the MHRA. Although it is possible to extract data for individual subjects, this can only be done for a limited number of records and is time intensive. The access system is designed to run queries online, which avoids investment in hardware at the user's site but relies heavily on the stability of the technology in use.

Some researchers prefer the flexibility of working with raw data as opposed to conducting studies within an integrated system where the data sit behind a set of prewritten queries that run in the background and generate prespecified reports through which the data can be viewed. The GPRD data set is available in raw format from EPIC but is not updated beyond March 2002. An alternative to GPRD that includes updated data, uses the same data structure as GPRD, and permits working with raw data is offered by a newly created database, The Health Improvement Network (THIN).

REFERENCES

1. García Rodríguez LA, Pérez-Gutthann S, Jick S. The UK General Practice Research Database. In: Strom BL, ed., *Pharmacoepidemiology*, 3rd edn. Chichester: John Wiley & Sons, 2000; pp. 375–85.
2. Wood L, Coulson R. Revitalizing the General Practice Research Database: plans, challenges, and opportunities. *Pharmacoepidemiol Drug Saf* 2001; **10**: 379–83.
3. Lawson DH, Sherman V, Hollowell J. The General Practice Research Database. Scientific and Ethical Advisory Group. *Q J Med* 1998; **91**: 445–52.
4. Jick SS, Kaye JA, Vasilakis-Scaramozza C, Garcia Rodriguez LA, Ruigomez A, Meier CR, Schlienger RG, Black C, Jick H. Validity of the general practice research database. *Pharmacotherapy* 2003; **23**: 686–9.
5. Walley T, Mantgani A. The UK General Practice Research Database. *Lancet* 1997; **350**: 1097–9.

6. McKeever TM, Lewis SA, Smith C, Collins J, Heatlie H, Frischer M, Hubbard R. Siblings, multiple births, and the incidence of allergic disease: a birth cohort study using the West Midlands general practice research database. *Thorax* 2001; **56**: 758–62.

7. Jick H, Jick SS, Derby LE. Validation of information recorded on general practitioner based computerised data resource in the United Kingdom. *BMJ* 1991; **302**: 766–8.

8. Hollowell J. The General Practice Research Database: quality of morbidity data. *Popul Trends* 1997; **87**: 36–40.

9. Ruigomez A, Johansson S, Wallander MA, Rodriguez LA. Incidence of chronic atrial fibrillation in general practice and its treatment pattern. *J Clin Epidemiol* 2002; **55**: 358–63.

10. Jick H, Jick S, Derby LE, Vasilakis C, Myers MW, Meier CR. Calcium-channel blockers and risk of cancer. *Lancet* 1997; **349**: 525–8.

11. Derby L, Maier WC. Risk of cataract among users of intranasal corticosteroids. *J Allergy Clin Immunol* 2000; **105**: 912–16.

12. Soriano JB, Maier WC, Visick G, Pride NB. Validation of general practitioner-diagnosed COPD in the UK General Practice Research Database. *Eur J Epidemiol* 2001; **17**: 1075–80.

13. Lewis JD, Brensinger C, Bilker WB, Strom BL. Validity and completeness of the General Practice Research Database for studies of inflammatory bowel disease. *Pharmacoepidemiol Drug Saf* 2002; **11**: 211–18.

14. Lewis JD, Bilker WB, Brensinger C, Deren JJ, Vaughn DJ, Strom BL. Inflammatory bowel disease is not associated with an increased risk of lymphoma. *Gastroenterology* 2001; **121**: 1080–7.

15. Jick H, Derby LE, Gurewich V, Vasilakis C. The risk of myocardial infarction associated with antihypertensive drug treatment in persons with uncomplicated essential hypertension. *Pharmacotherapy* 1996; **16**: 321–6.

16. van Staa TP, Selby P, Leufkens HG, Lyles K, Sprafka JM, Cooper C. Incidence and natural history of Paget's disease of bone in England and Wales. *J Bone Miner Res* 2002; **17**: 465–71.

17. Jick SS, Terris BZ. Anticonvulsants and congenital malformations. *Pharmacotherapy* 1997; **17**: 561–4.

18. Margolis DJ, Knauss J, Bilker W. Hormone replacement therapy and prevention of pressure ulcers and venous leg ulcers. *Lancet* 2002; **359**: 675–7.

19. Nazareth I, King M, Haines A, Rangel L, Myers S. Accuracy of diagnosis of psychosis on general practice computer system. *BMJ* 1993; **307**: 32–4.

20. Jick SS, Dean AD, Jick H. Antidepressants and suicide. *BMJ* 1995; **310**: 215–18.

21. Lawrenson R, Todd JC, Leydon GM, Williams TJ, Farmer RD. Validation of the diagnosis of venous thromboembolism in general practice database studies. *Br J Clin Pharmacol* 2000; **49**: 591–6.

22. Gelfand JM, Berlin J, Van Voorhees A, Margolis DJ. Lymphoma rates are low but increased in patients with psoriasis: results from a population-based cohort study in the United Kingdom. *Arch Dermatol* 2003; **139**: 1425–9.

23. Rothman K, Greenland, S. *Modern Epidemiology*. Philadelphia, PA: Lippincott-Raven, 1988; pp. 93–115.

24. Lewis JD, Brensiger, C. Agreement between GPRD smoking data and a survey of general practitioners. *Pharmacoepidemiol Drug Saf* 2003; **12**: S60.

25. Hubbard R, Venn A, Lewis S, Britton J. Lung cancer and cryptogenic fibrosing alveolitis. A population-based cohort study. *Am J Respir Crit Care Med* 2000; **161**: 5–8.

26. Metlay JP, Kinman JL. Failure to validate pneumococcal pneumonia diagnoses in the General Practice Research Database. *Pharmacoepidemiol Drug Saf* 2003; **12**: S163.

27. Blumentals WA, Brown RR, Gomez-Caminero A. Antihypertensive treatment and erectile dysfunction in a cohort of type II diabetes patients. *Int J Impot Res* 2003; **15**: 314–17.

28. Wood SL, Jick H, Sauve R. The risk of stillbirth in pregnancies before and after the onset of diabetes. *Diabet Med* 2003; **20**: 703–7.

29. Huerta C, Zhao SZ, Garcia Rodriguez LA. Risk of acute liver injury in patients with diabetes. *Pharmacotherapy* 2002; **22**: 1091–6.

30. Kornegay CJ, Vasilakis-Scaramozza C, Jick H. Incident diabetes associated with antipsychotic use in the United Kingdom general practice research database. *J Clin Psychiatry* 2002; **63**: 758–62.

31. Jick H, Hall GC, Dean AD, Jick SS, Derby LE. A comparison of the risk of hypoglycemia between users of human and animal insulins. 1. Experience in the United Kingdom. *Pharmacotherapy* 1990; **10**: 395–7.

32. van Staa T, Abenhaim L, Monette J. Rates of hypoglycemia in users of sulfonylureas. *J Clin Epidemiol* 1997; **50**: 735–41.

33. Meier CR, Krahenbuhl S, Schlienger RG, Jick H. Association between body mass index and liver disorders: an epidemiological study. *J Hepatol* 2002; **37**: 741–7.

34. Ruigomez A, Wallander MA, Johansson S, Garcia Rodriguez LA. One-year follow-up of newly diagnosed irritable bowel syndrome patients. *Aliment Pharmacol Ther* 1999; **13**: 1097–102.

35. Johansson S, Wallander MA, Ruigomez A, Garcia Rodriguez LA. Incidence of newly diagnosed heart failure in UK general practice. *Eur J Heart Fail* 2001; **3**: 225–31.

36. Garcia Rodriguez LA, Varas C, Patrono C. Differential effects of aspirin and non-aspirin nonsteroidal antiinflammatory drugs in the primary prevention of myocardial infarction in postmenopausal women. *Epidemiology* 2000; **11**: 382–7.

37. Meier CR, Derby LE, Jick SS, Vasilakis C, Jick H. Antibiotics and risk of subsequent first-time acute myocardial infarction. *JAMA* 1999; **281**: 427–31.

38. Meier CR, Jick SS, Derby LE, Vasilakis C, Jick H. Acute respiratory-tract infections and risk of first-time acute myocardial infarction. *Lancet* 1998; **351**: 1467–71.

39. Marrie RA, Wolfson C, Sturkenboom MC, Gout O, Heinzlef O, Roullet E, Abenhaim L. Multiple sclerosis and antecedent infections: a case–control study. *Neurology* 2000; **54**: 2307–10.

40. Thorogood M, Armstrong B, Nichols T, Hollowell J. Mortality in people taking selegiline: observational study. *BMJ* 1998; **317**: 252–4.

41. Jick H, Derby LE, Vasilakis C, Fife D. The risk of seizures associated with tramadol. *Pharmacotherapy* 1998; **18**: 607–11.

42. Moser K. Inequalities in treated heart disease and mental illness in England and Wales, 1994–1998. *Br J Gen Pract* 2001; **51**: 438–44.

43. Kaye JA, Bradbury BD, Jick H. Changes in antipsychotic drug prescribing by general practitioners in the United Kingdom from 1991 to 2000: a population-based observational study. *Br J Clin Pharmacol* 2003; **56**: 569–75.

44. Haste F, Charlton J, Jenkins R. Potential for suicide prevention in primary care? An analysis of factors associated with suicide. *Br J Gen Pract* 1998; **48**: 1759–63.

45. Yang CC, Jick SS, Jick H. Lipid-lowering drugs and the risk of depression and suicidal behavior. *Arch Intern Med* 2003; **163**: 1926–32.

46. Seaman HE, de Vries CS, Farmer RD. Differences in the use of combined oral contraceptives amongst women with and without acne. *Hum Reprod* 2003; **18**: 515–21.

47. McKeever TM, Lewis SA, Smith C, Collins J, Heatlie H, Frischer M, Hubbard R. Siblings, multiple births, and the incidence of allergic disease: a birth cohort study using the West Midlands general practice research database. *Thorax* 2001; **56**: 758–762.

48. Margolis DJ, Bilker W, Knauss J, Baumgarten M, Strom BL. The incidence and prevalence of pressure ulcers among elderly patients in general medical practice. *Ann Epidemiol* 2002; **12**: 321–5.

49. Castellsague J, Garcia-Rodriguez LA, Duque A, Perez S. Risk of serious skin disorders among users of oral antifungals: a population-based study. *BMC Dermatol* 2002; **2**: 14.

50. Meier CR, Schmitz S, Jick H. Association between acetaminophen or nonsteroidal antiinflammatory drugs and risk of developing ovarian, breast, or colon cancer. *Pharmacotherapy* 2002; **22**: 303–9.

51. Kaye JA, Derby LE, del Mar Melero-Montes M, Quinn M, Jick H. The incidence of breast cancer in the General Practice Research Database compared with national cancer registration data. *Br J Cancer* 2000; **83**: 1556–8.

52. Garcia-Rodriguez LA, Huerta-Alvarez C. Reduced risk of colorectal cancer among long-term users of aspirin and nonaspirin nonsteroidal antiinflammatory drugs. *Epidemiology* 2001; **12**: 88–93.

53. Kaye JA, Myers MW, Jick H. Acetaminophen and the risk of renal and bladder cancer in the general practice research database. *Epidemiology* 2001; **12**: 690–4.

54. Andrews N, Miller E, Waight P, Farrington P, Crowcroft N, Stowe J, Taylor B. Does oral polio vaccine cause intussusception in infants? Evidence from a sequence of three self-controlled case series studies in the United Kingdom. *Eur J Epidemiol* 2001; **17**: 701–6.

55. Black C, Kaye JA, Jick H. MMR vaccine and idiopathic thrombocytopaenic purpura. *Br J Clin Pharmacol* 2003; **55**: 107–11.

56. Kaye JA, del Mar Melero-Montes M, Jick H. Mumps, measles, and rubella vaccine and the incidence of autism recorded by general practitioners: a time trend analysis. *BMJ* 2001; **322**: 460–3.

57. Tata LJ, West J, Harrison T, Farrington P, Smith C, Hubbard R. Does influenza vaccination increase consultations, corticosteroid prescriptions, or exacerbations in subjects with asthma or chronic obstructive pulmonary disease? *Thorax* 2003; **58**: 835–9.

58. Lawrence M, Jones L, Lancaster T, Daly E, Banks E. Hormone replacement therapy: patterns of use studied through British general practice computerized records. *Fam Pract* 1999; **16**: 335–42.

59. Varas-Lorenzo C, Garcia-Rodriguez LA, Perez-Gutthann S, Duque-Oliart A. Hormone replacement therapy and incidence of acute myocardial infarction. A population-based nested case–control study. *Circulation* 2000; **101**: 2572–8.

60. Perez Gutthann S, Garcia Rodriguez LA, Castellsague J, Duque Oliart A. Hormone replacement therapy and risk of venous thromboembolism: population based case–control study. *BMJ* 1997; **314**: 796–800.

61. Seshadri S, Zornberg GL, Derby LE, Myers MW, Jick H, Drachman DA. Postmenopausal estrogen replacement therapy and the risk of Alzheimer disease. *Arch Neurol* 2001; **58**: 435–40.

62. Ruigomez A, Garcia Rodriguez LA, Johansson S, Wallander MA. Is hormone replacement therapy associated with an increased risk of irritable bowel syndrome? *Maturitas* 2003; **44**: 133–40.

63. Meier CR, Sturkenboom MC, Cohen AS, Jick H. Postmenopausal estrogen replacement therapy and the risk of developing systemic lupus erythematosus or discoid lupus. *J Rheumatol* 1998; **25**: 1515–19.

64. Schlienger RG, Jick H, Meier CR. Use of nonsteroidal antiinflammatory drugs and the risk of first-time acute myocardial infarction. *Br J Clin Pharmacol* 2002; **54**: 327–32.

65. Watson DJ, Rhodes T, Cai B, Guess HA. Lower risk of thromboembolic cardiovascular events with naproxen among patients with rheumatoid arthritis. *Arch Intern Med* 2002; **162**: 1105–10.

66. Langman MJ, Cheng KK, Gilman EA, Lancashire RJ. Effect of anti-inflammatory drugs on overall risk of common cancer: case–control study in general practice research database. *BMJ* 2000; **320**: 1642–6.

67. Hernandez-Diaz S, Garcia-Rodriguez LA. Epidemiologic assessment of the safety of conventional nonsteroidal anti-inflammatory drugs. *Am J Med* 2001; **110** (suppl 3A): 20S–27S.

68. Garcia Rodriguez LA, Hernandez-Diaz S. Nonsteroidal antiinflammatory drugs as a trigger of clinical heart failure. *Epidemiology* 2003; **14**: 240–6.

69. Garcia Rodriguez LA, Duque A, Castellsague J, Perez-Gutthann S, Stricker BH. A cohort study on the risk of acute liver injury among users of ketoconazole and other antifungal drugs. *Br J Clin Pharmacol* 1999; **48**: 847–52.

70. Jick SS, Kremers HM, Vasilakis-Scaramozza C. Isotretinoin use and risk of depression, psychotic symptoms, suicide, and attempted suicide. *Arch Dermatol* 2000; **136**: 1231–6.

71. Seaman HE, Lawrenson RA, Williams TJ, MacRae KD, Farmer RD. The risk of liver damage associated with minocycline: a comparative study. *J Clin Pharmacol* 2001; **41**: 852–60.

72. Soriano JB, Vestbo J, Pride NB, Kiri V, Maden C, Maier WC. Survival in COPD patients after regular use of fluticasone propionate and salmeterol in general practice. *Eur Respir J* 2002; **20**: 819–25.

73. Smeeth L, Boulis M, Hubbard R, Fletcher AE. A population based case–control study of cataract and inhaled corticosteroids. *Br J Ophthalmol* 2003; **87**: 1247–51.

74. Hubbard RB, Smith CJ, Smeeth L, Harrison TW, Tattersfield AE. Inhaled corticosteroids and hip fracture: a population-based case–control study. *Am J Respir Crit Care Med* 2002; **166**: 1563–6.

75. Wallace H, Shorvon S, Tallis R. Age-specific incidence and prevalence rates of treated epilepsy in an unselected population of 2,052,922 and age-specific fertility rates of women with epilepsy. *Lancet* 1998; **352**: 1970–3.

76. Derby LE, Tennis P, Jick H. Sudden unexplained death among subjects with refractory epilepsy. *Epilepsia* 1996; **37**: 931–5.

Part IIIc

Other Approaches to Pharmacoepidemiology Studies

23

Other Approaches to Pharmacoepidemiology Studies

BRIAN L. STROM

University of Pennsylvania School of Medicine, Philadelphia, Pennsylvania, USA.

INTRODUCTION

As described in Chapter 3, although pharmacoepidemiology studies use the traditional study designs of epidemiology, they pose a special problem. Inasmuch as most drugs are studied in between 500 and 3000 individuals prior to marketing, postmarketing surveillance cohort studies will not be able to detect rarer drug effects reliably unless they include at least 10 000 exposed individuals. Postmarketing surveillance case–control studies need to accumulate diseased cases and undiseased controls from a target population of sufficient size to have included 10 000 exposed patients if a cohort study had been performed. The need to study populations this large without incurring undue costs represents an unusual logistical challenge.

Some of the major approaches useful for addressing this challenge have been presented in Chapters 9 through 22. There are a number of other approaches as well. Several of these are derived from one or more of the approaches presented earlier, but some represent important potential resources that the reader should be aware of. Thus, the purpose of this chapter is to describe them. The approaches will be presented according to the study designs they usually utilize, in order of the hierarchy of study designs presented in Chapter 2. Approaches will be presented that involve performing analyses of secular trends, case–control studies, cohort studies, and randomized clinical trials. None of these approaches involves analyzing case reports. Case series will be discussed under case–control and cohort studies, since exposed (or diseased) patients in case series should generally be compared to unexposed (or undiseased) controls.

DATA SOURCES FOR ANALYSES OF SECULAR TRENDS

As described in Chapter 2, analyses of secular trends examine trends in an exposure and trends in a disease and explore whether the trends coincide. These trends can be examined over time or over geographic area. In other words, one could analyze data from a single country or region and examine how the exposure and the disease have changed over time. Alternatively, one could analyze data from a single time period, exploring how the prevalence of the exposure

Pharmacoepidemiology, Fourth Edition   Edited by B.L. Strom
© 2005 John Wiley & Sons, Ltd

and the incidence of the disease differ from region to region or country to country.

The advantages and disadvantages of this study design are presented in Chapter 2. Analyses of secular trends in pharmacoepidemiology are *ad hoc* studies, i.e., there are no ongoing systems for performing such studies. In order to perform such studies, however, one obviously needs data on both the frequency of the exposure and the incidence of the disease. Thus, this discussion will focus on the data sources available for performing such studies in pharmacoepidemiology.

DRUG UTILIZATION DATA

In pharmacoepidemiology studies, the primary exposure of interest is drug use. Thus, in order to perform analyses of secular trends, one needs to have one or more sources of data on drug utilization. In the US, and in many other countries, the major sources of data on drug utilization are several private companies that specialize in collecting these data and then selling them to pharmaceutical manufacturers for use in marketing studies.

Probably the best-known source of such data is IMS HEALTH, a leading data resource on the sales of pharmaceuticals worldwide. IMS conducts a number of different ongoing surveys of drug use, which it then sells to pharmaceutical manufacturers and to government agencies, as well as other categories of clients. Perhaps the most useful of these for pharmacoepidemiologic research is the National Disease and Therapeutic Index™ (NDTI™), an ongoing medical audit that provides insight into disease and treatment patterns of office-based physicians. A rotating panel of over 3500 of the approximately 400 000 office-based US physicians reports four times each year on all contacts with patients during a 48-hour period. Data are collected on the drug prescribed and its quantity, the diagnosis the drug was prescribed for, the action desired, concomitant drugs, concomitant diagnoses, and whether the prescription in question was the first time the patient received the drug or whether it was for continuing therapy. Demographic data about the patient and the prescriber are also collected. Periodic reports are prepared, including reports organized by drug and by diagnosis. In addition, special analyses can be performed using the data.

Although the physician panel is relatively small compared to the overall total of office-based physicians in the US, NDTI™ data are projected to the national level using statistical methodology. The sample of physicians used for the NDTI™ is a thin one, i.e., it contains relatively few individuals, relative to the number of individuals that are being generalized to and the number of variables that are being studied. Nevertheless, the results obtained using the NDTI™ tend to be relatively stable over time,[1] and agree fairly well with other sources of drug utilization information.[2] NDTI™ has proven itself very useful, and it has been used often for pharmacoepidemiologic research.

A few of the other IMS databases are: (i) the National Prescription Audit Plus™ (NPA Plus™), a study of pharmacy sales from retailers, mail order, and long-term care facilities, based on a panel of computerized pharmacies which submit data on dispensed prescriptions to IMS electronically, (ii) LifeLink™, a patient longitudinal database of medical and pharmacy claims, and (iii) IMS National Sales Perspective™—Retail and National Sales Perspective™—Non-Retail, two audits that provide national sales dollar estimates of pharmaceutical products purchased by retail drug stores, food stores, mass merchandise, closed wall health maintenance organizations (HMOs), non-Federal hospitals, Federal facilities, clinics and long-term care facilities. The IMS National Sales Perspective™, based on data from both audits, covers over 90% of drug sales. The existence of these and other IMS databases changes over time, as new products are developed and old products are discontinued. These and other IMS databases can sometimes be useful for pharmacoepidemiologic research, but the NDTI™ is generally the most useful. Generously, IMS is often willing to make its data available to academic investigators at little or no cost.

There are other commercial sources of drug utilization data in the US, although these have not been used as frequently for academic research. In addition, as part of its National Ambulatory Medical Care Survey, the US National Center for Health Statistics has been studying drug use, providing data very similar to that included in IMS America's NDTI. A summary of these results used to be published in an annual publication entitled *Highlights of Drug Utilization in Office Practice*,[3] and other studies have been published from them since.[4–8] Other special analyses can be requested as well. Other potential sources of drug utilization data include all of the databases described in Chapters 13 through 22.

A new source of drug utilization data is the Slone Survey.[9] This is based on an ongoing telephone random survey of the non-institutionalized population in the continental US. Its first report contained data on 3180 participants interviewed in 1998 and 1999. It is an excellent new source of information about the US use of prescription drugs, but also non-prescription drugs, vitamins/minerals, and herbals/supplements. Its limitations, of course, are nonparticipation, although the participation rate was an excellent 72%, and the uncertain and variable validity of the data obtained via a telephone interview with selective memory prompts (see Chapter 45).

Finally, in a number of countries other than the US, true national data are available on drug sales. For example, Sweden's Apoteksbolaget (now called Apotek AB), the National Corporation of Swedish Pharmacies, provides pharmacy services for the entire country.[10] It retains remarkable data on the drugs dispensed in Sweden, regionally or nationally. Through analyses of this type of data, Scandinavian investigators have become the world's leaders in studies of drug utilization (see Chapter 27).

It is important to note that, with the exception of data derived from the databases described earlier in the book, all of the drug utilization databases are useful for descriptive studies only, not for analytic studies. In some drug utilization data sets, information on subsequent diagnoses is unavailable. For example, in NDTI the patients who happen to be seen in any given 48-hour cycle are unlikely to be the same as those in the preceding or subsequent 48-hour cycles. In some drug utilization data sets information *is* available on diagnoses, but may be inappropriate. For example, the diagnosis data in NDTI includes the indication for treatment rather than the results of treatment. Finally, in some drug utilization data sets the information on drugs cannot be linked to disease outcome. For example, the excellent Swedish drug data cannot be linked to the excellent Swedish hospitalization data, as the former are retained in aggregate only; that is, without individual patient identification numbers. Thus, this type of data can only be used for descriptive studies or aggregate analyses, such as those performed for analyses of secular trends. More information on drug utilization studies is provided in Chapter 27.

DISEASE INCIDENCE DATA

Data Sources

The major source of disease incidence information useful for this type of study are the vital statistics maintained by most countries in the world. Most countries, for example, maintain mortality statistics, derived from the death certificates completed by physicians at the time of death. Importantly, these death certificates include information on causes of death. In the US, these death certificates are collected and maintained by the states. However, the National Center for Health Statistics then obtains magnetic tapes of a portion of these data from the states' vital statistics offices. These have been compiled into the National Death Index, which can be used for research purposes at a modest cost.[11] Data are available beginning in 1979. The index contains the following information for each of those who died: last name, first name, middle initial, social security number, date of birth,

state of birth, father's surname, sex, race, marital status, and state of residence. It also contains the name of the state, the death certificate number, and the date of death. To obtain cause of death information, an investigator must request a death certificate directly from the state. A similar data resource in Canada is the Canadian Mortality Database.[12]

US death data are also available from the Social Security Administration, as the "Social Security death tapes." These arise out of the government's need to know of deaths, in order to avoid paying social security benefits to individuals who have died.

Other types of vital statistics that are recorded by most countries include birth data, marriage data, divorce data, and so on. These are less likely to be useful for pharmacoepidemiologic research.

Morbidity data can be more problematic. There is no comprehensive source of morbidity data in most countries, comparable to mortality data. However, many specific types of data are available. A large number of countries maintain cancer registries, collecting all cases of cancer in one or more defined populations.[13–15] These can be used to calculate incidence rates of cancer. Other specialized registries can also exist. For example, in the US the Centers for Disease Control maintains a registry of children born with birth defects in the Atlanta metropolitan area[16] (see Chapter 32).

In addition, many developed countries maintain "population laboratories," defined and stable populations which have been observed over time, with multiple measurements made of both exposures and diseases. The classic population laboratory in the US has been Framingham, Massachusetts, which has been the source of an enormous amount of knowledge about risk factors for cardiovascular disease, as well as other diseases.[17]

Many developed countries also conduct periodic health surveys, in order to explore trends in exposures and diseases. For example, the US National Center for Health Statistics conducts a periodic Health Interview Study as a study of illnesses reported by patients. The National Center for Health Statistics also conducts a periodic Health Examination Survey, including physical examinations and laboratory tests. The National Ambulatory Medical Care Survey, mentioned above, investigates samples of office-based physicians. The Health Records Survey (no longer being conducted) and the Institutional Population Survey (no longer being conducted) investigated samples of institutionalized patients. The Hospital Discharge Survey investigates samples of patients discharged from acute care hospitals. As a last example, the National Natality and Mortality Surveys collect additional data on individuals sampled from vital statistics data.

Finally, many countries have selected "reportable diseases." These are diseases of particular interest to the local public health authorities, and are often infectious diseases. Sometimes reporting is "required," although enforcement is difficult. Sometimes reporting is just requested. In either case, however, reporting is not complete, and so it can be difficult to disentangle trends in disease incidence from trends in reporting.

Potential Problems

This type of data can be extremely useful in performing analyses of secular trends, and has been used to address a number of important questions in pharmacoepidemiology.[18] However, whenever one uses data that were not collected specifically for the study at hand, one must be very careful to be aware of its limitations. Each of the data sources described presents its own problems. Mortality data are the most likely to be used for analyses of secular trends, and the problems of these data represent good illustrations of the types of problems one must consider when using any of the data sources. As such, they will be discussed in more detail.

Overall, in using mortality data one is limited by the care, or lack of care, taken by physicians in completing death certificates. This is particularly a problem for studies that rely on information about the cause of death. Physicians may not know the cause of death accurately or, even if they do, they may not be careful in recording it. This is unlikely to create false findings in analyses of secular trends, unless there is a systematic change in these errors over time or across geographic areas. Unfortunately, however, these systematic changes can occur in many ways.

First, one can see changes in physicians' index of suspicion about any given disease. This can lead to trends in how frequently patients are diagnosed with the disease. For example, pulmonary emboli frequently are not detected.[19] As physicians have become aware of this problem, one would expect that a larger proportion of patients with this disease would be diagnosed.

Second, diagnostic methods can change over time. This, too, can create false trends. For example, clinical diagnoses of pulmonary emboli have been shown to be wrong over 50% of the time.[20] As lung scanning procedures became widely available, one would expect that a larger proportion of patients with pulmonary embolism received correct diagnoses.

Third, diagnostic terminology can change over time. For example, with the development of the extractable nuclear antigen serologic test, patients previously diagnosed with other conditions are now being diagnosed as having mixed connective tissue disease.

Fourth, there can be changes in coding systems. A blatant example is the periodic shift from an older version of the International Classification of Diseases to a more recent one, such as from ICD-8 to ICD-9. Less obvious changes can cause major problems as well. For example, in a study of methyldopa and biliary carcinoma using data from multiple international cancer registries, all but one showed no association between drug sales and disease incidence or mortality.[21] In one, however, a marked increase shortly after drug marketing was seen in cancer of the biliary tract, excluding the code for cancer of the biliary tract—part unspecified. A complementary pattern was seen for the excluded code. Further investigation revealed that a change in coding policy was instituted in that registry in 1966. After that date, more specific coding was to be used. This resulted in an apparent increase in the incidence rates of the diseases of specified sites, accompanied by an apparent decrease in the incidence rates of diseases with unspecified sites.[22]

Fifth, there can be changes in population demographics. The aging of the US population now under way would obviously dictate a shift in mortality from diseases of the young to diseases of the old. Age-specific analyses could be performed to control for this trend, but other trends cannot be adjusted for as easily, for example migration.

Finally, using mortality data one cannot differentiate between a change in the incidence rate of a disease and a change in the case-fatality rate of a disease. For example, we know that cardiovascular mortality is decreasing in much of the developed world.[23] However, we do not know whether that decrease is because fewer people are developing coronary artery disease or whether the same proportion of the population is developing the disease, but they are living longer with the disease before dying.

DATA SOURCES FOR CASE–CONTROL STUDIES

REGISTRY DATA

As discussed above, there are a number of registries available, each comprised of cases of selected diseases. Usually these are just a collection of cases, without controls. However, if there is a registry extant that has a collection of cases of a disease one wishes to study, then this can be useful for performing a case–control study of that disease. One needs to be careful, however, about whether the registry collected all cases of a disease in a defined population or just some of them. If the latter, then one needs to consider whether the method of recruitment might introduce some bias into the study.

One particular registry, which is often forgotten in this context, is the spontaneous reporting system maintained by regulatory bodies throughout the world (see Chapters 9 and 10). These represent sources of cases of adverse drug reactions and can be used for case finding for case–control studies. As a specific example, a study used this approach to investigate the pathophysiology of the suprofen-induced flank pain syndrome. Cases with the acute flank pain syndrome were compared to controls without the syndrome, both groups exposed to suprofen. This provided interesting information on risk factors for the acute flank pain syndrome among those who have been exposed to suprofen.[24]

OLMSTED COUNTY MEDICAL RECORDS

Another approach to performing case–control studies takes advantage of the unique medical record system in Olmsted County, Minnesota.[25,26] The Mayo Clinic and its affiliated clinics and hospitals provide the medical care for most of the 125 000 residents of Olmsted County. These data have been supplemented since 1966 by information on diagnostic and surgical procedures from the other medical groups and hospitals in Olmsted County, as well as the few independent practitioners who were not part of the Mayo Clinic system. This database now covers the medical care delivered to County residents from 1909 through the present. These records represent an extremely useful and productive resource for epidemiologic studies, including case finding for case–control studies.[27–31] For pharmacoepidemiology studies, however, drug exposure data must usually be gathered de novo.

MANITOBA

The Canadian province of Manitoba maintains computerized files for its clients, as a by-product of its provincial health plan.[32] This administrative database has 1.1 million people, starting in 1970. Data can be accessed from four computerized databases maintained by Manitoba Health Services Insurance Plan (MHSIP). These linked databases include: (i) registration files, containing a record for every individual registered to receive insured health services, (ii) records of physician reimbursement claims for medical care provided, containing information on patient diagnosis and physician specialty, (iii) records of hospital discharge abstracts, and (iv) records of prescriptions dispensed in retail pharmacies, containing data on the date of prescription dispensing, drug name, dosage form, quantity dispensed, and a drug identification number.[33–37]

AD HOC CASE–CONTROL STUDIES

Finally, case–control studies can be performed as ad hoc studies as well. Cases can then be recruited from whatever source is appropriate for that disease, whether hospitals, outpatient practices, or some other source. Investigators in some geographic areas maintain ongoing relationships with a number of hospitals, to permit case finding for case–control studies.

Case definitions must, of course, be clear. Cases should be "incident cases," that is individuals who have recently developed the disease, so one can inquire about exposures that precede the onset of the disease. All individuals who meet the case definition should be enrolled, if possible, to decrease the risk of a selection bias. Finally, if all cases can be identified in a defined population, then the incidence of the disease in the population can be determined.

Controls can then be recruited from either the site of medical care for the cases or from the community where the cases come from. The latter is now generally perceived as a better approach than the former. Community controls can be recruited from friends of the cases, from neighbors of the cases, from a reverse telephone directory, by using random digit dialing, or from some comprehensive listing of the target population. The last is generally the best approach, although it often is not available. Exceptions are selected geographic areas in which the government maintains such a list, organized medical care programs which can provide listings of eligible individuals, such as general practitioners' patient lists in the United Kingdom and the other programs described in Chapters 13 through 22, and other special situations. An example would be a study limited to the elderly, which could obtain listings of those eligible for Medicare in the local area.

Friend controls are convenient, but risk overmatching; friends may be similar in personal habits, and this can be problematic if these are risk factors of importance in the study. Reverse telephone directories list individuals by address, rather than by name. They can be useful for choosing community controls that are matched for neighborhood and, thereby, crudely matched for socioeconomic status. However, the use of reverse telephone directories to recruit controls is problematic in areas where a large proportion of the population has unlisted telephone numbers. This is becoming common in major metropolitan areas in the US. Thus, random digit dialing is often the best method available for the selection of community controls. As shown by results from a recently published study,[38] despite concerns about low participation rates in random digit dialing surveys, drug utilization information provided by study participants may be representative of the utilization practices of the nonpartici-pants. As part of a methodologic study designed to compare agreement between women's reports of their utilization of hormone replacement therapy (HRT) and the information available for these women in a claims database about drugs dispensed to them,[38] selection bias was tested by assessing the difference in utilization of HRT between responders and nonresponders. Women aged 50–79 years old were contacted to ask them to participate in a telephone interview about their hormone use. An initial screening telephone call was administered in order to recruit them into the study and to arrange the time for the main telephone interview to be administered. The contact experience with the study sub-jects was designed to be similar to that for typical random digit dialing. Out of a random sample of 213 women selected from the claims database who were contacted, 154 (72.3%) women agreed to participate and 59 (32.7%) women refused. Among the 154 women who agreed to par-ticipate, 79 (51.3%, 95% CI: 43.1–59.4%) were shown by the claims database to have been dispensed an HRT during a 15-month period. Among the 59 women who refused to participate, 30 (50.8%, 95% CI: 37.5–64.1%) were shown by the database to have been dispensed an HRT during the same period.[38] Thus, this study showed that use of HRT was almost identical in responders and nonresponders.

However, patient refusals are becoming an increasing problem for random digit dialing. While it is difficult to compare response rates among studies because of variations in calculating and reporting these rates, there is a sense in the field that recent rates are lower than rates reported in earlier studies.[39–41] Further, the growing use of cell phones instead of landlines may make this problematic in the future as well, if the cell phone numbers remain inaccessible to researchers.

The validity of exposure data collected from patients as part of *ad hoc* case–control studies is discussed in Chapter 45.

Of course, many other details must be considered in plan-ning a case–control study. A more extensive discussion of this is beyond the scope of this book. The interested reader is referred to a standard epidemiology textbook and/or to one of the books now available which specifically discuss case–control studies.[42–44] Overall, the advantages and disadvantages of this approach are identical to those of case–control surveillance, described in Chapter 11. The major additional advantages of the latter are that it has a large database of potential controls and a standardized procedure, which can expedite the study process. However, *ad hoc* studies have more flexibility in their design, allowing one to use community controls and to tailor the data collection effort to the question at hand.

DATA SOURCES FOR COHORT STUDIES

The major logistic issues in performing pharmacoepidemi-ology studies using a cohort design are, first, how to identify a cohort of patients exposed to a drug of interest and one or more control groups without exposure to the drug and, second, how to determine their clinical outcome. The major sources of information about drug exposures are billing claims, physicians, pharmacies, and patients. To date, the last has been considered relatively unreliable, and most approaches have used one of the other three sources. Examples of each will be presented below. As to clinical outcomes, the major source of information must be the physician, directly or indirectly, through the medical record. Patients can be used as a partial source of this information, but confirmatory and supplementary information will generally be needed from physicians. The validity of disease outcome data collected from different sources is discussed in more detail in Chapter 45.

PHARMACY-BASED POSTMARKETING SURVEILLANCE STUDIES

A relatively underused method of recruiting patients into pharmacoepidemiology studies is through the pharmacy that dispenses the drug. One approach to this would be to collect data on drug exposures from computerized pharmacies. This would be similar to a billing data source. Alternatively, one could obtain the participation of the pharmacist, asking him to solicit patient recruitment. Finally, one could enclose recruitment information in a drug's packaging, requesting that patients return an enclosed business reply card to enroll in the study.

The major pioneer in the use of pharmacy-based methods of pharmacoepidemiology was the pharmacoepidemiology group at what used to be Upjohn Pharmaceuticals. The results of a feasibility study using this approach were published.[45] Briefly, the study consisted of the identification and follow-up of 21 372 patients treated between July 1975 and July 1977 with oral antibacterials in an ambulatory care setting. Participating centers were limited to those which combined medical care delivery sites with on-site pharmacies, excluding large hospital outpatient clinics and large referral centers. The pharmacists at participating sites were asked to invite a patient to participate if he or she received a drug of interest. The patient was given an explanatory brochure, which was supplemented by a discussion with the pharmacist, if needed. The brochure included a "Release of Information" statement, which was retained by the pharmacist. At weekly intervals, the pharmacist sent the coordinating center a list of all antibacterials dispensed, information about each prescription, and information about the patients who agreed to participate. The pharmacists were paid for the time this involved. Data on health outcomes were collected from the patients using a questionnaire mailed to them one month later. This was supplemented by telephone follow-up when needed. Reports of hospitalizations or deaths were confirmed at the place of treatment.

Pharmacy-based surveillance was used by Upjohn in other studies as well.[46] In general, the approach remained the same, although computer-assisted telephone interviews were used to collect outcome data, rather than mailed questionnaires. People who could not be contacted by telephone were sent certified letters, asking them to telephone the research center. If they signed the receipt for the certified letter, but still could not be contacted, they were classified as alive.

The advantages of this approach are that it is free of the selection bias inherent in using physicians to recruit patients. Also, this approach does not interfere with prescribing practices, it allows one to collect information about patients' use of concomitant drugs other than those any given physician may be aware of, it allows one to study outcomes which need not come to medical attention, and, compared to studies that recruit patients via prescribers, it is less expensive—it is free of the large cost of reimbursing the prescriber for his cooperation. The disadvantages of the approach are the potential for a volunteer bias and the extensive resources and time needed for site recruitment and data collection. Overall, however, this appears to be a very effective, although underused, approach to performing cohort studies in pharmacoepidemiology.

As another approach to pharmacy-based surveillance, the Center for Medication Monitoring at the University of Texas Medical Branch in Galveston has been performing postmarketing surveillance using patient self-monitoring.[47,48] Patients filling a prescription for a target medication are presented with an announcement of the study along with their prescription. Patients who agree to participate are then asked to report during the next month on any changes in their health status. While they are mailed two questionnaires to obtain demographic and medication usage information, patients are asked to telephone the Center to report any new clinical events.[47,48] This is a variation on pharmacy-based surveillance, which relies on patients to self-report new events. While this type of approach raises concerns about the representativeness of patients agreeing to participate, that may not be a problem since there is a control group subject to the same selection process. Unless willingness to participate was somehow different among the groups of study subjects being compared, no bias should result. Perhaps

more serious, however, is the risk of missing many clinical events by relying on patient initiative to report them, and that the degree of incomplete reporting could easily be related to study group or, alternatively, sufficiently severe to mask any real result due to nondifferential misclassification.

Finally, pharmacy-based surveillance was used to conduct a massive study of parenteral ketorolac.[49–51] A retrospective cohort study between November 18, 1991 through August 31, 1993, identified subjects from 35 hospitals in the Delaware Valley Case–Control Network. Included were 9907 inpatients given 10 279 courses of parenteral ketorolac and 10 248 inpatients given parenteral narcotics and no parenteral ketorolac, matched on hospital, admission service, and date of initiation of therapy. Patients were enrolled by identifying users of these drugs, from the hospital pharmacies. The source of data on these patients was then chart review, using computer-assisted chart abstracting forms. The study concluded that the adverse event profiles of ketorolac and narcotics appeared different, mostly in the pattern predicted, with ketorolac having an increased risk of gastrointestinal bleeding, especially in the elderly, associated with higher doses, and with use greater than 5 days, and with narcotics having a higher risk of respiratory depression, but without a difference in risk in many other outcomes. Overall, the risk/benefit balance of parenteral ketorolac versus parenteral opiates was deemed to be similar, but that improving the use of ketorolac (e.g., duration <5 days) would improve risk/benefit balance further, and that the choice of the optimal drug needs to be made on a patient-specific basis. Extensive changes were made to the drug's labeling in response to these results, and these changes protected the drug's availability in some markets where concerns had been raised.

AD HOC COHORT STUDIES

The "traditional" approach to recruiting patients into pharmacoepidemiology cohort studies has been for pharmaceutical manufacturers to use their sales representatives (also known as "detail men") to solicit physicians to enroll the next few patients for whom they prescribe the drug in question. The physicians then provide follow-up information on the results of this treatment. For example, in the Phase IV postmarketing drug surveillance study conducted of prazosin, the investigators collected a series of over 20 000 newly exposed subjects, recruited through the manufacturer's sales force. The goal of this study was to quantitate better the incidence of first-dose syncope, which was a well-recognized adverse effect of this drug.[52] As another example, when cimetidine was first marketed there was a concern over whether it could cause agranulocytosis, since it was chemically closely related to metiamide, another H_2 blocker which had been removed from the market in Europe because it caused agranulocytosis. This study also collected 10 000 subjects, using a similar design, and found no cases of agranulocytosis.[53]

Although this is the "standard" approach to this type of study, it suffers from a number of important problems. First, it is extremely expensive. The studies mentioned above cost over $1 million each, without counting in this cost the considerable time of the pharmaceutical representatives.[54]

Second, these studies did not include any control group. A control group was not necessary for them to provide useful information about the questions they were designed to answer. They were designed to quantitate the frequency of a defined medical event in those who were exposed to the drug, rather than to test hypotheses about whether the drug caused particular outcomes. However, in general, the absence of a control group is a major problem. Without a control group, one cannot determine whether the observed frequency of any medical event is larger or smaller than would have been expected. Thus, one would expect that such studies would provide little new information, despite their cost, and this is what has been observed.[55]

It often would be difficult or impossible to enroll appropriate controls for a new drug in this type of study. For example, no other H_2 blocker was available on the market at the time cimetidine was marketed. When a United Kingdom postmarketing surveillance study was performed that compared users of cimetidine to the next eligible patient in their general practitioners' offices, differences were seen which were likely to be due to the underlying disease for which the cimetidine was being administered, rather than the cimetidine.[56] Whether or not recruiting a valid control group would be possible, however, it would double the already considerable cost of a study of this type.

Finally, the physicians recruited into a study via a pharmaceutical company's sales representatives are unlikely to be representative of all physicians. In addition, there is no way to monitor whether the physicians select patients who are representative of all their patients, recruit patients sequentially, or even provide complete information on the patients selected. For all of these reasons, there is a considerable potential for biased results.

Thus, although this method continues to be used, this is mainly for its marketing potential rather than for the scientific information it will gather. In fact, some so-called postmarketing surveillance studies that are designed in this way are in fact pure marketing efforts, with no real attempt to gather useful scientific information. These are described to participants as pharmacoepidemiology studies, when in fact they are market-seeding studies. This practice is unfortunate, however, and should be abandoned. In addition to being of questionable integrity, this practice is troublesome, as physicians could become jaded as well as disillusioned with and skeptical about postmarketing surveillance studies in general, jeopardizing future studies which could make important contributions.[57]

OTHER APPROACHES

Other approaches to recruiting patients for cohort postmarketing surveillance studies are more opportunistic. As an example, most of the databases described in earlier chapters can be used to identify individuals exposed to selected drugs (see Chapters 13–22).

As another example, in a United Kingdom postmarketing surveillance study, the Prescription Pricing Bureau and local pharmacies in four geographic areas were used to identify individuals prescribed cimetidine by their general practitioners. Controls were selected from the general practitioners' practice file, as the next patient in the file of the same sex, age (by decade), and who had attended the practice within the prior 12 months. Outcome data were collected by visiting the general practitioner again 15 months later and reviewing his/her records for any intervening care received by the patient.[58]

Finally, other approaches can be considered as well, such as by systematically approaching physicians who are likely to be prescribing the drug. For example, to evaluate cimetidine one could solicit via mail the cooperation of all gastroenterologists. As another example, to evaluate a new vaccine one could approach city health clinics that administer the vaccine, and one could solicit the cooperation of pediatricians.

USING RANDOMIZED CLINICAL TRIALS AS POSTMARKETING SURVEILLANCE STUDIES

For the reasons described in Chapter 2, randomized clinical trials do not have as large a role in postmarketing studies as they do in premarketing studies.[59] They are artificial and raise logistical problems. Perhaps most importantly, however, they are often unnecessary, because of the studies performed premarketing. In fact, however, most studies performed after drug marketing *are* randomized clinical trials.[60] Most of those are intended to address specific questions about drug efficacy, and are conducted as if they were premarketing studies. A few are designed to study drug safety.[61] However, there is a relative lack of postmarketing surveillance randomized clinical trials that take advantage of the fact that they are studying an approved drug.

Specifically, pharmacoepidemiology techniques can be used to conduct postmarketing clinical trials in ways that could be less costly and less artificial. An example is the Group Health Cooperative of Puget Sound's randomized clinical trial comparing the toxicity of microencapsulated versus wax-matrix formulations of oral potassium chloride.[62]

Since these are both FDA-approved products and are theoretically interchangeable formulations of the same active drug, this HMO randomly allocated its pharmacies to dispense either the wax-matrix formulation or the microencapsulated formulation.

As another example, one could conduct a large-scale double-blind randomized clinical trial of two different drugs in the same drug class, using participating prescribers to enlist the patients. The study would be performed by mail. After obtaining patient consent, participating prescribers would use special preprinted prescription pads for the "study drug." These prescriptions would be telephoned, and later mailed, into the coordinating center, which would then express mail the drug to the patient, who would not have to pay for the drug. Data collection would be performed by questionnaires mailed to the patients and by obtaining copies of the physicians' medical records. The incentives needed to obtain physician participation should be much less than those used in classical premarketing clinical trials, because of the markedly decreased amount of work being requested. This would be explored within a pilot study to be conducted first.

Thus, postmarketing randomized clinical trials can be conducted in innovative ways that take advantage of the postmarketing setting, rather than simply performing a premarketing randomized trial after marketing. This is uncommonly done, however. Much more is presented in Chapter 39, on the use of randomized clinical trials for pharmacoepidemiology studies.

ADDITIONAL DATABASES USEFUL FOR PHARMACOEPIDEMIOLOGIC RESEARCH

Finally, there are a number of other databases potentially useful for pharmacoepidemiologic research. In addition, new databases are continuously under development. In general these, of course, can be used for either cohort or case–control studies. Most have been used only rarely for pharmacoepidemiology, but could be used more often, especially if expanded.

One of these is the medical record linkage system used in Finland. The Finnish Cancer Registry, Congenital Malformation Register, and Hospital Discharge Register can each be linked to the Register of Persons Entitled to Free Drugs.[63] The particular advantages of this system are that it collects nationwide data and some of the notifications are mandatory. The particular disadvantages are the relatively small population size. Finland's population is only 5.2 million in total. There are now only 1.2 million individuals in the register (406 000 with 100% reimbursement, and 800 000 at 75% reimbursement). Nevertheless, it has been used on occasion for formal analytic research in pharmacoepidemiology. For example, a paper reported a case–control study, which did not confirm the initial reports of an association between reserpine and breast cancer.[64] As another example, some epidemiologic studies have been conducted by combining information with data from other registers. For example, the total medication pattern of diabetic patients was studied by identifying diabetic patients through the database maintained by the Social Insurance Institution of Finland—where individuals with specified chronic diseases (about 50 diseases) are entitled to special reimbursement for drug treatment costs—and by linking this information to prescription data in the same database, including all details and costs of medications prescribed, purchased, and reimbursed.[65] Matched controls were chosen from the population registry, identified by the section of the population *not* entitled to special reimbursement for diabetes and who did not purchase antidiabetic medications.

Another database occasionally being used for pharmacoepidemiologic research is the longstanding Regenstrief Medical Record System.[66,67] This database contains all laboratory, pharmacy, and appointment information for a network of inner city facilities in Indianapolis, including 5 large hospitals, 44 outpatient clinics, 13 homeless care sites, and the county and state health departments, all of which are located in and around Indianapolis. It has been used for many studies, although only a few pharmacoepidemiology studies.[68–73]

Although it is a uniquely deep data resource, e.g., in its availability of laboratory data, for the purposes of pharmacoepidemiology studies, it suffers from a relatively small population, and incomplete ascertainment of outcomes, i.e., patients who go to other facilities in Indianapolis for some of their care will not have the associated care recorded. This means that key exposures or outcomes could be missed, as well as important confounders.

Another database used for pharmacoepidemiologic research, very different from Regenstrief, is IMS America's MediPlus database. IMS HEALTH maintains de-identified, population-based, longitudinal patient databases for the UK, Germany, France, and Austria (IMS Disease Analyzer-Mediplus, formerly MediPlus), the information recorded being dependent on the local health care system. IMS Disease Analyzer—Mediplus UK contains full records from around 125 computerized general practices. There are approximately 560 partners at participating practices, over 2 million patient records (~1 million active) and over 95 million prescriptions. Of active patients (i.e., currently registered with a panel GP), nearly 400 000 have prescription history of more than 10 years. The earliest live data entry was in 1991, histories before that date being summarized. This is a UK medical record database, very similar to the General Practice Research Database described in detail in Chapter 22. One difference is the lack of an attempt to add hospital outcome data to these data, so it is mostly useful for studies of outpatient prescribing patterns and of events that do not result in hospitalization.[74–78] IMS Disease Analyzer—Mediplus Germany contains patient records from 400 practices (290 GPs and 110 internal specialists) since 1992. There are over 4 million patients and over 66 million issued prescriptions recorded. Approximately 45% of patients in the German database have over 3 years of history although, due to the constraints of the health care system, their records may be incomplete. The German database also allows access to panels of specialists, including gynecologists, pediatricians, urologists, orthopedic surgeons, ENT doctors, dermatologists, surgeons, and neurologists. For Disease Analyzer—Mediplus France, clinical information on over 1 million patients with approximately 22 million prescriptions is collected from around 450 GPs working in a computerized environment. In-depth information on the management of a patient's diagnosis and its treatment can be obtained. In Austria, the database contains about 100 practices (GPs and internists), almost 500 000 patients, and over 11 million prescriptions in total. Though all four databases are primary care-based, participating doctors themselves record hospital admission, specialist referral, and other information that is necessary for a complete clinical record, such as laboratory tests (differences according to country). The databases are increasingly used in research for publication.[77–85]

Yet another, very different, type of database that has been available for a number of years is the Health Evaluation through Logical Processing (HELP) System at LDS Hospital, Salt Lake City, Utah (540 beds).[86,87] This is a computerized hospital information system designed to provide administrative, financial, and clinical hospital services. There is patient-based information on the drugs administered, which can be linked to events, other therapies, and procedures. HELP is an integrated expert system that conducts evaluations and provides recommendations on the care of each patient. HELP collects information from admissions, diagnostic laboratories, the pharmacy, nursing care documentation, and more, by cross-checking and analyzing critical information from various departments of Intermountain Healthcare Hospitals. The epidemiologic applications of the HELP system at first have been primarily in the area of infectious diseases and antibiotic use, and have been expanded to other areas as well.[88–94] Another application of the HELP system has been for computerized surveillance of adverse drug events.[95,96] The adverse drug event monitoring system combined "enhanced" voluntary reporting by hospital personnel through entry of potential adverse events at any computer terminal in the hospital, with automated detection of adverse drug events through signal events, e.g., sudden discontinuation of a drug, an order for an antidote, certain laboratory tests, and abnormal results. Using this system, 36 653 patients were monitored over an 18-month period. Of these patients, 648 experienced 731 adverse drug events. Before initiation of this program, only 10–20 adverse drug events were reported on a voluntary basis annually. The investigators were able to determine the patient populations at risk for an adverse drug event and those drug classes most often associated with an adverse event.[97]

A number of databases are emerging from Italy as well. There is one in particular, from the Italian region of Friuli Venezia Giulia (FVG), which has been productive of a number of papers in the international literature.[98–103] All Italian residents are registered with the national health service, which provides free medical care (including hospitalizations) through all of the public and most of the private providers. FVG is a region in the northeastern part of Italy, at the border with Slovenia and Austria. The region is divided into four provinces, with a total of 1.2 million residents with age and sex distributions comparable to those of the rest of Italy. Since 1976 the Regional Directorate of Health in FVG has developed a large automated database (Sistema Informativo Sanitario Regionale, SISR), in which data on all hospitalizations and prescriptions filled in the region are collected, in addition to demographic information and a variety of specialized medical and administrative files.

Drug data have been collected since 1991 or 1992, depending on the province within FVG. The *hospital record file* has accumulated information about all hospitalizations in public and private hospitals within the region since 1985. Since January 1, 1998 an *outpatient file* has collected information on encounters with specialists (including contacts with in-hospital emergency care), laboratory tests, and diagnostic and treatment procedures reimbursed by the national health service.

CONCLUSIONS

In summary, there are a number of other approaches to pharmacoepidemiology studies, in addition to the ones described in detail earlier. No approach to pharmacoepidemiology studies is ideal. Each available approach has its advantages and its disadvantages. In the next chapter, we will place all of these options in perspective, discussing how one chooses among the available alternatives.

REFERENCES

1. IMS Research Group. *A Special Analysis of the National Disease and Therapeutics Index Service for the Pharmaceutical Industry*. Ambler, PA: IMS America, 1979.

2. Knapp D. *Comparisons of NAMCS, NDTI, and Medicaid Data*. Washington, DC: US Food and Drug Administration, 1983.

3. *Highlights of Drug Utilization in Office Practice—National Ambulatory Medical Care Survey, 1985*. Advance Data Number 137. Hyattsville, MD: National Center for Health Statistics, 1987.

4. Cherry DK, Burt CW, Woodwell DA. National Ambulatory Medical Care Survey: 2001 summary. *Adv Data* 2003; **337**: 1–44.

5. Burt CW. National trends in use of medications in office-based practices 1985–1999. *Health Aff* 2000; **21**: 206–14.

6. Burt CW, Bernstein AB. Trends in use of medications associated with women's ambulatory care visits. *J Womens Health* 2003; **12**: 213–17.

7. McCaig LF, Besser RE, Hughes JM. Antimicrobial drug prescription in ambulatory care settings, United States, 1992–2000. *Emerg Infect Dis* 2003; **9**: 432–7.

8. Aparasu RR, Mort JR, Sitzman S. Psychotropic prescribing for the elderly in office-based practice. *Clin Ther* 1998; **20**: 603–16.

9. Kaufman DW, Kelly JP, Rosenberg L, Anderson TE, Mitchell AA. Recent patterns of medication use in the ambulatory adult population of the United States: the Slone Survey. *JAMA* 2002; **287**: 337–44.

10. Lilja J. The nationalization of the Swedish pharmacies. *Soc Sci Med* 1987; **24**: 423–9.

11. Edlavitch SA, Feinleib M, Anello C. A potential use of the National Death Index for postmarketing drug surveillance. *JAMA* 1985; **253**: 1292–5.

12. Johnson KC. Canadian health databases relevant to Great Lakes Basin research. *Toxicol Ind Health* 1996; **12**: 551–5.

13. Weir HK, Thun MJ, Hankey BF, Ries LAG, Howe HL, Wingo PA *et al*. Annual report to the nation on the status of cancer, 1975–2000, featuring the uses of surveillance data for cancer prevention and control. *J Natl Cancer Inst* 2003; **95**: 1276–99.

14. US Cancer Statistics Working Group. *United States Cancer Statistics: 2000 Incidence*. Atlanta, GA: Department of Health and Human Services, Centers for Disease Control and Prevention and National Cancer Institute, 2003.

15. Parkin DM, Whelan SL, Ferlay J, Teppo L, Thomas DB, eds. *Cancer Incidence in Five Continents*, vol. VIII. Lyon, France: IARC Scientific Publications, 2003.

16. Oakley GP. Population and case–control surveillance in the search for environmental causes of birth defects. *Public Health Rep* 1984; **99**: 465–8.

17. Dawber TR. *The Framingham study. The Epidemiology of Atherosclerotic Disease*. Cambridge, MA: Harvard University Press, 1980.

18. Stolley PD. The use of vital and morbidity statistics for the detection of adverse drug reactions and for monitoring of drug safety. *J Clin Pharmacol* 1982; **22**: 499–504.

19. Dalen JE, Alpert JS. National history of pulmonary embolism. *Prog Cardiovasc Dis* 1975; **517**: 259–70.

20. Hull RD, Raskob GE, Hirsh J. The diagnosis of clinically suspected pulmonary embolism. *Chest* 1986; **89** (suppl 5): S417–25.

21. Strom BL, Hibberd PL, Stolley PD. No evidence of association between methyldopa and biliary carcinoma. *Int J Epidemiol* 1985; **14**: 86–90.

22. Stolley PD, Strom BL. Evaluating and monitoring the safety and efficacy of drug therapy and surgery. *J Chron Dis* 1986; **39**: 1145–55.

23. Gillum RF, Folsom AR, Blackburn H. Decline in coronary heart disease mortality. Old questions and new facts. *Am J Med* 1984; **76**: 1055–65.

24. Strom BL, West SL, Sim E, Carson JL. Epidemiology of the acute flank pain syndrome from suprofen. *Clin Pharmacol Ther* 1989; **46**: 693–9.

25. Kurland LT, Molgaard CA. The patient record in epidemiology. *Sci Am* 1981; **245**: 54–63.

26. Melton LJ. History of the Rochester Epidemiology Project. *Mayo Clin Proc* 1996; **71**: 266–74. Available at: http://www.mayo.edu/research/mir/topic_1029.html.

27. Doran MF, Crowson CS, O'Fallon WM, Hunder GG, Gabriel SE. Trends in the incidence of polymyalgia rheumatica over a 30 year period in Olmsted County, Minnesota, USA. *J Rheumatol* 2002; **29**: 1694–7.

28. Roberts RO, Bergstralh EJ, Bass SE, Lightner DJ, Lieber MM, Jacobsen SJ. Incidence of physician-diagnosed interstitial cystitis in Olmsted County: a community-based study. *Br J Urology* 2003; **91**: 181–5.

29. Bower JH, Maraganore DM, Peterson BJ, McDonnell SK, Ahlskog JE, Rocca WA. Head trauma preceding PD: a case–control study. *Neurology* 2003; **60**: 1610–15.

30. Conio M, Cameron AJ, Romero Y, Branch CD, Schleck CD, Burgart LJ *et al*. Secular trends in the epidemiology and outcome of Barrett's oesophagus in Olmsted County, Minnesota. *Gut* 2001; **48**: 304–9.

31. Benedetti MD, Maraganore DM, Bower JH, McDonnell SK, Peterson BJ, Ahlskog JE *et al*. Hysterectomy, menopause, and estrogen use preceding Parkinson's disease: an exploratory case–control study. *Mov Disord* 2001; **16**: 830–7.

32. Roos LL, Nicol JP. Building individual histories with registries. *Med Care* 1983; **21**: 955–69.

33. Kozyrskyj AL, Mustard CA, Cheang MS, Simons FE. Income-based drug benefit policy: impact on receipt of inhaled corticosteroid prescriptions by Manitoba children with asthma. *Can Med Assoc J* 2001; **165**: 897–902.

34. Kozyrskyj A. Prescription medications in Manitoba children: are there regional differences? *Can J Public Health* 2002; **93** (suppl 2): S63–9.

35. Kozyrskyj A, Hildes-Ripstein GE. Assessing health status in Manitoba children: acute and chronic conditions. *Can J Public Health* 2002; **93** (suppl 2): S44–9.

36. Brownell M, Kozyrskyj A, Roos NP, Friesen D, Mayer T, Sullivan K. Health service utilization by Manitoba children. *Can J Public Health* 2002; **93** (suppl 2): S57–62.

37. Metge CJ, Blanchard JF, Peterson S, Bernstein CN. Use of pharmaceuticals by inflammatory bowel disease patients: a population-based study. *Am J Gastroenterol* 2001; **96**: 3348–55.

38. Strom BL, Schinnar R. Participants and refusers in a telephone interview about hormone replacement therapy were equally likely to be taking it. *J Clin Epi* 2004; **57**: 624–6.

39. Marelich WD, Berger DE, McKenna RB. Gender differences in the control of alcohol-impaired driving in California. *J Stud Alcohol* 2000; **61**: 396–401.

40. Weiss KB, Grant EN, Li T. The effects of asthma experience and social demographic characteristics on responses to the Chicago Community Asthma Survey-32. Chicago Asthma Surveillance Initiative Project Team. *Chest* 1999; **116** (suppl 1): S183–9.

41. Funkhouser E, Macaluso M, Wang X. Alternative strategies for selecting population controls: comparison of random digit dialing and targeted telephone calls. *Ann Epidemiol* 2000; **10**: 59–67.

42. Schlesselman JJ. *Case–Control Studies—Design, Conduct, Analysis*. New York: Oxford University Press, 1982.

43. Ibrahim MA, Spitzer WO. The case control study: the problem and the prospect. *J Chron Dis* 1979; **32**: 139–44.

44. Breslow NE, Day NE. *Statistical Methods in Cancer Research: The Analysis of Case–Control Studies*, vol. 1. Lyon, France: IARC Scientific Publications, 1980.

45. Borden EK, Lee JG. A methodologic study of postmarketing drug evaluation using a pharmacy-based approach. *J Chron Dis* 1982; **35**: 803–16.

46. Luscombe FA. Methodologic issues in pharmacy-based post-marketing surveillance. *Drug Inf J* 1985; **19**: 269–74.

47. Fisher S, Bryant SG. Postmarketing surveillance of adverse drug reactions: patient self-monitoring. *J Am Board Fam Pract* 1992; **5**: 17–25.

48. Fisher S, Bryant SG, Kent TA. Postmarketing surveillance by patient self-monitoring: trazodone versus fluoxetine. *J Clin Psychopharmacol* 1993; **13**: 235–42.

49. Strom BL, Berlin JA, Kinman JL, Spitz RW, Hennessy S, Feldman H *et al*. Parenteral ketorolac and risk of gastrointestinal and operative site bleeding: a postmarketing surveillance study. *JAMA* 1996; **275**: 376–82.

50. Feldman HI, Kinman JL, Berlin JA, Hennessy S, Kimmel SE, Farrar J *et al*. Parenteral ketorolac: the risk for acute renal failure. *Ann Intern Med* 1997; **126**: 193–9.

51. Hennessy S, Kinman JL, Berlin JA, Feldman HI, Carson JL, Kimmel SE *et al*. Lack of hepatotoxic effects of parenteral ketorolac in the hospital setting. *Arch Intern Med* 1997; **157**: 2510–14.

52. Graham RM, Thornell IR, Gain JM, Bagnoli C, Oates HF, Stokes GS. Prazosin: the first dose phenomenon. *BMJ* 1976; **2**: 1293–4.

53. Gifford LM, Aeugle ME, Myerson RM, Tannenbaum PJ. Cimetidine postmarket outpatient surveillance program. *JAMA* 1980; **243**: 1532–5.

54. Joint Commission on Prescription Drug Use. *Final Report*. Washington, DC: 1980.

55. Rossi AC, Knapp DE, Anello C, O'Neill RT, Graham CF, Mendelis PS *et al*. Discovery of adverse drug reactions. A comparison of selected Phase IV studies with spontaneous reporting methods. *JAMA* 1983; **249**: 2226–8.

56. Colin-Jones DG, Langman MJS, Lawson DH, Vessey MP. Postmarketing surveillance of the safety of cimetidine: 12 month mortality report. *BMJ* 1983; **286**: 1713–16.

57. Strom BL, and members of the ASCPT Pharmacoepidemiology Section. Position paper on the use of purported postmarketing drug surveillance studies for promotional purposes. *Clin Pharmacol Ther* 1990; **48**: 598.

58. Colin-Jones DG, Langman MJS, Lawson DH, Vessey MP. Cimetidine and gastric cancer: preliminary report from post-marketing surveillance study. *BMJ* 1982; **285**: 1311–13.

59. Bell RL, Smith EO. Clinical trials in postmarketing surveillance of drugs. *Control Clin Trials* 1982; **3**: 61–7.

60. Mattison N, Richard BW. Postapproval research requested by the FDA at the time of NCE approval, 1970–1984. *Drug Inf J* 1987; **21**: 309–29.

61. Bradford RH, Shear CL, Chremos AN, Dujovne C, Downton M, Franklin FA *et al*. Expanded clinical evaluation of Lovastatin (EXCEL) study results. *Arch Intern Med* 1991; **151**: 43–9.

62. Jick H, Jick SS, Walker AM, Stergachis A. A comparison of wax matrix and microencapsulated potassium chloride in relation to upper gastrointestinal illness requiring hospitalization. *Pharmacotherapy* 1989; **9**: 204–6.

63. Idanpaan-Heikkila J. Finland. In: Inman HW, ed., *Monitoring for Drug Safety*. Boston, MA: MTP Press, 1986; pp. 83–92.

64. Aromaa A, Hakama M, Hakulinen T, Saxen E, Teppo L, Ida lan-Heikkila J. Breast cancer and use of rauwolfia and other antihypertensive agents in hypertensive patients: a nation-wide case–control study in Finland. *Int J Cancer* 1976; **18**: 727–38.

65. Reunanen A, Kangas T, Martikainen J, Klaukka T. Nationwide survey of comorbidity, use, and costs of all medications in Finnish diabetic individuals. *Diabetes Care* 2000; **23**: 1265–71.

66. McDonald CJ, Tierney WM, Overhage JM, Martin DK, Wilson GA. The Regenstrief Medical Record System: 20 years of experience in hospitals, clinics, and neighborhood health centers. *MD Comput* 1992; **9**: 206–17.

67. McDonald CJ, Overhage JM, Tierney WM, Dexter PR, Martin DK, Suico JG *et al*. The Regenstrief Medical Record System: a quarter century experience. *Int J Med Inform* 1999; **54**: 225–53.

68. Williams CL, Johnstone BM, Kesterson JG, Javor KA, Schmetzer AD. Evaluation of antipsychotic and concomitant medication use patterns in patients with schizophrenia. *Med Care* 1999; **37** (suppl 4): S81–6.

69. MacDonald CJ, Tierney WM, Overhage JM, Martin DK, Smith B, Wodniak C *et al*. The Regenstrief Medical Record System— experience with MD order entry and community-wide extensions. In: Ozbolt JG, ed., *Proceedings of the 18th Annual Symposium on Computer Applications in Medical Care*, Washington, DC, November, 1994. Philadelphia, PA: Hanley & Belfus, 1994; p. 1059.

70. Tierney WM, Miller ME, Overhage JM, McDonald CJ. Physician inpatient order writing on microcomputer workstations. Effects on resource utilization. *JAMA* 1993; **269**: 379–83.

71. Gregor KJ, Overhage JM, Coons SJ, McDonald RC. Selective serotonin reuptake inhibitor dose titration in the naturalistic setting. *Clin Ther* 1994; **16**: 306–15.

72. Williams CL, Johnstone BM, Kesterson JG, Javor KA, Schmetzer AD. Evaluation of antipsychotic and concomitant medication use patterns in patients with schizophrenia. *Med Care* 1999; **37** (suppl 4): S81–6.

73. Liu GC, Cunningham C, Downs SM, Marrero DG, Fineberg N. A spatial analysis of obesogenic environments for children. In: Kohane IS, ed., *Proceedings of the AMIA Annual Symposium*, San Antonio, TX, November, 2002. Philadelphia, PA: Hanley & Belfus, 2002; pp. 459–63.

74. Qizilbash N, Kiri V, Boudiaf N, Feudjo-Tepie M. Statins and Alzheimer's disease: why specificity should be a necessary criterion for trusting aetiological analyses from observational databases. *Pharmacoepidemiol Drug Saf* 2003; **12** (suppl 1): S62–3.

75. Langman M, Kong SX, Zhang Q, Kahler KH, Finch E. Safety and patient tolerance of standard and slow-release formulations of NSAIDs. *Pharmacoepidemiol Drug Saf* 2003; **12**: 61–6.

76. Hasford J, Mimran A, Simons WR. A population-based European cohort study of persistence in newly diagnosed hypertensive patients. *J Hum Hypertens* 2002; **16**: 569–75.

77. van der Linden PD, Sturkenboom MCJM, Herings RMC, Leufkens HGM, Stricker BH. Fluoroquinolones and risk of Achilles tendon disorders: case–control study. *BMJ* 2002; **324**: 1306–7.

78. Melia J, Moss S. Survey of the rate of PSA testing in general practice. *Br J Cancer* 2001; **85**: 656–7.

79. Dietlein G, Schröder-Bernhardi D. Doctors' prescription behaviour regarding dosage recommendations for preparations of kava extracts. *Pharmacoepidemiol Drug Saf* 2003; **12**: 417–21.

80. Schröder-Bernhardi D, Dietlein G. Lipid-lowering therapy: do hospitals influence the prescribing behavior of general practitioners? *Int J Clin Pharmacol Ther* 2002; **40**: 317–21.

81. Mockenhaupt M, Schlingmann J, Schröder-Bernhardi D, Schöpf E. Linking registry data on severe skin reactions with patient data from computerized medical practices: experience of a pilot study. *Pharmacoepidemiol Drug Saf* 2002; **11** (suppl 1): S102.

82. Dietlein G, Schröder-Bernhardi D. Use of the Mediplus patient database in healthcare research. *Int J Clin Pharmacol Ther* 2002; **40**: 130–3.

83. Schröder-Bernhardi D, Dietlein G. Compliance with prescription recommendations by physicians in practices. *Int J Clin Pharmacol Ther* 2001; **39**: 477–9.

84. Perez E, Schröder-Bernhardi D, Dietlein G. Treatment behavior of doctors regarding *Helicobacter pylori* infections. *Int J Clin Pharmacol Ther* 2002; **40**: 126–9.

85. Farmer RD, Todd JC, Lewis MA, MacRae KD, Williams TJ. The risks of venous thromboembolic disease among German women using oral contraceptives: a database study. *Contraception* 1998; **57**: 67–70.

86. Classen DC, Burke JP. The computer-based patient record: the role of the hospital epidemiologist. *Infect Control Hosp Epidemiol* 1995; **16**: 729–36.

87. Gardner RM, Pryor TA, Warner HR. The HELP hospital information system: update 1998. *Int J Med Inform* 1999; **54**: 169–82.

88. Evans RS, Pestotnik SL, Classen DC, Clemmer TP, Weaver LK, Orme JF Jr *et al*. A computer-assisted management program for antibiotics and other antiinfective agents. *N Engl J Med* 1998; **338**: 259–60.

89. Classen DC, Burke JP, Pestotnik SL, Lloyd JF. Clinical and financial impact of intravenous erythromycin therapy in hospitalized patients. *Ann Pharmacother* 1999; **33**: 669–73.

90. Burke JP, Pestotnik SL. Antibiotic use and microbial resistance in intensive care units: impact of computer-assisted decision support. *J Chemother* 1999; **11**: 530–5.

91. Mullett CJ, Evans RS, Christenson JC, Dean JM. Development and impact of a computerized pediatric anti-infective decision support program. *Pediatrics* 2001; **108**: E75.

92. Fiszman M, Chapman WW, Aronsky D, Evans RS, Haug PJ. Automatic detection of acute bacterial pneumonia from chest X-ray reports. *J Am Med Inform Assoc* 2000; **76**: 593–604.

93. Pestotnik SL, Classen DC, Evans RS, Burke JP. Implementing antibiotic practice guidelines through computer-assisted decision support: clinical and financial outcomes. *Ann Int Med* 1996; **124**: 884–90.

94. Classen DC, Pestotnik SL, Evans RS, Lloyd JF, Burke JP. Adverse drug events in hospitalized patients: excess length of stay, extra costs, and attributable mortality. *JAMA* 1997; **277**: 301–6.

95. Oderda GM, Evans RS, Lloyd J, Lipman A, Chen C, Ashburn M *et al*. Cost of opioid-related adverse drug events in surgical patients. *J Pain Symptom Manage* 2003; **25**: 276–83.

96. Lazarus HM, Fox J, Evans RS, Lloyd JF, Pombo DJ, Burke JP *et al*. Adverse drug events in trauma patients. *J Trauma* 2003; **54**: 337–43.

97. Classen DC, Pestotnik SL, Evans RS, Burke JP. Computerized surveillance of adverse drug events in hospital patients. *JAMA* 1991; **266**: 2847–51.

98. Varas-Lorenzo C, Garcia-Rodriguez LA, Cattaruzzi C, Troncon MG, Agostinis L, Perez-Gutthann S. Hormone replacement therapy and the risk of hospitalization for venous

thromboembolism: a population-based study in southern Europe. *Am J Epidemiol* 1998; **147**: 387–90.

99. Garcia Rodriguez LA, Cattaruzzi C, Troncon MG, Agostinis L. Risk of hospitalization for upper gastrointestinal tract bleeding associated with ketorolac, other nonsteroidal anti-inflammatory drugs, calcium antagonists, and other antihypertensive drugs. *Arch Intern Med* 1998; **158**: 33–9.

100. Cattaruzzi C, Troncon MG, Agostinis L, Garcia Rodriguez LA. Positive predictive value of ICD-9th codes for upper gastrointestinal bleeding and perforation in the Sistema Informativo Sanitario Regionale database. *J Clin Epidemiol* 1999; **52**: 499–502.

101. Castellsague J, Garcia-Rodriguez LA, Perez-Gutthann S, Agostinis L, Cattaruzzi C, Troncon MG. Characteristics of users of inhaled long-acting beta 2-agonists in a southern European population. *Respir Med* 1999; **93**: 709–14.

102. Sturkenboom MC, Romano F, Simon G, Correa-Leite ML, Villa M, Nicolosi A *et al.* The iatrogenic costs of NSAID therapy: a population study. *Arthritis Rheum* 2002; **47**: 132–40.

103. Borgnolo G, Simon G, Francescutti C, Lattuada L, Zanier L. Antibiotic prescription in Italian children: a population-based study in Friuli Venezia Giulia, north-east Italy. *Acta Paediatrica* 2001; **90**: 1316–20.

24

How Should One Perform Pharmacoepidemiology Studies? Choosing Among the Available Alternatives

BRIAN L. STROM

University of Pennsylvania School of Medicine, Philadelphia, Pennsylvania, USA.

INTRODUCTION

As discussed in the previous chapters, pharmacoepidemiology studies apply the techniques of epidemiology to the content area of clinical pharmacology. Between 500 and 3000 individuals are usually studied prior to drug marketing. Most postmarketing pharmacoepidemiology studies need to include at least 10 000 subjects, or draw from an equivalent population for a case–control study, in order to contribute sufficient new information to be worth their cost and effort. This large sample size raises logistical problems. Chapters 9 through 23 presented each of the different data collection approaches and data resources that have been developed to perform pharmacoepidemiology studies efficiently, despite the need for these very large sample sizes. This chapter is intended to synthesize this material, to assist the reader in choosing among the available approaches.

CHOOSING AMONG THE AVAILABLE APPROACHES TO PHARMACOEPIDEMIOLOGY STUDIES

Once one has decided to perform a pharmacoepidemiology study, one needs to decide which of the data collection approaches or data resources described in the earlier chapters of this book should be used. Although, to some degree, the choice may be based upon a researcher's familiarity with given data resources and/or the investigators who have been using them, this author feels strongly that it is important to tailor the choice of pharmacoepidemiology resource to the question to be addressed. One may want to use more than one data collection strategy or resource, in parallel or in combination. If no single resource is optimal for addressing a question, it can be useful to use a number of approaches that complement each other. Indeed, this is probably the preferable approach for addressing important questions.

Pharmacoepidemiology, Fourth Edition   Edited by B.L. Strom
© 2005 John Wiley & Sons, Ltd

Regardless, investigators are often left with a difficult and complex choice.

In order to explain how to choose among the available pharmacoepidemiologic data resources, it is useful to synthesize the information from the previous chapters on the relative strengths and weaknesses of each of the available pharmacoepidemiology approaches, examining the comparative characteristics of each (see Table 24.1). One can then examine the characteristics of the research question at hand, in order to choose the pharmacoepidemiology approach best suited to addressing that question (see Table 24.2). The assessment and weights provided in this discussion and in the accompanying tables are arbitrary. They are not being represented as a consensus of the pharmacoepidemiology community, but represent the judgment of this author alone, based on the material presented in earlier chapters of this book. Nevertheless, I think that most would agree with the general principles presented, and even many of the relative ratings. My hope is that this synthesis of information, despite some of the arbitrary decisions inherent in it, will make it easier for the reader to synthesize the large amount of information presented in the prior chapters.

COMPARATIVE CHARACTERISTICS OF PHARMACOEPIDEMIOLOGIC DATA RESOURCES

Table 24.1 lists each of the different pharmacoepidemiologic data resources that were described in earlier chapters, along with some of their characteristics.

The *relative size* of the database refers to the population it covers. Only spontaneous reporting systems, The Netherlands Automated Pharmacy Record Linkage System, and Prescription-Event Monitoring in the UK cover entire countries or large fractions thereof. Medicaid databases are next largest, with UnitedHealth Group approaching that, with over 16 million persons. The GPRD database has a population of about 3 million individuals. Then, Kaiser in Northern California currently includes 2.8 million subscribers, Kaiser in Southern California about 2 million, and Kaiser Northwest about 440 000. The Saskatchewan database includes about 1 million currently active individuals. The other data resources are generally smaller. Case–control surveillance, as conducted by the Slone Epidemiology Unit, can cover a variable population, depending on the number of hospitals and metropolitan areas they include in their network for a given study. The population base of registry-based case–control studies depends on the registries used for case finding. *Ad hoc* studies can be whatever size the researcher desires for the study at hand.

As to *relative cost*, studies that collect new data are most expensive, especially randomized trials and cohort studies, for which sample sizes generally need to be large and follow-up may need to be prolonged. In the case of randomized trials, there are additional logistical complexities. Studies that use existing data are least expensive, although their cost increases when they gather primary medical records for validation purposes. Studies that use existing data resources to identify subjects but then collect new data about those subjects are intermediate in cost.

As regards *relative speed* to completion of the study, studies that collect new data take longer, especially randomized trials and cohort studies. Studies that use existing data are able to answer a question most quickly, although considerable additional time may be needed to obtain primary medical records for validation purposes. Studies that use existing data resources to identify subjects but then collect new data about those subjects are intermediate in speed.

Representativeness refers to how well the subjects in the data resource represent the population at large. Prescription-Event Monitoring in the UK, the health databases in Saskatchewan, the Automated Pharmacy Record Linkage in the Netherlands, and the Tayside Medicines Monitoring Unit in Scotland each include entire countries, provinces, or states and, so, are typical populations. Spontaneous reporting systems are drawn from entire populations, but of course the selective nature of their reporting could lead to less certain representativeness. Medicaid programs are limited to the disadvantaged, and so include a population that is least representative of a general population. Randomized trials include populations skewed by the various selection criteria plus their willingness to volunteer for the study. The GPRD uses a nonrandom large subset of the total UK population, and so may be representative. The Group Health Cooperative, the HMO Research Network, Kaiser Permanente, and UnitedHealth include HMO populations. These are closer to representative populations than a Medicaid population would be, although they include a largely working population and, so, include few patients of low socioeconomic status. Some of the remaining data collection approaches or resources are characterized in Table 24.1 as "variable," meaning their representativeness depends on which hospitals are recruited into the study. *Ad hoc* studies are listed in Table 24.1 "as desired," because they can be designed to be representative or not, as the investigator wishes.

Table 24.1. Comparative characteristics of pharmacoepidemiologic data resources[a]

Pharmacoepidemiology approach	Relative size	Relative cost	Relative speed	Representativeness	Population-based	Cohort studies possible	Case–control studies possible
Spontaneous reporting	+++	+	+++	++	−	−	+
Group Health Cooperative	+	+	++++	+++	+	+	+
Kaiser Permanente Medical Care Programs	++	+	++++	+++	+	+	+
The HMO Research Network	+++	+	+++	+++	+	+	+
UnitedHealth Group	+++	+	++++	+++	−	+	+
Medicaid databases	+++	+	++++	+	+	+	+
Health databases in Saskatchewan	++	+	++++	++++	+	+	+
Netherlands	+++	+	++++	++++	+	+	+
Tayside	+	+	++++	++++	+	+	+
GPRD	+++	+	+++	+++	−	−	+
Ad hoc analyses of secular trends	As desired	+	+++	As desired	−	−	−
Case–control surveillance	Variable	+++	+	Variable	−	−	+
Registry-based case–control studies	Variable	++	++	Variable	Variable	−	+
Ad hoc case–control studies	As desired	+++	+	As desired	Variable	−	+
Prescription-Event Monitoring	+++	++	++	++++	−	+	−
Pharmacy-based surveillance: outpatient	++	++	++	Variable	−	+	−
Ad hoc cohort studies	As desired	+++	−	As desired	−	+	−
Pharmacoepidemiology randomized trials	As desired	++++	−	−	−	+	−

Table 24.1. (Continued)

Pharmacoepidemiology approach	Validity of exposure data	Validity of outcome data	Control of confounding	Inpatient drug exposure data	Outpatient diagnosis data	Dates of available data	Loss to follow-up
Spontaneous reporting	++	++	—	+	+++	Fall 1969 to date	N/A
Group Health Cooperative	++	+ to +++	+++	+	—	1972 to date	15%/y×2 y, then 5%/y
Kaiser Permanente Medical Care Programs	++	+ to +++	+++	—	—	—b	3%/y after 2y
The HMO Research Network	++	+ to +++	++	+/−	++	Varies	14%/y
UnitedHealth Group	+	− to +++	++	—	++	1990 to date	Unknown
Medicaid databases	+++	− to +++	++	—	++	—c	20–25%/y
Health databases in Saskatchewan	+++	− to +++	++	—	+	9/75–6/87, 1/89 to date	Nil
Netherlands	+++	+ to +++	+	—	—	1987 to date	Nil
Tayside	+++	+ to +++	++	—	+	1989 to date	Nil
GPRD	++	++ to +++	++	+/−	+++	1990 to date	5%
Ad hoc analyses of secular trends	Variable	Variable	—	Variable	+	As desired	N/A
Case–control surveillance	+ to ++	+++	+++	—	+	1975 to date	N/A
Registry-based case–control studies	+ to ++	+++	++		Variable	Variable	N/A
Ad hoc case–control studies	+ to ++	+++	+++	+	+	As desired	N/A
Prescription-Event Monitoring	+++	+++	++	—	+++	Variable	25%
Pharmacy-based surveillance: outpatient	+++	+++	+++	—	+	As desired	Variable
Ad hoc cohort studies	+++	+++	+++	+	+++	As desired	Variable
Pharmacoepidemiology randomized trials	+++	+++	+++	+	++++	As desired	Variable

a See the text of this chapter for descriptions of the column headings, and previous chapters for descriptions of the data resources.
b Varies by Kaiser site.
c Varies by state and data vendor.

Whether a database is *population-based* refers to whether there is an identifiable population, all of whose medical care would be included in that database, regardless of the provider. This allows one to determine incidence rates of diseases, as well as being more certain that one knows of all medical care that any given patient receives. As an example, assuming little or no out-of-plan care, the Kaiser programs are population-based. One can use Kaiser data, therefore, to study medical care received in and out of the hospital, as well as diseases which may result in repeat hospitalizations. For example, one could study the impact of the treatment initially received for venous thromboembolism on the risk of subsequent disease recurrence. In contrast, hospital-based case–control studies are not population-based: they include only the specific hospitals that belong to the system. Thus, a patient diagnosed with and treated for venous thromboembolism in a participating hospital could be readmitted to a different, nonparticipating, hospital if the disease recurred. This recurrence would not be detected in a study using such a system. The data resources that are population-based are those which use data from organized medical systems. Registry-based and *ad hoc* case–control studies can occasionally be conducted as population-based studies, if all cases in a defined geographic area are recruited into the study,[1] but this is unusual (see also Chapters 2 and 23).

Whether *cohort studies are possible* within a particular data resource would depend on whether individuals can be identified by whether or not they were exposed to a drug of interest. This would be true in any of the population-based systems, as well as any of the systems designed to perform cohort studies.

Whether *case–control studies are possible* within a given data resource depends on whether patients can be identified by whether or not they suffered from a disease of interest. This would be true in any of the population-based systems. Data from spontaneous reporting systems can be used for case finding for case–control studies, although this has been done infrequently.[2]

The *validity of the exposure data* is most certain in hospital-based settings, where one can be reasonably certain of both the identity of a drug and that the patient actually ingested it. Exposure data in spontaneous reporting systems come mostly from health care providers and, so, are probably valid. However, one cannot be certain of patient compliance in these data. Exposure data from organized systems of medical care are unbiased data recorded by pharmacies, often for billing purposes, a process that is closely audited as it impacts on reimbursement. These data are likely to be accurate, therefore, although again one cannot assure compliance. In addition, in health maintenance organizations (HMOs) there are drugs that may fall beneath a patient's deductibles, or not be on formularies. For UnitedHealth Group, since Medicare drug benefits vary depending on the plan, pharmacy files may not capture all prescribed drugs if beneficiaries reach the drug benefit limit. In GPRD, drugs prescribed by physicians other than the general practitioner could be missed, although continuing prescribing by the general practitioner would be detected. Case–control studies generally rely on patient histories for exposure data. These may be very inaccurate, as patients often do not recall correctly the medications they are taking.[3] However, this would be expected to vary, depending on the type of drug taken, the questioning technique used, etc.[3–11] (see Chapter 45).

The *validity of the outcome data* is also most certain in hospital-based settings, in which the patient is subjected to intensive medical surveillance. It is least certain in out-patient data from organized systems of medical care. There are, however, methods of improving the accuracy of these data, such as using drugs and procedures as markers of the disease and obtaining primary medical records. The outcome data from automated databases are listed as variable, therefore, depending on exactly which data are being used, and how. GPRD analyzes the actual medical record, rather than claims, and can access additional questionnaire data from the general practitioner as well.

Control of confounding refers to the ability to control for confounding variables. The most powerful approach to controlling for confounding is the randomized clinical trial. As discussed in Chapter 2, the randomized clinical trial is the only way of controlling for unknown, unmeasured, or unmeasurable confounding variables. Approaches that collect sufficient information to control for known and measurable variables are next most effective. These include Group Health, GPRD, Kaiser, case–control surveillance, *ad hoc* case–control studies, and *ad hoc* cohort studies. The health databases in Saskatchewan, UnitedHealth Group, Tayside, Medicaid (sometimes), and the HMO Research Network can obtain primary medical records, but not all information necessary is always available in those records. They generally are unable to contact patients to obtain supplementary information that might not be in a medical record. Medicaid databases have considerable additional data available, but are no longer as certain to be able to access medical records. Finally, spontaneous reporting systems and analyses of trends do not provide for control of confounding.

Relatively few of the data systems have data on *inpatient drug use*. The exceptions include spontaneous reporting systems, Group Health (only since 1989, and not yet used for research), Harvard Pilgrim Health Care (within the HMO Research Network), *ad hoc* studies, and the rare analyses of trends designed to study inpatient drug use.

Only a few of the data resources have sufficient *data on outpatient diagnoses* available without special effort, to be able to study them as outcome variables. *Ad hoc* studies can be designed to be able to collect such information. In the case of *ad hoc* randomized clinical trials, this data collection effort could even include tailored laboratory and physical examination measurements. In some of the resources, the outpatient outcome data are collected observationally, but directly via the physician, and so are more likely to be accurate. Included are spontaneous reporting systems, GPRD, the HMO Research Network, Prescription-Event Monitoring, and some *ad hoc* cohort studies. Other outpatient data come via physician claims for medical care, including Medicaid databases, UnitedHealth Group, and the health databases in Saskatchewan. The latter include outpatient data, but only to three digits of the ICD-9 coding system. Finally, other data resources can access outpatient diagnoses only via the patient, and so they are less likely to be complete; although the diagnosis can often be validated using medical records, it generally needs to be identified by the patient. These include most case–control studies and outpatient pharmacy-based monitoring.

The *start dates and duration* of the available data differ substantially among the different resources, as does the degree of *loss to follow-up*. They are specified in Table 24.1.

CHARACTERISTICS OF RESEARCH QUESTIONS AND THEIR IMPACT ON THE CHOICE OF PHARMACOEPIDEMIOLOGIC DATA RESOURCES

Once one is familiar with the characteristics of the pharmaco-epidemiology resources available, one must then examine more closely the research question, to determine which resources can best be used to answer it (see Table 24.2).

Pharmacoepidemiology studies can be undertaken to generate hypotheses about drug effects, to strengthen hypotheses, and/or to test *a priori* hypotheses about drug effects. *Hypothesis-generating studies* are studies designed to raise new questions about possible unexpected drug effects, whether adverse or beneficial. Virtually all studies can and do raise such questions, through incidental findings in studies performed for other reasons. In addition, virtually any case–control study could be used, in principle, to screen for possible drug causes of a disease under study, and virtually any cohort study could be used to screen for unexpected

outcomes from a drug exposure under study. In practice, however, the only approaches that have attempted to do this systematically have been Kaiser Permanente, case–control surveillance, Prescription-Event Monitoring, and Medicaid databases, none of which have resulted in notable new findings. To date, the most productive source of new hypotheses about drug effects has been spontaneous reporting.

Hypothesis-strengthening studies are studies designed to provide support for, although not definitive evidence for, existing hypotheses. The objective of these studies is to provide sufficient support for, or evidence against, a hypothesis to permit a decision about whether a subsequent, more definitive, study should be undertaken. As such, hypothesis-strengthening studies need to be conducted rapidly and inexpensively. Hypothesis-strengthening studies can include crude analyses conducted using almost any data set, evaluating a hypothesis which arose elsewhere. Because potentially confounding variables would not be controlled, the findings could not be considered definitive. Alternatively, hypothesis-strengthening studies can be more detailed studies, controlling for confounding, conducted using the same data resource that raised the hypothesis. In this case, because the study is not specifically undertaken to test an *a priori* hypothesis, the hypothesis-testing type of study can only serve to strengthen, not test, the hypothesis. Spontaneous reporting systems are useful for raising hypotheses, but are not very useful for providing additional support for those hypotheses. Conversely, randomized trials can certainly strengthen hypotheses, but are generally too costly and logistically too complex to be used for this purpose. Of the remaining approaches, those that can quickly access, in computerized form, both exposure data and outcome data are most useful. Those that can rapidly access only one of these data types, only exposure or only outcome data, are next most useful, while those that need to gather both data types are least useful, because of the time and expense that would be entailed.

Hypothesis-testing studies are studies designed to evaluate in detail hypotheses raised elsewhere. Such studies must be able to have simultaneous comparison groups and must be able to control for most known potential confounding variables. For these reasons, spontaneous reporting systems cannot be used for this purpose, as they cannot be used to conduct studies with simultaneous controls (with rare exceptions—see Strom *et al.*).[2] Analyses of trends cannot be used to test hypotheses as they cannot control for confounding. The most powerful approach, of course, is a randomized clinical trial, as it is the only way to control for unknown or unmeasurable confounding variables. Techniques which allow access to patients and their medical

Table 24.2. Characteristics of research questions and their impact on the choice of pharmacoepidemiologic data resource[a]

Pharmacoepidemiology approach	Hypothesis generating[b]	Hypothesis strengthening[c]	Hypothesis testing[d]	Study of benefits (versus risks)	Incidence rates desired	Low incidence outcome
Spontaneous reporting	++++	+	—	+	—	++++
Group Health Cooperative	+	+++	+++	+	+++	+
Kaiser Permanente Medical Care Programs	++	++	+++	+	+++	+++
The HMO Research Network	+	++++	++++	+	++++	++++
UnitedHealth Group	+	++++	++++	+	++++	++++
Medicaid databases	++	++++	+	+	++++	++++
Health databases in Saskatchewan	+	++++	+++	+	++++	++
Netherlands	+	++	+++	+	++++	++++
Tayside	+	++++	+++	+	++++	+
GPRD	+	++++	+++	+	++++	++
Ad hoc analyses of secular trends	+	+++	—	+	—	++++
Case–control surveillance	++	+++	+++	+	—	++++
Registry-based case–control studies	+	+++	+++	+	+	+++
Ad hoc case–control studies	+	++	++++	+	+	++++
Prescription-Event Monitoring	+	++	++++	+	+++	++++
Pharmacy-based surveillance: outpatient	+	++	+++	+	+++	++
Ad hoc cohort studies	+	++	+++	+	+++	++
Pharmacoepidemiology randomized trials	+	+	++++	++++	++	+

Table 24.2. (Continued)

Pharmacoepidemiology approach	Low prevalence exposure	Important confounders	Drug use inpatient (versus outpatient)	Outcome does not result in hospitalization	Outcome does not result in medical attention	Outcome a delayed effect	Exposure a new drug	Urgent question
Spontaneous reporting	+++	+	++++	++++	+	+	++++	++++
Group Health Cooperative	+	+++	−	−	−	+++	++	++++
Kaiser Permanente Medical Care Programs	+++	+++	+/−	+	−	++	++	+++
The HMO Research Network	+++	++	+/−	+	−	++	++	++
UnitedHealth Group	++++	++	−	+++	−	−	+++	+++
Medicaid databases	++	+	−	+++	−	+	++	+++
Health databases in Saskatchewan	++++	+−	−	++	−	++++	+++	++++
Netherlands	+	+	−	−	−		+++	+++
Tayside	++	+	−	−	−	−	+++	+++
GPRD	−	++	+/−	++++	−	−	+++	++
Ad hoc analyses of secular trends	+	−	−	−	−	++	+	+ to ++++
Case-control surveillance	+	++	−	−	−	++	+	+
Registry-based case–control studies	+	++	−	+	+	++	+	+
Ad hoc case–control studies	++++	+++	++++	+++	−	++	+	+ to ++++
Prescription-Event Monitoring	+++	++	−	++++	++	+	++++	+
Pharmacy-based surveillance: outpatient	+++	+++	−	++++	++	++	++++	+
Ad hoc cohort studies	++	+++	+	+++	+++	++	+++	+
Pharmacoepidemiology randomized trials	+++	+++	+	++++	++++	+	++++	+

a See the text of this chapter for descriptions of the column headings, and previous chapters for descriptions of the data resources.
b Hypothesis-generating studies are studies designed to raise new questions about possible unexpected drug effects, whether adverse or beneficial.
c Hypothesis-strengthening studies are studies designed to provide support for, although not definitive evidence for, existing hypotheses.
d Hypothesis-testing studies are studies designed to evaluate in detail hypotheses raised elsewhere.

records are the next most powerful, as one can gather information on potential confounders that might only be reliably obtained from one of those sources or the other. Techniques which allow access to primary records but not the patient are next most useful.

The research implications of questions about the *beneficial effects* of drugs are different, depending upon whether the beneficial effects of interest are expected or unexpected effects. Studies of *unexpected beneficial effects* are exactly analogous to studies of unexpected adverse effects, in terms of their implications to one's choice of an approach; in both situations one is studying side effects. Studies of *expected beneficial effects*, or drug efficacy, raise the special methodologic problem of confounding by the indication: patients who receive a drug are different from those who do not in a way which usually is related to the outcome under investigation in the study. This issue is discussed in detail in Chapter 40. As described there, it *is* sometimes possible to address these questions using nonexperimental study designs. Generally, however, the randomized clinical trial is far preferable, when feasible.

In order to address questions about the *incidence of a disease* in those exposed to a drug, one must be able to quantitate how many people received the drug. This information can be obtained using any resource that can perform a cohort study. Techniques that need to gather the outcome data *de novo* may miss some of the outcomes if there is incomplete participation and/or reporting of outcomes, such as with Prescription-Event Monitoring, *ad hoc* cohort studies, and outpatient pharmacy-based cohort studies. On the other hand, *ad hoc* data collection is the only way of collecting information about outcomes that need not come to medical attention (see below). The only approaches that are free from either of these problems are the hospital-based approaches. Registry-based case–control studies and *ad hoc* case–control studies can occasionally be used to estimate incidence rates, if one obtains a complete collection of cases from a defined geographic area. The other approaches listed cannot be used to calculate incidence rates.

To address a question about a *low incidence outcome*, one needs to study a large population (see Chapter 3). This can best be done using spontaneous reporting, Prescription-Event Monitoring, the Netherlands system, or *ad hoc* analyses of secular trends, which can or do cover entire countries. Alternatively, one could use UnitedHealth Group, the HMO Research Network, or Medicaid databases, which cover a large proportion of the United States, or GPRD in the UK. Kaiser in Northern California includes 2.8 million subscribers, Kaiser in Southern California over 2 million, and Kaiser Northwest about 440 000. Saskatchewan contains a population of about one million. Pharmacy-based surveillance methods and *ad hoc* cohort studies could potentially be expanded to cover equivalent populations. Group Health Cooperative includes fewer individuals and so would be less useful to answer questions about uncommon outcomes. Tayside is also small. Case–control studies, either *ad hoc* studies, studies using registries, or studies using case–control surveillance, can also be expanded to cover large populations, although not as large as the previously mentioned approaches. Because case–control studies recruit study subjects on the basis of the patients suffering from a disease, they are more efficient than attempting to perform such studies using analogous cohort studies. Finally, randomized trials could, in principle, be expanded to achieve very large sample sizes, but this would be very difficult and costly.

To address a question about a *low prevalence exposure*, one also needs to study a large population (see Chapter 3). Again, this can best be done using spontaneous reporting, the Netherlands system, or Prescription-Event Monitoring, which cover entire countries. Alternatively, one could use UnitedHealth Group, the HMO Research Network, or Medicaid databases, which cover a large proportion of the United States, or GPRD in the UK. Pharmacy-based surveillance methods and *ad hoc* cohort studies could also be used to recruit exposed patients from a large population. Analogously, randomized trials, which specify exposure, could assure an adequate number of exposed individuals. Case–control studies, either *ad hoc* studies, studies using registries, or studies using case–control surveillance, could theoretically be expanded to cover a large enough population, but this would be difficult and expensive. *Ad hoc* analyses of trends would not be useful, as a change in the prevalence of a rare exposure is unlikely to affect the general burden of disease enough to be detectable.

When there are *important confounders* that need to be taken into account in order to answer the question at hand, then one needs to be certain that sufficient and accurate information is available on those confounders. Spontaneous reporting systems and analyses of trends cannot be used for this purpose. The most powerful approach is a randomized trial, as it is the only way to control for unknown or unmeasurable confounding variables. Techniques which allow access to patients and their medical records are the next most powerful, as one can gather information on potential confounders that might only be reliably obtained from one of those sources or the other. Techniques which allow access to primary records but not the patient are the next most useful.

If the research question involves *inpatient* drug use, then the data resource must obviously be capable of collecting data on inpatient drug exposures. The number of approaches that have this capability are limited, and include spontaneous reporting systems, Harvard Pilgrim Health Care (part of the HMO Research Network), and inpatient pharmacy-based surveillance systems. *Ad hoc* studies could also, of course, be designed to collect such information in the hospital.

When the *outcome under study does not result in hospitalization, but does result in medical attention*, the best approaches are randomized trials and *ad hoc* studies which can be specifically designed to be sure this information can be collected. Prescription-Event Monitoring and GPRD, which collect their data from general practitioners, are excellent sources of data for this type of question. Reports of such outcomes are likely to come to spontaneous reporting systems as well. Medicaid databases can also be used, as they include outpatient data, although one must be cautious about the validity of the diagnosis information in outpatient claims. Saskatchewan is similar, although outpatient data is more limited. Finally, registry-based case–control studies could theoretically be performed, if they included outpatient cases of the disease under study.

When the *outcome under study does not result in medical attention at all*, the approaches available are much more limited. Only randomized trials can be specifically designed to be certain this information is collected. *Ad hoc* studies can be designed to try to collect such information from patients. Finally, occasionally one could collect information on such an outcome in a spontaneous reporting system, if the report came from a patient or if the report came from a health care provider who became aware of the problem while the patient was visiting for medical care for some other problem.

When the *outcome under study is a delayed drug effect*, then one obviously needs approaches capable of tracking individuals over a long period of time. The best approach for this is the health databases in Saskatchewan. Drug data are available for more than 25 years, and there is little turnover in the population covered. Thus, this is an ideal system within which to perform such long-term studies. Group Health Cooperative, Kaiser Permanente, and parts of the HMO Research Network have even longer follow-up time available. However, as HMOs they suffer from some turnover, albeit more modest after the first few years of enrollment. Analogously, any of the methods of conducting case–control studies can address such questions, although one would have to be especially careful about the validity of the exposure information collected many years after the exposure. Medicaid databases have been available since 1973. However, the large turnover in Medicaid programs, due to changes in eligibility with changes in family and

employment status, makes studies of long-term drug effects problematic. Similarly, one could conceivably perform studies of long-term drug effects using *ad hoc* analyses of secular trends, Prescription-Event Monitoring, outpatient pharmacy-based surveillance, *ad hoc* cohort studies, or randomized clinical trials, but these approaches are not as well suited to this type of question as the previously discussed techniques. Theoretically, one also could identify long-term drug effects in a spontaneous reporting system. This is unlikely, however, as a physician is unlikely to link a current medical event with a drug exposure long ago.

When *the exposure under study is a new drug*, then one is, of course, limited to data sources that collect data on recent exposures, and preferably those that can collect a significant number of such exposures quickly. *Ad hoc* cohort studies or a randomized clinical trial are ideal for this, as they recruit patients into the study on the basis of their exposure. Spontaneous reporting is similarly a good approach for this, as new drugs are automatically and immediately covered, and in fact reports are much more common in the first three years after a drug is marketed. The major databases are next most useful, especially Medicaid databases, the HMO Research Network, and UnitedHealth, as their large population bases will allow one to accumulate a sufficient number of exposed individuals rapidly, so one can perform a study sooner. In some cases, there is a delay until the drug is available on the program's formulary, however. *Ad hoc* analyses of secular trends and case–control studies, by whatever approach, must wait until sufficient drug exposure has occurred that it can affect the outcome variable being studied.

Finally, if *one needs an answer to a question urgently*, potentially the fastest approach, if the needed data are included, is a spontaneous reporting system; drugs are included in these systems immediately, and an extremely large population base is covered. Of course, one cannot rely on any adverse reaction being detected in a spontaneous reporting system. The computerized databases are also useful for these purposes, depending on the speed with which the exposures accumulate in that database; of course, if the drug in question is not on the formulary in question, it cannot be studied. Analyses of secular trends can be mounted faster than other *ad hoc* studies, and so these can be useful sometimes when an alternative approach will not work. The remaining approaches are of limited use, as they take too long to address a question. One exception to this is Prescription-Event Monitoring, if the drug in question happens to have been a subject of one of its studies.

The other, and more likely, exception is case–control surveillance, if the disease under study is available in adequate numbers in its database, either because it was the topic of a prior study or because there were a sufficient number of individuals with the disease collected to be included in control groups for prior studies.

EXAMPLES

As an example, one might want to explore whether nonsteroidal anti-inflammatory drugs (NSAIDs) cause upper gastrointestinal bleeding and, if so, how often. One could examine the manufacturer's premarketing data from clinical trials, but the number of patients included is not likely to be large enough to study clinical bleeding, and the setting is very artificial. Alternatively, one could examine premarketing studies using more sensitive outcome measures, such as endoscopy. However, these are even more artificial. Instead, one could use any of the databases to address the question quickly, as they have data on drug exposures that preceded the hospital admission. Some databases could only be used to investigate gastrointestinal bleeding resulting in hospitalization (e.g., Kaiser Permanente, except via chart review, or Tayside). Others could be used to explore inpatient or outpatient bleeding (e.g., Medicaid, Saskatchewan). Because of confounding by cigarette smoking, alcohol, etc., which would not be well measured in these databases, one also might want to address this question using case–control or cohort studies, whether conducted *ad hoc* or using any of the special approaches available, for example case–control surveillance or Prescription-Event Monitoring. If one wanted to be able to calculate incidence rates, one would need to restrict these studies to cohort studies, rather than case–control studies. One would be unlikely to be able to use registries, as there are no registries, known to this author at least, which record patients with upper gastrointestinal bleeding. One would not be able to perform analyses of secular trends, as upper gastrointestinal bleeding would not appear in vital statistics data, except as a cause of death. Studying death from upper gastrointestinal bleeding is problematic, as it is a disease from which patients usually do not die. Rather than studying determinants of upper gastrointestinal bleeding, one would really be studying determinants of complications from upper gastrointestinal bleeding, diseases for which upper gastrointestinal bleeding is a complication, or determinants of physicians' decisions to withhold supportive transfusion therapy from patients with upper gastrointestinal bleeding, for example age, terminal illnesses, etc.

Alternatively, one might want to address a similar question about nausea and vomiting caused by NSAIDs. Although this question is very similar, one's options in addressing it would be much more limited, as nausea and vomiting often do not come to medical attention. Other than a randomized clinical trial, for a drug that is largely used on an outpatient basis one is limited to outpatient pharmacy-based surveillance systems which request information from patients, or *ad hoc* cohort studies.

As another example, one might want to follow up on a signal generated by the spontaneous reporting system, designing a study to investigate whether a drug which has been on the market for, say, five years is a cause of a relatively rare condition, such as allergic hypersensitivity reactions. Because of the infrequency of the disease, one would need to draw on a very large population. The best alternatives would be Medicaid databases, the HMO Research Network, United Health Group, *ad hoc* analyses of trends, case–control studies, or Prescription-Event Monitoring. To expedite this hypothesis-testing study and limit costs, it would be desirable if it could be performed using existing data. Prescription-Event Monitoring and case–control surveillance would be excellent ways of addressing this, but only if the drug or disease in question, respectively, had been the subject of a prior study. Other methods of conducting case–control studies require gathering exposure data *de novo*.

As a last example, one might want to follow up on a signal generated by a spontaneous reporting system, designing a study to investigate whether a drug which has been on the market for, say, three years is a cause of an extremely rare but serious illness, such as aplastic anemia. One's considerations would be similar to those above, but even Medicaid databases would not be sufficiently large to include enough cases. One would have to gather data *de novo*. Assuming the drug in question is used mostly by outpatients, one could consider using Prescription-Event Monitoring or a case–control study.

CONCLUSION

Once one has decided to perform a pharmacoepidemiology study, one needs to decide which of the resources described in the earlier chapters of this book should be used. By considering the characteristics of the pharmacoepidemiology resources available as well as the characteristics of the question to be addressed, one should be able to choose those resources that are best suited to addressing the question at hand.

REFERENCES

1. Anonymous. Risks of agranulocytosis and aplastic anemia. A first report of their relation to drug use with special reference to analgesics. The International Agranulocytosis and Aplastic Anemia Study. *JAMA* 1986; **256**: 1749–57.
2. Strom BL, West SL, Sim E, Carson JL. Epidemiology of the acute flank pain syndrome from suprofen. *Clin Pharmacol Ther* 1989; **46**: 693–9.
3. Klemetti A, Saxen L. Prospective versus retrospective approach in the search for environmental causes of malformations. *Am J Public Health* 1967; **57**: 2071–5.
4. Glass R, Johnson B, Vessey M. Accuracy of recall of histories of oral contraceptive use. *Br J Prev Soc Med* 1974; **28**: 273–5.
5. Stolley PD, Tonascia JA, Sartwell PE, Tockman MS, Tonascia S, Rutledge A *et al.* Agreement rates between oral contraceptive users and prescribers in relation to drug use histories. *Am J Epidemiol* 1978; **107**: 226–35.
6. Paganini-Hill A, Ross RK. Reliability of recall of drug usage and other health-related information. *Am J Epidemiol* 1982; **116**: 114–22.
7. Rosenberg MJ, Layde PM, Ory HW, Strauss LT, Rooks JB, Rubin GL. Agreement between women's histories of oral contraceptive use and physician records. *Int J Epidemiol* 1983; **12**: 84–7.
8. Schwarz A, Faber U, Borner K, Keller F, Offermann G, Molzahn M. Reliability of drug history in analgesic users. *Lancet* 1984; **2**: 1163–4.
9. Coulter A, Vessey M, McPherson K. The ability of women to recall their oral contraceptive histories. *Contraception* 1986; **33**: 127–39.
10. Mitchell AA, Cottler LB, Shapiro S. Effect of questionnaire design on recall of drug exposure in pregnancy. *Am J Epidemiol* 1986; **123**: 670–6.
11. Persson I, Bergkvist L, Adami HO. Reliability of women's histories of climacteric oestrogen treatment assessed by prescription forms. *Int J Epidemiol* 1987; **16**: 222–8.

Part IV

SELECTED SPECIAL APPLICATIONS OF PHARMACOEPIDEMIOLOGY

25

National Medicinal Drug Policies: Their Relationship to Pharmacoepidemiology

SUZANNE HILL and DAVID A. HENRY

Faculty of Medicine and Health Sciences, The University of Newcastle, NSW, Australia.

INTRODUCTION

Pharmacoepidemiology exists primarily to quantify the effects of medicinal drugs in communities. Drug policies are the instruments used by governments (with varying degrees of success) to control the development, distribution, subsidization, pricing, and use of drugs in communities. Pharmacoepidemiologic methods, such as pharmacoeconomics, drug utilization studies, adverse drug reaction monitoring, and formal analytical designs, are some of the tools that can be used to plan, monitor, and evaluate medicinal drug policies. It can be seen that drug policies are very relevant to pharmacoepidemiology, and vice versa.

Although there are obviously numerous different policy issues in relation to medicines, in this chapter we wish to concentrate on national medicinal drug policies (NMDP), which have become a topical subject in recent years. A comprehensive NMDP covers four aspects: ensuring the *quality* of pharmaceuticals that are available in a given setting, enabling *access* to affordable medicines, ensuring *appropriate use* of medicines, and ensuring a viable and appropriate pharmaceutical industry. A number of developing and developed countries now have comprehensive written policies that are implemented to varying degrees. It must also be recognized that many countries have made significant progress in controlling the supply and use of modern drugs without recourse to written policies. However, national governments, district health authorities, and managed care organizations around the world have to deal with the rising costs of modern drugs, and the results of the suboptimal prescribing and consumption patterns that are common in so many communities. National policies that set standards to be followed by manufacturers, health care organizations, health professionals, and patients are very valuable, even in an era of "small government." Such policies have to operate in an environment shaped by budgetary pressures, community expectations, medical politics, corporate lobbying, and media coverage.

This chapter can do no more than scratch the surface of this complex subject; many specific issues are covered in more detail in other chapters (e.g., adverse reaction detection, drug utilization studies, and pharmacoeconomics). Readers who wish to learn more are referred to the website of the World Health Organization/Essential Drugs and Medicines

Pharmacoepidemiology, Fourth Edition   Edited by B.L. Strom
© 2005 John Wiley & Sons, Ltd

(WHO/EDM) (www.who.int/medicines), which has an extensive range of technical reports, and to an excellent publication *Managing Drug Supply*.[1] We have drawn extensively on this work when compiling this chapter.

CLINICAL PROBLEMS TO BE ADDRESSED BY PHARMACOEPIDEMIOLOGIC RESEARCH

The "problem" that needs to be addressed in relation to drug policies has been succinctly defined by Sven Hamrell[2] in a study of drug policy in South-East Asia.

> 'The problem isn't so much in the drugs, which are medicines used to relieve sickness or cure disease. The problem lies in the way these drugs are dispensed, manufactured and marketed. The problem can be put simply: there is a disparity between the world's health needs and what drugs the world actually gets.'

It is a sad indictment of our attempts to improve the health of the world's populations that, while the technologies and treatments needed to save lives and reduce suffering are technically feasible and available in many countries, they are denied to too many of those who need them most. The reasons are a lack of political will, an international desire to protect the commercial interests of some of the world's most profitable corporations, and significant failures of national drug policy development and implementation in many developing countries.

The problems that beset developing countries can be categorized under four broad and overlapping headings, that reflect the components needed in an NMDP:

- poor quality and counterfeit drugs;
- lack of availability of essential drugs for a population;
- poor quality use of pharmaceuticals (e.g., overuse, misuse, polypharmacy);
- the effects of international activities, particularly the development of trade agreements and law on intellectual property.

It is entirely appropriate to give priority to the policy needs of developing countries. However, there are many examples of policy failures in developed countries as well, and we will highlight some of these in this chapter in addition.

POOR QUALITY AND COUNTERFEIT DRUGS

Drugs must be produced according to appropriate standards of good manufacturing practice (GMP). Such standards have been developed and implemented in most developed countries, and are widely promulgated by the World Health Organization and include controls on all aspects of the manufacturing process for pharmaceuticals. Notwithstanding the systems for assessing GMP that are in place in many developed countries, counterfeit and poor quality products are an increasing problem. In the US in 2002, substandard erythropoietin (i.e., inadequate active ingredient) was identified, and in 2003, counterfeit atorvastatin (branded as Lipitor) was identified from adverse reaction reports of bitter tasting tablets that caused a burning sensation on the tongue.[3]

Many developing countries do not have the technical, financial, or human resources required for the implementation of GMP, and the quality problems, including counterfeit products, in these countries are significantly worse. Essential medicines such as quinine, amoxicillin, aspirin, and prednisolone have been found to be substandard in many ways (including inadequate active ingredient, and incorrect excipients) in many settings.[4-6] Often criticized for their promotional activities in developing countries, transnational pharmaceutical manufacturers have high quality manufacturing practices and can help maintain standards in developing countries. However, because many drugs are unaffordable (at international prices), there are major incentives for the development of local producers. Lack of technical expertise, and ineffective government inspection, may lead to substandard products being sold, and in some circumstances contaminated or counterfeit products becoming available. Hanif *et al.*[7] and O'Brien *et al.*[8] provide the two most recent descriptions of "epidemics" of renal failure in children due to diethylene glycol contamination of acetaminophen syrup (perhaps mistaken for the nontoxic propylene glycol). There are many other reports of diethylene glycol poisonings, dating back to the 1937 "epidemic" in the United States.[9-13] In all cases, the contamination has been a result of the failure of manufacturing practice, or the failure of regulatory and surveillance systems to adequately control manufacturing practices.

Counterfeit drugs are another manifestation of problems of inadequate regulation and control of the quality of pharmaceuticals. A recent example was the release of a counterfeit meningococcal vaccine during an epidemic of meningitis in Niger.[14,15] As described by Pecoul *et al.*[16] the problem was first noted when a team from Médecins Sans Frontières working with local health workers noticed that vaccines from Nigeria, labeled as a product from Pasteur Merieux, had an unusual appearance. Subsequent investigations identified them as counterfeit. It was estimated that approximately 60 000 persons were vaccinated with the false vaccine; the scale of the production would have required a large-scale manufacturing facility. In other words, this was large-scale organized crime, certainly not an isolated example.

There seem to be two general groups of counterfeit products—organized illegal circuits that manufacture copies of known trademarked products, and nonorganized production of small quantities of inadequate or substandard products, including generic drugs. Shakoor et al.[17] described a study of chloroquine products available in Thailand and Nigeria which found that 36.5% of the products sampled were substandard. In general, this appeared to be due to substandard manufacturing processes and problems with decomposition of the products, rather than fraudulent manufacturing. Nazerali and Hogerzeil[18] described a similar problem in an investigation of the quality of essential drugs in Zimbabwe; they identified initial quality problems with ampicillin, retinol, and ergometrine, as well as problems with the stability of ergometrine injections over time.

Ensuring that pharmaceutical products are of satisfactory quality does not only require adequate controls on manufacturing. Systems of GMP if appropriately implemented may provide some certainty about manufacturing processes, but in addition there should be systems that monitor and control the pharmaceutical market in a country, including controls over distribution and sale of a product. An adequate distribution system for drugs is critical to ensure that drugs reach the user in good condition. Degradation of products during distribution has been most extensively documented for vaccines; this has been a problem in both developed and developing countries. Standards for vaccine handling have been developed by WHO, initially to allow for the transport of the most fragile of the essential vaccines, oral polio vaccine.[19] Studies in South Africa,[20] Italy,[21] Australia,[22–25] Malaysia,[26] India,[27] and Nigeria[28] document the difficulties of maintaining an adequate cold chain in different environments. The problems that were identified ranged from the central storage facility having inadequate monitoring systems, to refrigerators in pharmacies and doctors' practices being inadequate for storage of vaccines immediately prior to their administration.

Serious problems can also occur during bulk transport. Hogerzeil et al.[29] examined drugs that were shipped by sea or land from a donor agency to recipient countries. They found that the drugs in the shipment were exposed to much higher temperatures and humidity than was recommended by their manufacturers. However, this only affected the clinical effectiveness of two of the products.

In general, ensuring that quality pharmaceuticals are available in a country requires that there is a competent drug regulatory authority. Although developed countries generally have competent regulatory authorities, the expense and technical skills required mean that developing countries' authorities are often unable to provide the full range of functions needed to ensure adequate quality of medicines available.

ACCESS: LACK OF AVAILABILITY OF ESSENTIAL MEDICINES

The chronic mismatch between drugs that are available in developing countries and the diseases and populations requiring treatment led to the development of the "essential drugs" concept. The history of this important movement has been described in detail by Kanji et al.[30] "Essential drugs," as defined by WHO in 1975, are "those considered to be of utmost importance and hence basic, indispensable and necessary for the health needs of the population. They should be available at all times, in the proper dosage forms, to all segments of society." The first model list of essential drugs was prepared by WHO in 1977; it is now in its 13th edition and listed in full at www.who.int/medicines/organization/par/edl/expcom13/eml13_en.pdf. Despite the policy having been adopted in many countries, Pecoul et al.[16] consider that access to essential drugs of adequate quality appears to be getting worse, not better, in many settings. This is illustrated when one considers the consumption of pharmaceuticals in various countries. Developed countries account for approximately 16% of the world's population, and in 1990, accounted for approximately 72% of consumption, with the US and EU being the largest markets. Developing countries account for approximately 77% of the world's population, and in 1990, consumed 19% of the pharmaceuticals. This has declined from 24% in 1975.[31]

There have been many studies that describe the lack of availability of essential drugs in developing and developed countries. In Rwanda, for example, Habiyambere and Wertheimer[32] estimated that 70% of the population did not have access to essential drugs. Another manifestation of this problem can be excessive and unregulated supply of the wrong drugs, as described by Luechai[33] in Thailand. The reasons for lack of essential drugs may vary from setting to setting, ranging from lack of production because the drug is unprofitable (such as meglumine antimoniate for leishmaniasis),[16] to because the drugs are too expensive, such as the widely discussed antiretrovirals for the treatment of HIV. Other more complex reasons have been described by Foster[34] and may relate to the structure of the local pharmaceutical market and the various components of the supply and distribution chain.

The mismatch between what is available and what is needed can lead to a range of strategies to obtain essential drugs. Kandela[35] illustrates this with the example of the effect of the economic embargo on Iraq. As the supply there of essential drugs became compromised, residents with relatives and friends overseas ensure that any visitor's suitcase contains supplies of basic drugs such as antibiotics and thyroxine. Kent and Glatzer[36] noted the chaos that developed in Bosnia, with the media coverage determining the supply of particular medicines. If the story of the week emphasized a shortage of anesthetic agents, the hospital concerned would be overwhelmed with inappropriate donation of expensive anesthetic agents at the expense of more essential products. (Drug donations are discussed in more detail below.)

Over the past 5 years, the WHO Model Essential Drugs List has been in the spotlight particularly in relation to the antiretrovirals used for the management of HIV/AIDS. Not only are these medicines generally expensive, but they are protected by patent and intellectual property rights. In particular, the agreement on Trade-Related Aspects of Intellectual Property Rights (TRIPS), which requires all member countries of the World Trade Organization to adhere to minimum standards of intellectual property protection, has significantly reduced access to new and essential medicines (see below for a more detailed discussion) and maintained high prices that keep them out of the reach of those who need them most.[37,38]

As described by Subramanian,[39] the TRIPS debate has also highlighted the large differences in prices of medicines between developed and developing countries. Sometimes low income countries end up paying higher prices than rich countries for patented medicines. This may accelerate the search for a new system of controls on patents that both provides incentives for creating knowledge and recovering the large fixed costs involved, but at the same time, allows maximum benefits from the diffusion and dissemination of the innovation.[39]

Lack of access to essential drugs is clearly not only a problem in developing countries. In developed countries, vulnerable populations can be without access to essential drugs, usually because of avoidable failures of government policy. The most spectacular examples of this are in the US, where a significant proportion of the population lacks guaranteed access to affordable supplies of the drugs that they need.[40] Attempts to contain drug costs at a state level or in managed care organizations can have unintended effects. In an earlier study, Soumerai et al.[41] described the impact of a three month prescription payment limit or "cap" on the use of psychotropic drugs and acute mental health

care by patients with schizophrenia. Not surprisingly, the "cap" resulted in an immediate reduction in the use of psychotropic medication by the population. With decreased consumption of essential medications, the use of acute mental health services (and the associated costs) increased. Rabon et al.[42] describe another manifestation of this type of problem in their survey of the availability of cancer medication in pharmacies in South Carolina. They found that only 25% of a list of cancer medications were available to be dispensed from 90% of the pharmacies surveyed.

In many cases, the lack of availability of essential drugs is due to the high prices being requested by manufacturers. This mismatch of demand and affordable supply is an important example of market failure, and the inadequacy of government intervention in many countries. International comparisons of prices of pharmaceuticals are difficult and are influenced by fluctuating exchange rates, variable purchasing power of currencies, and wages. However, Health Action International, a consumer organization that aims to promote the rational use of drugs, published price comparisons of 12 commonly used drugs in five Asian countries and Canada (HAI News, December 1995). Enormous price variation was documented. For example, the price of 100×150 mg ranitidine tablets ranged from $US3 in India to $US150 in Indonesia, presumably due to different manufacturers and suppliers negotiating different prices, plus the variability in retail systems.

Finally, it is important to recognize that "essential" drugs only deserve that title so long as they are used in an appropriate manner. There are many examples of the misuse of drugs on the WHO's model list, and ensuring appropriateness of use is just as important as establishing stable systems for selection, procurement, and distribution.

POOR QUALITY USE OF PHARMACEUTICALS

The third aspect of the policy problem that needs to be considered is the poor quality *use* of pharmaceuticals. This can be divided into three areas: overuse, underuse, and misuse. The problems of overuse have probably received most attention and there is an extensive literature in this field. The overuse and inappropriate use of antibiotics is a problem internationally.[43] Most surveys in developing countries show that antibiotics are prescribed in 35–60% of clinical visits, although they are appropriate in less than 20%.[44] The size of the antibiotic market in developing countries has been estimated to be double that of developed countries.[45] The factors that contribute to this include unregulated availability of products combined with poor prescribing and information. The resulting significant problems of antibiotic resistance have been extensively documented. Ironically, many patients are unable to afford more than 1 to 2 days' treatment. The perverse situation arises in which those who do not need the drugs receive a brief course, which may encourage antibiotic resistance, while those who really need antibiotics receive a totally inadequate course of treatment.

Overuse of drugs in developing countries is not restricted to antibiotics. Nonsteroidal anti-inflammatory drugs have been described as being inappropriately used in Brazil, where expenditure on one agent (diclofenac) exceeds that on almost any other drug—a clear example of the misalignment of community needs and clinical practice.[46] Elzubier and Al-Shehry[47] have documented the excessive use of vitamins in diabetic patients in Saudi Arabia.

Medication practices vary not only by country, but by area within a country, so that descriptive studies of local prescribing patterns are essential to determine the precise nature of the problem in any given locality.

Hogerzeil et al.[48] have described a standard set of indicators that were developed for the measurement of drug use in developing countries, but these can also be applied to a developed country setting, and are summarized in Table 25.1.

In developed countries, there are other manifestations of the problems of overuse and polypharmacy. Use of greater numbers of drug therapies has been found to be associated with an increased risk of developing adverse drug reactions.[49] Polypharmacy in the elderly has been shown to be associated with urinary incontinence, delirium,[50] and syncope.[51] Studies in a variety of settings have shown that patients over 65 years of age use an average of 2–6 prescribed medications and

1–3.4 non-prescribed medications.[52] In nursing homes in particular, overuse of psychotropic drugs has been shown to be a problem.[53]

Equally problematic, however, is the *underuse* of appropriate medications in this population. This is probably best documented for the lack of use of β-blockers following myocardial infarction,[54] although it has also been suggested to be the case for the use of diuretics in hypertension,[55] and until the recent studies, the use of hormone replacement therapy.[56]

An NMDP, therefore, needs to include the development of strategies that improve the use of medicines. These might include academic detailing and education of prescribers, prescriber audit and feedback, legal restriction on prescription of products for certain indications, and, importantly, education of consumers. While the relative effectiveness of each of these strategies will vary, what is clear from experience to date is that a diversity of approaches is needed to have a sustained impact on prescribing behavior.

ADVERSE EFFECTS OF INTERNATIONAL ACTIVITIES

Although this chapter is primarily concerned with national drug policies, we cannot ignore the impact of some important global trends. As noted above, a key challenge for many countries is dealing with the impact of trade agreements and TRIPS (see below). An additional issue is the difficulty created for national governments, and aid workers, by unsolicited donations of drugs during national emergencies caused by natural disasters or acts of war. Although these donations are nearly always well intended, they can create many problems, as has been well documented.[57] Sometimes donated drugs have been close to expiry and in poor condition, labeled in foreign languages, and quite inappropriate to the recipient country's short- to medium-term needs. Hogerzeil et al.[57] give a number of examples, including seven truckloads of expired aspirin tablets delivered to Eritrea that took six months to burn, and the arrival of contact lens solution, appetite stimulants, and lipid-lowering drugs in a war zone in the Sudan. The work involved in disposing of unwanted pharmaceuticals can tie up key personnel for long periods, and may be very costly if it involves either burying the pharmaceuticals in concrete-filled drums or high temperature incineration.

The motives behind drug donations may be altruistic (although perhaps not always—see below), but good intentions do not invariably translate into good deeds. One perverse incentive is the tax relief in the US that can be earned on the commercial value of drug donations. This has led to the

Table 25.1. Core drug-use indicators

Prescribing indicators
Average number of drugs per encounter
Percentage of drugs prescribed by generic name
Percentage of encounters with an antibiotic prescribed
Percentage of encounters with an injection prescribed
Percentage of drugs prescribed from essential drugs list or formulary

Patient care indicators
Average consultation time
Average dispensing time[a]
Percentage of drugs actually dispensed
Percentage of drugs adequately labeled
Patients' knowledge of correct dosage

Health facility indicators
Availability of a copy of essential drugs list or formulary
Availability of key drugs

---

[a] Time that personnel dispensing drugs spend with patients.
Source: Hogerzeil et al.[48]. Reproduced by permission of Elsevier.

cynical view that some manufacturers can make more money by donating expiring stock than trying to sell it to their normal clients. One difficulty for recipients of donations is that they do not want to appear ungrateful as it may compromise future, more appropriate, aid, and so vociferous complaints are uncommon.

The World Health Organization, in collaboration with a number of agencies, has produced detailed guidelines for drug donations (WHO/DAP 1996), and for the safe disposal of unwanted pharmaceuticals (WHO/EDM 1999). The guidelines make it clear that the responsibility of donors is to ensure that the recipients have been allowed to specify their needs, that the donations are appropriate, in good condition, have a long shelf-life, and are labeled in a way that enables them to be used effectively and safely in the field. If in doubt, cash donations will always be acceptable. It is likely that countries with well-established national drug policies will be well positioned to make the best use of appropriate drug donations.

The second major international influence comes in the form of the agreements on Trade-Related Intellectual Property Rights (TRIPS) mediated by the World Trade Organization (WTO). Through these agreements, member states are expected to guarantee intellectual property rights for a period of 20 years.[58] These agreements have the potential to limit the access of developing countries to new health technologies at affordable prices, as they might be denied the right to manufacture drugs locally at prices much lower than will be demanded by transnational corporations. This issue received a great deal of publicity during 1999 because of attempts by the US pharmaceutical industry to block the local production of cheap antiretroviral drugs in South Africa, where the prevalence of AIDS is very high. Much of the argument has centered on the legal interpretation of the WTO treaty obligations. However, most observers considered that TRIPS did not actually remove the right of countries to force compulsory licensing, (i.e., forcing an international manufacturer to give a license to a local manufacturer to produce a drug that is essential to the national interest). This position was admitted by the US Trade Secretary in late July 1999, after an effective campaign by AIDS activists in the US that was aimed at Vice-President Al Gore. A coalition of organizations including the US-based Consumer Project on Technology, Médecins Sans Frontières, and Health Action International held a meeting in early 1999 to explore ways of introducing compulsory licensing more widely as a means of improving the access of developing countries to the drugs that they need.

In response to a growing international outcry, the World Trade Organization (WTO) Ministerial meeting in Doha in 2002 made a landmark declaration that the TRIPS agreement should be implemented in a manner "supportive of WTO members' right to protect public health, and in particular to promote access to medicines for all." The Doha declaration also asserted the rights of countries to issue compulsory licenses for diseases that constitute a threat to public health. There have been a number of problems in the implementation of the principles embodied in the Doha declaration, including the use of compulsory licensing in countries with limited or non-existent local manufacturing capacity. Another threat has come in the form of a series of bilateral trade agreements (for instance those between the United States of America and Jordan, Chile, and Australia), which have not been under the close scrutiny of the international community. These trade agreements include more restrictions on compulsory licensing than TRIPS and enforce greater levels of intellectual property protection. They seem to be designed to undermine the principles of the Doha agreement and are a threat to the development of national medicinal drug policies. Although this issue may be seen as one grounded in obscure interpretations of international law, these are clearly important issues that are likely to have major implications for national drug policies in the future.[59]

METHODOLOGIC PROBLEMS TO BE ADDRESSED BY PHARMACOEPIDEMIOLOGIC RESEARCH

DEFINING NATIONAL MEDICINAL DRUG POLICIES

Public "policies" can range from having written documents that express intent on particular issues, to a complex process in which values, interests, and resources compete through institutions to influence government actions. They should be distinguished from "politics," although increasingly politics influence policy, as the costs of drugs continue to rise and restrictive policies are seen to limit access to drugs and to reduce corporate profits.

Health policies should reflect, and ideally meet, health needs. As pharmaceuticals are recognized to play a major role in meeting health needs, medicinal drug policies need to be part of health policies and use of drugs in a community should be consonant with overall health goals. This requires "careful analysis of existing and desirable relationships between health needs, drug demands and drug sales, within fluctuating political, economic and social pressures. These are often in conflict with each other because of the different and sometimes competing interests of the groups involved."[60]

Since the mid-1970s, NMDPs have been developed in many countries to ensure access to pharmaceutical products of adequate quality, safety, efficacy, and cost-effectiveness. These developments have received strong encouragement, and great practical support, from the World Health Organization, through its Action Program on Essential Drugs (recently restructured as the "Program for Essential Drugs and other Medicines"). As a result, drug policy development has become recognized as a legitimate topic for study, not just the preserve of governments.

Ideally, NMDPs should provide the framework to coordinate the activities of the pharmaceutical sector, the public and private sectors, NGOs, donors, and other stakeholders. They have been described as a "guide for action."[1] It is not only developing countries that should pursue such an approach; many developed countries have similar aims, but few have produced formal documents. Increasingly, experts are advocating that a policy document, even where the elements of a comprehensive NMDP already exist, can be of value, especially as part of any evaluation process.

OBJECTIVES OF NATIONAL MEDICINAL DRUG POLICIES

The objectives of an NMDP will vary from setting to setting, but in general terms, are likely to include the following:[1]

- to make essential drugs available and affordable to those who need them;
- to ensure the safety, efficacy, and quality of all medicines provided to the public;
- to improve prescribing and dispensing practices and to promote the correct use of medicines by health care workers and the public;
- to ensure an appropriate balance of local production and importation of pharmaceutical products;
- to build and maintain human capacity to ensure the sustainability of the NMDP.

Clearly, the extent to which these components are included in an individual country's NMDP will vary depending on the country's particular needs, and there are many examples of this variation. This is illustrated by Table 25.2, which summarizes the core objectives of national medicinal drug policies in a developing and developed country (using Australia as an example).

It is immediately apparent that there are similarities and differences between these two sets of NMDP objectives. Assuring the efficacy, safety, and quality of medicines is a common goal, but is much easier to achieve in developed

Table 25.2. Comparison of policy objectives in developing and developed countries

Developing country[1]	Developed country (Australia)
• To make essential drugs available and affordable to those who need them	• To achieve affordable access to a satisfactory range of cost-effective drugs
• To ensure the safety, efficacy, and quality of all medicines provided to the public	• To ensure the safety, efficacy, and quality of all medicines provided to the public
• To improve prescribing and dispensing practices and promote the correct use of medicines by health workers and the public	• To achieve quality use of medicines
	• To encourage the development of a successful pharmaceutical industry

countries because of the high quality of production facilities that usually exist in these countries. Both quality assurance procedures (maintenance of good manufacturing practices, close examination of data packages) and testing of samples can be carried out in a rigorous manner. As noted earlier, failure of these systems in developing countries may lead to drug contamination, substandard drugs, or counterfeit drugs. However, these processes are labor intensive, and expensive, and a large investment may not be a priority when the health budget is insufficient to meet the most basic needs of the community.

Relevant to this consideration is the objective of any industry policy that is in place. This is explicit in the Australian policy. Most governments in developed countries appear to give a high priority to investment by large pharmaceutical manufacturers (although sometimes the reasons for this lack clarity), and also encourage the local production of generics. In some cases, the large international companies own the generic manufacturers. The situation in developing countries is different. It is often unclear whether a government should encourage local generic manufacture (risking quality failures), investment in manufacturing capacity by international companies (which may provide employment but do little to meet the health needs of the local community), or the development of sound procurement practices using the international market for essential drugs (many suppliers are based in Europe, but increasingly supplies are from India and Brazil).

The affordability and accessibility of important drugs is an essential issue in any drug policy. Most developed countries (the US is a notable exception) have universal insurance programs that guarantee access to heavily subsidized drugs. Generally, the distribution and sales of drugs within such programs are handled fairly efficiently by the private sector.

Insurance programs are less common in developing countries, however, largely because of their great expense, and distribution systems that are taken for granted in developed countries often fail. A variety of procurement and distribution systems has been employed, with technical details that are beyond this scope of this chapter (see Quick *et al.*[1] for details). Finding the right public/private sector mix is a challenge: poor quality manufacture, theft, improper storage, and expiration due to poor stock control can lead to losses of 40% or more of the total value of purchases.[1]

Achieving quality use of medicines (a less pejorative term than "rational drug use") must be a priority in both developing and developed countries. In the former, the targets for educational campaigns and behavior change strategies include a wide range of health workers (including unlicensed drug sellers) and the public. In developed countries, most programs are aimed at prescribing doctors, and a few at consumers. However, essentially the aims are the same: to reduce the adverse effects associated with excessive drug use, to ensure that adequate treatment is given to those that need it, and to contain expenditures. In many ways, developing countries are more advanced in investigating and implementing techniques for improving drug use practices.[61] General methods for modifying physician prescribing are discussed in Chapter 28, and Chapter 29 discusses the use of drug utilization review as a specific and common technique used toward that end. In the remainder of this chapter, we will discuss the use of NMDPs for this and other purposes.

CURRENTLY AVAILABLE SOLUTIONS

THE IMPLEMENTATION OF NATIONAL MEDICINAL DRUG POLICIES

The components that are necessary to implement NMDPs have been defined by WHO:[62]

- an appropriate legislative and regulatory framework
- a system for choosing appropriate drugs
- a mechanism for ensuring supply and distribution
- a program for improving rational use of drugs
- appropriate economic strategies for the pharmaceutical sector
- the development of human resources
- a system for monitoring and evaluating the impact of the policy
- research—drug research and development, and operational (R&D).

As mentioned in the section on the objectives of NMDPs, the correct policy mix will vary according to the stage of development and economic state of a country. However, experience indicates that successful implementation requires a strong central group with the necessary expertise, concentration on some key issues (it is not possible to achieve everything), public endorsement by senior politicians (the president/prime minister or health minister should "launch" the policy), international support, and a thick skin (the industry and local medical association may object on the grounds that the policy will reduce profits and clinical freedom).

A number of the features of NMDPs have been covered in previous sections of this chapter and there is insufficient space to do justice to all of the topics listed above. However, we would like to cover some selected implementation issues, including the growing interest in the use of formal economic analyses in the selection and pricing of drugs within an NMDP.

Legislative and Regulatory Frameworks

A key step for national drug policies is the drafting and implementation of an appropriate law that regulates the supply of pharmaceuticals. In developed countries, drug laws have usually evolved over many years. For example, in the US, the first national drug law was passed in 1906 and this was then modified following public health "disasters" such as the contamination of sulfonilamide in 1938 and thalidomide in the early 1960s (see also Chapter 1). The aims of most drug laws are similar: to regulate the supply of pharmaceuticals (including import and export), and to ensure that the forms in which pharmaceuticals are supplied meet accepted standards. Most drug laws do not try to regulate the way in which pharmaceuticals are used, by either the prescriber or the consumer.

In developing countries, drug laws have often been developed in the recent past, based on the WHO Model Drugs Law, for example in Laos and some of the eastern European countries. To be effective, such legislation has to be supported by appropriate enforcement strategies. This may appear to be self-evident, but there are many examples where legislation has been implemented without enforcement, particularly relating to provisions about who can supply pharmaceuticals to the consumer. In Thailand and Vietnam, for example, despite the existence of national drug laws, there is as yet no effective control over the supply of antibiotics to the consumer, which contributes to major problems of inappropriate use.

It is not altogether clear what makes drug regulation effective. The WHO estimates that, of its member states, only 1/6 have an "effective" drug regulatory system.[63] It is possible to identify some factors that will contribute to ineffective drug regulation, such as lack of appropriate technical expertise, and inefficient or corrupt administration. Solutions to these problems are more difficult.

Systems for Choosing Appropriate Drugs and Ensuring Access

The Essential Drugs Program has probably been the most effective solution that has been implemented for choosing appropriate drugs. The advantages of using a limited list are summarized in Table 25.3. For example, Hogerzeil *et al.*[64] documented the impact of the introduction of an Essential Drugs Program in Yemen, showing improved availability, use, and knowledge in relation to a selection of essential medicines. One of the difficulties, however, has been that in many settings, industry has not accepted the Essential Drugs Program and it has not been prepared to produce essential drugs at affordable prices.[65]

At the International Conference on National Medicinal Drug Policies held in Manly, Australia in 1995, the policy options for improving access to essential drugs were discussed. The options identified included price control, price competition, price awareness, and health insurance.[66] Although a number of examples appeared to be successful, the conditions for success of any particular strategy are still not fully understood.

Systems for choosing between drugs are developing. The "VEN classification" proposed by the WHO[67] represents a logical approach, as it provides a basis for choosing between a range of medications, of different types, and for

Table 25.3. Advantages of adopting a limited list of essential drugs[1]

Supply
- Easier procurement storage and distribution
- Lower stocks
- Easier dispensing

Prescribing
- Training more focused and therefore easier
- More experience with fewer drugs
- No irrational treatment alternatives
- Focused drug information
- Better recognition of adverse drug reactions

Cost
- Lower prices, more competition

Patient Use
- Focused education efforts
- Reduced confusion and increased adherence to treatment
- Improved drug availability

different indications, when working under budgetary constraints. Briefly, drugs are classified as Vital, Essential, or Non-essential, and this establishes a hierarchy for managing choices. When drugs are genuinely different from each other, those that are classified as "vital" should be selected ahead of those that are "essential." When drugs are similar in their actions and indications (i.e., in the same VEN category), the decision should be based on an assessment of their comparative cost-effectiveness (see Chapter 41). When the drugs are identical, the only decision criterion is the acquisition cost. As will be seen in the section on economic considerations, this approach, advocated by the WHO for use in developing countries, is very similar to the selection processes used in the operation of the Australian Pharmaceutical Benefits Scheme.

In 1999, the WHO decided to update its methods for choosing drugs for its Model Essential Drugs list. The Expert Committee in that year expressed concern at the lack of evidence provided to the committee to justify revisions, and asked for summaries of appropriate evidence to be presented to support applications for additions and deletions. Over the next two years a new process was developed that included assessment of not only the quality, safety, and comparative efficacy of a medicine, but an assessment of its public health relevance and cost-effectiveness as well. Introduction of the new guidelines was challenged by the US, particularly in relation to cost considerations, but eventually the new procedure was adopted and has been used in all subsequent revisions of the list.[68]

A Program for Achieving Quality Use of Medicines

A key component of any NMDP is a program to encourage the quality use of medicines. Factors that influence use of pharmaceuticals are complex and may be culture-specific. A number of strategies for changing professional practice have been studied, for example the provision of standard treatment guidelines, the use of educational seminars, and more intensive approaches such as "academic detailing." The most recent reviews of the various approaches suggest that a combination of methods is usually required to have sustained impact on practice.[69,70] (See also Chapters 28 and 29.) The methods for changing consumer practices are still being defined.

The provision of adequate information about the efficacy and safety of pharmaceuticals is regarded as an important component of any program that is aimed at improving use of pharmaceuticals. Premarketing evaluation of drugs can help provide information about the efficacy of products, but it is well recognized that premarketing data do not provide the complete picture of the safety of products (see also Chapter 1). Surveillance systems for adverse drug reactions can be an important contributor to the information base as well as to other aspects of national medicinal drug policies. For example, spontaneous reporting systems can contribute to the education of prescribers and hopefully improve the quality of use of pharmaceuticals (see Chapters 9 and 10). In Australia, the hepatic side effects of flucloxacillin that were identified through the spontaneous reporting system were publicized in the quarterly adverse drug reactions bulletin. Formal investigation of the problem (using case–control methodology) identified the dose and duration of therapy and the age of the patients as major risk factors for developing the reaction.[71] This allowed appropriate advice to be issued regarding the usage of the product, and eventually there was a marked decline in usage.

Appropriate Economic Strategies for the Pharmaceutical Sector: The Example of Australia

The use of formal economic analysis (see Chapter 41) in the selection and pricing of drugs has been a controversial issue for a number of years. Increasingly, a number of countries are considering the implementation of an approach that uses pharmacoeconomics and have published guidelines to assist the pharmaceutical industry in making applications for listing new products on national formularies.

Most experience of using pharmacoeconomics in formulary management has been gained during the operation of the Australian Pharmaceutical Benefits Scheme (PBS). The PBS and the processes used for evaluating drugs have been described in a number of articles.[72,73] The use of economic analysis in the choice and pricing of pharmaceuticals is a central activity of the Australian national drug policy.

The PBS is a comprehensive, publicly funded, insurance program that reimburses pharmacists for the costs of a selected range of prescription drugs. Drugs are placed in different categories of access (restricted benefit, authority required), based on evidence of their comparative efficacy and cost-effectiveness in defined patient groups. The decisions to place new drugs in the PBS are made by the Commonwealth Health Minister on the advice of the Pharmaceutical Benefits Advisory Committee (PBAC). The PBAC receives advice from an economics subcommittee regarding the validity of the economic analyses contained in submissions from the pharmaceutical industry. The PBAC has a strong preference for using data from randomized controlled clinical trials as the basis of its judgment about the comparative efficacy of drugs. The guidelines for economic analysis released by the Department of Health and Aged Care

(DHAC)[74] encourage the sponsors of new drugs to conduct a preliminary economic analysis, based on the results of randomized trials, before conducting an analysis using an economic model in which assumptions are made about long-term health effects and costs when the drugs are used in Australia. The database of submissions to the PBS that is maintained by the DHAC contains details of more than 300 submissions from the industry. Eighty-six percent of submissions were based on the results of randomized clinical trials, of which one quarter included the results of meta-analyses[75] (see Chapter 44). This is the most extensive experience in the world of the use of trial data in the assessment of the comparative efficacy and cost-effectiveness of any health care intervention.

The key decisions that have to be made when a drug is considered for listing are whether it is superior to its comparators in clinical terms (improved efficacy, greater safety, both, or neither). The net costs associated with its use are then related to the assessment of comparative clinical performance. If there is no worthwhile difference in efficacy or safety, the new drug will receive the same price as the comparator (an established drug for the same indication). If the new drug is superior, the additional clinical benefits have to be related to the net costs in an incremental cost-effectiveness ratio. Whether this ratio represents "value for money" is the judgment of the advisory committee, and the decisions are sometimes quite controversial. It should be noted that factors other than cost-effectiveness are considered in the decision making process, such as clinical need, equity of access, "rule of rescue," and total cost to the health care system. The complexity of this process reflects the true difficulties of making this sort of decision, and the provision of evidence at different stages helps to make the issues more clear-cut.

Decision making based on pharmacoeconomics has recently been implemented in South Africa and the Baltic States. In South Africa, the initial emphasis has been on the development of a system of price controls using international reference pricing comparison as well as reference pricing by pharmacological class. In the Baltic States, the three countries of Latvia, Estonia, and Lithuania have produced joint guidelines for the pharmaceutical industry and are combining their technical capacity to consider economic evaluations of new products. These two examples illustrate different ways a rational decision making system can be implemented in settings with limited resources and capacity, and are likely to be models for other countries considering adopting a similar approach.

The overall impact of this policy is difficult to judge, but one effect on drug pricing is fairly clear. The use of "cost minimization" to eliminate cost differences between very similar drugs has considerable social value, as it reduces expenditure that has no prospect of bringing greater health benefits. It also minimizes the need for educational efforts directed at doctors that are intended to shift prescribing between very similar drugs for purely economic reasons. An example of the effect of this policy is given in Figure 25.1, where the prices of commonly used (but very similar) nonsteroidal anti-inflammatory drugs in Australia and the United Kingdom are compared. The difference in average price is not the issue, as this is influenced by the exchange rate at the time the study was carried out. However, the notable difference between the two countries is in the price variation across this class of very similar compounds.

Undoubtedly, there are benefits to the community in pursuing a policy that minimizes price differences across classes of equivalent drugs. This will apply in both developing and developed countries.

The Australian PBS has been a successful example of a large buyer—a government—using its market power to exert leverage on prices. This has been an unpopular approach for some sectors of the pharmaceutical industry and there have been a number of challenges, both political and legal, to the operations of the program. At the time of this writing (June 2004) the main threat to the continued smooth operation of the Australian PBS comes in the form of the proposed free trade agreement between the USA and Australia. The text of the proposed agreement has a chapter on the PBS, which appears to be designed to weaken the price-setting mechanisms and extend patent life of originator brands in order to delay entry of generic products. The agreement has still to be passed by the US Senate and Australian parliament, so the full effects remain unclear.

THE FUTURE

As countries become increasingly concerned with costs of drugs and with their proper use, it is likely that there will be increasing attention paid to the development of national medicinal drug policies. The development of these policies will modify the types of research that pharmacoepidemiologists will be able to perform.

In addition, as these programs are expanded and developed, it is important that their effects are rigorously evaluated. There are several obvious roles for pharmacoepidemiologists in this process. These include drug utilization studies as part of a program to improve the quality of use of medicines (see Chapter 27), designing interventions to improve prescribing (see Chapters 28 and 29), the conduct and evaluation of pharmacoeconomic studies (see Chapter 41), and identifying and quantifying adverse drug reactions (see Chapters 9–24). In developing countries, there is still a need for adverse reaction reporting as part of the process to identify failure in the quality of production. A range of indicators of quality drug use have been suggested by the WHO, and by some countries. However, as with any system of assessment, there are virtues in simplicity. Table 25.4 lists a few basic indicators that can be used to assess the degree of implementation of national drug policies. It should be stressed (again) that their use should not be confined to developing

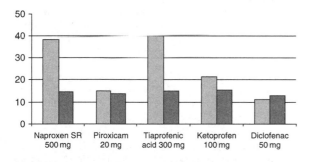

Figure 25.1. The impact of cost minimization on drug prices. A comparison of the prices of commonly used and similarly performing NSAIDs in Australia (dark shading) and the United Kingdom. The comparisons are based on the prices listed in the Australian Schedule and British National Formulary in the last quarter of 1997. The Australian prices were adjusted to the maximum quantities provided by a UK prescription. Prices are in $AU, using an exchange rate of $1AU = £0.40.

Table 25.4. Indicators used in the world drug situation to assess the effectiveness of national drug policies (modified from WHO, 1988)

Indicators of availability
- The existence and use of an essential drug list (or selective national formulary)
- The extent of an operating system for procurement
- The extent of an operating system for distribution
- The extent of quality assurance
- The extent of regulatory mechanisms
- The extent of coverage

Indicators of rational use of drugs
- The existence of a functioning and independent system that provides objective information on drugs to health workers and patients
- The existence of a system of continuing education for all types of personnel dealing with drugs
- The existence of a monitoring system for adverse drug reactions

Indicator of the commitment of government
- The existence of a national medicinal drug policy

countries—they have relevance across all stages of economic development and there are few countries that will perform well on all of these indicators.

Pharmacoepidemiologists also have the potential to make major contributions to policies, by recognizing policy issues in the environments in which they work, measuring the impact of NMDPs, and contributing to policy development. Many pharmacoepidemiologists already have considerable influence with governments and pharmaceutical manufacturers. That influence can be used to persuade governments to develop better policies, and to commit resources to policy research. It could also be used to persuade governments and manufacturers to respect the rights of developing countries and to recognize the legitimacy of their efforts to improve the access of their populations to essential drugs. Through these initiatives, both in research and policy, pharmacoepidemiologists can play an important role in improving the risk/benefit balance of drug use in their communities.

REFERENCES

1. Quick JD, Rankin JR, Laing RO, O'Connor RW, Hogerzeil HV, Dukes MGN, Garnett A., eds, *Managing Drug Supply: The Selection, Procurement, Distribution and Use of Pharmaceuticals*. 2nd edn. West Harford, CT: Kumarian Press, 1997.
2. Dag Hammarskjold Foundation. *Prescription for Change. National Drug Policies, Social Transformation and the Media*. Manila, The Philippines: Philippine Centre for Investigative Journalism, 1992.
3. Rudolf PM, Bernstein IBG. Counterfeit drugs. *N Engl J Med* 2004; **350**: 1384–6.
4. Risha PG, Shewiyo D, Msami A, Masuki G, Vergote G, Vervaet C, Remon JP. *In vitro* evaluation of the quality of essential drugs in the Tanzanian market. *Trop Med Int Health* 2002; **7**: 701-7.
5. Taylor RB, Shakoor O, Behrens RH, Everard M, Low AS, Wangboonskul J, Reid RG, Kolawole JA. Pharmacopoeial quality of drugs supplied by Nigerian pharmacies. *Lancet* 2001; **357**: 1933–6.
6. Afu S. Incidence of substandard drugs in developing countries [letter]. *Trop Med Int Health* 1999; **4**: 73.
7. Hanif M, Mobarak MR, Ronan A, Rahman D, Donovan JJ Jr, Bennish ML. Fatal renal failure caused by diethylene glycol in paracetamol elixir: the Bangladesh epidemic. *BMJ* 1995; **311**: 950–1.
8. O'Brien KL, Selanikio JD, Hecdivert C, Placide MF, Louis M, Barr DB *et al*. Epidemic of pediatric deaths from acute renal failure caused by diethylene glycol poisoning. *JAMA* 1998; **279**: 1175–80.
9. Geiling EMK, Cannon PR. Pathological effects of elixir of sulfonilamide (diethylene glycol) poisoning. *JAMA* 1938; **111**: 919–26.
10. Bowie MD, McKenzie D. Diethylene glycol poisoning in children. *S Afr Med J* 1972; **46**: 931–4.
11. Cantarell MC, Fort J, Camps J, Sans M, Piera L. Acute intoxication due to topical application of diethylene glycol. *Ann Intern Med* 1987; **106**: 478–9.
12. Pandya SK. An unmitigated tragedy. *BMJ* 1988; **297**: 117–19.
13. Okuonghae HO, Ighogboja IS, Lawson JO, Nwana EJC. Diethylene glycol poisoning in Nigerian children. *Ann Trop Paediatr* 1992; **12**: 235–8.
14. Pinel J, Varaine, F, Fermon F, Marchant G, Marioux, G. Des faux vaccins anti-meningocoque lors d'une epidemie de meningite au Niger. *Med Mal Infect* 1997; **27**: 1–563.
15. World Health Organisation. Fake drugs: a scourge on the system. *WHO Drug Inf* 1995; **9**: 127–9. Available at http://www.who.int/druginformation. Accessed November 2004.
16. Pecoul B, Chirac P, Trouiller P, Pinle J. Access to essential drugs in poor countries: a lost battle? *JAMA* 1999; **281**: 361–7.
17. Shakoor O, Taylor RB, Behrens RH. Assessment of the incidence of substandard drugs in developing countries. *Trop Med Int Health* 1997; **2**: 839–45.
18. Nazerali H, Hogerzeil H. The quality and stability of essential drugs in rural Zimbabwe: controlled longitudinal study. *BMJ* 1998; **317**: 512–13.
19. Zaffran M. Vaccine transport and storage: environmental challenges. *Dev Biol Stand* 1996; **87**: 9–17.
20. Shoub BD, Cameron NA. Problems encountered in the delivery and storage of OPV in an African country. *Dev Biol Stand* 1996; **87**: 27–32.
21. Grasso M, Ripabelli G, Sammarco ML, Manfredi Selvaggi TM, Quaranta A. Vaccine storage in the community: a study in central Italy. *Bull World Health Org* 1999; **77**: 352–5.
22. Guthridge SL, Miller NC. Cold chain in a hot climate. *Aust N Z J Public Health* 1996; **20**: 657–60.
23. Jeremijenko A, Kelly H, Sibthorpe B, Attewell R. Improving vaccine storage in general practice refrigerators. *BMJ* 1996; **312**: 1651–2.
24. Wawryk A, Mavromatis C, Gold M. Electronic monitoring of vaccine cold chain in a metropolitan area. *BMJ* 1997; **315**: 518–19.
25. Reimer RF, Lewis PR. Vaccine storage in pharmacies on the Central Coast of New South Wales. *Aust N Z J Public Health* 1998; **22**: 274–5.
26. Hanjeet K, Lye MS, Sinniah M, Schnur A. Evaluation of cold chain monitoring in Kelantan, Malaysia. *Bull World Health Org* 1996; **74**: 391–7.
27. John TJ. Vaccine stability in the context of vaccine delivery in a developing country: India. *Dev Biol Stand* 1996; **87**: 19–25.
28. Adu FD, Adedeji AA, Esan JS, Odusanya OG. Live viral vaccine potency: an index for assessing the cold chain system. *Public Health* 1996; **110**: 325–30.
29. Hogerzeil HV, Battersby A, Srdanovic V, Stjernstrom NE. Stability of essential drugs during shipment to the tropics. *BMJ* 1992; **304**: 210–12.
30. Kanji N, Hardon A, Harnmeijer JW, Mamdani M, Walt G. *Drugs Policy in Developing Countries*. Atlantic Highlands, NJ: Zed Books, 1992.

31. Ballance R, Pogany J, Forstner H. *The World's Pharmaceutical Industries*. Aldershot: Edward Elgar Publishing, 1992.

32. Habiyambere V, Wertheimer AI. Essential drugs should be accessible to all people. *World Health Forum* 1993: **14**: 140–4.

33. Luechai S-N. Drug abundance: situation of drugs and drug distribution in the villages of rural Thailand. *Asia Pac J Public Health* 1996–7: **9**: 18–23.

34. Foster S. Supply and use of essential drugs in Sub-Saharan Africa: some issues and possible solutions. *Soc Sci Med* 1991: **32**: 1201–18.

35. Kandela P. Shortages distort the social fabric of Iraq. *Lancet* 1998: **351**: 1711–12.

36. Kent D, Glatzer M. Inappropriate drug-donation practices in Bosnia and Herzegovina [letter]. *N Engl J Med* 1998: **338**: 1472–4.

37. Goemaere E, Kaninda A, Ciaffi L, Mulemba M, t'Hoen E, Pecoul B. Do patents prevent access to drugs for HIV in developing countries ?[letter] *JAMA* 2002: **287**: 841–2.

38. Henry D, Lexchin J. The pharmaceutical industry as a medicines provider. *Lancet* 2002; **360**: 1590–5.

39. Subramanian A. Medicines, patents and TRIPS. *Finance Dev* 2004; March: 22–25.

40. Soumerai SB, Ross-Degnan D. Inadequate prescription-drug coverage for Medicare enrollees—a call for action. *N Engl J Med* 1999: **340**: 722–8.

41. Soumerai SB, McLaughlin TJ, Ross-Degnan D, Casteris CS, Bollini P. Effects of limiting Medicaid drug-reimbursement benefits on the use of psychotropic agents and acute mental health services by patients with schizophrenia. *N Engl J Med* 1994: **331**: 650–5.

42. Rabon PG, Linette DC, Gonzalez MF, Garrison S, McGee KH. Limited availability of medications for cancer patients. *South Med* J 1993: **86**: 914–18.

43. Wise R, Hart T, Cars O, Streulens M, Helmuth R, Huovinen P, Sprenger M. Antimicrobial resistance is a major threat to public health [editorial]. *BMJ* 1998: **317**: 609–10.

44. Trostle J. Inappropriate distribution of medicines by professionals in developing countries. *Soc Sci Med* 1996: **42**: 1117–20.

45. Rodruguez-Noriega E, Morfin-Otero R, Esparza-Ahumada S. The use of quinolones in developing countries. *Drugs* 1993: **45**: 42–5.

46. Ferraz MB, Pereira RB, A Paiva JG, Atra E, Dos Santos JQ. Availability of over-the-counter drugs for arthritis in Sao Paulo, Brazil. *Soc Sci Med* 1996: **42**: 1129–31.

47. Elzbier AG, Al-Shehry SZ. Too many vitamins for diabetics. *World Health Forum* 1997: **18**: 73–4.

48. Hogerzeil HV, Bimo, Ross-Degnan D, Laing RO, Ofori-Adjei D, Santoso B *et al*. Field tests for rational drug use in twelve developing countries. *Lancet* 1993: **342**: 1408–10.

49. Gurwitz JH, Avorn J. The ambiguous relation between aging and adverse drug reactions. *Ann Intern Med* 1991: **114**: 956–66.

50. Hogan DB. Revisiting the O complex: urinary incontinence, delirium and polypharmacy in elderly patients. *Can Med Assoc J* 1997: **157**: 1071–7.

51. Linzer M, Yang EH, Estes NA, Wang P, Vorperian VR, Kapoor WN. Diagnosing syncope. Part 1: value of history, physical examination and electrocardiography. *Ann Intern Med* 1997: **126**: 989–96.

52. Stewart RB, Cooper JW. Polypharmacy in the aged. Practical solutions. *Drugs Aging* 1994: **4**: 449–61.

53. Furniss L, Craig SK, Burns A. Medication use in nursing homes for elderly people. *Int J Geriatr Psychiatry* 1998: **13**: 433–9.

54. Soumerai SB, McLaughlin TJ, Spiegelman D, Hertzmark E, Thibault G, Goldman L. Adverse outcomes of under use of beta-blockers in elderly survivors of acute myocardial infarction. *JAMA* 1997: **277**: 115–21.

55. Moser M. Why are physicians not prescribing diuretics more frequently in the management of hypertension? *JAMA* 1998: **297**: 1813–16.

56. Rochon PA, Gurwitz JH. Prescribing for seniors. Neither too much nor too little. *JAMA* 1999: **282**: 113–15.

57. Hogerzeil HV, Couper MR, Gray R. Guidelines for drug donations. *BMJ* 1997: **314**: 737–40.

58. WHO/Action Program on Essential Drugs. *Globalization and Access to Drugs. Perspectives on the WTO/TRIPS Agreement*. Geneva: WHO, 1999.

59. Drahos P, Henry D. The free trade agreement between Australia and the United States. *BMJ* 2004; **328**: 1271–2.

60. Helling-Borda M. The role and experience of the World Health Organisation in assisting countries to develop and implement medicinal drug policies. *Australian Prescriber* 1997: **20**: 34–8.

61. Ross-Degnan D, Laing R. Improving use of medicines by health providers in primary care. In: International Conference on Improving Use of Medicines (ICIUM), Chiang Mai, Thailand, 1997.

62. WHO. *Report of the WHO Expert Committee on National Drug Policies*. Geneva: World Health Organization, 1995.

63. WHO. *Effective Drug Regulation: What Can Countries Do?* WHO working paper. Geneva: World Health Organization, 1999.

64. Hogerzeil HV, Wlaker GJ, Sallami AO, Fernando G. Impact of an essential drugs program on availability and rational use of drugs. *Lancet* 1989: **1**: 141–2.

65. Molina-Salzar RE, Rivas-Vilchis JE. Overpricing and affordability of drugs: the case of essential drugs in Mexico. *Cad Saude Publica* 1998: **14**: 501–16.

66. Quick J. Affordability and availability of drugs in the private market: promising experiences and cautions. *Australian Prescriber* 1997: **20**: 99–100.

67. Dumoulin J, Kaddar M, Velásquez G. *Guide to Drug Financing Mechanisms*. Geneva: World Health Organization, 1998.

68. Laing R, Waning B, Gray A, Ford N, 't Hoen E. 25 years of the WHO essential medicines lists: progress and challenges. *Lancet* 2003; **361**: 1723–9.

69. Grimshaw JM, Russell IT. Effect of clinical guidelines on medical practice: a systematic review of rigorous evaluations. *Lancet* 1993: **342**: 1317–22.

70. Bero LA, Grilli R, Grimshaw JM, Harvey E, Oxman AD, Thomson MA. Closing the gap between research and practice: an overview of systematic reviews of interventions to promote the implementation of research findings. *BMJ* 1998: **317**: 465–8.

71. Fairley CK, McNeil JJ, Desmond P, Smallwood R, Young H, Forbes A, Purcell P, Boyd I. Risk factors for development of flucloxacillin associated jaundice. *BMJ* 1993: **307**: 1179.

72. Henry D. Economic analysis as an aid to subsidisation decisions. *Pharmacoeconomics* 1992: **1**: 54–67.

73. Sketris IS, Hill S. The Australian national publicly subsidized Pharmaceutical Benefits Scheme: any lessons for Canada? *Can J Clin Pharmacol* 1998: **5**: 111–18.

74. Commonwealth of Australia. *Guidelines for the Pharmaceutical Industry on Preparation of Submissions to the Pharmaceutical Benefits Advisory Committee, Including Major Submissions Involving Economic Analyses*. Canberra: Department of Human Services and Health, 1995.

75. Hill S, Mitchell AM, Henry D. Problems in the conduct of pharmacoeconomic evaluations. *JAMA* 2000; **283**: 2116–21.

26

Premarketing Applications of Pharmacoepidemiology

HARRY A. GUESS

University of North Carolina, Chapel Hill, North Carolina, USA.

INTRODUCTION

While most of the interest in pharmacoepidemiology has centered on its role in the evaluation of drug safety after marketing (see Chapter 1),[1-3] epidemiology is increasingly recognized as an essential research discipline for drug and vaccine development.[4] These applications of epidemiology represent the expanded scope of premarketing pharmacoepidemiology as it is practiced today at several major pharmaceutical companies (see Chapter 7).

To help prioritize early drug development programs it is important to characterize potential treatment populations and to estimate market size. If effective drug therapy is already available and the new drug is simply one for which an incremental improvement in tolerability, dosing interval, or efficacy is expected, then market research data will often suffice. However, when the disease is one for which there is no effective drug therapy, epidemiologic information is generally needed.[5,6] At the earliest stages of drug development one needs to understand the biochemical pathways affected by a drug so as to anticipate likely intended and unintended effects. Epidemiology, genetics, biology, and pharmacology

help inform such evaluations (see Chapters 2, 4, and 37). This work is needed to design human proof of concept studies and special animal and human studies to characterize specific aspects of safety, tolerability, and efficacy. These early Phase I and II studies are used to make decisions about which drug candidates to take forward into the large and very expensive late Phase II and III studies and how to establish program priorities.

Epidemiologists also develop new measurement scales, especially those involving patient-reported outcomes for efficacy[7] and tolerability,[8-10] and they supply methodologic expertise in developing, refining, and standardizing clinical measurement techniques[11,12] (see Chapter 42). It is essential for this work to be undertaken very early in drug development so that the measurement techniques and the patient-reported outcome measures can be pilot tested in early (Phase II-A) studies. The pilot testing is used to establish statistical properties of the measurements and to develop versions in multiple languages. All this must be done in time to permit use in the Phase II-B and Phase III efficacy trials. Epidemiologists are often members of the team responsible for the design and operation of clinical efficacy trials. For example, epidemiologists may establish procedures to ensure completeness of case ascertainment and endpoint adjudication procedures to improve validity. Epidemiologists can play a leading role in the design of both prespecified efficacy analyses combining data from several trials[13] and pooling analyses to evaluate safety hypotheses.[14]

These activities go beyond anticipating and evaluating potential safety concerns. The latter applications of premarketing pharmacoepidemiology are similar in many ways to analyses of postmarketing pharmacoepidemiology. Two important differences are that: (i) safety questions arising in premarketing clinical trials typically require answers in a matter of days rather than weeks or months, and (ii) the threshold for either the manufacturer or a regulatory agency to decide to halt human exposure to a drug is much lower before market approval than after approval.

This chapter will first review the clinical and regulatory context relevant for epidemiologic research supporting pre-approval drug and vaccine development. Next, some of the methodologic issues and approaches will be reviewed. Finally, several examples will be provided. This chapter should be of interest not only to epidemiologists, clinical researchers, and biostatisticians in the pharmaceutical industry and in regulatory agencies, but also to students and faculty members in academic departments of epidemiology.

CLINICAL PROBLEMS TO BE ADDRESSED BY PHARMACOEPIDEMIOLOGIC RESEARCH

CHARACTERIZING THE TARGET POPULATION

Estimates of the age- and sex-specific prevalence of a disease may be obtained from the literature with little effort. These may be used to develop rough estimates of the potential target population for a new drug. However, such estimates may prove overly optimistic if one does not take into account which patients with the disease are likely to be candidates for drug therapy.[5,6] For such more detailed estimates one needs information on the expected safety and efficacy profile of the drug, available therapeutic options, and medical practices in different countries. Producing useful estimates often requires epidemiologic, clinical, and economic collaboration and may sometimes require additional data collection. For example, it required considerable information about the timing and causes of preterm labor to conclude that the maximum possible reduction in preterm labor one could expect from a safe and effective tocolytic was relatively modest because many pregnancies with early preterm labor have contraindications to tocolytics.[15]

DEVELOPING AND STANDARDIZING CLINICAL ASSESSMENT METHODS

Epidemiologists have long played a role in standardizing anthropomorphic measurements, blood pressure measurements, and other clinical assessments (see Chapter 42). Methods of clinical assessment used in clinical practice are often not precise enough for use in clinical or epidemiologic research. Hence when a drug is developed it is important to review existing assessment methods to determine whether they are sufficiently accurate, precise, reliable, and robust for use in the proposed development program. If they are not, it will be necessary to refine existing measures or to develop new ones; in either case it will be necessary to establish statistical properties, and create training materials in time to support drug development.

DEVELOPING, PILOT TESTING, AND VALIDATING PATIENT-REPORTED OUTCOME MEASURES

Patient-reported outcome measures are increasingly used to help assess how new therapies benefit patients (see Chapter 42). Such measures include not only symptom scales but also scales to measure how therapies affect patients' physical, emotional, social, and occupational functioning. In the development of a rizatriptan for treatment of migraine, such a broader patient-reported outcome scale provided some of the earliest evidence of dose–response.[16] More recently, a patient-reported outcome scale was used to help assess the impact of chemotherapy-induced nausea and vomiting on patients' daily lives and the effectiveness of anti-emetic therapy in reducing the impact.[17] Because Phase II-B and III drug development programs often involve clinical trials in 20–30 different countries, all patient-reported outcome measures need to be available in many different languages. Accepted standards for translation and linguistic piloting patient-reported outcome measures need to take into account cultural differences and to convey the psychometric constructs consistently in different languages and cultures.[18] Developing new instruments, establishing statistical properties, and carrying out cross-cultural adaptations in time to permit their application in drug development can be a daunting challenge.

DESIGNING ANALYSES OF COMBINED DATA FROM SEVERAL CLINICAL TRIALS

Phase II-B and III clinical trials that are sufficient to provide safety and efficacy data for drug approval are often not adequately powered to demonstrate improvement in clinical outcomes. However, the totality of all Phase II-B and III randomized clinical trials combined may sometimes provide sufficient patient-days of therapy to support a combined prespecified analysis of the effects of therapy on clinical outcomes. Such a study is a meta-analysis where all of the individual patient data are available and where the set of studies included in the analysis is specified in advance[13] (see Chapter 44). Meta-analyses of clinical trial data within a drug development program are also useful in addressing questions of tolerability or safety.[14]

CONTRIBUTING TO PREMARKETING RISK ASSESSMENTS AND RISK MANAGEMENT PLANS

Risk management (see Chapter 33) has been defined in an FDA report as a process which "encompasses processes for identifying and assessing the risks of specific health hazards, implementing activities to eliminate or minimize those risks, communicating risk information, and monitoring and evaluating the results of the interventions and communications."[19] Risk assessment has been defined as, "identifying and characterizing the nature, frequency, and severity of the risks associated with the use of a product."[20]

A recent set of FDA draft guidances discussed premarketing risk assessment,[20] development and use of risk minimization action plans,[21] and good pharmacovigilance practices and pharmacologic assessment.[21] Premarketing pharmacoepidemiology is an essential component of premarketing risk assessment. This is true whether premarketing pharmacoepidemiology is considered broadly as encompassing all applications of epidemiology in supporting premarketing drug development or narrowly as encompassing only anticipation and evaluation of potential drug risks.

METHODOLOGIC PROBLEMS TO BE ADDRESSED BY PHARMACOEPIDEMIOLOGIC RESEARCH

DEVELOPING AND STANDARDIZING CLINICAL AND PATIENT-REPORTED OUTCOME MEASURES

The application of epidemiologic methods in drug development poses a number of methodologic challenges and has provided the motivation for new methodologic developments. Development, validation, and cross-cultural adaptation of new measurement scales make use of methods from psychometrics[23] and clinical epidemiology.[24] Qualitative

research methods include use of focus group methodology; interviews with patients, care-givers, and health care professionals; reviews of existing measures; construct development; item development; and design of validation studies. The statistical methods include factor analysis and other techniques for domain definition, assessment of internal consistency, reliability, discriminant validity, and responsiveness.[23] Methods for evaluation of measurement scales for classification or diagnosis make use of likelihood ratios and receiver operating characteristic curves.[25]

The Consolidated Standards for Reporting Trials (CONSORT statement) is a widely accepted set of standards for reporting randomized clinical trials in medical journals.[26] It has also become a standard for designing clinical trials. One of the topics mentioned (Item 6b) is methods to enhance the quality of measurements. Examples included validation of measurement scales and use of clinical endpoint adjudication committees for assessing clinical outcomes in a blinded manner. Epidemiologists often play a major role in designing and implementing these interventions both in epidemiologic studies and in clinical trials, while making use of expert clinicians for the actual endpoint adjudications.

Assessing Causality of Adverse Events in Pre-approval Clinical Trials

Clinical investigators and clinical monitors continually review reports of adverse events occurring in pre-approval clinical trials. Investigators are asked to provide a clinical assessment as to the causality of each event. Such assessments are a necessary part of safety monitoring in clinical research, although they are known to be subjective and imprecise[27] (see also Chapter 36). Criteria to help guide causality assessments have been published by the FDA.[28] These criteria are most useful when there are well-defined differences in clinical features of drug-related and non-drug-related cases of the adverse event. However, for serious, uncommon adverse events where the clinical features of the drug-related cases could be similar to those of non-drug-related cases, it can sometimes be helpful to supplement clinical causality assessments of individual cases by epidemiologic assessment criteria based on comparisons between groups of patients.

The epidemiologic literature provides several sets of criteria for helping to decide whether an empirical association is likely to be causal. The best known criteria are those proposed in 1965 by Hill to help evaluate evidence linking cigarette smoking with lung cancer[29] (see also Chapter 2). The nine Hill criteria are discussed briefly below as they relate to evaluation of adverse experiences in premarketing clinical trials:

Strength of Association

This is commonly quantified in terms of a suitably adjusted hazard-function ratio or risk ratio (relative risk), rather than a p-value. In general, the farther the ratio is from unity, the less likely it could be entirely attributable to imbalances in risk factors between groups. An exception to this occurs when the ratio is based on very small numbers or is highly influenced by only a few cases.

In addition, it is worth noting that with the large number of different kinds of adverse events often seen in large clinical trials, it is quite likely that some risk ratios far from unity will occur by chance alone. Multiple comparisons not only distort p-values, but can also bias risk ratios and their confidence intervals away from unity.[30] Because pre-approval reviews of drug safety use the same set of data for identifying potentially drug-related events and for providing preliminary estimates of the risk, the relative risk estimates can be biased away from unity.

It is also important to recognize that the absence of any association between a drug and any given adverse event has to be judged in the context of the limited amount of patient exposure in pre-approval clinical trials. This topic is reviewed in ICH Guideline E1A, which addresses the extent of population exposure needed to assess clinical safety for drugs intended for long-term treatment of non-life-threatening conditions.[31]

Consistency

The original wording was, "Has [the association] been repeatedly observed by different persons, in different places, circumstances and times?" This is a useful criterion for assessing adverse experiences in a program of several clinical trials. Results that show a consistently elevated risk associated with a drug in each of several studies are generally more convincing than those in which the elevated risk is largely due to one study. It has been noted by FDA, however, that an apparent lack of consistency among trials may simply reflect differences in trial design, making the event less likely in some trials than others.[27]

Temporality

In both epidemiologic and clinical assessments of causality, it is important to distinguish between events having onset before a drug was started and those having onset after drug therapy was started. Especially in the evaluation of adverse experiences from studies without a comparison group, it sometimes occurs that early symptoms of a disease which is present but not yet recognized lead a patient to be prescribed a drug, which then appears to be the cause of the disease when it is eventually diagnosed. This has been called "proto-pathic bias" and is similar to, but not synonymous with, "confounding by indication" (see also Chapter 40).[32]

Another way in which the concept of temporality plays a role in the evaluation of adverse experiences is whether the timing of the reaction in relation to duration of exposure is consistent with the proposed mechanism. Thus, an elevated incidence of cancer in patients who had been taking a drug for many years would be of more concern than would an elevated incidence in the first year of therapy. Timing plays a major role in the evaluation of adverse events that are thought to be due to immune mechanisms or hypersensitivity (e.g., anaphylaxis, angioedema, hemolytic anemia, serum-sickness), altered metabolism, or drug interactions.[28]

Dose–response

Adverse effects caused by exaggerated pharmacological actions of a drug are often dose dependent. Examples include hypotension resulting from the use of antihypertensive drugs and gastrointestinal hemorrhage from nonsteroidal anti-inflammatory drugs. For such adverse events it is especially important to characterize how the incidence of the event varies with dose in different patient populations. This is not only important in assessing causality and quantifying inci-dence, but also in understanding the mechanism and providing guidance to clinicians. The case of renal failure in patients with congestive heart failure treated with the angiotensin converting enzyme (ACE) inhibitor enalapril provides an excellent example of where a drug shown in clinical trials to reduce mortality in patients with congestive heart failure when properly dosed was capable of causing renal failure in such patients when started at too high a dose.[33,34] While ACE inhibitors improve survival in patients with congestive heart failure, too high a dose can shut off renal function, because angiotensin-II is part of the compensatory process for maintaining adequate renal perfusion pressure in the face of low cardiac output.[35] This example illustrates the importance of understanding both pathophysiology and dose–response relationships in evaluating drug safety.

Experimental Evidence

Evidence from animal experiments or from previous human clinical trials can be especially important in helping to interpret adverse experiences. Well-designed animal studies can be especially helpful in determining the extent to which animal results are applicable to humans. On the other hand, poorly designed animal studies may produce misleading results, which can require carefully designed further experiments to correct.

Biological Plausibility

In the original statement of biological plausibility as one of the considerations in judging causality, Hill noted:

> It will be helpful if the causation we suspect is biologically plausible. But this is a feature I am convinced we cannot demand. What is biologically plausible depends on the biological knowledge of the day.

He went on to note, among other examples, that the role of rubella in causing congenital malformations was initially doubted on the basis of presumed lack of biological plausibility.[29] As important as we consider biological plausibility to be, it is equally important to realize that it can mislead in either direction. It is worth noting, however, that some epidemiologists have expressed the view that too little attention is currently paid to biological plausibility in reviews of epidemiologic evidence.[36]

Coherence

The postulated cause-and-effect interpretation should not seriously conflict with what is known of the natural history and biology of the event. In this regard, biological and laboratory evidence may strengthen a causal interpretation, but lack of it cannot be used to nullify one.

Analogy

Reasoning by analogy often serves as a basis for having a lower threshold for judging an adverse event to be causally related to one drug in a class when the same effect is considered to be causally related to another drug in the class. Such reasoning can be misleading when applied uncritically to individual drugs. However, it is important to anticipate potential mechanism-based toxicity based on considerations including experience with similar drugs and to design the drug development program to address concerns that can reasonably be anticipated and tested.[20,31]

Specificity

The finding that an adverse event has a very specific presentation or is associated with a specific histopathology can be useful evidence in favor of causality. Absence of specificity in an epidemiologic study often manifests itself as elevation in positive associations between an exposure and a large number of unrelated outcomes. Such a finding raises the possibility of uncontrolled confounding or selection bias.

In summary, while the Hill criteria were originally proposed for use in interpreting evidence from observational studies, they also provide a good framework for evaluating evidence from unplanned comparisons of adverse experiences in pre-approval clinical trials.

Another approach to assessing causality is through Bayesian causality assessment,[37,38] which provides a framework for using clinical and epidemiologic information to compute a probability that a specific drug caused a specific set of events in a specific patient. In Bayesian causality assessments the statement that a given drug D *caused* an event E is defined to mean that the event would not have happened as and when it did, if drug D had not been administered. Using this definition, a Bayesian causality assessment begins by decomposing the calculation of a probability of causation into a number of sub-calculations, some of which make use of epidemiologic information and others of which make use of pharmacologic and medical information specific to the case. Thus, rather than being alternatives to epidemiologic assessments, Bayesian causality assessments *require* epidemiologic assessments as a (somewhat hidden) part of a process which yields a numerical probability of causation. Bayesian analysis is discussed in more detail in Chapter 36.

STATISTICAL ANALYSIS METHODS IN PREMARKETING AND POSTMARKETING PHARMACOEPIDEMIOLOGY

While both cohort and case–control study designs are commonly used in postmarketing pharmacoepidemiology, premarketing studies typically involve only cohort designs. One of the most common problems in premarketing pharmacoepidemiology is to compare the incidence of a given adverse event in the cohort of patients exposed to the study drug to the incidence in a suitably chosen cohort of historical controls. Here *incidence* is used in the epidemiologic sense, where the numerator refers to the number of events (counting only the initial event in each patient) and the denominator often refers to the total *person-time at risk* during exposure to the study drug, sometimes referred to as incidence density. Person-time at risk is typically measured in *person-days*, where each patient contributes one person day for each day he or she is on the study drug and is at risk for the given adverse event. The person-time of exposure for each patient is thus most commonly measured from the day of first exposure to the study drug, up to the earlier of: (i) the date of last follow-up for the patient, or (ii) the day that the patient first experienced the adverse event. When analyzing incidence it is important to review the data for any evidence of temporal trends in relation to start of therapy.[39,40] This may occur, for example, through depletion of susceptibles.[41] When such trends are found, it may be necessary to produce separate risk computations for different windows of time-on-therapy.

Events in relation to person-time can be analyzed by Cox regression, Poisson regression, or by stratified incidence density computations using standard software packages, such as Stata® or SAS®. When the sample sizes are very small confidence intervals on the stratified relative risk estimates may be computed by exact methods.[42,43] Analytic methods and their limitations are further discussed in standard references.[44,45] Issues that often arise include calculation of point and interval estimates of standardized morbidity or mortality ratios (SMRs), [46, p. 65] comparing adjusted risk ratios for different groups of patients, [46, pp. 106–9] and testing for heterogeneity (representing potential effect modification) and dose–response trend. [46, p. 110] As with all epidemiologic studies, it is essential to approach these analyses with recognition of the biological and clinical aspects of the problem, as well as with an understanding of the meaning and limitations of the formal computational methods.

INFORMATION TECHNOLOGY REQUIREMENTS

Effective premarketing pharmacoepidemiology requires considerable advanced planning to make sure that information can be assembled, analyzed, summarized, reviewed, and reported in hours or days. For historical data to be useful, it must be either available in sufficient detail from published sources or from existing data sets that can be accessed, analyzed, and checked for errors within a day or two. This can only be done if one can anticipate at least some types of problems likely to arise with the drug and have appropriate sources of epidemiologic information readily accessible.

In addition, the clinical trials data management organization has to be able to produce accurate, suitably detailed patient exposure information from many different trials in a number of different countries. This is more difficult than it might initially appear to be. Because of regulatory reporting requirements, adverse experience information (the numerator) will typically be current to within a few days, while the patient exposure information (the denominator) may be weeks behind and may not yet have essential covariate information and demographics in accurately retrievable form.

Getting new drugs approved in a timely manner can depend on the ability to answer safety questions rapidly and accurately, and that can depend on the way in which data management is staffed, organized, and equipped. One of the rate-limiting factors in securing timely approval is the manpower needed to process worldwide clinical trial data on thousands of patients from many different countries accurately. This entails producing both standard efficacy and safety analyses and special *ad hoc* safety analyses required for responding to questions raised by reviewers at drug regulatory agencies. The data management problems posed by the need to answer *ad hoc* safety questions rapidly are different from those posed by the need for the formal statistical analyses of efficacy required for drug approval. To be successful, the data management organization and systems must meet both challenges.

CURRENTLY AVAILABLE SOLUTIONS

Drug development for treatment of facial acne illustrates several aspects of clinical and patient-reported outcome measure development. When this development program was initially undertaken no standardized assessment measures or patient-reported outcome measures suitable for clinical trial use were available in the literature. Lucky and colleagues developed a clinical assessment tool for acne and established intra- and inter-observer agreement.[11] The statistical sampling design used a 12 by 12 Latin Square to account for first-, second-, and third-order effects with observers, patients, and assessment order.[11] Girman and colleagues developed the patient-reported outcome measure starting with patient focus groups to assess what aspects of facial acne were important to patients.[47] A cross-sectional validation study was conducted to show that the patient-reported outcome measurements for patients with different levels of clinician-assessed acne severity showed the hypothesized relationship.[48] Later Fehnel and colleagues showed that the instrument was highly responsive in detecting patient-reported outcome improvement in response to therapy with a clinically effective drug.[49]

Development of patient- and parent-reported measures for use in asthma clinical trials illustrates approaches to outcome measure development for pediatric trials. Santanello and colleagues developed and validated asthma patient-reported outcome measures for use in children 6–14 years old and a care-giver diary for use in clinical trials of children 2–5 years old.[50,51]

Patient-reported and parent-reported outcome measures are used not only to assess efficacy but also to help assess tolerability and safety. Examples include a patient-reported outcome measure of tolerability of topical ophthalmic medications,[10] a male sexual function index,[8] and a standardized reporting measure for assessing symptoms following vaccine administration.[9] The FDA draft guidance on premarketing risk assessment[20] recommends use of targeted safety questionnaires or other patient-reported outcome measurements for certain types of safety assessments which may not be adequately measured by routine adverse event monitoring in clinical trials.

In addition to these specific examples, the CONSORT statement,[26] discussed above, provides an online checklist with more than 200 references describing clinical trial methodology, including several key references illustrating methods for developing and validating measurement scales and enhancing quality of trial measurements.

Epidemiologic investigation of premarketing drug safety problems is a collaborative undertaking that requires the ability not only to respond to inquiries promptly and accurately, but also to recognize and answer questions that should have been asked but were not. Sometimes the initial request from the clinical or regulatory group in a pharmaceutical company to the epidemiology group asks for a specific tabulation or calculation, which may not in fact represent the most appropriate way to approach the problem. Requests transmitted through several intermediaries often change in meaning, so that what finally reaches the person responsible for the analysis may be quite different from what was originally asked. When the original request is a written inquiry (e.g., from a regulatory agency), it is important to read the actual written question and the surrounding context before attempting to answer a paraphrased version of it.

As with all epidemiologic and statistical consulting, the best way to approach a request for consultation on a potential safety problem with a premarketing investigational drug is to first understand the broader context surrounding the immediate inquiry. This includes gaining at least a basic understanding of the pharmacology, mechanism of action, preclinical toxicity profile, and clinical safety profile of the compound. It also entails understanding the characteristics and comorbidities of the patient population in which the drug has been studied. Finally, it requires knowing how and in what context the question arose.

One example, which illustrates the interplay between clinical pharmacology and epidemiology, involved seizures in seriously ill hospitalized patients with systemic gram-negative infections being treated with the β-lactam antibiotic imipenem/cilastatin.[52,53] During initial randomized clinical trials few seizures were reported, either with imipenem/cilastatin or with control antibiotics. In subsequent noncomparative studies many more seizures were noted, often in patients with predisposing factors, such as compromised renal function, that could alter drug metabolism and affect serum levels of the antibiotic. An association of seizure risk with antibiotic level was biologically plausible, in light of known epileptogenic properties of β-lactam antibiotics. At the time these studies were conducted, laboratory

techniques to measure serum levels had not yet become widely available and so serum levels of these patients were rarely known.

To study seizure risk in relation to serum level, clinical pharmacology studies were reviewed to determine how serum levels varied with dose, body weight, gender, age, and renal function. An equation was developed to predict serum level as a function of these parameters. The predicted serum levels were then used as one variable in an analysis of seizure risk in the noncomparative clinical trial patients. It was found that risk of seizures was strongly and independently related to predicted serum level, after controlling for several non-drug-related seizure risk factors.[52] At the same time, however, the other factors found to be related to seizure risk in patients receiving imipenem/cilastatin were also found to be risk factors for seizures in patients who had not received imipenem/cilastatin. These factors included a history of seizures, central nervous system insults, and renal impairment.[53] Age was not found to be predictive of seizures when adjustment for the above factors was made.

This study illustrates the concept of *pharmaco*epidemiology in a study where methods of clinical pharmacology and epidemiology were both brought into play to investigate and solve a problem that arose during the course of premarketing clinical trials. It also illustrates the important point that merely quantifying risk and identifying patients at increased risk would not have been sufficient. What was needed was to identify measures to help reduce the risk and to help educate physicians on the need for dosage adjustments. The investigation into seizure risk led to improved prescribing information with better recommendations for dosage adjustments in the presence of impaired renal function.

A recent example of a problem involving both premarketing and postmarketing pharmacoepidemiology is that of evaluating drug-induced hepatotoxicity. In early 2001, the FDA and PhRMA held a conference to review current approaches to detect and avoid drug-induced liver injury (DILI) and to outline a program of research to develop improved approaches.[54] One of the problems identified in the postmarketing White Paper, available on the conference website,[54] and equally applicable to premarketing studies, is that when screening for a rare disease, nearly all abnormal tests will be false positives unless the test is almost perfectly specific. For example, even if transaminases were 99.5% specific and 100% sensitive, about 96% of all positive tests would be false positives if serious DILI occurred in only 1 in every 5000 patients treated (Figure 26.1). Thus, when periodic monitoring with transaminases is recommended for drugs for which serious DILI is rare, nearly all the positives will be false positive. Patients may be led to

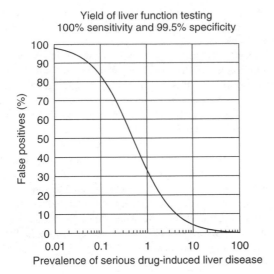

Figure 26.1. Diagnostic yield of liver function testing in a population of users of a drug. The hypothetical test is assumed to have 100% sensitivity and 99.5% specificity. The graph shows that nearly all of the abnormal test results are false positive when the prevalence of serious drug-induced liver disease is very rare among users of the drug.

discontinue effective therapy and may have to undergo additional evaluation.

At the conference several research initiatives were undertaken to develop additional information about mechanisms of DILI and to identify better screening modalities. One promising result in the latter direction grew out of a research collaboration between a hepatologist at the FDA and a statistician at Merck to determine whether the combination of elevated transaminases and elevated bilirubin could improve specificity with little or no loss in sensitivity for detecting serious DILI.[55] This combination of >3-fold elevation above the upper limit of normal (ULN) in either serum alanine (ALT) or aspartate (AST) aminotransferase together with >2-fold elevation above ULN in total bilirubin is known as "Hy's Rule" after the late Hyman Zimmerman.[54] The FDA and Merck investigators used the placebo group ($n = 3248$) from a randomized double blind placebo-controlled clinical trial in which patients were followed with periodic transaminase and bilirubin monitoring, for up to five years. The investigators found that use of Hy's Rule, instead of requiring either ALT or AST >3-fold ULN, improved specificity from 98.8% (3204/3243) to 99.97% (3242/3243). Although sensitivity was 83.3% for each measure, this was only based on 6 cases of DILI. Further studies would be needed to confirm that sensitivity is not impaired.

If sensitivity is preserved, use of Hy's Rule instead of transaminase elevations alone to screen for potential hepatotoxicity has the potential for reducing false positives. For example, if the sensitivity of 83.3% for both tests were confirmed in larger studies and if the specificities of 98.8% and 99.97% found in this study were also confirmed, then for a drug with a prevalence of serious DILI in one in every 5000 treated, the positive predictive value for serious DILI using transaminases alone would be only 1.4%, while that using Hy's Rule would be 35.7%.

THE FUTURE

Premarketing and postmarketing applications of pharmacoepidemiology differ in the speed of response required and in the fact that the threshold for halting human exposure to a drug is lower before market approval than after market approval. In addition, premarketing pharmacoepidemiology uses cohort study designs almost exclusively, while postmarketing pharmacoepidemiology often uses case–control study designs as well. Safety monitoring in clinical trials can be improved by anticipating potential questions and organizing data resources in advance to answer them as rapidly as possible. Having a responsive data management system is as essential to premarketing applications of pharmacoepidemiology as it is to the entire process of drug development. Epidemiology is an essential discipline for drug development and should be involved in planning early human studies. Premarketing pharmacoepidemiology is also an important component of premarketing risk assessment and risk management planning. These activities require having access to appropriate databases and to highly qualified epidemiologists capable of making efficient and valid use of these resources. It also requires undertaking epidemiologic studies far enough in advance of clinical trials to be able to contribute to clinical trial planning and analysis. Finally, it requires that the epidemiologic group maintains an awareness of pertinent research findings in areas relevant to the diseases under study and to the types of measurements and analytic techniques likely to be needed.

ACKNOWLEDGMENT

This research was funded (or funded in part) by the Agency for Healthcare Research and Quality as part of the UNC Center for Education and Research on Therapeutics (Harry Guess, CERTs PI; award number 2 U18 HS10397-05).

REFERENCES

1. Lawson DH. Pharmacoepidemiology: A new discipline. *BMJ* 1984; **289**: 940–1.

2. Tilson HH. Pharmacoepidemiology: the future. *Drug Intell Clin Pharm* 1988; **22**: 416–21.

3. Guess HA. Adverse and beneficial effects in pharmacoepidemiology. In: Armitage P, Colton T, eds, *Encyclopedia of Biostatistics*. New York: John Wiley & Sons, 1998; pp. 3332–8.

4. Guess HA, Stephenson WP, Sacks ST, Gardner JS. Beyond pharmacoepidemiology: the larger role of epidemiology in drug development. *J Clin Epidemiol* 1988; **41**: 995–6.

5. Epstein RS, Feng W, Hirsch LJ, Kelly M. Intervention thresholds for the treatment of osteoporosis: comparison of different approaches to decision-making. *Osteoporos Int* 1998; **8** (suppl 1): 22–7.

6. Jacobsen SJ, Girman CJ, Guess HA, Oesterling JE, Lieber MM. New diagnostic and treatment guidelines for benign prostatic hyperplasia. Potential impact in the United States. *Arch Intern Med* 1995; **155**: 477–81.

7. Santanello NC, Barber BL, Reiss TF, Friedman BS, Juniper EF, Zhang J. Measurement characteristics of two asthma symptom diary scales for use in clinical trials. *Eur Respir J* 1997; **10**: 646–51.

8. O'Leary MP, Fowler FJ, Lenderking WR, Barber B, Sagnier PP, Guess HA *et al*. A brief male sexual function inventory for urology. *Urology* 1995; **46**: 697–706.

9. Coplan P, Chiacchierini L, Nikas A, Shea J, Baumritter A, Beutner K *et al*. Development and evaluation of a standardized questionnaire for identifying adverse events in vaccine clinical trials. *Pharmacoepidemiol Drug Saf* 2000; **9**: 457–71.

10. Barber BL, Strahlman ER, Laibovitz R, Guess HA, Reines SA. Validation of a questionnaire for comparing the tolerability of ophthalmic medications. *Ophthalmology* 1997; **104**: 334–42.

11. Lucky AW, Barber BL, Girman CJ, Williams J, Ratterman J, Waldstreicher J. A multirater validation study to assess the reliability of acne lesion counting. *J Am Acad Dermatol* 1996; **35**: 559–65.

12. Ross PD, He YF, Davis JW, Epstein RS, Wasnich RD. Normal ranges for bone loss rates. *Bone Miner* 1994; **26**: 169–80.

13. Hirsch LJ, Pryor-Tillotson S. An overview of the results of clinical trials with alendronate, a promising treatment of osteoporosis in postmenopausal women. *Ann Ital Med Int* 1995; **10** (suppl): 22–8.

14. Rojas C, Coplan PM, Rhodes T, Robertson MN, DiNubile MJ, Guess HA. Indinavir did not further increase mean triglyceride levels in HIV-infected patients treated with nucleoside reverse transcriptase inhibitors: an analysis of three randomized clinical trials. *Pharmacoepidemiol Drug Saf* 2003; **12**: 361–9.

15. West SL, Yawn BP, Thorp JM, Korhonen MJH, Savitz DA, Guess H. Tocolytic therapy for preterm labor: assessing its potential for reducing preterm delivery. *Paediatr Perinat Epidemiol* 2001; **15**: 243–51.

16. Santanello NC, Polis AB, Hartmaier SL, Kramer MS, Block GA, Silberstein SD. Improvement in migraine-specific quality of life in a clinical trial of rizatriptan. *Cephalalgia* 1997; **17**: 867–72.

17. Martin AR, Pearson JD, Cai B, Elmer M, Horgan K, Lindley C. Assessing the impact of chemotherapy-induced nausea and vomiting on patients' daily lives: a modified version of the Functional Living Index—Emesis (FLIE) with 5-day recall. *Support Care Cancer* 2003; **11**: 522–7.

18. Guillemin F, Bombardier C, Beaton D. Cross-cultural adaptation of health-related quality of life measures: literature review and proposed guidelines. *J Clin Epidemiol* 1993; **46**: 1417–32.

19. US Food and Drug Administration. Task Force on Risk Management. *Managing the Risks from Medical Product Use—Creating a Risk Management Framework*. May 1999, Part 4, p. 73. Available at: http://www.fda.gov/oc/tfrm/riskmanagement.pdf. Accessed: June 6, 2004.

20. US Food and Drug Administration. Guidance for Industry. *Pre-marketing Risk Assessment*. Draft Guidance. Available at: http://www.fda.gov/cder/guidance/5765dft.pdf. Accessed: June 6, 2004.

21. US Food and Drug Administration. Guidance for Industry. *Development and Use of Risk Minimization Action Plans*. Draft Guidance. Available at: http://www.fda.gov/cder/guidance/5766dft.pdf. Accessed: June 6, 2004.

22. US Food and Drug Administration. Guidance for Industry. *Good Pharmacovigilance Practices and Pharmacoepidemiologic Assessment*. Draft Guidance. Available at: http://www.fda.gov/cder/guidance/5767dft.pdf. Accessed: June 6, 2004.

23. Streiner DL, Norman GR. *Health Measurement Scales—A Practical Guide to their Development and Use*, 3rd edn. New York: Oxford University Press, 2003.

24. Guyatt G, Rennie D. *Users' Guides to the Medical Literature—A Manual for Evidence-Based Clinical Practice*. Chicago, IL: AMA Press, 2001.

25. Pepe MS. *The Statistical Evaluation of Medical Tests for Classification and Prediction*. New York: Oxford University Press, 2003.

26. Moher D, Schulz KF, Altman DG. The CONSORT statement: revised recommendations for improving the quality of reports of parallel-group randomized trials. *Ann Intern Med* 2001; **134**: 657–62.

27. US Food and Drug Administration. Center for Drug Evaluation and Research. *Conducting a Safety Review of a New Product Application and Preparing a Report on the Review*. Available at: http://www.fda.gov/cder/guidance/issrvg08.pdf. Accessed: June 6, 2004.

28. Food and Drug Administration. Staff College. *MedWatch Continuing Education Article—Clinical Therapeutics and the Recognition of Drug-Induced Disease*. June 1995. Available at: http://www.fda.gov/medwatch/articles/dig/rcontent.htm. Accessed: June 6, 2004.

29. Hill AB. The environment and disease: association or causation. *Proc R Soc Med* 1965; **58**: 295–300.

30. Guess HA. Invited commentary: vasectomy and prostate cancer. *Am J Epidemiol* 1990; **132**: 1062–5.

31. International Conference on Harmonisation of Technical Requirements for Registration of Pharmaceuticals for Human Use (ICH). The Extent of Population Exposure to Assess Clinical Safety for Drugs Intended for Long-Term Treatment of Non-Life-Threatening Conditions, E1. ICH, 1994. Available at: http://www.ich.org.Accessed June 6, 2004.

32. Salas M, Hofman A, Stricker BH. Confounding by indication: an example of variation in the use of epidemiologic terminology. *Am J Epidemiol* 1999; **149**: 981–3.

33. The CONSENSUS Trial Study Group. Effects of enalapril on mortality in severe congestive heart failure. Results of the Cooperative North Scandinavian Enalapril Survival Study (CONSENSUS). *N Engl J Med* 1987; **316**: 1429–35.

34. Speirs CJ, Dollery CT, Inman WH, Rawson NS, Wilton LV. Postmarketing surveillance of enalapril. II: investigation of the potential role of enalapril in deaths with renal failure. *BMJ* 1988; **297**: 830–2.

35. Badr KF, Ichikawa I. Prerenal failure: a deleterious shift from renal compensation to decompensation. *N Engl J Med* 1988; **319**: 623–9.

36. Weed DL, Hursting SD. Biologic plausibility in causal inference: current method and practice. *Am J Epidemiol* 1998; **147**: 415–25.

37. Lane DA. The Bayesian approach to causality assessment: an introduction. *Drug Inf J* 1986; **20**: 455–61.

38. Hutchinson TA. Bayesian assessment of adverse drug reactions. *Can Med Assoc J* 2000; **163**: 1463–4.

39. Guess HA. Behavior of the exposure odds ratio in a case control study when the hazard function is not constant over time. *J Clin Epidemiol* 1989; **42**: 1179–84.

40. Ray WA. Evaluating medication effects outside of clinical trials: new-user designs. *Am J Epidemiol* 2003; **158**: 915–20.

41. Yola M, Lucien A. Evidence of the depletion of susceptibles effect in non-experimental pharmacoepidemiologic research. *J Clin Epidemiol* 1994; **47**: 731–7.

42. Guess HA, Thomas JE. A rapidly converging algorithm for exact binomial confidence intervals about the relative risk in follow-up studies with stratified incidence density data. *Epidemiology* 1990; **1**: 75–7.

43. Martin DO, Austin H. An exact method for meta-analysis of case–control and follow-up studies. *Epidemiology* 2000; **11**: 255–60.

44. Greenland S, Rothman KJ. Introduction to stratified analysis. In: Rothman KJ, Greenland S, eds, *Modern Epidemiology*, 2nd edn. Philadelphia, PA: Lippincott-Raven, 1998; pp. 253–79.

45. Kleinbaum DG, Kupper LL, Morgenstern H. *Epidemiologic Research: Principles and Quantitative Methods*. Belmont, CA: Lifetime Learning, 1982; p. 163.

46. Breslow NE, Day NE. *Statistical Methods in Cancer Research*, vol. II *The Design and Analysis of Cohort Studies*. International Agency for Research on Cancer Scientific Publication No. 82. Lyon, France: World Health Organization, 1987.

47. Girman CJ, Hartmaier S, Thiboutot D, Johnson J, Barber B, Demuro-Mercon C *et al.* Evaluating health-related quality of life in patients with facial acne: development of a self-administered questionnaire for clinical trials. *Qual Life Res* 1996; **5**: 481–90.

48. Martin AR, Lookingbill DP, Botek A, Light J, Thiboutot D, Girman CJ. Health-related quality of life among patients with facial acne—assessment of a new acne-specific questionnaire. *Clin Exp Dermatol* 2001; **26**: 380–5.

49. Fehnel SE, McLeod LD, Brandman J, Arbit DI, McLaughlin-Miley CJ, Coombs JH *et al.* Responsiveness of the acne-specific quality of life questionnaire (acne-QoL) to treatment for acne vulgaris in placebo-controlled clinical trials. *Qual Life Res* 2002; **11**: 809–16.

50. Santanello NC, Demuro-Mercon C, Davies G, Ostrom N, Noonan M, Rooklin A *et al.* Validation of a pediatric asthma caregiver diary. *J Allergy Clin Immunol* 2000; **106**: 861–6.

51. Santanello NC, Davies G, Galant SP, Pedinoff A, Sveum R, Seltzer J *et al.* Validation of an asthma symptom diary for interventional studies. *Arch Dis Child* 1999; **80**: 414–20.

52. Calandra G, Lydick E, Carrigan J, Weiss L, Guess H. Factors predisposing to seizures in seriously ill infected patients receiving antibiotics: experience with imipenem/cilastatin. *Am J Med* 1988; **84**: 911–18.

53. Guess HA, Resseguie LJ, Melton LJ III, Kurland LT, Lydick EG, Wilson WR. Factors predictive of seizures among intensive care unit patients with gram-negative infections. *Epilepsia* 1990; **31**: 567–73.

54. US Food and Drug Administration. *Drug Induced Liver Toxicity*. Available at: http://www.fda.gov/cder/livertox/default.htm/. Accessed: June 6, 2004.

55. Senior JR, Tipping RW. Serum transaminase elevations alone lack specificity for detecting rare serious liver disease (abstract 1132). *Hepatology* 2003; **38** (suppl 1): 701A.

27

Studies of Drug Utilization

DAVID LEE[1] and ULF BERGMAN[2]

[1] Center for Pharmaceutical Management, Management Sciences for Health, Arlington, Virginia, USA; [2] Karolinska Institute, Stockholm, Sweden.

INTRODUCTION

DEFINITIONS

Drug utilization was defined by the World Health Organization (WHO) as the "marketing, distribution, prescription and use of drugs in a society, with special emphasis on the resulting medical, social, and economic consequences."[1] Some authors have suggested that the development of drugs relative to health priorities should also be included.[2] This broad definition differs from the more narrow one which appeared in the North American literature, "the prescribing, dispensing and ingesting of drugs."[3,4]

In both of the above definitions, recognition is granted, explicitly or implicitly, of the non-pharmacologic (socio-anthropological, behavioral, and economic) factors influencing drug utilization. Studies of the process of drug utilization focus on the factors influencing and events involved in the prescribing, dispensing, administration, and taking of medication. However, the broader definition of the WHO goes beyond the "process" or "pharmacokinetic" aspect of drug utilization—that is, the movement of drugs along the therapeutic drug chain—to include consideration of the various "outcomes" or "pharmacodynamics" of drug use.[5] According to this definition, studies of drug utilization include not only studies of the medical and nonmedical aspects influencing drug utilization, but also the effects of drug utilization at all levels. Studies of how drug utilization relates to the effects of drug use, beneficial or adverse, are usually labeled analytic pharmacoepidemiologic research. These two aspects of the study of drug utilization have developed along parallel lines, but may now be regarded as interrelated and part of a continuum of interests and methodologies.[6]

As stated by Lunde and Baksaas,[7] the general objectives of drug utilization studies are:

> problem identification and problem analysis in relation to importance, causes, and consequences; establishment of a weighted basis for decisions on problem solution; assessment of the effects of the action taken. These objectives are relevant to problems and decision making throughout the drug and health chain. The approaches may vary according to the purpose and the needs of the users. Those include the health authorities, the drug manufacturers, the academic and clinical health professionals, social scientists, and economists as well as the media and the consumers.

This chapter focuses on the current status of descriptive epidemiological approaches to the study of the processes (or "pharmacokinetics") of drug utilization. The epidemiological approaches to the study of the effects (or "pharmacodynamics") of drug utilization, both beneficial and harmful, are covered in other chapters of this book.

TYPES OF DRUG UTILIZATION STUDIES AND THEIR USES

Drug utilization studies may be *quantitative* or *qualitative*. In the former, the objective of the study is to quantify the present state, the developmental trends, and the time course of drug usage at various levels of the health care system, whether national, regional, local, or institutional. Routinely compiled drug statistics or drug utilization data that are the result of such studies can be used to estimate drug utilization in populations by age, sex, social class, morbidity, and other characteristics, and to identify areas of possible over- or underutilization. They also can be used as denominator data for calculating rates of reported adverse drug reactions, to monitor the utilization of specific therapeutic categories where particular problems can be anticipated (e.g., narcotic analgesics, hypnotics and sedatives, and other psychotropic drugs), to monitor the effects of informational and regulatory activities (e.g., adverse events alerts, delisting of drugs from therapeutic formularies), as markers for very crude estimates of disease prevalence (e.g., antiparkinsonian drugs for Parkinson's disease), to plan for drug importation, production, and distribution, and to estimate drug expenditures.[2]

Qualitative studies, on the other hand, assess the appropriateness of drug utilization, usually by linking prescription data to the reasons for the drug prescribing (see also Chapters 28 and 29). The crucial difference between these studies and quantitative drug utilization studies is that they include the concept of appropriateness.[8] Explicit predetermined criteria are created against which aspects of the quality, medical necessity, and appropriateness of drug prescribing may be compared. Drug use criteria may be based upon such parameters as indications for use, daily dose, and length of therapy. Other possible criteria for poor drug prescribing include the failure to select a more effective or less hazardous drug if available, the use of a fixed combination drug when only one of its components is justified, or the use of a costly drug when a less costly equivalent drug is available.[9] In North America, these studies are known as *drug utilization review* (DUR) or *drug utilization review studies*. For example, a large number of studies in North America have documented the extent of inappropriate

prescribing of drugs, in particular antibiotics, and the associated adverse clinical, ecological, and economic consequences.[10–18]

In Spain, the appropriateness of drug utilization has been assessed on the basis of adequate evidence for the clinical efficacy ("high intrinsic value") of the most commonly sold drugs. The analysis revealed a striking proportion of drugs of "doubtful, no, or unacceptable value," among the 400 top pharmaceutical products in sales, albeit a trend toward more rational consumption as reflected in consumption of drugs of "high intrinsic value."[19] This approach has been used to assess prescribing patterns in France, Germany, Great Britain, and Italy,[20] appropriateness of non-prescription drug sales in Brazil,[21] and drug prescribing in Spanish primary care centers.[22,23]

Another approach analyzed the number of drugs that accounted for 90% of drug utilization (DU90%) and the percentage of these drugs that adhered to the evidence-based guideline issued by the Drug Committee in the catchment area.[24] The 90% level was arbitrarily selected to focus on the bulk of prescribing, yet allow some degree of individual variation. The number of different products in the DU90% segment varied between 117 and 194 among 38 primary health care centers in Stockholm; adherence to the guideline varied between 56% and 74%. The Swedish Medical Quality Council has recommended the DU90% method for assessing quality in drug prescribing. DU90% has also been used to compare nonsteroidal anti-inflammatory drug prescribing in Denmark, Italy, Croatia, and Sweden,[25,26] and antibiotics in Denmark and Italy.[27]

DUR and DUR studies are not interventions but rather activities aimed at problem detection and quantification. They should be distinguished, therefore, from DUR *programs* (Table 27.1) (see also Chapter 29). DUR studies are usually one-time projects, not routinely conducted. They provide for only minimal feedback to the involved prescribers and, most importantly, do not include any follow-up measures to ascertain whether any changes in drug therapy have occurred. A DUR program, on the other hand, is an intervention in the form of an authorized, structured, and *ongoing system* for improving the quality of drug use within a given health care institution. The quality of drug prescribing is evaluated by employing predetermined standards for initiating administrative or educational interventions to modify patterns of drug use which are not consistent with these standards. The measurement of the effectiveness of these interventions is an integral part of the program.[8,28]

In the US, DUR programs (commonly known in hospitals as drug use evaluation or DUE programs) are part of the

Table 27.1. Drug utilization studies in perspective: operational concepts

	Drug statistics	Drug utilization study	Drug utilization review program
Synonyms (therapeutic)	Drug utilization data	Drug utilization review or drug utilization review study	Drug audit
Quantitative approach	Yes	Usually	Usually
Qualitative approach	No	Maybe	Yes
Continuous (ongoing)	Usually	No	Yes

quality assurance activities required by Medicaid–Medicare regulations, the Joint Commission on Accreditation of Healthcare Organizations (JCAHO), the former Professional Standards Review Organizations (PSRO), and Section 4401 of the Omnibus Budget Reconciliation Act of 1990[28] (see Chapter 29). In Europe, DUR programs have been proposed as periodic "therapeutic audits" performed at various levels (patient, prescriber, hospital, county, municipality, country, and groups of countries), assessing not only the clinical consequences of drug utilization, but also the social and economic consequences. These studies are to be followed by whatever feedback is felt to be necessary and appropriate to effect changes in therapeutic practices.[29–31] Most commonly, these therapeutic audits have been based on aggregate data analysis of medicines consumption at a national level, and interventions, usually regulatory or informational and educational, are aimed accordingly at whole populations or subgroups, rather than specific individuals.

CLINICAL PROBLEMS TO BE ADDRESSED BY PHARMACOEPIDEMIOLOGY RESEARCH

In order for a drug to be marketed, it must be shown that it can effectively modify the natural course of disease or alleviate symptoms when used appropriately—that is, for the right patient, with the right disease, in the proper dosage and intervals, and for the appropriate length of time. However, used inappropriately, drugs fail to live up to their potential, with consequent morbidity and mortality. Even when used appropriately drugs have the potential to cause harm. However, a large proportion of their adverse effects is predictable and preventable.[32]

Adverse drug reactions and drug noncompliance are important causes of adult and pediatric hospital admissions[33–35] (see also Chapters 34, 35, and 46). Many of these drug-related admissions are preventable, through the application of existing principles and data.[35] The situations that may lead to preventable adverse drug reactions and drug-induced illness include the use of a drug for the wrong indication, the use of a potentially toxic drug when one with less risk of toxicity would be just as effective, the concurrent administration of an excessive number of drugs, thereby increasing the possibility of adverse drug interactions, the use of excessive doses, especially for pediatric or geriatric patients, and continued use of a drug after evidence becomes available concerning important toxic effects. Many contributory causes have been proposed: excessive prescribing by the physician, failure to define therapeutic endpoints for drug use, the increased availability of potent prescription and non-prescription drugs, increased public exposure to drugs used or produced industrially that enter the environment, the availability of illicit preparations, and prescribers' lack of knowledge of the pharmacology and pharmacokinetics of the prescribed drugs.[32] Increased morbidity or mortality due to medication error,[36] poor patient compliance,[37] discontinuation of therapy,[38–40] and problems in communication resulting from modern day fragmentation of patient care are also to be considered. The failure of physicians to prescribe an effective drug or effective doses for a treatable disease is a significant concern. For example, in a geographic area of Sweden with a higher suicide rate than average for the country, sales of antidepressant drugs were about half of that in other areas.[41] In the US, the underuse of β-blockers in elderly patients with myocardial infarction was associated with an increased risk of death.[42] Other studies have documented significant underuse of antithrombotic drugs,[43–45] lipid-lowering therapy,[40,46,47] β-blockers,[48] aspirin,[49] and thrombolytics[50] in patients with appropriate indications, but the outcomes were not assessed.

Therapeutic practice, as recommended, is based predominantly on data available from premarketing clinical trials. Complementary data from studies in the postmarketing period are needed to provide an adequate basis for improving drug therapy.[51,52] Regardless, drug utilization studies address the relationship between therapeutic practice as recommended and actual clinical practice.[53]

METHODOLOGIC PROBLEMS TO BE ADDRESSED BY PHARMACOEPIDEMIOLOGY RESEARCH

A considerable amount of drug use data may be obtainable or are already available, the usefulness of which depends on the purpose of the study at hand. All have certain limitations in their direct clinical relevance.[54] For quantitative studies, the ideal is a count of the number of patients in a defined population who ingest a drug of interest during a particular time frame. The data available are only approximations of this, and thereby raise many questions about their presentation and interpretation. For qualitative studies, the ideal is a count of the number of patients in a defined population who use a drug inappropriately during a particular time frame, of all those who received the drug in that population during that time frame. Again, the data available are suboptimal—both the exposure data and the diagnosis data. In addition, the criteria to be used to define "appropriate" are arbitrary.

Since most statistics on drug consumption were compiled for administrative or commercial reasons, the data are usually expressed in terms of cost or volume (see Table 27.2). First, data on drug utilization can be available as total costs or unit cost, such as cost per package, tablet, dose, or treatment course. Although such data may be useful for measuring and comparing the economic impact of drug use, these units do not provide information on the amount of drug exposure in the population. Moreover, cost data are influenced by price fluctuations over time, distribution channels, inflation, exchange rate fluctuations, price control measures, etc.[55]

Volume data are also available, as the overall weight of the drug that is sold or the unit volume sold—that is, the number of tablets, capsules, or doses sold. This is closer to the number of patients exposed. However, tablet sizes vary, making it difficult to translate weight into even the number of tablets. Prescription sizes also vary, so it is difficult to translate number of tablets into the number of exposed patients.

Table 27.2. Types of drug utilization data available

(1)	Cost or unit cost
(2)	Weight
(3)	Number of tablets, capsules, doses, etc.
(4)	Number of prescriptions
(5)	Number of patients ingesting drug[a]

[a] Generally not available.

The number of prescriptions is the measure most frequently used in drug utilization studies. However, different patients receive a different number of prescriptions in any given time interval. To translate the number of prescriptions into the number of patients, one must divide by the average number of prescriptions per patient, or else distinctions must be made between first prescriptions and refill prescriptions. The latter is, of course, better for studies of new drug therapy, but will omit individuals who are receiving chronic drug therapy. Additional problems may be posed by differences in the number of drugs in each prescription. Finally, it should be noted that all these units represent approximate estimates of true consumption. The latter is ultimately modified further by the patients' actual drug intake, that is, their degree of compliance.

In the context of DUR, drug utilization data may be presented in the form of profiles of physicians according to the number, monetary value, and even type of prescription ordered during a given time period. Pharmacies may be ranked according to the number, cost, and type of prescription dispensed for similar intervals. However, these gross measures of prescription activity and drug use are very limited in their capacity to reflect the wide spectrum of specific problems in prescribing. For example, they ignore problems such as the wrong drug for the indication, the wrong drug for the patient, the wrong dose, the wrong interval, and the wrong duration of therapy. Also, one's deviation from the practices of the mean practitioner is not a good measure of one's "appropriateness" as a provider. Purely quantitative data characterizing prescribers as "high" or "low" may be driven, for example, by the number of patients seen by the physician and the type and severity of the patients' diseases. Likewise, cost profiles are not indicative of appropriateness, whether high or low relative to the mean.

From a quality of care perspective, to interpret drug utilization data appropriately, there is a need to relate the data to the reasons for the drug usage. Data on morbidity and mortality may be obtained from national registries (general or specialized), national samples where medical service reimbursement schemes operate, *ad hoc* surveys and special studies, hospital records, physician records, and patient or household surveys. "Appropriateness" of use must be assessed relative to indication for treatment, patient characteristics (age-related physiological status, sex, habits), drug dosage (over- or under-dosage), concomitant diseases (that might contraindicate or interfere with chosen therapy), and the use of other drugs (interactions). However, no single source is generally available for obtaining all this information. Moreover, because of incompleteness, the medical record may not be a very useful source of drug use data.[56,57]

Generally agreed upon standards or criteria for appropriateness, based upon currently available knowledge, are essential elements of the drug utilization review process. These criteria must be based on scientifically established evidence, updated regularly according to new scientific evidence, explicitly stated (to ensure consistency in the evaluations), and applicable to a given setting.[58] The development and standardization of these criteria are major undertakings. Finally, for drug utilization review programs, even the strategy to be used to optimize one's intervention is still unclear (see Chapter 29).

CURRENTLY AVAILABLE SOLUTIONS

THE EVOLUTION OF DRUG UTILIZATION STUDIES

The current growth of interest in drug utilization studies began on both sides of the Atlantic in the early 1960s. Previously, drug utilization studies had been conducted mostly for marketing purposes and data were not widely available for use by academic researchers or health authorities. The increased interest resulted from recognition of the virtual explosion in the marketing of new drugs, the wide variations in the patterns of drug prescribing and consumption, the growing concern about the delayed adverse effects, and the increasing concern about the cost of drugs, as reflected in the increase in both the sales and the volume of prescriptions of drugs.[59,60] However, the development of pharmacoepidemiologic methods can be characterized by two different lines of work (drug utilization studies as performed in Europe versus as performed in the US), currently approaching each other from opposite directions, strongly influenced by the varied availability and accessibility of data sources.

Drug utilization studies at the national and international levels have been more developed in Europe, where this line of research was pioneered by the Scandinavian countries, Scotland, and Northern Ireland. Under the auspices of the WHO Regional Office for Europe, a Drug Utilization Research Group was established in the 1970s to stimulate interest in comparative studies with a common methodology.[59] Factors which contributed greatly to this line of development, primarily in the countries of northern Europe, have been the relatively small size of the populations involved, the limited number of pharmaceutical products on the market (2000–3000 in Norway and Sweden), and the availability of centralized statistics on sales or prescriptions.[59] Drug utilization studies in Europe have been predominantly quantitative, describing

and comparing patterns of utilization of specific groups of drugs according to geographic regions and time. For example, international studies have documented wide variations in the utilization of antidiabetic,[59,61] psychotropic,[29] NSAIDs,[25,26] antihypertensive drugs,[29,59] antibiotic drugs,[62] and lipid-lowering drugs[63] among European and other countries. Follow-up studies on the utilization of antidiabetic and antihypertensive drugs among some of these countries indicate that the differences cannot be explained only by differences in the prevalence of disease.[64–66] National studies have also revealed striking variations in drug utilization among regions and communities within the same country.[29,59] One study addressed the relation between variations in drug sales and treatment outcomes. For example, the degree of good metabolic control, as defined by the authors (body mass index and glycosylated hemoglobin A value), in diabetic subjects in three Swedish areas with high, medium, and low sales of antidiabetic drugs was achieved among only 16%, 17%, and 12% of subjects, respectively.[67] These findings were confirmed in a Nordic survey of the marked differences in the use of antidiabetic drugs in the Nordic countries. It was concluded that differences in morbidity were one important factor to explaining the differences. Other factors included differences in age structure, therapeutic traditions, reimbursement systems, and prevalence of obesity, emphasizing the importance of non-pharmacologic treatment (such as weight reduction and exercise).[68]

In the US, drug utilization research has developed on a smaller scale, primarily at institutional or local health program levels. Factors which have hindered studies at a national level have been the size of the population, the number of pharmaceutical products on the market (20 000–30 000), and the lack of an all-encompassing pharmaceutical data collection system.[69] Data on drug use are more readily available from prepaid health plans, health delivery institutions, and public health care programs. For example, early studies of physician prescribing showed that prescribing patterns varied greatly among physicians, according to their place and type of practice and the community in which they prescribed.[70] In US drug utilization research, greater emphasis had been placed initially on the study of the quality of physician prescribing habits, in particular with respect to antibiotics, in both hospital and outpatient settings.[10–18] More recently, many studies have targeted medications for cardiovascular diseases.[42–50] However, studies of the national patterns of drug utilization and expenditures in the US have also been published.[69]

Because of the critical importance of the decision making process in drug prescribing, a number of studies have addressed the factors which influence this decision: education, advertising, colleagues, working circumstances, personality, control and regulatory measures, and demands from society and patients.[71,72] Some controversy exists concerning the relative impact of the various sources of influence on prescribing behavior, particularly the influence of pharmaceutical advertising. In studies of hospital practice the following factors have been stated to contribute to excessive or inappropriate prescribing: simple errors of omission, physician ignorance of cost issues in prescribing, failure to review medication orders frequently and critically, inability to keep up to date with developments in pharmacology and therapeutics, insulation of physicians and patients from cost considerations because of third-party coverage, and lack of communication between physicians and pharmacists.[73]

The intervention strategies aimed at improving prescribing behavior in hospital as well as in primary care settings have been critically reviewed.[74–77] These may include (discussed in Chapter 28) dissemination of printed educational materials alone, multimedia warning campaigns, drug utilization audit followed by mailed or interactive feedback of aggregated results, group education through lectures or rounds, use of computerized reminder systems, use of opinion leaders to informally "endorse" or support specific behavior change interventions, one-to-one education initiated by a drug utilization expert, required consultation or justification prior to the use of specific drugs, and use of clinical guidelines.

CURRENT DATA SOURCES

Currently available computer databases for studies of drug utilization may be classified as non-diagnosis-linked and diagnosis-linked (see Table 27.3). Most of these data sources lack information on morbidity and are mostly used for generating drug statistics and descriptive studies of patterns of drug consumption. Some collect data in the form of drug sales (e.g., the Danish Medicines Agency, the National Agency for Medicines and Social Insurance in Finland, the Norwegian Institute of Public Health, and the National Corporation of Pharmacies in Sweden) (published regularly on the respective websites: www.laegemiddelstyrelsen.dk, www.nam.fi, www.legemiddelforbruk.no, www.apoteket.se), drug movement at various levels of the drug distribution channel (IMS America's National Prescription Audit, US Pharmaceutical Market—Hospitals, US Pharmaceutical Market—Drugstores) (www.imshealth.com), pharmaceutical or medical billing data (Prescription Pricing Authority in the UK, Spain's Drug Data Bank, Medicaid Management Information

Table 27.3. Some computer databases for drug utilization studies

Not diagnosis-linked	Diagnosis-linked
North America	
National Prescription Audit[a]	National Disease and Therapeutic Index[a]
US Pharmaceutical Market—Drugstores[a]	Kaiser Permanente Medical Plan[a]
US Pharmaceutical Market—Hospitals[a]	Group Health Cooperative[b]
Medicaid Management Information Systems	The Slone Survey[c]
Saskatchewan Health Plan[b]	
Europe	
Swedish National Corporation of Pharmacies	Sweden's Community of Tierp Project
Sweden's County of Jämtland Project	United Kingdom's General Practice Research Database
Norwegian Institute of Public Health	The Netherlands' Integrated Primary Care Information Database
United Kingdom's Prescription Pricing Authority	
Spain's Drug Data Bank (National Institute of Health)	
Denmark's Odense Pharmacoepidemiologic Database	
Denmark's County of North Jutland Pharmacoepidemiologic Prescription Database	

[a] IMS America, Ltd.
[b] Patient-specific data available for longitudinal studies.
[c] Reason for use.

System),[59,60,78,79] or all prescriptions dispensed (National Corporation of Pharmacies in Sweden) (www.apoteket.se).

The County of Jämtland Project (Sweden) is of interest for longitudinal patient-specific studies of drug utilization.[41,80,81] All drug prescriptions dispensed to 14% of the Jämtland population (approximately 17 000) have been continuously monitored since 1970. The recorded information includes the patient's unique identity number; name, dosage, quantity, and price of the drug; date of dispensing; dispensing pharmacy; and prescribing physician. Information relating to morbidity (diagnoses), however, is missing. Unfortunately, because of sensitivity to the issue of data confidentiality in Sweden, the correspondingly recorded data relative to individual patients in other parts of Sweden is not available for use in health care audits.[56] Similar individual-linked drug use data is also available from many local health systems covering populations of 300 000–500 000 inhabitants in Italy; these databases may provide data on incidence and prevalence of drug use.[27]

The Odense Pharmacoepidemiologic Database (OPED) and the Pharmacoepidemiologic Prescription Database of the County of North Jutland are two similar databases that include about half a million inhabitants in Denmark.[82] These databases contain all dispensed prescriptions since the early 1990s. The following information is captured for each prescription: a unique person identifier, the date of dispensing, identification of the dispensed product, the pharmacy, and the prescriber. The databases do not include information on over-the-counter medications (laxatives, analgesics, ibuprofen, antihistamines, antitussives, and certain anti-ulcer drugs) and non-subsidized drugs (oral contraceptives, hypnotics, and sedatives). They have been used for a number of population-based pharmacoepidemiologic surveys such as the use of the new antidepressants,[83] inappropriate use of inhaled steroids in asthma treatment,[84] inappropriate use of sumatriptan,[85] hemorrhagic complication during oral anticoagulant therapy,[86] and low use of long-term hormone replacement therapy.[87] The OPED database has also been used to develop a graphical approach to reduce the overwhelming volume of data in population-based pharmacoepidemiologic databases to a few parameters and a "waiting time distribution" that can be used to screen for certain unusual or unexpected patterns of drug use.[40,88] Based on prescriptions dispensed to individual patients, key parameters such as incidence, one-year and point prevalence, duration of treatment, relapse rate, and seasonality have a visual correlate.

In the US, several databases that contain both drug and morbidity data have been used to a relatively limited extent for this type of study, as opposed to hypothesis-testing research. These include data from the Group Health Cooperative and the Kaiser Permanente Medical Care Programs, described in more detail in Chapters 14 and 15, respectively. The Tayside Medicines Monitoring Unit (MEMO) and the General Practice Research Database (GPRD) in the United Kingdom (see Chapters 21 and 22) are databases that have been developed primarily for drug safety studies, but have also been used to study drug utilization.[89,90]

The National Disease and Therapeutic Index (NDTI), by IMS America, is an ongoing study of physician prescribing which is conducted mainly for use by pharmaceutical companies in their marketing activities.[91] This study employs a rotating sample of office-based physicians who record all patient encounters and corresponding "drug mentions" for two-day periods four times a year. A special prescription form is used to collect information on the drug (specific product, dosage form, new versus continuing therapy), patient characteristics (sex), prescriber (specialty, location, region), type of consultation (first versus subsequent), concomitant drugs and diagnoses, and the desired pharmacological action.[69] Data have been made available to academic researchers and the US Food and Drug Administration.[69] Although useful for studies of prescribing, longitudinal patient-specific studies are not possible with this database.

Similar to IMS America's NDTI, the Swedish Diagnosis and Therapy Survey was a collaborative project run by Swedish Pharmaceutical Data Ltd (LSAB), the National Corporation of Pharmacies (Apoteket AB), the Swedish Medical Association, and the National Board of Health and Welfare. Drug utilization data from this ongoing survey, in combination with overall sales statistics, are prepared yearly by the National Corporation of Pharmacies and have been available for research.[92] However, because of increasing physician nonparticipation in this community survey, it has been suspended and future prescribing data will be obtained from the computerized medical records that are increasingly used in Sweden.

The Community of Tierp Project is run by the Center for Primary Care Research, University of Uppsala, Sweden. Prescription and morbidity data are routinely collected from all pharmacies and the health center within the community for all residents since 1972.[93] The database has been used to study the use of antidepressant drugs,[93] antidiabetic medications,[94,95] and benzodiazepines.[96] It has also been used to study the impact of over-the-counter nasal sprays on sales, prescribing, and physician visits.[97] Limitations of this database are the size of the population covered (21 000 persons) and questions regarding the representativeness of this community for the whole of Sweden.

The Integrated Primary Care Information (IPCI) database, established at Erasmus University in The Netherlands, consists of the computer-based patient records of 150 general practitioners. To date the database has accumulated data on approximately 500 000 patients. The records are coded to ensure the anonymity of the patients; data include patient demographics, symptoms (in free text), diagnoses (based on the International Classification for Primary Care and free text), clinical examination findings, referrals, laboratory test results, hospitalizations, and physician-linked drug prescriptions and dosage regimen. This database has been used to study the use of preventive strategies in patients receiving nonsteroidal anti-inflammatory agents[98] and trends in primary care prescribing for heart failure.[99] Other Dutch computer databases are discussed in Chapter 20.

In Canada, the province of Saskatchewan has a series of computerized databases describing health services paid for by the provincial Department of Health, including prescription drugs.[100] A variety of drug utilization studies have been performed using these data, which are described in more detail in Chapter 19.

In the US, Medicaid medical and pharmaceutical billing data have been available for drug utilization studies. The most frequently used databases for academic pharmacoepidemiologic research are discussed in Chapter 18. The Protocare Sciences Proprietary Medicaid Database (formerly COMPASS®) and DURbase®, both originally developed by Health Information Designs, Inc., are examples of databases that are used for drug utilization review programs serviced by commercial firms. Drug utilization studies performed using COMPASS® have been limited.[101,102] Medicaid data are now frequently obtained from sources other than these commercial vendors (see Chapter 18). With the skewed population included in Medicaid, however, the generalizability of the results is a concern.

The Slone Epidemiology Unit of Boston University has developed a novel population-based database that includes prescription and non-prescription drugs, vitamins/minerals, and herbals/supplements.[103] Since 1998, the Slone Epidemiology Unit has been conducting an ongoing telephone survey of a random sample of the non-institutionalized continental US population (48 states and the District of Columbia). The survey excludes individuals without telephones, those residing temporarily in vacation homes, nursing homes, or rehabilitation hospitals, and individuals in prisons, military barracks, or college/university dormitories without telephones in individual rooms. Information is collected on each medication used at any time during the seven days preceding the phone interview, the reason for use, number of days that medication was taken, and total duration of use. Information on dose and number of pills taken is collected for medications containing acetylsalicylic acid, acetaminophen, ibuprofen, or conjugated estrogens. Other information elicited includes age, sex, race (based on 1990 US census categories), Hispanic origin, years of education, income (in ranges), health insurance prescription coverage, ZIP code of residence, and for women between 18 and 50 years of age, the pregnancy status, including due date or last menstrual period. Data from over 3000 interviews in the first three years of the survey suggested that more than 80% of the US adult population took one prescription or non-prescription medication and 25% took multiple products; 40% took vitamins/minerals, while 16% took herbals/supplements.[103]

Although the use of health insurance databases has also been reported in countries outside North America and Europe,[104–106] medical and pharmaceutical databases are generally not available in most developing countries.

An indicator-based approach, developed in the early 1990s by the International Network for Rational Use of Drugs (INRUD) and WHO,[107] has facilitated the study of drug utilization in developing countries. It includes recommendations on minimum sample sizes, sampling methods, and data collection techniques, depending on study objectives. The methodology recommends 12 core indicators and 7 complementary indicators to study drug use in health facilities (Table 27.4). These indicators can be used to describe prescribing practice,[108] conduct monitoring and supervision,[109] and assess the impact of interventions.[110–112] To date, researchers in more than 30 countries of Africa, Asia, and Latin America and the Caribbean have used this methodology.

UNITS OF MEASUREMENT

The defined daily dose (DDD) methodology was developed in response to the need to convert and standardize readily available volume data from sales statistics or pharmacy inventory data (quantity of packages, tablets, or other dosage forms) into medically meaningful units, to make crude estimates of the number of persons exposed to a particular

Table 27.4. WHO/INRUD drug use indicators

Core indicators
Prescribing indicators
Average number of drugs per encounter
Percentage of drugs prescribed by generic name
Percentage of encounters with an antibiotic prescribed
Percentage of encounters with an injection prescribed
Percentage of drugs prescribed from essential drugs list or formulary
Patient care indicators
Average consultation time
Average dispensing time
Percentage of drugs actually dispensed
Percentage of drugs adequately labeled
Patient's knowledge of correct dosage
Facility indicators
Availability of copy of essential drugs list or formulary
Availability of key drugs
Complementary indicators
Percentage of patients treated without drugs
Average drug cost per encounter
Percentage of drug costs spent on antibiotics
Percentage of drug costs spent on injections
Prescription in accordance with treatment guidelines
Percentage of patients satisfied with care they received
Percentage of health facilities with access to impartial drug information

medicine or class of medicines.[59,60,113] The DDD is the assumed average daily maintenance dose for a drug for its main indication in adults. Expressed as DDDs per 1000 inhabitants per day, for chronically used drugs, it can be interpreted as the proportion of the population that may receive treatment with a particular medicine on any given day. For use in hospital settings, the unit is expressed as DDDs per 100 bed-days (adjusted for occupancy rate); it suggests the proportion of inpatients that may receive a DDD. For medicines that are used for short-term periods, such as antimicrobials, the unit is expressed as DDDs per inhabitant per year; this provides an estimate of the number of days for which each person is treated with a particular medication in a year. The method has been useful in describing and comparing patterns of drug utilization,[29,59,60] providing denominator data to estimate reported adverse drug reaction rates,[114] performing epidemiologic screening for problems in drug utilization,[31] and monitoring the effects of informational and regulatory activities.[115] Recently, the methodology has been used to study variations in antimicrobial utilization[62] and their correlation with antimicrobial resistance in outpatient[116] and inpatient[117] settings in Europe.

The DDD methodology is useful for working with readily available gross drug statistics, allows comparisons between drugs in the same therapeutic class and between different health care settings or geographic areas, and evaluations of trends over time, and is relatively easy and inexpensive to use. The methodology is firmly established in Europe and Scandinavia and is increasingly used by researchers in other regions.[115,118–124] A recently published WHO manual on drug utilization research provides an overview of the methodology.[125]

The DDD methodology should be used and interpreted with caution. The DDD is not a recommended or a prescribed dose, but a technical unit of comparison; it is usually the result of literature review and available information on use in various countries. Thus, the DDDs may be high or low relative to actual prescribed doses. Moreover, the DDD refer to use in adults. Since children's doses are substantially lower than the established DDDs, if unadjusted, this situation will lead to an underestimation of population exposures, which may be significant in countries with a large pediatric population. Although pediatric DDDs have also been proposed,[126] the concept and its applicability have not been incorporated into the WHO methodology.[125] Finally, DDDs do not, of course, take into account variations in compliance.

The prescribed daily dose (PDD) is another unit, developed as a means to validate the DDDs. The PDD is the average daily dose prescribed, as obtained from a representative sample of prescriptions.[127] Problems may arise in calculating the PDD due to a lack of clear and exact dosage indication in the prescription, as is often the case with the prescribing of insulin. Prescriptions for chronic therapy, as in the case of insulin, may be refilled many times and the dosage may be altered verbally between prescribing events.[128] For certain groups of drugs, such as the oral antidiabetics, the mean PDD may be lower than the corresponding DDDs. Up to two-fold variations in the mean PDD have been documented in international comparisons.[127] Higher PDDs have been observed in the US relative to Sweden for commonly prescribed drugs, such as hydrochlorothiazide, diazepam, and oxazepam.[129–131] In risk assessments of antidepressants among suicides, a refined person-year of use estimate was obtained from adjusting the DDD by the average PDD for individual antidepressants.[132] Although the DDD and the PDD may be used to estimate population drug exposure "therapeutic intensity," the methodology is not useful to estimate incidence and prevalence of drug use or to quantify or identify patients who receive doses lower or higher than those considered effective and safe.

CLASSIFICATION SYSTEMS

The Anatomic Therapeutic Chemical (ATC) classification system is generally used in conjunction with the DDD methodology.[113,125] It was originally developed by the Norwegian Medicinal Depot, which became a WHO Collaborating Centre for Drug Statistics Methodology; the center is now located at the Norwegian Institute of Public Health (www.whocc.no). The ATC system is based on the main principles of the Anatomical Classification system developed by the European Pharmaceutical Marketing Research Association (EPhMRA) and the International Pharmaceutical Market Research Group (IPMRG).

The ATC system consists of five hierarchical levels: a main anatomical group, two therapeutic subgroups, a chemical–therapeutic subgroup, and a chemical substance subgroup. The coding of furosemide preparations is used to illustrate the ATC classification structure in Table 27.5. The first three levels are modifications of the three-level EPhMRA and IPMRG classification system. The fourth and fifth levels are extensions that are developed and updated by the WHO Collaborating Centre for Drug Statistics Methodology. Ongoing discussions aim to identify differences in the two classification systems and harmonize the first three levels. Statistics reported with the ATC system should not be directly compared with figures prepared with the EPhMRA system.

Table 27.5. ATC and IDIS classification and coding structures for furosemide

---

ATC Classification (C03CA01)

C   Cardiovascular system
     (first level, main anatomical group)

  03   Diuretics
        (second level, main therapeutic group)

     C   High ceiling diuretics
          (third level, therapeutic subgroup)

        A   Sulfonamides, plain
             (fourth level, chemical therapeutic
             subgroup)

          01   Furosemide
                (fifth level, chemical substance)

IDIS Classification (40280401)

40   Electrolyte solutions
      (first level, main therapeutic group)

  28   Diuretics
        (second level, therapeutic subcategory)

     04   Loop-diuretics
           (third level, therapeutic subcategory)

        01   Furosemide
              (fourth level, chemical substance)

Medicinal products are classified according to the main therapeutic indication for the principal active ingredient. Most products are assigned only one ATC code. However, some active medicinal substances may have more than one ATC code, if the drug has different uses at different strengths (acetylsalicylic acid as a platelet aggregation inhibitor and as an analgesic–antipyretic), dosage forms (timolol to treat hypertension and to treat glaucoma), or both (medroxyprogesterone for cancer therapy and as a sex hormone). Prednisolone is an example of a drug that has six different codes. Fixed-dose combination products pose classification difficulties. For example, a combination product that contains an analgesic and a tranquilizer is classified as an analgesic, even though it also contains a psychotropic substance. Because the ATC codes and DDDs may change over time with regular revisions, researchers must carefully document which version of the classification and DDD assignment is used, so that the resulting drug statistics may be adequately interpreted.[133]

The European Drug Utilization Research Group (Euro-DURG), formerly WHO Drug Utilization Research Group and currently an association of European national Drug Utilization Research Groups, recommends the use of the ATC classification system for reporting drug consumption statistics and conducting comparative drug utilization research.

Australia (www.health.gov.au), Denmark (www.laegemiddelstyrelsen.dk), Finland (www.nam.fi), Iceland (see www.nam.fi), Norway (www.legemiddelforbruk.no), and Sweden (www.apoteket.se) produce annual reports on drug consumption and make them available in print and/or web-based electronic versions. The WHO International Drug Monitoring Program uses the system for drug coding in adverse drug reaction monitoring (www.who-umc.org). Some developing countries have begun to use the ATC system to classify their essential drugs; this may eventually lead to preparation of drug utilization statistics.[134,135]

In the US, the Iowa Drug Information System (IDIS) is a hierarchical drug coding system that is based on the three therapeutic categories of the American Hospital Formulary Society (AHFS), to which a fourth level was added to code individual drug ingredients.[136] The IDIS code has eight numeric digits, two digits per level (see Table 27.5). This coding system was used in the Established Populations for Epidemiologic Studies of the Elderly survey.[136] Other coding systems, such as the National Drug Code and the Veterans' Administration Classification,[137] do not provide unique codes for drug ingredients.

INTERVENTION STRATEGIES BASED ON DRUG UTILIZATION DATA

Numerous studies have described interventions aimed at improving prescribing by the use of drug utilization data obtained from qualitative drug utilization studies, and are discussed more in Chapter 28. Two innovative intervention strategies exemplify different approaches to the use of drug utilization data available from computer databases of office practice.

In a randomized clinical trial, Avorn and Soumerai[138] used data from the Medicaid Management Information System to identify physicians who were prescribing drugs that were assessed as inappropriate (based on considerations of documented efficacy, relative efficacy, and relative cost). These physicians were targeted for educational or information activities, as either face-to-face contacts or written drug information. Schaffner *et al.*[139] and Ray *et al.*[140] used a similar approach in another controlled intervention study comparing different strategies aimed at modifying physician prescribing behavior: written drug information versus personal visits by pharmacists versus personal visits by physician educators. These two studies demonstrated the efficacy of face-to-face methods in improving drug prescribing.

The second approach uses claims data to perform computerized screening for patients who may be at increased risk for drug-induced illness, using patient-specific medical and drug histories.[102,141,142] Health professionals then evaluate profiles of patients with possibly inappropriate drug use. If drug use is indeed considered inappropriate, a letter is sent to the prescriber providing a profile of the patient's relevant computerized claims record and a warning of the potential for drug-induced disease. Often the problem is a concomitant drug or diagnosis that the prescriber was unaware of. This approach is obviously much less expensive than the face-to-face approach. Using before and after comparisons, a significant reduction in drug-induced hospitalizations has been noted.[141] However, the interpretation of these results is hampered by the use of a nonexperimental design. A simultaneously controlled trial is needed to adequately assess the value of this approach. (See Chapter 29 for more information about computerized claims-based drug utilization review programs.)

Many other studies have described intervention strategies based on providing drug utilization data feedback, alone or in combination with printed material and/or other "educational strategies," for example group discussions, lectures, seminars, or personal visits by "experts." The results from these studies are conflicting. Some suggest that methods that involve only feedback of drug utilization data or audit results are ineffective. Others suggest a transient effectiveness for those that combine the use of drug utilization review data with group discussions, lectures, and visits by "experts." However, these are difficult to interpret because of limitations in their research designs.[73]

Conceptually, DUR programs are aimed at the improvement of medical care and cost-containment. However, in practice traditional approaches have focused on the control of abuse or overuse of drugs, polypharmacy, or patients obtaining prescriptions from many different prescribers. Moreover, most DUR studies have emphasized process measures of quality of care, for example the use of clinical laboratory tests to monitor for adverse effects during chloramphenicol or aminoglycoside therapy. The approach described by Strom and Morse,[102] Morse et al.,[141] and Groves[142] was a significant advance in DUR programs, as it was primarily aimed at improving measurable patient outcomes. Also, it does not impose arbitrary restrictions on drug use, potentially impairing patient care, but seeks to reduce costs by improving patient care. In seeking to reduce the financial impact of drug use, it does not focus on the drug costs themselves, but on the effects of the drugs. By reducing the need for medical care through the beneficial effects of drugs, or by increasing the need for remedial medical care because of drug toxicity, pharmaceuticals can have a financial impact on the health care system which is much larger than the cost of the drugs themselves. (This is discussed more in Chapter 41.)

Despite their appeal, the role of DUR programs still remains to be established. A recent study of six Medicaid programs failed to identify an effect of retrospective drug utilization review on the rate of potential prescribing errors and clinical outcomes.[143] Another study did not find effects of two state prospective DUR interventions on the frequency of drug problems, utilization of prescription drugs and other health services, and clinical outcomes.[144] (See Chapter 29 for a detailed discussion of DUR.)

THE FUTURE

OPPORTUNITIES

From a public health perspective, the observed differences in national and international patterns of drug utilization require much further study. The medical consequences as well as the explanations for such differences are still not well documented. Analysis of medicine use by gender and age group may suggest important associations, as in a recent study on antidepressant medication use and decreased suicide rates.[145] The increasing availability of population-based data resources will facilitate studies of incidence and prevalence of medicine use by age and gender, such as those conducted in Sweden and Denmark.

Numerous studies have addressed the factors influencing drug prescribing. However, the relative importance of the many determinants of appropriate prescribing still remains to be adequately elucidated. Further research is needed to better define to what degree and which determinants of inappropriate prescribing are susceptible to modification and what might be an appropriate mix of interventions to achieve optimal impact. Although regulation is effective, it is not possible to regulate all aspects of the clinical decision making process to ensure optimal drug prescribing.[146] Other approaches in addition to educational and informational measures need to be explored.

Many strategies aimed at modifying prescribing behavior have been proposed and adopted. The evidence to date indicates that mailed educational materials alone are not sufficient to modify prescribing behavior.[74,75] Recent studies conducted in Australia[147] and Denmark[148] concluded that mailed, unsolicited, centralized, government-sponsored feedback, one based on aggregate prescribing data and the other with a clinical guideline, had no impact on physician prescribing. For interventions that have been shown to be effective in improving drug prescribing (discussed in Chapter 28), there is a need to further define their relative efficacy and proper role in a comprehensive strategy for optimizing drug utilization. Questions yet to be addressed through proper methodology deal with the role of printed drug information such as drug bulletins, the duration of effect of educational interventions such as group discussions, lectures, and seminars, each in both the outpatient as well as the inpatient settings, and the generalizability of face-to-face methods as described by Avorn and Soumerai,[138] Schaffner et al.,[139] and Ray et al.[140]

More clinically applicable approaches to drug utilization review programs, such as the computerized screening of patient-specific drug histories in outpatient care to prevent drug-induced hospitalizations, still require further development and assessment (see Chapter 29). Although numerous studies have described the results of these and other novel programs,[141,142,149,150] adequate documentation of their efficacy in improving quality of care is an important subject for future work. Patient outcome measures as well as process measures of quality of drug utilization have to be included in such studies. To be effective and efficient, health care policy options should be based on sound scientific evidence.[151]

PROBLEMS

The use of computerized databases has greatly facilitated the study of drug utilization. Although useful, most of these databases are far from ideal, as they have been set up mainly for administrative purposes, such as reimbursement, and drug utilization data are obtained as "spin off" information. The model information system that will suit both medical and administrative needs[152] is not to be expected in the near future, although there is increasing interest in computerizing medical records for routine practice in countries such as Sweden and The Netherlands. Existing medical and pharmaceutical databases, with all their described limitations, will continue to be the main resources for these drug utilization studies.

Confidentiality of patient records has been successfully handled at the technical level. However, in many countries political acceptance may be much more difficult to achieve. For example, although patient-specific information is captured in the current national prescription database in Sweden, due to legal restrictions this valuable information is not saved or stored and, thus, not available for health services research. EuroDURG researchers reported difficulties arising from confidentiality laws in five of ten European countries.[153] It was feared that implementation of Directive 95/46/EC of 24 October 1995, on the protection of individuals with regard to the processing of personal data and on the free movement of such data in the European Union, may adversely affect researcher access to patient health data (see also Chapter 38). The ethical issues in pharmacoepidemiology have been discussed in a recent special issue of *Pharmacoepidemiology and Drug Safety*.[154]

In an era of increased interest in cost-containment and cost-effectiveness, research is usually not awarded high priority, resulting in reduced opportunities for financing much needed drug utilization research. Moreover, the recruitment and training of researchers for this relatively new field may be hampered by limitations in funding, as well as limitations in career opportunities. These two problems will impose significant constraints on the future development of studies in drug utilization. However, despite this, the search must continue for simple and relatively inexpensive methods for conducting descriptive studies of drug utilization and effective intervention strategies that may contribute to the optimization of drug therapy. Fortunately, the increasing commitment to drug utilization research is reflected in the development and growth of international groups such as the International Society for Pharmacoepidemiology (ISPE) (www.pharmacoepi.org),[155] the International Clinical Epidemiology Network (INCLEN) (www.inclentrust.org),[156] the European Drug Utilization Research Group (EuroDURG) (www.eurodurg.com),[157] the Latin American Group for Drug Epidemiology (DURG-LA),[158] and the International Network for Rational Use of Drugs (INRUD) (www.msh.org/INRUD).[159,160]

In summary, the study of drug utilization continues to evolve. The development of large computerized databases that allow the linkage of drug utilization data to diagnoses, albeit subject to some inherent limitations, is contributing to expand this field of study. The WHO/INRUD indicator-based approach to drug utilization studies is facilitating the development of drug utilization research in developing countries. Many strategies have already been proposed and are being implemented to improve the quality of drug prescribing. Drug utilization review programs, particularly approaches that take into primary consideration patient outcome measures, merit further rigorous study. Opportunities for the study of drug utilization continue to be virtually unexplored, but the political issue regarding the confidentiality of medical records, as well as the shortage of funds and manpower in the current era of cost-containment, will determine the pace of growth of drug utilization research.

REFERENCES

1. WHO Expert Committee. *The Selection of Essential Drugs*, technical report series no. 615. Geneva: World Health Organization, 1977.
2. Lunde PKM, Andrew M, Baksaas I. Drug utilization—an instrument in drug research. In: Kewitz H, Roots I, Voight K, eds,

Epidemiological Concepts in Clinical Pharmacology. Berlin: Springer-Verlag, 1987; pp. 57–72.

3. Brodie DC. *Drug Utilization and Drug Utilization Review and Control*, NCHS-RD-70-8. Rockville: Department of Health, Education, and Welfare, National Center for Health Services Research and Development, Health Services and Mental Health Administration, 1970.

4. Conley BE. *Social and Economic Aspects of Drug Utilization Research*. Hamilton: Drug Intelligence Publications, 1976.

5. Baksaas I, Lunde PKM. Drug utilization: pharmacokinetics in the community. *Trends Pharmacol Sci* 1981; **2**: 5–7.

6. Laporte JR, Tognoni G, eds. *Principios de epidemiología del medicamento*, 2nd edn. Barcelona: Ediciones Científicas y Técnicas, 1993.

7. Lunde PKM, Baksaas I. Epidemiology of drug utilization—basic concepts and methodology. *Acta Med Scand Suppl* 1988; **721**: 7–11.

8. Stolar MH. Drug use review: operational definitions. *Am J Hosp Pharm* 1978; **35**: 76–8.

9. Lee PR. America is an overmedicated society. In: Lasagna L, ed., *Controversies in Therapeutics*. Philadelphia, PA: W. B. Saunders, 1980; pp. 4–15.

10. Scheckler NE, Bennet JV. Antibiotic usage in seven community hospitals. *JAMA* 1970; **213**: 264–7.

11. Roberts WA, Visconti AJ. The rational and irrational use of systemic antimicrobial drugs. *Am J Hosp Pharm* 1972; **29**: 828–34.

12. Castle M, Wilfert CM, Cate TR, Osterhout S. Antibiotic use at Duke University Medical Center. *JAMA* 1977; **237**: 2819–22.

13. Perry TL, Guyatt GH. Antimicrobial drug use in three Canadian hospitals. *Can Med Assoc J* 1977; **116**: 253–6.

14. Achong MR, Hauser BA, Krusky JL. Rational and irrational use of antibiotics in a Canadian teaching hospital. *Can Med Assoc J* 1977; **116**: 256–9.

15. Shapiro M, Townsend TR, Rosner B, Kass EH. Use of antimicrobial drugs in general hospitals. II. Analysis of patterns of use. *J Infect Dis* 1979; **139**: 698–706.

16. Townsend TR, Shapiro M, Rosner B, Kass EH. Use of antimicrobial drugs in general hospitals. IV. Infants and children. *Pediatrics* 1979; **64**: 573–8.

17. Schollenberg E, Albritton WL. Antibiotic misuse in a pediatric teaching hospital. *Can Med Assoc J* 1980; **122**: 49–52.

18. Naqvi SH, Dunkle LM, Timmerman KJ, Reichley RM, Stanley DL, O'Connor D. Antibiotic usage in a pediatric medical center. *JAMA* 1980; **242**: 1981–4.

19. Laporte JR, Porta M, Capellá D. Drug utilization studies: a tool for determining the effectiveness of drug use. *Br J Clin Pharmacol* 1983; **16**: 301–4.

20. Garattini S, Garattini L. Pharmaceutical prescriptions in four European countries. *Lancet* 1993; **342**: 1191–2.

21. Heineck I, Schenkel EP, Vidal X. Medicamentos de venta libre en el Brasil. *Rev Panam Salud Pública* 1998; **3**: 385–91.

22. Casado Zuriguel I. Intervención para mejorar la calidad de prescripción de antibióticos en una area básica de salud. *Aten Primaria* 1993; **11**: 37–9.

23. Mata Cases M, Avellana Revuelta E, Davins Miralles J, Calvet Junoy S, Hortelano García MA, Martín López A. Mejora continua de la calidad de la prescripción crónica en un centro de atención primaria: seguimiento de 5 años. *Aten Primaria* 1994; **13**: 172–6.

24. Wettermark B, Pehrsson Å, Jinnerot D, Bergman U. Drug utilization 90% profiles—a useful tool for quality assessment of prescribing in primary health care in Stockholm. *Pharmacoepidemiol Drug Saf* 2003; **12**: 499–510.

25. Bergman U, Andersen M, Vaccheri A, Bjerrum L, Wettermark B, Montanaro N. Deviations from evidence-based prescribing of non-steroidal anti-inflammatory drugs in three European regions. *Eur J Clin Pharmacol* 2000; **56**: 269–72.

26. Vlahovic-Palcevski V, Wettermark B, Bergman U. Quality of non-steroidal anti-inflammatory drug prescribing in Croatia (Rijeka) and Sweden (Stockholm), *Eur J Clin Pharmacol* 2002; **58**: 209–14.

27. Vaccheri A, Bjerrum L, Resi D, Bergman U, Montanaro N. Antibiotic prescribing in general practice: striking differences between Italy (Ravenna) and Denmark (Funen). *J Antimicrob Chemother* 2002; **50**: 989–97.

28. Todd M. Drug use evaluation. In: Brown TR, ed., *Handbook of Institutional Pharmacy Practice*, 3rd edn. Bethesda, MD: American Society of Hospital Pharmacists, 1992; pp. 261–71.

29. Sjöqvist F, Agenäs I, eds. Drug utilization studies: implications for medical care. *Acta Med Scand* 1984; suppl 683.

30. Baksaas I, Lunde PKM. National drug policies: the need for drug utilization studies. *Trends Pharmacol Sci* 1986; **7**: 331–4.

31. Westerholm B. Therapeutic auditing at the national and international level. *Br J Clin Pharmacol* 1986; **22** (suppl 1): 55–9.

32. Melmon KL. Preventable drug reactions: causes and curcs. *N Engl J Med* 1971; **284**: 1361–3.

33. Impicciatore P, Choonara I, Clarkson A, Provasi D, Pandolfini C, Bonati M. Incidence of adverse drug reactions in paediatric in/out-patients: a systematic review and meta-analysis of prospective studies. *Br J Clin Pharmacol* 2001; **52**: 77–83.

34. Runciman WB, Roughead EE, Semple SJ, Adams RJ. Adverse drug events and medication errors in Australia. *Int J Qual Health Care* 2003; **15** (suppl 1): 49–59.

35. Davidsen F, Haghfelt T, Gram LF, Brøsen K. Adverse drug reactions and drug non-compliance as primary causes of admission to a cardiology department. *Eur J Clin Pharmacol* 1988; **34**: 83–6.

36. Bates DW. Medication errors: how common are they and what can be done to prevent them? *Drug Saf* 1996; **15**: 303–10.

37. Haynes RB, Taylor DW, Sackett DL, eds. *Compliance in Health Care*. Baltimore, MD: Johns Hopkins University Press, 1979.

38. Andrade SE, Walker AM, Gottlieb LK, Hollenberg NK, Testa MA, Saperia GM *et al*. Discontinuation of antihyperlipidemic drugs—do rates reported in clinical trials reflect rates in primary care settings? *N Engl J Med* 1995; **332**: 1125–31.

39. Avorn J, Monette J, Lacour A, Bohn RL, Monane M, Mogun H *et al*. Persistence of use of lipid-lowering medications: a cross-national study. *JAMA* 1998; **279**: 1458–62.

40. Larsen J, Vaccheri A, Andersen M, Montanaro N, Bergman U. Lack of adherence to lipid-lowering drug treatment. A comparison

of utilization patterns in defined populations in Funen, Denmark and Bologna, Italy. *Br J Clin Pharmacol* 2000; **49**: 463–71.

41. Isacsson G, Boëthius G, Bergman U. Low level of antidepressant prescription for people who later commit suicide: 15 years of experience from a population-based drug database in Sweden. *Acta Psychiatr Scand* 1992; **85**: 444–8.

42. Soumerai SB, McLaughlin TJ, Spiegelman D, Hertzmark E, Thibault G, Goldman L. Adverse outcomes of underuse of beta-blockers in elderly survivors of acute myocardial infarction. *JAMA* 1997; **277**: 115–21.

43. Whittle J, Wickenheiser L, Venditti LN. Is warfarin underused in the treatment of elderly persons with atrial fibrillation? *Arch Intern Med* 1997; **157**: 441–5.

44. Antani MR, Beyth RJ, Covinsky KE, Anderson PA, Miller DG, Cebul RD *et al.* Failure to prescribe warfarin to patients with nonrheumatic atrial fibrillation. *J Gen Intern Med* 1996; **11**: 713–20.

45. Albers GW, Yim JM, Belew KM, Bittar N, Hattemer CR, Phillips BG *et al.* Status of antithrombotic therapy for patients with atrial fibrillation in university hospitals. *Arch Intern Med* 1996; **156**: 2311–16.

46. Mendelson G, Aronow WS. Underutilization of measurement of serum low-density lipoprotein cholesterol levels and of lipid-lowering therapy in older patients with manifest atherosclerotic disease. *J Am Geriatr Soc* 1998; **46**: 1128–31.

47. Aronow S. Underutilization of lipid-lowering drugs in older persons with prior myocardial infarction and a serum low-density lipoprotein cholesterol >125 mg/dl. *Am J Cardiol* 1998; **82**: 668–9, A6, A8.

48. McLaughlin TJ, Soumerai SB, Willison DJ, Gurwitz JH, Borbasi C, Guadagnoli E *et al.* Adherence to national guidelines for drug treatment of suspected acute myocardial infarction: evidence for undertreatment in women and the elderly. *Arch Intern Med* 1996; **156**: 799–805.

49. Krumholtz HM, Radford MJ, Ellerbeck EF, Hennen J, Meehan TP, Petrillo M *et al.* Aspirin in the treatment of acute myocardial infarction in elderly Medicare beneficiaries. Patterns of use and outcomes. *Circulation* 1995; **92**: 2841–7.

50. O'Connor GT, Quinton HB, Traven ND, Ramunno LD, Dodds TA, Marciniak TA *et al.* Geographic variation in the treatment of acute myocardial infarction: the Cooperative Cardiovascular Project. *JAMA* 1999; **281**: 627–33.

51. Slone D, Shapiro S, Miettinen OS, Finkle WD, Stolley PD. Drug evaluation after marketing. *Ann Intern Med* 1979; **90**: 257–61.

52. Strom BL, Melmon KL, Miettinen OS. Postmarketing studies of drug efficacy. *Arch Intern Med* 1985; **145**: 1791–4.

53. Lasagna L. A plea for the naturalistic study of medicines. *Eur J Clin Pharmacol* 1974; **7**: 153–4.

54. Rucker TD. Data, sources, and limitations. *JAMA* 1974; **230**: 888–90.

55. Anonymous. *Consumption of drugs: Report on a Symposium. Euro 3102.* Copenhagen: WHO Regional Office for Europe, 1970.

56. Bergman U. Pharmacoepidemiology—from description to quality assessment. A Swedish perspective. *Nor J Epidemiol* 2001; **11**: 31–6.

57. Strom BL, Carson JL, Halpern AC, Schinnar R, Snyder ES, Stolley PD *et al.* Using a claims database to investigate drug-induced Stevens–Johnson syndrome. *Stat Med* 1991; **10**: 565–76.

58. Rucker TD. Drug utilization review: guidelines for program development. In: Alloza JL, ed., *Clinical and Social Pharmacology. Postmarketing Period.* Aulendorf: Cantor, 1985; p. 57.

59. Bergman U, Grímsson A, Wahba AHW, Westerholm B, eds. *Studies in Drug Utilization*, European series no. 8. Copenhagen: WHO Regional Office for Europe; 1979.

60. Dukes MNG, ed. *Drug Utilization Studies: Methods and Uses*, European series no. 45. Copenhagen: World Health Organization, Regional Office for Europe, 1993.

61. Bergman U, Elmes P, Halse M, Halvorsen T, Hood H, Lunde PK *et al.* The measurement of drug consumption: drugs for diabetes in Northern Ireland, Norway and Sweden. *Eur J Clin Pharmacol* 1975; **8**: 83–9.

62. Cars O, Mölstad S, Melander A. Variation in antibiotic use in the European Union. *Lancet* 2001; **357**: 1851–3.

63. Magrini N, Einarson T, Vaccheri A, McManus P, Montanaro N, Bergman U. Use of lipid-lowering drugs from 1990 to 1994: an international comparison among Australia, Finland, Italy (Emilio Romagna Region), Norway and Sweden. *Eur J Clin Pharmacol* 1997; **53**: 185–9.

64. WHO Drug Utilization Research Group (DURG). Validation of observed differences in the utilization of antihypertensive and antidiabetic drugs in Northern Ireland, Norway and Sweden. *Eur J Clin Pharmacol* 1985; **29**: 1–8.

65. WHO Drug Utilization Research Group (DURG). Therapeutic traditions in Northern Ireland, Norway and Sweden. I. Diabetes. *Eur J Clin Pharmacol* 1986; **30**: 513–19.

66. WHO Drug Utilization Research Group (DURG). Therapeutic traditions in Northern Ireland, Norway and Sweden. II. Hypertension. *Eur J Clin Pharmacol* 1986; **30**: 521–5.

67. Stålhammar J, Bergman U, Boman K, Dahlen M. Metabolic control in diabetic subjects in three Swedish areas with high, medium, and low sales of antidiabetic drugs. *Diabetes Care* 1991; **14**: 12–19.

68. Groop P-H, Klaukka T, Reunanen A, Bergman U, Borch-Johnsen K, Damsgaard E-M *et al. Diabetesläkemedel i Norden. Analys av orsaker till variationen i förbrukningen.* [Antidiabetic drugs in the Nordic countries. Reasons for variation in their use.] Social Insurance Publication ML 105. Helsinki: Social Insurance Institution, 1991.

69. Baum C, Kennedy DL, Forbes MB, Jones JK. Drug use and expenditures in 1982. *JAMA* 1985; **253**: 382–6.

70. Stolley PD, Lasagna L. Prescribing patterns of physicians. *J Chronic Dis* 1969; **22**: 395–405.

71. Hemminki E. Review of literature on the factors affecting drug prescribing. *Soc Sci Med* 1975; **9**: 111–15.

72. Christensen DB, Bush PJ. Drug prescribing: patterns, problems and proposals. *Soc Sci Med* 1981; **15**: 343–55.

73. Soumerai SB, Avorn J. Efficacy and cost-containment in hospital pharmacotherapy: state of the art and future directions. *Milbank Mem Fund Q* 1984; **62**: 447–74.

74. Soumerai SB, McLaughlin TJ, Avorn J. Improving drug prescribing in primary care: a critical analysis of the experimental literature. *Milbank Q* 1989; **67**: 268–317.

75. Anderson GM, Lexchin J. Strategies for improving prescribing practice. *Can Med Assoc J* 1996; **154**: 1013–17.

76. Freemantle N, Harvey EL, Wolf F, Grimshaw JM, Grilli R, Bero LA. Printed educational materials: effects on professional practice and health care outcomes. *Cochrane Database Syst Rev* 2000; **2**: CD000172.

77. Grimshaw JM, Russell IT. Effect of clinical guidelines on medical practice: a systematic review of rigorous evaluations. *Lancet* 1993; **342**: 1317–22.

78. Gómez LA, Lobato CI. Evolución de las bases de datos de medicamentos del Ministerio de Sanidad y Consumo. *Inf Ter Seg Soc* 1987; **11**: 229.

79. Avorn J, Soumerai SB. Use of computer-based Medicaid drug data to analyze and correct inappropriate medication use. *J Med Syst* 1982; **6**: 377–8.

80. Boëthius G, Wiman F. Recording of drug prescriptions in the county of Jämtland, Sweden. I. Methodological aspects. *Eur J Clin Pharmacol* 1977; **12**: 31–5.

81. Henriksson S, Boëthius G, Håkansson J, Isacsson G. Indications for and outcome of antidepressant medication in a general population: a prescription database and medical record study, in Jämtland county, Sweden, 1995. *Acta Psychiatr Scand* 2003; **108**: 427–31.

82. Hallas J. Conducting pharmacoepidemiologic research in Denmark. *Pharmacoepidemiol Drug Saf* 2001, **10**: 619–23.

83. Rosholm J-U, Gram LF, Isacsson G, Hallas J, Bergman U. Changes in the pattern of antidepressants use upon the introduction of the new antidepressants: a prescription database study. *Eur J Clin Pharmacol* 1997; **52**: 205–9.

84. Gaist D, Hallas J, Hansen N-CG, Gram LF. Are young adults with asthma treated sufficiently with inhaled steroids? A population-based study of prescription data from 1991 and 1994. *Br J Clin Pharmacol* 1996; **41**: 2885–9.

85. Gaist D, Tsiropoulos I, Sindrup SH, Hallas J, Rasmussen BK, Kagstrup J *et al*. Inappropriate use of sumatriptan: population based register and interview study. *BMJ* 1998; **316**: 1352–3.

86. Steffensen FH, Kristensen K, Ejlersen E, Dahlerup JF, Sorensen HT. Major hemorrhagic complications during oral anticoagulant therapy in a Danish population-based cohort. *J Intern Med* 1997; **242**: 497–503.

87. Olesen C, Steffensen FH, Sorensen HT, Nielsen GL, Olsen J, Bergman U. Low use of long-term hormone replacement therapy in Denmark: a 5-year population-based survey. *Br J Clin Pharmacol* 1999; **47**: 323–8.

88. Hallas J, Gaist D, Bjerrum L. The waiting time distribution as a graphical approach to epidemiologic measures of drug utilization. *Epidemiology* 1997; **8**: 666–70.

89. Donnan PT, Steinke DT, Newton RW, Morris AD; DARTS/ MEMO Collaboration. Changes in treatment after the start of oral hypoglycaemic therapy in type 2 diabetes: a population-based study. *Diabet Med* 2002; **19**: 606–10.

90. Bromley SE, de Vries CS, Farmer RD. Utilisation of hormone replacement therapy in the United Kingdom: a descriptive study using the general practice research database. *Br J Obstet Gynaecol* 2004; **111**: 369–76.

91. Nash D. National Drug and Therapeutic Index. *P & T* 2002; **27**: 530.

92. Sanz E, Bergman U, Dahlström M. Pediatric drug prescribing— a comparison between Tenerife (Canary Islands, Spain) and Sweden. *Eur J Clin Pharmacol* 1989; **37**: 65–8.

93. Bingefors K. Computerised data bases on prescription drug use and health care in the community of Tierp, Sweden: experiences and challenges from a study of antidepressant-treated patients. *Nor J Epidemiol* 2001; **11**: 23–9.

94. Isacson D, Ståhlhammar J. Prescription drug use among diabetics—a population study. *J Chronic Dis* 1987; **40**: 651–60.

95. Ståhlhammar J, Berne C, Svärdsudd K. Do guidelines matter? A population-based study of diabetes use during 20 years. *Scand J Prim Health Care* 2001; **19**: 163–9.

96. Isacson D, Carsjö K, Bergman U, Blackburn JL. Long-term use, mortality and migration among benzodiazepine users in a Swedish community: an eight year follow-up. *J Clin Epidemiol* 1992; **45**: 429–36.

97. Lundberg L, Isacson D. The impact of over-the-counter availability of nasal sprays on sales, prescribing, and physician visits. *Scand J Prim Health Care* 1999; **17**: 41–5.

98. Sturkenboom MCJM, Burke TA, Dieleman JP, Tangelder MJD, Lee F, Goldstein JL. Underutilization of preventive strategies in patients receiving NSAIDs. *Rheumatology* 2003; **42** (suppl 3): 23–31.

99. Pont LG, Sturkenboom MC, van Gilst WII, Denig P, Haaijer-Ruskamp FM. Trends in prescribing for heart failure in Dutch primary care from 1996 to 2000. *Pharmacoepidemiol Drug Saf* 2003; **12**: 327–34.

100. Blackburn JL. The use of automated databases in North America. In: Crommelin DJA, Midha KK, eds, *Topics in Pharmaceutical Sciences 1991: Proceedings of the 51st International Congress of Pharmaceutical Sciences of FIP*, September 1–6, 1991, Washington, DC. Stuttgart: Medpharm Scientific, 1992; pp. 405–13.

101. Strom BL, Carson JL, Morse ML, LeRoy AA. The Computerized On-line Medicaid Pharmaceutical Analysis and Surveillance System: a new resource for postmarketing drug surveillance. *Clin Pharmacol Ther* 1985; **38**: 359–64.

102. Strom BL, Morse ML. Use of computerized data bases to survey drug utilization in relation to diagnoses. *Acta Med Scand Suppl* 1988; **721**: 13–20.

103. Kaufman DW, Kelly JP, Rosenberg L, Anderson TE, Mitchell AA. Recent patterns of medication use in the ambulatory adult population of the United States: the Slone survey. *JAMA* 2002; **287**: 337–44.

104. Chen TJ, Chou LF, Hwang SJ. Trends in prescribing proton pump inhibitors in Taiwan: 1997–2000. *Int J Clin Pharmacol Ther* 2003; **41**: 207–12.

105. Pelaez-Ballestas I, Hernandez-Garduno A, Arredondo-Garcia JL, Viramontes-Madrid JL, Aguilar-Chiu. Use of antibiotics in

upper respiratory infections on patients under 16 years old in private ambulatory medicine. *Salud Publica Mex* 2003; **45**: 159–64.

106. Kahan E, Kahan NR, Chinitz DP. Urinary tract infection in women—physician's preferences for treatment and adherence to guidelines: a national drug utilization study in a managed care setting. *Eur J Clin Pharmacol* 2003; **59**: 663–8.

107. World Health Organization. *How to Investigate Drug Use in Health Facilities: Selected Drug Use Indicators*, WHO/DAP/93.1. Geneva: World Health Organization, 1993.

108. Trap B, Hansen EH, Hogerzeil HV. Prescription habits of dispensing and non-dispensing doctors in Zimbabwe. *Health Policy Plan* 2002; **17**: 288–95.

109. Sunartono. From research to action: the Gunungkidul experience. *Essent Drugs Monit* 1995; **2**: 21–2.

110. Santoso B, Suryawati S, Prawitasari JE, Ross-Degnan D. Small group intervention vs formal seminar for improving appropriate drug use. *Soc Sci Med* 1996; **42**: 1163–8.

111. Ofori-Adjei D, Arhinful DK. Effect of training on the clinical management of malaria by medical assistants in Ghana. *Soc Sci Med* 1996; **42**: 1169–76.

112. Hadiyono JE, Suryawati S, Danu SS, Sunartono, Santoso B. Interactional group discussion: results of a controlled trial using a behavioral intervention to reduce the use of injections in public health facilities. *Soc Sci Med* 1996; **42**: 1177–83.

113. Anonymous. *Guidelines for ATC Classification and DDD Assignment*, 7th edn. Oslo: WHO Collaborating Centre for Drug Statistics, 2004.

114. Bergman U, Boman G, Wiholm BE. Epidemiology of adverse drug reactions to phenformin and metformin. *BMJ* 1978; **2**: 464–6.

115. Lee D, Chaves Matamoros A, Mora Duarte J. Changing patterns of antibiotic utilization patterns in Costa Rica. *APUA Newslett* 1991; **9**: 7.

116. Bronzwaer SLAM, Cars O, Bucholz U, Mölstad S, Goettsch W, Veldhuijzen IK *et al*. A European study on the relationship between antimicrobial use and antimicrobial resistance. *Emerg Infect Dis* 2002; **8**: 278–82.

117. Gulbinovic J, Myrback K-E, Bytautiene J, Wettermark B, Struwe J, Bergman U. Marked differences in antibiotic use and resistance between university hospitals in Vilnius, Lithuania, and Huddinge, Sweden. *Microb Drug Resist* 2001; **7**: 383–8.

118. Nappo S, Carlini EA. Preliminary finding: consumption of benzodiazepines in Brazil during the years 1988 and 1989. *Drug Alcohol Depend* 1993; **33**: 11–17.

119. Chen L, Wang Y, Jin Y. [Study on drug use in elderly outpatients in Beijing]. *Zhonghua Liu Xing Bing Xue Za Zhi* 2001; **22**: 414–17.

120. Truter I, Wiseman K, Kotze TT. The defined daily dose as a measure of drug consumption in South Africa. A preliminary study. *S Afr Med J* 1996; **86**: 675–9.

121. Su TP, Chen TJ, Hwang SJ, Chou LF, Fan AP, Chen YC. Utilization of psychotropic drugs in Taiwan: an overview of outpatient sector in 2000. *Zhonghua Yi Xue Za Zhi* (Taipei) 2002; **65**: 378–91.

122. Vlahovic-Palevski V, Palcevski G, Mavric Z, Francetic I. Factors influencing antimicrobial utilization at a university hospital during a period of 11 years. *Int J Clin Pharmacol Ther* 2003; **41**: 287–93.

123. Ansari F. Use of systemic anti-infective agents in Iran during 1997–1998. *Eur J Clin Pharmacol* 2001; **57**: 547–51.

124. Mond J, Morice R, Owen C, Korten A. Use of antipsychotic medications in Australia between July 1995 and December 2001. *Aust N Z J Psychiatry* 2003; **37**: 55–61.

125. WHO International Working Group for Drug Statistics Methodology, WHO Collaborating Centre for Drug Statistics Methodology, WHO Collaborating Centre for Drug Utilization Research and Clinical Pharmacology. *Introduction to Drug Utilization Research*. Geneva: World Health Organization, 2003.

126. Stanulovic M, Milosev M, Jakovlojevic V, Roncevic N. Epidemiological evaluation of anti-infective drug prescribing for children in outpatient practice. *Dev Pharmacol Ther* 1987; **10**: 278–91.

127. Bergman U, Sjöqvist F. Measurement of drug utilization in Sweden: methodological and clinical implications. *Acta Med Scand* 1984; **105** (suppl 683): 15–22.

128. Bergman U. Utilization of antidiabetic drugs in the island of Gotland, Sweden: agreement between wholesale figures and prescription data. *Eur J Clin Pharmacol* 1978; **14**: 213–20.

129. Bergman U, Dahlström M. Användningen av blodtryckssänkande läkemedel i Sverige. [Use of antihypertensive agents in Sweden.] In: Berglund G, ed., *Hypertoni 87*. Mölndal: Lindgren & Söner, 1988; pp. 22–32.

130. Bergman U, Dahlström M. Benzodiazepine utilization in Sweden and other Nordic countries. In: Lader MH, Davies HC, eds, *Drug Treatment of Neurotic Disorders*. Edinburgh: Churchill Livingstone, 1986; pp. 43–52.

131. Juergens JP, Bergman U, Baum C, Kennedy DL, Dahlstrom M. Use of benzodiazepines in the USA and Sweden. Drug Information Association Annual Meeting, Washington, DC, June 4, 1986.

132. Isacsson G, Holmberg P, Druid H, Bergman U. The utilization of antidepressants—a key issue in the prevention of suicide. An analysis of 5281 suicides in Sweden 1992–1994. *Acta Psychiatr Scand* 1997; **96**: 94–100.

133. Rönning M, Salvesen Blix H, Harbo BT, Strom H. Different versions of the anatomical therapeutic chemical classification system and the defined daily dose—are drug utilization data comparable? *Eur J Clin Pharmacol* 2000; **56**: 723–7.

134. Departamento de Farmacoterapia. *Lista Oficial de Medicamentos*. Costa Rica: Caja Costarricense de Seguro Social, 2002.

135. The National Essential Drugs Committee. *Standard Treatment Guidelines and Essential Drugs List for Primary Health Care*, 2nd edn. Pretoria, South Africa: National Department of Health, 1998.

136. Pahor M, Chrischilles EA, Guralnik JM, Brown SL, Wallace RB, Carbonin P. Drug data coding and analysis in epidemiologic studies. *Eur J Epidemiol* 1994; **10**: 405–11.

137. Anonymous. Appendix IV: VA medication classification system. In: *USP Dispensing Information*, vol. I: *Drug*

Information for the Health Care Professional. Englewood, CO: Micromedex, 1999; pp. 3045–62.

138. Avorn J, Soumerai SB. Improving drug-therapy decisions through educational outreach: a randomized controlled trial of academically based "detailing." *N Engl J Med* 1983; **308**: 1457–63.

139. Schaffner W, Ray WA, Federspiel CF, Miller WO. Improving antibiotic prescribing in office practice. A controlled trial of three educational methods. *JAMA* 1983; **250**: 1728–32.

140. Ray WA, Schaffner W, Federspiel CF. Persistence of improvement in antibiotic prescribing in office practice. *JAMA* 1985; **253**: 1774–6.

141. Morse ML, LeRoy AA, Gaylord TA, Kellenberger T. Reducing drug therapy-induced hospitalization: impact of drug utilization review. *Drug Inf J* 1982; **16**: 199–202.

142. Groves R. Therapeutic drug-use review for the Florida Medicaid program. *Am J Hosp Pharm* 1985; **42**: 316–19.

143. Hennessy SM, Bilker WB, Zhou L, Weber AL, Brensinger C, Wang Y, Strom BL. Retrospective drug utilization review, prescribing errors, and clinical outcomes. *JAMA* 2003; **290**: 1494–9.

144. Kidder D, Bae J. Evaluation results from prospective drug utilization review: Medicaid demonstrations. *Health Care Financ Rev* 1999; **20**: 107–18.

145. Hall WD, Mant A, Mitchell PB, Rendle VA, Hickie IB, McManus P. Association between antidepressant prescribing and suicide in Australia, 1991–2000: trend analysis. *BMJ* 2003; **326**: 1008–12.

146. Soumerai SB, Avorn J, Ross-Degnan D, Gortmaker S. Payment restrictions for prescription drugs under Medicaid. *N Engl J Med* 1987; **317**: 550–6.

147. O'Connell DL, Henry D, Tomlins R. Randomised controlled trial of feedback on general practitioners prescribing in Australia. *BMJ* 1999; **318**: 507–11.

148. Söndergaard J, Andersen M, Stövring H, Kragstrup J. Mailed prescriber feedback in addition to a clinical guideline has no impact: a randomized, controlled trial. *Scand J Prim Health Care* 2003; **21**: 47–51.

149. Monane M, Mathias DM, Nagle BA, Kelly MA. Improving prescribing patterns for the elderly through an online-drug utilization review intervention: a system linking the physician, pharmacist, and computer. *JAMA* 1998; **280**: 1249–52.

150. Taylor L, Tamblyn R. Reasons for physician non-adherence to electronic drug alerts. *Medinfo* 2004; **2004**: 1101–5.

151. Anderson GM, Spitzer WO, Weinstein MC, Wang E, Blackburn JL, Bergman U. Benefits, risks, and costs of prescription drugs: a scientific basis for evaluating policy options. *Clin Pharmacol Ther* 1990; **48**: 111–19.

152. Schiff GD, Rucker TD. Computerized prescribing: building the electronic infrastructure for better usage. *JAMA* 1998; **279**: 1024–9.

153. Von Ferber C. Confidentiality Working Group questionnaire. *EURO DURG Bull* 1998; **3**: 3–4.

154. Merz JF. Introduction: a survey of international ethics practices in pharmacoepidemiology and drug safety. *Pharmacoepidemiol Drug Saf* 2001; **10**: 579–81.

155. Lewis MA. ISPE: present, past and future. *PharmacoEpidemiology Newsletter* 1997; **11**: 4.

156. Guess HA, Goldsmith C, Henry D, Strom BL. Pharmacoepidemiology as a focus for clinical epidemiology in developing countries. *J Clin Epidemiol* 1991; **44** (suppl): 101–5.

157. Haaijer-Ruskamp FM, Bergman U. Rational drug use in Europe—challenges for the 21st century. Report from the 1st meeting of EURO DURG, the European Drug Utilization Research Group. *Eur J Clin Pharmacol* 1997; **52** (suppl 2): I–VIII.

158. Buschiazzo H, Chaves A, Figueras A, Laporte J-R. Drug utilization in Latin America—the example of DURG-LA. *Essent Drugs Monit* 2003; **32**: 17–18.

159. Ross-Degnan D, Laing R, Quick J, Ali HM, Ofori-Adjei D, Salako L *et al.* A strategy for promoting improved pharmaceutical use: the International Network for Rational Use of Drugs. *Soc Sci Med* 1992; **35**: 1329–41.

160. Lee D. The International Network for Rational Use of Drugs. *Essent Drugs Monit* 1997; **24**: 7–8.

28

Evaluating and Improving Physician Prescribing

SUMIT R. MAJUMDAR[1], HELENE LEVENS LIPTON[2] and STEPHEN B. SOUMERAI[3]

[1] Department of Medicine, University of Alberta, Edmonton, Alberta, Canada; [2] School of Medicine, University of California at San Francisco, San Francisco, California, USA; [3] Harvard Medical School and Harvard Pilgrim Health Care, Boston, Massachusetts, USA.

'Research and clinical practice may be on parallel tracks headed in the same direction, but in contact only through rotting ties.'

P.P. Morgan, 'Are physicians learning what they read in journals?' 1985.

INTRODUCTION

The broad purposes of pharmacoepidemiology are to advance our knowledge of the risks and benefits of medication use in real-world populations, and to foster improved prescribing and patient health outcomes. If, however, physicians and other health practitioners fail to update their knowledge and practice in response to new and clinically important data on the outcomes of specific prescribing patterns, then the "fruits" of pharmacoepidemiologic research may have little impact on clinical practice.

It is for these reasons that a new discipline in the fields of health services research and clinical decision making has grown rapidly in importance—the science of assessing and improving clinical practices. The rapid growth of this new field, fueled by increasing research support from the National Institutes of Health and the Agency for Healthcare Quality and Research, is based on the recognition that passive knowledge dissemination (e.g., publishing articles, distributing practice guidelines) is generally insufficient to improve clinical practices without supplemental behavioral change interventions based on relevant theories of diffusion of innovations, persuasive communications, adult learning theory, and knowledge translation.[1-9]

This chapter reviews some of these developments as they relate to medication use, defines several types of drug prescribing problems, discusses several thorny methodologic problems in this literature, reviews existing pharmacoepidemiologic and other evidence on the effectiveness of common interventions to improve prescribing, and concludes with a discussion of future research needs. For a more detailed and comprehensive examination of the literature on prescribing

Pharmacoepidemiology, Fourth Edition   Edited by B.L. Strom
© 2005 John Wiley & Sons, Ltd

education, the role of the pharmacist as a change agent, disease management strategies for use in various settings, and the use of financial incentives and penalties to improve performance, the reader is advised to consult several previous works published elsewhere.[9–25] Portions of this chapter are derived from this body of work; in addition, we conducted computerized literature searches (published through early 2004), hand-searched our personal files and the cited references, and extensively consulted the Cochrane Library's Effective Practice and Organisation of Care (EPOC) Group, a rigorous and continuously updated registry and synthesis of available evidence on studies of interventions to change physician behaviors.[26] A substantial, if uneven, literature also exists on the intended and unintended impacts of cost-sharing and other reimbursement restrictions designed to control drug expenditures,[26–33] but it is also beyond the scope of this chapter and will not be reviewed here.

CLINICAL PROBLEMS TO BE ADDRESSED BY PHARMACOEPIDEMIOLOGIC RESEARCH

There is little doubt that the importance of suboptimal prescribing practice (both underuse and overuse) vastly outweighs the costs of medications themselves[34–36] (see also Chapter 41). Drug therapies are the most common treatments in medical practice and more than three-quarters of all visits to a physician terminate with the writing of a prescription; the potential for drug therapies for both alleviating and causing illness are illustrated throughout this book. As suggested by Lee,[37] in this chapter we take a broad view of the concept of prescribing errors, and consider issues related to underuse, overuse, and misuse as all contributing to the suboptimal utilization of pharmaceutical therapies. For example, we would consider as prescribing errors the following:

- use of toxic or addictive drugs when safer agents are available (e.g., barbiturates instead of benzodiazepines);
- use of drug therapy when no therapy is required (e.g., antibiotics for viral respiratory infections);
- use of an ineffective drug for a given indication (e.g., cerebral vasodilators for senile dementia or hormone therapy for prevention of cardiovascular disease in postmenopausal women);
- use of a costly drug when a less expensive preparation would be just as effective (e.g., newer calcium channel blockers or angiotensin-receptor blockers, instead of effective and inexpensive thiazide diuretics, for uncomplicated hypertension);

- misuse of effective agents (e.g., too low doses of narcotic analgesics or too high dosages of benzodiazepines, when indicated, for the elderly);
- failure to discontinue therapy when the drug is no longer needed (e.g., use of histamine-2 blockers or proton pump inhibitors for months to years in patients without documented gastroesophageal reflux disease);
- failure to introduce new and effective drugs into practice (e.g., inhaled corticosteroids for asthma or spironolactone for congestive heart failure);
- failure to prescribe necessary drug therapies (e.g., use of aspirin or β-blockers following acute myocardial infarction or use of bisphosphonates after an osteoporotic fracture);
- failure to achieve recommended therapeutic goals (e.g., systolic blood pressure levels below 140 mmHg or LDL cholesterol levels below 100 mg/dl for the secondary prevention of myocardial infarction and stroke).

Specific illustrations of the above problem categories are ubiquitous in the literature. For example, propoxyphene, a toxic and abusable narcotic analgesic, is often prescribed for mild to moderate pain when other safer, more effective analgesics are available.[38,39] In the outpatient setting, numerous studies have documented that as much as 50% of antibiotic use is potentially inappropriate with the unintended consequence that overuse of antibiotics may lead to the emergence of resistant pathogens.[40] A group at particular risk of iatrogenic injuries as a result of inappropriate medication exposure appears to be the frail elderly, whether they reside in the community or in nursing homes.[34,41,42]

Because of the absence of diagnostic data in most published drug utilization research, and because of the emphasis on cost containment within drug utilization review (DUR) programs, the existing literature may *underemphasize* the important problem of underuse of highly effective medications.[34–36] For example, Berlowitz *et al.* found that nearly 40% of patients with documented hypertension in the Veterans' Administration (VA) health care system had uncontrolled hypertension (>160/90 mmHg), despite adequate health care and prescription drug coverage and more than six hypertension-related primary care visits each year.[43] Indeed, changes in antihypertensive therapy occurred in less than 10% of all of these visits.[43] In another study of 623 outpatients treated for acute myocardial infarction at the Yale-New Haven Hospital, researchers found that one-third of patients meeting strict randomized controlled trial (RCT) eligibility criteria for use of β-blockers did not even receive a trial of therapy—contrary to existing guidelines. As a result, they experienced a 20–40% higher mortality rate post-myocardial infarction than may have been necessary.[44] There are many other examples of underuse and resultant unnecessary morbidity and mortality throughout the pharmacoepidemiology literature.

Why do these problems occur? Can a comprehensive theory of behavioral change or knowledge translation provide the basis for programs designed to improve prescribing? Such an ideal model must be complex given the diversity of economic, organizational, educational, psychological, social, informational and technological influences on daily prescribing practices.[1-9,45-52] Some of the factors responsible for suboptimal prescribing include the failure of clinicians to keep abreast of important new findings on the risks and benefits of medications,[6-8,45,52] excessive promotion of some drugs through pharmaceutical company advertising, sales representatives, or other marketing strategies,[45,52] lack of promotion of highly effective but nonprofitable medications (e.g., spironolactone for heart failure),[45,52] simple errors of omission,[8,23,25,48,52] negative attitudes toward issues of cost effectiveness of medications, direct-to-consumer marketing strategies and other competing influences,[49] patient and family demand for a particular agent, even when it is not scientifically substantiated,[49,50,52] physician overreliance on clinical experience in opposition to scientific data,[50,51] a skepticism toward, and distrust of, the literature and academia among some community-based physicians,[51] clinical inertia,[52] the need to take some definitive therapeutic action even when "watchful waiting" may be the most justifiable action,[50,52] and the influence from clinical opinion leaders or other health practitioners.[50-52] These diverse influences suggest the need for tailoring multifaceted intervention strategies to the key factors influencing a given clinical behavior based on models of behavioral change and knowledge translation. One promising model will be discussed in the section entitled "Currently Available Solutions."

METHODOLOGIC PROBLEMS TO BE ADDRESSED BY PHARMACOEPIDEMIOLOGIC RESEARCH

Research on the impact of educational and administrative interventions to improve drug prescribing presents numerous methodological challenges. This section will review several of the most important methodological problems and suggested solutions: internal validity, regression toward the mean, unit of analysis errors, logistical issues, ethical and legal problems, and the detection of effects on patient outcomes.

INTERNAL VALIDITY

As early as 1975, Gilbert, Light, and Mosteller established that poorly controlled studies produce misleading estimates of the effects of a variety of social programs.[53] Many nonintervention factors can affect medication use over time, such as marketing campaigns, mass media, state or Federal regulatory policies, seasonal effects, changing in staffing of health care organizations, other "competing" interventions, changes in eligibility for insurance programs, shifting demographics, and so on. Because RCTs are sometimes not feasible (e.g., contamination of controls within a single institution) or ethical (e.g., withholding quality assurance programs from controls), other strong quasi-experimental designs (e.g., interrupted time-series with or without comparison series, pre–post with concurrent comparison group studies) should be used instead of weak one-group post-only or pre–post designs that do not generally permit causal inferences. In fact, the Cochrane Collaboration's EPOC Group considers rigorously conducted time-series studies and pre–post studies with a concurrent comparison group to be sufficiently valid to merit inclusion within their systematic reviews.[26]

Interrupted time-series designs include multiple observations (often 10 or more) of study populations before and after intervention. Such designs permit investigators to control for pre-intervention secular changes in study outcomes and to estimate the size and statistical significance of sudden changes in the level or slope of the time-series occurring at initiation of the treatment. The availability of a comparison series collected from a similar, but unexposed, comparison group can further increase causal inferences if no simultaneous change in trend is observed for this group.[18,54]

Another popular design that can often lead to interpretable results is the *pre–post with comparison group design.* This design includes a single observation both before and after treatment in a nonrandomly selected group exposed to a treatment (e.g., physicians receiving feedback on specific prescribing practices), as well as simultaneous before and after observations of a similar (comparison) group not receiving treatment. Although this design controls for many threats to the validity of causal inferences (e.g., due to the effects of testing or maturation), it cannot control for unknown factors (e.g., a regulatory policy) which might result in pre-intervention differences in trends between study and comparison groups.[53,54]

The weakest, and not uncommon, design is the *one-group, post-only design*, which consists of making only one observation on a single group which has already been exposed to a treatment. The *one-group pre–post design* merely adds a single pre-intervention observation to the previous design. As described below, such weak designs are unlikely to produce valid or reliable estimates of the effects of interventions. Unfortunately, however, 60% of 76 studies designed to improve drug prescribing in primary care and inpatient settings used the weakest available nonexperimental designs.[9] Furthermore, many (if not most) studies of newer technology-based approaches to improving prescribing, such as computerized physician order entry and other types of computerized decision support, have used the post-only or one-group pre–post designs to evaluate their efficacy and effectiveness.[55,56]

Inadequately controlled studies may exaggerate the effectiveness of many interventions to improve prescribing. For example, as shown in Figure 28.1, inadequately controlled studies of the dissemination of print-only materials used alone (right-hand side) have all reported positive effects on behavior, while well-controlled studies of such strategies (left-hand side) all reported small or nonexistent changes in behavior. The "success" of uncontrolled studies is often due to the attribution of pre-existing trends in practice patterns to the studied intervention.

There are many examples of the potential bias involved in failing to account for prior trends. In one study, the naturally occurring trends in the use of 23 categories of medication were examined in a four-year study of 390 000 enrollees in the New Jersey Medicaid program.[57] The results indicated that 50% of the estimated one-year percent changes in prescriptions per 1000 enrollees exceeded +20.3% or −10.8% of baseline levels. Effect sizes reported in the drug utilization/intervention literature are similar to these natural fluctuations.[35,58] suggesting that changes in drug use attributed to such interventions could merely reflect these underlying secular trends. This is particularly noteworthy, because the effect sizes reported for valid intervention studies tend to be modest at best, with improvements in the quality of prescribing (as variously defined by investigators) usually reported on the order of a 10–20% absolute improvement over controls.

The above findings provide further support for more widespread application of RCTs or, when RCTs are not feasible, time-series and other valid comparison series designs to evaluate whether suddenly introduced interventions are associated with corresponding changes in the level or slope of the utilization series, after controlling for prior trends (see references 18, 30, 32, 38, 47 for examples). If the collection of time-series data is not feasible, investigators may consider using pre–post with comparison group designs, which also control for most threats of history, as described in respected texts on intervention research design.[53,54]

REGRESSION TOWARD THE MEAN

Regression toward the mean—the tendency for observations on populations selected on the basis of exceeding a predetermined threshold level to approach the mean on

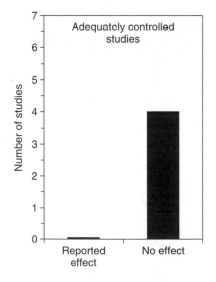
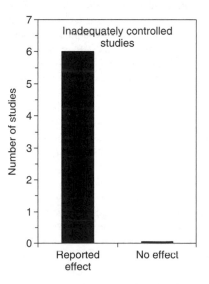

Figure 28.1. Reported effectiveness of dissemination of printed educational materials alone in well-designed versus inadequately controlled studies. Reprinted with permission from the *Milbank Quarterly*.[9]

subsequent observations—is a common and insidious problem in much of the drug utilization literature. For example, the most common Medicaid DUR programs typically screen prescribing data and eligibility files for possible co-occurrences of two interacting medications, or higher than recommended dosages for individual drugs. After case-by-case review by expert committees, letters are written to responsible physicians questioning the practice and asking for written responses. Unfortunately, however, the only published research evaluating this methodology used poorly controlled designs that are unable to control for regression to the mean. For example, in one often cited DUR study,[58] 50% of prescribing problems were absent several months after letters were sent, suggesting to the noncritical reader that the program was effective. However, it is equally plausible that the offending medications were withdrawn because the patients' conditions improved or because the physicians detected the error on their own (see Chapter 29 for a more detailed discussion of the DUR literature).

The likelihood that all screening algorithms employed in DUR programs are subject to regression toward the mean argues strongly for the need to conduct RCTs and well-controlled quasi-experiments (e.g., time-series with comparison series) to justify the efficiency and effectiveness of these interventions *before* they become a routine part of private and public quality improvement programs.[17,18,35] If regression effects are unavoidable—for example, due to selection of at-risk populations—investigators may consider including a "wash-out" period after selection and before pre- and post-intervention observations.[18,46]

UNIT OF ANALYSIS

A common methodological problem in studies of physician behavior is the incorrect use of the patient as the unit of analysis.[59–62] Such a practice violates basic statistical assumptions of independence because prescribing behaviors for individual patients are likely to be correlated within each physician's practice. There is also some data, primarily from studies based in the United Kingdom,[61] that the prescribing practices of physicians within a group practice are also not necessarily independent of each other. These various forms of hierarchical "nesting" or statistical "clustering" often lead to accurate point estimates of effect but exaggerated significance levels and inappropriately narrow confidence intervals when the correct unit of analysis ought to have been the physician or practice or health care facility.[60–62] As a result, interventions may appear to lead to "statistically significant" improvements in prescribing practices when in fact no such claim is warranted. For example, one review of articles on physicians' patient care behavior found that 70% of 54 articles incorrectly analyzed the data using the patient as the unit of analysis; among 19 reviewed studies of medication prescribing, 58% used the incorrect unit of analysis.[62]

The simplest, although sometimes overly conservative, solution to the problem of incorrect unit of analysis is to analyze data by facility or physician. Alternatively, new methods for analyzing clustered data are becoming increasingly available; such models can simultaneously control for clustering of observations at the patient, physician, and facility levels.[61–64] Such models allow aggregation at the patient level by controlling for correlation between patients cared for by the same provider or facility. The resulting significance levels for differences in prescribing rates between study and control groups are more conservative (i.e., confidence intervals are "wider") than assuming no intraclass correlation, but are still greater (i.e., confidence intervals "narrower") than the most conservative methods of analyzing at the provider or facility level. Much methodologic work remains to be done in terms of understanding what the appropriate unit of allocation and analysis is for various studies, how to best estimate power and sample sizes, and whether sensitivity analyses regarding unit of analysis need to be conducted or presented in the results of such studies.

LOGISTICAL ISSUES

While continuity of care is a goal in most settings, many patients, particularly those treated within academic medical centers, see multiple primary providers over time. For example, patients treated by residents may be reassigned to other residents at the end of the academic year. Providers may go on extended leave and transfer cases to other clinicians. Patients themselves may choose another primary care provider. In addition, many patients develop ongoing relationships with specialists as particular problems develop and are resolved.

While these changes may or may not improve patients' care, they almost always complicate and sometimes weaken research conducted in a clinical setting. Particularly in settings where providers may be assigned to both "intervention" and "control" patients, contamination problems are difficult to avoid. Even when interventions can be focused effectively on the intended patients or providers, informal communication among providers can lead to contaminated effects, thereby decreasing the likelihood of detecting significant changes.

Fortunately, solutions to the above problems exist. First, investigators should identify through baseline interviews and organizational records the extent to which patients are cared for by multiple providers, and the patterns of consultations and referrals between caregivers within and between facilities. If randomization of clinicians is likely to lead to contamination of controls, or if patient–provider pairs are frequently broken, the entire facility or subunit (e.g., the "firm" within an academic teaching hospital or the "primary care practice" in the community) should be assigned to the same study group. For instance, a quality improvement intervention randomized 37 hospitals in one state to intervention or control status.[65] However, when this strategy is not feasible, because it results in a small sample of facilities and inadequate statistical power, investigators are encouraged to collect data on medication use during multiple observation periods both before and after the intervention, and to use time-series regression methods that can often detect modest changes in utilization levels after as few as 6–12 months.

ETHICAL AND LEGAL PROBLEMS HINDERING THE IMPLEMENTATION OF RANDOMIZED CLINICAL TRIALS

Adequate control groups are essential for rigorous evaluation of results. Yet it has been argued that there are ethical and legal problems related to "withholding" interventions designed to improve drug prescribing practices. This is especially true in government-funded programs such as Medicaid. This argument explicitly assumes that the proposed interventions are known to be beneficial. In fact, the efficacy and effectiveness of many programs to improve drug use is the very question that should be under investigation. Some have argued, quite reasonably, that mandating such programs or interventions without adequate and valid proof of benefit is in fact unethical. For example, many researchers and policy makers have stated that computerized physician order entry (CPOE) does not need to be studied, and the Leapfrog advocacy group has gone so far as to state that not having CPOE compromises patient safety and quality of care.[66] What is important is to demonstrate that such interventions are safe, efficacious, and cost-effective *before* widespread adoption.[17,18,35,55] Even a safe and non-efficacious intervention is associated with opportunity costs; if this given intervention is widely adopted or legislatively mandated, many resources will have been diverted away from other parts of the health care delivery system.[17,18,35,55] In those very rare instances in which the intervention has shown unusual promise in similar populations, the

application of RCTs may be inappropriate but alternative research designs should still be considered to better define the absolute risks, benefits, and costs of the intervention. Feasible design alternatives are quasi-experimental designs such as interrupted time-series analysis or staged implementation in which the control population (or regions) receive the intervention after comparative data have been collected.[29,54,67,68]

DETECTING EFFECTS ON PATIENT OUTCOMES

While a number of studies have demonstrated positive effects of various interventions on prescribing practices, few large well-controlled studies have linked such changes in prescribing to improved patient outcomes. More recently, under the auspices of the Health Care Financing Administration, Marciniak *et al.*[69] conducted a controlled trial of guideline dissemination and feedback by peer-review organizations on seven quality (i.e., process) indicators for acute myocardial infarction care in Medicare patients in four states. This was a before (1992–93) and after (1995–96) intervention study, with a post-only comparison to a random national sample of patients from the other states. Almost 24 000 patient records were abstracted. Performance on all quality indicators improved in the intervention states compared to baseline; however, only the use of aspirin and β-blockers and counseling for smoking cessation were significantly greater than in the control states. An important strength of this study, beyond its size and scope, was an analysis of patient outcomes, namely mortality. There was no difference in mortality between intervention and control states in 1992–93, but after the intervention and consistent with documented improvements in process, mortality was approximately 1% lower (1 year mortality 30.4% versus 31.4% in the control states, $p = 0.004$) in the intervention states. Bearing in mind certain important threats to validity discussed in detail above (e.g., no baseline measurement of process indicators in control states, and possible lack of comparability between intervention and control states), this is one of the few studies that suggest a link between improvements in process and patient outcomes. These findings underline the difficulty of demonstrating statistically significant changes in patient outcomes in response to intervention. Explanations for the dissociation between improvements in prescribing and better patient outcomes include: (i) available clinical outcome measures may not be sensitive to the kinds of patient outcomes that might be affected by introduction or withdrawal of medications; (ii) changes in physician prescribing may lead to little or no change in patients' health status if patients do not adhere to the recommended regimens; and (iii) many medical therapies require months to years of continued adherence before clinical benefits become apparent.

Because of the above problems, sample sizes may need to be enormous to detect even very modest changes in patient outcomes (see Chapter 3 for a discussion of methods for determining statistical power). These problems are much less severe in standard drug trials because of experimenter control over the major independent variable—exposure to medications. However, process outcomes (e.g., use of recommended medications for acute myocardial infarction from evidence-based practice guidelines) are often sensitive, clinically reasonable, and appropriate measures of the quality of care,[63,67,69,70] and improvements in process should not be dismissed outright as surrogate outcomes. They may be important in and of themselves, as long as the processes are a measure of evidence-based and proven effective therapy.[63,67,69,70]

CURRENTLY AVAILABLE SOLUTIONS

CONCEPTUAL FRAMEWORK

A useful starting point for designing an intervention to improve prescribing is to develop a framework for organizing the clinical and nonclinical factors that could help or impede desired changes in clinical behaviors.[7,8,71] One such model—PRECEDE—was developed for adult health education programs by Green and Kreuter,[71] and proposes factors influencing three sequential stages of behavior change: predisposing, enabling, and reinforcing factors. *Predisposing* variables include such factors as awareness of a consensus guideline on appropriate use of a thrombolytic agent, knowledge of clinical relationships supporting such a guideline (e.g., major actions of thrombolytics in the artery), beliefs in the efficacy of treatment (e.g., probability of survival), attitudes or values associated with recommended behaviors (e.g., risk of intracranial hemorrhage associated with therapy), and a myriad of other potential factors.[8,52] However, while a mailed drug bulletin may predispose some physicians to new information (if they read it), behavior change may be impossible without new *enabling* skills (e.g., skills in administering a new therapy, or overcoming patient or family demand for unsubstantiated treatments). Once a new pattern of behavior is tried, multiple and positive *reinforcements* (e.g., through peers, reminders, or positive feedback) may be necessary to establish fully the new behavior. A number of recent thoughtful reviews of the literature have come to a similar conclusion: multifaceted interventions that encompass all stages of behavior change are most likely to improve physician prescribing.[6–12,19,20,24,35,52,72]

EMPIRICAL EVIDENCE ON THE EFFECTIVENESS OF INTERVENTIONS TO IMPROVE PRESCRIBING

Does existing empirical evidence on the effectiveness of alternative prescribing interventions provide any lessons on the key characteristics of successful approaches to this problem? Illustrative findings from several research syntheses will be used to evaluate the effectiveness of the most commonly studied or applied approaches. Because of severe biases introduced by uncontrolled designs which do not measure pre-existing trends in target drug use behaviors (see prior "Methodologic Problems" section), only studies using adequate experimental or quasi-experimental research designs (e.g., pre–post with comparison group and time-series designs) are discussed.

DISSEMINATION OF EDUCATIONAL MATERIALS AND CLINICAL PRACTICE GUIDELINES

Distributing printed educational materials aimed at improving prescribing practice remains the most ubiquitous form of prescribing education in the industrialized world. While the most sophisticated materials may incorporate visually arresting graphs, illustrations, and headlines to convey important behavioral and educational messages, such a strategy rests on assumptions that physicians will be exposed to the information, and that such rational information will be sufficiently persuasive to change clinical practices. Unfortunately, several reviews provide consistent evidence that use of disseminated educational materials *alone* (such as drug bulletins, self-education curricula, objective, graphically illustrated "un-advertisements," or other professionally prepared educational brochures) may affect some of the predisposing variables in the change process (e.g., knowledge or attitudes), but will have little or no effect on actual prescribing practice.[6,7,19,20,22,52,72–74]

A study of the effect of warning letters mailed to 200 000 physicians who were high prescribers of zomepirac sodium corroborates this previous literature.[39] As shown in Figure 28.2, the warning letters, which alerted these physicians to serious or fatal anaphylaxis associated with use of zomepirac, were not associated with any reduction in its use, especially in the face of stronger face-to-face pharmaceutical industry marketing campaigns which may have counteracted the warning messages.

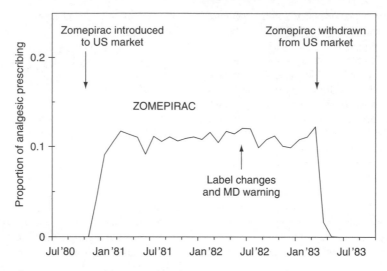

Figure 28.2. Time-series of zomepirac prescribing in Medicaid (as a proportion of total analgesic prescriptions) among 260 primary care physicians before and after warnings concerning possible severe adverse effects.[39] Reprinted with permission from *JAMA* 1993; **270**: 1937–42. Copyright 1993. American Medical Association. All rights reserved.

A distinct subset of educational materials are clinical practice guidelines. Although primarily educational in nature, they are also a codification of current best practice, and are intended to improve quality and decrease costs by minimizing unnecessary variations in practice. However, faith in the simple act of guideline dissemination presupposes that information alone, regardless of how reliable or how well referenced, can change behavior. When rigorously studied, guideline dissemination *alone* has not significantly influenced prescribing behavior or other clinical practices.[6–8,19–23,75–77] Given the proliferation and availability of numerous guidelines, dissemination of a particular guideline should be considered part of "usual care," and so unlikely to change practice as to provide a reasonable control "intervention" with which to compare more effective interventions or strategies.

In general, simple dissemination of educational materials does not appear to be effective by itself in altering prescribing patterns, but these materials may provide a necessary *predisposing* foundation for other *enabling* and *reinforcing* strategies.

MULTIMEDIA WARNING CAMPAIGNS

Occasionally, the discovery of important adverse effects of marketed drugs is accompanied by mailed educational materials to physicians as part of a broader warning campaign involving the medical and popular press, newspapers, television, and radio. When the adverse effects are severe and preventable, alternative agents exist, and the messages are simple enough to convey in mass communications, such multimedia campaigns may be effective in changing prescribing patterns in large populations. Previous examples include reductions in the use of chloramphenicol (aplastic anemia)[78] and calcium channel blockers (myocardial infarction) in response to widespread media warnings.[79] If one considers the prerelease, publication, and intense lay press associated with the results of the Women's Health Initiative RCT a form of multimedia campaign, it is noteworthy that the prescription of estrogen decreased by 38% within six months of widespread awareness of the findings of significant harm, and little benefit, associated with the use of hormone therapy.[80]

Figure 28.3 provides data from a US study suggesting that widespread reporting of the risk of Reye's syndrome associated with pediatric aspirin use by the medical and lay press was associated with declines in Reye's syndrome. This media campaign was conducted after Reye's syndrome was linked to aspirin use and antecedent viral illnesses in several epidemiological studies.[81] The authors concluded, based on this and other studies, that mass media warnings may be effective in changing both consumer and physician behavior when the illness is severe or life-threatening, the behavioral message is simple, no or few

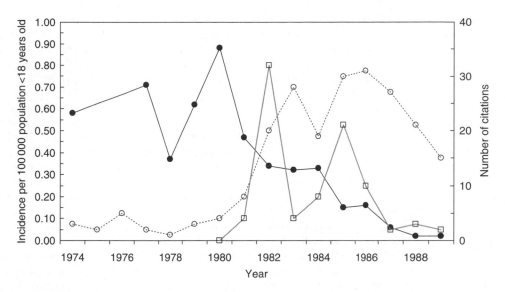

Figure 28.3. Trend in number of (○) medical and (□) lay press citations on aspirin and Reye's syndrome, and the (●) incidence of Reye's syndrome among children. Newspaper index limited to four continuously reporting national newspapers described in text. Reprinted with permission from *Milbank Quarterly*.[81]

barriers to alternative behaviors (e.g., acetaminophen versus aspirin) are present, and the campaign is comprehensive, involving both health professionals and consumers.

GROUP EDUCATION

Although rounds, seminars, and other group didactic educational programs are among the most universal methods for prescribing education, controlled studies of this approach are almost nonexistent in the literature, especially in nonteaching settings. Nevertheless, small group discussions conducted by clinical leaders in academic primary care settings have been shown to improve use of antibiotics[40] and agents for hypertension treatment and control.[82] These successful approaches have included reviews of patient records to establish the need for change and participatory methods based on adult learning theory, and have more in common with academic (individual or group) detailing than traditional modalities of continuing medical education. Traditional large-group, didactic continuing medical education seminars have not been as successful, by themselves, in improving physician performance.[19,20,83] The results of one early but important RCT of continuing medical education were summed up by the authors as follows: "Put simply, in terms of the effects of continuing education on the documented quality of care, wanting continuing education...was as good as getting it."[83]

PROFILING, AUDIT, AND FEEDBACK

During the last 20 years, an increasingly popular approach to improving physician performance has been some form of "feedback" of prescribing patterns to individuals or groups of physicians. One survey found that more than half of all US physicians received clinical or economic feedback regarding their prescribing practices.[21] While managers and health policy makers often assume that "feedback" is a unidimensional technique, its many variations have not been well defined or well studied.

One well-studied form of feedback, however, is the patient-level medication profile. It has frequently been hypothesized that simply making clinicians aware of all of the medications a patient may be prescribed might be an effective method for reducing use of excessive, duplicative, or interacting medications. The best controlled trials of this approach confirm that simply distributing such profiles, without explicit suggestions for changes in practices, has no detectable effect on prescribing practice.[84–86] Likely reasons for the failure of this intuitively appealing approach include: (i) much of the generated information was probably clinically irrelevant; (ii) unsynthesized and voluminous data may cause information "overload" and desensitization of busy clinicians; (iii) there was no provision of alternative measures to improve care; and (iv) the feedback was not derived from credible sources of information. This approach represents one of the few instances in which the volume of negative find-ings from methodologically rigorous studies strongly supports the exclusion of this strategy from future research.

Other forms of feedback may compare practice patterns with peers or predetermined standards such as practice guidelines. The former is typified by interventions of peer-comparison feedback, while DUR programs typify the latter (DUR is discussed extensively in Chapter 29 and will not be covered in detail here). A systematic review concluded that peer comparison feedback had a statistically significant, but clinically minimal, effect on prescribing or other physician behaviors.[21] Further, the authors doubted that such programs were likely to offset the costs of the intervention, much less lead to cost savings. The conclusions of this review were entirely supported by a more recent, methodologically rigor-ous, RCT of the effect of peer-comparison feedback on the prescription of five unrelated groups of medication.[87] These Australian investigators went so far as to conclude, based on their null results, that mailed "feedback is not worthwhile and should not be seen as a high priority by government agencies."[87]

In addition to the type or content of the feedback, a number of variables must be considered. Communication channels could be by letter, computer, or face-to-face encounter with a supervisor or colleague. The credibility of the source of the feedback information probably influences its effectiveness in changing behavior. For example, Eisenberg suggested that feedback of data is likely to work only when it is delivered by clinical leaders.[72] Thus, feedback programs operated by a government regulator or managed care organization may be less effective than professionally-based educational programs in which an ongoing relationship exists between the sender and receiver of information.[72,87-91]

The level at which feedback is given is another important issue that may differentiate successful and valid programs from questionable ones. For example, many existing DUR programs attempt to review the appropriateness of medica-tion prescribing for individual patients (e.g., drug interactions and dosage). Since the majority of feedback messages are likely to be clinically unimportant,[17,18,72,88] the clinically relevant messages could be unintentionally ignored. For this reason, a more valid method may be to compare patterns of prescribing by individual physicians with clinical guidelines or other more appropriate benchmarks.[89] Lastly, beyond the medium and the message, if physicians are not able to respond immediately to the feedback delivered, by altering prescribing during a specific patient encounter, they may not respond at all. It is not necessarily true that physicians will generalize behavior from one specific encounter to similar clinical situations.

One recent advance in the area of feedback, one that attempts to address many of the aforementioned problems, is the development of the concept of the "achievable benchmarks of care" by Kiefe *et al.*[89] The underlying theory is that viewing one's personal performance within the context of peers' performance should be a powerful motivator for change.[89] In essence, the achievable benchmark represents the average performance of the top 10% of local physicians being assessed.[89] By design, achievable benchmarks are higher than the group mean—and group mean data is what is provided in many audit and feedback programs. Kiefe *et al.* undertook a cluster-randomized controlled trial and allocated physicians ($N=97$) and their diabetic patients ($N \approx 2000$) to either "usual care" (in fact, it was a standard quality improvement intervention that profiled physicians and provided them with individual and group mean performance feedback on five different quality indicators such as influenza vaccination, foot examination, and measurement of glyco-sylated hemoglobin) or to an experimental intervention (usual care plus the provision of top 10% achievable bench-mark data). The intervention was associated with 15–57% relative improvements in all indicators compared with usual care; three out of five of these improvements were also statistically significant.[89] Unfortunately, there are few rigorous published evaluations of well-controlled studies in community populations such as this.

REMINDERS AND COMPUTERIZED DECISION SUPPORT SYSTEMS

Often, physicians are predisposed to certain therapeutic interventions, but simply omit them due to oversight or lack of coordination in the health care/communications system. In these cases, computerized reminder systems have been developed that enable physicians to reduce these errors of omission by issuing alerts to perform specific actions in response to patient-level information such as laboratory findings or diagnoses.

Several studies in hospitals, managed care organizations, and primary care settings have provided strong evidence that such systems can prevent the omission of essential preventive services such as deep venous thrombosis prophy-laxis, influenza immunization and others.[92-94] In general, prospective reminders are more effective than retrospective feedback; however, such systems are effective only as long as the reminders continue. Further, it is likely that such systems are only effective when clinicians are already pre-disposed to acting in concert with the protocols. Few data are available on the potential for such systems to reduce inappropriate drug prescribing in cases when physicians have strong beliefs in opposition to recommended practice and (for the most part) various reminder systems have only been studied with a few reminders at a time. "Reminder-fatigue" with concurrent bypassing of computer screens or generalized neglect of all alerts is an important possibility that has not been well documented or studied.

Finally, few well-controlled studies are available on the potential for such computerized systems to succeed beyond a "secretarial reminder" function, although early work using locally developed (i.e., homegrown) decision support systems at Brigham and Women's Hospital in Boston,[94–96] LDS Hospital in Salt Lake City,[94,97] and the Regenstrief Institute in Indianapolis,[48,93,94] show some promise in altering physicians' prescribing decisions in more complex areas such as dosage, schedule, suboptimal choices, and prevention of adverse drug events. This promise, however, should not be assumed. In the most rigorous study of advanced computer decision support conducted to date, Eccles *et al.* conducted a cluster-randomized controlled trial of 60 busy primary care practices in the UK.[98] These practices already had electronic records and electronic prescribing. Eccles *et al.* randomized these practices to a computerized guideline/decision support intervention that was fully integrated into the electronic clinic record; half of the practices were allocated to a symptomatic coronary disease guideline (*N* = 1415 intervention patients) and the other practices to an asthma guideline (*N* = 1200 intervention patients). After one year, there were no significant improvements in any one of more than 40 different quality indicators for either condition.[98] With this cautionary note, we refer the interested reader to a more detailed examination of adverse drug events in general, and the potential roles of CPOE and computerized decision support, in Chapter 34 of this textbook and recent systematic reviews.[92,94,95,99]

OPINION LEADERS OR EDUCATIONALLY INFLUENTIAL PHYSICIANS

The role of local opinion leaders in the adoption of new pharmaceutical agents has been well-documented by Coleman, Katz, and Menzel.[2] Their data indicated that after opinion leaders adopted drugs, other less integrated physicians eventually followed in a classic curve of technology diffusion. In several studies of diffusion of scientific information on treatment of arthritis and the inappropriate use of Cesarean sections,[100,101] local opinion leaders or educationally influential physicians have been identified and encouraged to consult informally with colleagues. These opinion leaders are approached frequently for clinical advice, are trusted by their colleagues to evaluate new medical practices in the context of local norms, have good listening skills, and are perceived as clinically competent and caring.[3,65,72,100–102] In addition to opinion-leader involvement, these interventions generally included brief orientation to research findings, printed educational materials, and encouragement to implement guidelines during informal "teachable moments" that occur naturally in their ongoing collegial associations. Success of these programs was attributed to "the importance of the local community's norms, the orientation of practitioners to locally credible individuals, and the need to translate the research findings into a locally applicable message."[102]

A more recent RCT demonstrated that opinion leaders could be used to improve prescribing in the treatment of acute myocardial infarction.[65] Hospitals in Minnesota (*N* = 37) were randomized to guideline dissemination, performance feedback, and opinion leaders (intervention), or guidelines and feedback alone (controls). Both the unit of randomization and the unit of analysis were the hospital. Clinical and process data were collected for a year before, and a year after, the intervention (which itself lasted about six months). The opinion leaders were asked to promote four separate practices, each consistent with national evidence-based guidelines: increased use of aspirin, increased use of β-blockers, increased use of thrombolytic therapy in elderly patients, and decreased routine use of lidocaine prophylaxis. Compared to controls, the intervention hospitals successfully increased the use of aspirin (absolute median improvement 13%, *p* = 0.04) and β-blockers (absolute median improvement 31%, *p* = 0.02; see Figure 28.4). However, there was no improvement in the use of thrombolytic therapy, and all hospitals decreased use of lidocaine by about 50%. This latter finding is evidence of a secular trend, a trend more powerful than the intervention itself, and one that would have been attributed to the intervention if a weaker study design had been employed. Although the recruitment and use of opinion leaders shows great promise in accelerating the adoption of evidence into practice, overall the results of rigorous opinion leader studies have been somewhat mixed,[103] and whether or not such interventions are reproducible across settings,[104] can improve prescribing for multiple conditions outside the hospital setting, and are cost effective, still remains to be determined.

FACE-TO-FACE EDUCATIONAL OUTREACH

A growing number of well-controlled studies support the conclusion that programs combining professionally illustrated educational materials with brief face-to-face visits (15–25 minutes) by university-based pharmacists (academic detailers) or physician counselors or peer-leaders are effective in

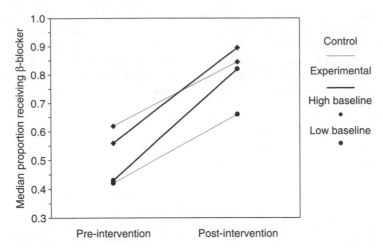

Figure 28.4. Change in proportion of eligible patients receiving β-blockers, stratified by hospitals above and below median baseline proportion. Median proportion was 0.49 (experimental group). The number of hospitals was 11 for the experimental group and 7 for the control group. Before and after change represents median change in proportion receiving β-blockers in each of the four strata.[65] Reprinted with permission from *JAMA* 1998; **279**: 1358–63. Copyright 1998. American Medical Association. All rights reserved.

reducing prescribing of contraindicated or marginally effective therapies in primary care settings. Similarly, several controlled studies of direct educational efforts by pharmacists have also documented improvements in targeted prescribing practices.[22,105,106] The principles and methods of this approach are described in detail elsewhere,[12] and include targeting of physicians with higher than average needs for education (e.g., through analyses of administrative data), conducting motivational research (e.g., surveys of focus group interviews) in advance of the intervention to understand the causes of suboptimal prescribing patterns, sponsorship by authoritative and credible medical organizations, two-way communication with prescribers to increase clinician involvement and relevance to different patient populations and settings, presentation and discussion of counterarguments to which physicians have been exposed, brevity, use of high-quality, graphical educational materials, repetition of major messages, and follow-up visits for positive reinforcement. Of course, pharmaceutical industry detailing also shares many of these principles and methods. What sets academic detailing apart from industry efforts is that the messengers and the messages of the former are independent, objective, and evidence-based.

Figure 28.5 provides an example of an educational leaflet briefly summarizing the main educational messages concerning the costs and lack of efficacy of propoxyphene that were emphasized in one RCT of a four-state academic detailing program.[74] A formal economic analysis of this study, conducted from a societal perspective (in this case,

a Medicaid program) concluded that targeting moderate to high prescribers of propoxyphene, cephalexin, and peripheral/cerebral vasodilators using administrative claims databases could lead to high benefit-to-cost ratios, even without considering positive spillover effects to nonparticipating physicians, improved quality of care, or possible cost savings due to elimination of adverse drug effects.[75]

If academic detailing is truly cost neutral (or even cost saving), the main barrier to more widespread use of the strategy is its *perceived* labor intensiveness. Nevertheless, academic detailing is the single most consistently effective method for changing physician practice that has been reported.[19,20,105–107] A number of controlled trials have attempted to replicate the positive results of face-to-face outreach with smaller group outreach sessions, often referred to as "group detailing."[22,67,108] Group detailing has the additional advantage of encouraging discussions within the group, which may enhance the diffusion of ideas and increase their impact. For example, in an RCT to improve the treatment of hyperlipidemia in Sweden, Diwan *et al.* randomized 134 health centers.[108] The intervention, for 67 of the health centers, consisted of printed guideline dissemination, an informational video, and four 30-minute group detailing sessions between all health center physicians and a clinical pharmacist, while the control centers only received printed information. Compared to baseline measurements, hyperlipidemia was treated more often for all patients in the intervention centers, although this reached conventional

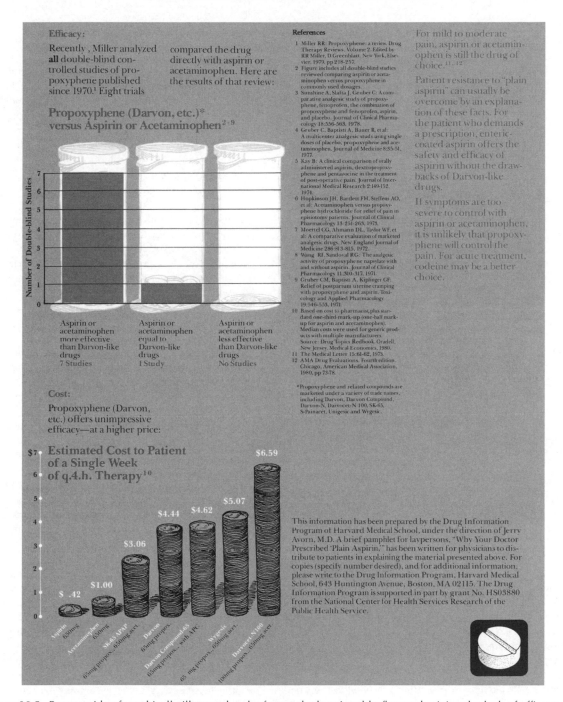

Figure 28.5. Reverse side of graphically illustrated and referenced educational leaflet emphasizing the lack of efficacy and high cost of propoxyphene in comparison to aspirin or acetaminophen. Leaflet was used in face-to-face academic detailing study.[12,74]

statistical significance only for women younger than 65 years of age. Moreover, "first-line prescribing" (use of specific agents in accordance with national guidelines) was 20% higher ($p = 0.03$) for the intervention centers.[108] It is likely that as long as the group size is kept relatively small (i.e., fewer than 5–10 participants), and the other precepts of academic detailing are adhered to,[12] group detailing is a reasonable alternative approach to individualized educational outreach. This is an area that merits further research.

FINANCIAL INCENTIVES AND PENALTIES

Although there are few studies of the effects of financial incentives or penalties on physician prescribing behavior *per se*,[22,109] numerous observational studies suggest that differing payment methods do affect the way that physicians practice medicine.[6,26–28,72] As a general rule, it has also been observed that financial incentives are consistently more powerful than penalties when it comes to changing behavior.[6,72]

In response to escalating drug costs, an increasing number of physician organizations in the US are entering into capitated drug risk-sharing arrangements with managed care organizations.[22,110] These innovative drug payment mechanisms are designed to control drug costs by encouraging physicians to prescribe "preferred" drug products (e.g., generic drugs or those that are on the health plan's formulary). Some analysts assert that capitation encourages physicians to examine their prescribing more critically, resulting in the choice of appropriate, effective, and low-cost medications.[28,110] This belief is based on a number of untested assumptions: (i) practices must be large enough to absorb risk, so that costly but appropriate prescribing decisions for the individual patient are not unduly affected; (ii) performance feedback to prescribers must be timely and provide specific advice about costs, risks, and possible substitutions; and (iii) physicians must understand and be sensitive to differences in drug pricing.[28] Because it is unlikely that these assumptions (in general) can be met, any intervention using financial incentives must be considered experimental. As such, any strategy employing financial incentives to change prescribing must be studied rigorously, with particular attention to the quality of prescribing, unintended consequences (e.g. cost-shifting), and patient outcomes. Reductions in prescribing costs, alone, are not appropriate or sufficient outcomes. As Bloor and Freemantle have noted, experimental or quasi-experimental studies are needed before sound evidence-based policies can be formulated.[27]

THE FUTURE

Based on this synthesis of the research literature, it is clear that our knowledge of the characteristics of successful interventions to improve prescribing is growing rapidly. Passive dissemination of drug information or practice guidelines is a necessary but insufficient method for improving most prescribing behaviors. In general, the achievement of long-term changes in practice will depend on inclusion of multiple strategies that predispose, enable, and reinforce desired prescribing behaviors. The following characteristics recur in successful interventions:

- identifying key factors influencing target and alternative prescribing decisions through surveys, focus groups, or in-depth interviews;
- targeting physicians in need of education (e.g., through review of prescribing data) to increase effectiveness and efficiency;
- recruitment and participation of local opinion leaders;
- use of credible and objective messengers and materials;
- face-to-face interaction, especially in primary care settings;
- audit and feedback (*if it is used at all*) that incorporates achievable benchmarks, comparisons with peers, and patient-specific data;
- repetition and reinforcement of a limited number of messages at one time;
- provision of acceptable alternatives to the practices that are deemed necessary to be extinguished;
- brief, graphic educational guidelines and evidence summaries to predispose and reinforce messages;
- use of multiple evidence-based strategies to address multiple barriers to best practice;
- an emphasis on the goal of improvement in the quality of prescribing and patient safety, not just cost minimization in the guise of quality improvement.

There is also a tremendous need for carefully controlled research of some existing and new methods for improving prescribing, and how best to combine various evidence-based strategies to allow for rapid local implementation of prescribing guidelines. New models are needed to predict the most effective types of intervention for specific problem types and a number of broader questions still need to be answered. What is the correct, or at least most reasonable, rate of adherence to a given prescribing guideline? Are face-to-face interventions (either one-on-one or in small groups) always necessary to address strongly held incorrect beliefs? What should we consider a "clinically important" improvement for a complex practice change strategy?

Can reminder systems that are so effective in correcting errors of omission change more resistant errors of commission? Even if single reminders are effective, is there a point of multiple reminder-fatigue and diminishing clinical returns? Lastly, are advanced computerized decision support systems safe and effective, and if so, are they worth the time, effort, and opportunity costs necessary to implement and use them?

Practice settings may also influence the choice of interventions to be evaluated. For example, organized systems of clinicians (e.g., medical groups, independent practice associations, integrated delivery systems) may be conducive to participatory approaches in which practicing physicians, and possibly patients, work with a facilitator/educator to explore current practices and barriers to change, and then develop or modify practice guidelines, along with methods to measure guideline adherence.[22,111,112] These group meetings also serve as vehicles for active learning and begin to converge with the strategy of group detailing described earlier. In addition, we believe more attention needs to be paid to the study of changing the behavior of busy physicians in community practice. Many successful strategies may not be transferable from a university hospital[94–97] to a busy ambulatory clinic.[98]

Most of the studies we reviewed were designed to assess only whether an intervention changed behavior; few studies have undertaken formal cost–benefit analyses.[22,107] One economic analysis of an RCT of academic detailing found that the intervention actually led to a net saving.[75] This is a clear illustration of what Eddy described as "getting more for less," the potential to improve quality and reduce costs simultaneously.[113] There are very few other well-controlled studies that compare the costs and benefits of alternative approaches to improving prescribing practice, and little has been published on when (or at what cost) it is reasonable to introduce an intervention to change physicians' practice.[107] This is another important research need.

Currently, we know that prescribing problems exist, but we know little about their prevalence or determinants.[41,42,114–120] This paucity of data is all the more remarkable considering three-quarters of all physician visits end in the prescription of a drug.[17] In a study of more than 30 000 hospital admissions, drug-related complications were common and accounted for 19% of all adverse events.[114] Bates *et al.* found that almost one-third of adverse drug events occurring in the hospital were preventable.[115] Less is known about the ambulatory setting,[41,42,116–118] with estimates of preventable adverse drug events ranging from 11% to 28%. One retrospective analysis of a New England malpractice insurance carrier observed that 6% of all malpractice claims were related to adverse drug events, and that half of these

claims occurred for events in the outpatient setting.[118] These investigators also estimated that three-quarters of these adverse drug events were preventable, and that most medication errors occurred as a result of system deficiencies (e.g., inadequate monitoring) or performance errors (e.g., wrong drug or wrong dose). Like most descriptions of adverse drug events, these studies documented only errors of commission; the extent of omission (e.g., underuse of effective therapies) has been extremely understudied. A notable exception is a study of 5332 elderly survivors of myocardial infarction, that found only 21% of eligible patients received a β-blocker, leading to an estimated 381 excess deaths among the 2952 eligible nonrecipients.[119]

Several factors determine the relative frequency of problems associated with the use of specific medications. Drugs such as the nonsteroidal anti-inflammatory agents, even if prescribed appropriately, are likely to be among the frequently implicated "problem" drugs simply because they are prescribed so commonly. Alternatively, medications such as the benzodiazepines are particularly difficult to monitor due to their variable rate of metabolism across patients and the fact that they are commonly prescribed along with other psychotropic agents. Moreover, many iatrogenic symptoms are nonspecific and difficult to discern from the complex clinical picture of patients with multiple chronic diseases. Consequently, drugs commonly prescribed to frail or clinically complex patients may be disproportionately implicated in studies of "inappropriate" prescribing.[116,117,120] Future research efforts need to describe in greater detail the nature, prevalence, rate of prescribing, and severity of prescribing problems associated with the overuse, misuse, and underuse of medications. A more detailed exploration of these and related issues is presented in Chapter 34.

Finally, studies examining the relationship between interventions and clinical outcomes would advance the field. While policy-induced reductions in use of essential medications have been associated with increased institutionalization[47] and emergency room visits and hospitalizations[32] among the frail elderly, and partial hospitalizations among schizophrenic patients,[30] few analogous patient outcomes studies exist in the literature on interventions to improve prescribing. Important effects of medications on many health outcomes have been demonstrated in clinical trials; therefore, it is reasonable to hypothesize that more appropriate use of some medications could reduce morbidity and mortality, increase patient functioning, and improve quality-of-life. Whether improved prescribing is a surrogate measure, or an outcome that directly leads to improved health outcomes, it remains a critically important area for study. Further, the promise of a comprehensive electronic patient record, one that is knowledge-generating and linked to prescriptions, clinical and laboratory information, and claims data, has yet to be fully realized.[94,95,121,122] Once there is widespread adoption of these technologies, the fields of health services research and pharmacoepidemiology will enter a new era when innovative measures to improve the quality of prescribing will be implemented and evaluated with heretofore unknown methodologic rigor.

REFERENCES

1. Morgan PP. Are physicians learning what they read in journals? *Can Med Assoc J* 1985; **133**: 263.

2. Coleman J, Katz E, Menzel H. *Medical Innovation: A Diffusion Study*. Indianapolis, IN: Bobbs-Merrill, 1966.

3. Rogers E. *Diffusion of Innovations*. New York: Free Press, 1995.

4. Kotler P, Roberto E. *Social Marketing. Strategies for Changing Public Behaviour*. New York: Free Press, 1989.

5. Fox R, Mazmanian P, Putnam RW. *Changing and Learning in the Lives of Physicians*. New York: Praeger, 1989.

6. Greco PJ, Eisenberg JM. Changing physicians' practices. *N Engl J Med* 1993; **329**: 1271–4.

7. Davis D, Evans M, Jadad A, Perrier L, Rath D, Ryan D *et al.* The case for knowledge translation: shortening the journey from evidence to effect. *BMJ* 2003; **327**: 33–5.

8. Cabana MD, Rand CS, Power NR, Wu AW, Wilson MH, Abboud PC *et al.* Why don't physicians follow clinical practice guidelines? *JAMA* 1999; **282**: 1458–65.

9. Soumerai SB, McLaughlin TJ, Avorn J. Improving drug prescribing in primary care: a critical analysis of the experimental literature. *Milbank Q* 1989; **67**: 268–317.

10. Gurwitz J, Soumerai SB, Avorn J. Improving medication prescribing and utilization in the nursing home. *J Am Geriat Soc* 1990; **38**: 542–52.

11. Lipton HL, Bird JA. Drug utilization review in ambulatory settings: state of the science and directions for outcomes research. *Med Care* 1993; **31**: 1069–82.

12. Soumerai SB, Avorn JL. Principles of educational outreach ("academic detailing") to improve clinical decision making. *JAMA* 1990; **263**: 549–56.

13. Soumerai SB. Factors influencing prescribing. *Aust J Hosp Pharm* 1988; **18**: 9–16.

14. Lipton HL, Lee PR. *Drugs and the Elderly: Clinical, Social and Policy Perspectives*. Stanford, CA: Stanford University Press, 1988.

15. Lipton HL, Byrns PH, Soumerai SB, Chrischilles EA. Pharmacists as agents of change for rational drug therapy. *Int J Technol Assess Health Care* 1995; **11**: 485–508.

16. Beney J, Bero LA, Bond C. Expanding the roles of outpatient pharmacists: effects on health services utilisation, costs, and patient outcomes (Cochrane Review). In: *The Cochrane Library*, Issue 4, 2003. Chichester: John Wiley & Sons.

17. Soumerai SB, Lipton HL. Computer based drug utilization review—risk, benefit, or boondoggle? *N Engl J Med* 1995; **332**: 1641–4.

18. Hennessy S, Bilker WB, Zhou L, Weber AL, Brensinger C, Wang Y *et al.* Retrospective drug utilization review, prescribing errors, and clinical outcomes. *JAMA* 2003; **290**: 1494–9.

19. Oxman AD, Thomson MA, Davis DA, Haynes RB. No magic bullets: a systematic review of 102 trials of interventions to improve professional practice. *Can Med Assoc J* 1995; **153**: 1423–31.

20. Grimshaw JM, Shirran L, Thomas R, Mowatt G, Fraser C, Bero L *et al.* Changing provider behavior: an overview of systematic reviews of interventions. *Med Care* 2001; **39**(suppl 2): 2–45.

21. Balas EA, Boren SA, Brown GD, Ewigman BG, Mitchell JA, Perkoff GT. Effect of physician profiling on utilization: meta-analysis of randomized clinical trials. *J Gen Intern Med* 1996; **11**: 584–90.

22. Pearson SA, Ross-Degnan D, Payson A, Soumerai SB. Changing medication use in managed care: a critical review of the available evidence. *Am J Manag Care* 2003; **9**: 715–31.

23. Worrall G, Chaulk P, Freake D. The effects of clinical practice guidelines on patient outcomes in primary care: systematic review. *Can Med Assoc J* 1997; **156**: 1705–12.

24. Weingarten SR, Henning JM, Badamgarav E, Knight K, Hasselblad V, Gano A Jr. *et al.* Interventions used in disease management programmes for patients with chronic illness—which ones work? Meta-analysis of published reports. *BMJ* 2002; **325**: 925–33.

25. Jamtvedt G, Young JM, Kristoffersen DT, Thomson O'Brien MA, Oxman AD. Audit and feedback: effects on professional practice and health care outcomes (Cochrane Review). In: *The Cochrane Library*, Issue 4, 2003. Chichester: John Wiley & Sons.

26. Alderson P, Bero LA, Grilli R, Grimshaw JM, McAuley LM, Oxman AD *et al.* eds, Effective Practice and Organisation of Care Group. In: *The Cochrane Library*, Issue 4, 2003. Chichester: John Wiley & Sons.

27. Bloor K, Freemantle N. Lessons from international experience in controlling pharmaceutical expenditure II: influencing doctors. *BMJ* 1996; **312**: 1525–7.

28. Soumerai SB, Ross-Degnan D. Prescribing budgets: economic, clinical, and ethical perspectives. *Aust Prescriber* 1997; **20**: 28–9.

29. Soumerai SB, Ross-Degnan D, Fortess EE, Abelson J. A critical analysis of studies of state drug reimbursement policies: research in need of discipline. *Milbank Q* 1993; **71**: 217–52.

30. Soumerai SB, McLaughlin TJ, Ross-Degnan D, Casteris CS, Bollini P. Effects of limiting Medicaid drug reimbursement benefits on the use of psychotropic agents and acute mental health services by patients with schizophrenia. *N Engl J Med* 1994; **331**: 650–6.

31. Smalley WE, Griffin MR, Fought RL, Sullivan L, Ray WA. Effect of a prior authorization requirement on the use of nonsteroidal anti-inflammatory drugs by Medicaid patients. *N Engl J Med* 1995; **332**: 1612–17.

32. Tamblyn R, Laprise R, Hanley JA, Abrahamowicz M, Scott S, Mayo N *et al.* Adverse events associated with prescription drug

cost-sharing among poor and elderly persons. *JAMA* 2001; **285**: 421–9.

33. Huskamp HA, Deverka PA, Epstein AM, Epstein RS, McGuigan KA, Frank RG. The effect of incentive-based formularies on prescription-drug utilization and spending. *N Engl J Med* 2003; **349**: 2224–32.

34. Gurwitz JH. Improving quality of medication use in elderly patients. *Arch Intern Med* 2002; **162**: 1670–2.

35. Majumdar SR, Soumerai SB. Why most interventions to improve physician prescribing do not seem to work. *Can Med Assoc J* 2003; **169**: 30–1.

36. McGlynn EA, Asch SM, Adams J, Kessey J, Hicks J, DeCristofaro A *et al*. The quality of health care delivered to adults in the United States. *N Engl J Med* 2003; **348**: 2635–45.

37. Lee TH. A broader concept of medical errors. *N Engl J Med* 2002; **347**: 1965–7.

38. Soumerai SB, Avorn J, Gortmaker S, Hawley S. Effect of government and commercial warnings on reducing prescription misuse: the case of propoxyphene. *Am J Public Health* 1987; **77**: 1518–23.

39. Ross-Degnan D, Soumerai SB, Fortess EE, Gurwitz J. Examining product risk in context: market withdrawal of zomepirac sodium as a case study. *JAMA* 1993; **270**: 1937–42.

40. Gonzales R, Steiner JF, Lum A, Barrett PH. Decreasing antibiotic use in ambulatory practice: impact of a multidimensional intervention on the treatment of uncomplicated acute bronchitis in adults. *JAMA* 1999; **281**: 1512–19.

41. Gurwitz JH, Field TS, Avorn J, McCormick D, Jain S, Eckler M *et al*. Incidence and preventability of adverse drug events in nursing homes. *Am J Med* 2000; **109**: 87–94.

42. Gurwitz JH, Field TS, Harrold LR, Rothschild J, Debellis K, Seger AC *et al*. Incidence and preventability of adverse drug events among older persons in the ambulatory setting. *JAMA* 2003; **289**: 1107–16.

43. Berlowitz DR, Ash AS, Hickey EC *et al*. Inadequate management of blood pressure in a hypertensive population. *N Engl J Med* 1998; **339**: 1957–63.

44. Horwitz RI, Viscoli CM, Clemens JD, Sadock RT. Developing improved observational methods for evaluating therapeutic effectiveness. *Am J Med* 1990; **89**: 630–8.

45. Majumdar SR, McAlister FA, Soumerai SB. Synergy between publication and promotion: comparing adoption of new evidence in Canada and the United States. *Am J Med* 2003; **115**: 467–72.

46. Soumerai SB, Avorn J, Ross-Degnan D, Gortmaker S. Payment restrictions for prescription drugs in Medicaid: effects on therapy, cost, and equity. *N Engl J Med* 1987; **317**: 550–6.

47. Soumerai SB, Ross-Degnan D, Avorn J, McLaughlin TJ, Choodnovskiy I. Effects of Medicaid drug-payment limits on admission to hospitals and nursing homes. *N Engl J Med* 1991; **325**: 1072–7.

48. McDonald CJ. Protocol-based computer reminders, the quality of care and the non-perfectibility of man. *N Engl J Med* 1976; **295**: 1351–5.

49. Mintzes B, Barer ML, Kravitz RL, Bassett K, Lexchin J, Kazanjian A *et al*. How does direct-to-consumer advertising (DTCA) affect prescribing? A survey in primary care environments with and without legal DTCA. *Can Med Assoc J* 2003; **169**: 405–12.

50. Schwartz RK, Soumerai SB, Avorn J. Physician motivations for non-scientific drug prescribing. *Soc Sci Med* 1989; **28**: 577–82.

51. Greer AL. The state of the art versus the state of the science: the diffusion of new medical technologies into practice. *Int J Technol Assess Health Care* 1988; **4**: 5–26.

52. Majumdar SR, McAlister FA, Furberg CD. From knowledge to practice in chronic cardiovascular disease—a long and winding road. *J Am Coll Cardiol* 2004; **43**: 1738–42.

53. Gilbert JR, Light RJ, Mosteller F. Assessing social innovations: an empirical base for policy. In: Bennett CH, Lumsdaine AA, eds, *Evaluation and Experiment: Some Critical Issues in Assessing Social Programs*. New York: Academic Press, 1975.

54. Cook TD, Campbell DT. *Quasi-Experimentation: Design and Analysis Issues for Field Settings*. Boston, MA: Houghton Mifflin, 1979.

55. Shojania KG, Duncan GW, McDonald KM, Wachter RM. Safe but sound: Patient safety meets evidence-based medicine. *JAMA* 2002; **288**: 508–13.

56. Leape LL, Berwick DM, Bates DW. What practices will most improve safety? Evidence-based medicine meets patient safety. *JAMA* 2002; **288**: 501–7.

57. Soumerai SB, Ross-Degnan D, Gortmaker S, Avorn J. Withdrawing payment for non-scientific drug therapy: intended and unexpected effects of a large-scale natural experiment. *JAMA* 1990; **263**: 831–9.

58. Groves R. Therapeutic drug-use review for the Florida Medicaid Program. *Am J Hosp Pharm* 1985; **42**: 316–19.

59. Donner A, Birkett N, Buck C. Randomization by cluster—samples size requirements and analysis. *Am J Epidemiology* 1981; **114**: 906–14.

60. Campbell MK, Mollison J, Grimshaw JM. Cluster trials in implementation research: estimation of intracluster correlation coefficients and sample size. *Stat Med* 2001; **20**: 391–9.

61. Freemantle N, Eccles M, Wood J, Mason J, Nazareth I, Duggan C *et al*. A randomized trial of evidence-based outreach: rationale and design. *Control Clin Trials* 1999; **20**: 479–92.

62. Divine GW, Brown JT, Frazier LM. The unit of analysis error in studies about physicians' patient care behavior. *J Gen Intern Med* 1992; **7**: 623–9.

63. Diggle PJ, Liang KY, Zeger SL. *Analysis of Longitudinal Data*. Oxford: Clarendon Press, 1996.

64. McCullagh P, Nelder JA. *Generalized Linear Models*, 2nd edn. London: Chapman & Hall, 1989.

65. Soumerai SB, McLaughlin TJ, Gurwitz JH, Guadagnoli E, Hauptman PJ, Borbas C *et al*. Effect of local medical opinion leaders on quality of care for acute myocardial infarction: a randomized controlled trial. *JAMA* 1998; **279**: 1358–63.

66. The Leapfrog Group for Patient Safety: Rewarding higher standards. Available at: http://www.leapfroggroup.org/consumer_intro2.htm. Accessed: January 11, 2004.

67. Majumdar SR, Guirguis LM, Toth EL, Lewanczuk RZ, Lee TK, Johnson JA. Controlled trial of a multifaceted intervention to improve the quality of care for rural patients with type-2 diabetes. *Diabetes Care* 2003; **26**: 3061–6.

68. Avorn J, Soumerai SB, Wessels M, Taylor W, Janousek J, Weiner M. Reduction of incorrect antibiotic dosing through a structured educational order form. *Arch Intern Med* 1988; **148**: 1720–4.

69. Marciniak TA, Ellerbeck EF, Radford MJ, Kresowik TF, Gold JA, Krumholz HM *et al.* Improving the quality of care for Medicare patients with acute myocardial infarction: results from the Cooperative Cardiovascular Project. *JAMA* 1998; **279**: 1351–7.

70. Brook RH, McGlynn EA. Measuring quality of care. *N Engl J Med* 1996; **335**: 966–9.

71. Green LW, Kreuter MW. *Health Promotion Planning: An Educational and Environmental Approach.* Mountain View, CA: HJ Kaiser Foundation, 1991.

72. Eisenberg JM. *Doctors' Decisions and the Cost of Medical Care.* Ann Arbor, MI: Health Administration Press Perspectives, 1986.

73. Schaffner W, Ray WA, Federspiel CF, Miller WO. Improving antibiotic prescribing in office practice: a controlled trial of three educational methods. *JAMA* 1983; **250**: 1728–32.

74. Avorn JL, Soumerai SB. Improving drug therapy decisions through educational outreach: a randomized controlled trial of academically-based "detailing." *N Engl J Med* 1983; **308**: 1457–63.

75. Soumerai SB, Avorn JL. Economic and policy analysis of university-based drug "detailing." *Med Care* 1986; **24**: 313–31.

76. Kosecoff J, Kanouse DE, Rogers WH, McCloskey L, Winslow CM, Brook RH. Effects of the National Institutes of Health consensus development program on physician practice. *JAMA* 1987; **258**: 2708–13.

77. Lomas J, Anderson GM, Domnick-Pierre K, Vayda E, Enkin MW, Hannah WJ. Do practice guidelines guide practice? The effect of consensus statements on the practice of physicians. *N Engl J Med* 1989; **321**: 1306–11.

78. Wade OL, Hood H. Prescribing of drugs reported to cause adverse reactions. *Br J Prev Soc Med* 1972; **26**: 205–11.

79. Maclure M, Dormuth C, Naumann T, McCormack J, Rangno R, Whiteside C *et al.* Influences of educational interventions and adverse news about calcium channel blockers on first line prescribing of antihypertensive drugs to elderly people in British Columbia. *Lancet* 1998; **352**: 943–8.

80. Hersh AL, Stefanick ML, Stafford RS. National use of postmenopausal hormone therapy: annual trends and response to recent evidence. *JAMA* 2004; **291**: 47–53.

81. Soumerai SB, Ross-Degnan D, Spira J. The effects of professional and media warnings about the association between aspirin use in children and Reye's syndrome. *Milbank Q* 1992; **70**: 155–82.

82. Inui TS, Yourtee EL, Williamson JW. Improved outcomes in hypertension after physician tutorials: a controlled trial. *Ann Intern Med* 1976; **84**: 646–51.

83. Sibley JC, Sackett DL, Neufeld V, Gerrard B, Rudnick KV, Fraser W. A randomized trial of continuing medical education. *N Engl J Med* 1982; **306**: 511–15.

84. Johnson RE, Campbell WH, Azevedo D, Christensen DB. Studying the impact of patient drug profiles in an HMO. *Med Care* 1976; **14**: 799–807.

85. Hershey CO, Porter DK, Breslau D, Cohen DI. Influence of simple computerized feedback on prescription changes in an ambulatory clinic: a randomized clinical trial. *Med Care* 1986; **24**: 472–81.

86. Koepsell TD, Gurtel A, Diehr PH, Temkin NR, Helfand KH, Gleser MA *et al.* The Seattle evaluation of computerized drug profiles: effects on prescribing practices and resource use. *Am J Public Health* 1983; **73**: 850–5.

87. O'Connell DL, Henry D, Tomlins R. Randomized controlled trial of effect of feedback on general practitioners' prescribing in Australia. *BMJ* 1999; **318**: 507–11.

88. Lipton HL, Bero LA, Bird JA, McPhee SJ. The impact of clinical pharmacists' consultations on physicians' geriatric drug prescribing: a randomized controlled trial. *Med Care* 1992; **30**: 646–58.

89. Kiefe CI, Allison JJ, Williams OD, Person SD, Weaver MT, Weissman NW. Improving quality improvement using achievable benchmarks for physician feedback: a randomized controlled trial. *JAMA* 2001; **285**: 2871–9.

90. Hershey CO, Goldberg HI, Cohen DI. The effect of computerized feedback coupled with a newsletter upon outpatient prescribing charges. A randomized controlled trial. *Med Care* 1988; **26**: 88–93.

91. Gehlbach SH, Wilkinson WE, Hammond WE, Clapp NE, Finn AL, Taylor WJ *et al.* Improving drug prescribing in a primary care practice. *Med Care* 1984; **22**: 193–201.

92. Balas EA, Weingarten S, Garb CT, Blumenthal D, Boren SA, Brown GD. Improving preventive care by prompting physicians. *Arch Intern Med* 2000; **160**: 301–8.

93. Dexter PR, Perkins S, Overhage JM, Maharry K, Kohler RB, McDonald CJ. A computerized reminder system to increase the use of preventive care for hospitalized patients. *N Engl J Med* 2001; **345**: 965–70.

94. Hunt DL, Haynes RB, Hanna SE, Smith K. Effects of computer-based clinical decision support systems on physician performance and patient outcomes: a systematic review. *JAMA* 1998; **280**: 1339–46.

95. Bates DW, Gawande AA. Improving patient safety with information technology. *N Engl J Med* 2003; **348**: 2256–34.

96. Bates DW, Leape LL, Cullen DJ, Laird N, Petersen LA, Teich JM *et al.* Effect of computerized physician order entry and a team intervention on prevention of serious medication errors. *JAMA* 1998; **280**: 1311–16.

97. Evans RS, Pestotnik SL, Classen DC, Clemmer TP, Weaver LK, Orme JF Jr *et al.* A computer assisted management program for antibiotics and other anti-infective agents. *N Engl J Med* 1998; **338**: 232–8.

98. Eccles M, McColl E, Steen N, Rousseau N, Grimshaw J, Parkin D *et al.* Effect of computerized evidence based guidelines

on management of asthma and angina in adults in primary care: a cluster randomized controlled trial. *BMJ* 2002; **325**: 941–8.

99. Kaushal R, Shojania KG, Bates DW. Effects of computerized physician order entry and clinical decision support systems on medication safety: a systematic review. *Arch Intern Med* 2003; **163**: 1409–16.

100. Stross JK, Bole GG. Evaluation of a continuing education program in rheumatoid arthritis. *Arthritis Rheum* 1980; **23**: 846–9.

101. Lomas J, Enkin M, Anderson G, Hannah WJ, Vayda E, Singer J. Opinion leaders vs. audit and feedback to implement practice guidelines. Delivery after previous cesarean section. *JAMA* 1991; **265**: 2202–7.

102. Lomas J. Teaching old (and not so old) docs new tricks: effective ways to implement research findings. In: Dunn EV, Norton PG, Stewart M, Bass MJ, Tudives F, eds, *Disseminating New Knowledge and Having an Impact on Practice*. New York: Sage, 1994.

103. Thomson O'Brien MA, Oxman AD, Haynes RB, Davis DA, Freemantle N, Harvey EL. Local opinion leaders: effects on professional practice and health care outcomes (Cochrane Review). In: *The Cochrane Library*, Issue 4, 2003. Chichester: John Wiley & Sons.

104. Berner ES, Baker CS, Funkhouser E, Heudebert GR, Allison JJ, Fargason CA Jr *et al.* Do local opinion leaders augment hospital quality improvement efforts? A randomized trial to promote adherence to unstable angina guidelines. *Med Care* 2003; **41**: 420–31.

105. Freemantle N, Nazareth I, Eccles M, Wood J, Haines A, Evidence-based OutReach trialists. A randomized controlled trial of the effect of educational outreach by community pharmacists on prescribing in UK general practice. *Br J Gen Practice* 2002; **52**: 290–5.

106. Thomson O'Brien MA, Oxman AD, Davis DA, Haynes RB, Freemantle N *et al.* Educational outreach visits: effects on professional practice and health care outcomes (Cochrane Review). In: *The Cochrane Library*, Issue 4, 2003. Chichester: John Wiley & Sons.

107. Mason J, Freemantle N, Nazareth I, Eccles M, Haines A, Drummond M. When is it cost effective to change behavior of health professionals? *JAMA* 2001; **286**: 2988–92.

108. Diwan VK, Wahlstrom R, Tomson G, Beermann B, Sterky G, Eriksson B. Effects of group detailing on the prescribing of lipid lowering drugs: a randomized controlled trial in Swedish primary care. *J Clin Epidemiol* 1995; **48**: 705–11.

109. Gosden T, Forland F, Kristiansen IS, Sutton M, Leese B, Giuffrida A *et al.* Capitation, salary, fee-for-service and mixed systems of payment: effects on the behaviour of primary care physicians (Cochrane Review). In: *The Cochrane Library*, Issue 4, 2003. Chichester: John Wiley & Sons.

110. Lipton HL, Kreling DK, Collins T, Hertz KC. Pharmacy benefit management companies: dimensions of performance. *Ann Rev Public Health* 1999; **20**: 361–401.

111. Gutierrez G, Guiscafre H, Munoz O. Strategies for improving the therapeutic patterns used in acute diarrhea in primary medical care units. X. Conclusions and research perspectives. *Arch Invest Med (Mex)* 1988; **19**: 437–43.

112. Hadiyono JEP, Suryawati S, Danu SS, Sunartono S, Santosa B. Interactional group discussion: results of a controlled trial using a behavioral intervention to reduce the use of injections in public health facilities. *Soc Sci Med* 1996; **42**: 1177–83.

113. Eddy D. Rationing resources while improving quality: how to get more for less. *JAMA* 1994; **272**: 817–24.

114. Leape LL, Brennan TA, Laird NA, Lawthers AG, Localio AR, Barnes BA *et al.* The nature of adverse events in hospitalized patients. *N Engl J Med* 1991; **324**: 377–83.

115. Bates DW, Cullen DJ, Laird N, Petersen LA, Small SD, Servi D *et al.* Incidence of adverse drug events and potential adverse drug events: implications for prevention. *JAMA* 1995; **274**: 29–34.

116. Gandhi TK, Weingart SN, Borus J, Seger AC, Peterson J, Burdick E *et al.* Adverse drug events in ambulatory care. *N Engl J Med* 2003; **348**: 1556–64.

117. Tierney WM. Adverse outpatient drug events—a problem and an opportunity. *N Engl J Med* 2003; **348**: 1587–9.

118. Rothschild JM, Federico FA, Gandhi TK, Kaushal R, Williams DH, Bates DW. Analysis of medication related malpractice claims—causes, preventability, and costs. *Arch Intern Med* 2002; **162**: 2414–20.

119. Soumerai SB, McLaughlin TJ, Spiegelman D, Hertzmark E, Thibault G, Goldman L. Adverse outcomes of underuse of beta blockers in elderly survivors of acute myocardial infarction. *JAMA* 1997; **277**: 115–21.

120. Lesar TS, Briceland LL, Delcoure K, Parmalee JC, Masta-Gornic V, Pohl H. Medication prescribing errors in a teaching hospital. *JAMA* 1990; **263**: 2329–34.

121. Schiff GD, Rucker TD. Computerized prescribing: building the infrastructure for better medication usage. *JAMA* 1998; **279**: 1024–9.

122. Tamblyn R, Huang A, Perreault R, Jacques A, Roy D, Hanley J *et al.* The medical office of the 21st century (MOXXI): effectiveness of computerized decision-making support in reducing inappropriate prescribing in primary care. *Can Med Assoc J* 2003; **169**: 549–56.

29

Drug Utilization Review

SEAN HENNESSY[1], STEPHEN B. SOUMERAI[2], HELENE LEVENS LIPTON[3]
and BRIAN L. STROM[1]

[1] University of Pennsylvania School of Medicine Philadelphia, Pennsylvania, USA; [2] Harvard Medical School and Harvard Pilgrim Health Care, Boston, Massachusetts, USA; [3] School of Medicine, University of California at San Francisco, San Francisco, California, USA.

INTRODUCTION

Drug utilization review (DUR) programs have been defined as "structured, ongoing initiatives that interpret patterns of drug use in relation to predetermined criteria, and attempt to prevent or minimize inappropriate prescribing."[1] In this chapter, we distinguish DUR programs from other efforts to improve the quality and reduce the costs of drug therapy, describe the conceptual framework that underlies DUR, review the history of DUR, and describe the DUR process and its application in different settings. We then describe the clinical and methodologic problems to be addressed by pharmacoepidemiologic research in this area, critically evaluate the evidence regarding the effectiveness of DUR programs, and look to the future of DUR.

DUR has many synonyms, including *drug use review*, *drug use evaluation*, and *medication use evaluation*. DUR programs differ from *drug utilization studies* (see Chapter 27), which are time-limited investigations that measure drug use, but do not necessarily assess appropriateness or attempt to change practice.

DUR programs operate alongside other approaches whose goal is to improve the quality or reduce the cost of drug therapy. One such program is the formulary system, which makes use of *formularies*, or enumerated lists of drugs which may be prescribed (and, by exclusion, those which may not be prescribed). Many formularies also include economic incentives to consumers to promote use of less expensive medications over more expensive ones. Other administrative measures that affect medication use include the imposition of limits ("caps") on the monetary cost of prescription medications or on the number of prescriptions that will be paid per person per time period, required copayments by consumers, mandatory generic drug substitution, and requirements for prior approval for particular drugs. Because DUR programs use explicit criteria, they are distinct from monthly, Federally-mandated drug regimen reviews performed by pharmacists in US nursing homes. Because of their use of explicit criteria. DUR programs are also distinct from routine pharmacy practice, which involves implicit review of patient-specific information (i.e., a patient profile) maintained by the individual pharmacy.[2]

Pharmacoepidemiology, Fourth Edition   Edited by B.L. Strom
© 2005 John Wiley & Sons, Ltd

DUR programs are categorized by the timing of interventions within the drug use process, with *prospective* DUR occurring before the patient receives the medication (i.e., during the prescribing or dispensing processes) and *retrospective* DUR occurring after the patient has received the medication (e.g., by alert letter after a medication has been prescribed and dispensed). In recent years, the use of clinical decision support within computerized prescriber order entry (CPOE) programs has risen dramatically. The use of such programs to improve prescribing can be considered a form of prospective DUR in which prescribers are the targets of interventions. Such programs are discussed in Chapter 34. Other methods of changing prescribing, such as academic detailing, when part of an ongoing program, can be considered a form of DUR. Academic detailing is discussed in Chapter 28.

CONCEPTUAL FRAMEWORK UNDERLYING DUR

In 1993, Lipton and Bird proposed a conceptual framework underlying DUR,[3] which is presented schematically in Figure 29.1. According to this conceptual model, prospective and retrospective DUR programs affect either current or future prescribing and dispensing practices within the context of other important factors. These factors can be categorized as patient and family influences, prescriber characteristics, and system factors (Figure 29.1). Patient and family influences include demographic characteristics, cultural beliefs, willingness to take needed drugs, and demands for unnecessary drugs (e.g., demands for antibiotics in the setting of viral infections, which do not respond to antibiotics). Prescriber characteristics include knowledge about pharmacology, knowledge of drug prices, and imperfect memory. System factors include drug reimbursement policies, formularies, organization of the medical care system, influence of pharmaceutical companies, abundance of drug therapy options, and lack of data on comparative safety and efficacy among therapeutic alternatives.

DUR programs are hypothesized to affect many of the undesirable influences of patient, prescriber, and system factors. Also reflected in this model is the fact that both prospective and retrospective DUR might influence care for patients identified in the alerts, the care of future patients (called the "spillover effect"), or both.

HISTORY OF DUR

The literature evaluating DUR interventions has historically emanated predominantly from North America, although studies from other countries have become more common in recent years.[4–6] Several developments are viewed as having sentinel importance in the emergence of DUR. One such factor is the growth of insurance coverage for outpatient prescriptions that took place in the 1970s and 1980s,[7] which created both the financial interest to minimize prescription drug costs and the computerized patient-level data needed to conduct such programs. Technical feasibility within the US Medicaid program (see Chapter 18) was enhanced in the early- to mid-1960s, when the US Department of Health, Education and Welfare (DHEW, predecessor of the present US Department of Health and Human Services—DHHS) collaborated with state Medicaid agencies to develop computerized information systems to perform administrative functions within Medicaid. The first published reference to DUR was a 1969 background paper by the DHEW's Task Force on Prescription Drugs,[8] which was charged with evaluating the feasibility and implications of providing prescription drug coverage to beneficiaries of the US Medicare system. As part of this evaluation, the Task Force evaluated the possibility of using claims data to improve the quality and reduce the cost of drug therapy. Although the Task Force perceived that outpatient DUR appeared promising, it believed that evidence of effectiveness was needed before implementation, and recommended further study of DUR rather than its widespread adoption.[9] However, as described below, DUR programs proliferated without convincing evidence that they were effective in improving clinical outcomes.

In 1970, PAID Prescriptions, a private sector pharmaceutical benefit management company, began a formal DUR program that focused on cost issues in California's San Joaquin Valley Medicaid program.[10,11] By the mid-1970s, other US Medicaid programs and other third-party payers had begun collaborating with private companies, known as DUR vendors, to initiate outpatient DUR programs that focused on cost and quality of care issues. Based largely on the intuitive appeal and promise of DUR, DUR was enthusiastically advocated in a 1977 report that examined issues surrounding a drug benefit for a proposed US national health insurance program.[12] The Joint Commission on Accreditation of Health Care Organizations (JCAHO), which accredits health care facilities in the US, required hospitals to conduct inpatient DUR for antibiotics beginning in 1985, and for medications in general beginning in 1987. By that time, some hospitals had been performing DUR for over a decade.[13–16] A 1988 US Federal law mandated DUR as part of a law providing catastrophic benefits to US Medicare recipients.[17] However, this legislation was repealed the following year.[18] Probably the most significant event in the growth of outpatient DUR in the US has been the Omnibus Budget Reconciliation Act of 1990,[19] which required that all US states conduct both retrospective and prospective DUR on behalf of Medicaid enrollees.

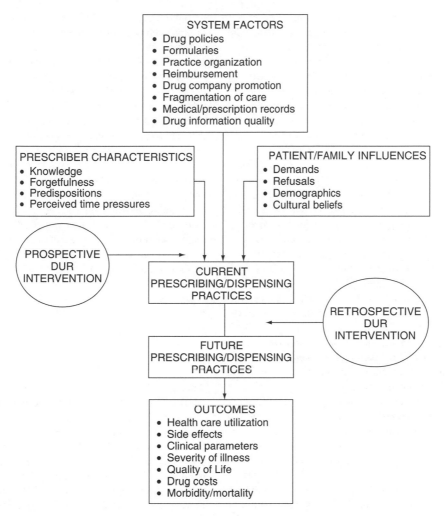

Figure 29.1. Relationship of DUR interventions to drug prescribing and dispensing. Reprinted with permission from Lipton HL, Bird JA. Drug utilization review in ambulatory settings: state of the science and directions for outcomes research. *Med Care* 1993; **31**: 1069–82. © Lippincott Williams & Wilkins.

THE DUR PROCESS

Although there is variation in how different authors specify the steps of the DUR process,[11,20–22] one general and widely accepted model for both retrospective and prospective DUR was described by Erwin:[21]

1. Design the basic structure.
2. Seek approval.
3. Construct criteria.
4. Apply criteria.
5. Evaluate and analyze yield (i.e., the frequency of exceptions).
6. Establish prescribing patterns.
7. Establish intervention strategies.
8. Re-apply criteria to databases.
9. Revise criteria as needed.

Although this basic model is applied differently in different settings, some characteristics are common across settings.

In general, the DUR process involves comparing actual behavior to explicit, prospectively established standards, referred to as *criteria*. For example, a commonly used criterion is that patients should not receive more than one nonsteroidal anti-inflammatory agent at any one time. Criteria have been developed to identify the following types of problems: drug–drug interactions, drug–disease interactions, drug–age interactions, drug–allergy interactions, use of too high or too low a dose, duplication of therapeutic class, excessive duration of therapy, obtaining prescription refills sooner or later than should be needed, failure to prescribe a known effective agent in patients with certain conditions, abuse of psychoactive medications, and use of a more costly agent when a less costly agent is available. However, it has been observed that DUR programs tend to focus on overuse of medications, e.g., prolonged use of histamine H-2 receptor antagonists (H2RAs), giving less attention to problems of underuse, e.g., failure to use β-blockers in patients who have had a myocardial infarction.[23]

Naturally, a criterion must be *valid* in order for the application of that criterion to improve clinical outcomes. In this context, we define validity as the ability of a DUR criterion to detect instances in which a change in therapy would ultimately benefit the patient. However, there is good reason to withhold judgment on the validity of any DUR criterion until it has been demonstrated empirically. This is because the current state of knowledge in drug therapy is such that what is considered to be "good care" is supported by levels of evidence that range from case reports, to reasoning based in pharmacologic theory, to randomized trials. Even when DUR criteria are based on the results of randomized trials (i.e., the best case scenario), it still remains uncertain that the criteria will identify patients whose care will improve if therapy is changed. For example, the use of β-blockers has been conclusively shown to improve average survival in patients who have had a heart attack.[24–26] Thus, a very reasonable criterion would be that patients with a history of myocardial infarction and no evidence of contraindication (e.g., chronic obstructive lung disease) should receive a β-blocker. However, it is conceivable that applying this criterion in practice would identify patients who, because of some measured or unmeasured characteristics, would fail to benefit from β-blocker therapy. This is because populations in whom criteria are violated may well be different from the population in whom β-blockers were tested, or may represent subgroups that did not derive benefit. Thus, the only way to know for certain whether a given criterion is valid in a particular population is to measure the clinical effectiveness of a DUR program that employs that criterion.

The next step in the DUR process is to measure adherence to explicit criteria by examining individual-level data. Instances in which medication use does not agree with criteria are called *exceptions*. Next, interventions are implemented where appropriate, often following an implicit review. Although the general model for DUR does not require that practitioners be made aware of individual exceptions occurring in their patients (that is, interventions can be made based on aggregate rather than individual findings), this step usually involves alerting the physician and/or pharmacy of record as to the occurrence of the specific exception. Naturally, the intervention needs to be successful in achieving a *beneficial* change in therapy (rather than *any* change in therapy, or even the *desired* change in therapy) for a DUR program to be effective in its primary goal of improving clinical endpoints. For example, a DUR program might lead to a reduction in use of H2RAs (the desired change in prescribing), but result in an increased rate of peptic ulcer disease events.

Differences in how the general DUR model is applied in different settings will now be discussed.

Outpatient Retrospective DUR Programs

Although US Federal law requires outpatient retrospective DUR programs only for Medicaid patients, most private sector outpatient drug benefit plans in the US also perform retrospective DUR. Because of the large number of patients, virtually all outpatient retrospective DUR programs use computerized administrative data (i.e., data maintained for billing and other administrative purposes) to identify exceptions. Some DUR programs use both pharmacy and medical claims data, while others use pharmacy claims only.

Although the frequency of exceptions varies with the criteria employed, one study showed that, each year, 3–7% of persons who filled a prescription had an exception to a set of 61 DUR criteria.[27] In most outpatient retrospective DUR programs, computer-generated exceptions are reviewed by a physician or pharmacist, or by a committee of health professionals, and result in an intervention only when the exception does not meet some additional implicit or subjective criterion. The proportion of exceptions that results in an alert varies considerably. For example, one study of six Medicaid programs found that the alerts were issued for 1–25% of exceptions.[28] At least part of this variability is due to constraints in the availability of reviewers to examine specific exceptions on a case-by-case basis.

Most outpatient retrospective DUR programs intervene by mailing an alert letter to the physician, and sometimes to the pharmacist of record. This alert letter typically describes the DUR program and the criterion, and provides literature references supporting the criterion and a patient profile demonstrating that the criterion was violated. A few outpatient retrospective DUR programs use telephone calls or face-to-face meetings to convey alerts. An ongoing development in outpatient retrospective DUR is the use of data grouped at the level of the prescriber (an approach known as "physician profiling") to make decisions regarding interventions, rather than making intervention decisions by viewing each criterion exception in isolation.[29,30]

Outpatient Prospective DUR Programs

Prospective DUR includes efforts that occur before or during the prescribing process, or during the dispensing process. Thus, the use of computerized decision support for either prescribing or dispensing can be considered a form of prospective DUR. The evidence for the effectiveness of computerized decision support in improving prescribing in CPOE programs is described in Chapter 34.

Many outpatient prospective DUR programs intervene by conveying computer alerts to the pharmacist filling the prescription. These alerts can be generated either by the pharmacy's own computer or by the computer of the pharmaceutical benefit management company that reimburses the pharmacy for dispensing the prescription. The responsibility of resolving the potential problem then belongs to the pharmacist, who must contact the prescriber if the prescription is to be changed. The fact that the alert is conveyed to the pharmacist rather than the physician (who is in a better position to change therapy) would be expected to reduce the effectiveness of pharmacy-based prospective DUR programs relative to physician-based interventions. Computer-aided review of patient profiles may have advantages over manual review by virtue of increased sensitivity in detecting potential problems. However, computer review systems that are based on overly inclusive criteria for producing alerts produce a large number of apparently trivial alerts, and may thus foster disregard of alerts, reducing the effectiveness of such systems. For example, one study found that more than 10% of all outpatient prescriptions led to an alert to the pharmacist.[31] Pharmacists initially overrode 88% of such alerts, and overrode an additional 9% of the alerts after consulting with the patient, physician, or pharmaceutical benefit manager.

Thus, only 3% of prospective DUR alerts led to a change in therapy.

Hospital DUR Programs

Hospitalized patients are sicker, and take more numerous and more toxic medications than community-dwelling individuals. Hospitals are also characterized by more centralized decision making and better availability of clinical data than is present in most outpatient environments. Therefore, it is not surprising that DUR practice originated in hospitals, where it is both more acutely needed and more politically and logistically feasible.

Hospital DUR programs are usually conducted by the pharmacy department acting in conjunction with and by the authority of a medical staff committee, such as the pharmacy and therapeutics ("P&T") committee. Hospital DUR programs often use the same overall process that is described above, although, unlike most outpatient DUR programs, they generally have access to primary medical records. Hospital DUR programs also tend to perform series of discrete evaluations rather than ongoing evaluations, and often include elements of both prospective and retrospective review.

Because of more centralization in decision making authority, hospital DUR programs often are able to use regulatory interventions that are unavailable to many outpatient DUR programs. These interventions can include formulary deletions, restriction of a medication for use in particular circumstances, restriction of a medication for use by certain specialists, and mandatory drug order forms, all of which tend to be more effective than nonregulatory interventions in affecting prescribing.[32] Regulatory interventions are discussed in Chapter 28.

Therapeutic areas that have received recent attention by hospital DUR programs include antimicrobials,[33–61] analgesics,[62–68] sedative–hypnotics,[62,63,67–71] and anti-ulcer drugs.[72–75] Some hospitals have implemented ongoing antibiotic management programs in which patients meeting certain criteria have their therapy reviewed by an infectious disease specialist, who makes treatment recommendations to the prescribing physician when therapy is deemed to be suboptimal.[76]

There are a number of barriers in assessing the effectiveness of inpatient DUR progress programs. First, studies of the impact of in-hospital DUR programs tend to focus on process measures such as prescribing rather than clinical outcome measures. Second, the problems identified and the interventions available in a particular institution may be specific to that institution, making poor generalizability an issue. Third, successful efforts may be more likely to be published by authors and journals, which would lead to publication bias. For these reasons, this chapter will not review in detail studies examining the effectiveness of in-hospital DUR programs. (See also Chapter 35.)

CLINICAL PROBLEMS TO BE ADDRESSED BY PHARMACOEPIDEMIOLOGIC RESEARCH

While the entire process of DUR can be seen as an application of pharmacoepidemiology *practice*, the primary role for pharmacoepidemiologic *research* in the area of DUR is to evaluate the effectiveness of these programs in meeting their stated goals. Namely, to what degree do they change prescribing, improve clinical outcomes, and reduce costs?

Clarifying the mechanisms by which DUR acts is also important. For example, if DUR is effective in altering prescribing, does it do so by changing prescribing for patients identified in alerts, by changing prescribing in future patients ("spillover" effects), or both? What features of DUR programs influence their effectiveness, and how might programs be made more effective?

METHODOLOGIC PROBLEMS TO BE ADDRESSED BY PHARMACOEPIDEMIOLOGIC RESEARCH

BARRIERS TO RANDOMIZED TRIALS

There are a number of challenges to studying the effectiveness of DUR programs. Although it is well recognized that randomized experiments provide the most convincing evidence for the effectiveness of an intervention, significant barriers exist to the conduct of randomized trials to evaluate DUR programs. One important barrier is that in the US, Medicaid programs are required by Federal law to perform DUR, making randomized trials of entire DUR programs impossible within Medicaid. However, this would not preclude randomized trials of specific components of DUR programs.

A barrier to randomized trials outside of Medicaid is the fact that some agencies appear interested in DUR primarily as a means to reduce drug costs, and thus have little or no incentive to study the clinical effects of DUR. Another major barrier is that some private sector programs consider both DUR criteria and the data needed to measure effectiveness to be proprietary information, and thus secret.[77] Despite these barriers, one experimental trial of an overall DUR program and a number of experimental trials of individual drug use audits have been conducted, although most have looked at process measures such as drug utilization rather than clinical endpoints.

CLUSTERED OBSERVATIONS

When randomized experiments have been performed, the need to keep the intervention and control groups free from cross-contamination has necessitated the randomization of *clusters*, or units such as physicians, pharmacies, or geographic regions, rather than the randomization of individual patients. Randomization by cluster[78–86] results in fewer randomized units, and thus reduced statistical power.[87] However, unless clustering is correctly accounted for in the analysis, the results will tend to overstate the true precision of the data. This means that ignored clustering can artificially reduce p-values and the width of confidence intervals. Although statistical methods to account for clustering have been developed,[80,81] they have not been used widely in studies of DUR.

RARE OUTCOMES

An additional challenge to research in this area is that the serious clinical outcomes that DUR programs are intended to prevent (for example, serious gastrointestinal bleeding caused by nonsteroidal anti-inflammatory drugs) are relatively rare on a population basis. Thus, in most settings, the relatively small effect that DUR programs are likely to have on clinical outcome measures such as all-cause and even cause-specific hospitalizations is likely to be overwhelmed by underlying variability in the rates of these events. Therefore, studies attempting to show clinical effects of DUR programs need to be enormous in size.

POTENTIALLY NONCOMPARABLE STUDY GROUPS

Challenges associated with the use of nonrandomized study designs to make causal inferences are a central theme throughout pharmacoepidemiology (see Chapters 2, 23, 39, 40, 47, and 48). Not surprisingly, they are central to the interpretation of nonrandomized studies of DUR programs as well. That is, the validity of any nonrandomized study is subject to threat by many factors, the most prominent of which is unmeasured baseline differences between treated and untreated subjects.

Nonrandomized studies of programmatic interventions like DUR are best described using the terminology of program evaluation ("quasi-experimentation") literature (e.g., interrupted time series, pre–post with comparison group) as developed by Campbell and Stanley[88] and Cook and Campbell,[89] and summarized in Chapter 28. As described elsewhere[88,89] and in Chapter 28, there is a general hierarchy that ranks quasi-experimental designs with respect to scientific rigor and the strength of the casual inferences that can be drawn from them.

CURRENTLY AVAILABLE SOLUTIONS

FRAMEWORK FOR EVALUATING THE EFFECTIVENESS OF DUR

As noted above, the true effectiveness of the DUR model can be evaluated only by examining the effects of real-life DUR programs. Thus, it is possible that a given DUR program is ineffective as *currently implemented*, but that it might be effective if it were implemented differently, or under different circumstances.

Real-world DUR programs operate by performing individual drug use audits, which are either discrete or ongoing. Thus, each criterion or small group of related criteria used by a DUR program can be considered to be a distinct drug use audit. Studies focusing on the effects of specific drug use audits (i.e., the application of an individual criterion or small group of related criteria) are more specific, and thus more credible than evaluations of overall DUR programs.

Similarly, evidence for more effects on process measures, such as changes in prescribing, tends to be more credible than evidence for clinical outcomes such as reductions in the rate of all-cause hospital admission. This is because there is greater potential for external factors to influence the rate of clinical outcomes.

In addition to being more credible, demonstrating an effect of DUR on process measures such as prescribing is also *easier* than showing an effect on clinical outcome measures, since such effects are more proximal to the intervention than the clinical effects that DUR programs are intended to produce. However, this increased credibility and relative ease in showing an effect comes at the price of reduced importance. That is, an effect on prescribing, even if it is the desired effect, may not result in an improvement in clinical outcomes. Further, many DUR interventions are intended not to improve clinical outcomes, but rather to reduce drug costs.

Because one of the goals of DUR programs is to reduce health care costs (both drug costs and, because of effects on clinical outcomes, medical costs such as for hospital admissions), their ability to do so is frequently evaluated.[90] In fact, every US Medicaid program is required to estimate the cost savings of their retrospective and prospective DUR programs each year.[19] Moore *et al.* used econometric methods to evaluate the economic impact of retrospective DUR programs in Medicaid from 1985 to 1992.[91] They found evidence that such programs reduced drug costs; however, they failed to observe any reduction in non-drug costs, such as would occur if DUR programs led to fewer hospitalizations.[91]

Inpatient DUR programs often use approaches to change prescribing that are not typically used by outpatient programs, including special order forms, making drugs unavailable, restriction of drugs to particular clinical specialties, and educational efforts by clinical opinion leaders.[22] The effectiveness of these interventions in changing prescribing is reviewed in detail in Chapter 28. In general, these approaches can be successful in changing prescribing, although studies evaluating their effects on clinical outcomes are lacking.

EVIDENCE FOR THE EFFECTIVENESS OF OUTPATIENT RETROSPECTIVE DUR PROGRAMS IN CHANGING PRESCRIBING FOR THE PATIENT IDENTIFIED IN THE ALERT

Zimmerman *et al.*[92] used a nonrandomized, pre–post design with control group to evaluate the effectiveness of an intervention to reduce overuse of H2RAs within the Wisconsin Medicaid DUR program. H2RAs are used for acid-peptic disorders, and have been the focus of many cost minimization interventions because of perceived overuse. In the study by Zimmerman *et al.*, patients who received acute dose therapy for more than 90 days were assigned to intervention or control status based on whether their prescribing physician cared for three or more such patients (intervention group) or two or fewer such patients (control group). The intervention consisted of a packet mailed to the prescriber that included a letter explaining the concerns of chronic full-dose H2RA therapy, profiles of patients with an exception, and references to the peer-reviewed literature. H2RA use was measured 6 months pre- and 12 months post-intervention. Although treatment assignment was based on physician (i.e., cluster of patients), clustering was ignored in the analysis. Therefore, the precision of the effect measures presented by the authors may overestimate the true precision.

Both groups reduced their use of H2RAs during the 12-month post-intervention period. Among patients in long-term care facilities, the pre–post reduction was 16% greater in the intervention group than in the control group, although this difference was not statistically significant. Among ambulatory patients, the pre–post reduction was 30% greater in the intervention group than in the control group, a difference that was statistically significant. Thus, despite possibly incomparable treatment and control groups, and potential overstatement of the degree of precision, this study provides some evidence that a retrospective drug use audit aimed at reducing chronic use of acute-dose H2RA therapy can have a small to moderate effect on prescribing for identified patients. Clinical endpoints were not examined in this study.

Okano and Rascati[93] performed a randomized controlled trial to examine the effectiveness of an intervention aimed at reducing duplicative peptic ulcer therapy within the Texas Medicaid population. The intervention consisted of a mailed alert letter that included a patient profile. Physicians practicing within a given small town were randomized as a single unit. Thus, randomization was by cluster, although the analysis ignored clustering, which may have resulted in overstatement of the precision of the results. The outcome measure was the continued presence of duplicative therapy six months after the intervention.

The desired outcome (discontinuation of at least one component of the duplicative therapy) was seen in 42% of patients in the intervention group and 33% of patients in the control group, for a risk ratio of the desired outcome of 1.70 (95% confidence interval, 1.12–2.59). Thus, these data appear to support the conclusion that a drug use audit that uses a mailed alert letter can have a modest effect on duplicative therapy. However, the true precision of the effect estimate may be less than that reported by the investigators.

Collins et al.[94] performed an experimental study to evaluate the effectiveness of an intervention designed to reduce dipyridamole use among patients not receiving concomitant warfarin. Dipyridamole is a vasodilator and antiplatelet that was commonly used for a variety of conditions for which there was inadequate support. The intervention consisted of a mailed alert letter containing patient profiles, and was performed within the Wisconsin Medicaid DUR program. The state was divided into four geographic regions, with each region assigned to one of the following study groups: no intervention, alert letters mailed to pharmacies, alert letters mailed to physicians, and alert letters mailed to both physicians and pharmacies. Because of logistical constraints, one region was assigned to the control group, while the remaining three regions were assigned using random allocation. Subjects were followed for six months following the intervention. The proportion of patients in whom dipyridamole was discontinued was compared among study groups. Clustering by region was not accounted for in the analysis.

In patients residing in long-term care facilities, the adjusted odds ratios for discontinuation of therapy (with 95% confidence intervals) compared with the control group were: pharmacy only: 0.92 (0.55–1.55); physician only: 1.31 (0.83–2.08); pharmacy+physician: 2.10 (1.63–3.68). In ambulatory care patients, the corresponding odds ratios were: pharmacy only: 1.67 (0.89–3.14); physician only: 2.22 (1.16–4.24); pharmacy+physician: 3.81 (2.10–6.93). Predictably, the magnitude of effect appears highest in the group in which both the physician and pharmacist received the intervention, followed by the physician-only and pharmacist-only groups, in that order.

The difference between the physician+pharmacist group and the physician-only group was not statistically significant. In contrast, the difference between the physician+pharmacist group and the pharmacist-only group was statistically significant. Together, these data support the hypothesis that letters sent to physicians had a greater effect than those sent to pharmacists. In summary, these data provide some support for the hypothesis that alert letters to physicians were effective in reducing the chronic use of a possibly ineffective medication. However, the true precision of the effect measures (as measured by the width of the 95% confidence intervals) may be less than that reported in the paper.

Sleath et al.[95] conducted a randomized trial to determine whether sending intervention materials to both pharmacies and physicians was more effective than sending them only to physicians. However, because the authors reported only pre–post comparisons within each group, and did not include any between-group comparisons of pre–post differences, the study is difficult to interpret. Farris et al.[96] studied the effectiveness of a DUR intervention designed to reduce the use of broad-spectrum antibiotics and first-line use of nonsedating antihistamines in a health maintenance organization (HMO). The intervention group consisted of physicians at two family practice clinics, and two control groups were assembled from the remaining pool of physicians within the HMO. However, because this study included only three experimental units, and there appeared to be substantial differences in baseline characteristics among the three, the study results are difficult to interpret.

Smith et al.[97] conducted a randomized trial to measure the effect of an intervention aimed at reducing the use of five benzodiazepines for which the only US Food and Drug Administration approved indication was insomnia. This drug use audit was conducted as part of the Washington State Medicaid DUR program, and focused on those who had received one of the target medications at a dose of at least one tablet per day for at least one year. Thus, the DUR program targeted patients whose treatment was well outside of published guidelines.[98,99] The intervention consisted of a mailed alert letter to the prescriber that contained guidelines on sedative–hypnotic use, the claims profiles of patients treated by that prescriber, and physician-specific measures of sedative hypnotic prescribing. Contamination of the control group by exposure to the intervention was avoided by randomizing physicians rather than individual patients. The effect of clustering on inferential statistics was eliminated by including in the analysis only one randomly selected patient per physician. The amount of sedative–hypnotic drug dispensed in the three-month post-intervention period was the outcome measure of interest.

Patients in the intervention group reduced their use of target drugs by 28%, while those in the control group reduced their use by 8%, a difference that was statistically significant. The study results also suggested that some undesirable use of non-targeted sleep agents may have resulted. In addition, despite advice to the contrary, some prescribers appeared to have immediately discontinued sedative–hypnotic medications, potentially placing patients at risk of withdrawal. As well, anecdotal responses from physicians in the intervention group suggested that, despite the investigators' attempt to use well-accepted criteria to identify a group of patients for whom therapy was clearly inappropriate, even careful discontinuation of sedative–hypnotic therapy may not have been in the best interest of some medically complicated patients. That is, despite great care in developing apparently clear-cut criteria, they may not have been valid, as defined above. Thus, this study provides strong evidence that a DUR program that identifies patients on long-term therapy can have a moderate effect on prescribing and dispensing for the identified patient. It also points to the possibility that even carefully chosen criteria can have appropriate exceptions, and that unintended responses to alerts are possible.

Raisch and Sleath[100] performed an experimental trial to measure the effectiveness of an intervention designed to reduce inappropriate prescription of anti-ulcer drugs, including H2RAs in the New Mexico Medicaid DUR program. The intervention consisted of a mailed alert letter containing a fact sheet on prescription of anti-ulcer agents, and patient profiles. Contamination was avoided by excluding patients who were seen by physicians in both study groups. Dispensing of anti-ulcer agents in the three-month post-intervention period was measured.

Forty-three percent of patients in the intervention group had no exceptions to anti-ulcer criteria in the follow-up period, compared to 28% in the control group (unadjusted odds ratio for the desired outcome = 1.98, 95% confidence interval, 1.23–3.18). Anti-ulcer agents were not dispensed during the follow-up period for 33% of intervention patients and 18% of control patients (odds ratio = 2.29, 95%

confidence interval, 1.35–3.87). Clustering of patients within physician practice was not accounted for in the analysis, which may have spuriously reduced confidence interval widths. Regardless, this study provides relatively strong evidence that a DUR program using mailed alert letters can have a moderate effect on prescribing of chronically administered medications for patients identified in the alert letters.

A report by Abt Associates Inc.[27] presented results from four studies that evaluated the hypothesis that alert letters sent to prescribers can affect the drug therapy of patients identified in alert letters. According to the report, the results suggested that patient-specific DUR intervention letters sent to prescribers were effective in: (i) increasing the prescription of misoprostil to patients receiving nonsteroidal anti-inflammatory agents; (ii) increasing the use of short-acting bronchodilators in patients receiving salmeterol (a long-acting β-agonist bronchodilator); and (iii) reducing long-term therapy with acute-dose ranitidine. However, these studies have not been published in peer-reviewed journals, and the final report does not present sufficient detail of the methods and results to enable a critical evaluation of these studies.

In summary, the available evidence indicates that alert letters containing patient-specific profiles mailed to physicians may have a small but measurable effect on prescribing practices for the patient identified in the alert. There is some evidence suggesting that sending a similar letter to the pharmacy of record augments the effect of the letter to the prescriber, but this evidence is equivocal. Many published outpatient DUR efforts have focused on cost rather than quality issues. Failure to account for clustering in the analysis of studies with clustered treatment assignment is common, and results in spuriously narrow confidence intervals. Publication of original research findings in peer-reviewed journals should be encouraged by those who fund policy research.

EVIDENCE FOR THE EFFECTIVENESS OF OUTPATIENT RETROSPECTIVE DUR PROGRAMS TO CHANGE DRUG THERAPY IN PATIENTS NOT IDENTIFIED IN ALERTS ("SPILLOVER" EFFECTS)

Three studies described in the report by Abt Associates[27] evaluated the hypothesis that DUR intervention letters can affect prescribing for patients other than those who were identified in alert letters. The report concluded that there was no evidence of spillover effects of an intervention designed to increase the prescription of misoprostil in patients receiving nonsteroidal anti-inflammatory agents, or in an intervention designed to increase prescription of short-acting bronchodilators in patients receiving salmeterol. In contrast, the report found evidence suggestive of a spillover effect of an intervention designed to reduce long-term therapy with acute-dose ranitidine. Because of the absence of baseline information on patients included in this analysis, the authors acknowledge that caution is needed in the interpretation of their results.

Hennessy *et al.* conducted an ecologic analysis that examined the frequency of DUR exceptions in six Medicaid programs, as a function of implementation of retrospective DUR programs in those states.[28] The six Medicaid programs varied by size and geography, but all used the same software for their DUR programs, and all used alert letters to the physician as the primary way of communicating alerts. The frequency of exceptions in the Medicaid populations did not appear to decline following DUR implementation, as would be expected if there were an important spillover effect of DUR intervention letters. This finding argues against an important spillover effect of the retrospective DUR programs studied. As described below, this study also examined effects on clinical outcomes.

EVIDENCE FOR THE EFFECTIVENESS OF OUTPATIENT RETROSPECTIVE DUR PROGRAMS IN IMPROVING CLINICAL OUTCOMES

Jay *et al.*[101] conducted a controlled trial of the effectiveness of the California Medicaid DUR program. The DUR program can be considered conventional, as it used a typical structure (expert review of computer-identified exceptions, leading to mailed alert letters to physicians and pharmacists), and examined typical DUR criteria. The study compared two counties that implemented the same retrospective DUR to two counties that did not, over a 24-month pre-intervention period and a 12-month post-intervention period. It examined trends in indices of health services use such as hospital admissions, physician visits, and drug expenditures in the Medicaid population. The study did not examine the program's effectiveness in altering prescribing. The investigators observed no materially important or statistically significant changes in health services use attributable to the program, suggesting that the California program may have been ineffective in improving clinical outcomes. The results of this study have also not been reported in the peer-reviewed literature. Given that the study was performed within a single state, and examined the program's effect in the overall population rather than in any of the specific subgroups of the population that were most likely to benefit (such as those identified in an exception or those at highest risk of

hospitalization), it seems likely that the results can exclude the existence of only large effects. In addition, the investigators cite a number of weaknesses of the DUR program (such as the unavailability of diagnosis data, the small proportion of exceptions that resulted in alerts, and the inability to identify prescribers in about one-fourth of exceptions) that also may have contributed to the absence of demonstrable effect.

The previously described study by Zimmerman *et al.*[92] of a DUR intervention designed to reduce overuse of histamine-2 receptor antagonists (H2RAs) also looked for an increase in the rate of hospitalization for gastrointestinal ulcer or bleeding, which might occur if the intervention resulted in the discontinuation of H2RAs in patients who actually needed them. The investigators did not detect an effect of the DUR intervention on GI hospitalizations, although the study was large enough only to detect very large effects. Thus, this study provides some evidence that a DUR intervention that aimed to reduce H2RA use did not greatly increase the occurrence of serious gastrointestinal ulcer and bleeding.

Hennessy *et al.* performed an observational study comparing clinical outcomes in patients with exceptions before versus after DUR implementation in three Medicaid DUR programs.[28] After adjusting for a wide array of potential confounding factors, they found no evidence that retrospective DUR reduced all-cause hospitalization or cause-specific hospitalization for diagnoses specifically related to the criteria being studied (warfarin + gastrointestinal acid/peptic disorders; warfarin + aspirin; nonsteroidal anti-inflammatory drug (NSAID) + NSAID; beta-agonist + angina pectoris). These findings argue against a meaningful clinical effect of DUR programs among patients with exceptions, although the study does not exclude the possibility of an effect in patients for whom an alert was actually issued.

EVIDENCE FOR THE EFFECTIVENESS OF OUTPATIENT PROSPECTIVE DUR PROGRAMS IN CHANGING DRUG THERAPY AND IMPROVING CLINICAL OUTCOMES

Chrischilles *et al.*[27,102] performed a randomized trial to evaluate the effectiveness of an online prospective drug utilization review program. The results of this trial have not appeared in the peer-reviewed literature. The study was conducted within the Iowa Medicaid program, and recruited pharmacies through newsletters, recruitment letters, and articles in the state pharmacy association journal. Eligible pharmacies were grouped into clusters based on shared prescribers in order to reduce contamination of study groups. Clusters were randomized to intervention or control status.

Pharmacies in the intervention group received online, point-of-service DUR messages that resulted from computerized reviews of prescription medication (but not diagnosis) data. Pharmacies in the control group received no online messages, but still could have received alerts from in-pharmacy computer systems. Pharmacies in both groups documented nondispensing activities such as patient counseling (i.e., "cognitive services") performed for Medicaid beneficiaries.

The rate of nondispensing activities was not statistically different between groups. The investigators also evaluated the effect of the intervention on: (i) use of health care services; (ii) use and cost of prescription drugs; (iii) occurrence of subsequent exceptions; and (iv) occurrence of adverse events related to use of angiotensin converting enzyme inhibitors, antidepressants, antipsychotics, benzodiazepines, calcium channel blockers, digoxin, and nonsteroidal anti-inflammatory drugs. They found no consistent evidence that the intervention had an effect on any of these measures.

Thus, the available data do not appear to support the hypothesis that providing pharmacists with computerized DUR messages based on patients' overall prescription profile impacts drug therapy or clinical outcomes versus in-pharmacy messages. It remains possible that a system that uses diagnosis data derived from medical claims to identify drug–disease interactions and omitted-but-necessary therapy might have a demonstrable effect, although this hypothesis needs to be evaluated empirically.

Monane *et al.*[103] evaluated a prospective DUR program performed by 13 mail order pharmacies owned by a pharmaceutical benefit management company. The DUR program identified prescriptions that were presented for elderly patients that violated one of 11 prespecified clinical criteria, such as use of long-acting benzodiazepines in the elderly, excessive dose of short-acting benzodiazepines, or use of a nonsteroidal anti-inflammatory drug in a patient with prescriptions for drugs used for peptic ulcer disease. The intervention consisted of attempted telephone contact of the prescriber, with a pharmacist-initiated discussion of therapeutic alternatives. Pharmacists performing the telephone intervention successfully contacted the prescriber in 56% of cases and were successful in persuading the prescriber to change the target prescription in 8% of all cases. However, the "DUR change rate" of 24% presented in the paper is overly optimistic, since it: (i) includes as successes cases in which the prescriber did not change the prescription, but rather stated an intention to review the patient's therapy at the next visit; and (ii) included in the denominator only cases in which the physician was successfully contacted, rather than all attempted contacts. Because no concurrent control group was studied, it is not known how many

prescriptions would have been intervened upon by pharmacists in the normal course of pharmacy practice, and how many of the physicians would have stopped the therapy on their own.[104] Therefore, the degree to which this program represents an incremental benefit over standard pharmacy practice is unknown.

SUMMARIZING THE EVIDENCE

Retrospective and prospective DUR are both mandated in the US for Medicaid programs, and are widely employed outside of Medicaid. Although there is evidence that some forms of retrospective DUR can have a modest impact on prescribing, there is no evidence that it achieves its primary objective of improving clinical outcomes, and some evidence that it does not. Further, there is some evidence suggesting that even thoughtfully considered and well-intentioned interventions aimed at improving care might have unintended consequences that need to be uncovered through rigorous research. Prospective DUR, while intuitively appealing, lacks evidence that it provides an incremental benefit over standard pharmacy practice. Although the conduct of rigorous research in this area is challenging, continued support for these programs as a means to improve clinical care should be based on empiric evidence. More than three decades after outpatient DUR programs were first proposed, the only available evidence suggests the absence of an observable effect on clinical outcomes.

There are a number of plausible explanations for the apparent lack of effect of DUR programs as currently implemented. One is the unknown validity of many DUR criteria. For example, most information about drug–drug interactions comes from either case reports or controlled studies of effects on serum drug concentrations—a surrogate endpoint. Both types of evidence have limited utility for inferring causal effects on clinical outcomes; as a result, there is a striking amount of disagreement among standard drug interaction references regarding which drug combinations need to be avoided. A second plausible explanation is that systems that provide too many alerts (especially those that are perceived to be baseless or clinically unimportant) result in user fatigue and disregard of alerts, and thus reduce effectiveness of the systems. There is evidence for this in the setting of prospective DUR.[31]

THE FUTURE

There is now a reasonable body of research suggesting that outpatient prospective and retrospective DUR programs have not produced a large or even measurable improvement in clinical outcomes on a population basis. However, unless there is a change in US Federal legislation, DUR will continue to be used in Medicaid programs. Given the increasing use of CPOE programs that permit the incorporation of computerized decision support (including prospective DUR with alerts presented to the prescriber at the time of prescribing), we should expect the use of CPOE-based DUR to grow. However, given that major perceived flaws of existing DUR programs include criteria with questionable validity and alert rates that are unacceptably high, it would be naïve to expect that applying standard criterion sets to CPOE-based DUR would improve clinical outcomes. Indeed, prescribers are unlikely to be any more tolerant of apparently invalid alerts presented with high frequency than are pharmacists.

It remains unclear what, if any, the proper role for letter-based DUR should be in an environment in which CPOE-based DUR is available. We believe that those implementing CPOE-based DUR should use a slow, incremental approach to building a criterion set, starting with apparently unambiguous criteria such as absolutely contraindicated therapies (e.g., drugs contraindicated in pregnant women). Although exceptions to such criteria will hopefully be rare, a high frequency of exceptions should not be a goal. The effects of implementing specific criteria should be measured on appropriate endpoints. As well, the knowledge base underlying potential criteria needs to be strengthened before they are implemented. For example, most information about drug–drug interactions takes the form of case reports or drug concentrations. The utility of both of these types of information for inferring causal effects on clinical outcomes is limited. We also need research into the best way to communicate alerts.

The clinical and economic costs of suboptimal medication use are enormous, which is why DUR programs were first envisioned and implemented. We look forward to the development and testing of even more creative approaches to this important program in the years to come.

REFERENCES

1. Soumerai SB, Lipton HL. Computer-based drug-utilization review—risk, benefit, or boondoggle? *N Engl J Med* 1995; **332**: 1641–5.
2. Lesshafft Jr CT. Ambulatory patient care. In: Osol A, Chase G, Gennaro AR, Gibson MR, Granberg CB, Harvey SC *et al.*, eds, *Remington's Pharmaceutical Sciences*. Easton, PA: Mack, 1980; pp. 1631–40.
3. Lipton HL, Bird JA. Drug utilization review in ambulatory settings: state of the science and directions for outcomes research. *Med Care* 1993; **31**: 1069–82.
4. Richards MJ, Robertson MB, Dartnell JG, Duarte MM, Jones NR, Kerr DA *et al.* Impact of a web-based antimicrobial approval system on broad-spectrum cephalosporin use at a teaching hospital. *Med J Aust* 2003; **178**: 386–90.
5. Rogers JE, Wroe CJ, Roberts A, Swallow A, Stables D, Cantrill JA *et al.* Automated quality checks on repeat prescribing. *Br J Gen Pract* 2003; **53**: 838–44.
6. Sondergaard J, Andersen M, Stovring H, Kragstrup J. Mailed prescriber feedback in addition to a clinical guideline has no impact: a randomised, controlled trial. *Scand J Prim Health Care* 2003; **21**: 47–51.
7. Kralewski J, Wertheimer A, Ratner E. Prescription drug utilization review in the private sector. *Health Care Manage Rev* 1994; **19**: 62–71.
8. *Approaches to Drug Insurance Design: Background Papers by the Task Force on Prescription Drugs*. Washington, DC: US Government Printing Office, 1969.
9. *Final Report of the Task Force on Prescription Drugs*. Washington, DC: US Government Printing Office, 1969.
10. Baylis RD. Drug utilization review: a description of use for a Medicaid population (Maryland) 1986–1994. *J Law Med Ethics* 1994; **22**: 247–51.
11. Knoben JE. Drug use review. In: McLeod DC, Miller WA, eds, *The Practice of Pharmacy: Institutional and Ambulatory Pharmaceutical Services*, 1st edn. Cincinnati, OH: Harvey Whitney Books, 1981; pp. 83–93.
12. Silverman M, Lydecker M. *Drug Coverage Under National Health Insurance: Policy Options*. DHEW publication no. (HRA) 77-3189. US Department of Health, Education, and Welfare, 1977.
13. Brodie DC. Drug utilization review-planning. *Hospitals* 1972; **46**: 103–12.
14. Ebel JA. Drug utilization review—selective surveillance. *Hospitals* 1972; **46**: 108–14.
15. Pierpaoli PG, Bowman GK. Drug utilization review/implementation. *Hospitals* 1972; **46**: 95–104.
16. Rucker TD. The role of computers in drug utilization review. *Am J Hosp Pharm* 1972; **29**: 128–34.
17. *Medicare Catastrophic Coverage Act of 1988*. Public Law 100–360, 1988.
18. *Medicare Catastrophic Coverage Repeal Act of 1989*. Public Law 101-234, 1989.
19. *Omnibus Budget Reconcilliation Act of 1990*. Public Law 101-508, 1990.
20. *Primer on Drug Use Review*. 5-7-1992. Pharmaceutical Manufacturers Association/American Medical Association/American Pharmaceutical Association.
21. Erwin WG. The definition of drug utilization review: statement of issues. *Clin Pharmacol Ther* 1991; **50**: 596–9.
22. Hennessy S, Strom BL. Issues in hospital-based drug use evaluation. *P&T* 1992; **17**: 733–54.
23. Moore WJ. Medicaid drug utilization review: a critical appraisal. *Med Care Rev* 1994; **51**: 1–37.

24. Beta-Blocker Heart Attack Research Group. A randomized trial of propranolol in patients with acute myocardial infarction. I. Mortality results. *JAMA* 1982; **247**: 1707–14.

25. Lau J, Antman EM, Jimenez-Silva J, Kupelnick B, Mosteller F, Chalmers TC. Cumulative meta-analysis of therapeutic trials for myocardial infarction. *N Engl J Med* 1992; **327**: 248–54.

26. The Norwegian Multicenter Study. Timolol-induced reduction in mortality and reinfarction in patients surviving acute myocardial infarction. *N Engl J Med* 1981; **304**: 801–7.

27. Abt Associates. *Evaluation of Drug Use Review Demonstration Projects: Final Report*, October 28, 1998. Cambridge, MA: Abt Associates, 1998.

28. Hennessy S, Bilker WB, Zhou L, Weber AL, Brensinger C, Wang Y *et al*. Retrospective drug utilization review, prescribing errors, and clinical outcomes. *JAMA* 2003; **290**: 1494–9.

29. Avorn J, Soumerai SB. Use of a computer-based Medicaid drug data to analyze and correct inappropriate medication use. *J Med Syst* 1982; **6**: 377–86.

30. Avorn J, Soumerai SB. Improving drug-therapy decisions through educational outreach. A randomized controlled trial of academically based "detailing." *N Engl J Med* 1983; **308**: 1457–63.

31. Chui MA, Rupp MT. Evaluation of online prospective DUR programs in community pharmacy practice. *J Manag Care Pharm* 2000; **6**: 27–32.

32. Soumerai SB, Avorn J. Efficacy and cost-containment in hospital pharmacotherapy: state of the art and future directions. *Milbank Mem Fund Q Health Soc* 1984; **62**: 447–74.

33. Aseffa A, Desta Z, Tadesse I. Prescribing pattern of antibacterial drugs in a teaching hospital in Gondar, Ethiopia. *East Afr Med J* 1995; **72**: 56–9.

34. Ashkenazi S, Samra Z, Konisberger H, Drucker MM, Leibovici L. Factors associated with increased risk in inappropriate empiric antibiotic treatment of childhood bacteraemia. *Eur J Pediatr* 1996; **155**: 545–50.

35. Beidas S, Khamesian M. Vancomycin use in a university medical center: comparison with hospital infection control practices advisory committee guidelines [letter]. *Infect Control Hosp Epidemiol* 1996; **17**: 773–4.

36. Belliveau PP, Rothman AL, Maday CE. Limiting vancomycin use to combat vancomycin-resistant *Enterococcus faecium*. *Am J Health Syst Pharm* 1996; **53**: 1570–5.

37. Cira LM, Briceland LL, Lesar TS. Pitfalls of using antimicrobial order forms to evaluate drug use [letter]. *Am J Hosp Pharm* 1970; **51**: 700.

38. DesHarnais S, Simpson KN, Paul JE. Variations in practice patterns: antiviral drug use in hospitalized patients with herpes infections. *Am J Med Qual* 1996; **11**: 33–42.

39. Evans ME, Kortas KJ. Vancomycin use in a university medical center: comparison with hospital infection control practices advisory committee guidelines. *Infect Control Hosp Epidemiol* 1996; **17**: 356–9.

40. Fonseca SN, Ehrenkranz RA, Baltimore RS. Epidemiology of antibiotic use in a neonatal intensive care unit. *Infect Control Hosp Epidemiol* 1994; **15**: 156–62.

41. Fraser GL, Stogsdill P, Dickens JD Jr, Wennberg DE, Smith RP Jr, Prato BS *et al*. Antibiotic optimization. An evaluation of patient safety and economic outcomes. *Arch Intern Med* 1997; **157**: 1689–94.

42. Goeckner BJ, Hendershot E, Scott K, Drake M. A vancomycin monitoring program at a community hospital. *Jt Comm J Qual Improv* 1998; **24**: 379–85.

43. Gutierrez F, Wall P, Cohen J. An analysis of the trends in the use of antifungal drugs and fungal isolates in a UK university hospital [letter]. *J Hosp Infect* 1995; **31**: 149–52.

44. Harbarth S, Pittet D, Gabriel V, Garbino J, Lew D. Cefepime—assessment of its need at a tertiary care center. *J Clin Pharm Ther* 1998; **23**: 11–17.

45. Janknegt R, Wijnands WJ, Caprasse M, Brandenburg W, Schuitenmaker MG, Stobberingh E. Antimicrobial drug use in hospitals in The Netherlands, Germany and Belgium. *Eur J Clin Microbiol Infect Dis* 1993; **12**: 832–8.

46. Jozefiak ET, Lewicki JE, Kozinn WP. Computer-assisted antimicrobial surveillance in a community teaching hospital. *Am J Health Syst Pharm* 1995; **52**: 1536–40.

47. Lee KR, Leggiadro RJ, Burch KJ. Drug use evaluation of antibiotics in a pediatric teaching hospital. *Infect Control Hosp Epidemiol* 1994; **15**: 710–12.

48. LeMire M, Wing L, Gordon DL. An audit of third generation cephalosporin prescribing in a tertiary care hospital. *Aust N Z J Med* 1996; **26**: 386–90.

49. Logsdon BA, Lee KR, Luedtke G, Barrett FF. Evaluation of vancomycin use in a pediatric teaching hospital based on CDC criteria. *Infect Control Hosp Epidemiol* 1997; **18**: 780–2.

50. Natsch S, Conrad C, Hartmeier C, Schmid B. Use of amoxicillin-clavulanate and resistance in *Escherichia coli* over a 4-year period. *Infect Control Hosp Epidemiol* 1998; **19**: 653–6.

51. Rahal JJ, Urban C, Horn D, Freeman K, Segal-Maurer S, Maurer J *et al*. Class restriction of cephalosporin use to control total cephalosporin resistance in nosocomial Klebsiella. *Chest* 1998; **280**: 1233–7.

52. Redding PJ, Taylor A, Smith AM. Audit of parenteral antimicrobial agents and infusion fluids. *Health Bull (Edinb)* 1995; **53**: 110–14.

53. Rovers JP, Bjornson DC. Assessment of methods and outcomes: using modified inpatient ciprofloxacin criteria in community-based drug use evaluation. *Ann Pharmacother* 1994; **28**: 714–19.

54. Singer MV, Haft R, Barlam T, Aronson M, Shafer A, Sands KE. Vancomycin control measures at a tertiary-care hospital: impact of interventions on volume and patterns of use. *Infect Control Hosp Epidemiol* 1998; **19**: 248–53.

55. Soto J. Strategies for rationing the use of antibiotics in hospitals. *Enferm Infecc Microbiol Clin* 1996; **14**: 576–7 (in Spanish).

56. Speirs GE, Fenelon LE, Reeves DS, Speller DC, Smyth EG, Wilcox MH *et al*. An audit of ciprofloxacin use in a district general hospital. *J Antimicrob Chemother* 1995; **36**: 201–7.

57. Thomas M, Govil S, Moses BV, Joseph A. Monitoring of antibiotic use in a primary and tertiary care hospital. *J Clin Epidemiol* 1996; **49**: 251–4.

58. van der Hoek W. Prescription audit for antibiotics in a district hospital (letter). *Trop Doct* 1994; **24**: 85–6.

59. Wright SW, Wrenn KD. Appropriateness of vancomycin use in the emergency department. *Ann Emerg Med* 1998; **32**: 531–6.

60. Zadik PM, Moore AP. Antimicrobial associations of an outbreak of diarrhoea due to *Clostridium difficile*. *J Hosp Infect* 1998; **39**: 189–93.

61. Zaran FK, Weingarten CM, Rybak MJ, Stevenson JG. Effect of constructive feedback on pharmacist handling of orders for monitored antimicrobials. *Am J Health Syst Pharm* 1996; **53**: 2196–8.

62. Dasta JF, Fuhrman TM, McCandles C. Patterns of prescribing and administering drugs for agitation and pain in patients in a surgical intensive care unit. *Crit Care Med* 1994; **22**: 974–80.

63. Dasta JF, Fuhrman TM, McCandles C. Use of sedatives and analgesics in a surgical intensive care unit: a follow-up and commentary. *Heart Lung* 1995; **24**: 76–8.

64. Friedland LR, Kulick RM. Emergency department analgesic use in pediatric trauma victims with fractures. *Ann Emerg Med* 1994; **23**: 203–7.

65. Tholl DA, Wager MS, Sajous CH, Myers TF. Morphine use and adverse effects in a neonatal intensive care unit. *Am J Hosp Pharm* 1994; **51**: 2801–3.

66. Turner R, Clark J, Root T, McElligott L, Hardy J. An audit of morphine prescribing in a specialist cancer hospital. *Palliat Med* 1994; **8**: 5–10.

67. Woolard DJ, Terndrup TE. Sedative–analgesic agent administration in children: analysis of use and complications in the emergency department. *J Emerg Med* 1994; **12**: 453–61.

68. Zisselman MH, Rovner BW, Kelly KG, Woods C. Benzodiazepine utilization in a university hospital. *Am J Med Qual* 1994; **9**: 138–41.

69. Alran C, Damase-Michel C, Celotto N, Durand MC, Montastruc JL. Consumption of benzodiazepines in a French university hospital between 1980 and 1991. *Fundam Clin Pharmacol* 1993; **7**: 319–23.

70. Stone P, Phillips C, Spruyt O, Waight C. A comparison of the use of sedatives in a hospital support team and in a hospice. *Palliat Med* 1997; **11**: 140–4.

71. Yuen EJ, Zisselman MH, Louis DZ, Rovner BW. Sedative–hypnotic use by the elderly: effects on hospital length of stay and costs. *J Ment Health Adm* 1997; **24**: 90–7.

72. Wyncoll DL, Roberts PC, Beale RJ, McLuckie A. H2 blockers in the intensive care unit: ignoring the evidence? Telephone survey. *BMJ* 1997; **314**: 1013.

73. Barnhart MR. Effect of physician education on omeprazole use at a small public hospital [letter]. *Am J Health Syst Pharm* 1336; **53**: 1334.

74. Brandhagen DJ, Pheley AM, Onstad GR, Freeman ML, Lurie N. Omeprazole use at an urban county teaching hospital. *J Gen Intern Med* 1995; **10**: 513–15.

75. Segal R, Russell WL, Oh T, Ben-Joseph R. Use of i.v. cimetidine, ranitidine, and famotidine in 40 hospitals. *Am J Hosp Pharm* 1993; **50**: 2077–81.

76. John JFJ, Fishman NO. Programmatic role of the infectious diseases physician in controlling antimicrobial costs in the hospital. *Clin Infect Dis* 1997; **24**: 471–85.

77. Lipton HL. Pharmacy benefit management companies: dimensions of performance. *Annu Rev Public Health* 1999; **20**: 361–401.

78. Donner A, Brown KS, Brasher P. A methodological review of non-therapeutic intervention trials employing cluster randomization, 1979–1989. *Int J Epidemiol* 1990; **19**: 795–800.

79. Donner A. Sample size requirements for stratified cluster randomization designs. *Stat Med* 1992; **11**: 743–50.

80. Donner A, Klar N. Confidence interval construction for effect measures arising from cluster randomization trials. *J Clin Epidemiol* 1993; **46**: 123–31.

81. Donner A, Klar N. Methods for comparing event rates in intervention studies when the unit of allocation is a cluster. *Am J Epidemiol* 1994; **140**: 279–89.

82. Kerry SM, Bland JM. The intracluster correlation coefficient in cluster randomisation. *BMJ* 1998; **316**: 1455.

83. Kerry SM, Bland JM. Trials which randomize practices II: sample size. *Fam Pract* 1998; **15**: 84–7.

84. Kerry SM, Bland JM. Trials which randomize practices I: how should they be analysed?. *Fam Pract* 1998; **15**: 80–3.

85. Kerry SM, Bland JM. Sample size in cluster randomisation. *BMJ* 1998; **316**: 549.

86. Kerry SM, Bland JM. Analysis of a trial randomised in clusters. *BMJ* 1998; **316**: 54.

87. Bland JM, Kerry SM. Statistics notes. Trials randomised in clusters. *BMJ* 1997; **315**: 600.

88. Campbell DT, Stanley JC. *Experimental and Quasi-Experimantal Designs for Research*. Boston, MA: Houghton Mifflin, 1966.

89. Cook TD, Campbell DT. *Quasi-Experimentation: Design and Analysis for Field Studies*. Boston, MA: Houghton Mifflin, 1979.

90. Kreling DH, Mott DA. The cost effectiveness of drug utilisation review in an outpatient setting. *Pharmacoeconomics* 1993; **4**: 414–36.

91. Moore WJ, Gutermuth K, Pracht EE. Systemwide effects of Medicaid retrospective drug utilization review programs. *J Health Polit Policy Law* 2000; **25**: 653–88.

92. Zimmerman DR, Collins TM, Lipowski EE, Sainfort F. Evaluation of a DUR intervention: a case study of histamine antagonists. *Inquiry* 1994; **31**: 89–101.

93. Okano GJ, Rascati KL. Effects of Medicaid drug utilization review intervention letters. *Clin Ther* 1995; **17**: 525–33.

94. Collins TM, Mott DA, Bigelow WE, Zimmerman DR. A controlled letter intervention to change prescribing behavior: results of a dual-targeted approach. *Health Serv Res* 1997; **32**: 471–89.

95. Sleath B, Collins T, Kelly HW, McCament-Mann L, Lien T. Effect of including both physicians and pharmacists in an asthma drug-use review intervention. *Am J Health Syst Pharm* 1997; **54**: 2197–200.

96. Farris KB, Kirking DM, Shimp LA, Opdycke RA. Design and results of a group counter-detailing DUR educational program. *Pharm Res* 1996; **13**: 1445–52.

97. Smith DH, Christensen DB, Stergachis A, Holmes G. A randomized controlled trial of a drug use review intervention for sedative hypnotic medications. *Med Care* 1998; **36**: 1013–21.

98. Ashton H. Guidelines for the rational use of benzodiazepines. When and what to use. *Drugs* 1994; **48**: 25–40.

99. Gillin JC. The long and the short of sleeping pills. *N Engl J Med* 1991; **324**: 1735–7.

100. Raisch DW, Sleath BL. Influencing the use of anti-ulcer agents in a Medicaid program through patient-specific prescribing feedback letters. *J Gen Intern Med* 1999; **14**: 145–50.

101. Jay DE, Eynon BP, Javitz HS. *The Medi-Cal Therapeutic Drug Utilization Review Project.* Menio Park, CA: SRI International, 1991.

102. Chrischilles EA. *The Iowa Medicaid OPDUR Demonstration Project Annual Report.* Des Moines, IA: Iowa Department of Human Services, 1997.

103. Monane M, Mathias DM, Nagle BA, Kelly MA. Improving prescribing patterns for the elderly through an online drug utilization review intervention: a system linking the physician, pharmacist, and computer. *JAMA* 1998; **280**: 1249–52.

104. Soumerai SB, Lipton HL. Improving prescribing patterns for the elderly through an online drug utilization review program [letter]. *JAMA* 1999; **281**: 1168–9.

30

Special Methodological Issues in Pharmacoepidemiology Studies of Vaccine Safety

ROBERT T. CHEN[1], ROBERT L. DAVIS[2] and PHILIP H. RHODES[1]

[1] Immunization Safety Branch, National Immunization Program, Centers for Disease Control and Prevention, Atlanta, Georgia, USA; [2] Associate Professor, Pediatrics and Epidemiology, University of Washington, Seattle, Washington, USA.

INTRODUCTION

Vaccines are among the most cost-effective and prevalent public health interventions.[1,2] Where immunizations are widely practiced, morbidity and mortality attributable to vaccine-preventable diseases have declined considerably.[3] No vaccine is perfectly safe or effective, however.[4] With high rates of vaccinations and a low incidence of vaccine-preventable diseases, adverse events after immunizations are understandably of concern, and have received increasing attention from the medical community and the public.[5-8] Unfortunately, this concern has often affected the stability of immunization programs.

For example, widespread publicity raising questions about the safety of pertussis vaccine in Japan and elsewhere during the 1970s led to fewer pertussis vaccinations, which were followed by epidemics of pertussis.[9] Similar concerns in the United States during the early 1980s led to an outbreak of lawsuits, substantial increases in the price of vaccines, the loss of vaccine manufacturers,[10] and the potential deterrent to the development of new vaccines.[11] More recently, concerns about the safety of mercury-based thimerosal preservative used in vaccines[12,13] and the safety of anthrax[14] and smallpox vaccines[15,16] have impacted on the stability of civilian and military immunization programs in the United States, respectively. Similarly, the pubic acceptance of measles–mumps–rubella (MMR) vaccine in the United Kingdom[17] and hepatitis B vaccine in France have been affected by safety concerns.[18]

As noted in an extensive review of vaccine safety in the early 1990s by the Institute of Medicine (IOM) in the United States,[19,20] however, knowledge and research capacity has been limited by: (i) inadequate understanding of biologic mechanisms underlying adverse events; (ii) insufficient or

Pharmacoepidemiology, Fourth Edition   Edited by B.L. Strom
© 2005 John Wiley & Sons, Ltd

inconsistent information from case reports and case series; (iii) inadequate size or length of follow-up of many population-based epidemiologic studies; (iv) limitations of existing surveillance systems to provide persuasive evidence of causation; and (v) few experimental studies published relative to the total number of epidemiologic studies published. The IOM concluded, "if research capacity and accomplishments (are) not improved, future reviews of vaccine safety (will be) similarly handicapped."

In ensuing attempts to overcome these gaps and limitations, epidemiology has been vital in providing the scientific methodology for assessing the safety of vaccines.[21,22] Many research and knowledge gaps continue to be identified in each IOM review of specific immunization safety controversies since 2001, ranging from autism to unexpected infant deaths.[14,23–29] In this chapter, we discuss the major differences between vaccines and other pharmaceutical products in how epidemiology is applied, with respect to both policy and methodology.

CLINICAL PROBLEMS TO BE ADDRESSED USING PHARMACOEPIDEMIOLOGIC RESEARCH

POLICY ISSUES

Vaccines share many characteristics with other pharmaceuticals, such as their phased development and licensure, but differ fundamentally in many ways. Understanding these differences is important in appreciating the policy context of vaccine safety and the possible role of pharmacoepidemiology. Vaccines, for example, are biological products that are inherently more complex than most (physico-chemical) drugs in terms of both constituent components and the production process.[30,31] Each component of the vaccine formulation—the immunogen, preservative, adjuvant, stabilizer, diluent, and other excipients—has its respective safety considerations (e.g., sourcing, production, quality assurance, safety profile), individually as well as combined.[32] The safety of injection can also be a concern, especially in developing countries.[33,34]

A higher standard of safety is also expected of vaccines. In contrast to pharmaceuticals, most of which are administered to ill persons for curative purposes, vaccines are generally given to healthy persons to prevent disease. In the public's eye, tolerance of adverse reactions to products given to healthy persons—especially healthy babies—is substantially lower than to products administered to persons who are already sick. This lower risk tolerance for vaccines

translates into a need to investigate the possible causes of much rarer adverse events following vaccinations than would be acceptable for other pharmaceuticals. Events that occur at ~$1/10^5$–$1/10^6$ doses, such as acute encephalopathy after whole cell pertussis vaccine,[19,35] Guillain–Barré syndrome (GBS) after swine influenza vaccine,[36] and oral polio vaccine-associated paralytic polio (VAPP),[37] are of concern for vaccines. In contrast, side effects are essentially universal for cancer chemotherapy and gastrointestinal side effects are very common (10–30%) among persons on high dose aspirin therapy.[38]

The cost and the difficulty of studying events increase with their rarity, however (see Chapter 3). Furthermore, the ability to provide definitive conclusions from epidemiologic studies of rare events is poor. Attributable risks on the order of $1/10^5$–$1/10^6$ are on the margin of resolution for epidemiologic methods.[19,39] Perhaps not surprisingly, but adding to the confusion, the bulk of the published literature to date on vaccine safety has been in the form of case reports and case series, rather than controlled studies with adequate power.[19,20] As an example of how difficult it is to study extremely rare events following vaccination, the UK organized a very large case–control study in an attempt to assess the possible association between pertussis vaccination and encephalopathy.[40] Enrolled in the study were all children 2 to 35 months of age in England, Scotland, and Wales hospitalized for a variety of neurological illnesses during a 36-month period ($N=1167$). The finding of a significant association between vaccine and permanent brain damage was based on only seven exposed cases;[35] the validity of this study finding generated much controversy in and out of the courts.[19,41]

Despite considerably more robust data linking GBS with the swine influenza vaccine,[36] subsequent controversy[42,43] resulted in a court-ordered independent re-examination of the data[44] and ultimately partial redo of the study confirming the initial findings.[45] Robust results of recent studies on rhesus rotavirus vaccine and intussusception[46,47] have also been challenged,[48,49] despite evidence to the contrary.[50] Even when two independent large controlled studies showed that the relative risk of intussusception exceeded 30 after the first dose of the rhesus rotavirus vaccine (RRV),[46,47] some have argued this finding was an artifact of "triggering" based on uncontrolled ecologic evidence,[48,49] despite evidence to the contrary.[50]

A higher standard of safety is also required for vaccines because of the large number of persons who are exposed, some of whom are compelled to do so by law or regulation for public health reasons.[51] Such requirements were implemented by public health authorities because vaccine-preventable diseases are generally highly infectious (e.g., measles, pertussis). Vaccinations protect individual vaccinees and may also confer protection indirectly to other susceptible persons in the population, by limiting the spread of disease organisms (so-called *herd immunity*).[52] Without such mandates, a "tragedy of the commons" may occur where high vaccine coverage is reached and the individual risk/benefit ratio becomes less than the societal risk/benefit ratio.[53,54] Persons may attempt to avoid the risks of vaccination while being protected by the herd immunity resulting from others being vaccinated. However, this commons provided by herd immunity may disappear if too many persons avoid vaccination, with the resulting tragedy that outbreaks return. A similar policy consideration occurs for some mandatory military vaccinations like anthrax[14] and smallpox,[15,16] where a higher vaccine reaction rate may be accepted in exchange for battlefield readiness.

Due to the need for almost universal exposure to many vaccines, the medical maxim "first do no harm" applies even more in public health than in clinical medicine (where decisions affect many fewer persons). Inadequately inactivated polio vaccine was administered to about 400 000 persons in the "Cutter Incident," resulting in 260 polio cases.[55] Other incidents similar in tragedy if not in scope have occurred due to errors in production.[4] Recent concerns that (i) polio vaccine contaminated by simian virus 40 may have been received by millions of persons during the 1950s,[26,56] (ii) some vaccines may have contained gelatin stabilizers produced in cattle infected with bovine spongiform encephalopathy,[57] and (iii) some US children were exposed to high levels of ethyl mercury from thimerosal preservatives in vaccines,[13] further highlight the importance of ensuring the safety of a relatively universal human-directed "exposure" like immunizations. These concerns are the basis for strict regulatory control and other oversight of vaccines by the FDA[30] and the World Health Organization.[58]

Very high standards of accuracy and timeliness are needed because vaccine safety studies have extremely narrow margins for error. Unlike many classes of drugs for which other effective therapy may be substituted, vaccines generally have few alternative strains or types (oral and inactivated poliovirus vaccines being the best known exception). The decision to withdraw a vaccine[42] or switch between strains may also have wide ramifications.[37,59] In 1992, the United Kingdom withdrew the license of mumps vaccines containing the Urabe strain after studies suggested a high rate of vaccine-associated meningitis.[60] The manufacturers subsequently withdrew this product worldwide, leaving those countries where the Urabe strain had been the sole mumps vaccine licensed without an alternative vaccine.[61,62] Safety concerns led more recently to the withdrawal of the only licensed

vaccines against rotavirus[48] and Lyme[63] in the US, rendering these vaccines unavailable anywhere. Establishing associations of adverse events with vaccines and prompt definition of the attributable risk are critical in placing adverse events in the proper risk/benefit perspective. An erroneous association or attributable risk can undermine confidence in a vaccine and have disastrous consequences for vaccine acceptance and disease incidence. On the other hand, denials of association despite accumulating evidence can backfire.[62,64]

Because many vaccinations are mandated for public health reasons and no vaccine is perfectly safe, several countries have established compensation programs for persons who may have been injured by vaccination.[65] Accurate assessment of whether adverse events can be caused by specific vaccines is essential to a fair and efficient vaccine injury compensation program.[66] In the United States, for example, the Vaccine Injury Table contains the vaccines, adverse events, and intervals after which no-fault decisions are made in favor of the claimants.[67] Periodic revisions of the Vaccine Injury Table are necessary to reflect the best scientific information on associations between vaccines and adverse events. Furthermore, because the compensation program reduces the product liability incentive for improving vaccines by manufacturers in the US, this shifts even greater responsibility for vaccine safety monitoring to the government.

Finally, recommendations for use of vaccines represent a dynamic balancing of risks and benefits. Vaccine safety monitoring is necessary to weigh this balance accurately. When diseases are close to eradication, data on complications due to vaccine relative to that of disease may lead to discontinuation or decreased use of the vaccine, as was done in the past with smallpox vaccine[68] and with the shift to either inactivated polio[59,69] or sequential inactivated/live oral polio vaccine schedules.[37] With the renewed fears of bioterrorism, however, stopping immunizations and thereby creating a lacunae in herd immunity no longer seems advisable.[70]

Almost all immunizations will therefore be needed indefinitely, with their attendant adverse reactions and potential for loss of public confidence. Due to the success of immunizations in the near elimination of their target diseases, however, most health providers (let alone parents) will increasingly have not ever seen a case of the wild vaccine-preventable disease. Each future generation will therefore have to be convinced to be immunized based on increasingly ancient experience of wild disease but fear of contemporary vaccine adverse event. A credible and effective immunization safety system (applying pharmacoepidemiologic principles) will therefore be critical to maintaining public confidence in continuing immunizations.

Research in vaccine safety can help to distinguish true vaccine reactions from coincidental events,[19,20] estimate their attributable risk,[35,36,47,71–74] identify risk factors that may permit development of valid contraindications,[35,75] and if the pathophysiologic mechanism becomes known, develop safer vaccines.[76–79] Equally importantly, such research demonstrates a commitment to reducing disease from all causes, vaccine-preventable and vaccine-induced, and may help to maintain public confidence in immunizations and the credibility of immunization programs.

CLINICAL ISSUES

Vaccines, like other pharmaceutical products, undergo extensive safety and efficacy evaluations in the laboratory, in animals, and in phased human clinical trials before licensure.[80] Phase I trials usually number their subjects in the tens and can only detect extremely common adverse events. Phase II trials generally enroll hundreds of subjects. When carefully coordinated, as in the comparative infant diphtheria–tetanus–acellular pertussis (DTaP) trials, important conclusions such as the relationship between concentration of antigen, number of vaccine components, formulation technique, effect of successive doses, and profile of common reactions[81] can be drawn. Such studies can affect the choice of the candidate vaccine chosen for Phase III.[82,83]

Sample sizes for Phase III vaccine trials are generally larger than those for drugs. In the most extreme example, more than 200 000 vaccinees were enrolled in the famous Francis field trial of inactivated Salk poliovirus vaccine.[84] Conjugate *Haemophilus influenzae* type b vaccine trials have enrolled 30 000–50 000 vaccinees.[85,86] Nevertheless, sample sizes for Phase III vaccine trials are principally based on efficacy considerations. Inferences on safety are drawn to the extent possible based on the sample size ($\sim 10^2$–10^5) and the duration of observation (often <30 days).[82] This usually means that observations of the common local and systemic reactions (e.g., injection site swelling, fever, fussiness) have been possible. Due to the experimental randomized, double-blind, placebo-controlled design of clinical trials, inferences on the causal relationship of an adverse event with the vaccine are relatively straightforward.[19,20]

Better standardization of safety evaluations in Phase III trials is needed, however, so that safety data across trials and vaccines can be compared (see also subsection on "Classifications and case definitions"). In the Phase III trials for infant DTaP, a standard case definition was developed for efficacy, but ironically not for safety—the main reason for the development of DTaP.[87] For example, definitions of high fever across trials varied by the temperature (39.5 °C versus

40.5 °C), the mode of measurement (oral versus rectal), and time after vaccination measured (48 versus 72 hours).[88] Major differences in detected rates of hypotonic–hyporesponsive episodes after the same whole cell pertussis vaccine used in the Swedish and Italian trials highlight the difficulty of standardizing assessment of rarer events across cultures and health systems, however.[89] The finding of delayed excess mortality in some recipients of high titer measles vaccine in developing countries,[240] now believed by some to be due to a change in sequence of vaccinations,[91] has also raised difficult questions about design of future vaccine trials.[92,93]

By virtue of vaccines being relatively universal exposures, despite the relative rarity of serious true vaccine reactions, the absolute number of clinically significant vaccine adverse event reports received annually in the US now averages ~15 000 reports. The medical science of how to diagnose, manage, prevent, or treat such adverse events remain at a relatively rudimentary stage, however. The reasons are multifold and the challenges are as much logistical as scientific. Modern medicine cannot make progress on rare disorders like leukemia (or serious vaccine adverse events) by relying on primary care providers alone. Instead, subspecialties with adequate referral base and research funds (e.g., hematology/oncology) are needed. With the exception of certain regions in Italy[94] and Australia,[95,96] a similar well-organized, well-identified subspecialty infrastructure has been missing for the study of rare vaccine safety outcomes in most countries. The diversity of vaccine exposures (active/passive, live/killed, single/combined, etc.) combined with the range of adverse event outcomes (in essence the entire medical textbook, including some not yet defined) means that the new subspecialty will need to play a "case manager" role of drawing upon other subspecialty expertise as needed. In the US, insurance reimbursement and liability are also potential barriers.

METHODOLOGIC PROBLEMS TO BE ADDRESSED USING PHARMACOEPIDEMIOLOGIC RESEARCH

SIGNAL DETECTION

Because vaccines are biologic rather than chemical in nature, variation in rate of adverse events by manufacturer or even lot might be expected.[97–99] Surveillance systems need to detect such potential aberrations in a timely manner. Some factors make identification of true signals difficult, however. Many vaccines are administered early in life, at a time when the baseline risk is constantly evolving and may be affected by other perinatal events. Furthermore, by definition, if vaccination rates are high, most persons with adverse medical events will have had a history of vaccination. Distinguishing causal from coincidental events on a case-by-case basis is rarely possible. Since many vaccinations are administered to individuals either simultaneously or as combination vaccine, unless the number of persons who also receive that exact permutation of vaccine exposures (including manufacturer and lot number) is known, it may be difficult if not impossible to know if an aberration has occurred.[100]

Unlike most public health surveillance systems, which focus on either a single exposure (e.g., lead) or single disease outcome (e.g., measles), vaccine safety surveillance systems need to examine multiple exposures (e.g., different vaccine antigens, manufacturers, lot numbers) and multiple disease outcomes. Until the recent advent of data mining methods, detection of a vaccine safety signal occurred as much due to a persistent patient[101] as it did on data analysis.[102] The trade-off between sensitivity and specificity depends critically on whether the goal of the surveillance is the detection of a previously unknown illness or syndrome (sensitivity > specificity) or tracking a known disease (specificity > sensitivity). Vaccine safety surveillance systems are asked to monitor *both* previously known and previously unknown adverse events in the same system, however.[103]

STANDARD DEFINITIONS AND EVALUATIVE PROTOCOLS

Case definitions can be used at the time of reporting or at the time of analysis to improve specificity. Applying definitions at the time of reporting may reduce the number of reports processed and lower the operating cost (e.g., Canadian Vaccine Associated Adverse Event).[104] The sensitivity of surveillance may be lower and the difficulty of assessing misclassification greater, however. Alternatively, if the reporting form is open-ended, this may increase the sensitivity of surveillance but only at the cost of sorting through many nonspecific reports (e.g., US Vaccine Adverse Event Reporting System).[105] Definitions can be applied at the time of analysis. But substantial variation in diagnostic work-up and description of events makes classification difficult without additional follow-up information, which in turn is usually costly.

Historically, it was difficult if not impossible to compare and collate vaccine safety data across trials or surveillance systems in a valid manner due to lack of standard case definitions. This gap represents a major "missed opportunity" to advance our scientific knowledge of immunization safety overall, but is especially unfortunate in the pre-licensure setting where maximizing yield of safety data despite

limited sample size is most needed. The Brighton Collaboration (see "Classifications and case definitions") is beginning to address this gap.

ASSESSMENT OF CAUSALITY

Assessing whether any adverse event was actually caused by vaccine is generally not possible unless a vaccine-specific clinical syndrome (e.g., myopericarditis in healthy young adult recipients of smallpox vaccine[16]), recurrence upon rechallenge (e.g., alopecia and hepatitis B vaccination[101]), or a vaccine-specific laboratory finding (e.g., Urabe mumps vaccine virus isolation[106]) can be identified. Whenever the adverse event can also occur in the absence of vaccination (e.g., seizure), epidemiologic studies are necessary to assess whether vaccinated persons are at higher risk than unvaccinated persons. When multiple vaccinations are administered simultaneously, determining whether events are attributable to particular antigens or one of several combinations is frequently difficult if not impossible.

EXPOSURE

Misclassification of exposure status may occur if there is poor documentation of vaccinations. Such errors are more likely if there is substantial mobility between health care providers. Documentation of exposure status has been fairly good through school age, due to entry requirements linked to vaccinations. Substantial difficulty may be encountered in ascertaining vaccination status in older persons, however. In the United States, recent and likely future increases in the number of licensed vaccines, the relative lack of combination vaccines, plus the high mobility between immunization providers (up to 25% annually) due to changes in health insurance plans, are leading to a potential confusing maze of vaccination history misclassifications.[107]

For example, even though an infant may have actually received the DTaP or the combined diphtheria–tetanus–pertussis–*Haemophilis influenzae* type b (DTPH) vaccine, the immunization card recorder may, due to habit, have erroneously recorded "DTP." An infant may have started their immunization series with one provider who uses DTaP vaccine primarily, but due to change in parental health insurance, switched to another provider to complete the series, who uses DTPH primarily. Add in the complexity of whether other vaccines like polio or hepatitis B vaccines are administered simultaneously or not, at different dose series in the schedule, at different ages, using different lots of vaccine and the number of permutations of vaccine exposures that need assessment for potential safety concerns quickly becomes formidable.[108] The rare availability of complete documentation of vaccine exposure on a large cohort of children in the Vaccine Safety Datalink (VSD) project allowed the evaluation of the safety of thimerosal preservatives.[13]

OUTCOME

Because the events being assessed are frequently extremely rare (e.g., encephalopathy, GBS), identifying enough cases for a meaningful interpretation of study findings can be a major challenge. Even when technically feasible, a study may be logistically infeasible or the findings likely to be too inconclusive to justify the resources. This was the conclusion of an Institute of Medicine committee that evaluated whether the UK's National Childhood Encephalopathy Study should be replicated in the United States.[39] The difficulty with adequate study power is further compounded in assessing rare events in populations less frequently exposed (e.g., vaccines given to travelers or subpopulations with special indications). Studies of GBS after influenza vaccination required the active surveillance of over 20 million persons for several months.[109,110] Identifying risk factors of such rare associations imposes an additional (and possibly prohibitive) level of sample size requirements.

Many adverse events hypothesized to be caused by vaccines are poorly defined clinical syndromes that are diagnoses of exclusion, e.g., encephalopathy,[111] GBS,[36] chronic fatigue syndrome,[112] and sudden infant death syndrome (SIDS)[113]. Our scientific understanding of these diseases is frequently limited in the absence of vaccination, let alone with vaccination. This poor understanding plus the lack of diagnostic tools for these syndromes severely limits clinical and epidemiologic studies of these illnesses. Furthermore, in highly vaccinated populations, risk-interval analyses may be the only epidemiologic study design possible (see "Analyses"). Determining the onset of illness is critical in calculating the risk interval. For certain hypothesized vaccine adverse events, there is no known biological mechanism to allow definition of the risk interval. Diseases with insidious or delayed onset like autism,[114] inflammatory bowel disease,[115] and multiple sclerosis[116] do not permit determination of the risk interval and are therefore also difficult to study.

ANALYSES, CONFOUNDING, AND BIAS

The possibility that vaccines could be responsible for a myriad of outcomes leads one to consider cohort studies in which events and person-times at risk are enumerated in strata formed by various age group and exposure windows. When outcomes are rare, however, cohort studies can be prohibitively expensive, unless all requisite information is automated and linkable.

Because adverse events are rare, studies typically sample the source population of the cases, identify an appropriate control group, assess the exposure status of both groups, and use the ratio of exposure odds among the cases and controls to estimate the risk associated with exposure. Because childhood vaccines are generally administered on schedule and children may have developmental dispositions to particular events, age may confound exposure–outcome relations, e.g., DTP vaccine and febrile seizures or SIDS.[117] Consequently, such factors must be controlled, generally by matching, as well as in the analysis.

More difficult to control are factors leading to delayed vaccination or nonvaccination.[90] Such factors (e.g., low socio-economic status) may confound studies of vaccine adverse events (AEs) and lead to underestimates of the true relative risks. The extent of bias introduced by confounding can be examined as a function of six variables (Table 30.1). Relatively little is known about the nature, frequency, and implications of these variables, however. Vaccination rates are generally high in populations in which vaccine AEs have become a concern. Those who have not been vaccinated may differ substantially from the vaccinated population in risks of AEs and thus be unsuitable as a reference group in epidemiologic studies. The unvaccinated may be persons for whom vaccination is medically contraindicated, or they may have other risks (e.g., they may be members of low socio-economic groups) for the outcome being studied.[90]

Sometimes the biases in studies are difficult to characterize and to adequately control for, and special studies may be needed to resolve controversies that arise from observational data. For example, a recent very large study of the safety of

Table 30.1. Variables determining the extent of bias attributable to confounding in studies of vaccine adverse events[90]

Variable	Description
S	Risk of AE in unvaccinated children who lack the contraindication
R	True relative risk of AE associated with vaccination
D	Relative risk of AE associated with the contraindication
C	Proportion of children with the contraindication
V	Proportion vaccinated among children without the contraindication
P	Proportion vaccinated among children with the contraindication

thimerosal in vaccines gave contradictory findings with regards to a potential relationship with various childhood neurodevelopmental outcomes.[13] Because of inherent limitations in the observational data that were available to study this issue, a follow-up study is under way which incorporates extensive in-person evaluation of neurodevelopmental status along with detailed exposure information.[118]

CURRENTLY AVAILABLE SOLUTIONS

PRE-LICENSURE

Given the need to appreciate better the safety of vaccines given universally to healthy babies and the methodologic difficulties of assessing safety post-licensure, some have argued that larger experimental trials may be needed to better assess rarer serious vaccine risks. This could be done either with larger pre-licensure trials, as has been done for antipyretics in children[119–121] and the post-rhesus-rotavirus vaccine trials,[122] or in some organized manner post-licensure prior to universal recommendation of the vaccine for entire birth cohorts (e.g., registry of first million vaccinations).[120] Even with these measures, separate large-scale long-term randomized intervention trials would theoretically be the only way to study unforeseen delayed vaccine adverse effects or nonspecific effects on mortality;[123] for example, that seen with killed or high titer measles vaccines.[124–126] Such trials would have to overcome major concerns about the ethics of withholding efficacious vaccines from persons in need, however. Therefore a more likely way forward probably lies in maximizing both the pre- and post-licensure assessment processes, as discussed in this chapter.

In addition to standardized case definitions for safety, Data and Safety Monitoring Boards (DSMBs) represent another area of potential improvements in the pre-licensure process. Currently, such DSMBs are constituted uniquely for each clinical trial. If instead there is greater overlap across pre-licensure trials for the same vaccine, the DSMB may have better ability to oversee the safety data for the experimental vaccine. Furthermore, despite its name, there are currently no requirements that the DSMB includes someone with safety experience. For vaccine trials, this means someone with rare disease (versus infectious disease) epidemiology skills, usually fine tuned from post-licensure safety monitoring experience. Infectious disease experts are used to dealing with hundreds if not thousands of cases and are therefore prone to dismissing "just a couple of cases" of an adverse event. In contrast, someone with rare disease experience may be more inclined to think that seeing two rare adverse events is worth looking into. These suggested

changes in DSMB may help prevent another rotavirus vaccine–intussusception scenario where Chi-square rather than person-time analysis was used.[127]

POST-LICENSURE

Spontaneous Reporting Systems

Informal or formal passive surveillance or spontaneous reporting systems (SRS) have been the cornerstone of most vaccine safety monitoring systems, because of their relative low cost of operations.[128] The national reporting of vaccine adverse events can be done through the same reporting channels as those used for other adverse drug reactions,[129] as is the practice in France,[130] Japan,[131] New Zealand,[132] Sweden,[133] and the United Kingdom[134] (see also Chapters 9 and 10). An increasing number of countries are collecting safety data specific to vaccinations either with reporting forms and/or surveillance systems different from the drug safety monitoring systems. These countries include Australia,[60] Canada,[83,135] Cuba,[136] Denmark,[137] India,[138] Italy,[139] Germany,[140] Mexico,[128] The Netherlands,[141] Sao Paulo State in Brazil,[142] and the United States.[105] Vaccine manufacturers also maintain SRS for their products, which are usually forwarded subsequently to appropriate national regulatory authorities.[30,128,143]

Because of their importance in infectious disease control, a significant proportion of vaccines in many countries is purchased or administered by national public health authorities. For example, the public sector (Federal, state, and local governments) in coordination with the Centers for Disease Control and Prevention (CDC) purchases over half of the childhood vaccines administered in the US. In many developing countries, the Ministry of Health in conjunction with WHO's Expanded Programme on Immunization (EPI) administers almost all vaccines. Potential vaccine adverse events commonly are first reported to the health care providers who administered the vaccine. In many countries, such health workers also participate in surveillance for other diseases. These health authorities (e.g., CDC) therefore commonly lead or collaborate with the vaccine licensure and regulatory agency (e.g., the US FDA) in developing vaccine adverse event reporting systems. A similar model is followed in Canada.[144]

The US Experience

The US National Childhood Vaccine Injury Act of 1986 mandated for the first time that health providers report certain adverse events after immunizations (Table 30.2).[145] The Vaccine Adverse Event Reporting System (VAERS) was implemented jointly by the CDC and FDA in 1990 to provide an unified national focus for collection of all reports of clinically significant adverse events, including but not limited to those mandated for reporting.[105] The creation of VAERS also provided an opportunity to correct some shortcomings of the predecessor CDC Monitoring System for Adverse Events Following Immunizations (MSAEFI) and FDA Adverse Drug Reaction Reporting System.[75]

To increase sensitivity, the VAERS form is designed to permit narrative descriptions of adverse events. All

Table 30.2. Table of reportable events following vaccination, United States

Vaccine/toxoid	Event	Interval from vaccination
Tetanus in any combination; DTaP, DTP, DTP-HiB, DT, Td, TT	A. Anaphylaxis or anaphylactic shock B. Brachial neuritis C. Any sequela (including death) of above events D. Events described in manufacturer's package insert as contraindications to additional doses of vaccine	7 days 28 days No limit See package insert
Pertussis in any combination; DTaP, DTP, DTP-HiB, P	A. Anaphylaxis or anaphylactic shock B. Encephalopathy (or encephalitis) C. Any sequela (including death) of above events D. Events described in manufacturer's package insert as contraindications to additional doses of vaccine	7 days 7 days No limit See package insert
Measles, mumps and rubella in any combination; MMR, MR, M, R	A. Anaphylaxis or anaphylactic shock B. Encephalopathy (or encephalitis) C. Any sequela (including death) of above events D. Events described in manufacturer's package insert as contraindications to additional doses of vaccine	7 days 15 days No limit See package insert
Rubella in any combination; MMR, MR, R	A. Chronic arthritis B. Any sequela (including death) of above events C. Events described in manufacturer's package insert as contraindications to additional doses of vaccine	42 days No limit See package insert
Measles in any combination; MMR, MR, M	A. Thrombocytopenic purpura B. Vaccine-strain measles viral infection in an immunodeficient recipient C. Any sequela (including death) of above events D. Events described in manufacturer's package insert as contraindications to additional doses of vaccine	7–30 days 6 months No limit See package insert
Oral polio (OPV)	A. Paralytic polio B. Vaccine-strain polio viral infection C. Any sequela (including death) of above events D. Events described in manufacturer's package insert as contraindications to additional doses of vaccine	30 days/6 months 30 days/6 months No limit See package insert
Inactivated polio (IPV)	A. Anaphylaxis or anaphylactic shock B. Any sequela (including death) of above events C. Events described in manufacturer's package insert as contraindications to additional doses of vaccine	7 days No limit See package insert
Hepatitis B	A. Anaphylaxis or anaphylactic shock B. Any sequela (including death) of above events C. Events described in manufacturer's package insert as contraindications to additional doses of vaccine	7 days No limit See package insert
Hemophilus influenzae type b	A. Events described in manufacturer's package insert as contraindications to additional doses of vaccine	See package insert

Varicella	A. Events described in manufacturer's package insert as contraindications to additional doses of vaccine	See package insert
Rotavirus	A. Intussusception	30 days
	B. Any sequela (including death) of the above event	Not applicable
	C. Events described in manufacturer's package insert as contraindications to additional doses of vaccine	See package insert
Pneumococcal conjugate	A. Events described in manufacturer's package insert as contraindications to additional doses of vaccine	See package insert

The Reportable Events Table (RET) reflects what is reportable by law (42 USC 300aa-25) to the Vaccine Adverse Event Reporting System (VAERS) including conditions found in the manufacturer's package insert. In addition, individuals are encouraged to report **any** clinically significant or unexpected events (even if you are not certain the vaccine caused the event) for **any** vaccine, whether or not it is listed on the RET. Manufacturers are also required by regulation (21CFR 600.80) to report to the VAERS program all adverse events made known to them for any vaccine. Effective date August 26, 2002.

persons, including patients or their parents and not just health professionals, are permitted to report to VAERS, especially clinically significant events. (However, as of 2004, <5% of VAERS reports come directly from consumers.) There are no restrictions set on interval between vaccination and onset of illness nor that a patient must have medical care to be reported. Annual reminders about VAERS are mailed to physicians likely to administer vaccines. The form is pre-addressed and postage-paid so that after completion it can be folded and mailed. Report forms, assistance in completing the form, or answers to other questions about the VAERS are available by calling a 24-hour toll-free telephone number (1-800-822-7967).

Web-based reporting also became available beginning in 2002; experience to date has shown it to be more complete and timely,[146] and it was therefore heavily used during the 2003 US smallpox vaccination campaign.[147] Work is also under way to integrate VAERS reporting modules with computerized immunization registries. Since the vaccine exposure and patient identifier information can be transferred automatically, this would result in more accurate, complete, efficient, and timely transmission of VAERS reports. Other eventual enhancements include timely notification of the report of available protocols for standardized evaluation of adverse events (see "Standardized clinical assessment protocols and centers"), and reporting of denominators from the registry to allow calculation of VAERS reporting rates.[148] The latter is especially important to overcome the problem of interpreting VAERS data in the face of increasing heterogeneity of vaccine exposures in the US.

Other enhancements to VAERS passive surveillance since its inception have included novel reporting channels such as patient safety organizations, capability for near-real-time report review by CDC and FDA medical officers, integration of reports from complementary (e.g., denominator) databases, in addition to frequent review and dissemination of safety data. "Enhanced passive" surveillance via VAERS has been successfully utilized to date in safety surveillance for rotavirus,[149] yellow fever,[150] and smallpox vaccines,[151] and would likely be implemented in any counter-bioterrorism-related wide-scale vaccine use.[152]

Approximately 15 000 VAERS reports are now received annually, about 15% of which are defined as serious (death, life-threatening illness, disability, hospitalization).[153] A contractor, under CDC and FDA supervision, distributes, collects, codes (using the Coding Symbols for a Thesaurus of Adverse Reaction Terms (COSTART)[154] currently, and Medical Dictionary for Regulatory Activities (MedDRA)[155] in the future) and enters VAERS reports in a database. Reporters of selected serious events receive medical follow-up from trained nurses to provide additional information about the VAERS report, including patient's recovery status. The CDC and FDA have online access to the VAERS database and focus their efforts on analytical tasks of interest to the respective agencies. These data (without personal identifiers) are also available to the public at www.vaers.org.

Other National Experiences

Several other countries also have substantial experience with passive surveillance for vaccine safety. In 1987, Canada developed the Vaccine Associated Adverse Event (VAAE) reporting system.[104] Reporting forms have check-off boxes for specific events with accompanying case definitions. Provision is also made for an "other" category. To supplement the VAAE, an active, pediatric hospital-based surveillance system that searches all admissions for possible relationships to immunizations, known as the Immunization Monitoring Program—Active (IMPACT), has been operational since

1990.[156] An Advisory Committee on Causality Assessment, consisting of a panel of experts, has also been formed to review the serious VAAE reports.[157] The Netherlands also convenes an annual panel to categorize their reports, which are then published.[141] The UK and most members of the former Commonwealth use the "yellow card" system, where a reporting form is attached to officially issued prescription pads.[129,158] Data on adverse drug (including vaccine) events from about 40 nations are compiled by the WHO Collaborating Centre for International Drug Monitoring in Uppsala.[159]

A field guide for implementation of monitoring of Adverse Events Following Immunizations (AEFI) has recently been developed by the WHO.[160] The primary focus is on detection of correctable programmatic errors like injection site abscesses (suggestive of inadequate sterilization), and development of a rapid response/assessment team for clusters of more serious events (e.g., toxic shock syndrome from contamination of vaccine vials[138] or deaths from confusing other medications for vaccines[161]). As of 2004, however, only 67 (35%) of 192 national EPIs have a functioning program for monitoring AEFIs (personal communications, Adwoa Bentsienchilla, WHO, 2004).

Classifications and Case Definitions

Vaccine adverse events can be classified by frequency (common, rare), extent (local, systemic), severity (hospitalization, disability, death), causality, and preventability (intrinsic to vaccine, faulty production, faulty administration). Wilson developed the first classification system with focus on errors of production (e.g., bacterial, viral, toxin contamination) and administration (e.g., nonsterile apparatus).[4] A more recent classification divides adverse events after vaccinations into:[162,163] (i) *vaccine-induced*: due to the intrinsic characteristic of the vaccine preparation and the individual response of the vaccinee, these events would not have occurred without vaccination (e.g., vaccine-associated paralytic poliomyelitis); (ii) *vaccine-potentiated*: would have occurred anyway, but were precipitated by the vaccination (e.g., first febrile seizure in a predisposed child); (iii) *programmatic error*: due to technical errors in vaccine preparation, handling, or administration; and (iv) *coincidental*: associated temporally with vaccination by chance or due to underlying illness. The distinction between vaccine-induced and vaccine-potentiated has recently been clarified for DTP and DT vaccine and infantile spasm, perhaps best observed in Figure 30.1.[164]

Because the simultaneous administration of vaccines is common and multiple adverse events may be reported,

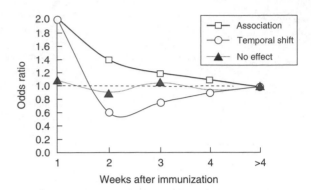

Figure 30.1. Three theoretical models of the temporal relationship between immunization and an adverse effect: (1) Association: the risk exceeds 1 at all time windows post-immunization; (2) temporal shift: the risk exceeds 1 initially but then falls below 1 but coming back to 1 eventually, such that the area under the curve above and below 1 is similar; and (3) no effect: the risk stays around 1.[164]

the Dutch system further classifies reports as: (i) *simple*—a single vaccine injection and a single major reaction; (ii) *compound*—a single vaccine injection and more than one major reaction (each major reaction is counted separately); (iii) *multiple*—>1 vaccine injection in the same person and one major reaction; or (iv) *compound–multiple*—>1 vaccine injection in the same person and >1 major reaction.[165] In the future, to better identify potential solutions, it will probably be useful to classify vaccine safety incidents as they do in aviation safety by whether they are: (i) *procedural* (e.g., unsafe injections[166] or errors in production[99,167]); (ii) *engineered* (e.g., intussusception after rotavirus vaccine,[46,47] Bell's palsy after intranasal influenza vaccine[74]); or (iii) *system* (e.g., excessive mercury exposure due to thimerosal in vaccine schedule[12]).

Case definitions of certain vaccine adverse events were first developed in Brazil,[142] Canada,[168] India,[138] and the Netherlands.[165] To improve comparability of data across reporting systems, the Workshop on Standardization of Definitions for Postmarketing Surveillance of Adverse Vaccine Reactions was held in October 1991. Definitions for approximately 20 local, central nervous system, and other adverse reactions were adopted by the workshop participants.[168] These case definitions are printed on the Canadian VAAE form as guidance for what should be reported. The proportion of VAAE reports meeting the case definition criteria has increased from 69% to 87%.[104] Alternatively, in a more open reporting system like VAERS, these definitions can be applied to reports to develop a case series for further investigation.[169,170] Real progress in implementation of similar standards across national boundaries has only begun to be realized recently, however, with the advent of the International Conference on Harmonization (ICH)[171] and the Brighton Collaboration.[172]

With the increase in interest in vaccine safety globally, the lack of a standard vocabulary was hindering scientific progress in vaccine safety. To meet this need, the Brighton Collaboration, an international voluntary effort to facilitate the development, evaluation, and dissemination of standardized case definitions of adverse events following immunizations, was launched in 2000.[172] Global workgroups of experts are convened to develop draft case definitions that are then reviewed by relevant Reference Groups. The Brighton case definitions for each adverse event are arrayed by the level of evidence presented (insufficient, low, intermediate, and highest); therefore they can also be used in settings with a range of resources (e.g., from pre-licensure trials to post-licensure surveillance, or from developing to developed country settings). The first six Brighton case definitions on fever, seizure, hypotonic–hyporesponsive episode, intussusception, nodule at injection site, and persistent crying are now available for use, with 50–100 additional definitions planned.

Standardized Clinical Assessment Protocols and Centers

More recently, there has been an increasing awareness that the utility of SRS as a potential disease registry and the immunization safety infrastructure can be usefully augmented by tertiary clinical centers. The US initiated its Clinical Immunization Safety Assessment (CISA) network with four (now seven) sites in 2001, bringing together infectious disease epidemiologists, immunologists, dermatologists, and other subspecialists as needed.[173] Among their tasks will be the standardized assessment of persons who suffered a true vaccine reaction (e.g., anaphylaxis, intussusception) to improve our scientific understanding of the pathophysiology and risk factors of the reaction. Since most persons are vaccinated without such complications, these persons are clearly outliers in a biologic Gaussian spectrum. New understanding of the human genome, pharmacogenomics, and immunology may now make it possible for us to truly understand the reaction (see also Chapter 37).[95,174]

Second, standardized assessment protocols will be developed to examine patients with similar adverse events to see if they may constitute a previously unrecognized clinical syndrome. If so, a case definition could then be developed that would permit the identification of cases for follow-up

validation studies examining the potential role of vaccination in causing this syndrome.

Third, for patients who had an adverse event that is not contraindicating but generates enough concern to interfere with completion of the series, the CISA centers can provide assessment and management under protocols, as was done with hypotonic–hyporesponsive episodes.[95] Finally, the CISA centers can provide regional referral and advice services— with the major difference that whenever advice is provided, follow-up and documentation of compliance and outcome will be done so that this rare experience is added to our scientific knowledge. Ultimately, many of the above protocols will be made available on the web for other clinicians to use (and contribute their experience).[175] During its first years, the CISA network is focusing on studies such as assessing severe limb swelling after DTaP,[176] alopecia following hepatitis B vaccination[101] and adverse events following smallpox vaccination.[16]

Assessment of Causality

The formal process of assessing causality of an adverse event and an exposure (e.g., vaccine) is a complex process that can be considered in terms of the answers to three questions: (i) *Can It?*, (ii) *Did It?*, and (iii) *Will It?*[177] The answer to *Can It?* was the focus of the Institute of Medicine reviews.[19,20] It is usually based on population level inferences drawn from epidemiologic studies and the following considerations: (i) strength of association, (ii) analytic bias, (iii) biologic gradient/dose–response, (iv) statistical significance, (v) consistency, and (vi) biologic plausibility/coherence.[178]

For individual case reports, the *Did It?* question is more relevant. If the answer is yes, then *Can It?* is also answered in the affirmative. It is natural to suspect vaccine to be the cause when an adverse event occurs in temporal association following vaccination. To base causal inference purely on temporal association, however, is to fall for the logical fallacy of *post hoc ergo propter hoc* ("after this, therefore because of this").[20] Information useful for assessing causality in individual case reports includes: (i) previous general experience with vaccine (e.g., duration of licensure, number of vaccinees, whether similar events have been observed among other vaccinees or nonvaccinees, whether animal models exist to test vaccine as a cause); (ii) alternative etiologies; (iii) individual characteristic of the vaccinee that may increase the risk of the adverse event; (iv) timing of events; (v) characteristic of the event (e.g., laboratory findings); and (vi) re-challenge[179,180] (see also Chapter 36).

When a vaccine *can* cause an adverse event, the *Will It?* refers to the probability that an individual will experience the event, or, for populations, the proportion that will experience it (i.e., the attributable risk). These data are critical for developing valid contraindications for the individuals at high risk and risk/benefit policy decisions for the population. The *Will It?* is usually very difficult to answer, however, as it can only be answered based on epidemiologic studies.[20] Furthermore, the sample sizes of such studies may be large enough to establish whether vaccine can cause a given event but yet inadequate to stratify by subgroups to examine risk factors that can help delineate potential contraindications.

Specific adverse events can usually be said to be caused by a specific vaccine if the event is associated with a unique: (i) laboratory finding, and/or (ii) clinical syndrome. For example, Urabe mumps vaccine virus was implicated as a cause of aseptic meningitis because mumps virus was isolated from the cerebrospinal fluid (a normally sterile body site) and was shown to be vaccine and not wild strain by genetic sequencing.[106] Demonstrations that severe local swelling following tetanus toxoid tended to occur in persons with extremely high levels of circulating antitoxin (due to excessive tetanus boosters) support the proposed mechanism of an Arthus reaction.[181] Acute flaccid paralysis is almost pathognomonic of vaccine-associated paralytic polio in countries where wild polio virus is unlikely to be circulating, especially shortly after receipt (or contact with a recipient) of oral polio vaccine.[37,182] Similarly, acute myopericarditis in otherwise healthy recent smallpox vaccinees also supports causal relationship.[15,16] Causality can also usually be inferred if a specific and uncommon clinical finding occurs after each vaccination (i.e., challenge/re-challenge), as in cases of alopecia after hepatitis B vaccination.[101]

If the adverse event is known to be associated with the wild vaccine-preventable disease (e.g., acute arthritis and idiopathic thrombocytopenic purpura after rubella), its association with the attenuated vaccine at a lesser frequency is not surprising.[19] This relationship is not universal, however, as pregnant women who receive rubella vaccine, unlike those exposed to wild rubella, have not been shown to have illness compatible with congenital rubella syndrome.[183] Clustering of events in time after vaccination can also suggest causation if "reporting bias" can be ruled out. Such bias may occur as parents and doctors are most likely to link adverse events with vaccinations the shorter the time interval between the two. Febrile seizures associated with killed bacterial vaccines tend to occur within a day of vaccination while those due to live viral vaccines are delayed by about a week due to viral replication.[71,184] Onset of GBS after the swine influenza vaccination was delayed up to 6 weeks as autoimmune demyelination is a slower process.[36] The pattern of the risk by time since vaccination may suggest that the relationship to vaccination is more one of temporal shift or triggering of an underlying susceptibility (Figure 30.1).[164,185]

Unfortunately, most serious reported vaccine adverse events lack these unique features that permit easy inferences on causality. Adverse events like autism, chronic fatigue syndrome, SIDS, seizures, and GBS either have multiple or as yet unknown etiologies. For these outcomes, vaccination is clearly never the principal "cause" *per se*. Otherwise, given the large number of vaccinations, we would see many more such cases. The question is more whether the association with vaccination can either potentiate the outcome or induce it in a "high risk" subpopulation, or alternatively, the association is purely coincidental and vaccination is blamed because it is a highly distinctive, painful, and memorable event usually followed by some true local and systemic vaccine reactions like injection site swelling and fever. For such adverse events, possible link with vaccination is usually based on a process of elimination, ruling out all other possible causes. Unfortunately, even after this is done, only a relatively unsatisfying nondefinitive conclusion can be drawn on any individual case report because other etiologies may not yet be discovered. The uncertainty in determining the cause of illness in individual cases has led to much confusion, controversy, and litigation.[67] With non-unique clinical syndromes or laboratory findings, epidemiologic studies have to be relied upon to ascertain likelihood of association and attributable fraction.

Another approach to causality is to make a blanket assumption that all adverse events occurring within particular periods after vaccination are caused by the vaccine, irrespective of whether they were truly causal or just coincidental. This approach to causality is used in some vaccine injury compensation programs to simplify the proceedings.[67]

In some countries, expert committees of specialists in relevant disciplines (e.g., pediatrics, infectious disease, neurology) review reports. This "global introspection" approach[186] has been used in both Canada[157] and the Netherlands[141] to classify reports of adverse events in gradations of probable association to vaccination (see also Chapter 36). The CISA network is piloting a standard protocol for individual case reviews of adverse events, building on the lessons of the Canadian ACCA. Classifications are based on the reported symptoms, the interval between vaccination and onset of symptoms, and a set of case definitions. Because opinions of experts play such a major role in this form of causality assessment, the results are less satisfying than results obtained from rigorously conducted scientific studies.

The global introspection method can be improved by the use of branched logic tree algorithms[187] or Bayesian analysis[188] (see also Chapter 36). In both, each expert's degree of belief in the key considerations of the plausibility of vaccine causation is made explicit and measured quantitatively. The algorithm requires the assessor to answer a series of questions which are then scored. The Bayesian analysis calculates the posterior probability of vaccine causation based on applying prior probability that the vaccine can cause the adverse event to the facts of an individual case. Advantages of these approaches include accountability and the possibility of recalculating the probability of causation if the quality of data improves. Disadvantages include, however, the resources required and the frequent lack of information to construct the prior probabilities. This approach was piloted in a review of MSAEFI cases[162] and used by the Institute of Medicine to review case reports,[20] but has not yet been adopted for routine use.

Signal Detection

Identifying a potential new vaccine safety problem ("signal") requires a mix of clinical intuition and epidemiologic expertise.[189] As indicated above, unusual clinical features and/or clustering by time or space usually suggest that something may be awry. No illness other than GBS was reported more commonly in the second and third week than in the first week after swine influenza vaccination, leading to further validation studies.[36,190,191] Traditionally, raising the alarm relies on some kind of calculation that the observed number exceeds the number of cases expected by chance alone for the specific data source. For vaccines, to minimize risk of a false positive alarm, this probability is frequently set at 95%. Detecting nonrandom clustering of onset intervals (e.g., via the scan statistic which tests for randomness or not), however, may allow earlier detection of a possible signal when the adverse event is rare, not seasonal, serious enough to require emergency care, and there is little change in age over time, relative to any age-dependence of the rate for the event.[192]

Recent events in the United States and elsewhere have underscored the importance of rapidly identifying and responding to serious adverse events identified secondary to new vaccines or newly reintroduced vaccines. Passive reports to VAERS of intussusception among children vaccinated with rhesus rotavirus vaccine was the first post-licensure signal of a problem,[149] leading to several studies to verify these findings.[46,47] A report by a concerned mother of recurrent alopecia after successive hepatitis B vaccinations in her child led to a review of VAERS data that showed several other similar reports.[101] Similarly, initial reports to VAERS of a previously unrecognized serious yellow fever vaccine-associated viscerotropic disease,[193,194] and neurotropic disease[150] have since been confirmed

elsewhere.[195] Acute myopericarditis has been a relatively unexpected finding among recent smallpox vaccines in the US.[16,151] Oculorespiratory syndrome was found among recent influenza vaccines from one Canadian manufacturer in one season.[196] Bell's palsy was detected in recipients of a new Swiss intranasal influenza vaccine.[74]

Because of the success in detecting these signals, there have been various attempts to automate screening for signals using SRS reports. Historically this has been relatively unsuccessful,[197] largely due to inherent methodologic problems of spontaneous reports (see above and Chapters 9 and 10). New tools developed recently for pattern recognition in extremely large databases are beginning to be applied, however.[198–201] VAERS is one of the largest registries for rare vaccine adverse events in the world. By the end of 2003 it had accumulated over 170 000 reports. Because of its continuously increasing size and the need to monitor a large number of vaccine–symptom combinations, there has been a substantial effort made in recent years to apply various computer-assisted techniques for automated detection of unusual trends and patterns. Among different "data mining" methods that have been evaluated, tools that utilize various types of disproportionality analysis seem to be most suitable for SRS databases.[202–204]

The idea of comparing safety profiles (proportional morbidity distributions) is simple. It involves calculation of proportions of particular symptoms out of the total number of events for a given vaccine, and then comparing the results with the proportions of similar symptoms observed among reports for another vaccine or group of vaccines.[205,206] Due to its ease of implementation and interpretation, the proportional reporting rate ratio (PRR) method is the most widely used disproportionality measure in VAERS for prospective and retrospective signal generation.[153,199,207] Association rule discovery (ARD), which is essentially a more general example of PRR methodology, has also been applied to VAERS data for detection of multisymptom syndromes and symptom interactions that are seen proportionally more frequently following specific vaccines.[202] This methodology has been widely used in market research and genetics, and appears to be suitable for some SRS data analyses. Rational approaches to prioritizing the large numbers of potential signals generated using ARD may involve utilization of complementary approaches, such as data visualization.

A promising future direction for PRR, ARD, and related methods is the development of automated algorithms to efficiently screen the entire database and perform safety profile comparisons as periodic (monitoring) activity. It has been shown previously that different measures of disproportionality used in performing this task are largely comparable.[204,208] Automated signaling techniques used in SRS data screenings have several limitations. For example, automated signal generation will not flag events that are not uniquely coded (e.g., the coding system may lack a specific term for Sjogren's disease or other rare conditions). Ultimately, these methods do represent a useful adjunct to, not a substitute for, traditional methods of scrutinizing spontaneous reports in increasingly complex databases such as VAERS.[199]

A new initiative has been formed by the CDC Vaccine Safety Datalink project (see "Automated large-linked databases" below) to rapidly analyze safety data on new vaccines and the yearly flu vaccine strain. This initiative utilizes the strengths of the VSD with its ability to gather automated vaccination and medical care utilization data from enrolled members in eight managed care organizations, and incorporates new data management to collect and analyze the safety profile of each successive week's cohort of vaccinated children. Sequential probability ratio testing is used to detect safety signals based on prespecified limits, while accurately accounting for repeated testing of the data. To date the project has successfully simulated a rapid-cycle approach to routinely collected VSD data, and has been able to detect an increased safety profile with the new acellular pertussis vaccines (e.g., a decreased risk for seizures and other neurologic events compared to the old whole-cell pertussis vaccines).[209]

Where one is data mining large data sets, by whatever methodologies, for signals not leading to immediate conclusion but to further investigation, the real issue is minimizing false negatives, while false positives are not an issue as long as they are manageable in terms of the available man hours to investigate them.

Mass Immunization Campaigns

Whenever a very large number of vaccine doses are administered over a well-defined short time interval, this can result either in more prominent clusters of vaccine adverse events, or by their absence demonstrate their safety. Note that this occurs irrespective of whether the vaccine exposure is part of a planned mass immunization campaign or not. For example, the links drawn between MMR and autism in the UK,[114] thimerosal and autism in the US, and hepatitis B vaccine and demyelinating disease in France[18] are arguably examples of the latter. Surveillance of vaccine adverse events around the time of mass immunization campaigns have therefore been extremely useful in generating signals, either positive (e.g., GBS with swine influenza vaccine,[36] GBS after oral polio vaccine,[210] allergic reactions after Japanese encephalitis vaccine,[211] neuropathy after rubella vaccine[212]) or negative (e.g., events after meningococcal

vaccine,[213] GBS after measles[134]). Such signals still require validation, however, since some, after more careful scientific studies, turn out to be incorrect (e.g., GBS after oral polio vaccine).[214]

Lessons Learned to Date

Several lessons are beginning to emerge from spontaneous reporting systems like VAERS.[153,215–217] Such systems worldwide have successfully detected previously unrecognized reactions and helped to obtain data to evaluate whether these events are causally linked to vaccines.[74,101,149–151,196] VAERS has also successfully served as a source of cases for further investigation of idiopathic thrombocytopenic purpura after MMR,[218] anaphylaxis after MMR,[219] and syncope after immunization.[220] VAERS has been of great value for answering routine public queries such as "has adverse event X ever been reported after vaccine Y?" and describing the safety profile of new vaccines.[221,222]

When denominator data on doses are available from other sources (e.g., net doses distributed, vaccine coverage surveys, immunization registries), VAERS can be used to evaluate changes in reporting rates over time or when new vaccines replace old vaccines. For example, VAERS showed that after millions of doses had been distributed, the reporting rate for serious events like hospitalization and seizures after DTaP in toddlers was one-third that after DTP.[205] Reports of vaccine-associated paralytic polio to VAERS disappeared after shifting away from oral polio vaccine in the US.[153] VAERS is also currently the only surveillance system that covers the entire US population and the data are available on a relatively timely basis. It is, therefore, the major means available currently to detect possible new, unusual, or extremely rare adverse events, including whether certain lots of vaccines are associated with unusually high rates of adverse events,[223,224] especially when combined with modeled estimates of lot use denominator.[225]

VAERS type of data has helped to identify potential risk factors for vaccine adverse events, ranging from advanced age associated with yellow fever vaccine complications,[194] personal and family history of convulsions in pertussis vaccinees,[75] and post-vaccinial syncope-related injuries.[220]

The reporting efficiency or sensitivity of a spontaneous reporting system can be estimated by capture–recapture methods (examining the proportion of subjects present in two or more independent data sources) or if expected rates of adverse events generated from carefully executed studies are available. An estimated 47% of rhesus rotavirus vaccine attributable cases of intussusception were reported to VAERS.[226] A higher proportion of serious events like seizures that follow vaccinations are likely to be reported to

VAERS than milder events like rash or delayed events requiring laboratory assessment such as thrombocytopenic purpura after MMR vaccination (Table 30.3).[227] Although formal evaluation has been limited, the probability that a serious event reported to VAERS has been accurately diagnosed (i.e., predictive value positive) is likely to be high. Of 26 patients reported to VAERS who developed GBS after influenza vaccination during the 1990–91 season, whose hospital charts were reviewed by an independent panel of neurologists blinded to immunization status, the diagnosis of GBS was confirmed in 22 (85%).[109]

Despite the above uses, spontaneous reporting systems for drug and vaccine safety have a number of major methodologic weaknesses (see also Chapters 9 and 10) and pitfalls for the unwary user of public use data sets.[217] Under-, biased, and incomplete reporting are inherent to all such spontaneous reporting systems and potential safety concerns may be missed.[189,227] Aseptic meningitis associated with the Urabe mumps vaccine strain, for example, was not detected by spontaneous reporting systems in most countries during routine use until this vaccine was used during mass campaigns.[71,228] Most importantly, however, the information content of such spontaneous reports represents just cell "a" of a 2×2 table of vaccination versus adverse event (Figure 30.2), and an underreported and biased content at that. It is therefore less than one fourth of the information necessary to complete an epidemiologic analysis of a vaccine adverse event. Use of data from spontaneous reporting systems is further complicated by lack of specific clinical syndromes being evaluated, absence of laboratory confirmation of many of the events, and simultaneous vaccinations, which make proper attribution of the causal vaccine difficult.

Current spontaneous reporting systems are also prone to detecting increases in adverse events that are not true increases. Instead, they may be due to an increase in (i) reporting efficiency, (ii) vaccine coverage, or (iii) other causes of the adverse event. Spontaneous reporting systems are usually unable to sort out causally related from coincidentally related adverse events because of inherent methodologic weaknesses. For example, an increase in GBS reports after 1993–94 influenza vaccination was found to be due to improvements in vaccine coverage and increases in GBS independent of vaccination.[110] An increased reporting rate of an adverse event following one hepatitis B vaccine compared to a second brand was likely due to differential distribution of brands in the public versus private sectors, which have differential VAERS reporting rates (higher in the public sector).[229]

These studies highlight the crude nature of the "signal" generated by VAERS and the difficulty in ascertaining which vaccine safety concerns warrant further investigation. Not only are there problems with reporting efficiency and potentially biased reporting, but also precise denominators for calculating true rates are usually not available. Instead, crude measures such as doses distributed must often be used as surrogates for doses administered. Due to these difficulties, the requirement for manufacturers to notify the FDA whenever they receive an increased number of reports has been dropped.[230]

Historically, most countries have relied on spontaneous reporting systems alone for post-licensure vaccine safety monitoring. The inadequacy of scientific information on vaccine safety found by the Institute of Medicine is related to these methodologic weaknesses inherent to spontaneous reporting systems. The establishment of new population-based immunization registries, in which all vaccines administered are entered, may provide more timely submission of spontaneous reports as well as more accurate and specific denominators for doses administered, providing information necessary to calculate more accurate adverse event rates.[231,232]

Table 30.3. Reporting efficiencies for selected outcomes, two passive surveillance systems for vaccine adverse events, US[227]

Adverse event	Vaccine	Reporting efficiency(%)		
		MSAEFI[a]	VAERS[a] (overall)	VAERS[a] (public sector)
Vaccine-associated polio	Oral polio vaccine (OPV)	72	68	[b]
Seizures	Diphtheria–tetanus–pertussis (DTP)	42	24	36
Seizures	Measles–mumps–rubella (MMR)	23	37	49
Hypotonic–hyporesponsive episodes	DTP	4	3	4
Rash	MMR	<1	<1	5
Thrombocytopenia	MMR	<1	4	<1

[a] MSAEFI, Monitoring System for Adverse Events Following Immunizations; VAERS, Vaccine Adverse Event Reporting System.
[b] Public and private sector information is missing on these cases.

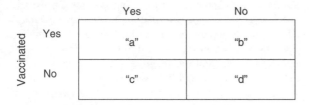

Figure 30.2. "2 × 2" table necessary for epidemiological analysis of causality between vaccine and an adverse event.
Rate of adverse event following vaccination = a/a + b.
Rate of adverse event in the absence of vaccination = c/c + d.
Reports to passive surveillance systems for vaccine adverse events (e.g., Vaccine Adverse Event Reporting System) represent just partial information (due to under- and biased reporting) for cell "a" of the table.
Epidemiologic studies aim to gather information for all four cells of this table in an unbiased manner.

Clinical Trials

Post-Licensure Clinical Trials

Immunization programs are in a dynamic relationship with their target diseases.[233] To optimize vaccine use, clinical trials may be conducted after vaccine licensure to assess the effects of changes in vaccine formulation,[234] vaccine strain,[235] age at vaccination,[236] the number and timing of vaccine doses,[237] simultaneous administration,[238] and interchangeability of vaccines from different manufacturers[239] on vaccine safety and immunogenicity. The importance of such trials was demonstrated when studies showed an unanticipated differential mortality among recipients of high and regular titer measles vaccine in developing countries,[240] albeit lower than among unvaccinated children.[241] This finding resulted in a change in recommendations by WHO for the use of such vaccines.[242] The development of automated large-linked databases (see below) may permit improved ability to monitor the safety of such post-licensure changes in vaccine use without necessarily conducting such clinical trials.

Phase IV Surveillance Studies

To improve the ability to detect adverse events that are not detected during pre-licensure trials, most recently licensed vaccines in developed countries have undergone formal Phase IV surveillance studies on populations with sample sizes of ~10[5]. These studies have usually used cohorts in health maintenance organizations supplemented by diary or telephone interview. These methods were first extensively used after the licensure of polysaccharide and conjugated Hib vaccines.[243–245] Post-licensure studies on safety and efficacy of infant DTaP are also continuing.[87] Extensive Phase IV evaluation of varicella vaccine includes multi-year evaluation for disease incidence, herpes zoster, and a pregnancy registry.[246,247] Requirements for Phase IV evaluation have even been extended to less frequently used vaccines, like Japanese encephalitis vaccine.[248] A large post-licensure randomized trial for this vaccine was also completed in China recently to improve the available data on its short-term safety.[249]

Ad Hoc Epidemiologic Studies

Historically, *ad hoc* epidemiologic studies have been employed to assess signals of potential adverse events generated by spontaneous reporting systems, the medical literature, or other mechanisms. Traditional analyses of secular trends (ecologic studies), cohort, and case–control studies have been used to gather information necessary to measure or compare risks of an adverse event following vaccination with risk in the absence of vaccination. Occasionally, data collected for other study outcomes may be reanalyzed to see if vaccine was causally related or not.[250] Examples of *ad hoc* follow-up studies to signals of vaccine safety issues are the investigations of poliomyelitis after inactivated[55] and oral[182] polio vaccines; SIDS after DTP vaccination;[19,113,251–253] encephalopathy after DTP vaccination;[40,254] meningoencephalitis after mumps vaccination;[106,255] injection site abscesses post-vaccination;[256] and GBS after influenza vaccine.[36,109,110] Many such studies have been compiled and reviewed by the Institute of Medicine.[19,20,23,25–29] While automated large-linked databases (see below) provide a more cost-effective and flexible framework for hypothesis testing, *ad hoc* epidemiologic studies may still be needed in settings without automated large-linked databases,[74,196] or where the power of the automated large-linked databases may be inadequate to answer a question in a timely manner.[109,110]

Automated Large-Linked Databases

Ad hoc epidemiologic studies of vaccine safety, while potentially informative about vaccine causality, are costly, time-consuming, and usually limited to assessment of a single event. As with drug safety research (see Chapters

13–22), efforts have increasingly turned to record linkage between automated exposure (immunization records in lieu of pharmacy) files and outcome medical files. The CDC participated in two pilot vaccine safety studies using automated large-linked databases in Medicaid and HMO populations, respectively, during the late 1980s.[257,258] While validating this approach for vaccine safety studies and providing scientifically rigorous results, these studies were limited by their relatively small sample sizes, retrospective design, and focus on the most severe reactions.[19] These limitations, the constraints of VAERS, and the recognition of the need for improved monitoring of vaccine safety prompted the CDC to initiate the Vaccine Safety Datalink (VSD) project in 1990.[184,259,260] To help overcome the previously identified shortcomings, the VSD study prospectively collects vaccination, medical outcome (e.g., hospital discharge, outpatient visits, emergency room visits, and deaths), and covariate data (e.g., birth certificates, census) under joint protocol at multiple HMOs. Selection of staff model prepaid health plans also minimized potential biases for more severe outcomes resulting from data generated from fee-for-service claims.

Originally, the VSD conducted active surveillance on approximately 500 000 children from birth through 6 years of age (75 000 birth cohort, approximately 2% of US population in these age groups).[184] Expansion to eight HMOs (including data on all age groups at three HMOs) was accomplished in 2000. The VSD focused its initial efforts on examining potential associations between immunizations and 34 serious neurologic, allergic, hematologic, infectious, inflammatory, and metabolic conditions. The VSD is also being used to test new *ad hoc* vaccine safety hypotheses that may arise from the medical literature,[261] from VAERS,[229] from changes in immunization schedules,[262] or introduction of new vaccines.[47] The size of the VSD population may also permit separation of the risks associated with individual vaccines from those associated with vaccine combinations, whether given in the same syringe or simultaneously at different body sites. Such studies will be especially valuable in view of the new combined pediatric vaccines currently in development.[263]

When the VSD identifies an adverse event as being caused by vaccine, data on the incidence rate attributable to vaccine is available, permitting accurate risk/benefit assessment by both the public and policy makers.[264] Subgroup analyses may permit identification of risk factors for adverse events, which may be useful in identifying contraindications to vaccinations. Data from VSD have been useful in calculating background rates of illnesses in the absence of vaccination that can serve as expected rates when comparing rates of vaccine-associated events in SRS. Also, incidence rates of vaccine-associated adverse events derived from VSD can be used to evaluate the sensitivity of passive reporting systems. The VSD data also aids the FDA in its evaluation of VAERS data[265] and the Vaccine Injury Compensation Program in determinations of what events should be compensated as vaccine "injuries."[67]

Amid these promises, a few caveats are appropriate. While diverse, the population in the HMOs currently in the VSD is not wholly representative of the US in terms of geography or socioeconomic status. More importantly, due to the high coverage attained in the HMOs for most vaccines, few non-vaccinated controls are available. The VSD must therefore rely predominantly on some type of "risk-interval" analysis[257,258,266] (Box 30.1). The capability of this approach to assess associations between vaccination and adverse events with delayed or insidious onset (e.g., neurodevelopmental or behavioral outcomes) is limited.[13] Many of these outcomes are either under-ascertained or mis-ascertained in medical settings. Additionally, many diagnoses of these outcomes will be given at well-child care visits and/or vaccination visits, which may lead to a spurious positive observed relationship between measures based on completion of a vaccine series or overall on-time vaccination. The VSD also cannot easily assess adverse events not currently captured in existing HMO databases, because they do not result in a health care consultation (e.g., fever).[184] The current VSD is also not large enough to examine the risk of extremely rare events such as Guillain–Barré syndrome after each season's influenza vaccine. Finally, because the VSD relies on epidemiologic methods, it may not successfully control for confounding and bias in each analysis[90] and inferences on causality may be limited.[267]

Despite these potential shortcomings, the VSD provides an essential, powerful, and relatively cost-effective complement to ongoing evaluations of vaccine safety in the US. In view of the methodologic and logistical advantages offered by automated large-linked databases, the UK[71,106,268,269] and Canada[270] have also developed automated large-linked databases linking immunization registries with medical files. The first such pilot database in a less developed setting has been established in Vietnam.[271] Because of the relatively limited number of vaccines used worldwide, however, and the costs associated with establishing and operating them, it is unlikely that all countries will be able to or need to establish their own automated large-linked databases. They should be able to draw upon the scientific base established by the existing automated large-linked databases for vaccine safety and, if the need arises, conduct *ad hoc* epidemiologic studies.

(1) Define "risk interval" for adverse event after vaccination (e.g., 30 days after each dose).

(2) Partition observation time for each child in the study into periods within and outside of risk intervals, and sum respectively (e.g., for a child observed for 365 days during which three doses of vaccine were received; total risk interval time = 3 × 30 person-days = 90 person-days; total non-risk interval time = 365 − 90 = 275 person-days).

```
o————————x════—————————x════————————x════————//———>|
Birth           Dose 1              Dose 2              Dose 3                       365 days
```

(3) Add up (i) total risk interval and non-risk interval observation times for each child in the study (= person-time observed; for mathematical convenience, the example below uses 100 and 1000 person-months of observation), and (ii) adverse events occurring in each time period to complete 2 × 2 table (for illustration, the example below uses 3 and 10 cases):

	Adverse event yes	Person-time observed (months)	Incidence rate
Vaccinated in risk interval yes	3	100	0.03
Vaccinated in risk interval no	10	1000	0.01
Total	13	1100	

Incidence rate adverse event$_{vaccinated}$ = 3/100 = 0.03
Incidence rate adverse event$_{unvaccinated}$ = 10/1000 = 0.01
Relative risk vaccinated: unvaccinated = 0.03/0.01 = 3.0
Probability finding due to chance: <5/100
Conclusion: There is a three-fold increase in risk for developing the adverse event within the interval following vaccination.

Box 30.1 Example of method for risk-interval analysis of association between a universally recommended three-dose vaccine (with few unvaccinated persons for comparision) and adverse event.

METHODOLOGIC APPROACHES

Exposures

In countries where vaccinations are required for entry into daycare, kindergarten, schools, and/or colleges, documentation (e.g., vaccination cards or medical records) is usually available and of good quality for most infants and children. In the US, documentation of the vaccine type, date of vaccination, manufacturer, lot number, and vaccine provider in a permanent medical record has been required since 1988 for certain routine childhood vaccinations.[145] This requirement, along with improvements in technology, has prompted many organizations to automate their vaccination records.[232]

Although vaccination records can be manually retrieved and reviewed for any study design, automated vaccination records greatly ease the logistics of organizing such studies. Whenever sampling is necessary in the design, automated records also ease the selection of samples that are representative. Assessing the accuracy of such automated data is important in any study.[272,273] When persons receive their vaccinations from a variety of providers (as they commonly do in the US), their exposure status may be misclassified.[274] This error could be minimized if a centralized National Vaccination Registry were implemented to track all vaccinations from birth. Such a registry has been implemented in most of the UK,[231] and regional registries are under development in the US,[232] Canada,[275] and Australia.[276]

The availability and quality of vaccination records generally decrease as people age. Some vaccines for older people (e.g., tetanus–diphtheria boosters in emergency rooms, hepatitis B vaccinations for health care workers) may be administered in settings other than primary health care. In addition to review of primary medical records, interviews or a review of data from secondary vaccination sites may therefore be necessary to accurately ascertain exposure status in adverse event studies of these vaccines in older populations. To increase the accuracy of exposure data in a study of adverse reactions to plasma-derived hepatitis B vaccine among Alaskan natives,[277] medical records from the village, the hospital, and the regional public health nurse, in addition to the automated vaccination record, were reviewed.[277,278] Recent studies of GBS and influenza vaccine relied on both patient/family interview and validation with health provider for exposure ascertainment.[109] Interestingly, reliance on provider verification may lead to under-ascertainment of vaccination status, either due to poor record keeping[274] or to concerns about liability in vaccine safety studies.[110]

To further improve the accuracy and efficiency of transfer of vaccine identification information from the vaccine vial to either automated or paper immunization records, the CDC has organized the Vaccine Identification Standards

Initiative (VISI).[107] Working with a coalition of industry, immunization providers, and other Federal agencies, the Initiative seeks to develop standards for: (i) abbreviations for new vaccine antigens and vaccine manufacturers, (ii) peel-off labels, (iii) bar codes, (iv) lot numbers, (v) immunization records, and (vi) presentation of key identifier information on vaccine packaging (as on the nutrition label). All of these should contribute to minimizing exposure misclassification for any vaccine-related study.

Outcomes

To ensure both high sensitivity and specificity, a sequential approach is usually required. The initial screening definition is highly sensitive but less specific. For a study of neurologic illness following DTP immunization, a combination of hospitalization codes and prescriptions of any drug that might have been used to treat such illnesses were used for case finding.[279] The medical records of these patients were then reviewed (sometimes after chart abstraction) to see if they met the study case definition. In difficult diagnoses like GBS, a panel of specialists may also be asked to review the charts after exposure status has been masked.[45] For outcomes with insidious onset like multiple sclerosis, multiple dates (e.g., first symptom, first medical visit, first diagnosis) and sources of information (patient recall, medical chart) may need to be collected and analyzed.[280,281]

The primary focus during the study of a new possible association is usually on avoiding a false positive conclusion by ensuring that only cases meeting the most specific case definition are included in the analysis. Doing so may miss the broader safety profile of the vaccine, however. For example, adverse neurologic outcomes other than GBS were reported among swine flu vaccinees.[282] Follow-up analyses of rhesus rotavirus vaccine reports to VAERS suggest that intussusception[149] may have been just the tip of the "iceberg" of a broader syndrome.[221] Unfortunately, the association between these outcomes and the vaccine of interest remains unknown and controversial, as formal studies have not been done.

Should the concern be a new previously undescribed syndrome, analyses of existing databases may be inadequate. A recent study of "Gulf War syndrome" and vaccinations relied on a thorough interview of patients meeting a de novo complex case definition before linkage with vaccination history.[283]

Analyses

Different analytical strategies are needed depending on how a vaccine is used in the population. For low frequency use vaccines for which the vaccinees are generally no different than the nonvaccinees (e.g., travel vaccines), comparison between the two groups with adequate matching or adjustment is relatively straightforward. For vaccines that are almost universally recommended (e.g., most childhood vaccines), however, too few persons are "unexposed" to compare adverse outcomes among vaccinated and unvaccinated (i.e., typical cohort study) or vaccination among cases and non-cases (i.e., typical case–control study). Therefore, an alternative definition of "exposure" is used in most post-licensure vaccine safety studies. A "window of risk" after vaccination for the specific event of interest is defined a priori based on current understanding of the most plausible biologic mechanism should such an association actually exist (Box 30.1). Incidence rates inside ("exposed") and outside ("unexposed") the risk window (or recent exposures among cases and non-cases) are then compared. To allow for the possibility of delayed reactions, multiple risk windows may be defined (e.g., 1, 2–3, 4–7, 8–14, 15–30, 31 or more days, or even longer for autoimmune demyelinating diseases like GBS), preferably a priori. Several calculations typically should be performed by using different intervals, or windows, to identify the window in which the rate ratio or other estimate of risk is greatest. For evaluating hypothesized causes and for establishing new hypotheses, this information is invaluable.

Most members of populations under active surveillance contribute little to analysis because few experience adverse events, but the per capita cost of information is more or less constant. Thus, investigators sometimes use the case–cohort method, which requires information only about the cases and samples of the population to which they belong, the latter of which can be used repeatedly with different outcomes (i.e., fewer people must be studied). Efficiency is even further increased for the case-crossover method (i.e., there are no controls). Both of these designs are discussed in more detail in Chapter 48.

The case-crossover[284,285] or case-series approaches are gaining popularity in vaccine safety studies.[46,73,74,286] Unlike conventional analyses of studies involving matching, to which only discordant pairs contribute, all exposed cases contribute to case-series analyses, increasing their potential efficiency. Because cases serve as their own controls, moreover, this design controls within-individual variation perfectly. There are some caveats, however. All relevant information for the cases and factors that can change over the observation period and affect the occurrence of the event of interest still needs to be collected for the entire observation period of interest. For example, controlling for age and calendar time is needed for: (i) young children in the first six months of life when many vaccines are received and rates of many medical events change considerably over the course of one month of age, and (ii) influenza vaccination, with its narrow seasonal window of receipt in mid- to late autumn, and many outcomes have a seasonal variation with an upswing in incidence at about or just past the time of receipt of influenza vaccine. Note also that the presence of an interaction between age or calendar time and any demographic factor such as gender would then require controlling for the interaction as well. Thus, constant factors may still need to be taken into account. This is, of course, difficult to do for those pesky, unmeasured factors. Standard cohort methods employing a Cox survival regression methodology that use age or calendar time as the basic time scale and then stratify on the other time scale plus other factors such as sex may control for a very large number of time-dependent factors that are often overlooked in a case-series analysis.

Confounding and Bias

Once a universally recommended vaccine is licensed, it is usually unethical to withhold the vaccine in subsequent randomized trials as a means to minimize confounding and bias. If further assessment of short-term safety is critical, however, it may be possible to do a randomized trial post-licensure in certain settings, as long as the controls also receive the vaccine after a relatively short observation period.[249] Assessing whether vaccines have nonspecific effects on mortality will similarly require study designs that avoid selection factors for vaccination (e.g., randomized trial, time–series designs, comparison of mortality in carefully selected populations who receive vaccines in sequential order).[123]

To minimize recall bias, it is best to rely on data sources that gather information on outcomes and vaccine exposure independently. This is one of the major advantages of record linkage studies.[184,287] In a recent study of GBS and influenza vaccine, for example, all GBS cases meeting predefined case definition were ascertained from statewide hospital discharge data sets.[110] The cases were then interviewed for a range of risk factors for GBS, including vaccination. Only when patients reported that they were vaccinated, were they asked which type. The patients are unaware of the specific hypothesis being evaluated (influenza vaccine and GBS) throughout the interview. A separate random digit dialing survey was conducted to ascertain the comparison influenza vaccination rate in the general population. Similarly, within the VSD, data on exposure are collected from automated databases created originally for

billing purposes, and hence are unbiased with regards to the timing of any particular outcome or disease.

Control for potential confounders may be addressed routinely by obtaining the necessary information and adjusting for them at the time of analysis. For the CDC Vaccine Safety Datalink project, sources of covariates include birth certificates and the decennial census (linked via postal zip codes of the children). Alternatively, the case-series design[286] or assessment of unusual clustering in onset intervals may provide additional information on possible causal association with minimal confounding. The case-series design focuses on changes in disease events through time within individuals, with measured changes pooled over individuals. It has nearly as much statistical power as the full cohort approach if a high percentage of the population has been vaccinated. Since only known vaccinated cases are used in the analysis, there is no exposure misclassification bias. On the negative side, the case-series design is still subject to confounding by "within-person" variables that change through time. For example, no epidemiologic method yet can address the "healthy child" bias resulting from avoiding vaccinations during transient illness. Also, research questions may not be limited to events that are time-varying (e.g., gender, race/ethnicity).[288]

THE FUTURE

Many persons look to vaccines as the "magic bullet" solution to a number of public health problems, which range from acquired immunodeficiency syndrome (AIDS) to malaria. Rapid advances in biotechnology have brought the promise of these new vaccines closer to reality.[289] Novel delivery technologies such as DNA vaccines and new adjuvants are being explored to permit more antigens to be combined, reducing the number of injections.[263,290] These changes in vaccines and vaccine delivery will continue to provide additional challenges in proving their safety to an increasingly skeptical and risk-averse public, however.[291] Combined with methodologic difficulties associated with studying rare, delayed, or insidious vaccine safety allegations, well-organized anti-vaccine organizations, media eagerness for controversy,[292] and relatively rare individual encounters with wild vaccine-preventable diseases like measles, vaccine safety concerns are unlikely to "go away" in mature immunization programs.[6]

Ironically, just as the need for a credible and effective immunization safety system is at its greatest in human history, and the needed infrastructure to study rare adverse events has been or is being built in some countries,[71,105,172,293–295] several nonscientific challenges are accumulating, especially an increasingly acrimonious atmosphere that may destroy the viability of this important research. The push for transparency and data sharing have resulted in claimed results or publications based on questionable analysis and interpretation of public use data sets.[217] Various "credible" bodies (e.g., IOM,[23–29] World Health Organization Global Advisory Committee on Vaccine Safety[296]) are being asked to review immunization safety studies. The credibility of government-sponsored vaccine safety studies has been questioned by some, less because of the scientific merits, but based on perceived conflict of interest since the vaccine safety researchers are located within national immunization programs that "promote" immunizations.[297] The credibility of researchers from the "other side" has also been questioned, due to their failure to disclose source of study funding from legal sources.[298–300] A large class action lawsuit on thimerosal and autism with its associated extensive "discovery" burdens may ironically not only interfere/deter timely conduct of the needed studies but also the viability of the immunization enterprise itself.[301]

It is clear that a larger societal dialogue is needed to articulate the characteristics of a sustainable, credible, and effective immunization safety system that will meet the needs of this "brave new world" where vaccine-induced immunity will increasingly replace wild-disease-induced immunity and the "post-modern" populace is increasingly risk aversive.[302,303] Immunizations may have much to learn from the aviation safety system, where the best of separation and integration occurs.[5,304] The duties of risk assessment by the National Transportation Safety Board (NTSB) are clearly separate from the risk management duties of the manufacturer, regulatory body, or the airline. Yet using the "parties" model, the NTSB has the power to convene and lead an investigation team consisting of the appropriate stakeholders with the relevant knowledge for the investigation (versus excluding them due to concerns about perceived conflict of interest).[305] The NTSB model has also been proposed for drug safety,[306] patient safety,[307] and recently, for vaccine safety.[304]

Concomitantly, vaccine safety concerns have also "emerged" as an issue in EPI's developing countries.[8] The high titer measles vaccine mortality experience highlighted the importance of improving quality control and evaluating the safety of vaccines used in developing countries.[91,235,240] Plans to eliminate neonatal tetanus and measles via National Immunization Days where millions of persons receive parenteral immunizations over a period of days[308] pose substantial challenges to ensuring injection safety.[166]

The increasing computerization and centralization of health care services may facilitate epidemiologic studies to reassure the public about the safety of future vaccines. Like other arenas concerned with safety (e.g., aviation, food, blood), a comprehensive "systems" design approach to minimize risk and promote safety is needed. Developments in biotechnology may continue to offer better, safer vaccines.[289] The availability of computerized immunization registries may permit optimal implementation of immunization policies at the individual level, ensuring receipt of indicated vaccines, avoiding extra vaccinations, and assuring appropriate observance of valid contraindications to vaccinations.[232] On a longer horizon, vaccine safety research combined with genetic epidemiology may permit better characterization of risk groups for vaccine reactions.[309,310] Integrated with immunization registries for both children and adults, this may ultimately offer the possibility for better prevention of both vaccine-preventable and vaccine-induced diseases.

ACKNOWLEDGMENT

The authors wish to thank Drs Vitali Pool, Margaret Kolczak, and John Sawyer for their contributions to the section on Signal Detection, Alison Howard and Tamera Murphy for their assistance in preparing the manuscript, and Dr James Baggs with the reference software.

REFERENCES

1. World Bank. *World Development Report 1993: Investing in Health*. New York: Oxford University Press, 1993.
2. England S, Loevinsohn B, Melgaard B, Kou U, Jha P. *The Evidence Base for Interventions to Reduce Mortality from Vaccine-Preventable Diseases in Low and Middle-Income Countries*. World Health Organization Commission on Macroeconomics and Health, working paper series, paper no. WG5, 10. Geneva: WHO, 2001.
3. Centers for Disease Control and Prevention. Achievements in public health, 1900–1999: impact of vaccines universally recommended for children—United States, 1990–1998. *MMWR Morb Mortal Wkly Rep* 1999; **48**: 243–8.
4. Wilson GS. *The Hazards of Immunization*. London: Athlone Press, 1967.

5. Chen RT. Vaccine risks: real, perceived and unknown. *Vaccine* 1999; **17**(suppl 3): S41–6.

6. Plotkin SA. Lessons learned concerning vaccine safety. *Vaccine* 2001; **20**(suppl 1): S16–19.

7. Freed GL, Clark SJ, Hibbs BF, Santoli JM. Parental vaccine safety concerns. The experiences of pediatricians and family physicians. *Am J Prev Med* 2004; **26**: 11–14.

8. Duclos P, Delo A, Aguado T, Bilous J, Birmingham M, Kieny MP *et al.* Immunization safety priority project at the World Health Organization. *Semin Pediatr Infect Dis* 2003; **14**: 233–9.

9. Gangarosa EJ, Galazka AM, Wolfe CR, Phillips LM, Gangarosa RE, Miller E *et al.* Impact of anti-vaccine movements on pertussis control: the untold story. *Lancet* 1998; **351**: 356–61.

10. Orenstein WA. DTP vaccine litigation, 1988. *Am J Dis Child* 1990; **144**: 517.

11. Institute of Medicine. Liability for the production and sale of vaccine. In: Sanford JP, ed., *Vaccine Supply and Innovation*. Washington, DC: National Academy Press, 1985; pp. 85–122.

12. Ball LK, Ball R, Pratt RD. An assessment of thimerosal use in childhood vaccines. *Pediatrics* 2001; **107**: 1147–54.

13. Verstraeten T, Davis RL, DeStefano F, Lieu TA, Rhodes PH, Black SB *et al.* Safety of thimerosal-containing vaccines: a two-phased study of computerized health maintenance organization databases. *Pediatrics* 2003; **112**: 1039–48.

14. Joellenbeck LM, Zwanziger LL, Durch JS, Strom BL, eds., Committee to Assess the Safety and Efficacy of the Anthrax Vaccine. *The Anthrax Vaccine: Is it safe? Does it work?* Washington, DC: National Academy Press, 2002.

15. Chen RT, Lane JM. Myocarditis: the unexpected return of smallpox vaccine adverse events. *Lancet* 2003; **362**: 1345–6.

16. Halsell JS, Riddle JR, Atwood JE, Gardner P, Shope R, Poland GA *et al.* Myopericarditis following smallpox vaccination among vaccinia-naive US military personnel. *JAMA* 2003; **289**: 3283–9.

17. Spooner MH. Measles outbreak in UK linked to fears about MMR vaccine. *CMAJ* 2002; **166**: 1075.

18. Balinska MA. L'affaire hepatite B en France. *Espirit* 2001; **276**: 34–48.

19. Howson CP, Howe CJ, Fineberg HV, eds, *Adverse Effects of Pertussis and Rubella Vaccines: A Report of the Committee to Review the Adverse Consequences of Pertussis and Rubella Vaccines*. Washington, DC: National Academy Press, 1991.

20. Stratton KR, Howe CJ, Johnston RB, eds, *Adverse Events Associated with Childhood Vaccines: Evidence Bearing on Causality*. Washington, DC: National Academy Press, 1994.

21. Miller E, Waight P, Farrington P. Safety assessment post-licensure. *Dev Biol Stand* 1998; **95**: 235–43.

22. Johnston RB Jr. Do vaccines cause harm? The need for open-minded analysis based on science and reason. *Adv Pediatr* 2003; **50**: 231–44.

23. Stratton K, Gable A, McCormick M, eds, Immunization Safety Review Committee. *Immunization Safety Review: Thimerosal–Containing Vaccines and Neurodevelopmental Disorders*. Washington, DC: National Academy Press, 2001.

24. Stratton K, Gable A, Shetty PMM, eds, Immunization Safety Review Committee. *Immunization Safety Review: Measles–Mumps–Rubella Vaccine and Autism*. Washington, DC: National Academy Press, 2001.

25. Stratton K, Wilson CB, McCormick M, eds, Immunization Safety Review Committee. *Immunization Safety Review: Multiple Immunizations and Immune Dysfunction*. Washington, DC: National Academy Press; 2002.

26. Stratton K, McCormick M, eds, Immunization Safety Review Committee. *Immunization Safety Review: SV40 Contamination of Polio Vaccine and Cancer*. Washington, DC: National Academy Press, 2002.

27. Stratton K, Almario D, McCormick M, eds, Immunization Safety Review Committee. *Immunization Safety Review: Hepatitis B Vaccine and Demyelinating Neurological Disorders*. Washington, DC: National Academy Press, 2002.

28. Stratton K, Almario DA, Wizeman TM, McCormick MC, eds, Immunization Safety Review Committee. *Immunization Safety Review: Vaccinations and Sudden Unexpected Death in Infancy*. Washington, DC: National Academy Press, 2003.

29. Stratton K, Almario DA, Wizeman TM, McCormick MC, eds, Immunization Safety Review Committee. *Immunization Safety Review: Influenza Vaccines and Neurological Complications*. Washington, DC: National Academy Press, 2003.

30. Baylor NW, Midthun K. Regulation and testing of vaccines. In: Plotkin S, Orenstein WA, eds, *Vaccines*, 4th edn. Philadelphia, PA: W.B. Saunders, 2003; pp. 1539–81.

31. Ellis RW. Technologies for making new vaccines. In: Plotkin S, Orenstein WA, eds, *Vaccines*, 4th edn. Philadelphia, PA: W.B. Saunders, 2003; pp. 1177–97.

32. Offit PA, Jew RK. Addressing parents' concerns: do vaccines contain harmful preservatives, adjuvants, additives, or residuals? *Pediatrics* 2003; **112**: 1394–7.

33. Hutin YJ, Hauri AM, Armstrong GL. Use of injections in healthcare settings worldwide, 2000: literature review and regional estimates. *BMJ* 2003; **327**: 1075.

34. Dziekan G, Chisholm D, Johns B, Rovira J, Hutin YJ. The cost-effectiveness of policies for the safe and appropriate use of injection in healthcare settings. *Bull World Health Organ* 2003; **81**: 277–85.

35. Miller D, Wadsworth J, Diamond J, Ross E. Pertussis vaccine and whooping cough as risk factors in acute neurologic illness and deaths in young children. *Dev Biol Stand* 1985; **61**: 389–94.

36. Schonberger LB, Bregman DJ, Sullivan-Bolyai JZ, Keenlyside RA, Ziegler DW, Retailliau HF *et al.* Guillain–Barre syndrome following vaccination in the National Influenza Immunization Program, United States, 1976–1977. *Am J Epidemiol* 1979; **110**: 105–23.

37. Centers for Disease Control and Prevention. Poliomyelitis prevention in the United States: introduction of a sequential vaccination schedule of inactivated poliovirus vaccine followed by oral poliovirus vaccine. Recommendations of the Advisory Committee on Immunization Practices (ACIP). *MMWR Morb Mortal Wkly Rep* 1997; **46**: 1–25.

38. McGoldrick MD, Bailie GR. Nonnarcotic analgesics: prevalence and estimated economic impact of toxicities. *Ann Pharmacother* 1997; **31**: 221–7.

39. Marcuse EK, Wentz KR. The NCES reconsidered: summary of a 1989 workshop. National Childhood Encephalopathy Study. *Vaccine* 1990; **8**: 531–5.

40. Alderslade R, Bellman MH, Rawson NSB, Ross EM, Miller DL. The National Childhood Encephalopathy Study. In: *Whooping Cough: Reports from the Committee on the Safety of Medicines and the Joint Committee on Vaccination and Immunisation*. Department of Health and Social Security. London: HM Stationery Office, 1981; pp. 79–169.

41. Wentz KR, Marcuse EK. Diphtheria–tetanus–pertussis vaccine and serious neurologic illness: an updated review of the epidemiologic evidence. *Pediatrics* 1991; **87**: 287–97.

42. Neustadt RE, Fineberg HV. *The Swine Flu Affair: Decision-Making on a Slippery Disease*. Washington, DC: US Government Printing Office, 1978.

43. Kurland LT, Wiederholt WC, Kirkpatrick JW, Potter HG, Armstrong P. Swine influenza vaccine and Guillain–Barre syndrome. Epidemic or artifact? *Arch Neurol* 1985; **42**: 1089–90.

44. Langmuir AD, Bregman DJ, Kurland LT, Nathanson N, Victor M. An epidemiologic and clinical evaluation of Guillain–Barre syndrome reported in association with the administration of swine influenza vaccines. *Am J Epidemiol* 1984; **119**: 841–79.

45. Safranek TJ, Lawrence DN, Kurland LT, Culver DH, Wiederholt WC, Hayner NS *et al.* Reassessment of the association between Guillain–Barre syndrome and receipt of swine influenza vaccine in 1976–1977: results of a two-state study. Expert Neurology Group. *Am J Epidemiol* 1991; **133**: 940–951.

46. Murphy TV, Gargiullo PM, Massoudi MS, Nelson DB, Jumaan AO, Okoro CA *et al.* Intussusception among infants given an oral rotavirus vaccine. *N Engl J Med* 2001; **344**: 564–72.

47. Kramarz P, France EK, DeStefano F, Black SB, Shinefield H, Ward JI *et al.* Population-based study of rotavirus vaccination and intussusception. *Pediatr Infect Dis J* 2001; **20**: 410–16.

48. Simonsen L, Morens D, Elixhauser A, Gerber M, Van Raden M, Blackwelder W. Effect of rotavirus vaccination programme on trends in admission of infants to hospital for intussusception. *Lancet* 2001; **358**: 1224–9.

49. Hall AJ. Ecological studies and debate on rotavirus vaccine and intussusception. *Lancet* 2001; **358**: 1197–8.

50. Murphy TV, Gargiullo PM, Wharton M. More on rotavirus vaccination and intussusception. *N Engl J Med* 2002; **346**: 211–12.

51. Schumacher W. Legal/ethical aspects of vaccinations. *Dev Biol Stand* 1979; **43**: 435–8.

52. Fine PE. Herd immunity: history, theory, practice. *Epidemiol Rev* 1993; **15**: 265–302.

53. Hardin G. The tragedy of the commons. *Science* 1968; **162**: 1243–8.

54. Fine PE, Clarkson JA. Individual versus public priorities in the determination of optimal vaccination policies. *Am J Epidemiol* 1986; **124**: 1012–20.

55. Nathanson N, Langmuir AD. The Cutter incident. Poliomyelitis following formaldehyde-inactivated poliovirus vaccination in the United States during the spring of 1955. I. Background. *Am J Hyg* 1963; **78**: 16–18.

56. Shah KV. Simian virus 40 and human disease. *J Infect Dis* 2004; **190**: 2061–4.

57. Food and Drug Administration. Bovine-derived materials: Agency letters to manufacturers of FDA-regulated products. *Fed Reg* 1994; **59**: 44591–4.

58. Milstien J, Dellepiane N, Lamert S, Belgharbi L, Rolls C, Knezevic I *et al.* Vaccine quality—can a single standard be defined? *Vaccine* 2002; **20**: 1000–3.

59. Centers for Disease Control and Prevention. Poliomyelitis prevention in the United States: updated recommendations of the Advisory Committee on Immunization Practices (ACIP). *MMWR Morb Mortal Wkly Rep* 2000; **49**: 1–25.

60. Anonymous. Two MMR vaccines withdrawn. *Lancet* 1992; **340**: 922.

61. Schmitt HJ, Just M, Neiss A. Withdrawal of a mumps vaccine: reasons and impacts. *Eur J Pediatr* 1993; **152**: 387–8.

62. Kimura M, Kuno-Sakai H, Yamazaki S, Yamada A, Hishiyama M, Kamiya H *et al.* Adverse events associated with MMR vaccines in Japan. *Acta Paediatr Jpn* 1996; **38**: 205–11.

63. Lathrop SL, Ball R, Haber P, Mootrey GT, Braun MM, Shadomy SV *et al.* Adverse event reports following vaccination for Lyme disease: December 1998–July 2000. *Vaccine* 2002; **20**: 1603–8.

64. Singleton JA, Lloyd JC, Mootrey GT, Salive ME, Chen RT. An overview of the vaccine adverse event reporting system (VAERS) as a surveillance system. *Vaccine* 1999; **17**: 2908–10.

65. Evans G. Vaccine injury compensation programs worldwide. *Vaccine* 1999; **17**(suppl 3): S25–35.

66. Evans G. Vaccine liability and safety: a progress report. *Pediatr Infect Dis J* 1996; **15**: 477–8.

67. Evans G, Harris D, Levine EM. Legal issues. In: Plotkin S, Orenstein WA, eds, *Vaccines*, 4th edn. Philadelphia, PA: W.B. Saunders, 2003; pp. 1591–617.

68. Centers for Disease Control and Prevention. Public Health Service recommendations on smallpox vaccination. *MMWR Morb Mortal Wkly Rep* 1971; **20**: 339–45.

69. Bottiger M. The elimination of polio in the Scandinavian countries. *Public Health Rev* 1993; **21**: 27–33.

70. Henderson DA. Countering the posteradication threat of smallpox and polio. *Clin Infect Dis* 2002; **34**: 79–83.

71. Farrington P, Pugh S, Colville A, Flower A, Nash J, Morgan-Capner P *et al.* A new method for active surveillance of adverse events from diphtheria/tetanus/pertussis and measles/mumps/rubella vaccines. *Lancet* 1995; **345**: 567–9.

72. Dourado I, Cunha S, Teixeira MG, Farrington CP, Melo A, Lucena R *et al.* Outbreak of aseptic meningitis associated with mass vaccination with a urabe-containing measles–mumps–rubella vaccine: implications for immunization programs. *Am J Epidemiol* 2000; **151**: 524–30.

73. Ki M, Park T, Yi SG, Oh JK, Choi B. Risk analysis of aseptic meningitis after measles–mumps–rubella vaccination in Korean children by using a case-crossover design. *Am J Epidemiol* 2003; **157**: 158–65.

74. Mutsch M, Zhou W, Rhodes P, Bopp M, Chen RT, Linder T *et al.* Use of the inactivated intranasal influenza vaccine and the risk of Bell's palsy in Switzerland. *N Engl J Med* 2004; **350**: 896–903.

75. Stetler HC, Orenstein WA, Bart KJ, Brink EW, Brennan JP, Hinman AR. History of convulsions and use of pertussis vaccine. *J Pediatr* 1985; **107**: 175–9.

76. Robbins JB, Pittman M, Trollfors B, Lagergard TA, Taranger J, Schneerson R. Primum non nocere: a pharmacologically inert pertussis toxoid alone should be the next pertussis vaccine. *Pediatr Infect Dis J* 1993; **12**: 795–807.

77. Brown EG, Dimock K, Wright KE. The Urabe AM9 mumps vaccine is a mixture of viruses differing at amino acid 335 of the hemagglutinin-neuraminidase gene with one form associated with disease. *J Infect Dis* 1996; **174**: 619–22.

78. Kew OM, Nottay BK. Molecular epidemiology of polioviruses. *Rev Infect Dis* 1984; **6**(suppl 2): S499–S504.

79. Plotkin SA, Rupprecht CE, Koprowski H. Rabies vaccine. In: Plotkin SA, Mortimer EA, eds, *Vaccines*, 4th edn. Philadelphia: W.B. Saunders, 2003; pp. 1011–38.

80. Mathieu M. *Biologics Development: A Regulatory Overview*, 4th edn. Waltham, MA: Parexel, 2004.

81. Decker MD, Edwards KM, Steinhoff MC, Rennels MB, Pichichero ME, England JA *et al.* Comparison of 13 acellular pertussis vaccines adverse reactions. *Pediatrics* 1995; **96**: 557–66.

82. Rosenthal KL, McVittie LD. The clinical testing of preventive vaccines. In: Mathieu M, ed., *Biologics Development: A Regulatory Overview*. Waltham, MA: Parexel, 1993; pp. 119–30.

83. Pinichiero ME. Acellular pertussis vaccine: towards an improved safety profile. *Drug Experience* 1996; **15**: 311–24.

84. Francis T, Korns R, Voight R. An evaluation of the 1954 poliomyelitis vaccine trials: summary report. *Am J Public Health* 1955; **45**: 1–63.

85. Eskola J, Kayhty H, Takala A. A randomized, prospective field trial of a conjugate vaccine in the protection of infants and young children against invasive *Haemophilus influenzae type b* disease. *N Engl J Med* 1990; **323**: 1381–7.

86. Black SB, Shinefield HR, Lampert D, Fireman B, Hiatt RA, Polen M *et al.* Safety and immunogenicity of oligosaccharide conjugate *Haemophilus influenzae type b* (HbOC) vaccine in infancy. The Northern California Kaiser Permanente Vaccine Study Center Pediatrics Group. *Pediatr Infect Dis J* 1991; **10**: 92–6.

87. Chen RT. Safety of acellular pertussis vaccine: follow-up studies. *Dev Biol Stand* 1997; **89**: 373–5.

88. Bonhoeffer J, Kohl K, Chen R, Duclos P, Heijbel H, Heininger U *et al.* The Brighton Collaboration: addressing the need for standardized case definitions of adverse events following immunization (AEFI). *Vaccine* 2002; **21**: 298–302.

89. Heijbel H, Ciofi degli Atti MC, Harzer E, Liese J, Preziosi MP, Rasmussen F *et al.* Hypotonic hyporesponsive episodes in eight pertussis vaccine studies. *Dev Biol Stand* 1997; **89**: 101–3.

90. Fine PE, Chen RT. Confounding in studies of adverse reactions to vaccines. *Am J Epidemiol* 1992; **136**: 121–35.

91. Aaby P, Jensen H, Samb B, Cisse B, Sodemann M, Jakobsen M *et al.* Differences in female–male mortality after high-titre measles vaccine and association with subsequent vaccination with diphtheria–tetanus–pertussis and inactivated poliovirus: reanalysis of West African studies. *Lancet* 2003; **361**: 2183–8.

92. Hall AJ, Cutts FT. Lessons from measles vaccination in developing countries. *BMJ* 1993; **307**: 1294–5.

93. Cutts FT, Fine PE. Caution—mortality ratios ahead. *Lancet* 2003; **361**: 2169–70.

94. Zanoni G, DNTG. *Fourth Report on the Green Channel Activities and the Monitoring System of Reactions to Vaccines in the Veneto Region: Analysis of the Three Year Period 1997–1999, General Summary 1992–99.* University of Verona, Immunology Section, 2000.

95. Goodwin H, Nash M, Gold M, Heath TC, Burgess MA. Vaccination of children following a previous hypotonic–hyporesponsive episode. *J Paediatr Child Health* 1999; **35**: 549–52.

96. Gold MS. Hypotonic–hyporesponsive episodes following pertussis vaccination: a cause for concern? *Drug Saf* 2002; **25**: 85–90.

97. Baraff LJ, Cody CL, Cherry JD. DTP-associated reactions: an analysis by injection site, manufacturer, prior reactions, and dose. *Pediatrics* 1984; **73**: 31–6.

98. Baraff LJ, Manclark CR, Cherry JD, Christenson P, Marcy SM. Analyses of adverse reactions to diphtheria and tetanus toxoids and pertussis vaccine by vaccine lot, endotoxin content, pertussis vaccine potency and percentage of mouse weight gain. *Pediatr Infect Dis J* 1989; **8**: 502–7.

99. Centers for Disease Control and Prevention. Notice to readers: manufacturer's recall of human rabies vaccine—April 2, 2004. *MMWR Recomm Rep* 2004; **53**: 1–2.

100. Chen RT, Pool V, Takahashi H, Weniger BG, Patel B. Combination vaccines: postlicensure safety evaluation. *Clin Infect Dis* 2001; **33**(suppl 4): S327–33.

101. Wise RP, Kiminyo KP, Salive ME. Hair loss after routine immunizations. *JAMA* 1997; **278**: 1176–8.

102. Centers for Disease Control and Prevention. Intussusception among recipients of rotavirus vaccine—United States, 1998–1999. *MMWR Morb Mortal Wkly Rep* 1999; **48**: 577–81.

103. Chen RT. Surveillance for vaccine adverse events and public health disease: similarities and differences. *Pharmacoepidemiol Drug Saf* 1996; **5**: S45.

104. Division of Immunization. Vaccine-associated adverse events in Canada, 1992 Report. *Can Commun Dis Rep* 1995; **21**: 117–28.

105. Chen RT, Rastogi SC, Mullen JR, Hayes SW, Cochi SL, Donlon JA *et al.* The Vaccine Adverse Event Reporting System (VAERS). *Vaccine* 1994; **12**: 542–50.

106. Miller E, Goldacre M, Pugh S, Colville A, Farrington P, Flower A *et al.* Risk of aseptic meningitis after measles, mumps, and rubella vaccine in UK children. *Lancet* 1993; **341**: 979–82.

107. CDC. Vaccine Identification Standards Initiative. Available at: http://www.edc.gov/nip/visi/default.htm.

108. Halsey NA. An update on pediatric immunization. *Adv Pediatr Infect Dis* 1995; **10**: 187–225.

109. Chen RT, Kent JH, Rhodes PH, Simon P, Schonberger LS. Investigation of a possible association between influenza vaccination and Guillain–Barre syndrome in the United States, 1990–1991. *Post Marketing Surveillance* 1992; **6**: 5–6.

110. Lasky T, Terracciano GJ, Magder L, Koski CL, Ballesteros M, Nash D *et al*. The Guillain–Barre syndrome and the 1992–1993 and 1993–1994 influenza vaccines. *N Engl J Med* 1998; **339**: 1797–1802.

111. Miller D, Wadsworth J, Diamond J, Ross E. Pertussis vaccine and whooping cough as risk factors in acute neurological illness and death in young children. *Dev Biol Stand* 1985; **61**: 389–94.

112. Laboratory Centre for Disease Control. Report of the working group on the possible relationship between hepatitis B vaccination and the chronic fatigue syndrome. *Can Med Assoc J* 1993; **149**: 314–19.

113. Bernier RH, Frank JA Jr, Dondero TJ Jr, Turner P. Diphtheria–tetanus toxoids–pertussis vaccination and sudden infant deaths in Tennessee. *J Pediatr* 1982; **101**: 419–21.

114. Wakefield AJ, Murch SH, Anthony A, Linnell J, Casson DM, Malik M *et al*. Ileal-lymphoid-nodular hyperplasia, non-specific colitis, and pervasive developmental disorder in children. *Lancet* 1998; **351**: 637–41.

115. Thompson NP, Montgomery SM, Pounder RE, Wakefield AJ. Is measles vaccination a risk factor for inflammatory bowel disease? *Lancet* 1995; **345**: 1071–4.

116. Expanded Programme on Immunization. Lack of evidence that hepatitis B vaccine causes multiple sclerosis. *Wkly Epidemiol Rec* 1997; **72**: 149–56.

117. Mortimer EA, Jones P, Adelson L. DTP and SIDS [letter]. *Pediatr Infect Dis* 1983; **2**: 492–3.

118. Goodson BD. How will we know if thimerosal leads to neurodevelopmental problems? 38th National Immunization Conference, Nashville, TN, May 14, 2004.

119. Ray WA, Griffin MR. Re: "Confounding in studies of adverse reactions to vaccines". *Am J Epidemiol* 1994; **139**: 229–30.

120. Ellenberg SS. Safety considerations for new vaccine development. *Pharmacoepidemiol Drug Saf* 2001; **10**: 411–15.

121. Lesko SM, Mitchell AA. The safety of acetaminophen and ibuprofen among children younger than two years old. *Pediatrics* 1999; **104**: e39.

122. Glass RI, Bresee JS, Parashar UD, Jiang B, Gentsch J. The future of rotavirus vaccines: a major setback leads to new opportunities. *Lancet* 2004; **363**: 1547–50.

123. Cooper WO, Boyce TG, Wright PF, Griffin MR. Do childhood vaccines have non-specific effects on mortality? *Bull World Health Organ* 2003; **81**: 821–6.

124. Scott TF, Bonanno DE. Reactions to live-measles-virus vaccine in children previously inoculated with killed-virus vaccine. *N Engl J Med* 1967; **277**: 248–50.

125. Kristensen I, Aaby P, Jensen H. Routine vaccinations and child survival: follow up study in Guinea-Bissau, West Africa. *BMJ* 2000; **321**: 1435–8.

126. Bennett JV, Cutts FT, Katz SL. Edmonston–Zagreb measles vaccine: a good vaccine with an image problem. *Pediatrics* 1999; **104**: 1123–4.

127. Rennels MB. The rotavirus vaccine story: a clinical investigator's view. *Pediatrics* 2000; **106**: 123–5.

128. Rastogi SC, ed., *International Workshop: Harmonization of Reporting of Adverse Events Following Vaccination*. Rockville, MD: Food and Drug Administraion/CBER, 1993.

129. Wilholm B-E, Olsoon S, Moore N, Wood S. Spontaneous reporting systems outside the US. In: Strom BL, ed., *Pharmacoepidemiology*, 2nd edn. Chichester: John Wiley & Sons, 1994; pp. 139–55.

130. Jonville-Bera AP, Autret E, Galy-Eyraud C, Hessel L. Thrombocytopenic purpura after measles, mumps and rubella vaccination: a retrospective survey by the French regional pharmacovigilance centres and Pasteur-Merieux Serums et Vaccins. *Pediatr Infect Dis J* 1996; **15**: 44–8.

131. Takahashi H. Need for improved vaccine safety surveillance. *Vaccine* 2000; **19**: 1004.

132. Mansoor O, Pillans PI. Vaccine adverse events reported in New Zealand 1990–5. *N Z Med J* 1997; **110**: 270–2.

133. Taranger J, Holmberg K. Urgent to introduce countrywide and systematic evaluation of vaccine side effects. *Lakartidningen* 1992; **89**: 1691–3.

134. da Silveira CM, Salisbury DM, de Quadros CA. Measles vaccination and Guillain–Barre syndrome. *Lancet* 1997; **349**: 14–16.

135. Duclos P. Surveillance of secondary effects of vaccination. *Sante* 1994; **4**: 215–20.

136. Galindo Santana BM, Galindo Sardina MA, Perez RA. Adverse reaction surveillance system for vaccination in the Republic of Cuba. *Rev Cubana Med Trop* 1999; **51**: 194–200.

137. Andersen MM, Ronne T. Side-effects with Japanese encephalitis vaccine. *Lancet* 1991; **337**: 1044.

138. Sokhey J. Adverse events following immunization: 1990. *Indian Pediatr* 1991; **28**: 593–607.

139. Squarcione S, Vellucci L. Adverse reactions following immunization in Italy in the years 1991–93. *Ig Mod* 1996; **105**: 1419–31.

140. Fescharek R, Arras-Reiter C, Arens ER, Quast U, Maass G. [Oral vaccines against poliomyelitis and vaccination-related paralytic poliomyelitis in Germany. Do we need a new immunization strategy?] *Wien Med* 1997; **147**: 456–61 (in German).

141. Vermeer-de Bondt PE, Wesselo C, Dzaferagic A, Phaff TAJ. *Adverse Events Following Immunisation under the National Vaccination Programme of the Netherlands. Part VIII: Reports in 2001*. Bilthoven: RIVM, 2003.

142. Brito GS. *System of Investigation and Notification of Adverse Events Following Imunization*, preliminary report. Sao Paolo, Brazil: Health Department, 1991.

143. Sokhey J, Sarkars. Vaccines: quality issues. *J Indian Med Assoc* 2000; **98**: 22–3.

144. Duclos P, Hockin J, Pless R, Lawlor B. Reporting vaccine-associated adverse events. *Can Fam Physician* 1997; **43**: 1551–6.

145. Centers for Disease Control. National Childhood Vaccine Injury Act. Requirements for permanent vaccination records and for reporting of selected events after vaccination. *MMWR Morb Mortal Wkly Report* 1988; **37**: 197–200.

146. Haber P, Rashidee A, Zhou W, English R. Web-based Reporting: 10 months experience in the VAERS. *Pharmacoepidemiol Drug Saf* 2003; **12**: S1–S189.

147. Centers for Disease Control and Prevention. Smallpox vaccine adverse events monitoring and response system for the first stage of the smallpox vaccination program. *MMWR Morb Mort Wkly Rep* 2003; **52**: 88–9, 99.

148. Rashidee AH, Chen RT, Lugg M, Black S. Integrating vaccine safety initiatives in immunization registry/systems. *Pharmacoepidemiol Drug Saf* 2002; **11**: (suppl 1), S195.

149. Zanardi LR, Haber P, Mootrey GT, Niu MT, Wharton M. Intussusception among recipients of rotavirus vaccine: reports to the vaccine adverse event reporting system. *Pediatrics* 2001; **107**: E97.

150. Centers for Disease Control and Prevention. Adverse events associated with 17D-derived yellow fever vaccination United States 2001–2002. *CDC Morb Mort Wkly Rep* 2002; pp. 989–93.

151. Centers for Disease Control and Prevention. Cardiac adverse events following smallpox vaccination—United States, 2003. *MMWR Morb Mort Wkly Rep* 2003; **52**: 248–50.

152. Centers for Disease Control and Prevention. Surveillance for adverse events associated with anthrax vaccination—U.S. Department of Defense, 1998–2000. *MMWR Morb Mort Wkly Rep* 2000; **49**: 341–5.

153. Zhou W, Pool V, Iskander JK, English-Bullard R, Ball R, Wise RP *et al.* Surveillance for safety after immunization: Vaccine Adverse Event Reporting System (VAERS)—United States, 1991–2001. *MMWR Surveill Summ* 2003; **52**: 1–24.

154. Food and Drug Administration. *COSTART—Coding Symbols for Thesaurus of Adverse Reaction Terms*, 3rd edn. Rockville, MD: FDA, 1989.

155. Brown EG, Wood L, Wood S. The Medical Dictionary for Regulatory Activities (MedDRA). *Drug Saf* 1999; **20**: 109–17.

156. Scheifele D, Duval B, De Serres G, Skowronski DM. Unique roles of a data and safety monitoring board in vaccine safety trials with compressed timelines and urgent implications. *Control Clin Trials* 2003; **24**: 99–104.

157. Collet JP, MacDonald N, Cashman N, Pless R. Monitoring signals for vaccine safety: the assessment of individual adverse event reports by an expert advisory committee. Advisory Committee on Causality Assessment. *Bull World Health Organ* 2000; **78**: 178–85.

158. *1996 Immunisation Against Infectious Disease*. London: HMSO, 1996.

159. Lindquist M, Edwards IR. The WHO Programme for International Drug Monitoring, its database, and the technical support of the Uppsala Monitoring Center. *J Rheumatol* 2001; **28**: 1180–7.

160. World Health Organization. *Surveillance of Adverse Events Following Immunization*, WHO/EPI/TRAM/93.02 Rev. 1. Geneva: WHO, 1997.

161. World Health Organization. Vaccine supply and quality: surveillance of adverse events following immunization. *Weekly Epidemiology Rec* 1996; **71**: 237–42.

162. Fenichel GM, Lane DA, Livengood JR, Horwitz SJ, Menkes JH, Schwartz JF. Adverse events following immunization: assessing probability of causation. *Pediatr Neurol* 1989; **5**: 287–90.

163. Wassilak SGF, Sokhey J. *Monitoring of Adverse Events Following Immunization in the Expanded Programme on Immunization*. 91.2, 1-29. Geneva: World Health Organization/EPI/GEN, 1991.

164. Goodman M, Lamm SH, Bellman MH. Temporal relationship modeling: DTP or DT immunizations and infantile spasms. *Vaccine* 1998; **16**: 225–31.

165. Health Council of the Netherlands. Committee on Adverse Reactions to Vaccinations. *Adverse Reactions to Vaccines in the National Immunization Programme in 1993*, publication no. 1995/08E. The Hague: Health Council of the Netherlands, 1995.

166. Simonsen L, Kane A, Lloyd J, Zaffran M, Kane M. Unsafe injections in the developing world and transmission of blood-borne pathogens: a review. *Bull World Health Organ* 1999; **77**: 789–800.

167. Nathanson N, Langmuir AD. The Cutter incident. Poliomyelitis following formaldehyde-inactivated poliovirus vaccination in the United States during the spring of 1955. II. Relationship of poliomyelitis to Cutter vaccine. 1963. *Am J Epidemiol* 1995; **142**: 109–40.

168. *Proceedings of a Workshop on the Standardization of Definitions for Post-Marketing Surveillance of Adverse Vaccine Reactions*, Ottawa, Canada, October 30–31, 1991. Ottawa, Canada: Laboratory Centre for Disease Control, 1992.

169. Braun MM, Terracciano G, Salive ME, Blumberg DA, Vermeer-de Bondt PE, Heijbel H *et al.* Report of a US public health service workshop on hypotonic–hyporesponsive episode (HHE) after pertussis immunization. *Pediatrics* 1998; **102**: E52.

170. Ball R, Halsey N, Braun MM. Development of case definitions for acute encephalopathy, encephalitis, and multiple sclerosis reports to the Vaccine Adverse Reporting System. *J Clin Epidemiol* 2002; **55**: 821–30.

171. Food and Drug Administration. International Conference on Harmonisation: Guideline on clinical safety data management: Periodic safety update reports for marketed drugs. *Fed Reg* 1997; **62**: 27470–6.

172. Kohl K, Bonhoeffer J, Chen R. The Brighton Collaboration: enhancing comparability of vaccine safety data. *Pharmacoepidemiol Drug Saf* 2003; **12**: 335–40.

173. Chen RT. Evaluation of vaccine safety after the events of 11 September 2001: role of cohort and case–control studies. *Vaccine* 2004; **22**: 2047–53.

174. Phillips KA, Veenstra DL, Oren E, Lee JK, Sadee W. Potential role of pharmacogenomics in reducing adverse drug reactions: a systematic review. *JAMA* 2001; **286**: 2270–9.

175. Sim I, Sanders GD, McDonald KM. Evidence-based practice for mere mortals: the role of informatics and health services research. *J Gen Intern Med* 2002; **17**: 302–8.

176. Rennels MB. Extensive swelling reactions occurring after booster doses of diphtheria–tetanus–acellular pertussis vaccines. *Semin Pediatr Infect Dis* 2003; **14**: 196–198.

177. Kramer MS, Lane DA. Causal propositions in clinical research and practice. *J Clin Epidemiol* 1992; **45**: 639–49.

178. Hill AB. The environment and disease: association or causation. *Proc Roy Soc Med* 1965; **58**: 295–300.

179. Kramer MS. Difficulties in assessing the adverse effects of drugs. *Br J Clin Pharmacol* 1981; **11**: 105–10.

180. Jones JK. Determining causation from case reports. In: Strom BL, ed., *Pharmacoepidemiology*, 3rd edn. Chichester: John Wiley & Sons, 2000; pp. 525–38.

181. Edsall G, Elliott MW, Peebles TC, Eldred MC. Excessive use of tetanus toxoid boosters. *JAMA* 1967; **202**: 111–13.

182. Henderson DA, Witte JJ, Morris L *et al.* Paralytic disease associated with oral polio vaccines. *JAMA* 1964; **190**: 153–60.

183. Centers for Disease Control and Prevention. Rubella vaccination during pregnancy—United States, 1971–1988. *MMWR Morb Mort Wkly Rep* 1989; **38**: 289–93.

184. Chen RT, Glasser JW, Rhodes PH, Davis RL, Barlow WE, Thompson RS *et al.* Vaccine Safety Datalink project: a new tool for improving vaccine safety monitoring in the United States. The Vaccine Safety Datalink Team. *Pediatrics* 1997; **99**: 765–73.

185. Cherry JD. Pertussis and the vaccine controversy. In: Roote RK, Griffiss JM, Warren KS *et al.*, eds, *Immunization*. New York: Churchill Livingstone, 1989; pp. 47–63.

186. Lane DA. A probabilist's view of causality assessment. *Drug Inform J* 1984; **18**: 323–30.

187. Venuiet J, Berneker G-C, Ciucci AG. *Assessing Causes of Adverse Drug Reactions with Special Reference to Standardized Methods*. London: Academic Press, 1982.

188. Lane DA, Kramer MS, Hutchinson TA *et al.* The causality assessment of adverse drug reactions using a Bayesian approach. *Pharmaceut Med* 1987; **2**: 265–83.

189. Finney DJ. The detection of adverse reactions to therapeutic drugs. *Stat Med* 1982; **1**: 153–61.

190. Retailliau HF, Curtis AC, Storr G, Caesar G, Eddins DL, Hattwick MA. Illness after influenza vaccination reported through a nationwide surveillance system, 1976–1977. *Am J Epidemiol* 1980; **111**: 270–8.

191. Bate A, Lindquist M, Edwards IR, Olsson S, Orre R, Lansner A *et al.* A Bayesian neural network method for adverse drug reaction signal generation. *Eur J Clin Pharmacol* 1998; **54**: 315–21.

192. Wallenstein S, Gould MS, Kleinman M. Use of the scan statistic to detect time–space clustering. *Am J Epidemiol* 1989; **130**: 1057–64.

193. Martin M, Tsai TF, Cropp B, Chang GJ, Holmes DA, Tseng J *et al.* Fever and multisystem organ failure associated with 17D-204 yellow fever vaccination: a report of four cases. *Lancet* 2001; **358**: 98–104.

194. Martin M, Weld LH, Tsai TF, Mootrey GT, Chen RT, Niu M *et al.* Advanced age a risk factor for illness temporally associated with yellow fever vaccination. *Emerg Infect Dis* 2001; **7**: 945–51.

195. Chan RC, Penney DJ, Little D, Carter IW, Roberts JA, Rawlinson WD. Hepatitis and death following vaccination with 17D-204 yellow fever vaccine. *Lancet* 2001; **358**: 121–2.

196. Skowronski DM, Strauss B, De Serres G, MacDonald D, Marion SA, Naus M *et al.* Oculo-respiratory syndrome: a new influenza vaccine-associated adverse event? *Clin Infect Dis* 2003; **36**: 705–13.

197. Carson JL, Strom BL, Maislin G. Screening for unknown effects of newly marketed drugs. In: Stom BL, ed., *Pharmacoepidemiology*, 2nd edn. Chichester: John Wiley & Sons, 1994; pp. 431–47.

198. Walker AM. Pattern recognition in health insurance claims databases. *Pharmacoepidemiol Drug Saf* 2001; **10**: 393–7.

199. Ball R. Methods for ensuring vaccine safety. *Expert Rev Vaccines* 2002; **1**: 161–8.

200. Zhou W, Pool V, DeStefano F, Iskander JK, Haber P, Chen RT. A potential signal of Bell's palsy after parenteral inactivated influenza vaccines: reports to the Vaccine Adverse Event Reporting System (VAERS) US 1991–2001. *Pharmacoepidemiol Drug Saf* 2004; **13**: 505–510.

201. Haber P, Iskander J, English-Bullard R. Use of proportional reporting rate ratio in monitoring vaccine adverse event reports. *Pharmacoepidemiol Drug Saf* 2002; **11**: S229.

202. Pool V, Chen RT. Association rule discovery as a signal generation tool for the Vaccine Adverse Event Reporting System. *Pharmacoepidemiol Drug Saf* 2003; **11**: S57.

203. Niu MT, Erwin DE, Braun MM. Data mining in the US Vaccine Adverse Event Reporting System (VAERS): early detection of intussusception and other events after rotavirus vaccination. *Vaccine* 2001; **19**: 4627–34.

204. Banks D, Woo EJ, Burwen D, Perucci P, Braun MM, Ball R. Comparison of 4 data mining methods in the US Vaccine Adverse Event Reporting System (VAERS). *Pharmacoepidemiol Drug Saf* 2003; **12**: S138.

205. Rosenthal S, Chen R, Hadler S. The safety of acellular pertussis vaccine vs whole-cell pertussis vaccine. A postmarketing assessment. *Arch Pediatr Adolesc Med* 1996; **150**: 457–60.

206. Finney DJ. The design and logic of a monitor of drug use. *J Chronic Dis* 1965; **18**: 77–98.

207. Evans SJ, Waller PC, Davis S. Use of proportional reporting ratios (PRRs) for signal generation from spontaneous adverse drug reaction reports. *Pharmacoepidemiol Drug Saf* 2001; **10**: 483–6.

208. van Puijenbroek EP, Bate A, Leufkens HG, Lindquist M, Orre R, Egberts AC. A comparison of measures of disproportionality for signal detection in spontaneous reporting systems for adverse drug reactions. *Pharmacoepidemiol Drug Saf* 2002; **11**: 3–10.

209. Davis RL, Kolczak M, Lewis E, Nordin J, Goodman M, Shay DK, Platt R, Black S, Shinefield H, Chen RT. Active

surveillance of vaccine safety: a system to detect early signs of adverse events. *Epidemiology* 2005; **16**: 336–41.

210. Uhari M, Rantala H, Niemela M. Cluster of childhood Guillain–Barre cases after an oral poliovaccine campaign. *Lancet* 1989; **2**: 440–1.

211. Berg SW, Mitchell BS, Hanson RK, Olafson RP, Williams RP, Tueller JE *et al.* Systemic reactions in U.S. Marine Corps personnel who received Japanese encephalitis vaccine. *Clin Infect Dis* 1997; **24**: 265–6.

212. Kilroy AW, Schaffner W, Fleet WF Jr, Lefkowitz LB Jr, Karzon DT, Fenichel GM. Two syndromes following rubella immunization. Clinical observations and epidemiological studies. *JAMA* 1970; **214**: 2287–92.

213. Yergeau A, Alain L, Pless R, Robert Y. Adverse events temporally associated with meningococcal vaccines. *Can Med Assoc J* 1996; **1154**: 503–7.

214. Rantala H, Cherry JD, Shields WD, Uhari M. Epidemiology of Guillain–Barre syndrome in children: relationship of oral polio vaccine administration to occurrence. *J Pediatr* 1994; **124**: 220–3.

215. Braun MM, Ellenberg SS. Descriptive epidemiology of adverse events after immunization: reports to the Vaccine Adverse Event Reporting System (VAERS), 1991–1994. *J Pediatr* 1997; **131**: 529–35.

216. Singleton JA, Lloyd JC, Mootrey GT, Salive ME, Chen RT. An overview of the vaccine adverse event reporting system (VAERS) as a surveillance system. VAERS Working Group. *Vaccine* 1999; **17**: 2908–17.

217. Varricchio F, Iskander J, DeStefano F, Pless R, Braun MM, Chen RT. Understanding vaccine safety information from the Vaccine Adverse Event Reporting System. *Pediatr Infect Dis J* 2004; **23**: 287–94.

218. Beeler J, Varricchio F, Wise R. Thrombocytopenia after immunization with measles vaccines: review of the vaccine adverse events reporting system (1990 to 1994). *Pediatr Infect Dis J* 1996; **15**: 88–90.

219. Pool V, Braun MM, Kelso JM, Mootrey G, Chen RT, Yunginger JW *et al.* US Vaccine Adverse Event Reporting System. Prevalence of anti-gelatin IgE antibodies in people with anaphylaxis after measles–mumps–rubella vaccine in the United States. *Pediatrics* 2002; **110**: e71.

220. Braun MM, Patriarca PA, Ellenberg SS. Syncope after immunization. *Arch Pediatr Adolesc Med* 1997; **151**: 255–9.

221. Haber P, Chen RT, Zanardi LR, Mootrey GT, English R, Braun MM. An analysis of rotavirus vaccine reports to the Vaccine Adverse Event Reporting System: more than intussusception alone? *Pediatrics* 2004; **113**: e353–9.

222. Wise RP, Salive ME, Braun MM, Mootrey GT, Seward JF, Rider LG *et al.* Postlicensure safety surveillance for varicella vaccine. *JAMA* 2000; **284**: 1271–9.

223. Rastogi SC, Wise RP. Exploring associations between vaccine lot potencies and human safety experience. *Pharmacoepidemiol Drug Saf* 1996; **5**: S75.

224. Ellenberg SS, Chen RT. The complicated task of monitoring vaccine safety. *Public Health Rep* 1997; **112**: 10–20.

225. Dayan G, Iskander JK, English-Bullard R, Glasser J, Chen RT. Tracking the lifecycle of vaccines and vaccine lots via the Vaccine Adverse Event Reporting System (VAERS). *Pharmacoepidemiol Drug Saf* 2002; **11**(suppl 1): S117.

226. Verstraeten T, Baughman AL, Cadwell B, Zanardi L, Haber P, Chen RT. Enhancing vaccine safety surveillance: a capture–recapture analysis of intussusception after rotavirus vaccination. *Am J Epidemiol* 2001; **154**: 1006–12.

227. Rosenthal S, Chen R. The reporting sensitivities of two passive surveillance systems for vaccine adverse events. *Am J Public Health* 1995; **85**: 1706–9.

228. Lloyd JC, Chen RT. The Urabe mumps vaccine: lessons in adverse event surveillance and response. *Pharmacoepidemiol Drug Saf* 1996; **5**: S45.

229. Niu MT, Rhodes P, Salive M, Lively T, Davis DM, Black S *et al.* Comparative safety of two recombinant hepatitis B vaccines in children: data from the Vaccine Adverse Event Reporting System (VAERS) and Vaccine Safety Datalink (VSD). *J Clin Epidemiol* 1998; **51**: 503–10.

230. Food and Drug Administration. Postmarketing expedited adverse experience reporting for human drug and licensed biological products; increased frequency reports. *Fed Reg* 1997; **62**: 34166–8.

231. Begg NT, Gill ON, White JM. COVER (cover of vaccination evaluated rapidly): description of the England and Wales scheme. *Public Health* 1989; **103**: 81–9.

232. Freeman VA, DeFriese GH. The challenge and potential of childhood immunization registries. *Annu Rev Public Health* 2003; **24**: 227–46.

233. Chen RT, Orenstein WA. Epidemiologic methods in immunization programs. *Epidemiol Rev* 1996; **18**: 99–117.

234. Patriarca PA, Laender F, Palmeira G, Oliveira MJ, Lima FJ, Dantes MC *et al.* Randomised trial of alternative formulations of oral poliovaccine in Brazil. *Lancet* 1988; **1**: 429–33.

235. Bhargava I, Chhaparwal BC, Phadke MA, Irani SF, Chakladhar BK, Maheshwari CP. Reactogenecity of indigenously produced measles vaccine. *Indian Pediatr* 1996; **33**: 827–31.

236. Orenstein WA, Markowitz L, Preblud SR, Hinman AR, Tomasi A, Bart KJ. Appropriate age for measles vaccination in the United States. *Dev Biol Stand* 1986; **65**: 13–21.

237. Booy R, Taylor SA, Dobson SR, Isaacs D, Sleight G, Aitken S *et al.* Immunogenicity and safety of PRP-T conjugate vaccine given according to the British accelerated immunisation schedule. *Arch Dis Child* 1992; **67**: 475–8.

238. Deforest A, Long SS, Lischner HW, Girone JA, Clark JL, Srinivasan R *et al.* Simultaneous administration of measles–mumps–rubella vaccine with booster doses of diphtheria–tetanus–pertussis and poliovirus vaccines. *Pediatrics* 1988; **81**: 237–46.

239. Scheifele D, Law B, Mitchell L, Ochnio J. Study of booster doses of two *Haemophilus influenzae* type b conjugate vaccines including their interchangeability. *Vaccine* 1996; **14**: 1399–1406.

240. Garenne M, Leroy O, Beau JP, Sene I. Child mortality after high-titre measles vaccines: prospective study in Senegal. *Lancet* 1991; **338**: 903–7.

241. Aaby P, Samb B, Simondon F, Knudsen K, Seck AM, Bennett J et al. A comparison of vaccine efficacy and mortality during routine use of high-titre Edmonston–Zagreb and Schwarz standard measles vaccines in rural Senegal. *Trans R Soc Trop Med Hyg* 1996; **90**: 326–30.

242. Expanded programme on immunization (EPI). Safety of high titer measles vaccines. *Wkly Epidemiol Rec* 1992; **67**: 357–61.

243. Black SB, Shinefield HR. b-CAPSA I *Haemophilus influenzae*, type b, capsular polysaccharide vaccine safety. *Pediatrics* 1987; **79**: 321–5.

244. Meekison W, Hutcheon M, Guasparini R. Post-marketing surveillance of adverse events following PROHIBIT vaccine in British Columbia. *Can Dis Wkly Rep* 1989; **15**: 143–5.

245. Vadheim CM, Greenberg DP, Marcy SM, Froeschle J, Ward JI. Safety evaluation of PRP-D *Haemophilus influenzae* type b conjugate vaccine in children immunized at 18 months of age and older: follow-up study of 30000 children. *Pediatr Infect Dis J* 1990; **9**: 555–61.

246. Centers for Disease Control and Prevention. Unintentional administration of varicella virus vaccine—United States, 1996. *MMWR Morb Mort Wkly Rep* 1996; **45**: 1017–18.

247. Black S, Shinefield H, Ray P, Lewis E, Hansen J, Schwalbe J et al. Postmarketing evaluation of the safety and effectiveness of varicella vaccine. *Pediatr Infect Dis J* 1999; **18**: 1041–6.

248. Centers for Disease Control and Prevention. Inactivated Japanese encephalitis virus vaccine. Recommendations of the Advisory Committee on Immunization Practices (ACIP). *MMWR Morb Mort Wkly Rep* 1993; **42**: 1–15.

249. Liu ZL, Hennessy S, Strom BL, Tsai TF, Wan CM, Tang SC et al. Short-term safety of live attenuated Japanese encephalitis vaccine (SA14–14–2): results of a randomized trial with 26,239 subjects. *J Infect Dis* 1997; **176**: 1366–9.

250. Heijbel H, Chen RT, Dahlquist G. Cumulative incidence of childhood-onset IDDM is unaffected by pertussis immunization. *Diabetes Care* 1997; **20**: 173–5.

251. Solberg LK. *DTP Vaccination, Visit to Child Health Center and Sudden Infant Death Syndrome (SIDS): Evaluation of DTP Vaccination*. Report to the Oslo Health Council 1985. Besthesda, MD: NIH Library Translation, 1985; pp. 85–152.

252. Bouvier-Colle MH, Flahaut A, Messiah A, Jougla E, Hatton F. Sudden infant death and immunization: an extensive epidemiological approach to the problem in France—winter 1986. *Int J Epidemiol* 1989; **18**: 121–6.

253. Mitchell EA, Stewart AW, Clements M. Immunisation and the sudden infant death syndrome. New Zealand Cot Death Study Group. *Arch Dis Child* 1995; **73**: 498–501.

254. Gale JL, Thapa PB, Wassilak SG, Bobo JK, Mendelman PM, Foy HM. Risk of serious acute neurological illness after immunization with diphtheria–tetanus–pertussis vaccine. A population-based case-control study. *JAMA* 1994; **271**: 37–41.

255. Fullerton KE, Reef SE. Commentary: Ongoing debate over the safety of the different mumps vaccine strains impacts mumps disease control. *Int J Epidemiol* 2002; **31**: 983.

256. Simon PA, Chen RT, Elliott JA, Schwartz B. Outbreak of pyogenic abscesses after diphtheria and tetanus toxoids and pertussis vaccination. *Pediatr Infect Dis J* 1993; **12**: 368–71.

257. Walker AM, Jick H, Perera DR, Thompson RS, Knauss TA. Diphtheria–tetanus–pertussis immunization and sudden infant death syndrome. *Am J Public Health* 1987; **77**: 945–51.

258. Griffin MR, Ray WA, Livengood JR, Schaffner W. Risk of sudden infant death syndrome after immunization with the diphtheria–tetanus–pertussis vaccine. *N Engl J Med* 1988; **319**: 618–23.

259. DeStefano F. The Vaccine Safety Datalink project. *Pharmacoepidemiol Drug Saf* 2001; **10**: 403–6.

260. Verstraeten T, DeStefano F, Chen RT, Miller E. Vaccine safety surveillance using large linked databases: opportunities, hazards and proposed precautionary measures. *Expert Rev Vaccines.* 2003; **2**: 21–9.

261. Ray P, Black S, Shinefield H, Dillon A, Schwalbe J, Holmes S et al. Risk of chronic arthropathy among women after rubella vaccination. Vaccine Safety Datalink Team. *JAMA* 1997; **278**: 551–6.

262. Davis RL, Marcuse E, Black S, Shinefield H, Givens B, Schwalbe J et al. MMR2 immunization at 4 to 5 years and 10 to 12 years of age: a comparison of adverse clinical events after immunization in the Vaccine Safety Datalink project. The Vaccine Safety Datalink Team. *Pediatrics* 1997; **100**: 767–71.

263. Williams JC, ed, *Combined Vaccines and Simultaneous Administration: Current Issues and Perspective.* New York, NY: Academy of Sciences, 1995.

264. Hinman AR, Rodewald LE, Orenstein WA. Immunizations in the United States. In: Plotkin SA, Orenstein WA, eds, *Vaccines*, 4th edn. Philadelphia, PA: W.B. Saunders, 2003; pp. 1357–86.

265. Niu MT, Salive ME, Ellenberg SS. Neonatal deaths after hepatitis B vaccine: the vaccine adverse event reporting system, 1991–1998. *Arch Pediatr Adolesc Med* 1999; **153**: 1279–82.

266. Griffin MR, Ray WA, Mortimer EA, Fenichel GM, Schaffner W. Risk of seizures and encephalopathy after immunization with the diphtheria–tetanus–pertussis vaccine. *JAMA* 1990; **263**: 1641–5.

267. Rothman KJ. *Causal Inference*. Chestnut Hill, MA: Epidemiology Resources, 1988.

268. Andrews N, Miller E, Waight P, Farrington P, Crowcroft N, Stowe J et al. Does oral polio vaccine cause intussusception in infants? Evidence from a sequence of three self-controlled cases series studies in the United Kingdom. *Eur J Epidemiol* 2001; **17**: 701–6.

269. Kaye JA, Mar Melero-Montes M, Jick H. Mumps, measles, and rubella vaccine and the incidence of autism recorded by general practitioners: a time trend analysis. *BMJ* 2001; **322**: 460–3.

270. Roberts JD, Roos LL, Poffenroth LA, Hassard TH, Bebchuk JD, Carter AO et al. Surveillance of vaccine-related adverse events in the first year of life: a Manitoba cohort study. *J Clin Epidemiol* 1996; **49**: 51–8.

271. Ali M, Canh DG, Clemens JD, Park JK, von Seidlein L, Thiem VD *et al.* The vaccine data link in Nha Trang, Vietnam: a progress report on the implementation of a database to detect adverse events related to vaccinations. *Vaccine* 2003; **21**: 1681–6.

272. Griffin MR, Ray WA, Fought RL, Foster MA, Hays A, Schaffner W. Monitoring the safety of childhood immunizations: methods of linking and augmenting computerized data bases for epidemiologic studies. *Am J Prev Med* 1988; **4** (suppl 2): 5–13.

273. Mullooly J, Drew L, DeStefano F, Chen R, Okoro K, Swint E *et al.* Quality of HMO vaccination databases used to monitor childhood vaccine safety. Vaccine Safety DataLink Team. *Am J Epidemiol* 1999; **149**: 186–94.

274. Wilton R, Pennisi A. Evaluating the accuracy of transcribed computer-stored immunization data. *Pediatrics* 1994; **94**: 902–6.

275. Boulianne N, Hemon YA, Mawhinney T, Strong D, Gemmill I, Dobson S *et al.* National eligible, due, and overdue guidelines for immunization registries: draft recommendations from the Canadian Immunization Registry Network, Data Standards Task Group. *Can Commun Dis Rep* 2004; **30**: 53–9.

276. Hull BP, Lawrence GL, MacIntyre CR, McIntyre PB. Immunisation coverage in Australia corrected for under-reporting to the Australian Childhood Immunisation Register. *Aust N Z J Public Health* 2003; **27**: 533–8.

277. McMahon BJ, Helminiak C, Wainwright RB, Bulkow L, Trimble BA, Wainwright K. Frequency of adverse reactions to hepatitis B vaccine in 43,618 persons. *Am J Med* 1992; **92**: 254–6.

278. Street RL Jr. Information-giving in medical consultations: the influence of patients' communicative styles and personal characteristics. *Soc Sci Med* 1991; **32**: 541–8.

279. Walker AM, Jick H, Perera DR, Knauss TA, Thompson RS. Neurologic events following diphtheria–tetanus–pertussis immunization. *Pediatrics* 1988; **81**: 345–9.

280. DeStefano F, Verstraeten T, Jackson LA, Okoro CA, Benson P, Black SB *et al.* Vaccinations and risk of central nervous system demyelinating diseases in adults. *Arch Neurol* 2003; **60**: 504–9.

281. Ascherio A, Zhang SM, Hernan MA, Olek MJ, Coplan PM, Brodovicz K *et al.* Hepatitis B vaccination and the risk of multiple sclerosis. *N Engl J Med* 2001; **344**: 327–32.

282. Poser CM. Neurological complications of swine influenza vaccination. *Acta Neurol Scand* 1982; **66**: 413–31.

283. Hotopf M, David A, Hull L, Ismail K, Unwin C, Wessely S. Role of vaccinations as risk factors for ill health in veterans of the Gulf war: cross sectional study. *BMJ* 2000; **320**: 1363–7.

284. Maclure M. The case-crossover design: a method for studying transient effects on the risk of acute events. *Am J Epidemiol* 1991; **133**: 144–53.

285. Confavreux C, Suissa S, Saddier P, Bourdes V, Vukusic S. Vaccinations and the risk of relapse in multiple sclerosis. Vaccines in Multiple Sclerosis Study Group. *N Engl J Med* 2001; **344**: 319–26.

286. Farrington CP, Nash J, Miller E. Case series analysis of adverse reactions to vaccines: a comparative evaluation. *Am J Epidemiol* 1996; **143**: 1165–73.

287. Strom BL, Carson JL. Use of automated databases for pharmacoepidemiology research. *Epidemiol Rev* 1990; **12**: 87–107.

288. Gargiullo PM, Kramarz P, DeStefano F, Chen RT. Principles of epidemiological research on drug effects. *Lancet* 1999; **353**: 501.

289. Poland GA, Murray D, Bonilla-Guerrero R. New vaccine development. *BMJ* 2002; **324**: 1315–19.

290. Russo S, Turin L, Zanella A, Ponti W, Poli G. What's going on in vaccine technology? *Med Res Rev* 1997; **17**: 277–301.

291. Ward BJ. Vaccine adverse events in the new millennium: is there reason for concern? *Bull World Health Organ* 2000; **78**: 205–15.

292. Freed GL, Katz SL, Clark SJ. Safety of vaccinations. Miss America, the media, and public health. *JAMA* 1996; **276**: 1869–72.

293. Chen RT, DeStefano F, Davis RL, Jackson LA, Thompson RS, Mullooly JP *et al.* The Vaccine Safety Datalink: immunization research in health maintenance organizations in the USA. *Bull World Health Organ* 2000; **78**: 186–94.

294. Pless R, Casey CG, Chen RT. Improving the evaluation, management and understanding of adverse events possibly related to immunizations. Available at: http://www. partnersforimmunization.org/cisa.pdf. Accessed: April 1, 2004.

295. Zanoni G, Nguyen TM, Valsecchi M, Gallo G, Tridente G. Prevention and monitoring of adverse events following immunization: the "Green Channel" of the Veneto region in Italy. *Vaccine* 2003; **22**: 194–201.

296. WHO Vaccine Safety Advisory Committee. Vaccine safety. *Wkly Epidemiol Rec* 1999; **74**: 337–40.

297. Weldon D. Before The Institute of Medicine, February 9, 2004. Available at: http://www.iom.edu/includes/DBFile.asp?id=19029. Accessed: April 1, 2004.

298. Murch SH, Anthony A, Casson DH, Malik M, Berelowitz M, Dhillon AP *et al.* Retraction of an interpretation. *Lancet* 2004; **363**: 750.

299. Horton R. The lessons of MMR. *Lancet* 2004; **363**: 747–9.

300. Horton R. A statement by the editors of The Lancet. *Lancet* 2004; **363**: 820–1.

301. Rock A. Toxic tipping point. *Mother Jones* 2004; March/April: 70–7.

302. Gellin BG, Maibach EW, Marcuse EK. Do parents understand immunizations? A national telephone survey. *Pediatrics* 2000; **106**: 1097–102.

303. Slovic P. The risk game. *J Haz Materials* 2001; **86**: 17–24.

304. Salmon DA, Moulton LH, Halsey NA. Enhancing public confidence in vaccines through independent oversight of postlicensure vaccine safety. *Am J Public Health* 2004; **94**: 947–50.

305. National Transportation Safety Board. *We Are All Safer: NTSB-Inspired Improvements in Transportation Safety.* Washington, DC: NTSB, 1998.

306. Wood AJ, Stein CM, Woosley R. Making medicines safer—the need for an independent drug safety board. *N Engl J Med* 1998; **339**: 1851–4.

307. Committee on Quality of Health Care in America. Kohn LT, Corrigan JM, Donaldson MS, eds, *To Err Is Human: Building a Safer Health System*. Washington, DC: National Academy Press, 2000.

308. Pless RP, Bentsi-Enchill AD, Duclos P. Monitoring vaccine safety during measles mass immunization campaigns: clinical and programmatic issues. *J Infect Dis* 2003; **187**(suppl 1): S291–8.

309. Pope J, Stevens A, Howson W, Bell D. The development of rheumatoid arthritis after recombinant hepatitis B vaccination. *J Rheumatol* 1998; **25**: 1687–93.

310. Khoury MJ. Genetics and genomics in practice: the continuum from genetic disease to genetic information in health and disease. *Genet Med* 2003; **5**: 261–8.

31

Pharmacoepidemiologic Studies of Devices

ROSELIE A. BRIGHT

Center for Devices and Radiological Health, Food and Drug Administration, Rockville, Maryland, USA.

INTRODUCTION

In early 1990, the Food and Drug Administration (FDA) Center for Devices and Radiological Health (CDRH) received reports of two rapid deaths associated with barium enemas (used to provide X-ray contrast media for colon imaging). The interesting feature was that the middle-aged women, in different parts of the country, had suffered their reactions after the barium enema cuffs were put in place, but before barium had been introduced. The reactions were clearly consistent with anaphylaxis, although in one instance, the reporter called it a vasovagal reaction. The medical community was already familiar with allergy to barium, and the Center for Drug Evaluation and Research (CDER) already had many such reports on hand. However, in these two cases, the only potential allergens were the lubricants or the cuffs.

The scope of investigation was widened to look at all reports associated with barium enemas in the files of both Centers and the manufacturer of the cuff, which held most of the market. The FDA had received, from all sources, reports of 5 deaths and 28 very serious reactions, all of an allergic nature (except for one death due to aspiration of oral barium). All of the

deaths occurred in 1989 or 1990. There was a preponderance of middle-aged female victims.

A literature search found a fatality immediately after and attributed to a single contrast colonic infusion reported in 1989,[1] and a 1990 publication reporting 7 reactions among 6918 barium enema infusions at one hospital from January 1987 to March 1989, attributed to some unknown new additive in the barium enema infusion.[2]

At this point, the evidence implicated the cuff rather than the lubricant. However, just as with other problems with therapeutic products, there were still many other questions to consider:

- Was the problem specific to the manufacturer, the cuff, or the material?
- Could the problem be mitigated by changing manufacturing procedures?
- If the cuff were to be recalled, would substitute products be available?
- Was this a trend or an isolated, fixable problem?
- What were the public health implications?

Epidemiology has the potential to address the first, fourth, and fifth questions. During the 1990s, it became apparent that the culprit was the material, latex, which is more or less allergenic depending on the manufacturing process.[3] Humans contact latex in many different devices, including condoms, diaphragms, anesthetic gas masks (many reactions attributed to gas may have been to latex, instead), airway tubes, catheter tip occluders, dental dams, tympanostomy tubes, and gloves. Allergenic particles are more readily exposed to immune cells through surgical wounds or mucous membranes than through intact skin, and one can see that many of the listed devices have direct contact with the former.[3] Furthermore, the health care profession and patient population had been experiencing greater latex exposure throughout the 1980s with the introduction of universal precautions[4] and promotion of condom use. The stage had been set for a serious latex allergy problem.

So, where are the numbers? How many people are or were exposed to latex? What is or was the extent of exposure? Does anatomical site of exposure matter in the way that was hypothesized? What are the rates of mild moderate, severe, and fatal reactions? Are recommendations that have been made (elimination of powder from gloves, reduction of latex in parts of devices that have body contact) having a mitigating effect? Medical device epidemiology has begun to answer these questions.[4–8] The rest of this chapter will present some of the challenges to, and successes of, good medical device epidemiology, emphasizing features that differ from medications epidemiology.

CLINICAL PROBLEMS TO BE ADDRESSED BY PHARMACOEPIDEMIOLOGIC RESEARCH

WHAT ARE MEDICAL DEVICES?

The term "medical devices" covers such a broad range of entities that it is difficult to define simply. However, in a regulated environment, one way of defining medical devices is to resort to a legal definition. The definition, for example, given by the United States Congress[9] is:

The term "device" ... means an instrument, apparatus, implement, machine, contrivance, implant, in vitro reagent, or other similar or related article, including any component, part, or accessory, which is recognized in the official National Formulary, or the United States Pharmacopeia, or any supplement to them, intended for the use in the diagnosis of disease or other conditions, or in the cure, mitigation, treatment, or prevention of disease, in man or other animals, or intended to affect the structure or function of the body of man or other animals, and which does not

achieve its primary intended purposes through chemical action within or on the body of man or other animals and which is not dependent upon being metabolized for the achievement of its primary intended purposes.

The definition offered by the European Union[10] is somewhat different:

(a) "medical device" means any instrument, apparatus, appliance, material or other article, whether used alone or in combination, including the software necessary for its proper application intended by the manufacturer to be used for human beings for the purpose of:

• diagnosis, prevention, monitoring, treatment or alleviation of disease,
• diagnosis, monitoring, treatment, alleviation of or compensation for an injury or handicap,
• investigation, replacement or modification of the anatomy or of a physiological process,
• control of conception,

and which does not achieve its principal intended action in or on the human body by pharmacological, immunological or metabolic means, but which may be assisted in its function by such means;

(b) "accessory" means an article which whilst not being a device is intended specifically by its manufacturer to be used together with a device to enable it to be used in accordance with the use of the device intended by the manufacturer of the device;

(c) "device used for in vitro diagnosis" means any device which is a reagent, reagent product, kit, instrument, equipment or system, whether used alone or in combination, intended by the manufacturer to be used in vitro for the examination of samples derived from the human body with a view to providing information on the physiological state, state of health or disease, or congenital abnormality thereof.

The Canadian government's[11] definition of a medical device is:

any article, instrument, apparatus, or contrivance, including a component, part or accessory thereof, manufactured, sold or represented for use in

(a) the diagnosis, treatment, mitigation or prevention of a disease, disorder or abnormal physical state, or its symptoms, in human beings or animals,
(b) restoring, correcting or modifying a body function or the body structure of human beings or animals,
(c) the diagnosis of pregnancy in human beings or animals, or
(d) the care of human beings or animals during pregnancy and at and after birth of the offspring,

and includes a contraceptive device but does not include a drug.

In Australia,[12] the regulatory definition is:

> any instrument, apparatus, appliance, material or other article (whether used alone or in combination, and including the software necessary for its proper application) intended by the person under whose name it is to be supplied, to be used for human beings for the purposes of one or more of the following:
>
> - diagnosis, prevention, monitoring, treatment or alleviation of disease,
> - diagnosis, monitoring, treatment, alleviation of or compensation for an injury or handicap,
> - investigation, replacement or modification of the anatomy or of a physiological process,
> - control of conception,
>
> and does not achieve its principal intended action in or on the human body by pharmacological, immunological or metabolic means, but which may be assisted in its function by such means; or an accessory to such an instrument, apparatus, appliance, material or other article.

The Japanese government's[13] definition is:

> instruments and apparatus which are intended for use in the diagnosis, cure or prevention of diseases in man or animals, or intended to affect the structure or any function of the body of man or other animals, and which are designated by Cabinet Order.

Although the wording and level of detail is quite different for these five definitions, the overall meaning is obviously quite similar.

The main regulatory purpose of categorizing medical devices is to vary the level of premarket information required before marketing may begin, according to the potential risk posed by the particular device. This is an approach used in the European Union,[10] United States,[14] Canada,[15] and Australia,[12] and encouraged by the Global Harmonization Task Force.[16] The highest level of control is to require randomized controlled clinical trials before applying for approval to market the device. This is, obviously, similar to the expectations for a new drug. In contrast, if a new device is very similar to several that have already been cleared for marketing, then the device sponsor may need to demonstrate equivalence to the earlier devices, or attest that the device conforms with an international standard recognized by the regulatory agency. Further, a very large category of devices receives minimal regulation; the sponsor simply must register itself and the device with the agency and is expected to follow general guidelines. A device may be moved to less regulated categories over time as clinical experience with its use expands, depending on the comfort of the agency with the regulatory history of the device.

Once a device is marketed, sponsors must follow Good Manufacturing Practices and monitor the safety of their products.[10,12,15,17] They are subject to inspections by the regulatory agency or a proxy. The safety of most devices is monitored by keeping a complaint file at the manufacturer level. The manufacturer must then forward reports of "malfunctions," "serious injuries," and deaths, using criteria specified in regulations, to the regulatory agency. More intensive safety efforts involve bench testing returned products, offering free replacements for returned products, and sponsoring registries of users.

Regulatory agencies participating in the Global Harmonization Task Force monitor the safety of devices by reviewing adverse event reports from users, sponsors, or the scientific literature.[13] The US FDA also has a regulatory tool unique among members of the Global Harmonization Task Force;[18] it may require the sponsor of a marketed device to conduct a "postmarketing surveillance study" of safety and/or effectiveness, if warranted by public health considerations.[19]

The nature of the medical device manufacturers themselves also varies extensively, from ownership by large pharmaceutical companies, to long-term establishment as large developers of cutting-edge technology, to very small entrepreneurial operations. This variation in size naturally results in variations in safety and epidemiologic expertise, as well. The large number of small companies involved is reflected organizationally at the US FDA by the Division of Small Manufacturers, International and Consumer Assistance in the CDRH, which is charged with helping small companies understand regulatory requirements.[20]

While governments classify medical devices for the sake of varying the level of control over different categories, epidemiologists may find other classification schemes to be more useful, e.g., the different use patterns of devices (see Table 31.1). Distinct epidemiologic problems, in the sense of hypotheses to be tested and challenges to study validity, derive from each of these categorizations. Table 31.2 shows a classification scheme that combines elements of the use patterns above, with consequent study hypotheses that might be entertained, challenges to validity, and example devices. There are several types of study hypotheses that are appropriate for epidemiologic studies of medical devices. Short-term safety and efficacy issues apply to all the device categories listed in Table 31.2, except for diagnostics. Long-term safety and efficacy hypotheses readily apply to reused and durable equipment, and long-term implants. Human error issues related to proper use, and perhaps maintenance, pertain to all types of devices. The consequences of device reuse are worth studying for equipment (whether designed to be reused or durable, or reused in spite of being designed for

Table 31.1. Spectrum of different use patterns for devices

Number of patients exposed to a particular device
- one
- multiple

Number of times a particular device is used
- once
- multiple times

Extent of direct patient exposure to the device
- none (as in laboratory analysis of a specimen)
- intact skin contact
- intact mucous membrane contact
- intact endothelium contact
- penetration of tissue
- penetration by energy or particles emitted by the device (such as ultrasound or X-rays)

Nature of device effect
- mechanical
- electronic
- chemical (e.g., diagnostic devices)

Permanence of a particular device
- used for a few minutes
- used for a few days
- used up to a year
- used several years
- "permanent" (used over 10 years)

Setting of device use
- hospital
- emergency vehicle
- clinic
- long-term care facility
- private home

Device user
- doctoral care provider such as physician or dentist
- nurse
- other allied health professional
- family member
- patient

single-use only). Finally, hypotheses regarding the validity of the test result are appropriate for diagnostic devices.

INDIVIDUAL SAFETY

Because randomized clinical trials have the power to demonstrate clinically significant efficacy (a positive effect must be demonstrated in a substantial proportion of patients), but little power to assure safety (because adverse effects affect a much smaller fraction of patients), safety has become largely the domain of epidemiology. The body of safety data includes private studies by the device manufacturer, adverse event reports to government agencies (redacted portions are publicly available), and epidemiologic studies reported in the scientific literature. Only high-risk and some other new devices are subject to a clinical trial requirement. Devices that are similar to

well-established devices simply have to be demonstrated as meeting a standard, or being similar to a marketed device; if the predicate device was never studied in a randomized clinical trial (in the US, many devices marketed before the 1976 Medical Device Amendment have never been subjected to the requirement), gaps in human safety and efficacy data exist. Furthermore, the definition of "similar" is such that incremental changes are allowed; after an accumulation of such changes, the latest device may be quite different from the original predicate device.

PUBLIC HEALTH IMPACT

If epidemiologic evidence points to a safety problem with a device, further information is then required to evaluate the public health impact of various options, such as doing nothing, taking an action, or perhaps taking an alternative action. Available epidemiologic evidence of both the effectiveness and extent of device use, as well as the availability of alternative therapies, have a bearing on the decision. For example, medical gloves are made of either latex or vinyl; vinyl is less likely to cause allergic reactions, but latex is far more flexible and durable and is still used in most situations.[21]

DIFFERENTIAL EFFECTS

Another problem that is amenable to epidemiology is the study of the differential effects of devices by some cofactor, such as gender or a concomitant therapy. In other words, epidemiology can help identify patients at higher risk of complications from a device. Two examples are the higher risk of ventilator-associated pneumonia in men and in patients receiving a paralyzing agent.[22]

METHODOLOGIC PROBLEMS TO BE SOLVED BY PHARMACOEPIDEMIOLOGIC RESEARCH

RECOGNITION AND CHARACTERIZATION OF NEW SYNDROMES OR ADVERSE EVENTS

Sometimes, as with the latex barium enema cuff example, the discovery of a device's role in causing a well-recognized outcome is difficult, partly because devices are generally taken to be benign. At other times, a new outcome must be defined. An example is first use syndrome occurring during hemodialysis. As the name implies, this syndrome only occurs when a device, such as a dialysis membrane (which may be routinely reused many times), is brand new.[23,24] Where controversy exists over the establishment of a definition

Table 31.2. A device categorization scheme, with implications for epidemiologic study designs

Category	Applicable types of study hypotheses	Challenges to study validity	Examples
Disposable equipment	Short-term safety and efficacy; human error issues related to proper use; reuse consequences	Device use must be inferred from procedures and knowledge of standard care, if studied retrospectively in a health care facility. Otherwise, must use interviews. Device may be part of a system that includes disposable, reusable, and durable equipment	Barium enema cuffs, gloves
Equipment reused for the same patient and discarded within the first year of use	Short- and long-term safety and efficacy; human error issues related to proper use; reuse consequences	If used in a clinic, record keeping likely to be good. At home, records could be available. Otherwise, must use interviews. Device may be part of a system that includes disposable, reusable, and durable equipment	Extended wear soft contact lenses
Durable equipment used for many patients and many years	Short- and long-term safety and efficacy; human error issues related to proper use; reuse consequences	The particular device is uniquely identifiable only if just one is used by the facility. The type of device used must be inferred from procedure codes and knowledge of standard practice. Otherwise, must use interviews. Equipment may be refurbished or certain components may have been replaced with parts from another manufacturer. Device may be part of a system that includes disposable, reusable, and durable equipment	Ventilators
Implants that remain in the body short-term	Short-term safety and efficacy; human error issues related to proper placement and maintenance	The unique device is generally not identifiable. The type of device used often must be inferred from procedure codes and knowledge of standard practice. Device may be part of a system that includes disposable, reusable, and durable equipment	Catheters
Implants that remain in the body long-term	Short- and long-term safety and efficacy, human error issues related to proper implantation and maintenance	Operating room notes and patient charts have detailed data; forming a cohort and following patients can be challenging, especially if the follow-up physician is not the implanting physician. Some registries exist	Pacemakers
Diagnostics	Validity of test result; human error issues related to proper use and maintenance	Patient charts generally report results, not type of device. Home tests may be unrecorded. Device may be part of a system that includes disposable, reusable, and durable equipment	Home pregnancy test kits

of a new syndrome, as is the case with the possibility of a new connective tissue disease that may be associated with silicone gel breast implants, the situation is even murkier.[25] In all of these circumstances, epidemiologists can contribute to improved methodology to detect and characterize adverse events and syndromes.

INDIVIDUAL EXPOSURE ASSESSMENT

For epidemiologists, it is a given that a determination of exposure and outcome status at the level of the individual study subject is critical to making confident assessments of the relationship between the two. The general ways to do

this for medical device studies are to consult a medical record or to ask the subject.

Almost all of the challenges to medical device study validity that are listed in Table 31.2 relate to individual exposure assessment. The brand, model, or exact unit used for a particular patient are generally not explicitly written for disposable or durable equipment or short-term implants, but the type of device can generally be inferred from the recorded procedures and knowledge of standard care. For instance, a barium enema cuff is likely to have been used for a barium enema procedure, but the brand and model will not have been recorded. In the case of durable equipment, if only one was available at the facility, it is possible to get detailed information on the device. Equipment reused by the same patient may be well recorded in a clinic setting and less well recorded in a home setting. Another problem to be considered with equipment and short-term implants is that device systems (such as for hemodialysis or ventilation) are constructed of many different components, and may include disposable, reused, or durable equipment, a diagnostic device, or a short-term implant. These components may or may not be the same brand; this is relevant because the performance of a particular component may be affected by the brands of other components. Assessing the critical device for the study hypothesis may require accounting for all the other components in the device system. A piece of durable equipment may present this exposure–assessment dilemma in itself; over time, it may have acquired updated parts from the same or a different manufacturer during repair or refurbishment.

For long-term implants, operating room notes and patient data generally have detailed data on the implant. Registries have been formed for a variety of implants, although patients may resist registration if the implant is of a socially sensitive nature. Long-term follow-up, furthermore, can be challenging, especially if the physician following the patient is not the physician inserting the implant.

In the case of diagnostic devices, patient charts generally record the results but not the device used. Depending on the test, home test kit use may go unrecorded.

Prospective studies to confirm the methodology of inferring the particulars of device use need to be conducted, especially in light of the fact that until recently there was no universally accepted nomenclature for devices that was comparable to the National Drug Code for drugs. Two old schemes, the FDA's Medical Device Product Code[26] (still in use by the FDA) and ECRI's Universal Medical Device Nomenclature System,™ [27] were based on intended use and do not specify brand, model, or other details that may be relevant, such as size or material. The newly developed scheme, the Global Medical Device Nomenclature (GMDN), is intended to provide a standard nomenclature for all countries and manufacturers to use.[28] Many countries have adopted it for use.[29] The GMDN classifies all devices into one of 12 "device categories" (code and term):

1. Active implantable devices
2. Anaesthetic and respiratory devices
3. Dental devices
4. Electromechanical medical devices
5. Hospital hardware
6. In vitro diagnostic devices (IVD)
7. Non-active implantable devices
8. Ophthalmic and optical devices

9. Reusable instruments
10. Single use devices
11. Technical aids for disabled persons
12. Diagnostic and therapeutic radiation devices.

The GMDN database includes the device category, unique five-digit code chosen by the manufacturer, preferred specific term, template term (groups of preferred terms), and synonym terms.[30] The manufacturer has the option, but not requirement, to choose a five-digit code that reflects the model or other device particulars. However, none of the Global Harmonization or member countries' regulations require the device code to be on the device itself.

When asking the subject about medical device use, recall can be a problem because the patient may not have taken particular note of many of the details. Furthermore, some devices, such as breast implants or impotence devices, are associated with social discomfort, so may be underreported.[31] The interviewer must take special care to encourage full disclosure.

As an example of some of these methodologic problems, consider the case of extended use of soft contact lenses. Because these lenses are relatively inexpensive, they may be purchased out of pocket from a source outside of the subject's normal health plan. Consequently, full contact lens information is often not available in the subject's main medical records, making exposure assessment difficult to measure from records alone. In their studies of corneal ulcer, exposure was assessed by Poggio et al.[32] with a population survey, and by Schein et al.[33] with a structured interview of all cases and controls. The different methods used in each study were probably valid because they resulted in similar effect estimates: relative risks for corneal ulcer of 5.2 (95% confidence interval of 3.5–7.7) by Poggio et al. and 3.9 (95% confidence interval of 2.4–6.5) by Schein et al.

NATIONAL POPULATION EXPOSURE ASSESSMENT

Once a regulator has discovered a likely relationship between exposure and outcome, he or she needs to determine the extent of population exposure. Public sources of device exposure data include market data, medical care claims, medical records, and population survey data. Market data firms derive their information in various ways, from polling health care providers[34,35] to collecting device purchase information from a nationally representative set of health care facilities and providers.[36] Market data may express incident or prevalent exposure data. A nationally representative hospital claims database provides national incidence estimates for devices that can be adequately measured by hospital procedure codes.[37,38] Other medical care claims records can also be a source of procedure codes that may be used to infer device use. Exposure estimates can also be made by consulting a sample of medical records or by surveying the population. The limitations of measuring device exposure with medical data sources that are discussed above in the section on individual exposure assessment also apply to these methodologies. The Medical Device Implant Supplement to the 1988 National Health Interview Survey of households provided the first population exposure prevalence assessment of a variety of implants.[31,39,40] In general, these information sources are much less abundant, reliable, or detailed than comparable types of drug exposure information.

CURRENTLY AVAILABLE SOLUTIONS

This section describes observational and descriptive epidemiologic tools currently available for studying medical device use.

SAFETY SURVEILLANCE

In the US, general safety surveillance is done by the FDA through voluntary and mandatory reporting of suspected adverse events due to devices. Manufacturers must report malfunctions, serious injuries, and deaths. Health care facilities must report deaths.[41] Anyone can make a voluntary report. The FDA receives reports of more than 120 000 adverse device events per year[42] (compared to about 250 000 for drugs[43]). They are recorded and reviewed in a manner similar to drug reports, although the reviewers are largely nurses, as opposed to pharmacists, because nurses generally have the most extensive clinical experience with devices. Reports are assigned to individual reviewers based largely on the organ system related to the device's intended use, so that each reviewer is responsible for a large variety of types of devices. Reviewers may ask the reporters or manufacturers for more information. The FDA has taken actions that include recalls, public alerts, required changes to device labeling, and required epidemiologic studies.

Although medical device adverse event reporting is also required by Canada, Japan, Australia, and the European Union, very little public information is available about these systems, besides what is specified in their regulations. All of these countries have mandatory reporting by device sponsors and voluntary reporting by anyone. The types of reportable events are very similar to those in the US. None of these other countries require reporting by health care facilities.[13]

The general discussions of reporting systems found elsewhere in this book also apply to adverse *device* event reports. Whether adverse events due to medical devices are more or less likely to be reported than those due to medications is unknown. In the US, two programs have been started to address some of the deficiencies in the current safety surveillance system. The Medical Product Surveillance Network (MedSun)[44] was started in 2002. Designated representatives (usually risk managers or biomedical engineers) of member hospitals and nursing homes file extensive reports on actual and potential adverse medical device events with a contractor, using a web system or the phone. The contractor works with the reporter to complete as many details as possible. The report is then made available to the FDA. Reporters receive quick feedback on the completeness of the report, as well as newsletters and posters for use in their facilities. Annual conferences among the members, contractor staff, and FDA staff are used for training and networking. As of September 2003 MedSun included 180 hospitals and nursing homes. Plans for 2004 included the first recruitment of members from west of the Mississippi to bring the total number of participants to 240.

The second new surveillance program builds on the National Electronic Injury Surveillance System (NEISS) administered by the Consumer Product Safety Commission (CPSC).[45] The FDA effort for devices is based on the core of NEISS: trained and audited reporters at each of 64 US hospitals search all the emergency visit records and abstract the records of injuries related to devices. The abstracted data are sent to CPSC, which has a statistical scheme for weighting the data to produce national estimates. This new effort started in the summer of 2003 and is the first systematic active surveillance of adverse medical device events that occur outside of hospitals. A pilot study, conducted July 1999–June 2000, showed the value of the system.[46] That year, the estimated total number of emergency visits related to device injury was 450 000, of which 59 000 were serious enough to result in death or hospitalization and 190 000 occurred in home environments.

SURVEYS

The population-based surveys conducted by the US National Center for Health Statistics have provided a variety of data on medical devices, including the Medical Device Implant Supplement to the 1988 National Health Interview Survey[47] mentioned above, the 1988 National Maternal and Infant Health Survey,[48] the National Health and Nutrition Examination Survey series,[49] the 1993 Mortality Followback Survey,[50] and the 1996 National Home and Hospice Care Survey.[51] These are summarized in Table 31.3.

Table 31.3. Some surveys conducted by the US National Center for Health Statistics that include medical device information

Title	General and Device information	Sample size
Medical Device Implant Supplement (MDIS) to the 1988 National Health Interview Survey[39,47]	"The . . . National Health Interview Survey . . . is based on . . . a continuing nationwide survey by household interview." The survey collects data on demographics and health conditions.[47] The MDIS was administered only in 1988, and collected information on medical implants in all household members.[39]	The sample included 122 000 members of about 47 000 households. The net MDIS response rate was 92%.[39]
1988 National Maternal and Infant Health Survey (NMIHS)[48]	"The NMIHS data file consists of three independent national files of live births, fetal deaths, and infant deaths; and a small supplementary sample of Hispanic live births, fetal deaths, and infant deaths in Texas, and a supplementary sample of live births for urban American Indians. Each mother named on those vital records was mailed a 35-page mother's questionnaire." The data include prenatal and perinatal tests and procedures, such as ultrasound examination. "The 1988 NMIHS can be merged with the 1991 Longitudinal Follow-up." Information about some devices, such as home apnea monitors, is included.	The data file is based on the responses of 10 000 mothers of live births, 3300 mothers of late fetal deaths, and 5300 mothers of infant deaths.
National Health and Nutrition Examination Survey (NHANES)[49]	The data consists of standardized questionnaires, physical examinations, and laboratory testing regarding health and nutrition status and behaviors. Serum latex allergy (IgE) was tested in the 1999–2001 sample of 12–59 year olds[52] using the AlaStat Microplate method.[53]	10 000 people participated in NHANES 1999–2000 (part of NHANES 1999–2004).[54]
1993 Mortality Followback Survey[50]	"The Mortality Followback Survey Program . . . uses a sample of United States residents who die in a given year to supplement the death certificate with information from the next of kin or another person familiar with the decedent's life history . . . The 1993 survey samples [22 957] individuals aged 15 years or over who died in 1993." The focus areas of the 1993 survey included risk factors for death, disability, unintentional death, and access to and utilization of health care in the last year of life. It provides information on devices used in the home (hospital beds, blood glucose meters, infusion pumps, dialysis machines, etc.).	Almost 23 000 subjects.
2000 National Home and Hospice Care Survey (NHHCS)[51]	"The sampling frame for the 2000 National Home and Hospice Care Survey (NHHCS) consisted of 15 451 agencies classified as agencies providing home health and hospice care." The survey asked about various devices used in home care, including assistive (such as wheelchairs), therapeutic (such as oxygen delivery systems), and diagnostic (such as blood glucose meters) devices.	The sample consisted of 1800 "agencies providing home health and hospice care" services at the time of the survey. Of these, 1425 agreed to participate.

The Medical Device Implant Supplement to the 1988 National Health Interview Survey[47] mentioned above was used to generate the first overall national prevalence estimates of implants.[39] More extensive reports were generated for the particular devices. Examples include one on breast implants,[31] which demonstrated that using a general medically-oriented screening question asked of a household representative may not elicit all socially sensitive or cosmetic implants for all household members. Another example was an analysis of pacemakers,[40] showing that there were about 456 000 non-institutionalized implant recipients; about 15% of the prevalent implants were replacements. Prevalence rose steeply with recipient age and was higher for men, whites, and those reporting an activity limitation. Geographic region, income, and educational level were not related to pacemaker prevalence.

The 1988 National Maternal and Infant Health Survey was used to generate national statistics on home pregnancy test use among women who carried their pregnancies to term.[55] It was estimated that a third of such women used the test, and that they were more likely to be white, married, older, more educated, and wealthier than the other mothers.

Hefflin used the 1993 Mortality Followback Survey to conclude that "older persons who had initial pacemakers implanted during their final year of life . . . [were] relatively independent, physically functional candidates who frequently died unexpectedly," indicating that expert guidelines for pacemaker implantation were generally followed. Eighteen percent of the estimated 79 000 elderly recipients of pacemakers who had died in 1993 had received the implant for the first time during their final year of life.[56]

Ad hoc surveys are also used to study specific devices, such as latex gloves. Table 31.4 shows the features of five example studies.[4–8] All of these latex studies were occupationally based, on the assumption that sensitivity rates would be higher in these groups. Studies directed to understanding risk factors and testing candidate interventions are statistically relatively powerful in these occupational groups, and the results will presumably be applicable to patients.

As described in an earlier section of this chapter, *ad hoc* studies were required to measure the use and complications from extended wear soft contact lenses.[32] Poggio *et al.* surveyed the general population to measure exposure to extended wear soft contact lenses and combined the results with their survey of all ophthalmologists to estimate corneal ulcer rates.

Table 31.4. Features of five example studies of sensitivity to latex gloves

Author and year of study	Surveyed population	Latex sensitivity assessment method	Sensitivity rate	Sensitivity predictors
Turjanmaa 1987[5]	All operating room and laboratory employees in a Finnish hospital. Also, 130 consecutive patients who were due for routine scratch testing.	Scratch test for latex, vinyl, 20 common inhalant allergens with histamine, and diluent. Glove use test with latex and with vinyl.	Employees: 2.8%. Patients: 0.8%. $p < 0.01$.	Atopy, hand eczema, operating room work, physician.
Sussman *et al.* 1995[4]	All 71 housekeeping staff in a Canadian hospital (70% participated). All wore unpowdered, unflocked latex gloves for 25 to 30 hours per week.	Questionnaire screen; positives were skin tested with latex, eight common inhalant and food allergens, and histamine.	8%.	
Kaczmarek *et al.* 1996[6]	915 emergency room workers (nurses, physicians, emergency medical technicians) in 9 hospitals; 42% completed all sensitivity measures.	Questionnaire and test of serum for IgE antibodies to latex.	6%, by serum test.	Any allergy history, nonwhite race.
Brown *et al.* 1998[7]	All 171 health care employees of an anesthesiology and critical care department of a hospital. Excluded provocation tests for those with recent unstable asthma or interfering medications, or pregnancy. 168 provided history and blood; 154 provided the skin test.	History; blood test for latex, three fruits, and a combination of eight common allergens; skin test to latex, glycerinated saline, histamine, and nonammoniated latex; and glove provocation test.	20% by history. 12.5% by blood test.	Atopy; food allergies; specific allergies to banana, kiwi, or avocado.
Sussman *et al.* 1998[8]	Phase I: 2062 health care workers at two sites of a hospital (1351 participated). Phase II: introduction of powder-free gloves at one site; continuance of powdered gloves at the other. Of 479 eligible workers negative at baseline, 435 completed follow-up.	1 year prospective follow-up. Skin test with latex, noncompounded ammoniated latex, several food and inhalant allergens, and saline used to measure new sensitivity.	1.0% in powdered; 0.9% in nonpowdered glove group.	Atopy.

REGISTRIES

Registries are sometimes formed to establish cohorts of patients with particular device exposures. Several registries form the basis of pacemaker studies. Examples include the Implantable Lead Registry, formed by six North American hospitals in 1979,[57] the Fyn County registry in Denmark formed in 1964,[58] and the Danish Pacemaker Register for all of Denmark begun in 1982.[59] In addition, Kawanishi et al.[60] used data from four registries: the Bilitch Registry of pacemaker pulse generators, operating from 1973 to 1993, with 3–6 sites, 22 786 devices, and 16 903 patients;[60] the Implantable Lead Registry of pacemaker leads, operating from 1979 to 1989, with the same sites as the Bilitch Registry and 7311 patients; the United States Veterans Administration Registry of Pacemaker Leads, still operating in 1992 at 182 facilities, with 8612 patients; and the Cleveland Clinic Lead Registry, operating from 1980 to 1991. Device life could be estimated by type, brand, model, and reason for replacement.[57,59] If a registry is population based, the incidence of device implantation, prevalence of implant recipients, and mortality rates for recipients can also be calculated.[58]

MEDICAL CARE CLAIMS

An example of a large medical care claims database suitable for some medical device epidemiologic topics is the Healthcare Cost and Utilization Project (HCUP) Nationwide Inpatient Sample (NIS), which has been made available by the Agency for Healthcare Research and Quality.[37] This database is updated periodically:

- NIS is the largest all-payer inpatient care database in the United States. It contains data from approximately 7 million hospital stays.
- NIS 2001 contains all discharge data from 986 hospitals located in 33 States, approximating a 20-percent stratified sample of U.S. community hospitals.
- The sampling frame for the NIS 2001 is a sample of hospitals that comprises about 85 percent of all hospital discharges in the United States.
- NIS data are available from 1988 [for 8 states] to 2001 [33 states] . . .
- NIS's large sample size enables analyses of rare conditions, such as congenital anomalies; uncommon treatments, such as organ transplantation; and special patient populations, such as children.

NIS includes hospital identifiers that permit linkages to the American Hospital Association's database and county identifiers that permit linkages to the Area Resource File.

Since NIS data consist of discharge claims, studies of devices depend on the adequacy of procedure codes for capturing device exposure. Within this limitation, studies of the extent of use, adverse events in the same hospitalization, or longitudinal trends can be performed, as was done for pacemaker implantations.[38] US census data adjusted to the year 1992 was used along with the national pacemaker implantation estimates from NIS, to calculate 5-year age group and gender specific implantation rates for the US. The investigators were also able to analyze the principal diagnoses, associated diagnoses, whether the implant was a replacement, and death before discharge.

MEDICAL RECORDS

Medical records are a resource for medical device epidemiology to the extent that they note the use of devices. Medical record systems vary from entirely paper-based, to partially systematized, to fully automated. An international effort is under way to create uniform standards for storing and transmitting health-related data;[61] US participation has been encouraged by the National Academy of Science's Institute of Medicine.[61]

Paper-based medical record systems were used to measure outcomes for some pacemaker studies. Rubin et al.[62] reported their retrospective review of 287 patients at one clinic in the southeastern US who had been actively followed. They calculated generator life, complications, replacements, and patient mortality. Another example is from Mueller et al.,[63] who reported on patients who had been implanted and regularly followed at an Austrian cardiology department. They were able to analyze by gender, age at implantation, indication, patient survival (compared to the general Austrian population), and cause of death.

A partially systematized system is used at the Mayo Clinic, where another pacemaker survival study was conducted.[64] The Mayo Clinic has access to all data regarding medical care provided in Olmsted County, Minnesota, USA.[65] A card system was available to identify pacemaker recipients, but other medical information was obtainable from the full paper medical record. Shen et al.[64] defined a group of patients and followed them through time with the medical records and death certificates. Patient survival was calculated in comparison to the North Central white population at a comparable time, and stratified by demographics, clinical history, heart disease type, and some comorbid conditions. Another Mayo Clinic study with a similar data collection strategy investigated transtracheal oxygen catheters.[66] Records of patients receiving the device were reviewed for demographics, reason for placement, complications, reason for removal, and duration of use.

Some of the major managed care providers, such as Harvard Pilgrim Health Care (see Chapter 16), have a fully automated patient record system. At LDS Hospital, part of Intermountain Health Care, a study of adverse medical device events was recently conducted by relying on electronic records of various types.[67] While the use of electronic records detected two orders of magnitude higher rates of adverse events than the incident reports database, in instances where the same events should have been detected by different mechanisms, the overlap was small. The overall incidence of adverse medical device events detected by at least one of several methods was 83.7 (95% confidence interval: 78.8–88.6) per 1000 admissions. These findings suggest that documentation of adverse medical device events is either quite incomplete, or located in some files that the authors did not examine.

As demonstrated by the examples, the assessment of medical device exposure depends on the nature of facility-specific practices regarding the extent of notes or logs.

NEW DATA COLLECTION

New study-specific data collection is also an option that may be crucial to study success. It is often the only option for studies of devices used in the home, because broad surveys may not sample enough device users to be informative and medical records may not capture the information that is required. A case in point is soft contact lens use, as described earlier in this chapter,[32,33] where only the subject can reliably provide the exposure (length of wear times) and some covariate information (such as cleaning practices).

COMBINATIONS OF TECHNIQUES

At times, as for other epidemiologic situations, a combination of study techniques may be used to strengthen the results. In a study of pacemaker use, Greenspan *et al.*[68] presumably used Medicare claims obtained by a Professional Standards Review Organization in the US to identify patients; the remainder of the information was collected via extensive chart review. The authors evaluated the appropriateness of implantation of Medicare-reimbursable pacemakers.

A new program, the Medicare Patient Safety Monitoring System, is being sponsored by the US Centers for Medicare and Medicaid Services (CMS).[69] Claims are being used to select a random sample of hospitalizations. The patient charts are being abstracted for specific types of adverse events, including some that are related to medical devices. The claims data are being used to follow the patients after discharge to note rehospitalization or death within 30 days. CMS plans to continue this program indefinitely to measure progress in patient safety and investigate new issues.

Another example of multiple techniques is the use of different survey types as well as complementary study designs (case–control and case–cohort) to address the same primary and complementary secondary questions. During the 1980s, the ophthalmology and regulatory communities became suspicious that long-term wear of extended wear soft contact lenses increased the risk of corneal ulcer. The complementary epidemiologic studies were designed together and incorporated both a random sample survey of a population and of all ophthalmologists serving the population,[32] as well as case selection with both hospital and population controls.[33] The first study established the incidence rate of corneal ulcer and the second demonstrated several risk factors. It appeared that risk rose with each day of wear but varied among individuals (some people could not tolerate even one night of extended wear, while others experienced no trouble with a week). Based on these studies, FDA found it prudent to have eye care professionals set individual patient maximum wear times, subject to an overall limit of 7 days.[70] More recently, FDA has approved lenses made of more highly permeable material for wear up to 30 days.[71]

THE FUTURE

TRENDS IN MEDICAL DEVICE TECHNOLOGY

Medical devices are becoming more sophisticated, smaller, more precise, and easier to use in the home.[72] As applications have increased, medical device nomenclatures that are based on intended use have become cumbersome. As described in an earlier section, an international effort is currently under way to standardize and adopt a new nomenclature.[28–30] Once the new nomenclature is fully accepted, a useful future step would be to universally use this nomenclature in individual patient records to help define device exposure.

Another trend is the ever speedier introduction of new generations of devices.[73] In some cases, new technology is in use before an epidemiologic study of the older technology can be completed. This problem will need to be addressed by faster epidemiologic techniques, such as quicker assemblage of an exposed cohort after a device is introduced to the market, for observing long-term safety and effectiveness.

TRENDS IN EPIDEMIOLOGIC RESOURCES

Increasing uniformity and automation of medical records will improve the prospects for medical device epidemiology.[61,74–76] Some observers believe the Internet will enhance the conduct of records-based studies.[77–80] However, new privacy laws are restricting access by researchers,[75,81–83] and causing confusion over just how restrictive health care providers need to be.[84] Acceptable standard methods may be developed to address confidentiality concerns while allowing rigorous epidemiologic research.[85] Nonetheless, full access to records will be most useful when both device exposure and problems related to devices are completely documented.

TRENDS IN MEDICAL DEVICE EPIDEMIOLOGY

Awareness of medical devices as an object of epidemiologic study has been growing. It is my hope that as the field grows, recognition of medical devices as an influence on health will expand, thereby allowing major advances in both resources and methodology.

DISCLAIMER

The opinions expressed in this chapter are those of the author and do not necessarily represent the official policies of the US Food and Drug Administration.

REFERENCES

1. Feczko PJ, Simms SM, Bakirci N. Fatal hypersensitivity reaction during a barium enema. *Am J Roentgenol* 1989; **153**: 275–6.
2. Feczko PJ. Increased frequency of reactions to contrast materials during gastrointestinal studies. *Radiology* 1990; **174**: 367–8.
3. Tomazic VJ, Withrow TJ, Fisher BR, Dillard SF. Short analytical review: latex-associated allergies and anaphylactic reactions. *Clin Immunol Immunopathol* 1992; **64**: 89–97.
4. Sussman GL, Lem D, Liss G, Beezhold D. Latex allergy in housekeeping personnel. *Ann Allergy Asthma Immunol* 1995; **74**: 415–18.
5. Turjanmaa K. Incidence of immediate allergy to latex gloves in hospital personnel. *Contact Dermatitis* 1987; **17**: 270–5.
6. Kaczmarek RG, Silverman BG, Gross TP, Hamilton RG, Kessler E, Arrowsmith-Lowe JT *et al.* Prevalence of latex-specific IgE antibodies in hospital personnel. *Ann Allergy Asthma Immunol* 1996; **76**: 51–6.
7. Brown RH, Schauble JF, Hamilton RG. Prevalence of latex allergy among anesthesiologists: identification of sensitized but asymptomatic individuals. *Anesthesiology* 1998; **89**: 292–9.
8. Sussman GL, Liss GM, Deal K, Brown S, Cividino M, Siu S *et al.* Incidence of latex sensitization among latex glove users. *J Allergy Clin Immunol* 1998; **101**: 171–8.
9. Federal Food, Drug, and Cosmetic Act, Sec. 201. [321]. Definitions. (h).
10. The Council of the European Communities Directive 93/42/EEC of 14 June 1993 concerning medical devices. Document # 393L0042. Available at: http://europa.eu.int/smartapi/cgi/sga_doc?smartapi!celexapi!prod!CELEXnumdoc&lg=EN&numdoc=31993L0042&model=guichett. Accessed: December, 2003.
11. Food and Drugs Act Chapter F-27, Section 1. Available at: http://laws.justice.gc.ca/en/F-27/59736.html. Accessed: December, 2003.
12. Australian Medical Devices Guidelines. An Overview of the New Medical Devices Regulatory System. Guidance Document Number 1. Version 1.6. Available at: http://www.health.gov.au/tga/docs/pdf/devguid1.pdf. Accessed: December, 2003.
13. Comparison of the Device Adverse Reporting Systems in USA, Europe, Canada, Australia & Japan: Final Document. Global Harmonization Task Force Study Group 2. May 21, 2002. Available at: http://www.ghtf.org/sg2/inventorysg2/sg2-n6r3.pdf. Accessed: December, 2003.
14. United States Code of Federal Regulations, Title 21—Food and Drugs, Part 860—Medical Device Classification Procedures. April 1, 1998.
15. Therapeutic Products Programme, Health Canada. Food and Drugs Act Medical Devices Regulations P.C. 1998-783, May 7, 1998. Updated April 30, 2003. Available at: http:// laws.justice.gc.ca/en/F-27/SOR-98-282/126598.html. Accessed: December, 2003.
16. Global Harmonization Task Force Study Group 1. SG1/N015R22: Principles of Medical Devices Classification. Proposed Document, November 17, 2003. Available at: http://www.ghtf.org/sg1/inventorysg1/pd_sg1_n015r22.pdf/. Accessed: September, 2004.
17. Medical Device Quality Systems Manual. January 7, 1997. Available at: http://www.fda.gov/cdrh/qsr/contnt.html. Accessed: January 1, 2003.
18. Global Harmonization Task Force Study Group 2. Précis—GHTF Study Group 2: Vigilance and Postmarket Surveillance. Working Draft, SG2 N12 R9, March 1, 2002. Available at: http://www. ghtf.org/sg2/inventorysg2/sg2-n12r9.pdf. Accessed: January, 2004.
19. Food and Drug Administration Modernization Act of 1997. Sec. 212. Postmarket Surveillance. Available at: http://www.fda.gov/cder/guidance/s830enr.txt. Accessed: December, 2003.
20. Industry Support: Assistance for Small Manufacturers and Other Domestic and Foreign Producers of Medical Devices and Radiation- Emitting Electronic Products. June 17, 2003. Available at: http://www.fda.gov/cdrh/industry/support/index.html. Accessed: January, 2004.
21. Therapeutic Products Programme, Health Canada. Glove barrier protection and latex allergy: minimizing the risk. *Med Devices Bull* 1998; **4**: 16–17.
22. Cook DJ, Walter SD, Cook RJ, Griffith LE, Guyatt GH, Leasa D *et al.* Incidence of and risk factors for ventilator-associated pneumonia in critically ill patients. *Ann Intern Med* 1998; **129**: 433–40.

23. Nicholls AJ, Platts MM. Anaphylactoid reactions due to haemo-dialysis, haemofiltration, or membrane plasma separation. *BMJ* 1982; **285**: 1607–9.

24. Hakim RM, Breillatt J, Lazarus JM, Port FK. Complement activation and hypersensitivity reactions to dialysis membranes. *N Engl J Med* 1984; **311**: 878–82.

25. Silverman BG, Brown SL, Bright RA, Kaczmarek RK, Arrowsmith-Lowe JB, Kessler DA. Reported complications of silicone gel breast implants: an epidemiologic review. *Ann Intern Med* 1996; **124**: 744–56.

26. Product Code Classification Database, Center for Devices and Radiological Health, Food and Drug Administration. Available at: http://www.fda.gov/cdrh/prodcode.html. Accessed: January, 2004.

27. Universal Medical Device Nomenclature System™ (UMDNS™). Available at: http://www.ecri.org/Products_and_Services/Products/UMDNS/Default.aspx. Accessed: January, 2004.

28. Nordan J, Moore R, Naito M. The advantages gained by using a common classification and nomenclature for medical devices. Available at: http://www.uib.no/ood/advrep/Doc/GMDN_from_NKKN.pdf. Accessed: January, 2004.

29. Global Medical Device Nomenclature (GMDN) Homepage. Available at: http://www.gmdn.org. Accessed: December, 2003.

30. A short technical introduction to the GMDN. Version 2002. Available at: http://www.gmdn.org/GMDN_Introductory.pdf. Accessed: December, 2003.

31. Bright RA, Jeng LL, Moore RM. National survey of self-reported breast implants: 1988 estimates. *J Long Term Eff Med Implants* 1993; **3**: 81–9.

32. Poggio EC, Glynn RJ, Schein OD, Seddon JM, Shannon MJ, Scardino VA *et al*. The incidence of ulcerative keratitis among users of daily-wear and extended-wear soft contact lenses. *N Engl J Med* 1989; **321**: 779–83.

33. Schein OD, Glynn RJ, Poggio EC, Seddon JM, Kenyon KR. The relative risk of ulcerative keratitis among users of daily-wear and extended-wear soft contact lenses. A case-control study. *N Engl J Med* 1989; **321**: 773–8.

34. Bernstein AD, Parsonnet V. Survey of cardiac pacing and defibrillation in the United States in 1993. *Am J Cardiol* 1996; **78**: 187–96.

35. Parsonnet V, Bernstein AD, Galasso D. Cardiac pacing practices in the United States in 1985. *Am J Cardiol* 1998; **62**: 71–7.

36. IMS America. Hospital Supply Index 1998. Available at: http://www.imshealth.com. Accessed: January, 2004.

37. Nationwide Inpatient Sample (NIS): Powerful Database for Analyzing Hospital Care. United States Agency for Healthcare Research and Quality, July 2003. Available at: http://www.ahrq.gov/data/hcup/hcupnis.htm. Accessed: January, 2004.

38. Daley WR, Kaczmarek RG. The epidemiology of cardiac pacemakers in the older US population. *J Am Geriatr Soc* 1998; **46**: 1016–19.

39. Moss AJ, Hamburger S, Moore RM, Jeng LL, Howie LJ. Use of selected medical device implants in the United States, 1988. Advance Data from Vital and Health Statistics, no. 191. National Center for Health Statistics, Hyattsville, MD, 1990.

40. Silverman BG, Gross TP, Kaczmarek RG, Hamilton P, Hamburger S. The epidemiology of pacemaker implantation in the United States. *Public Health Rep* 1995; **110**: 42–6.

41. Title 21 Code of Federal Regulations, Chapter I, Part 803—Medical Device Reporting.

42. Feigal DW, Gardner SN, McClellan M. Ensuring safe and effective medical devices. *N Engl J Med* 2003; **348**: 191–2.

43. CDER Organizational Components: Office of Drug Safety. Available at: http://www.fda.gov/cder/Offices/ODS/default.htm. Accessed: January, 2004.

44. MedSun: playing a vital role in ensuring medical device safety. Available at: https://www.medsun.net. Accessed: January, 2004.

45. US Consumer Product Safety Commission: National Electronic Injury Surveillance System (NEISS) online. Available at: http://www.cpsc.gov/library/neiss.html. Accessed: January, 2004.

46. Hefflin B, Gross TP, Schroeder TJ. Estimates of medical device-associated adverse events from emergency departments. *Am J Prev Med* 2004; **27**: 246–53.

47. Adams PF, Hardy AM. Current estimates from the National Health Interview Survey, United States, 1988. National Center for Health Statistics. *Vital Health Stat* 1989; **10**(173). Available at: http://www.cdc.gov/nchs/data/series/sr_10/sr10_173.pdf. Accessed: January, 2003.

48. National Maternal and Infant Health Survey (NMIHS) public-use data file. Available at: http://www.cdc.gov/nchs/products/elec_prods/subject/mihs.htm. Accessed: January, 2004.

49. National Health and Nutrition Examination Survey. Available at: http://www.cdc.gov/nchs/about/major/nhanes/DataAccomp.htm. Accessed: January, 2004.

50. National Vital Statistics System: National Mortality Follow-back Survey. Available at: http://www.cdc.gov/nchs/about/major/nmfs/nmfs.htm. Accessed: January, 2004.

51. National Home and Hospice Care Survey. Available at: http://www.cdc.gov/nchs/about/major/nhhcsd/nhhcsd.htm. Accessed: January, 2004.

52. National Health and Nutrition Examination Survey: 1999–2004 Survey Content. September 2003. Available at: http://www.cdc.gov/nchs/data/nhanes/comp3.pdf. Accessed: January, 2004.

53. National Health and Nutrition Examination Survey: NHANES III serum latex allergy (IgE) data analysis issues. Available at: http://www.cdc.gov/nchs/about/major/nhanes/nhanes3/latex.htm. Accessed: January, 2004.

54. National Health and Nutrition Examination Survey. NHANES 1999–2000 data files: data, docs, codebooks, SAS code. November 4, 2003. Available at: http://www.cdc.gov/nchs/about/major/nhanes/NHANES99_00.htm. Accessed: January, 2004.

55. Jeng LL, Moore RM, Kaczmarek RG, Placek PJ, Bright RA. How frequently are home pregnancy tests used? Results from the 1988 National Maternal and Infant Health Survey. *Birth* 1991; **18**: 11–13.

56. Hefflin BJ. Final-year-of life pacemaker recipients. *J Am Geriatr Soc* 1998; **46**: 1396–400.

57. Furman S, Benedek ZM. Survival of implantable pacemaker leads. The Implantable Lead Registry. *Pacing Clin Electrophysiol* 1990; **13**: 1910–14.

58. Andersen C, Green A, Madsen GM, Arnsbo P. The epidemiology of pacemaker implantations in Fyn County, Denmark. *Pacing Clin Electrophysiol* 1991; **14**: 1614–21.

59. Moller M, Arnsbo P. Appraisal of pacing lead performance from the Danish Pacemaker Register. *Pacing Clin Electrophysiol* 1996; **19**: 1327–36.

60. Kawanishi DT, Song S, Furman S, Parsonnet V, Pioger G, Petitot JC *et al.* Failure rates of leads, pulse generators, and programmers have not diminished over the last 20 years: formal monitoring of performance is still needed. BILITCH Registry and STIMAREC. *Pacing Clin Electrophysiol* 1996; **19**: 1819–23.

61. Executive Summary for Aspden P, Corrigan JM, Wolcott J, Erickson SM, eds, *Patient Safety: Achieving a New Standard for Care*. Available at: http://books.nap.edu/execsumm_pdf/10863.pdf. Accessed: January, 2004.

62. Rubin JW, Killam HAW, Moore HV, Ellison RG. Permanent cardiac pacemakers: twelve-year experience with 287 patients. *Ann Thorac Surg* 1976; **22**: 74–9.

63. Mueller C, Cernin J, Glogar D, Laczkovics A, Mayr H, Scheibelhofer W *et al.* Survival rate and causes of death in patients with pacemakers: dependence on symptoms leading to pacemaker implantation. *Eur Heart J* 1988; **9**: 1003–9.

64. Shen WK, Hammill SC, Hayes DL, Packer DL, Bailey KR, Ballard DJ *et al.* Long-term survival after pacemaker implantation for heart block in patients > or =65 years. *Am J Cardiol* 1994; **74**: 560–4.

65. Kurland LT, Molgaard CA. The patient record in epidemiology. *Sci Am* 1981; **245**: 54–63.

66. Orvidas LJ, Kasperbauer JL, Staats BA, Olsen KD. Long-term clinical experience with transtracheal oxygen catheters. *Mayo Clin Proc* 1998; **73**: 739–44.

67. Samore MH, Evans RS, Lassen A, Gould P, Lloyd J, Gardner RM *et al.* Surveillance of medical device-related hazards and adverse events in hospitalized patients. *JAMA* 2004; **291**: 325–34.

68. Greenspan AM, Kay HR, Berger BC, Greenberg RM, Greenspon AJ, Gaughan MJS. Incidence of unwarranted implantation of permanent cardiac pacemakers in a large medical population. *N Engl J Med* 1988; **318**: 158–63.

69. Qualidigm. Medicare Patient Safety Monitoring System (MPSMS). Available at http://www.qualidigm.org/what_con_patientsafety.shtml. Accessed: September, 2004.

70. Villforth JC. New FDA recommendations and results of contact lens study. FDA Letter to Eyecare Practitioners, May 30, 1989.

71. List of FDA approved soft contact lenses for up to 30 days of wear available by entering product code "LPM" at "Search PMA Database (database updated December 2003)," Available at:http://www.accessdata.fda.gov/scripts/cdrh/cfdocs/cf PMA/pma.cfm. Accessed: January, 2004.

72. Spera G. CDRH predicts tomorrow's top technologies. *Med Device Diagnost Industry* 1998; **20**: 18, 20–1.

73. Padley K. Guidant's defibrillator wins race to market. *Saint Paul Pioneer Press*, September 10, 1998, p. 1.

74. Harman J. Topics for our times: new health care data—new horizons for public health. *Am J Public Health* 1998; **88**: 1019–21.

75. Coyne MM Jr. Information versus privacy: an imaginative look at the future. *Med Device Diagnost Industry* 1998; **20**: 24–6.

76. Longe K. How to implement a UPN system. *Med Device Diagnost Industry* 1998; **20**: 108–12.

77. Hjelm NM, Tong FFK. Patients' records on the Internet: a boost for evidence-based medicine. *Lancet* 1998; **351**: 1751–2.

78. Goldberg HI, Tarczy-Hornoch P, Stephens K, Larson EB, LoGerfo JP. Internet access to patients' records. *Lancet* 1998; **351**: 1811.

79. de Groen PC, Barry JA, Schaller WJ. Applying World Wide Web technology to the study of patients with rare diseases. *Ann Intern Med* 1998; **129**: 107–13.

80. Shortliffe EH. Health care and the next generation Internet. *Ann Intern Med* 1998; **129**: 138–40.

81. Melton LJ 3rd. The threat to medical-records research. *N Engl J Med* 1997; **337**: 1466–70.

82. Statement by Tommy G. Thompson, Secretary of Health and Human Services, regarding new Federal privacy regulations, April 11, 2003. Available at: http://www.hhs.gov/news/press/2003pres/20030411.html. Accessed: January, 2004.

83. US Department of Health and Human Services. HIPAA Privacy Rule Information for Researchers: Frequently Asked Questions. Available at: http://privacyruleandresearch.nih.gov/faq. asp. Accessed: January, 2004.

84. Parker L. Medical-privacy law creates wide confusion. *USA Today* October 17, 2003. Available at: http://www.usatoday. com. Accessed: October, 2003.

85. Rabinowitz J. A method for preserving confidentiality when linking computerized registries. *Am J Public Health* 1998; **88**: 836.

32

Studies of Drug-Induced Birth Defects

ALLEN A. MITCHELL

Slone Epidemiology Center, Boston University Schools of Public Health and Medicine, Brookline, Massachusetts, USA.

INTRODUCTION

Teratogenesis is a very different phenomenon from other drug-induced hazards, and it therefore requires special consideration. Although the fetus may experience a wide range of adverse effects as a result of antenatal drug exposure, such as mental/motor deficits and learning and behavioral problems, this chapter will confine itself to issues surrounding drug-induced physical malformations.

THE NATURE OF BIRTH DEFECTS AND THEIR RELATION TO DRUGS

Birth defects are part of the human condition, having been observed throughout history. Major birth defects, typically defined as those that are life threatening, require major surgery, or present a significant disability, affect approximately 3–4% of liveborn infants.[1,2] Minor malformations are of lesser clinical importance, and estimates of their prevalence vary considerably because of substantial differences in definition and detection.

Over the centuries, the "deformities" that characterize most birth defects have been viewed as a punishment to the mother or family for some fault on their part. This view was undoubtedly reinforced by the rarity of birth defects, their unpredictable occurrence, and the absence of known causes. Perhaps because these factors have not changed very much over time, elements of this primitive view persist today, largely in the form of guilt. Parents tend to search their memories to identify some factor—any factor—that might account for their misfortune. In developed societies, attention often focuses on drugs taken in pregnancy.

This concern, of course, is not without foundation. Less than 70 years ago it was believed that the placenta protected the fetus from noxious agents. That belief was shattered in 1941 by the recognition that maternal rubella infection in pregnancy produced a distinctive pattern of birth defects among exposed infants.[3] Two decades later, the thalidomide disaster demonstrated that drugs, too, could be teratogenic.[4] Many thousands of infants were born with major limb reductions and other defects, and the tragedy of this epidemic was etched into the consciousness of medical practitioners and the public alike. In the years that followed, other drugs were shown to be teratogenic, ranging from phenytoin to isotretinoin. Many additional drugs were alleged to be teratogenic, and although most of those allegations were unsupported by subsequent studies, they served to reinforce the general concern about the teratogenic effects of marketed drugs.

Teratogenesis is a unique kind of adverse drug effect, since it affects an organism (the fetus) other than the one for whom the drug was intended (the mother). In a benefit/risk consideration, the fetus may at best indirectly benefit from a medication given to its mother (e.g., by an improvement in the mother's health), but the fetus alone is at risk for birth defects. That "innocent bystander" status of the fetus raises profound medical, moral, and legal issues. It also poses serious concerns about the consequences of allegations that a given drug may be teratogenic.

CAN TERATOGENESIS BE PREDICTED PRIOR TO MARKETING A DRUG?

Under ideal circumstances, one would identify the teratogenic potential of drugs before they were used in humans. Unfortunately, our ignorance about the basic mechanisms of organ formation has constrained development of predictive *in vitro* tests. Testing in animals may be helpful in certain circumstances; for example, vitamin A and its congeners produce consistent patterns of malformations across many different species. However, for most known human teratogens (including thalidomide), results of animal tests vary so much as to seriously limit their predictive value.[5] Further, understanding of the structure/activity relationships of a particular agent can help predict that drug's efficacy and some adverse effects, but it does not necessarily help predict its teratogenic potential. Because there are no theoretical, *in vitro*, or animal models that can reliably provide meaningful information about the likelihood of human fetal risk, we are usually completely unaware of a given drug's teratogenic potential when it first appears on the market.

Clinical premarketing studies cannot be expected to provide this information either. Traditionally, women of childbearing age were excluded from early clinical studies, specifically because of concerns about potential teratogenicity; newer guidelines are designed to reverse these exclusions, but women entered into most clinical studies will, appropriately, be at minimal risk of becoming pregnant. Information derived from experience among nonpregnant adult women is not informative when the concern is teratogenesis, and might even provide a false sense of reassurance—it is worth recalling that thalidomide was used as a sedative in pregnant women specifically because of its "safety profile" in nonpregnant adults.

A NOTE ABOUT NON-PRESCRIPTION DRUGS

Non-prescription (or over-the-counter, OTC) drugs present a unique situation. Whatever caution physicians might exercise in their prescribing of drugs to pregnant women, they have little control over what consumers purchase over-the-counter or obtain from their friends, relatives, and neighbors. It can reasonably be assumed that women of childbearing age, like other consumers and their physicians, consider OTC drugs to be safer than prescription products, and they may assume the same is true for use of these drugs in pregnancy. This perception is based on the fact that prescription drugs tend to become available OTC on the basis of a history of wide use and safety. However, because there is little systematic information available on the human teratogenicity of most prescription drugs, the process of switching to OTC availability rarely takes account of a drug's risk or safety with respect to the fetus. This is particularly the case for drugs that became available OTC decades ago. As noted below, teratogenicity is more difficult to assess when a drug is used without prescription, and it is ironic that we may know less about the teratogenic hazard of drugs available OTC than we do about drugs available only by prescription.

The important reality is that we lack an understanding of the teratogenic effects of newly marketed and many other prescription drugs as well as most OTC drugs, and we typically lack an understanding even of their teratogenic potential; the opportunity to gain such knowledge comes from postmarketing experience, where pharmacoepidemiology can and must play a crucial role.

CLINICAL PROBLEMS TO BE ADDRESSED BY PHARMACOEPIDEMIOLOGIC RESEARCH

Like other adverse drug effects, teratogenesis is a critical aspect of a drug's benefit/risk profile, and such information obviously should be available to prescribers and consumers. Unlike other adverse drug effects, however, teratogenesis raises uniquely important and controversial clinical issues. First, the fetus is the "innocent bystander" with respect to its mother's therapy. Second, teratogenesis is not a concern limited to women who are pregnant when drug treatment is initiated; since roughly half of pregnancies (at least in the US) are unplanned, teratogenesis must also be a concern among women who might become pregnant while already taking a medication. Finally, unlike other adverse outcomes, teratogenic effects can be prevented by avoidance of pregnancy, and the birth of a malformed infant can be avoided by termination of pregnancy. Our understanding of a drug's teratogenic risk therefore has important consequences for how a given drug is used clinically.

DRUGS KNOWN TO BE TERATOGENIC

Experience has shown that human teratogens tend to fall into two broad categories.[6] Drugs that produce major defects in a high proportion (roughly, 25%) of exposed pregnancies can be considered "high risk" teratogens (e.g., thalidomide and isotretinoin). More common are "moderate risk" teratogens, which increase the rate of specific birth defects by perhaps 5–20-fold (e.g., carbamazepine and neural tube defects). In the latter situation, for example, the background rate of neural tube defects of 1 in 1000 pregnancies might be increased to 10 in 1000. The differences between high-risk and moderate-risk teratogens have relevance for how these drugs are considered in the clinical setting.

Broadly speaking, there are three approaches applied to the few drugs known to be human teratogens. In rare instances, such as was the case for thalidomide in most countries, a drug may be prohibited or removed from the general market once its teratogenicity becomes known; for thalidomide in the 1960s, this approach was justified by the fact that this high-risk teratogen posed a large absolute risk to the fetus but did not offer important or unique therapeutic benefits to the women using the drug.

Most known teratogens, such as phenytoin and valproic acid, pose moderate risks and are often considered to fill an important clinical need. For such drugs, information about teratogenicity is provided to physicians, who are expected to discuss the benefits and risks with their patients, who in turn can make informed decisions about their drug treatment. In some settings, a drug may be restricted to prescription by selected physicians; however, until follow-up data are available, the effectiveness of this approach remains unclear. It should be noted that considerations in these doctor–patient discussions may differ according to each woman's risk of becoming pregnant while on the drug.

The third approach utilizes a formal risk management program involving education of physicians and patients that is combined, in some cases, with restricted access to the drug (see Chapter 33). The educational component is intended to assure that physicians and their patients are informed about the drug's teratogenicity and the importance of avoiding pregnancy. The first such effort, in the US, was initiated in late 1988 by the manufacturer of isotretinoin (Accutane®), a high-risk teratogen that is uniquely effective in the treatment of severe acne.[7] Preliminary data from this voluntary "pregnancy prevention program" suggested some success in achieving both educational objectives, reducing the number of exposed pregnancies from about 4 per 1000 courses of therapy in 1989 to about 1 per 1000 in 2002.[8,9] Whether more restrictive approaches will further reduce the rate of pregnancy remains unclear.

In July, 1998, newly identified uses for thalidomide prompted the US Food and Drug Administration to approve, for the first time in the US, marketing of the drug (as Thalomid®), but only with an unprecedented FDA-regulated program sponsored by the drug's manufacturer, Celgene Corporation. This program included an educational component similar to that used for Accutane®, but also restricted prescription and distribution of the drug to registered prescribers and pharmacies, respectively; it also mandated that all patients participate in a follow-up survey designed to monitor and enhance compliance with the manufacturer's "System for Thalidomide Education and Prescribing Safety (STEPS)." Experiences derived from that effort led to a revision in the program in 2001, in which patients and prescribers complete a telephone-based screening before initial therapy and with each subsequent prescription. This screening provides an authorization number to the prescriber; that number, placed on the prescription and verified by the pharmacist, is designed to assure compliance with the risk management program. While this approach is more rigorous than those that were used for isotretinoin or other teratogens, it is important to recognize that most women of childbearing age who receive thalidomide have multiple myeloma and other resistant forms of cancer, and it is doubtful that the low rates of pregnancy encountered in this risk management program can be projected to other populations. It appears that no single formula for pregnancy prevention will apply to all human teratogens, but the efforts focused on isotretinoin and thalidomide will advance our understanding of how best to balance the therapeutic benefits of known human teratogens against the risks of fetal exposure.

DRUGS FOR WHICH TERATOGENIC RISK IS UNKNOWN

For reasons described above, the vast majority of prescription drugs and virtually all non-prescription drugs fall into the category of drugs for which teratogenic risk is unknown. Regulatory agencies or manufacturers in various countries may offer a general warning against unnecessary use in pregnancy, but such cautions hardly contribute to rational drug therapy. In settings where the true teratogenic risk is nil, these warnings serve to deny potentially useful drug therapy; where the true risk is elevated for a particular drug, the nonspecific and "standard" warnings offer little practical discouragement to its use in pregnancy.

DRUGS FOR WHICH TERATOGENESIS IS ALLEGED...AND CLINICAL CONSEQUENCES

At one time or another, a large number of drugs have been alleged to be teratogenic, and the clinical consequences can be profound. In one notorious situation, allegations of teratogenicity resulted in a widely used drug being withdrawn from the market. In the late 1970s and early 1980s, the antinausea drug Bendectin® (Debendox®, Lenotan®), used widely to treat nausea and vomiting of pregnancy, was alleged to cause a variety of birth defects; the history of this experience has been reviewed elsewhere.[10] Ironically, the aggregate data on the teratogenic hazards of Bendectin® have ultimately provided the strongest evidence of safety for any medication used in pregnancy. Despite that evidence, however, the manufacturer withdrew the drug from the market because of active and potential litigation. At least one study suggests that hospital admissions for hyperemesis gravidarum increased significantly following the drug's withdrawal,[11] and there is concern that, in the absence of Bendectin®, women are being treated with other antinausea drugs, for which the teratogenic risks are unknown.

There are other clinical aspects of unproven allegations, and these are too often ignored. Upon learning that a drug she took in pregnancy might be teratogenic, a woman who has given birth to a malformed infant may become overwhelmed with feelings of guilt. Further, a woman who is currently pregnant may develop considerable anxiety; that anxiety can lead to a number of clinical consequences, ranging from consultations with physicians, to diagnostic procedures (e.g., amniocentesis), to elective termination of the pregnancy. An experience in the mid-1970s involving a non-drug exposure is instructive. Following widely publicized allegations that spray glue adhesives (typically used to make Christmas decorations) were teratogenic, a US regulatory agency withdrew the product from the market. Although the allegations were subsequently found to be without basis, a survey conducted among genetic counseling centers identified 1100 inquiries from pregnant women prompted by concern about exposure to these agents; moreover, 11 underwent amniocenteses and because of this exposure, 9 women had therapeutic abortions (one had vague evidence of chromosomal damage and eight had no evidence of malformation).[12] These unique and potentially serious clinical consequences of false positive allegations argue for heightened attention to scientific rigor and caution in the teratologic assessment of drugs.

THE FALLACY OF "CLASS ACTION" TERATOGENESIS

Another clinically important concern specific to teratogenesis is the issue of "class action." It is widely recognized that an understanding of structure/activity relationships shared by members of a given drug class can be helpful in predicting a given class member's efficacy and adversity (indeed, this view is incorporated into regulatory action in the form of class labeling). However, class-based pharmacologic effects cannot be assumed to hold when the adversity at issue is teratogenesis. Given our ignorance about the causes of most birth defects, we cannot know whether it is the chemical structure common to the class that is responsible for teratogenesis or whether the responsible component is that part of the structure that differentiates one class member from another. For example, thalidomide and glutethimide (Doriden® and other brands) are both glutarimides, and both are sedative/hypnotics. Despite their structural and clinical similarities, thalidomide is clearly a high-risk teratogen and glutethimide is not.[13] Thus, we cannot assume that if one drug is a high-risk teratogen, all other members of its class will share that effect; conversely, we cannot assume that reassurance about the safety of one drug can be extended to other members of that drug's class.

METHODOLOGIC PROBLEMS TO BE ADDRESSED BY PHARMACOEPIDEMIOLOGIC RESEARCH

In many ways, the epidemiologic issues involved in the study of birth defects are similar to those of other adverse outcomes; these are considered in detail elsewhere in this text (see Chapters 2 and 3, and Part V). However, there are a number of considerations that are unique to birth defects or are sufficiently important to warrant particular attention. These have to do with sample size considerations, definitions of exposure and outcome, confounding, and biologic plausibility.

Although serious birth defects occur in approximately 3–4% of liveborn infants, we cannot consider "birth defects" as a single, homogeneous outcome. In fact, physical birth defects include a wide range of malformations that vary in many ways, including their gestational timing, embryologic tissue of origin, and mechanism of development. As examples of variations in timing of occurrence, chromosomal abnormalities generally predate conception; neural tube defects develop in the earliest weeks of gestation; cleft palate develops toward the end of the first trimester; and microcephaly can develop relatively late in pregnancy. As an illustration of variations in embryologic tissue of origin, some cardiovascular malformations (but not others) are derived from the neural crest cells that migrate from the area surrounding the primitive neural tube. Variations in mechanisms of development include inhibition, disruption, or alteration of the embryologic tissue that is responsible for normal structural development. From a theoretical perspective, then, one would predict that the malformations produced by a drug would vary according to the timing of exposure, the sensitivity of the end organ (i.e., embryologic tissue), and the mechanism of its teratogenesis.

Experience supports what would be predicted from biology. Even a brief review of known teratogens reveals a fact that is highly relevant in pharmacoepidemiologic studies: teratogens do not uniformly increase the rates of all birth defects, but rather increase rates of selected defects. Thus, the "classic" high-risk teratogen thalidomide produces defects in about 25% of exposed infants, but that overall increase is largely the result of increases in limb, spine, and central nervous system malformations;[14] another high-risk teratogen, isotretinoin, affects a similar proportion of liveborn infants, but again, that overall rate is the result of increases in rates of selected specific defects (ear, central nervous system, and cardiac).[15] Moderate-risk teratogens also increase the rate of specific defects (though to a lesser degree): valproic acid increases rates of neural tube defects,[16] warfarin increases the rate of cartilage defects,[17] and ACE inhibitors increase rates of renal defects.[18]

SAMPLE SIZE CONSIDERATIONS

The fact that pharmacoepidemiologic studies must consider rates of *specific* birth defects has a dramatic effect on sample size requirements, both for estimating risk and providing assurances of safety. With respect to risk in a population of women taking a given drug, a cohort study with a sample size of a few hundred exposed pregnancies might be sufficient to identify a doubling of the 3–4% overall rate of birth defects; ruling out a doubling of the overall rate would require larger numbers, but these would still be within the same order of magnitude. However, each specific defect (which in the aggregate form the overall category of "birth defects") occurs with far less frequency, ranging from about 1 per 1000 live births for oral clefts to 1 or fewer per 10 000 for biliary atresia. For a cohort study to *detect* a doubling of risk for a relatively common specific birth defect (e.g., 1/1000) requires a sample size of over 20 000 exposed

pregnancies (see Chapter 3 and Appendix A). To *rule out* a doubling of risk for the same defect, one would need a far larger sample size of exposed pregnancies.

EXPOSURE

There are two concerns regarding drug exposure that require special consideration in birth defects studies. One is the importance of non-prescribed drugs and the other is the issue of recall of drug exposure.

Non-Prescribed drugs

Most pharmacoepidemiologic research focuses attention on prescribed drugs, in part because many studies utilize data sources with inadequate information on non-prescribed drugs and in part because of the view that prescribed drugs pose the greater potential for risk (despite the fact, noted earlier, that there is no basis for believing that this is the case). Although the effects of non-prescription drugs on the fetus are largely unstudied, it is noteworthy that these agents have comprised a substantial proportion of drug exposures in pregnancy for decades.[19–21] The more recent increase in the use of herbal products by pregnant women[22] has raised additional concerns about potential teratogenesis, particularly given the unregulated nature of these agents and the fact that the precise contents and purity of these products are often unknown.

It is therefore important that pharmacoepidemiologic research include consideration of non-prescribed drugs. In this context, 'non-prescribed' can include not only OTC drugs, vitamins, and herbal products, but also prescription drug products that were not intended for the study subject but rather were obtained from friends, neighbors, and relatives: depending on the specific drug, we have found that more than 20% of exposure to prescription drugs can come from such "non-prescribed" sources.[23] For prescription drugs, one might argue about the validity of drug exposure information derived from records (medical, billing, insurance, etc.) versus that derived from patient interviews (see Chapters 11 and 45), but there is little question that information on the use of OTC, herbal, or non-prescribed prescription drugs must be obtained directly from the patient.

Illicit drugs represent a distinct but important subset of non-prescribed drugs. Use of these drugs is seriously underreported, whether information is drawn from records or interviews. Except in rare settings where exposure may be identified through systematic screening of biologic samples (e.g., urine, blood), epidemiologic studies have major limitations in identifying teratogenic (and confounding) effects of illicit drug use in pregnancy.

Recall Bias

Because of the sample size requirements described above, many researchers have turned to the case–control approach for the study of specific birth defects. Such studies generally (though not always) rely on maternal interviews for exposure information, and this approach raises concern both about the overall accuracy of recall (see also Chapters 11 and 45) and its susceptibility to bias. More than other drug-induced adverse outcomes, the birth of a malformed child carries an emotional burden and guilt that may affect recall of exposures in pregnancy. When compared to a mother of a normal child, the mother of a malformed infant may be more likely to recall carefully every possible act, event, and drug exposure in pregnancy.[24] This tendency is reinforced by repeated inquiries from physicians, nurses, genetic counselors, and relatives, as well as by media and legal attention on the subject of drug-induced birth defects. Thus, in a setting where drug exposure is in fact similar among mothers of normal and malformed infants, one might predict that recall of exposure will be more complete among the latter than among the former. Concern about recall bias is more than theoretical—such bias may well explain a number of drug–defect associations[25,26] that have subsequently been refuted.[27,28] On the other hand, evidence supporting the role of recall bias is inconsistent, and the issue of when and to what extent recall bias is present remains an unresolved controversy.

Despite this concern, the simple possibility of recall bias does not invalidate interview-based studies, and there are a number of approaches to reducing and dealing with this problem. These include the choice of controls, the design of the questions, and direct attempts to identify potentially biased recall.

There are differing schools of thought regarding what constitutes an appropriate control for a malformed infant—should controls be infants without malformations, or should they be infants with malformations other than the one under study? Some argue that normal infants should be used because of the possibility that a drug might increase the risk of all malformations, a finding that would be missed if only malformed controls were used.[29] Others argue that, since no known teratogen uniformly increases the risk of all malformations, normal controls may be unnecessary; further, use of normal controls might increase the opportunity for differential recall of exposure between mothers of normal and malformed infants. They argue that controls should comprise infants with a wide range of malformations other than the ones in the case series.[27] By assuring that the controls include a wide range of malformations, one reduces the likelihood that the control series will be biased by inclusion of a large proportion of defects that might be associated with the exposure under study. By restricting comparisons of exposures to those reported by mothers of malformed infants (whether cases or controls), one limits the likelihood of recall bias.

Both approaches are imperfect. Although no teratogen has yet been identified that uniformly increases the risk of all specific defects, the history of teratology is replete with examples of assumptions that proved to be false. We used to think that the fetus was protected by the placenta from noxious agents, and only 30 years ago it was inconceivable to some that a drug (diethylstilbestrol) could produce cancers in the adult offspring of exposed mothers, or birth defects in the children of women exposed to the drug *in utero*. In an effort to avoid such hubris, some researchers,[30] including ourselves, have elected to use two control series, one of malformed and one of normal infants. Since we believe that concern about recall bias exceeds concern about failing to identify an "across-the-board" teratogen, we usually give primary consideration to findings derived from comparisons with malformed controls.

By definition, recall bias cannot exist if reporting of drug exposure is complete among cases and controls. The closer one comes to that ideal, the less the likelihood of recall bias. It thus becomes critical how one elicits exposure information. Studies that use open-ended questions about drug exposure invite differential recall between mothers of malformed and normal infants.[25] As might be predicted, the more specifically one asks questions about drug use, the more likely is one to obtain complete information (see also Chapter 45). Recall is also substantially increased when women are asked about use according to various indications, and it is further increased when drugs are asked by specific names[23] (see also Chapter 45). This approach is not likely to result in exaggerated recall (i.e., false positives), as demonstrated by the fact that use of a specific drug ascertained by such a questionnaire was the same as that estimated from the manufacturer's marketing data; in addition, women do not tend to report exposure to a nonexistent drug.[27] In short, by improving ascertainment of drug exposure among both cases and controls, a carefully designed questionnaire can substantially reduce the opportunity for recall bias.

Unfortunately, the possibility of recall bias cannot be eliminated completely, either by the use of a malformed control group or by asking specific questions about drug use. In an effort to identify women who might be most at risk for biased recall, we began, in 1976, to ask routinely whether a woman has heard that any drug affects the risk of any defect.[27] (This question is asked at the end of the interview, so as not to itself affect reporting of exposures and events.) Our *a priori* assumption is that a woman who acknowledges that a particular drug causes (or prevents) a particular defect is more at risk for differential recall than one who does not. This approach has enabled us to identify indirect evidence of biased recall: in our study of the possible protective effects of folic acid on the development of neural tube defects, we observed different risk estimates when we stratified subjects according to their knowledge of the hypothesis.[31] By simply asking women about their perceptions of the teratogenic effects of drugs, one might obtain insight into the nature of biased recall in the study population.

OUTCOME

Given the etiologic heterogeneity of malformations, some have attempted to classify birth defects according to specific categories. We were among those who, more than two decades ago, classified defects by organ system, such as "musculoskeletal" or "cardiovascular."[1] However, classification in this way has little embryologic or teratologic basis, and a more appropriate approach is to create categories that reflect the embryologic tissue of origin. For example, neural crest cells in the earliest stages of embryogenesis migrate to form a variety of structures, including those of the face/ears, parts of the heart, and the neural tube.[32] Interference with the normal development of the neural crest would therefore be expected to produce malformations of tissues derived from neural crest, and that phenomenon has been observed in a number of animal experiments. In fact, these patterns have also been observed for certain human teratogens, the most striking example of which is the retinoid isotretinoin, which interferes with neural crest cell migration/development and leads to specific malformations of the ear, heart, and neural tube.[15] Similarly, certain defects are believed to result from disruption of the embryonic vasculature.[33,34] Although our ignorance about the origins of most birth defects may limit our ability to create categories which share a common etiology, it is preferable, whenever possible, to classify birth defects according to an understanding of their embryologic origins.[35]

CONFOUNDING

As with any other aspect of pharmacoepidemiologic research (see Chapters 2 and 47), confounding must be taken into account in studies focused on birth defects. Among those variables that require routine consideration are maternal age, race, geography, and socioeconomic status. An understanding of the epidemiology of a given defect or exposure often identifies other variables which

may act as confounders in a specific analysis. For example, ethnic background is strongly related to the risk of neural tube defects, maternal age is a strong risk factor for gastroschisis, and alcohol consumption has been associated with defects derived from neural crest. Since medication use may be associated with various other health behaviors (e.g., vitamin use is more common among nonsmokers than smokers), one may need to consider health behaviors, including nutrition, in studies of certain exposures and outcomes. Further, it may be critically important to separate the teratogenic risk of a drug from the underlying risk associated with the condition for which the drug is taken, something called "confounding by indication"[36] (see also Chapters 40 and 47).

Finally, an issue unique to the epidemiologic study of birth defects is the possibility of pregnancy termination. As more malformations become detectable at earlier stages of pregnancy (and as more such pregnancies are terminated), studies of liveborn and stillborn infants will increasingly underestimate the prevalence of such defects. In addition, there are a number of instances where this factor must be considered as a potential confounder (e.g., periconceptional vitamin exposure and neural tube defects).

BIOLOGIC PLAUSIBILITY

Our ignorance about the biologic mechanisms by which most human birth defects occur complicates our ability to determine when a finding may be biologically plausible. There are a few instances where *in vitro* and animal experiments support the biologic plausibility of drug–defect associations: these include the increased risk of defects derived from neural crest cells among infants exposed to retinoids,[15] the decreased risk of neural tube defects among infants exposed to folic acid[37] and the increased risks of those defects among infants exposed to folic acid antagonists,[38] and the increased risk of defects resulting from vascular disruption among infants exposed to aspirin and possibly pseudoephedrine.[39,40] However, biologic mechanisms remain unknown for most well-accepted drug–defect associations.

In light of this inconsistency, how does one evaluate the importance of biologic plausibility in relation to newly observed associations? On the one hand, a requirement that every association have an identifiable biologic mechanism would have led to dismissal of virtually every accepted human teratogen. On the other hand, some aspects of biologic plausibility must be met. For example, it is implausible that a defect could be caused by an exposure if that exposure first occurs after the gestational development of the defect has been completed. While less absolute, it is

unlikely to expect that an exposure would produce a range
of defects which span gestational timing from preconception to late pregnancy and which do not share embryologic
tissue of origin. Thus, we cannot dismiss hypotheses simply
because they lack a biologically plausible explanation;
however, until they are supported by subsequent studies,
such hypotheses must be considered more speculative than
hypotheses for which there is a strong biologic basis.

CURRENTLY AVAILABLE SOLUTIONS

There are a variety of approaches that are used to generate
and test hypotheses regarding drugs and birth defects. The
purpose of this section is not to list every available design
or data set, but rather to describe the types of resources and
their respective strengths and weaknesses. For convenience,
these may be divided into cohort and case–control designs.
Approaches that involve the monitoring of birth defects
without the systematic collection of exposure information
are not directly applicable to pharmacoepidemiologic study,
and are not considered in this chapter; interested readers are
referred to an excellent review.[41]

COHORTS

Broadly speaking, there are three types of cohorts relevant to the pharmacoepidemiologic study of birth defects.
These are studies designed to follow large populations
exposed to various agents, the use of data sets created
for other purposes, and follow-up studies of selected
exposures.

Studies Designed to Follow Large Populations Exposed to Various Agents

This approach involves the identification of a population of
pregnant women to be followed, with periodic collection of
information on demographic characteristics, exposures, and
potential confounders, as well as formal evaluation of the
offspring at birth and perhaps at some years later. A number
of studies of this kind have been conducted in various countries.[42–45] An example is the US Collaborative Perinatal
Project (CPP), which enrolled over 58 000 women between
1959 and 1965, obtained detailed information on their pregnancies, and followed the children until age 7.[1] More
recently, researchers in Denmark have similarly assembled
a cohort of 100 000 pregnancies.[46] The strength of this type
of approach lies in the prospective, systematic, and repeated
collection of information that includes exposure to a wide
variety of medications taken by a diverse population, many
potential confounding variables, and good outcome
information.

In the CPP, there was sufficient power for commonly
used drugs (such as aspirin in the 1960s) to assess risks for
malformations overall as well as for certain subgroups of
malformations.[47] However, despite the large number of
pregnancies in the database, a major weakness of even a
cohort this large is the small sample sizes of infants with
specific malformations. For example, there were approximately 2200 infants with any major malformation in over
50 000 pregnancies followed by the CPP. Among these,
however, there were only 31 with cleft palate (CP) and 11
with tracheoesophageal fistula (TEF). This weakness is further compounded by limited numbers of women exposed to
most drugs. For a commonly used drug, taken by as many
as 10% of the women, the expected number of exposed
infants with CP and TEF would be 3 and 1, respectively; if a
drug were used by 3% of pregnant women, the expected
intercepts would be 1 and 0.3. Such a cohort may be large
enough to identify some high-risk teratogens; however, as
experience with the CPP reflected, power is usually inadequate to identify moderate-risk teratogens among commonly
used drugs, and power is routinely inadequate to identify
such teratogens among the vast majority of other drugs.

Further, the inordinate costs of such intensive efforts
limit enrollment and data collection to a study period of no
more than a few years. Because of changing patterns of
drug use over time, the clinical relevance of the available
data diminishes.

Use of Data Sets Created for Other Purposes

In recent years, researchers have focused increasing
attention on cohorts identified from databases produced
for purposes other than for epidemiologic research by organizations or governments involved in medical care (see Part
IIIb). The strengths and weaknesses vary with the nature of
the specific data set. All have the advantage of identifying
exposures independent of knowledge of the outcome, some
may have good reporting of malformations, and some may
be derived from large populations. Like most other cohorts,
studies based on data from health maintenance organizations (HMOs) may be limited by their small samples of
specific malformations. For example, among almost 7000
pregnancies in which 33% of women filled a prescription
for Bendectin®, there were a total of 80 malformations
identified, of which only 24 were exposed to the drug *in
utero*.[48] For the more typical situation where a given drug
exposure is far less prevalent, sample size constraints are

even more striking: researchers reviewed 15 years of data and identified 215 women who delivered liveborn infants after presumed exposure to topical tretinoin, among whom there were 4 infants with a variety of malformations.[49] In both examples, the numbers of exposed infants with specific birth defects were too few to identify even substantial increases in the risk of these outcomes. Further, the definition of exposure was limited to receipt of a prescription for the drug during a given interval, birth defect rates among unexposed subjects were lower than expected, and information on confounding variables was largely absent.

In an effort to overcome sample size limitations, researchers have studied larger data sets. Among these are health insurance data. In a study of benzodiazepine abuse in pregnancy, researchers reviewed over 100 000 pregnancies in US Medicaid data and identified 80 women who received numerous prescriptions for the drugs of interest.[50] Unfortunately, records for the offspring could not be found for a substantial proportion of the study subjects, a problem not uncommon in such data sets.

Newer resources, and particularly the newer record linkage systems from Scandinavia,[51] offer promise of better information on exposure and outcome variables. Like other automated data sets, however, they lack important information on potential confounding variables (e.g., smoking, alcohol consumption, diet), and they are unlikely to identify exposure to non-prescription drugs, which may be of importance both as potential confounders and as primary exposures.

Follow-up of Selected Exposures

Various mechanisms may be used to identify cohorts of women exposed to specific drugs. Pregnant women can be enrolled in registries by physicians or by the women themselves, often on the basis of a call to a teratogen information service. The strength of such approaches lies in the ability to identify women exposed to a drug of interest early in pregnancy and, most importantly, to identify and enroll the woman before the pregnancy outcome is known. This design offers the additional advantage of providing an opportunity to prospectively collect other information, such as data relating to other exposures and potential confounding variables. These follow-up studies, often called pregnancy registries, have had strong support in the US from the Food and Drug Administration, and sponsors of selected new prescription drugs have been encouraged to establish such registries for those products.[52] The potential value of these cohorts is reflected in the dramatic observation among only 36 women who were followed after first-trimester exposure to isotretinoin:[15] there were 28

liveborn infants, and 5 (18%) were malformed. More striking than the overall rate of malformation was the distribution of defects: each of the five affected infants had at least one of the specific malformations hypothesized (from premarketing animal studies) to result from isotretinoin exposure (ear, palate, chin, certain heart, and certain brain defects). These findings have been supported by a subsequent study of 94 prospectively identified exposed pregnancies that resulted in live births.[53]

Cohorts of a few dozen to a few hundred exposed pregnancies are highly efficient and effective for identifying—and for ruling out—high-risk teratogens.[54] On the other hand, such cohorts are quite limited in their ability to identify a drug as a moderate-risk teratogen or to rule out such an effect. Two examples illustrate this point. In one, the manufacturer followed 276 prospectively identified pregnancies that had been exposed to alprazolam in the first trimester and resulted in a live birth; 13 malformations were found (4.7%), a rate comparable to that in the general population. The authors acknowledged, however, that their sample lacked power to detect 10–15-fold increases in specific common defects.[55] Similar issues surround data drawn from teratogen information services. For example, researchers from four such services identified 128 women who sought counseling because of first trimester exposure to fluoxetine. Among the 98 liveborn infants, there were two with major malformations.[56] For a specific defect (e.g., oral cleft) with a baseline rate of 1 in 1000 births, such a sample would easily miss increases in risk in the order of 30-fold.

Registries may be limited by problems of self-referral bias and losses to follow-up (with biases introduced if response to follow-up is related to whether the infant is malformed or normal). In addition, there may be difficulties in making comparisons between the drug-exposed cohort and those "unexposed." Some registry investigators compare observed rates of defects to rates reported in various other populations, and others compare the observed rates to those among pregnancies with exposures to no drugs or to other drugs (e.g., presumed "nonteratogenic" drugs); both are imperfect, and comparisons rarely if ever adequately take into account the risk of birth defects due to the condition for which the drug in question was taken.[36]

These methodologic concerns aside, all cohort studies have a common limitation: as is clear from the earlier discussion, cohorts are well suited to identify and rule out high-risk teratogens, but it is extremely difficult for such studies to achieve sample sizes sufficiently large to provide the broader range of critical information about a drug's risk or safety; such inquiry requires information not simply on the risk of birth defects overall, but also on risks of specific defects, most of which have background rates ranging from 1 per 1000 to 1 per 10 000. Thus, while a cohort of 100 or even 1000 exposed pregnancies might provide reassurance that the drug is not another thalidomide or isotretinoin, such a cohort cannot assure us that a drug is safe with respect to oral clefts, gastroschisis, or other specific birth defects.

CASE–CONTROL STUDIES

The rarity of birth defects in general, and of specific defects in particular, argues for the use of the case–control design in pharmacoepidemiologic studies of birth defects when there is a high enough prevalence of exposure to the drug(s) of interest. Of course, the strengths and limitations of these studies are similar to those for case–control studies of other outcomes (see Chapter 2), and will not be reviewed here. Such studies may be conducted on an *ad hoc* basis or within the context of case–control surveillance (see Chapter 11). Examples of the latter are few; in North America, two current examples include the longstanding "Birth Defects Study" conducted by our own group,[27] and the more recently established National Birth Defects Prevention Study, involving a number of state birth defects surveillance programs and coordinated by the US Centers for Disease Control and Prevention.[57]

From the unique perspective of birth defects, case–control studies can have the statistical power required for the assessment of both risk and safety. At the same time, however, they have the potential limitation of biased recall. There are numerous examples that illustrate both issues, but the following are among the most instructive.

In a study of spermicidal contraceptives, researchers using data from an HMO found the prevalence of birth defects among 763 infants born to exposed mothers to be 2.2% ($n = 17$), whereas the rate among infants born to non-exposed mothers was 1.0%. The excess was attributed to four different defects: chromosomal defects, limb reduction defects, hypospadias, and neoplasms.[58] Other investigators used different cohorts to test the hypothesis. Although two analyses involving populations of about 35 000 and 50 000 pregnant women failed to confirm an overall increase in malformation risk,[59,60] neither study had sufficient power to rule out, with reasonable confidence, an increased risk for each of the specific defects identified in the first study. Therefore, two case–control studies were mounted specifically to test the hypothesis. One identified about 100–400 cases of each of the outcomes of interest, and for a variety of exposure duration intervals found odds ratios close to unity; more importantly, the upper 95% confidence intervals were 2.2 or lower.[61] The other identified 151 fetuses with trisomy,

including 92 with trisomy 21; point estimates for various exposure duration intervals approximated unity, and the study had sufficient power to rule out more than a two-fold increase in the risk of trisomy in relation to spermicide use.[62]

While statistical power is a major strength of the case–control approach, power does not assure validity. There are numerous issues that relate to validity (see Chapters 11 and 45); in studies of birth defects, the one that requires particular consideration is recall bias. We previously cited a study of the protective effects of folic acid supplements in relation to neural tube defects, in which we found different risk estimates among women who reported, at the end of the interview, that they were aware of the hypothesis under study.[31] We believe that this study supports concern about recall bias. As stated above, however, the simple *possibility* of such bias does not necessarily invalidate a case–control study; rather, it requires that investigators consider its existence and make reasonable attempts both to minimize and identify it in their study population.

We cannot review issues in the epidemiologic study of birth defects without alluding to a concern that cuts across all study designs. Birth defects are complex outcomes, and the study of medications in relation to birth defects only adds to this complexity. For all the reasons described in the introduction to this chapter, the rigorous pharmacoepidemiologic evaluation of birth defects requires considerable understanding and experience not only of epidemiology, but also of related disciplines (e.g., pharmacology, embryology, teratology).

AN INTEGRATED APPROACH

As noted above, there are two broad concerns regarding teratogenesis. The first, both in theory and in practice, is to identify high-risk teratogens (exemplified by thalidomide and isotretinoin); the second is to identify moderate-risk teratogens (exemplified by phenytoin and valproic acid). Although not widely appreciated, a combination of the approaches described above can provide much of the information needed to respond to these concerns.[6] Cohorts of exposed subjects, preferably in the form of pregnancy registries, can identify high-risk teratogens in a timely way. In most instances, the extremely large risks associated with drugs such as thalidomide or isotretinoin tend to overwhelm the distinct methodologic limitations inherent in these approaches. If a drug makes it past that first line of defense, case–control surveillance (or focused case–control studies) can provide the power and rigor necessary to identify whether a drug is associated with specific defects. Simple sample size considerations will continue to limit our ability to demonstrate safety with respect to relatively rare exposures (or very rare outcomes), but an integrated approach that combines cohort and case–control surveillance offers an effective step towards resolving these two teratogenic concerns.

THE FUTURE

There are two important developments that have major implications for the future of pharmacoepidemiologic studies of birth defects. Our knowledge of teratogenicity can be dramatically enhanced by the increasing integration of epidemiology and biology, and it may be diminished by the legal and regulatory climate in which epidemiologists will operate.

INTEGRATION OF EPIDEMIOLOGY AND BIOLOGY

A major frustration among those who conduct epidemiologic studies of congenital malformations is the dearth of understanding of the mechanisms, both structural and molecular, by which defects occur. Advances in molecular biology (such as those related to understanding the role of retinoic acid) will markedly enhance our ability to classify defects in biologically meaningful categories. We may also see advances in the feasibility of using human tissue to identify antenatal drug exposures. Blood and urine have long been available for this purpose, but detection is largely limited to the interval shortly following exposure. For case–control studies in particular, where the mother is typically identified some time after delivery, such sampling is of no value for detecting exposures in early pregnancy. Researchers have explored the usefulness of other tissues, such as meconium[63] and hair[64] in which drugs or their metabolites may persist and accumulate. Although these techniques are still under evaluation and currently lack the ability to estimate timing precisely, they may enable researchers at least to confirm the presence or absence of certain exposures during pregnancy.

With respect to the role of drugs in the etiology of birth defects, there is no question that the most exciting biologic development is the rapid expansion of research focused on genetic polymorphisms of drug metabolizing enzymes (DMEs). It has puzzled many that known human teratogens do not produce malformations in all (or even most) exposed fetuses, and many believed that this "incomplete penetrance" was due to differences in host susceptibilities. In 1985, researchers demonstrated that such a phenomenon was likely to account for the inconsistent effect of at least

one such teratogen—phenytoin.[65] These workers found that a genetic variant in the detoxification of arene oxide (a radical metabolite of phenytoin) was strongly related to the risk of the major defects associated with phenytoin. Since then, the field has exploded, and polymorphic DMEs are being identified daily for a host of drugs and no doubt more will be identified in the future. In anticipation, we and others have added data banks of buccal cells or blood samples to ongoing studies of risk factors for birth defects. Improved understanding of genetic polymorphisms will dramatically enhance the identification of subsets of the population who are at increased risk for certain birth defects and the identification of drugs that might warrant particular study.

By analogy with the process of screening for rubella susceptibility or for genetic diseases, one can reasonably look forward to a time when women of childbearing age can be screened for genetic polymorphisms which may place them at particular risk for having a malformed infant if they are exposed to a particular drug. Information of this kind has obvious usefulness in selecting (and avoiding) specific drugs for the treatment of women who are pregnant or at risk for becoming pregnant. (See also Chapter 37 for a more detailed discussion of molecular pharmacoepidemiology.)

THE LEGAL AND REGULATORY CLIMATE

Whatever their design, studies of exposures in pregnancy in relation to birth defects ultimately depend on the ability to link exposure and outcome information. To accomplish such linkage, researchers require access to information that identifies women who have become pregnant, the outcomes of those pregnancies (including spontaneous and therapeutic abortions), and details as to the presence or absence of malformations. The issue of whether and how such information might be disclosed to researchers has become highly contentious in many countries. For case–control studies in particular, the enrollment of malformed and/or normal subjects requires that hospitals, other health providers, or government agencies make identifying information available to researchers, who then contact eligible subjects in order to invite them to participate in an interview.

At present, there is considerable public anxiety—and even anger—regarding the erosion of confidentiality, especially with respect to financial and related data. Parents of children with birth defects, and particularly those who have undergone therapeutic abortions, are exquisitely sensitive to the disclosure of information on their pregnancies and outcomes. Despite the fact that there is little evidence to suggest that medical researchers have compromised confidentiality, there is a real possibility that epidemiologic research into

drug-induced birth defects may be constrained or even eliminated by actions and laws intended to protect confidentiality,
without consideration to the substantially different societal
roles played by medical research and commercial interests.[66] It is therefore critical that the public be educated
about the extent to which epidemiologic research serves the
public health, and that they recognize that this benefit can
only be accomplished by the provision, under strict controls,
of limited confidential medical information to legitimate researchers. At the same time, the public must be
reassured—and researchers must accept—that violations of
this shared trust will be accompanied by serious penalties.
(See also Chapter 38 for a discussion of bioethics in
pharmacoepidemiology.)

HOPE FOR AN INTEGRATED APPROACH

Studies of birth defects in the future will undoubtedly focus
increased attention on issues of statistical power, validity,
and secular changes in exposures. The continuing concern
about isotretinoin and the relatively recent approval of thalidomide in the US will, one hopes, focus attention on not
only the high-risk teratogenic potential of prescription drugs
but the moderate-risk potential as well. One also hopes that
increased recognition of our ignorance regarding the safety
of OTC medications and herbal products will expand the
postmarketing research focus. Although the thalidomide
debacle did much to stimulate research attention on the
adverse effects of medications, it is ironic that the problem
identified by thalidomide—the teratogenic effects of
drugs—has failed to receive focused and systematic investigation. As a result, information available to pregnant
women and their health care providers about the safety of
drugs in pregnancy is not much better today than it was 50
years ago. As noted above and elsewhere,[6] this situation
need not persist—systematic approaches to pharmacoepidemiologic research in this important area can be established
simply by coordinating the various proven methodologies.
In the US, for example, our knowledge of each drug's risk
and safety to the fetus can be dramatically improved, in
a cost-efficient manner, by developing a comprehensive
surveillance system that combines the complementary strengths
of already established cohort and case–control surveillance
infrastructures.

ACKNOWLEDGMENTS

I wish to express my appreciation and thanks to Dennis
Slone, MD, Samuel Shapiro, MB, FRCP(E), Carol Louik,
ScD, Martha Werler, ScD, and Sonia Hernandez-Diaz, MD,
ScD, whose advice and close working relationships over the
years contributed to the issues covered and views expressed
in this chapter.

This work was supported in part by NIH Grants
HD27697 and HL58763; unrestricted additional support
to the SEC Birth Defects Study has been provided by
Aventis Pharmaceuticals, Inc., Glaxo-Wellcome Inc.,
and Pfizer Inc.

REFERENCES

1. Heinonen OP, Slone D, Shapiro S. The women, their offspring,
   and the malformations. In: Kaufman DW, ed., *Birth Defects
   and Drugs in Pregnancy*. Littleton, MA: Publishing Sciences
   Group, 1977; pp. 30–32.
2. CDC. *Congenital Malformations Surveillance Report: January
   1982–December 1985*. Atlanta, GA: US Department of Health
   and Human Services, Public Health Service, 1988.
3. Gregg NM. Congenital cataract following German measles in
   the mother. *Trans Ophthalmol Soc Aust* 1941; **3**: 35–46.
4. Lenz W. Thalidomide and congenital abnormalities. *Lancet*
   1962; **1**: 45.
5. Warkany J. Problems in applying teratologic observations in
   animals to man. *Pediatrics* 1974; **53**: 820.
6. Mitchell AA. Systematic identification of drugs that cause
   birth defects—a new opportunity. *N Engl J Med* 2003; **349**:
   2556–9.
7. Stern RS. When a uniquely effective drug is teratogenic: the
   case of isotreninoin. *N Engl J Med* 1989; **320**: 1007–9.
8. Mitchell AA, Van Bennekom C, Louik C. A pregnancy-
   prevention program in women of childbearing age receiving
   isotretinoin. *N Engl J Med* 1995; **333**: 101–6.
9. Mitchell AA, Van Bennekom C. *Isotretinoin Survey*. Presentation
   at FDA Advisory Committees. Gaithersburg, MD, February
   26, 2004.
10. Holmes LB. Teratogen update: Bendectin. *Teratology* 1983;
    27: 277–81.
11. Neutel CI, Johansen HL. Measuring drug effectiveness by
    default: the case of Bendectin. *Can J Pub Health* 1995; **86**:
    66–70.
12. Hook EB, Healy KB. Consequences of a nationwide ban on
    spray adhesives alleged to be human teratogens and mutagens.
    Science 1976; **191**: 566–7.
13. Heinonen OP, Slone D, Shapiro S. Sedatives, tranquilizers, and
    antidepressant drugs. In: Kaufman DW, ed., *Birth Defects and
    Drugs in Pregnancy*. Littleton, MA: Publishing Sciences
    Group, 1977; pp. 335–44.
14. Newman CGH. Teratogen update: clinical aspects of thal-
    idomide embryopathy—a continuing preoccupation. *Teratology*
    1985; **32**: 133–44.

15. Lammer EJ, Chen DT, Hoar RM, Agnish ND, Benke PJ, Braun JT *et al.* Retinoic acid embryopathy. *N Engl J Med* 1985; **313**: 837–41.

16. Robert E. [Example of teratogen detection using a birth defects registry: depakine and spina bifida.] *Rev Epidemiol Sante Publique* 1996; **44** (suppl 1): 78–81 (in French).

17. Whitfield MF. Chondrodysplasia punctata after warfarin in early pregnancy. *Arch Dis Child* 1980; **55**: 139–42.

18. Martin RA, Jones KL, Mendoza A, Barr M, Benirschke K. Effect of ACE inhibition on the fetal kidney: decreased renal blood flow. *Teratology* 1992; **46**: 317–21.

19. Werler MM, Mitchell AA, Shapiro S. First trimester maternal medication use in relation to gastroschisis. *Teratology* 1992; **45**: 361–7.

20. Rayburn W, Wible-Kant J, Bledsoe P. Changing trends in drug use during pregnancy. *J Reprod Med* 1982; **27**: 569–75.

21. Mitchell AA, Hernandez-Diaz S, Louik C, Werler MM. Medication use in pregnancy, 1976–2000. *Pharmacoepidemiol Drug Saf* 2001; **10**: S146.

22. Louik C, Werler MM, Hernandez-Diaz S, Mitchell AA. Use of herbal treatments in pregnancy. *Pharmacoepidemiol Drug Saf* 2003; **12**: S113.

23. Mitchell AA, Cottler LB, Shapiro S. Effect of questionnaire design on recall of drug exposure in pregnancy. *Am J Epidemiol* 1986; **123**: 670–6.

24. Werler MM, Pober BR, Nelson K, Holmes LB. Reporting accuracy among mothers of malformed and nonmalformed infants. *Am J Epidemiol* 1989; **129**: 415–21.

25. Rothman KJ, Fyler DC, Goldblatt A, Kreidberg MB. Exogenous hormones and other exposures of children with congenital heart disease. *Am J Epidemiol* 1979; **109**: 433–9.

26. Bingol N, Fuchs M, Diaz V, Stone RK, Gromisch DS. Teratogenicity of cocaine in humans. *J Pediatr* 1987; **110**: 93–6.

27. Mitchell AA, Rosenberg L, Shapiro S, Slone D. Birth defects related to Bendectin use in pregnancy. 1. Oral clefts and cardiac defects. *JAMA* 1981; **245**: 2311–14.

28. Slutsker L. Risks associated with cocaine use during pregnancy. *Obstet Gynecol* 1992; **79**: 778–89.

29. Bracken MB. Methodologic issues in the epidemiological investigation of drug-induced congenital malformations. In: Bracken MB, ed., *Perinatal Epidemiology*. New York: Oxford University Press, 1984.

30. Mills JL, Rhoads GG, Simpson JL, Cunningham GC, Conley MR, Lassman MR *et al.* The absence of a relation between the periconceptional use of vitamins and neural tube defects. *N Engl J Med* 1989; **321**: 430–5.

31. Werler MM, Shapiro S, Mitchell AA. Periconceptional folic acid exposure and risk of occurrent neural tube defects. *JAMA* 1993; **269**: 1257–61.

32. Johnston MC, Sulik KK. Some abnormal patterns of development in the craniofacial region. *Birth Defects Orig Artic Ser* 1979; **15**: 23–42.

33. Hoyme HE, Jones MC, Jones KL. Gastroschisis: abdominal wall disruption secondary to early gestational interruption of the omphalomesenteric artery. *Semin Perinatol* 1983; **7**: 294–8.

34. Werler MM, Sheehan JE, Mitchell AA. Association of vaso-constrictive exposures with risks of gastroschisis and small intestinal atresia. *Epidemiology* 2003; **14**: 349–54.

35. Khoury MJ, Moore CA, James LM, Cordero JF. The interaction between dysmorphology and epidemiology: methodologic issues of grouping and splitting. *Teratology* 1992; **45**: 133–8.

36. Slone D, Shapiro S, Miettinen OS, Finkle WD, Stolley PD. Drug evaluation after marketing. *Ann Intern Med* 1979; **90**: 257–61.

37. MRC Vitamin Study Research Group. Prevention of neural tube defects: results of the Medical Research Council Vitamin Study. *Lancet* 1991; **338**: 131–7.

38. Hernandez-Diaz S, Werler MM, Walker AM, Mitchell AA. Neural tube defects in relation to use of folic acid antagonists during pregnancy. *Am J Epidemiol* 2001; **153**: 961–8.

39. Martinez-Frias ML, Rodriguez-Pinilla E, Prieto L. Prenatal exposure to salicylates and gastroschisis: a case–control study. *Teratology* 1997; **56**: 241–3.

40. Werler MM, Sheehan JE, Mitchell AA. Maternal medication use and risks of gastroschisis and small intestinal atresia. *Am J Epidemiol* 2002; **155**: 26–31.

41. Khoury MJ, Holtzman NA. On the ability of birth defects monitoring to detect new teratogens. *Am J Epidemiol* 1987; **126**: 136–43.

42. Michaelis J, Gluck E, Michaelis H, Koller S, Degenhardt K-H. Teratogene Effekte von Lenotan. *Dtsch Arztebl* 1980; **23**: 1527–9.

43. Gibson GT, Colley DP, McMichael AJ, Hartshorne JM. Congenital anomalies in relation to the use of doxylamine/dicyclomine and other antenatal factors. *Med J Aust* 1981; **1**: 410–14.

44. Harlap S, Shiono PH, Ramcharan S, Golbus M, Bachman R, Mann J, Lewis JP. Chromosomal abnormalities in the Kaiser-Permanente Birth Defects Study, with special reference to contraceptive use around the time of conception. *Teratology* 1985; **31**: 381–7.

45. Czeizel A. Lack of evidence of teratogenicity of benzodiazepine drugs in Hungary. *Reprod Toxicol* 1988; **1**: 183–8.

46. Olsen J. Experiences from an existing birth cohort: the Danish National Birth Cohort. Presentation at Medicines Exposures Workshop (National Children's Study). Baltimore, MD, December 16, 2002.

47. Slone D, Siskind V, Heinonen OP, Monson RR, Kaufman DW, Shapiro S. Aspirin and congenital malformations. *Lancet* 1976; **1**: 1373–5.

48. Jick H, Holmes LB, Hunter JR, Madsen S, Stergachis A. First-trimester drug use and congenital disorders. *JAMA* 1981; **246**: 343–6.

49. Jick SS, Terris BZ, Jick H. First trimester topical tretinoin and congenital disorders. *Lancet* 1993; **341**: 1181–2.

50. Bergman U, Rosa FW, Baum C, Wiholm B-E, Faich GA. Effects of exposure to benzodiazepine during fetal life. *Lancet* 1992; **340**: 694–6.

51. Ratanajamit C, Skriver MV, Norgaard M, Jepsen P, Schonheyder HC, Sorensen HT. Adverse pregnancy outcome in users of sulfamethizole during pregnancy: a population-based observational study. *J Antimicrob Chemother* 2003; **52**: 837–41.

52. FDA. Guidance for industry: Establishing pregnancy exposure registries. Available at: http://www.fda.gov/cder/guidance/3626fnl.pdf.

53. Dai WS, LaBraico JM, Stern RS. Epidemiology of isotretinoin exposure during pregnancy. *J Am Acad Dermatol* 1992; **26**: 599–606.

54. Chambers C, Braddock SR, Briggs GG, Einarson A, Johnson YR, Miller RK *et al*. Postmarketing surveillance for human teratogenicity: a model approach. *Teratology* 2001; **64**: 252–61.

55. St Clair SM, Schirmer RG. First-trimester exposure to alprazolam. *Obstet Gynecol* 1992; **80**: 843–6.

56. Pastuszak A, Schick-Boschetto B, Zuber C, Feldkamp M, Pinelli M, Sihn S *et al*. Pregnancy outcome following first-trimester exposure to fluoxetine (Prozac). *JAMA* 1993; **269**: 2246–8.

57. Yoon PW, Rasmussen SA, Lynberg MC, Moore CA, Anderka M, Carmichael SL *et al*. The national birth defects prevention study. *Public Health Rep* 2001; **116** (suppl 1): 32–40.

58. Jick H, Walker AM, Rothman KJ, Hunter JR, Holmes LB, Watkins RN *et al*. Vaginal spermicides and congenital disorders. *JAMA* 1981; **245**: 1329–32.

59. Mills JL, Harley EE, Reed GF, Berendes HW. Are spermicides teratogenic? *JAMA* 1982; **248**: 2148–51.

60. Shapiro S, Slone D, Heinonen OP, Kaufman DW, Rosenberg L, Mitchell AA *et al*. Birth defects and vaginal spermicides. *JAMA* 1982; **247**: 2381–84.

61. Louik C, Mitchell AA, Werler MM, Hanson JW, Shapiro S. Maternal exposure to spermicides in relation to certain birth defects. *N Engl J Med* 1987; **317**: 474–8.

62. Warburton D, Neugut RH, Lustenberger A, Nicholas A, Kline J. Lack of association between spermicide use and trisomy. *N Engl J Med* 1987; **317**: 478–82.

63. Ostrea EM Jr, Romero A, Yee H. Adaptation of the meconium drug test for mass screening. *J Pediatr* 1993; **122**: 152–4.

64. Graham K, Koren G, Klein J, Schneiderman J, Greenwald M. Determination of gestational cocaine exposure by hair analysis. *JAMA* 1989; **262**: 3328–30.

65. Strickler SM, Dansky LV, Miller MA, Seni MH, Andermann E, Spielberg SP. Genetic predisposition to phenytoin-induced birth defects. *Lancet* 1985; **2**: 746–9.

66. Andrews EB, International Society for Pharmacoepidemiology. Data privacy, medical record confidentiality, and research in the interest of public health. *Pharmacoepidemiol Drug Saf* 1999; **8**: 247–60.

33

Pharmacoepidemiology and Risk Management

DAVID J. GRAHAM, ANDREW D. MOSHOLDER, KATE GELPERIN and MARK I. AVIGAN
Center for Drug Evaluation and Research, US Food and Drug Administration, Silver Spring, Maryland, USA.

INTRODUCTION

In business settings, risk management (RM) often refers to processes intended to limit financial liability. In industrial settings, RM can refer to policies, procedures, and engineering solutions intended to reduce or eliminate workplace injuries, often by containing the exposure.[1] The use of the term "risk management" in the setting of prescription drug safety is a relatively recent development and a consensus definition for it has not yet emerged. The concept has emerged and gradually developed, especially in response to the challenges created by accelerated review and approval times for marketed drugs, as well as drug product withdrawals for safety reasons in the US.[2] It represents a growing awareness of the need for continuing evaluation of risks related to drug products and the implementation of plans to minimize those risks after marketing. A US Food and Drug Administration (FDA) draft guidance described RM as an iterative process involving both the assessment and minimization of risk.[3] Often, RM represents those interventions that must be in place and must be effective in order to shift the balance of

benefit to risk from an unfavorable and unacceptable position to one that is favorable and acceptable. A corollary of this formulation is that, in these situations, in the absence of a successful RM program, the balance of benefit to risk for a drug requiring an RM program would be unfavorable and unacceptable. Regardless, the ultimate goal of RM is to enhance the safe use of medicines by optimizing the balance of benefit and risk. This can be accomplished by increasing the benefit and/or decreasing the risk associated with use of a drug product. Alternatively, it can be accomplished by limiting the use of the drug to those most likely to need it.

Underlying the concept of RM is the assumption that a drug product's benefit and its risks can and should be measured or estimated so that the balance between these can be favorably maximized. For most drugs and therapeutic indications, benefit is inferred from the Phase III clinical trials upon which marketing approval was based. Phase III trials are designed to permit statistical inferences about the biologic effects of a drug, in an ideal setting (efficacy). This is different from trials designed to assess the benefit of a therapy when applied to the population-at-large (effectiveness).

Pharmacoepidemiology, Fourth Edition Edited by B.L. Strom
© 2005 John Wiley & Sons, Ltd

(See also Chapter 40.) A drug's biologic effect measured as endpoints in a clinical trial may not translate to actual health benefit for patients when used in real-world settings outside the controlled and highly selective environment of Phase III clinical trials.[4]

Recent experience in the field of hypertension therapy illustrates this problem. The ALLHAT study was a 40 000 patient randomized controlled clinical trial comparing the occurrence of adverse health outcomes associated with hypertension among patients treated with four different antihypertension drugs, all approved by the FDA as "safe and effective."[5] For comparable levels of blood pressure control (efficacy), patients treated with the α-blocker doxazocin experienced significantly higher rates of stroke, congestive heart failure, and coronary revascularization, compared to patients treated with the diuretic chlorthalidone. In other words, despite equal efficacy in lowering blood pressure, doxazocin did not confer a comparable health benefit (effectiveness).

A number of interventions (sometimes referred to as "tools") have been employed to attempt to improve the balance of benefit to risk associated with use of specific drug products. The most traditional and common methods include professional labeling and package inserts, special letters sent to health care professionals, specific educational and training programs, and patient-package inserts and medication guides. These approaches emphasize communication, education, and outreach as the primary means of RM. Such strategies are often referred to as risk communication, and the specific components of these approaches may be varied according to the type of risk being targeted, e.g., warning prescribers about a drug–drug interaction versus warning female patients about a risk of teratogenicity.[6]

Other strategies have been used that go beyond the relatively passive transmission of information about risk. Frequently, more than one of these interventions will be employed as part of a product's "risk management program." These interventions include the signing of informed consent forms by patients prior to beginning drug therapy and prior registration of health care practitioners before they are "certified" to prescribe or dispense a particular drug. Other approaches have also been tried such as requiring that certain laboratory tests be performed with normal results prior to prescribing, and establishing registries of physicians, pharmacists, or patients who prescribe, dispense, or use a given drug product. Depending upon how these interventions are designed and used, access to the drug in question may be restricted. "Engineering" methods have also been applied in an effort to manage a drug's risk. The use of special packaging (e.g., blister packs), limitation of prescription size, and

reformulation of the drug product have also been used (e.g., change in tablet size/shape).

What types of information are needed to design an effective RM program? The answer may vary from issue to issue, but in general, several things are necessary, and the discipline of pharmacoepidemiology can contribute significantly and essentially to the RM process. The most frequent contribution has been in the sphere of risk identification and characterization after a drug has been marketed, based on activities pursued by national pharmacovigilance centers worldwide and by pharmaceutical companies. Understanding the nature, magnitude, and risk factors associated with experiencing a severe adverse drug effect has often formed the basis of risk communication efforts, product labeling, and regulatory policy formulation. Understanding how a drug product is used in the general population is also essential, because it provides insight into the magnitude of exposure and the particular vulnerabilities of the population being treated.

For pharmacoepidemiology to realize its potential vis-à-vis RM, it is important that each RM program have specific, clinically meaningful, and measurable goals to achieve. Pharmacoepidemiology can and should inform the goal setting process. These goals should be evidence based and directly relevant to the safety problem for which they were chosen. The goals should reflect the desired *health outcomes* of the RM program, rather than just process measures or surrogates for the health outcomes of interest. For example, if a drug has been found to increase the risk of developing congestive heart failure (CHF), the most appropriate goal of an RM program would be to reduce the risk of heart failure among patients treated with the drug. Components of the RM program might include contraindicating use of the product among patients with past history of or other risk factors for CHF. However, program success would be best judged by whether the risk of CHF was reduced to acceptable levels, not by whether there was merely compliance with RM plan process measures.

From an epidemiologic perspective, the design of the RM program should ensure that the appropriate data are collected so that the effect of the program on health outcomes can be determined in a timely fashion. The implementation of each new RM program is a public health intervention that can be viewed as analogous to a trial, subject to the rigors of experimental methodology, where an unproven intervention (the RM program) is tested in the population of patients and health professionals who use a given drug. Why do we suggest the construct of an experimental trial? The intended purpose of an RM program is the minimization of patient risk and optimization of a drug's balance between benefit and risk. Because there can be great uncertainty regarding the effectiveness of RM programs (to the extent that they are often unproven public health interventions), their use can be conceptualized as experimental in nature. However, for most RM programs implemented thus far, there has been little, if any, evidence to support a prior expectation of program success. For this reason, if no other, data collection is *essential* to testing whether an RM program has achieved its desired health benefit. With such monitoring it should be possible to evaluate both process endpoints, as well as other consequences for patients or the health care environment which are either intended or unintended. In this sense, RM programs provide a framework enabling measurements of simple quality assurance benchmarks as well as experimental analysis of complex social behaviors and health outcomes. The potential value of pharmacoepidemiology in this setting is great. In addition to documenting the health effects of an RM program, pharmacoepidemiology may contribute to providing useful information regarding the effect of individual factors or approaches within a more complex RM program.

CLINICAL PROBLEMS TO BE ADDRESSED BY PHARMACOEPIDEMIOLOGIC RESEARCH

RISK IDENTIFICATION AND CHARACTERIZATION

Assessment of drug safety and the extent to which therapeutic benefit offsets the known or suspected risks of medications requires careful synthesis of information from many sources. These include preclinical studies, pre- and postmarketing clinical trials, spontaneous adverse event reporting, published reports in the medical literature, and epidemiologic studies. Although randomized controlled trials (RCTs) are considered the gold standard of evidence-based clinical research and furnish the core clinical data used for marketing approval decisions (see Chapter 2), they have a number of limitations, especially in the area of drug safety. These limitations arise from the relatively small size and short duration of many RCTs and the highly selected, and hence unrepresentative, nature of the patients included in these studies.[7] As a result, different types of study designs are needed to answer different types of clinical questions.[8] Reliance on "evidence hierarchies" in an inflexible manner, whereby observational studies are discounted or ignored, may compromise patient safety because in many situations, well-designed epidemiologic studies offer the only way to characterize the safety risks associated with a given drug.[9]

At the same time, however, it is important to recognize that epidemiological approaches using health care databases may not be appropriate in a variety of settings, especially those requiring patient interviews or surveys for accurate data collection[10] (see also Chapter 45).

Premarketing

Sometimes, during clinical development of a new molecular entity, a safety signal of concern arises that cannot be well answered by available studies or data. In this setting, a large, simple, safety study (LSSS) could be considered (see Chapter 39). This may be particularly relevant when the product is being developed for use as a preventative measure in asymptomatic individuals or where extensive use is anticipated. An LSSS is a clinical study designed to assess relatively few outcomes in a large number of patients.[11] It incorporates the advantage conferred by randomization with the efficiency of an observational cohort study.

The difficulty of safety signal characterization prior to drug approval is illustrated by the clinical development program of the first vasopeptidase inhibitor to be extensively studied, omapatrilat. Preclinical and early clinical studies with this drug among patients with hypertension and CHF were promising.[12] However, larger Phase III clinical trials showed an excess rate of angioedema compared to an angiotensin converting enzyme inhibitor comparator. In response to concerns raised by the FDA during the review process, a large, multinational RCT was undertaken by the sponsor to compare the efficacy and safety of omapatrilat against enalapril in 25 000 patients with hypertension.[13] This study confirmed the magnitude of the safety signal for angioedema with omapatrilat (2.17%) compared to enalapril (0.68%).

Postmarketing

In the early stages of marketing experience with a new drug, observational studies using computerized databases (see Part IIIb) are often not practicable because there usually has not been sufficient patient exposure to the drug of interest. In most instances, exposure is not sufficient until several years after product launch. From a risk management perspective, this means that during the early postmarketing phase, most information about risk will be obtained from spontaneous or published case reports of adverse drug reactions, national drug surveillance programs, specialized patient registries, or *ad hoc* studies designed to answer these questions.

Product Usage

From the moment product marketing begins, drug use data can be monitored to identify patterns of use that might require intervention to maintain an acceptable balance of benefit and risk. Automated longitudinal databases are ideally structured to provide information about the demographics of drug users as well as the distribution of prescribed daily dose and duration of product use. Drug use in inappropriate age groups, or at higher doses, or for longer lengths of time than labeled might signal the emergence of a potential safety problem requiring RM intervention. The growth of off-label product use could also signal the presence of a situation warranting RM attention.

Case Reports

The essential role of case reports in the early identification of safety signals is well established[14] (see Chapters 9, 10, and 36). Global pharmaceutical companies have the opportunity and obligation to collect and analyze spontaneous reports of suspected adverse drug reactions, along with any published case reports, from every country in which their products are approved and marketed. Reporting rates of adverse drug reactions can be calculated based on the ratio of spontaneous reports received per number of prescriptions or other estimates of drug utilization for a given geographic location over a specified period of time. Importantly, reporting rates are not incidence rates and cannot be reliably used to compare one drug with another. This is due in large part to the well-described problem of underreporting.[15]

A variety of other epidemiologic techniques can be applied to case reports data in an effort to understand better the nature and magnitude of safety risks. Borrowing from the concept of standardized mortality ratios, an "observed to expected" ratio can be calculated if there are reliable estimates of the background rate for a particular outcome of interest. With this information and an estimate of the extent of drug usage, an "expected" number of cases can be derived and compared with the number of such cases actually reported for the drug. In the majority of instances, the number reported will fall far below the number predicted as due to background (chance). This situation is especially likely when the background rate for an event is relatively high (e.g., myocardial infarction). Also, given the extent of underreporting, the expected outcome of such an analysis is that no increase in risk will be found. Therefore, a negative finding using this method is not equivalent to the absence of increased risk. On the other hand, if the number reported approaches or exceeds the number expected, such a finding should be interpreted as evidence of a substantially increased risk, and could signify a problem requiring prompt attention

or intervention. A recent application of this method identified a greater than 100-fold increase in risk of fatal cardiomyopathy during the first month of treatment with clozapine.[16]

Another method for examining case reports involves the use of survival analysis methods.[17,18] Information regarding the persistency of drug use can be used to model the denominator of patients at risk of experiencing an adverse event with continued use of a drug product. The cases reported after varying lengths of product use can then be used to estimate time-specific reporting/hazard rates, providing insight into the contour of drug risk over time. Companies and regulators could use such information to design RM programs tailored to the profile of risk and its change over time.

Importantly, review of a well-documented series of case reports can provide useful insight into the spectrum, severity, and natural history of an adverse drug effect, as well as its reversibility, predictability, and preventability. Understanding these factors should be a critical component of any decision to design or implement an RM program.

Phase IV and *ad hoc* Postmarketing Epidemiologic Studies

Pharmacoepidemiology studies are sometimes relied upon to characterize further the nature and magnitude of safety signals arising during pre-approval clinical trials or, more commonly, from postmarketing spontaneous case reports. Limitations in the methods and design of these studies can undermine their power and utility, frequently leading to negative findings.[19]

Terodiline, an anticholinergic agent for the treatment of urinary frequency, was withdrawn from the European market in 1991 after a strong signal for torsade de pointes (TdP) was identified from spontaneous case reports.[20] Two subsequent studies, one using Prescription-Event Monitoring (PEM)[21] and the other, a retrospective study using the General Practice Research Database,[22] failed to confirm this signal, casting doubt on its validity. Subsequently, *in vitro* studies showed that terodiline blocked the rapid component of the delayed rectifier potassium current, the primary mechanism underlying QT interval prolongation and the initiation of TdP.[23] Also, clinical studies have shown that electrocardiographic monitoring of patients during clinical trials would have identified this problem had it been performed.[24]

A variety of biases may also compromise the utility of postmarketing pharmacoepidemiology safety studies. Misclassification bias arising from inaccurate or imprecise ICD-9-CM coding of hospital discharge diagnoses creates the potential for incorrect inferences to be drawn from studies using claims databases.[25] A study of drug-induced neutropenia, using Medicaid data from five states covering

3.8 million patients, defined cases based on an inpatient diagnosis of neutropenia (ICD-9-CM code 288.0).[26] Copies of medical records were reviewed for 198 of 549 potential cases. Although neutropenia was documented in 97% of these records, 13.5% of these had recurrent neutropenia and 9.9% had chronic neutropenia, neither of which was consistent with a drug-induced etiology. Had a careful review of medical records not been conducted, the study results would have suffered from substantial misclassification.

Similarly, as part of a case–control study of drug-induced Stevens–Johnson syndrome, a medical record review was performed of the cases identified using ICD-9-CM code 695.1, which includes Stevens–Johnson syndrome, erythema multiforme, and some other skin diseases such as staphylococcal scalded skin syndrome. Of the cases for which medical records were available (approximately 50%), only 14.8% actually had a diagnosis of Stevens–Johnson syndrome or erythema multiforme major.[27] It was also determined that erythema multiforme was frequently misdiagnosed by physicians in this sample, resulting in poor validity.

In some instances, observational studies have suggested the existence of unanticipated benefits that are not confirmed by large, randomized studies. Postmenopausal hormone replacement therapy (HRT) was thought to confer protection against cardiovascular disease based on several observational studies.[28] However, a large randomized primary prevention trial of HRT in healthy postmenopausal women (Women's Health Initiative) was terminated early due to increased risks of cardiovascular outcomes and breast cancer among women treated with HRT. A comprehensive review suggested that selection bias probably accounted for the cardiovascular benefits seen in previous observational studies.[29] Women who chose this therapy tended to be healthier, more affluent, and better educated than those who did not (healthy user bias). They were also more likely to follow medical advice (adherence bias), to have frequent contact with clinicians resulting in earlier detection of cardiovascular risk factors such as hypertension (surveillance bias), and to remain on HRT as long as their health remained otherwise good (survivor bias).

METHODOLOGIC PROBLEMS TO BE ADDRESSED BY PHARMACOEPIDEMIOLOGIC RESEARCH

RISK MANAGEMENT GOAL SETTING

Properly utilized, pharmacoepidemiology should contribute significantly to the process of RM goal setting. In many instances, the risk requiring minimization will be identified using pharmacoepidemiologic methods. During the process of risk characterization, estimates of absolute and relative risk may also be obtained, which can serve as initial benchmarks against which future performance of an RM program is judged.

A comprehensive understanding of factors contributing to the presence and magnitude of a drug safety risk is critical to establishing RM goals. High quality case reports are especially useful here because they detail the real-world circumstances surrounding the occurrence of a serious adverse effect and may thereby suggest junctures along the causal path where intervention might be useful and effective. In this regard, assessment of the case reports can be viewed as a type of failure mode and effect analysis, an approach widely practiced in industrial and business settings. Careful review of drug usage data may also contribute importantly to the goal setting process by documenting patterns of use that are intrinsically unsafe (e.g., concurrent use with contraindicated products), or that are off-label, where product risk may not be balanced by demonstrated effectiveness (benefit).

Understandably, different RM programs may have different goals. The goals of these programs should share certain characteristics, regardless of their particular differences. The primary goals of an RM program must be explicit, relevant, and measurable. An explicit goal is clear, unambiguous, and openly stated. It is something against which a comparison can be made and a judgment rendered with respect to program achievement or failure. A relevant goal is closely linked with the safety *event* of concern, and, usually, will be a direct health outcome immediately reflective of the *event* that the RM program is seeking to eliminate or minimize. In other words, a relevant goal will most often be framed in terms of a health outcome, a safety *event* that is the reason for the RM program in the first place.

An exception to this generalization might be the situation where off-label use contributes to the magnitude of adverse event occurrence. Here, one of the RM goals could be stated in terms of the health *event*/outcome of interest, while a second goal could be framed in terms of extent of off-label use. Health outcomes several steps removed from the safety *event* of concern and process goals that assess incremental aspects or components of an RM program would not be relevant. These are surrogate measures for the outcome of interest and usually will not accurately reflect the true effect of an RM program. Improved compliance with a particular component or process of an RM program does not answer the question about whether the occurrence of harm has been reduced. Finally, as the word suggests, a measurable goal is a health outcome that can be measured, an attribute that permits comparisons to be made and conclusions reached regarding goal achievement.

An RM plan will most often consist of one or more strategies or interventions, the purpose of which is achievement of the RM public health goal of minimizing drug-related harm and optimizing the ratio of benefit to harm. A variety of strategies are possible, though the ability to implement them and their ultimate effectiveness may be low. The following list is neither comprehensive nor exhaustive, but is intended to illustrate the population-based perspective that is critical to any RM program. If an adverse drug effect is reversible at an early stage, before it progresses to a serious or life-threatening outcome, early recognition of the adverse effect and prompt discontinuation of the drug might reduce patient harm. We are unaware of any examples where this has been demonstrated to be an effective strategy. If the adverse drug effect is serious and its occurrence cannot be predicted or prevented, efforts to minimize use of the drug product, such as relegating its use to "last-resort" status, might reduce the burden of harm. However, once marketing patterns and physician behaviors are established, and this often occurs quickly after initial marketing, it is nearly impossible to alter the manner of product use substantively without imposing a restricted distribution system of some sort. Similarly, although limiting use of a given product to patients with the most severe form of a particular disorder is intellectually appealing, in practice, product use may not remain confined only to severely affected patients in the absence of externally imposed restrictions.

RISK MANAGEMENT DESIGN AND EVALUATION

An RM program should be designed with its primary goal as the focus, and the design should facilitate the accomplishment of that explicit, relevant, and measurable goal. Ideally, this means that the primary health outcome(s) of importance will be specified in terms that permit accurate, reliable, and complete data collection and analysis to be performed. Risk management programs often represent interventions of uncertain and unknown effectiveness that will be applied to large numbers of patients within the "laboratory" of the postmarketing health care setting. To the extent that the impact of these interventions is unknown, RM programs could be viewed as experiments. The requirements of data quality and relevance should be an important design consideration and the role of the skilled pharmacoepidemiologist in this endeavor cannot be overstated.

For example, if the health outcome of interest is prevention of fetal exposure to a teratogen, accurate, reliable, and complete ascertainment of fetal exposure should be a design objective. An RM program that relies on voluntary participation to ascertain the occurrence of pregnancy exposure is highly unlikely to yield information that allows for an accurate and reliable assessment of the impact of the program. Volunteers are generally not representative of all patients, and underreporting of sensitive events such as pregnancy exposure is great.[30] If the design of an RM program does not foster the collection of accurate and reliable data on the health outcome of interest, there is no way to determine if the risk has been adequately managed and the balance of benefit to risk optimized. In this regard, closed-loop or restricted distribution systems offer the potential to create the environment within which one can best ensure that accurate and reliable data are collected.

CURRENTLY AVAILABLE SOLUTIONS

While RM may be considered to cover a broad range of safety issues and concerns, the above discussion implicitly addresses RM programs for the severe or serious end of the adverse effect spectrum, typically those that are potentially life threatening, or result in hospitalization, disability, or death. In these settings, the requirement that an RM program be implemented is a tacit admission that, without effective risk management, the balance of benefit to risk would be unacceptable. In this setting, implementation of an effective RM program is necessary to establish an acceptable balance. Examples of drug risks and efforts to manage them by minimizing harm have accrued over time. Those for which there are references in the literature are briefly presented below in alphabetical order (also see Table 33.1).

ACETAMINOPHEN PACKAGING IN THE UK

To reduce the incidence of acetaminophen (APAP) and aspirin overdosage and associated deaths, the UK implemented a law in 1998 that required packages of these drugs ordinarily available from pharmacies to contain no more than 32 tablets, and packages for sale in non-pharmacy retail stores no more than 16 tablets.[31] Several authors have studied the impact of this intervention. In the year following the package restrictions, investigators at the Royal Free Hospital in London found a 21% reduction in the number of APAP overdose cases at their hospital, and a 64% reduction in the number of overdoses requiring treatment with N-acetylcysteine or methionine.[32] Another study analyzed

Table 33.1. Summary of risk management programs and their effectiveness as qualitatively assessed by the authors

Drug	Safety concern	Risk management interventions	Effect of interventions
Acetaminophen	Overdose, acute liver failure, death	National law in UK mandating blister packs and sublethal package size	↓ hospitalizations, mortality, liver transplants[30,31,33,34]
All drugs	Pediatric overdose, death	National law mandating child-resistant packaging	↓ mortality from accidental poisoning[40,41]
Aspirin	Reye's syndrome	Prolonged multifaceted national campaign at Federal government level	↓ in incidence, mortality[35]
Bromfenac	Acute liver failure	Boxed warning in label, Dear HCP letter	No change in prescribing behaviors; continued reporting of liver failure[38]
Cisapride	Fatal cardiac arrhythmias	Multiple label changes and warnings, multiple Dear HCP letters, multiple articles in medical literature	±small changes in prescribing behavior; continued reports of TdP[42,45–47,49,50]
Clozapine	Agranulocytosis	Restricted access with mandatory linkage of normal lab result and registered prescription release	↓ incidence of agranulocytosis[51,52]
Isotretinoin	Pregnancy exposure	Multiple label changes and warnings, multiple Dear HCP letters, multiple public advisory meetings, multiple articles in medical literature, multiple intensive educational campaigns, signed informed consent, contraindicated use, qualification stickers, physician registry, pregnancy testing	No evidence of reduced pregnancy exposures; poor compliance with pregnancy testing; >2-fold increase in use of drug in women of child-bearing age (off-label use)[57,59,60]
Pemoline	Acute liver failure	Label changes, multiple Dear HCP letters, second-line therapy, liver enzyme monitoring	Persisting high level of 1st-line use; poor compliance with liver enzyme monitoring; no reliable data on liver failure occurrence[62]
Terfenadine	Fatal cardiac arrhythmias	Multiple label changes, multiple Dear HCP letters, replacement by non-cardiotoxic metabolite, fexofenadine	↓ co-prescribing with contraindicated macrolides and azole anti-fungals; persisting 1–3% same-day co-prescribing; continued reporting of cases of TdP[63–65]
Troglitazone	Acute liver failure	Multiple label changes, multiple Dear HCP letters, public advisory meeting, national media attention, liver enzyme monitoring. Removal from market in 2000	Poor compliance with liver enzyme monitoring; evidence that monitoring would not be effective had it been performed; continued reporting of liver failure[66,67]

referrals to a tertiary hepatology service for APAP toxicity, and referrals for liver transplantation following APAP poisoning to the UK transplant authority.[33] They found a statistically significant decrease in median monthly referrals for both outcomes following implementation of the packaging restrictions. In a study of admissions to five hospitals in Belfast for APAP poisoning during the first six months of 1998 and the first six months of 1999, a reduction in the estimated quantity of APAP ingested in overdose was found.[34] However, unlike the aforementioned studies, this study found no reduction in the incidence of liver failure following the restrictions. The impact of package restrictions on a number of outcomes in England and Wales was studied for the period September 1996–September 1999.[35] Statistically significant reductions in mortality due to poisoning with

APAP and salicylates were noted following the packaging changes, with decreases of 21% for APAP and 48% for salicylates. Other findings after the packaging changes included a 66% decrease in APAP-related liver transplantation among a sample of transplant centers and an 11% decrease in the number of cases of APAP overdosage treated at a sample of seven general hospitals. In another study, mortality from APAP poisoning in Scotland over the period 1994–2000 was examined, but no significant reduction was seen following the package changes.[36]

As can be seen, multiple different evaluations were performed by a variety of groups using different methods and patient settings. While individual results varied for impact on liver failure and deaths, these studies point to a decline in death due to APAP overdose and in the occurrence of liver transplantation and referral for transplantation following the changes in APAP packaging and marketing in the UK.

ASPIRIN AND REYE'S SYNDROME

Reye's syndrome, a frequently fatal neurologic disorder characterized by progressive encephalopathy and hepatic dysfunction in children, was associated with recent viral infections treated with aspirin. A national campaign was implemented to eliminate the use of aspirin in pediatric-aged children as a means of preventing Reye's syndrome. In 1980 the US Centers for Disease Control and Prevention (CDC) advised avoiding the use of aspirin in children with viral illnesses. This was followed in 1982 by a Surgeon General advisory on the subject, and in 1984 by labeling changes for aspirin products warning of the risk. Analysis of data from the CDC's National Reye Syndrome Surveillance System showed that the reported number of pediatric cases of Reye's syndrome decreased markedly, from a peak of 555 in 1980 to 2 or fewer cases per year throughout the mid-1990s. The steepest decline in the annual number of cases occurred in the early 1980s following the original CDC advisory, before product labeling was changed.[37] The success of this intervention likely depended on a combination of factors. The leading public health figure in the US (the surgeon general), and the agency most closely associated with public health (the CDC), initiated a national campaign to eliminate Reye's syndrome. The victims of this disorder were children and media coverage was extensive. Rapid uptake of the health message by pediatricians and their commitment to educating parents probably also contributed to the intervention's success. Finally, the availability of acetaminophen, an alternative antipyretic, in liquid form may also have been important.

BROMFENAC

Bromfenac is a nonsteroidal anti-inflammatory drug that was first marketed in the US in 1997 for treatment courses of less than 10 days duration. In premarketing clinical trials, longer-term use had been associated with elevations in liver enzymes.[38] In response to postmarketing reports of hepatitis and liver failure among patients using the drug for longer than 10 days, the manufacturer added a boxed warning to product labeling in February 1998.[39] Despite this, reports of hepatotoxicity among patients using the drug for longer than 10 days continued to accumulate. The drug was removed from the market in June 1998, after FDA concluded "further efforts to limit the use of the product to 10 days or less would not be practical or effective."[40] At the time of its

market withdrawal, 24 reports of serious hepatotoxicity had been received, including 4 fatal cases, and 8 resulting in liver transplant. The majority of reported cases occurred among the estimated 200 000–400 000 patients who received the drug for longer than 10 days, despite its labeling at the time.

CHILD-RESISTANT PACKAGING

The Poison Prevention Packaging Act of 1970 empowered the US Consumer Product Safety Commission to require child-resistant containers for a variety of toxic materials, including prescription drug products.[41] While this represented a public health intervention initiated at the highest levels of government, it can be viewed as an early example of RM. To evaluate the effectiveness of this intervention for prescription drugs, a study was performed using the US National Center for Health Statistics mortality data on deaths from unintentional ingestion of oral prescription drugs among children less than 5 years old, for the period 1964–92.[42] The analysis adjusted for trends in the use of prescription medications and general improvements in child safety during the study period, and compared mortality before and after implementation of child-resistant containers for prescription medications. It found a statistically significant 45% reduction in observed mortality over that predicted from accidental childhood poisonings with prescription drugs. Another study analyzed the impact of child-resistant packaging for mortality specifically associated with aspirin poisoning in children below 5 years of age, for the period 1958–1990.[43] As was done previously, adjustment was made for a variety of covariates, including trends in the amount of aspirin used in the US, general child safety trends, and discovery of the association of aspirin with Reye's syndrome in children. The analysis found a 34% reduction in aspirin overdose deaths following implementation of child-resistant packaging.

CISAPRIDE

Cisapride, a gastrointestinal pro-motility drug, was withdrawn from the general US market in 2000 after FDA receipt of a total of 341 reports of cardiac arrhythmias, with 80 fatalities.[44] Many of the postmarketing spontaneous reports of arrhythmias involved patients taking concomitant drugs known to interact with cisapride via inhibition of cytochrome P450 3A4 (CYP3A4), such as macrolide antibiotics or azole antifungal drugs.[45] Accordingly, warnings were issued to advise physicians of these drug–drug interactions, and of concomitant medical conditions that were contraindications to the use of cisapride.[46] A study was performed to assess the effectiveness of a June 1998 "Dear Health Care Provider" letter that contraindicated the use of cisapride in patients with pre-existing medical conditions or those taking certain interacting medications that predisposed them to cardiac arrhythmias. Data were collected from three separate health care databases for the period one year before and after the June 1998 letter.[47] Following the letter, there was an average decrease in contraindicated use of cisapride of only 2%, and the rate of contraindicated use remained at 24% or greater in all three databases.

A second US study analyzed co-dispensing of contraindicated drugs with cisapride in a single managed care database for the period July 1993–December 1998, during which several different warning letters were issued.[48] From a total of 141 119 prescriptions for cisapride dispensed to 48 485 patients, 3.4% overlapped with a prescription for at least one contraindicated medication, mostly macrolide antibiotics or azole antifungal drugs. For 50% of these overlapping contraindicated prescriptions, the same physician prescribed both medications, and for 89%, the same pharmacy filled both contraindicated drugs. Based on the latter finding, the authors suggested a risk management program directed at pharmacies. Another study using the same claims database focused on the temporal pattern of co-dispensing of contraindicated drugs, to determine the impact of individual warnings issued in February 1995, October 1995, and June 1998.[49] The authors showed that while there was generally a trend for less dispensing of contraindicated drugs with cisapride over time, only the June 1998 "Dear Health Care Professional" letter produced a statistically significant decrease in such co-dispensing. Nonetheless, even after the June 1998 letter, 3.1% of cisapride prescriptions were co-dispensed with contraindicated drugs. It should be noted that this study looked only at co-dispensing of contraindicated medications on the same day that cisapride was dispensed, and did not include time windows where contraindicated prescriptions dispensed on a different day overlapped in their days supply with cisapride. Also, this study did not look at contraindicated medical conditions. One other US study examined same-day dispensing of cisapride with a contraindicated medication in a large New England health insurer database.[50] No identifiable effect of the October 1995 warning was found, but a 66% decrease in contraindicated same-day co-dispensing after the June 1998 warning was noted.

Several studies were also conducted in Europe to examine the effect of regulatory risk management efforts with cisapride. In Italy, a study of trends in co-prescribing of contraindicated drugs with cisapride was performed, using the Italian National Health Service database for Umbria.[51] Over a four-year period, 4.5% of the cisapride prescriptions overlapped with a contraindicated drug, and half of these overlapping prescriptions occurred on the same day. There was no discernable impact of a 1998 "Dear Doctor" letter regarding contraindicated concomitant drugs. Using the Netherlands national health system PHARMO database, co-prescribing of drugs contraindicated with cisapride was examined for the period 1994–98.[52] The investigators estimated the expected extent of co-dispensing due to random chance, and compared this with the actual number of days that patients in the system were exposed to contraindicated concomitant medications. They found that the level of concomitant use of contraindicated drugs was less than expected by chance. However, the absolute number of days-at-risk did not decrease during this time, due to expanding overall use of the interacting drug products.

CLOZAPINE

Clozapine is an atypical antipsychotic drug approved for the treatment of patients with refractory schizophrenia. In clinical trials, its use was associated with a 1–2% risk of potentially fatal agranulocytosis.[53] Also, patients who developed neutropenia, but recovered after drug discontinuation, were at even greater risk of agranulocytosis if re-challenged with clozapine. Accordingly, before marketing was permitted in the US, the Clozapine National Registry (CNR) was established as the risk management system intended to ensure that weekly white blood cell (WBC) count monitoring be performed and that no patient with previous neutropenia on clozapine be re-exposed to it. Data from this registry for the years 1990–94 showed that of 99 502 clozapine-treated patients, there were 382 cases of agranulocytosis (with 12 fatalities) under the "no blood, no drug" risk management program, equivalent to a risk of agranulocytosis of 0.38%.[54] This compared favorably with the expected risk without the registry system from clinical trials. An analysis of fatal cases of clozapine-induced agranulocytosis from Europe, conducted at a time when the drug was marketed with WBC monitoring recommended but not obligatory, found that the majority of fatal cases involved noncompliance with recommended WBC monitoring, delayed discontinuation of clozapine treatment, or both.[55]

As an unanticipated by-product of collecting high quality outcome data by the CNR, it was possible to study mortality benefits among cohorts of current and former clozapine users.[56] Data from the CNR was linked to the National Death Index and the Social Security Administration Death Master File to obtain information on deaths and causes of death among patients ever treated with clozapine. For the years 1991–93, mortality from all causes was lower among current compared with former users. While there were higher mortality rates for deaths due to pulmonary embolism and respiratory disorders among current users, mortality from suicide was substantially reduced among current users, with a rate ratio of 0.17. This apparent benefit of clozapine treatment was later confirmed by the InterSePT study, a randomized, controlled trial, which showed that schizophrenic patients treated with clozapine had lower rates of suicidal behaviors than those treated with olanzapine.[57]

ISOTRETINOIN

Isotretinoin, a teratogenic retinoid, has been marketed in the US for treatment of severe recalcitrant nodular acne since 1982. Soon after marketing began, reports of fetal exposure and birth defects began to be reported. Despite several rounds of label revisions, boxed warnings, "Dear Doctor" letters, and FDA public advisory committee meetings, pregnancy exposures continued to occur. In 1988, an FDA advisory committee recommended the implementation of an intensive Pregnancy Prevention Program (PPP) to be directed at both prescribing physicians and patients. The purpose of the program was to eliminate the occurrence of pregnancy exposure and ensure that isotretinoin was not used in women of childbearing potential with a contraindication to its use.

A voluntary survey of women treated with isotretinoin was conducted to assess the effectiveness of the PPP.[58] During the period 1989–93, a total of 402 pregnancy exposures were identified by the survey, the majority of which were electively terminated. Pregnancy exposures to isotretinoin continued, leading to another FDA advisory committee meeting in 2000. During the period from 1989 to 1999, isotretinoin use in women increased about 250%, suggesting extensive off-label use for conditions other than severe recalcitrant nodular acne. In addition, the validity and generalizability of the PPP survey for identifying and counting pregnancy exposures was challenged because of its voluntary nature, low participation rate (estimated at about 30%), and the likelihood that abortion events would be underreported.[59] Also, despite more than a decade of educational outreach to physicians and patients, physicians (primarily dermatologists) continued to prescribe isotretinoin to substantial numbers of women without obtaining periodic pregnancy tests and without ensuring that the contraceptive recommendations outlined in labeling were being followed.[58] In response to these data, this advisory committee recommended that isotretinoin be available only within the framework of a comprehensive restricted distribution system. This was not implemented.

In 2002, the manufacturer of isotretinoin implemented a modified risk management program that centered on the use of a "qualification sticker" that, when affixed to a prescription, attested that the patient was qualified to use isotretinoin and that all risk management elements described in labeling had been followed.[60] Evaluation of this latest program found that reporting of pregnancy exposure to isotretinoin was unchanged from previous levels.[61] Critical data related to physician and patient behavior were obtained from a voluntary patient survey with a low participation rate of only 22–26%.[62] From this survey, 8–9% of sexually active women of childbearing age reported having no pregnancy tests performed during their five-month course of isotretinoin use and only 49% reported contraceptive use that complied with the risk management program recommendations. Importantly, use of a "qualification sticker" (present in 97% of prescriptions), a surrogate measure for the outcome of importance, did not correlate with compliance with contraceptive and pregnancy testing requirements. There was no difference among women reporting the presence or absence of a "qualification sticker" on their isotretinoin prescription with respect to these measures. Of note, this latest RM program did not directly measure the performance of pregnancy testing or the occurrence of pregnancy exposure to isotretinoin, but instead relied exclusively on surrogate process measures and volunteer surveys. An FDA advisory committee again recommended a restricted distribution system for isotretinoin in February 2004.

PEMOLINE

Pemoline is a psychostimulant, approved for the treatment of attention-deficit hyperactivity disorder (ADHD), and its use is associated with acute hepatic failure. In 1996, the product label was changed to designate pemoline as a second-line drug for ADHD. In 1999, recommendations for baseline and on-treatment liver enzyme monitoring were added to the label.[63] To assess the effectiveness of these risk management strategies, a retrospective cohort study was performed using a large health care database for the period January 1998 through March 2000.[64] For patients prescribed pemoline, the investigators looked for preceding prescriptions for first-line ADHD drugs. Out of 1308 patients in the cohort who received pemoline during the study period, only 34% had received a prescription for a first-line compound previously. In addition, only 11% of patients prescribed pemoline after the recommendation for liver enzyme monitoring had liver enzyme measurements prior to initiation of pemoline therapy. As a set of RM interventions, switching the product's indication to second-line status, and recommending that liver enzyme monitoring be performed monthly did not dramatically alter the way pemoline was prescribed by physicians. While there are no reliable patient outcome data regarding the occurrence of severe liver injury available to compare the pre- versus post-intervention periods, the process measures that were evaluated showed that physician behavior did not change meaningfully. Hence, the safety profile of pemoline is unlikely to have been altered by the interventions that were employed.

TERFENADINE

Terfenadine, a histamine H1 receptor antagonist, was associated with QT prolongation and QT-related cardiac arrhythmias when combined with inhibitors of cytochrome P-450 3A4 (CYP3A4). This prompted a number of "Dear Doctor" letters in the early 1990s, warning of the dangers of concomitant use of terfenadine with CYP3A4 inhibitors such as azole antifungal agents and macrolide antibiotics. Two studies examined the impact of these warnings on inappropriate dispensing of terfenadine with contraindicated concomitant drugs. Using pharmacy claims data from a large New England health plan, patients dispensed terfenadine during the period January 1990 through June 1994 were enumerated and the proportion with same-day dispensing or overlapping supply of an azole antifungal drug or macrolide antibiotic with terfenadine was determined.[65] The rate of same-day dispensing of contraindicated drugs was reduced by 84% over the study period, and that of contraindicated overlapping supply was decreased by 57%. Despite this improvement, the investigators estimated that 2–3% of all patients prescribed terfenadine during the first half of 1994 received an overlapping prescription for a macrolide antibiotic or azole antifungal drug. Another study examined dispensing of prescriptions for terfenadine and either erythromycin or ketoconazole within two days of each other, in two state Medicaid programs and a health maintenance organization, from 1988 to 1994.[66] The investigators reported substantial decreases in these inappropriate concomitant prescriptions, particularly in 1992. However, despite the decline in concomitant use of these drugs, nearly 1% of terfenadine prescriptions dispensed to patients in the two Medicaid plans were filled within two days of an erythromycin prescription at the end of the study period. In 1997, fexofenadine, a metabolite of terfenadine, was launched as a non-cardiotoxic alternative to terfenadine, which was withdrawn from the US market.[67]

TROGLITAZONE

Troglitazone is a thiazolidinedione compound that was marketed in the US for the treatment of diabetes from 1997 to 2000. In premarketing clinical trials, at least three patients developed jaundice or were hospitalized for acute liver injury. In the postmarketing environment, troglitazone was associated with acute hepatic failure within a few months of marketing. After a long series of labeling changes, boxed warnings, and "Dear Health Professional" letters, and after the marketing of other drugs in the same class that appeared to be free of this problem, it was removed from the US market.

A central component of the risk management strategy for the prevention of troglitazone-related acute liver failure was periodic liver enzyme monitoring. A large cohort study performed in a large managed care organization indicated that, despite four letters to physicians, these recommendations were disregarded for the majority of patients receiving troglitazone.[68] A larger question is whether liver enzyme monitoring would have reduced the number of cases of liver failure with troglitazone use had it been consistently performed. Analysis of 94 postmarketing reports of liver failure with troglitazone use found that in 19 cases with adequate data, irreversible liver injury developed within one month of initiating troglitazone use or of documented normal liver enzyme measurements.[69] Additionally, the mean time between the onset of clinical jaundice and hepatic encephalopathy, liver transplantation, or death was only 24 days. The investigators concluded that monthly liver enzyme monitoring was not likely to have prevented many, or perhaps any, cases of acute liver failure, even if it had been performed consistently.

EFFECTIVENESS OF RISK MANAGEMENT EFFORTS

As described, a variety of interventions and combinations of interventions have been used in an attempt to manage, that is, minimize, the occurrence of serious health risks with a variety of prescription and over-the-counter drug products. While the experience to date may be somewhat limited, several observations emerge from review of these examples (Table 33.2). Changes to product labeling and the posting of letters to health care providers about product risk, while absolutely necessary, do not alone appear to result in successful risk management, that is, optimized patient safety. In our view, such methods cannot be viewed as effective means to change physician or patient behaviors in a manner that optimizes the balance of benefit to risk. Even in the

Table 33.2. Classification and effectiveness of risk management approaches as qualitatively assessed by the authors

Intervention	Examples	Effectiveness
Legislation or national government campaign	APAP in the UK Aspirin—Reye's syndrome Childproof packaging	Generally good
Engineering-based	APAP: blister packs, limited tablet number Childproof packaging Clozapine: lab result linked to Rx dispensing Switch from terfenadine to fexofenadine	Generally good
Product labeling	Bromfenac, cisapride, isotretinoin, pemoline, terfenadine, troglitazone	Generally poor
Dear Health Care Provider letters	Bromfenac, cisapride, isotretinoin, pemoline, terfenadine, troglitazone	Generally poor
Public advisory meetings	Isotretinoin, troglitazone	Generally poor
Voluntary liver enzyme monitoring	Pemoline, troglitazone	Generally poor
Educational campaigns	Cisapride, isotretinoin	Generally poor
Signed informed consent	Isotretinoin	Generally poor

rare instance where these activities were associated with measurable improvements in prescribing behavior (terfenadine), the resultant changes were inadequate to sufficiently ensure safe marketing of the drug. In the terfenadine instance, despite a substantial reduction in contraindicated co-prescribing, there were still a large absolute number of patients experiencing the contraindicated use because of the extremely common prescribing of the contraindicated drugs in the first place. Also, the improvement that was noted occurred only after several different letters were mailed over a period of many months.

Likewise, public advisory committee meetings to discuss safety concerns such as those conducted in the US also do not appear to improve the safety profile of drug products. Such meetings, though not usually thought of as RM tools, may be considered as such if they engender substantial media coverage, and hence reach large numbers of people with a particular health or safety message. Multiple advisory committee meetings for isotretinoin, most with an accompanying high degree of media attention, did not lead to safer use of this teratogen.

Performance of liver enzyme monitoring and occurrence of liver failure cases with troglitazone were not meaningfully altered by another high-profile advisory committee meeting. Recommendations that periodic liver enzyme monitoring be performed are largely ignored. Additionally, in the case of troglitazone, monitoring probably would not have been effective even had it been reliably performed. This latter information became available subsequent to the issuance of the recommendation. Nonetheless, at the time of the monitoring recommendation, there was no reliable

evidence to support the idea that monitoring would be effective. Reliance on "educational campaigns" conducted by drug manufacturers and the use of signed informed consent with isotretinoin has not effected meaningful improvements in primary health outcomes.

Risk management programs supported by national legislation or a nationally coordinated comprehensive campaign, and those relying on "engineering-based" approaches have shown the greatest success at improving major health outcomes in the face of serious drug safety risks. By "engineering-based," we mean interventions that do not rely purely on patient or physician compliance, cooperation, or knowledge. A variety of approaches fall into this category, such as systems that regulate access to the drug product (as with mandatory laboratory testing with appropriately "safe" results), or which impose limits on access to dangerous quantities of the drug product (packaging, tablet quantity, tablet strength).

Manufacturing processes that physically alter or change the drug product to reduce or eliminate its intrinsic toxicity also are included here. Examples would include alendronate and loratadine with pseudoephedrine (24 hour extended release). After the start of marketing, cases of severe esophageal injury including ulceration and perforation with the use of alendronate were reported. The size and shape of the tablet were reformulated to decrease the risk of the drug becoming trapped in the mucosal folds of the esophagus. With loratadine plus pseudoephedrine (24 hour extended release), over 50 cases of esophageal obstruction, including some with upper airway obstruction and death, were reported to the FDA. The tablet size was large (~1 cm) and the surface of the tablet became sticky when moistened, perhaps increasing its tendency to stick to the esophageal mucosa when taken with water. The product was reformulated to streamline its shape and eliminate the problem of the sticky surface coating.[70] With each of these situations, formal evaluation of the impact of changing product size, shape, and surface coating was not performed. However, there was an abrupt decline in case reporting of these adverse events coincident with implementation of the product changes. Monitoring changes in case reporting after an RM intervention is not usually considered a reliable metric upon which to conclude that a safety problem has been remedied. However, in the loratadine example, there was a high-volume steady stream of case reports preceding the change that nearly completely disappeared afterwards.

THE FUTURE

The concept of RM has emerged as the latest response to the societal problem posed by the adverse health effects of medicines. Pharmacoepidemiology should be an intrinsic component of the RM process, from identification and characterization of product risk to evaluation of the success or failure of a product's RM program. For the latter to occur, the primary goals of the RM program must be clear, relevant, and measurable. Without this, patients may be needlessly harmed because no one can demonstrate that the program has "succeeded." As things currently stand, the absence of reliable evidence of success usually results in a default position favoring the *status quo*. This absence of evidence allows ineffective RM programs to continue while pharmaceutical companies and drug regulatory authorities assume that they have successfully mitigated a product's risk. Neither patient safety nor the balance of benefit to risk is improved under such circumstances.

Several broader questions also require examination. In the face of a serious drug safety issue, RM has sometimes been put forward as a means of preserving market availability of a product by shifting what has become an unfavorable balance of benefit to risk to one where this balance is acceptably shifted in favor of benefit. If a safety risk is serious enough to mandate a special RM program, several principles become operational. Borrowing from the world of clinical trials, new treatments are not tested in large numbers of patients without sufficiently strong evidence of efficacy to justify their experimental use in a study population. In the absence of promising results from a Phase II research program, exposing large numbers of patients to an apparently ineffective drug within a Phase III clinical trial would not be justified by the evidence. Similarly, in the situation of a serious or life-threatening illness, it is difficult to imagine an institutional review board approving the use of a completely untested therapy, or one that appears ineffective, in a clinical trial involving large numbers of subjects.

In the setting of RM, we propose that analogous principles should apply. Importantly, the number of patients "treated" with an RM program dwarfs that generally encountered with pre-approval clinical trials. When a serious postmarketing safety issue arises, involving tens if not hundreds of thousands of treated patients each year, the imperative to protect patients from harm becomes more urgent. Reliance on untested or unproven RM methods to mitigate risk, or optimize the balance of benefit to risk, could be considered inappropriate or even unethical in such circumstances.

The obligation to collect reliable, relevant, and analyzable data with which to determine whether an RM program is an effective "treatment" for the safety issue under consideration also rises in prominence. Again borrowing from the principles governing the conduct of clinical trials, subjecting patients to potential harm from a proven or unproven therapy, without collecting the appropriate data, would be considered scientifically inappropriate and unacceptable. Yet, to date, most enacted RM programs have failed to collect the appropriate data or even to insist that it be collected.[71] Implicit in the above construct is the expectation that the results of the assessments of RM programs would be published in the peer-reviewed literature.

The potential pitfalls of (i) relying on RM interventions that have little or no probability of success, or (ii) not collecting the right types of data to document optimization of the balance of benefit to risk, can all too easily threaten the value and integrity of the practice of RM. The effectiveness of RM programs cannot be assumed, but must be measured and documented. In a very real sense, RM programs function as public health trials that should be subject to the rigors of experimental methodology. The current paradigm is founded upon an opposite construct; namely, that one prove that optimization of the balance of benefit to risk has not occurred. This is a daunting, if not impossible task, for one cannot easily (if ever) disprove the negative. To be effective, RM needs to become a strategy that seeks first and foremost to protect the population of patients who may be treated with what has come to be recognized as an unsafe drug from unreasonable, unacceptable, or unnecessary risk of harm. Science-based efforts in this field must ensure that RM not become a strategy to enable the continued market availability of dangerous drugs, without addressing the underlying safety problem with an effective intervention.

A number of related questions immediately follow, most of which are beyond the scope of pharmacoepidemiology. What should be done if it is not possible to accurately measure a relevant health outcome? We believe it would be important to understand the nature of the "impossibility." If the safety problem is severe (as it most often is), we believe that the "burden of evidence" has shifted. In the absence of solid evidence that the balance of benefit to risk has been optimized, the assumption must be that it has not changed. The conclusion that follows would be that the drug product in question is no longer safe to be marketed.

Another difficult question relates to the use of surrogate measures of RM program performance (these may be process measures or behavioral measures) when relevant health outcome measures cannot be obtained. As a rule, the default presumption should be that these are insufficient to satisfy the "burden of evidence" requirement or to reject the null hypothesis, which states that the balance of benefit to risk has not been optimized.

In our view, risk management is very much an emerging field. The earliest example of a risk management intervention discussed in this chapter was from 1970 (child-resistant containers), but the majority were implemented during the past decade. In 1999, the FDA Task Force on Risk Management called for "better tools . . . to evaluate the effectiveness of FDA's risk management efforts."[2] We believe that careful, science-based application of pharmacoepidemiologic methods to the evaluation of RM interventions will help advance the nascent field of risk management in the context of modern therapeutic options.

DISCLAIMER

The views expressed are those of the authors and do not necessarily reflect those of the US Food and Drug Administration.

REFERENCES

1. Stematis DH. *Legal Approach to Liability. Failure Mode Effects Analysis: From Theory to Execution.* Milwaukee, WI: Quality Press, 2003; pp. 1–20.
2. FDA. *Managing the Risks from Medical Product Use: Creating a Risk Management Framework.* Available at: http://www.fda.gov/oc/tfrm/1999report.html. Accessed: August 11, 2004.
3. FDA. *Guidance for Industry (Draft): Development and Use of Risk Minimization Action Plans.* Available at: http://www.fda.gov/cder/guidance/5766dft.pdf. Accessed: July 13, 2004.
4. Piantadosi S. *Clinical Trials: A Methodologic Perspective.* New York: John Wiley & Sons, 1997; pp. 197–98, 521.
5. ALLHAT Investigators. Major cardiovascular events in hypertensive patients randomized to doxazosin vs chlorthalidone: the Antihypertensive and Lipid-Lowering Treatment to Prevent Heart Attack Trial. *JAMA* 2000; **283**: 1967–75.
6. Goldman SA. Communication of medical product risk: how effective is effective enough? *Drug Saf* 2004; **27**: 519–534.
7. Rogers AS, Israel E, Smith CR, Levine D, McBean AM, Valente C, Faich G. Physician knowledge, attitudes and behavior related to reporting adverse drug events. *Arch Intern Med* 1988; **148**: 1596–1600.
8. Glasziou P, Vandenbroucke J, Chalmers I. Assessing the quality of research. *BMJ* 2004; **328**: 39–41.
9. Ray WA. Population-based studies of adverse drug effects. *N Engl J Med* 2003; **349**: 1592–4.
10. Andrews EB, West SL. Rationale and organization for the ISPE mid-year symposium April 2000: the power and perils of health data used in epidemiologic and economic research. *Pharmacoepidemiol Drug Saf* 2001; **10**: 361–2.
11. Food and Drug Administration Concept Paper (Draft). *Premarketing Risk Assessment.* May 2004. Available at: http://www.fda.gov/cder/guidance/5765dft.htm.
12. Zanchi A, Maillard M, Burnier M. Recent clinical trials with omapatrilat: new developments. *Curr Hypertens Rep* 2003; **5**: 346–52.
13. Coats AJS. Omapatrilat—the story of Overture and Octave. *Int J Cardiol* 2002; **86**: 1–4.
14. Vandenbrouke JP. In defense of case reports and case series. *Ann Intern Med* 2001; **134**: 330–4.
15. Waller PC, Lee EH. Responding to drug safety issues. *Pharmacoepidemiol Drug Saf* 1999; **8**: 535–52.
16. La Grenade L, Graham DJ, Trontell A. Cardiomyopathy and myocarditis associated with clozapine use in the US [letter]. *New Engl J Med* 2001, **345**: 124–5.
17. Graham DJ, Green L, Senior JR, Nourjah P. Troglitazone-induced liver failure: clinical and epidemiologic aspects. *Am J Med* 2003; **114**: 299–306.
18. Bonnel RA, Graham DJ. Peripheral neuropathy in patients treated with leflunomide. *Clin Pharmacol Ther* 2004; **76**: 580–5.
19. Grimes DA, Schulz KF. Bias and causal associations in observational research. *Lancet* 2002; **359**: 248–52.
20. Shah RR. Withdrawal of terodiline: a tale of two toxicities. In: Mann RD, Andrews EB, eds, *Pharmacovigilance.* New York: John Wiley & Sons, 2002; pp. 135–54.
21. Inman W, Clarke J, Wilton L, Pearce G, Vendhuis GJ. PEM report no. 2: Terodiline. *Pharmacoepidemiol Drug Saf* 1993; **2**: 287–319.
22. Hall GC, Chukwujindu J, Richardson J, Lis Y, Wild RN. Micturin (terodiline) hydrochloride, torsades de pointe and other arrhythmias—a study using the VAMP database. *Pharmacoepidemiol Drug Saf* 1993; **2**: 127–32.
23. Jones SE, Ogura T, Shuba LM, McDonald TF. Inhibition of the rapid component of the delayed rectifier K+ current by

therapeutic concentrations of the antispasmodic agent terodiline. *Br J Pharmacol* 1998; **125**: 1138–43.

24. Thomas SH, Higham PD, Hartigan-Go K, Kamali F, Wood P, Campbell RW *et al*. Concentration dependent cardiotoxicity of terodiline in patients treated for urinary incontinence. *Br Heart J* 1995; **74**: 53–6.

25. Strom BL. Data validity issues in using claims data. *Pharmacoepidemiol Drug Saf* 2001; **10**: 389–92.

26. Strom BL, Carson JL, Schinnar R. Is cimetidine associated with neutropenia? *Am J Med* 1995; **99**: 282–90.

27. Strom BL, Carson JL, Halpern AC, Schinnar R, Snyder ES, Shaw M *et al*. A population-based study of Stevens–Johnson syndrome: incidence and antecedent drug exposures. *Arch Dermatol* 1991; **127**: 831–8.

28. Grodstein F, Stampfer MJ, Colditz GA, Willett WC, Manson JE, Joffe M *et al*. Postmenopausal hormone therapy and mortality. *N Engl J Med* 1997; **336**: 1769–75.

29. Grimes DA, Lobo RA. Perspectives on the Women's Health Initiative trial of hormone replacement therapy. *Obstet Gynecol* 2002; **100**: 1344–53.

30. Jones EF, Forrest JD. Contraceptive failure in the United States: revised estimates from the 1982 National Survey of Family Growth. *Fam Plann Perspec* 1989; **21**: 103–9.

31. Committee on Safety of Medicines, Medicines Control Agency. Paracetamol and aspirin. *Curr Prob Pharmacovigilance* 1997; **23**: 9.

32. Turvill JL, Burrourghs AK, Moore KP. Change in occurrence of paracetamol overdose in UK after introduction of blister packs. *Lancet* 2000; **355**: 2048–9.

33. Prince MI, Thomas SHL, James OFW, Hudson M. Reduction in incidence of severe paracetamol poisoning. *Lancet* 2000; **355**: 2047–8.

34. Robinson D, Smith AMJ, Johnston GD. Severity of overdose after restriction of paracetamol availability: retrospective study. *BMJ* 2000; **321**: 926–7.

35. Hawton K, Townsend E, Deeks J, Appleby L, Gunnell D, Bennewith O, Cooper J. Effects of legislation restricting pack sizes of paracetamol and salicylate on self poisoning in the United Kingdom: before and after study. *BMJ* 2001; **322**: 1–7.

36. Sheen CL, Dillon JF, Bateman DN, Simpson KJ, MacDonald TM. Paracetamol-related deaths in Scotland, 1994–2000. *Br J Clin Pharmacol* 2002; **54**: 430–2.

37. Belay ED, Bresee JS, Holman RC, Khan AS, Shahriari A, Schonberger LB. Reye's syndrome in the United States from 1981 through 1997. *N Engl J Med* 1999; **340**: 1377–82.

38. US Food and Drug Administration Talk Paper, June 22, 1998. Available at: http://www.fda.gov/bbs/topics/ANSWERS/ANS00879.html. Accessed: July 6, 2004.

39. US Food and Drug Administration Talk Paper, February 10, 1998. Available at: http://www.fda.gov/bbs/topics/ANSWERS/ANS00849.html. Accessed: July 6, 2004.

40. US Food and Drug Administration. Duract questions and answers, June 22, 1998. Available at: http://www.fda.gov/cder/news/duract/qa.htm. Accessed: July 6, 2004.

41. Poison Prevention Packaging Act of 1970. 15 USC 1471–6.

42. Rodgers GB. The safety effects of child-resistant packaging for oral prescription drugs: two decades of experience. *JAMA* 1996; **275**: 1661–5.

43. Rodgers GB. The effectiveness of child-resistant packaging for aspirin. *Arch Pediatr Adolesc Med* 2002; **156**: 929–33.

44. Henney JE. Withdrawal of troglitazone and cisapride. *JAMA* 2000; **283**: 2228.

45. Wysowski DK, Bacsanyi J. Cisapride and fatal arrhythmia. *N Engl J Med* 1996; **335**: 290–1.

46. Food and Drug Administration. Talk Paper T00-6, January 24, 2000. Available at: http://www.fda.gov/bbs/topics/ANSWERS/ANS00999.html/. Accessed: July 6, 2004.

47. Smalley W, Shatin D, Wysowski DK, Gurwitz J, Andrade SE, Goodman M *et al*. Contraindicated use of cisapride: impact of Food and Drug Administration regulatory action. *JAMA* 2000; **284**: 3036–9.

48. Jones JK, Fife D, Curkendall S, Goehring E Jr, Guo JJ, Shannon M. Coprescribing and codispensing of cisapride and contraindicated drugs. *JAMA* 2001; **286**: 1607–9.

49. Guo JJ, Curkendall S, Jones JK, Fife D, Goehring E, She D. Impact of cisapride label changes on codispensing of contraindicated medications. *Pharmacoepidemiol Drug Safe* 2003; **12**: 295–301.

50. Weatherby LB, Walker AM, Fife D, Vervaet P, Klausner MA. Contraindicated medications dispensed with cisapride; temporal trends in relation to the sending of "Dear Doctor" letters. *Pharmacoepidemiol Drug Safe* 2001; **10**: 211–18.

51. Raschetti R, Maggini M, Da Cas R, Popoli P, Rossi A. Time trends in the coprescribing of cisapride and contraindicated drugs in Umbria, Italy. *JAMA* 2001; **285**: 1840–1.

52. De Bruin ML, Panneman MJ, Leufkens HG, Hoes AW, Herings RM. Use of cisapride with contraindicated drugs in the Netherlands. *Ann Pharmacother* 2002; **36**: 338–43.

53. Clozaril [package insert]. Novartis Pharmaceuticals, East Hanover, New Jersey, 2003.

54. Honigfeld G, Arellano F, Sethi J, Bianchini A, Schein J. Reducing clozapine-related morbidity and mortality: 5 years of experience with the Clozaril National Registry. *J Clin Psychiatry* 1998; **59** (suppl 3): 3–7.

55. Krupp P, Barnes P. Leponex-associated granulocytopenia: a review of the situation. *Psychopharmacology* 1989; **99**: S118–S21.

56. Walker AM, Lanza LL, Arellano F, Rothman KJ. Mortality in current and former users of clozapine. *Epidemiology* 1997; **8**: 671–7.

57. Meltzer HY, Alphs L, Green AI, Altamura AC, Anand R, Bertoldi A *et al*. Clozapine treatment for suicidality in schizophrenia: International Suicide Prevention Trial (InterSePT). *Arch Gen Psychiatry* 2003; **60**: 82–91.

58. Mitchell AA, Van Bennekom CM, Louik C. A pregnancy-prevention program in women of childbearing age receiving isotretinoin. *N Engl J Med* 1995; **333**: 101–6.

59. Vega L. Accutane and pregnancy exposure. Presented at the FDA Dermatologic Drugs Advisory Committee Meeting. Gaithersburg, MD, September 18, 2004. Available

at: http://www.fda.gov/ohrms/dockets/ac/00/slides/3639s1.htm. Accessed: July 8, 2004.

60. Uhl K, Kennedy DL, Kweder SL. Risk management strategies in the Physicians' Desk Reference product labels for Pregnancy Category X drugs. *Drug Saf* 2002; **25**: 885–92.

61. Pitts M. Isotretinoin pregnancy exposures: spontaneous reports. Presented at the FDA Dermatologic Drugs Advisory Committee meeting. Gaithersburg, MD, February 26, 2004. Available at: http://www.fda.gov/ohrms/dockets/ac/04/slides/4017s1.htm. Accessed: July 8, 2004.

62. Brinker A. Isotretinoin pregnancy prevention program evaluation. Presented at the FDA Dermatologic Drugs Advisory Committee meeting. Gaithersburg, MD, February 26, 2004. Available at: http://www.fda.gov/ohrms/dockets/ac/04/slides/4017s1.htm. Accessed: July 8, 2004.

63. US Food and Drug Administration MedWatch Medical Product Safety Information. Available at: http://www.fda.gov/medwatch/safety.htm. Accessed: July 8, 2004.

64. Willy ME, Manda B, Shatin D, Drinkard CR, Graham DJ. A study of compliance with FDA recommendations for pemoline (Cylert). *J Am Acad Child Adolesc Psychiatry* 2002: **41**: 785–90.

65. Thompson D, Oster G. Use of terfenadine and contraindicated drugs. *JAMA* 1996; **275**: 1339–41.

66. Burkhart GA, Sevka MJ, Temple R, Honig PK. Temporal decline in filling prescriptions for terfenadine closely in time with those for either ketoconazole or erythromycin. *Clin Pharmacol Ther* 1997; **61**: 93–6.

67. US Food and Drug Administration Talk Paper, December 29, 1997. Available at: http://www.fda.gov/bbs/topics/ANSWERS/ANS00843.html. Accessed: July 8, 2004.

68. Graham DJ, Drinkard CR, Shatin D, Tsong Y, Burgess MJ. Liver enzyme monitoring in patients treated with troglitazone. *JAMA* 2001; **286**: 831–3.

69. Graham DJ, Green L, Senior JR, Nourjah P. Troglitazone-induced liver failure: a case study. *Am J Med* 2003; **114**: 299–306.

70. Honig PH, Graham DJ, Jenkins JK. Identification and risk management of upper gastrointestinal obstruction caused by an antihistamine-decongestant product [abstract]. *Clin Pharm Ther* 2000; **67**: 89.

71. Andrews E, Gilsenan A, Cook S. Therapeutic risk management interventions: feasibility and effectiveness. *J Am Pharm Assoc* 2004; **44**: 491–500.

34

The Use of Pharmacoepidemiology to Study Medication Errors

RAINU KAUSHAL and DAVID W. BATES

Division of General Internal Medicine and Primary Care, Brigham and Women's Hospital, and Harvard Medical School, Boston, Massachusetts, USA.

INTRODUCTION

Medications are the most commonly used form of medical therapy today. For adults, 75% of office visits to general practitioners and internists are associated with the continuation or initiation of a drug,[1] while in the hospital several medication orders tend to be written for each patient daily. Medication errors are frequent, though fortunately only a small proportion result in harm; these errors are referred to as preventable adverse drug events.[2] However, given the prevalence of prescription medication use, preventable adverse drug events are one of the most frequent types of preventable iatrogenic injuries. The IOM report, *To Err Is Human* suggested at least 44 000–98 000 deaths nationally from iatrogenic injury.[3] If accurate, this would mean that there are about 8000 deaths yearly from adverse drug events and 1 million injuries from drug use. This report stimulated public discussion of patient safety and several Federal policy initiatives, including increased funding for research, to improve patient safety.

SAFETY THEORY

Much of the framework for improving safety and understanding the causes of errors and accidents has been developed by groups outside medicine, for example by psychologists and human engineers. One frequent area of focus has been the man–machine interface, for example with nuclear reactors and aircraft.[4] These situations are similar to those faced in care today, when providers must make decisions using data from multiple monitoring systems while under stress and bombarded by interruptions.

Industrial quality theory suggests that most accidents occur because of problems with the production process itself, not the individuals operating it.[4,5] This theory suggests that blame for problems can be misplaced, and that

Pharmacoepidemiology, Fourth Edition   Edited by B.L. Strom
© 2005 John Wiley & Sons, Ltd

although "human errors" occur commonly, the true cause of accidents is often the underlying systems that allow an operator error to result in an accident. *Root cause* analysis is a tool that can be used to define the cause of the defect.[6] While sometimes an individual who makes repeated errors is to blame, most errors resulting in harm are made by workers whose overall work is good.[5] Nonetheless, the traditional medical approach to dealing with error has been to find the responsible individuals and punish them.[4] Not surprisingly, this has resulted in a culture in which medical personnel hide errors rather than discuss them. This makes detection of errors through approaches other than spontaneous reporting even more important than they might be otherwise.

To make the hospital a safer place, a key initial step is to eliminate the culture of blame,[4] and build a culture of safety. Errors and adverse outcomes should be treated as opportunities for improving the process of care through system changes, rather than a signal to begin disciplinary proceedings.

Systems changes for reducing errors can greatly reduce the likelihood of error, and probably in turn, of adverse outcomes. Within medicine, much of the research has come from anesthesia, which has made major improvements in safety. In medication delivery, one highly successful systems change was implementation of unit dosing, which resulted in an 82% decrease in medication errors in one study.[7] Similarly, computerized physician order entry is a systems change that reduced the serious medication error rate by 55%.[8] Other systems changes with great potential include barcoding of medications, and implementation of "smart pumps" which can recognize what medication is being delivered.

Some of these technologies—notably computer order entry, barcoding with computerized medication administration rates, and smart pumps—may be very useful to pharmacoepidemiologists who wish to study the epidemiology of medication errors. All of these can be used to track medication use, and more importantly, they can be set to track the frequencies and types of warnings as they go off.

Overall, the area of safety has a different philosophy and a number of different tools than classic epidemiology.[9] For improving safety, culture is extremely important, and tools such as root cause analysis and failure mode and effects analysis—which can be used to project what the problems with a process may be before they occur—are highly valuable. When combined with epidemiological data, such tools may be extremely powerful for improving the safety of care.

PATIENT SAFETY CONCEPTS, AS APPLIED TO PHARMACOEPIDEMIOLOGY

While the techniques of pharmacoepidemiology have most often been used to study the risks and benefits of drugs, they can also be used to study medication errors and preventable adverse drug events (i.e., those due to errors). *Medication errors* are defined as any mistake in the medication use process, including prescribing, transcribing, dispensing, administering, and monitoring.[10] *Adverse drug events* (ADEs) are harm resulting from medication use, and may be preventable or not. By definition, preventable ADEs are associated with an error, while nonpreventable ADEs are not. An example of a preventable ADE is a patient who is prescribed an antibiotic despite a known allergy and develops a rash, whereas a nonpreventable ADE would be a patient with no known drug allergies who is prescribed an antibiotic and develops a rash. To some people, nonpreventable ADEs are also referred to as adverse drug reactions, although this is a narrower definition than that used elsewhere in this book. Finally, *near misses* or *potential ADEs* are medication errors that have high potential for causing harm but did not, either because they were intercepted prior to reaching a patient or because the error reached the patient who fortuitously did not have any observable untoward sequelae. An example of the former is a prescription written for an overdose of a narcotic that is intercepted and corrected by a pharmacist prior to medication dispensing. An example of a non-intercepted near miss is a patient administered a two-fold overdose of a narcotic but without any consequence such as respiratory depression or sedation.

Several research study designs have been utilized to study medication errors. The early work was largely case reports and case-series. This was followed by larger and more rigorous epidemiological studies of errors.

Many of the early medication error and ADE studies were performed in the hospital setting.[2,11,12] In the inpatient adult setting, patients are vulnerable to medication errors because of their medical acuity, the complexity of their disease process, and medication regimens, as well as at times because of their age (e.g., the elderly are particularly susceptible).[2,11,12] One early study in adults demonstrated that medication errors were common, occurring at a rate of 5 per 100 medication orders.[2] Seven in 100 medication errors had significant potential for harm (i.e., near miss), and 1 in 100 actually resulted in an injury (i.e., preventable ADE).[2] The studies undertaken in a few hospitals have documented incidence rates of ADEs ranging from 2 to 7 per 100 admissions.[11,12] Pediatric inpatients have similar rates of ADEs, but a three-fold higher rate of near misses.[13]

There are several system-based factors in pediatric drug use that may contribute to this higher rate of near misses. These include the need for weight-based dosing and dilution of stock medicines, as well as decreased communication abilities of young children.

Increasing knowledge is being gained about errors in the ambulatory setting, although research in this area lags behind the inpatient setting due to the difficulties of accessing patients once they leave a doctor's office. In a recent study, Gandhi *et al.* found 25% of 661 adult outpatients had an adverse drug event.[14] Of these, 28% were ameliorable. Gurwitz *et al.* did a study of Medicare enrollees in the ambulatory clinical setting and documented 50 ADEs per 1000 person-years.[15] Comparison among these studies is difficult due to variations in methodology, analysis, and sometimes even in definitions. For example, the Gandhi *et al.* study included a patient survey while the Gurwitz *et al.* study did not. This is a particularly powerful tool to detect adverse drug events in the ambulatory setting and may have resulted in the apparent higher rates of errors in the Gandhi *et al.* study compared with the Gurwitz *et al.* one.

Finally, some work is emerging about errors at the point of transition from hospitals to ambulatory settings. Handoffs, in which the clinical care of a patient is transferred from one health provider or entity to another, are always vulnerable to errors. In one study of 400 patients discharged from a tertiary care hospital, 19% of patients had adverse events and of these 66% were adverse drug events.[16]

Most of these studies relied on primary data collection, including prescription and chart review, or direct observation by study staff of clinical care interactions primarily in the inpatient setting. Such data collection is very time and labor intensive. Typically it can only be successfully undertaken in the setting of research studies where large amounts of resources are available for data collection, including the training of data collectors to ensure inter-rater reliability. Comparisons among studies are challenging because of variations in data quality and methodology.

More recently, some work has been done using other types of pharmacoepidemiologic techniques, such as claims-based evaluations. For example, a recent study using this approach demonstrated that retrospective drug utilization review did not impact on rates of potential prescribing errors[17] (see also Chapter 29). Claims-based evaluations allow the ascertainment of errors in multiple parts of the medication use process, including ordering, transcribing, dispensing, and, in the outpatient setting, compliance. However, it is difficult to hone in on the actual stage at which an error occurred using solely claims-based data. For example, if a claims-based evaluation demonstrates that a patient was given an overdose of a medication, it is difficult to determine if this occurred due to a drug ordering, dispensing, or transcribing error.

In this chapter we address several aspects of pharmacoepidemiologic research into medication errors, including methodological issues that it needs to address, and its present strengths as well as future directions.

CLINICAL PROBLEMS TO BE ADDRESSED BY PHARMACOEPIDEMIOLOGIC RESEARCH

Medication errors can occur at any stage of the medication use process, including prescribing, transcribing, dispensing, administering, and monitoring.[10] Of these stages, prescribing errors in the hospital have most commonly been documented to cause harm,[11] although errors at any stage can do so, and monitoring errors (i.e., errors caused by lack of proper monitoring) are quite prominent outside the hospital.[14,15] The greater proportion of harmful errors at the drug ordering stage may be a consequence of the data collection methodology employed in these studies, which were multi-pronged but did not include direct observation, the most sensitive technique for administration error detection.

Important types of errors include dosing, route, frequency, drug-allergy, drug–drug interaction, drug–laboratory (including renal dosing), drug–patient characteristic, and drug administration during pregnancy. Although these errors occur most frequently at the drug ordering stage, they can occur at any stage in the medication use process.

In a number of studies, dosing errors have represented the most frequent category.[11,14,18,19] To determine whether or not a dosing error is present, most often some clinical context is needed, for example the patient's age, gender, weight, level of renal function, prior response to the medication (if it has been used previously), response to other similar medications, clinical condition, and often the indication for the therapy. While many of these data elements can be obtained from review of the medical chart, many are not typically available from claims data alone (see Chapters 13–21 for discussions of claims databases). Thus, while it is sometimes possible to state, based on claims data, that an extremely high dose is problematic, most studies that evaluate the adequacy of dosing include more clinical information, either from chart review or an electronic medical record (see Chapter 22).

Route of administration problems also represent a common type of error.[11] Many drugs can be given by one or a few routes and not by many others. Some such errors— such as giving benzathine penicillin that contains suspended solids intravenously instead of intramuscularly—would often be fatal, and though they have caused fatalities, are fortunately very rare. Other route errors—such as grinding up a sustained released preparation to give it via a jejunostomy tube—are much more frequent, and can have very serious consequences. Route errors are especially problematic at the administration stage of the medication use process, and administration errors are both difficult to detect and much less often intercepted than prescribing errors.[20] The best approach for detecting administration errors has long been direct observation, and Barker *et al.* have developed and refined an approach which reliably allows identification of these errors.[21]

Dosing frequency errors can occur either at the prescribing, dispensing, or administration stage. While overall these errors probably cause less harm cumulatively than dose or route errors, they can be problematic. Some frequency errors at the prescribing or dispensing stage can be detected even with claims or prescription data. Such errors have greater potential for harm when drugs are given with a greater frequency than intended. However, the therapeutic benefit may not be realized when given with too low frequency, and extremely negative effects can occur for some drugs, for example with antiretrovirals, to which resistance develops if they are given at a low frequency.

Allergy errors represent a particularly serious type of error, even though most of the time when a drug is given to a patient with a known allergy, the patient does well. For example, approximately two thirds of the time when a penicillin-allergic patient is given penicillin, they do well.[22] Allergy errors typically cannot be detected with claims data, since allergy information on patients is not available. Thus, these errors have to be detected either through chart review, which is laborious, or more often nowadays, through electronic record data.[23] Electronic medical records have made it much easier to collect large numbers of these errors, or at least instances in which patients were given a drug despite a known allergy or sensitivity. One of the findings that has emerged from these evaluations has been that the consequences of many such exposures may be less harmful than has been thought, with one recent study suggesting, for example, that the risk of allergic reactions to cephalosporins in patients with known penicillin allergy was no greater than for patients with allergies to other antibiotics.[24]

Drug–drug interaction exposures represent an interesting and difficult area, both for research and interventions to decrease errors.[19,25,26] While many interactions have been reported, the severity varies substantially from minor to life-threatening. If a conscious decision is made to give patients two medications despite the knowledge that they interact, this cannot be considered an error except in very limited circumstances, for example with meperidine and monoamine oxidase inhibitors. In addition, it is legitimate to give many medications together despite clear interactions with important consequences if there are no good alternatives, or if dose alterations are made, or if additional monitoring is carried out (for example, with warfarin and many antibiotics). However, the necessary alterations in dosing or additional monitoring are often omitted, which can have severe consequences. It is possible in large claims data sets to detect situations in which simultaneous exposures appear to have occurred, but not possible to determine if this actually occurred, as a physician may give patients instructions to cease the use of one of the drugs. It is also not possible to use claims data to assess the clinical rationale for the choice, and it is often difficult to determine whether or not adverse consequences have occurred from these data. Analyses that incorporate clinical decision making or include detailed outcomes typically require clinical data. Claims analyses of drug–drug interactions are exciting, however, because it is possible to assess millions of patients simultaneously, and as it becomes easier to link such data with more outcomes information it will undoubtedly become easier to assess the level of risk associated with specific interactions.

Drug–laboratory errors represent an important category of errors, but can be difficult to detect electronically because of poor interfaces between laboratory and pharmacy information.[27] When such information is available simultaneously, a number of categories of errors or problems can be identified (Table 34.1).[27] For example, digoxin is more risky when given when hypokalemia is present. Such errors are relatively straightforward to identify when large pharmacy and laboratory databases can be linked, although again assessment of clinical outcomes is difficult unless these data are also available.

Renal dosing errors represent a specific subtype of drug–laboratory errors and are probably especially important.[28] In one large inpatient study, nearly 40% of inpatients had at least mild renal insufficiency, and there are many medications that require dosing adjustment in the presence of decreased glomerular filtration.[28] In that study, without clinical decision support, patients received the appropriate dose and frequency of medication only 30% of the time. A number of other studies have identified this as a problem.[29–31]

Many studies of drug–patient characteristic checking have focused to date on the use of medications in the presence

Table 34.1. Ten ways laboratory and pharmacy can be linked to improve care

Category	Concept	Examples (drug–lab pair)[a]	Special role for the computer/linkages
Drug Selection	1. Lab *contraindicates* drug	+ Pregnancy test–ACE inhibitor ↑SUN/Cr–metformin hydrochloride	Prevents prescription writing or dispensing
	2. Lab suggests *indication* for drug	↑TSH–levothyroxine sodium ↑Cholesterol–lipid-lowering treatment	Generates timely reminders, tracking intervention
Dosing	3. Lab affecting drug *dose*	↑Creatinine–digoxin, vancomycin hydrochloride	Performs dose calculations based on age, sex, lab value, weight
	4. Drug requiring lab for *titration*	Warfarin sodium–PT/INR Anticonvulsants–drug levels	Statistical process control dosing adjustment charts
Monitoring	5. Abnormal lab *signaling* toxicity	Liver enzymes–isoniazid, glitazones ↓HCT, WBC–chloramphenicol	Triggers alert, assesses likelihood
	6. Drug warranting lab *monitoring* for *toxicity*	Clozapine–WBC Amphotericin B–creatinine	Oversees scheduling of both baseline and serial monitoring tests
Lab interpretation	7. Drug *influencing* or *interfering* with lab finding	Carbamazepine–free thyroxine Quinolones–false-positive urine opiates	Warns against/interprets false-positives and false-negatives
	8. Drug *impacting* on *response* to lab finding	Insulin–↓ or ↑glucose Penicillin–+RPR	Resets alarm threshold for treated patients
Improvement	9. Drug toxicity/effects *surveillance*	Detects signals of previously undocumented reaction (e.g. hepatotoxicity)	Data mining of lab and drug data to generate new hypotheses of drug effects
	10. Quality *oversight*	Treatment delay after abnormal results (↑TSH, ↑K+, +blood culture) and initiation of appropriate treatment	Monitors: time interval between lab testing and prescription change, adequacy/appropriateness of lab monitoring

Abbreviations: ACE, angiotensin-converting enzyme; Cr, creatinine; HCT, hematocrit; INR, international normalized ratio; K+, potassium; lab, laboratory; PT, prothrombin time; RPR, rapid plasma regain; SUN, serum urea nitrogen; TSH, thyrotropin; WBC, white blood cell count.
[a] Plus sign indicates positive.
Source: Reproduced from Schiff et al.[27] by permission of the American Medical Association.

of specific diseases, for example myasthenia gravis. However, in the future, genomic testing will undoubtedly dominate, as many genes have profound effects on drug metabolism (see Chapter 37). To date, few large data sets can be linked with genotype information, but this is becoming increasingly frequent in clinical trials and a number of cohorts are being established as well that include genotypic information, for example in Iceland and at the Marshfield Clinic in Wisconsin.[32]

Another important type of error is those that result inadvertently from system-based interventions such as the introduction of information technology. For example, automated pharmacy systems, featuring computer-controlled devices that package, dispense, distribute, and/or control medications, also have the potential to reduce administration errors. Although these systems in general reduce errors, one study demonstrated an increase in errors with a device that allowed nurses to obtain any medicine stored for any patient and did not integrate the computerized medication profiles of patients. The investigators attributed the increase in errors to nurses more commonly administering drugs from the automated device without checking them, compared with drugs taken from the patient's medication drawer.[33] This example highlights the importance of testing information technology interventions prior to widespread use and dissemination.

METHODOLOGIC PROBLEMS TO BE ADDRESSED BY PHARMACOEPIDEMIOLOGIC RESEARCH

There are several important methodological problems that need to be addressed by pharmacoepidemiologic research into medication errors, including information bias, sample size issues, and generalizability.

INFORMATION BIAS

In performing drug analyses, the present conventions preclude the determination of total daily dose in several ways. Physicians may prescribe a greater amount of medicine than is required for the time period prescribed. For example, if a patient requires 50 mg of atenolol per day, the doctor may actually write a prescription for 100 mg of atenolol per day and verbally convey instructions to the patient to divide the pills. This is particularly problematic with drugs that must be titrated to the appropriate therapeutic dose. If either physicians or pharmacists were required to document an accurate total daily dose, this would improve the ability to perform research.

Another important methodological issue is measurement of patient adherence to medications (see also Chapter 46). Since prescribing and dispensing data are seldom jointly available, determining patient adherence is extremely difficult. Improving clinician access to data from pharmacy benefit managers might be extremely useful, as might availability of electronic prescription data to pharmacies. It is widely known that patient non-adherence is a critical clinical problem with important medication safety consequences. However, the frequency of its occurrence and potential methods of addressing it are poorly understood.

Many medications are contraindicated in pregnancy, with notable examples being thalidomide, isotretinoin, and warfarin. Here, the greatest difficulty for the investigator is in assessing whether or not the patient is actually pregnant at the time of the exposure, although this can be assessed retrospectively by identifying the date of birth, assuming a term pregnancy, and then working backward. The outcomes of interest are often not represented in ways that make it easy to perform analyses, although data on medication exposures and on births are readily available and can often be linked.

Another important piece of clinical information for pediatrics is a child's weight. Most pediatric medications are dosed on the basis of weight. Standardized documentation of this information is unavailable, hindering not only analyses of pediatric dosing but also actual dosing by pediatricians.

A final issue is the coding of allergies.[22] It is important for both clinical care and research that allergies are differentiated from sensitivities or intolerances through codes rather than free text. Continued drug use in the presence of drug sensitivity may be perfectly appropriate, whereas the same treatment in the presence of an allergy is likely an error. It is particularly important that severe reactions, such as anaphylaxis, are clearly coded and identifiable in the medical records. New allergies need to be captured in better ways. For example, if it can be inferred that an allergic reaction may have occurred (e.g., after a new order for diphenhydramine is written), a prompt should be generated for clinicians to enter new allergies. The eventual aim is to have one universal allergy list in an electronic format for each patient, rather than multiple disparate lists.

SAMPLE SIZE ISSUES

Another important methodological issue is the small sample size often present in medication error and ADE studies, primarily due to the high costs of primary data collecting studies. Electronic databases will be an important tool to improve sample sizes in a cost effective manner. Computerized physician order entry systems, electronic health records, test result viewing systems, computerized pharmacy systems, barcoding systems, pharmacy benefit managers, and claims systems will all be important sources of such data. There will be important regulatory issues that will need to be addressed prior to actual construction and use of these systems.

GENERALIZABILITY

A final methodological issue is generalizability. Many existing medication error studies have limited generalizability due to their setting or methodology. For example, many studies have been performed in tertiary care, academic hospital settings. It is unclear how findings from this setting translate to other settings. In addition, methodologies vary widely from study to study, hindering comparisons.

CURRENTLY AVAILABLE SOLUTIONS

A number of data sources can be used to assess the frequency of medication errors. These include claims data, claims data linked with other types of clinical information such as laboratory data, electronic medical record information including that from computerized order entry or pharmacy systems, chart review, and direct observation. Spontaneous reporting can also be used, but underreporting is so great that it is only useful for getting samples of errors, and cannot be used to assess the underlying rate of medication errors in a population (see also Chapters 9 and 10).[2,34]

Claims data have the great advantage that they can be obtained for very large numbers of individuals; in the US this represents tens of millions of people, and in many other countries complete data for a population (such as the elderly in the province of Ontario) may be available. Weaknesses include the issue that it cannot be determined with certainty whether or not the patient actually consumed the medication, and clinical detail is often minimal, making it hard to ask questions that relate to a patient's clinical condition. Searches can be performed for specific diagnoses, but the accuracy of coding is limited for many of the diagnoses of interest, for example renal failure and depression, as well as for outcomes such as renal insufficiency. Nonetheless, many interesting questions can be asked about medication safety using such data. (See Chapters 13–21 for additional discussion of claims data.)

Linking claims and other types of data—in particular, laboratory results data—can substantially expand the range of medication errors that may be detected.[27] For example, it may be possible to assess what proportion of patients exposed to a certain medication has a serum creatinine above a specific level at the time of their initial exposure. Nonetheless, the lack of detailed clinical data can represent a problem.

Chart review can provide valuable additional clinical information, and can be done to supplement claims studies or studies that link claim information with laboratory information. With the chart, it is possible to understand the clinical context, for example the indication for starting a medication, which can sometimes be inferred but rarely determined with certainty with more limited data sources. The main problems with chart review are that it is time consuming and expensive, with the average chart review costing at least $20 for both chart retrieval and review.

Electronic medical records can provide the clinical detail available with paper-based chart review, but often at much lower cost. In addition, it is possible to search electronic medical records for specific diagnoses, laboratories, and key words suggesting the presence of outcomes. Such records are only used in a minority of outpatient offices today, but they have become the standard in many other countries in primary care, for example the United Kingdom.[35] It will be possible to use these records to detect both medication errors and adverse drug events at much lower costs than was

previously possible. (See also Chapter 22 for a discussion of a UK electronic records database.)

THE FUTURE

The future of pharmacoepidemiologic research will include large databases that allow linking of prescription information with clinical and claims data. These types of databases will facilitate the studies of medication errors and adverse drug events. They will also be a critical tool for detecting rare adverse drug events. Sources of data for these databases will include systems of computerized physician order entry, computerized pharmacy, barcoding, and pharmacy benefit managers.

Another important issue that is beginning to be addressed is standardized coding of data. In particular, drug names need to be coded in uniform ways to allow easy analysis, as well as drug doses and concentrations.

As mentioned above, other important issues that need to be addressed are representing prescriptions in ways that allow determination of total daily dose, joint documentation of prescriptions and dispensing data to allow determination of patient adherence, clear documentation of conditions like pregnancy or weights of pediatric patients, and improved coding of allergies.

Once such uniform large clinical databases are available, accurate determination of risks such as drug–drug interactions, drug–allergy exposures, and drug–laboratory interactions will be able to be determined. These events are relatively rare and difficult to ascertain at present, and this represents a major frontier in pharmacoepidemiology.

In the US today, there is much political activity striving to introduce information technology in health care as a means of improving quality and safety. These initiatives, already under way in other countries as well, have garnered bi-partisan support in the US, including recognition by President Bush in his January, 2004 State of the Union address that computerizing health records will reduce costs, improve care, and reduce the risk of medical mistakes. If health records do indeed become computerized nationwide, particularly with standardized terminology, the opportunities for pharmacoepidemiologic research into medication errors will increase immensely.

REFERENCES

1. Cypress BK. *Drug Utilization in Office Visits to Primary Care Physicians: National Ambulatory Medical Care Survey, 1980*. Washington, DC: US Department of Health and Human Services,

Public Health Service, National Center for Health Statistics, 1982; pp. 82–1250.

2. Bates DW, Boyle DL, Vander Vliet MB, Schneider J, Leape LL. Relationship between medication errors and adverse drug events. *J Gen Intern Med* 1995; **10**: 199–205.

3. Institute of Medicine. Kohn LT, Corrigan JM, Donaldson MS, eds, *To Err Is Human. Building a Safer Health System*. Washington, DC: National Academy Press, 1999.

4. Leape LL. Error in medicine. *JAMA* 1994; **272**: 1851–7.

5. Berwick DM. Continuous improvement as an ideal in health care. *N Engl J Med* 1989; **320**: 53–6.

6. Leape LL, Bates DW, Cullen DJ, Cooper J, Demonaco HJ, Gallivan T *et al*. Systems analysis of adverse drug events. *JAMA* 1996; **274**: 35–43.

7. Simborg DW, Derewicz HJ. A highly automated hospital medication system. Five years' experience and evaluation. *Ann Intern Med* 1975; **83**: 342–6.

8. Bates DW, Leape LL, Cullen DJ, Laird N, Petersen LA, Teich JM *et al*. Effect of computerized physician order entry and a team intervention on prevention of serious medication errors. *JAMA* 1998; **280**: 1311–16.

9. Leape LL, Berwick DM, Bates DW. What practices will most improve safety? Evidence-based medicine meets patient safety. *JAMA* 2002; **288**: 501–7.

10. Nadzam DM. Development of medication-use indicators by the Joint Commission on Accreditation of Health Care Organizations. *Am J Health Promot* 1991; **48**: 1925–30.

11. Bates DW, Cullen D, Laird N, Petersen LA, Small S, Servi D *et al*. Incidence of adverse drug events and potential adverse drug events: implications for prevention. *JAMA* 1995; **274**, 29–34.

12. Classen DC, Pestotnik SL, Evans RS, Lloyd JF, Burke JP. Adverse drug events in hospitalized patients. Excess length of stay, extra costs, and attributable mortality. *JAMA* 1997; **277**: 301–6.

13. Kaushal R, Bates DW, Landrigan C, McKenna KJ, Clapp MD, Federico F, Goldmann DA. Medication errors and adverse drug events in pediatric inpatients. *JAMA* 2001; **285**: 2114–20.

14. Gandhi TK, Weingart SN, Borus J, Seger AC, Peterson J, Burdick E *et al*. Adverse drug events in ambulatory care. *N Engl J Med* 2003; **348**: 1556–64.

15. Gurwitz JH, Field TS, Harrold LR, Rothschild J, Debellis K, Seger AC *et al*. Incidence and preventability of adverse drug events among older persons in the ambulatory setting. *JAMA* 2003; **289**: 1107–16.

16. Forster AJ, Murff HJ, Peterson JF, Gandhi TK, Bates DW. The incidence and severity of adverse events affecting patients after discharge from the hospital. *Ann Intern Med* 2003; **138**: 161–7.

17. Hennessy S, Bilker WB, Zhou L, Weber AL, Brensinger C, Wang Y *et al*. Retrospective drug utilization review, prescribing errors, and clinical outcomes. *JAMA* 2003; **290**: 1494–9.

18. Lesar TS, Briceland LL, Delcoure K, Parmalee JC, Masta-Gornic V, Pohl H. Medication prescribing errors in a teaching hospital. *JAMA* 1990; **263**: 2329–34.

19. Folli HL, Poole RL, Benitz WE, Russo JC. Medication error prevention by clinical pharmacists in two children's hospitals. *Pediatrics* 1987; **79**: 718–22.

20. Leape LL, Bates DW, Cullen DJ, Cooper J, Demonaco HJ, Gallivan T *et al*. Systems analysis of adverse drug events. ADE Prevention Study Group. *JAMA* 1995; **274**: 35–43.

21. Barker KN, Flynn EA, Pepper GA. Observation method of detecting medication errors. *Am J Health Syst Pharm* 2002; **59**: 2314–16.

22. Bates DW. Adverse drug reactions. In: Carruthers GS, Hoffman BB, Melmon KL, Nierenberg DW, eds, *Melmon and Morrelli's Clinical Pharmacology: Basic Principles in Therapeutics*, 4th edn. New York: McGraw Hill, 2000; pp. 1223–56.

23. Kuperman GJ, Gandhi TK, Bates DW. Effective drug-allergy checking: methodological and operational issues. *J Biomed Inform* 2003; **36**: 70–9.

24. Apter AJ, Kinman JL, Bilker WB, Herlim M, Margolis DJ, Lautenbach E *et al*. The cross-reactivity of penicillins and cephalosporins: investigation using a large electronic medical record database. Submitted.

25. Peterson JF, Bates DW. Preventable medication errors: identifying and eliminating serious drug interactions. *J Am Pharm Assoc* 2001; **41**: 159–60.

26. Hazlet TK, Lee TA, Hansten PD, Horn JR. Performance of community pharmacy drug interaction software. *J Am Pharm Assoc* 2001; **41**: 200–4.

27. Schiff GD, Klass D, Peterson J, Shah G, Bates DW. Linking laboratory and pharmacy: opportunities for reducing errors and improving care. *Arch Intern Med* 2003; **163**: 893–900.

28. Chertow GM, Lee J, Kuperman GJ, Burdick E, Horsky J, Seger DL *et al*. Guided medication dosing for inpatients with renal insufficiency. *JAMA* 2001; **286**: 2839–44.

29. Rind D, Safran C, Phillips RS, Wang Q, Calkins DR, Delbanco TL *et al*. Effect of computer-based alerts on the treatment and outcomes of hospitalized patients. *Arch Intern Med* 1994; **154**: 1511–17.

30. Falconnier AD, Haefeli WE, Schoenenberger RA, Surber C, Martin-Facklam M. Drug dosage in patients with renal failure optimized by immediate concurrent feedback. *J Gen Intern Med* 2001; **16**: 369–75.

31. Pillans PI, Landsberg PG, Fleming AM, Fanning M, Sturtevant JM. Evaluation of dosage adjustment in patients with renal impairment. *Intern Med J* 2003; **33**: 10–13.

32. Hakonarson H, Gulcher JR, Steffansson K, deCODE Genetics, Inc. *Pharmacogenomics* 2003; **4**: 209–15.

33. Barker KN, Allan EL. Research on drug-use-system errors. *Am J Health Syst Pharm* 1995; **52**: 400–3.

34. Cullen DJ, Bates DW, Small SD, Cooper JB, Nemeskal AR, Leape LL. The incident reporting system does not detect adverse drug events: a problem for quality improvement. *Jt Comm J Qual Improv* 1995; **21**: 541–8.

35. Bates DW, Ebell M, Gotlieb E, Zapp J, Mullins HC. A proposal for electronic medical records in U.S. primary care. *J Am Med Inform Assoc* 2003; **10**: 1–10.

35

Hospital Pharmacoepidemiology

BRIAN L. STROM and RITA SCHINNAR

University of Pennsylvania School of Medicine, Philadelphia, Pennsylvania, USA.

INTRODUCTION

Early studies that were performed in the hospital setting provided much of the initial experience in pharmacoepidemiology. Included in the early 1960s were a series of intensive hospital-based cohort studies performed at Johns Hopkins University, Boston Collaborative Drug Surveillance Program, Shands Hospital in Florida, and the Comprehensive Hospital Drug Monitoring Berne, in Switzerland. These efforts tracked the drugs administered to patients during their entire hospital stay and systematically recorded adverse events possibly linked to these exposures. The task of actually implementing these activities was not easy in a time before magnetic and electronic storage of data and automated processing became available.

These early efforts were followed by the creation of several inpatient databases, some quite comprehensive (e.g., IHS, Medimetrik) and some more selective (e.g., Brigham and Women's Hospital). Creation of these databases was made possible by the availability of computers capable of storing and processing voluminous data collected on large numbers of patients with large numbers of exposures over long periods of time.

Other initiatives followed (SUNY Buffalo Clinical Pharmacist Network, Joint Commission on Accreditation of Healthcare Organizations).

However, it was recognized that much of drug exposure was in the outpatient setting, and interest was growing in studying the effects of drugs in that setting. In time, with the increasing availability of claims databases and more recently medical record databases (see Chapters 13–22), research has shifted to the larger drug-exposed populations in the outpatient setting. This interest has dominated pharmacoepidemiologic research for several decades. However, a need for data on drug use and drug-related events in the hospital persists.

This chapter provides insights into clinical and methodological aspects relevant to pharmacoepidemiologic research in this setting, the evolution of hospital pharmacoepidemiology over the years, its current status, and future trends.

CLINICAL PROBLEMS TO BE ADDRESSED BY PHARMACOEPIDEMIOLOGIC RESEARCH

VOLUME AND CHARACTERISTICS OF HOSPITAL ADMISSIONS

A substantial proportion of the medical care provided in the US or elsewhere is in a hospital. As perspective, in the

Pharmacoepidemiology, Fourth Edition   Edited by B.L. Strom

© 2005 John Wiley & Sons, Ltd

US in 2002, there were 33.7 million hospital discharges (excluding newborn infants), or a hospital discharge rate of 1174.6 per 10 000 population, with an average length of stay of 4.9 days.[1] In that same year, 31% of total national health spending was for hospital care, totaling $486.5 billion[2] and, based on IMS data, 12% of all US drug sales were in hospitals.[3] Based on data from IMS MIDAS, in 2003 hospital drug use totaled $26 billion in the US, and $84.5 billion for the entire world, out of a total worldwide pharmaceutical market of $468 billion (personal communication from Lance Longwell, IMS Health, January 6, 2005).

Hospitalized patients are also, by definition, ill. Heart disease was the most common hospital discharge diagnosis in the US, at a rate of 154.8 per 10 000 population, and much more common in the elderly. Diseases of the respiratory system were present in 13% of all hospital stays for men, and over 9% of all stays for women.[1]

Variations in hospital care outcomes can be ascribed, to some degree, to the characteristics of the hospitals themselves as much as the characteristics of the patients admitted to them. One nationwide study[4] found that older patients who needed high-risk cardiovascular or cancer surgeries were more likely to survive in hospitals that performed a high volume of these complicated surgical procedures as compared to patients admitted to hospitals with little experience with these surgeries. Another study[5] reported fewer deaths among elderly Medicare patients hospitalized for first-time heart attack when staffing levels of registered nurses (RNs) were higher as opposed to substituting licensed practical nurses (LPNs) for RNs. Yet another study[6] found that elderly patients treated for heart attack at teaching hospitals were more likely to survive and receive better quality care than those treated at hospitals that do not train physicians.

CHARACTERISTICS OF HOSPITALIZED PATIENTS AND HOSPITAL DRUG USE

Hospitalized patients receive multiple drugs during their hospital stay, which is mostly warranted because these patients are older, sicker, and have multiple concurrent diseases.

The elderly population (aged 65 years old and older) in the US had grown to 35.3 million persons by 2001, 4.4 million of whom were aged 85 years or older.[7] Almost 40% (12.7 million) of all discharges from short-stay hospitals in 2002 involved patients aged 65 years and older.[1] Further, they are more likely to suffer complications from their care. As documented by one study,[8] major perioperative complications occurred in 4.3% of patients aged 59 years or younger, 5.7% of patients aged 60–69 years, 9.6% of patients aged 70–79 years, and 12.5% of patients aged 80 or older. Also,

in-hospital mortality was 2.6% in patients 80 years of age or older as compared to 0.7% in younger patients.[8] About 35% of women in the hospital and 31% of men have hypertension as a coexisting condition.[9]

The practice of polypharmacy, however, introduces the risks of unintended drug–drug interactions (e.g., using trimethoprim-sulfamethoxasole in patients receiving warfarin), prescribing suboptimal drug regimens (e.g., insufficiently aggressive dosing of heparin in patients presenting with pulmonary emboli), and inadequate laboratory monitoring of drug therapy (e.g., lack of monitoring of aminoglycoside levels). It is well documented that patients receiving multiple drugs during their hospital stay have higher rates of drug reactions.[10–15]

Another aspect of relevance to pharmacoepidemiologic research is the observation that most drug reactions tend to occur in the first five days on a drug;[16] therefore, active surveillance of drug use during this period is likely to detect most adverse reactions.[17]

These considerations illustrate that patient and hospital characteristics and practices need to be incorporated in study designs, analyses, and interpretations of data collected from hospital settings.

METHODOLOGIC PROBLEMS TO BE ADDRESSED BY PHARMACOEPIDEMIOLOGIC RESEARCH

There are multiple logistic and methodological issues that emerge from the attempt to perform studies specifically in the hospital setting.

LOGISTICAL ISSUES

Developing *complete information* on total drug exposure during a hospital stay is a major challenge for pharmacoepidemiologic research in the hospital setting. Hospitals are remarkably complex organizations, and drug use throughout a hospital is equally complex. In the hospital setting, patients are administered drugs at multiple sites, such as emergency rooms, operating rooms, radiology, and patient room beds. Drugs are also administered by multiple types of personnel, e.g., nurses, physicians, radiology technicians, etc. In addition, these administrations can be recorded in multiple different medical records forms, such as progress notes, pharmacy records, and nursing medication administration records. The task of measuring hospital drug exposure fully and accurately can therefore be daunting. Yet, without complete information about inpatient drug exposure, inferences about adverse drug reactions associated with particular exposures are impossible to make credibly.

Presumably, as hospitals increasingly implement comprehensive, linked, automated inpatient data systems, the capture of complete inpatient drug exposure will be addressed. Yet, even in hospitals that made the investment to adopt, for example, a Computerized Prescriber Order Entry (CPOE) system, many gaps remain in the completeness of information that could be useful and necessary for research purposes. CPOE data can be incomplete due to omitted high-risk populations, such as neonates or patients receiving chemotherapy; inability to handle selected complex clinical situations, e.g., patient-controlled analgesia and operating room medications; and CPOE systems that are not fully integrated with other medication system components, e.g., barcode point-of-care systems.[18] In addition, many CPOE systems are standalone products, without an interface with other institution-wide systems.[18]

METHODOLOGICAL ISSUES

In addition to the problem of measuring total exposure, there is the issue of uncertain *validity of the drug information* in the hospital medical record. Drugs dispensed from a pharmacy are not always administered to patients, actual drug administrations are not always recorded, and drugs ordered for a particular patient might be dispensed to a different patient.[19] Such errors of omission or commission need to be explored and assessed before relying on the hospital medical record as a sole source of information to answer questions about drug-associated risks.

The *validity of diagnosis information* in the hospital medical record may also be uncertain. Studies have found that diagnosed conditions, even those that were treated, were not always listed, and that procedures not performed in the operating room were often omitted from the chart.[20] (A fuller discussion of the methodologic problem of the validity of medical record information is presented in Chapter 45.) Of course, with electronic data entry medical records and with increasing linking of the pharmacy and clinical databases, this problem of incomplete or erroneous hospital data may diminish, though it is unlikely to be completely eliminated.

Another concern is the absence of *inpatient information that is linked to outpatient information*. An adverse event occurring in a hospital within a few days after admission may in fact be a reaction to a drug used prior to admission. Similarly, an adverse event occurring after discharge may in fact be due to a drug exposure during the hospital stay (e.g.,

post-gastrectomy anemia, hypothyroidism after radioiodine therapy).[17] Yet, these associations may be missed with inpatient data unless there is linkage to prior and follow-up data.

Another methodological problem is the *uniqueness of drug exposure* in the hospital setting. Hospitals generally use a restricted set of drugs as specified by their formularies. This limits the types of drugs that can be studied for adverse reactions. Another limitation for research is that hospitals use some drugs, dosages (often higher), and forms of administration (e.g., parenteral), which differ from those used in outpatient care. Also, drug usage in the hospital tends to be short-term in contrast to long-term drug use by outpatients. In addition, some hospitals choose some drugs, while others choose other drugs. The uniqueness of these patterns of inpatient drug use may have implications for the generalizability of findings from studies in particular hospitals. Also, because of small populations or the infrequent use of some drugs, it may not be possible to detect the rare adverse reactions to the majority of drugs.[21]

Another methodological problem is that hospitalized populations, as noted above, tend to be *more severely ill* than patients not requiring hospital admission. Because hospitalized patients are sicker than other people taking prescribed drugs, they are more likely to receive multiple drugs, and, consequently, more likely to experience an adverse drug event.[10] However, sicker patients tend to have more underlying medical problems, a fact that makes it more difficult for a physician to discern an adverse reaction to a drug from an event due to another cause.[22] Also, patients may react differently to the same drug, depending on various comorbidities, demographic profiles, and personal histories,[22] thereby further confounding a possible association between exposure and event.

In addition, because hospitalized patients tend to experience many events during the course of their stay, there may be a *tendency to record only the most extreme or dramatic events*. Therefore, certain mild adverse drug events (ADEs) may not be completely recorded, and would not be available for studies of drug effects.

When using hospital patients for a pharmacoepidemiology study one must be mindful also of the potential for *referral bias*. If an exposure is related to likelihood of hospitalization, then outcomes of hospitalization may falsely appear related to that exposure. Further, different hospitals get referrals of patients with different conditions, and each hospital uses different drugs. These can create or mask findings. Indeed, the problem inherent in using hospitalized controls for case–control studies (see Chapters 2 and 11) is related to this; patients need to be ill to be hospitalized, ill people are more likely to use drugs, so prior drug exposures tend to be higher in hospitalized patients than in the general population.

Relatedly, variations in hospital practices, such as ordering diagnostic or laboratory tests for patients on drugs, the effects of which are monitored, may produce an *ascertainment bias* and, with that, abnormally high or low rates of apparent ADEs.[23]

The definition of an *appropriate denominator for calculations of adverse drug reactions* depends on the question of interest.[24] The total quantity of drug received is the more useful denominator if one is interested in the incidence rate of adverse reaction for a specific drug. The total patient population is the appropriate denominator if one is interested in the overall rate of adverse drug reactions in a hospital.[24] The total number of patients exposed to a drug may be the most appropriate denominator, but is not always available.

A different methodologic problem emerges from problems in *hospital staff participation*. Hospitals are complex organizations with large numbers of organizational units and large numbers of personnel who function under stressful conditions in response to complex medical problems. Such convoluted activities involve complicated interactions among experts and technical support staff, such that in this milieu of busy people who concentrate on delivery of care, it is difficult to count on their cooperation for research activities. Approaching these already busy professionals with requests to identify and refer potentially eligible patients to the research team is an imposition that they tend to resist. It requires much effort on the part of the researcher to influence hospital physicians to agree to be participants in an epidemiologic study and to permit contacting their patients. It also requires lengthy negotiation and creative arrangements to get access to hospital admission logs, surgical logs, or patients' medical records. Concerns about privacy, of course, complicate the whole endeavor.

Finally, hospitals are huge bureaucracies obviously not created for research purposes. They collect vast amounts of information that can serve as rich resources for research but the information is collected for clinical care and administrative purposes rather than for research purposes. The implication of this is that *medical records are not organized for research*, i.e., in a fashion that makes it simple for an investigator to review and abstract the medical record for a particular research study. The medical record may not even contain certain information useful for an epidemiologic study (e.g., diet, exercise, occupational history). Missing information on important potential confounders may limit inferences about drug effects.

On the positive side, the study of inpatient drug effects is enhanced by the fact that there is a large amount of information recorded due to continuous monitoring and measurement of patients' conditions. Furthermore, there is less likely to be a problem of patient compliance with drug intake; therefore, the connection with a subsequent adverse reaction is more credible.

CURRENTLY AVAILABLE SOLUTIONS

INTENSIVE HOSPITAL-BASED SURVEILLANCE

Diseases of Medical Progress: A Survey of Diseases and Syndromes Unintentionally Induced as a Result of Properly Indicated, Widely-Accepted Therapeutic Procedures was the title of a 1959 book on risks associated with modern therapies,[25] and it was followed by a flurry of journal publications starting in the mid-1960s showing increasing interest and early initiatives in systematic monitoring of adverse reactions to drug therapy, mostly in hospital settings.

In Scotland, Finney[26] proposed in 1965 a framework for monitoring drug use and drug reactions that consisted of routine recording of demographic and clinical information on hospitalized patients, including all drugs administered throughout their hospital stay. Then, by comparing the rates of events occurring in these patients and performing cohort studies, one could detect adverse reactions, whether or not physicians suspected any associations between drugs and events.

Concurrently, an intensive inpatient drug monitoring program was developed at the Johns Hopkins University.[27] The cohort under surveillance was large—as it had to include a large at-risk population to be able to detect infrequent adverse reactions[21]—as was the amount of information that was systematically collected and recorded on patients in the cohort. The information collected in this early study was converted to a format suitable for electronic data entry and analysis by computer.[10,27–29] In fact, collecting drug usage data was started at Johns Hopkins by recording into the computer all drugs received by every hospitalized patient, initially for billing purposes and later for conducting epidemiologic studies. As noted by Seidl and colleagues,[27,28] the role of automatic data processing methods was vital because of the large number of drug charge bills processed each month. These drug charge bills provided the denominators of drug exposure. To get the numerator data of adverse drug reactions, they used multiple methods, including a report-of-drug-reaction-card attached to each patient's record on admission and completed at discharge; intensive surveillance of drug usage focused on either patients receiving a given drug, patients with a particular disease, or patients in a specific hospital area; retrospective chart review; and prospective studies of all patients receiving a particular drug or all patients on a particular service.[28]

One of this group's series of publications on studies on the epidemiology of adverse drug reactions[10] illustrates the amount of information collected on one hospital-based cohort in one of these early studies. For all patients admitted to a medical ward over a one-year period, the monitors recorded the name, age, race, sex, diagnosis, duration of hospital stay, condition at discharge, all drugs administered during the hospital stay, renal and liver function, presence or absence of infection, history of previous drug reactions, history of atopy, and information on suspected drug reactions, including a description of the reaction, organ system involved, probable mechanism, severity, drugs received prior to the reaction, hospital day on which the reaction occurred, and duration of therapy with the suspected drug before identification of the adverse reaction. In addition to collecting information from the hospital records, the method of ward surveillance involved daily visits by the research staff to the wards to question the head nurse and each house officer about adverse drug reactions occurring during the preceding 24 hours.[10]

In 1967, Hoddinott et al.[30] in Canada also reported on a drug monitoring study in a medical ward, but with several features that were different from those used by the Johns Hopkins group. The features used in the Hoddinott et al. study included: (i) developing specially tailored procedures for collecting all doctors' orders in the 31-bed ward and then carefully recording into a central logbook the information on drugs administered (specifically, the patient's name, drug name, dosage, and times of administration); (ii) requiring the nursing staff at the beginning of each shift to communicate to each other all information involving the use of medicines by patients during the previous shift; (iii) daily visits by the research staff to the ward to interview not only nurses and doctors but also the patients about possible adverse drug reactions; (iv) reviewing the nursing charts and comparing the doctors' orders with the nurses' records of the drugs given, to detect errors of omission or commission; (v) investigating immediately any suspected reactions and grading them as probable or possible; and (vi) analyzing the data on adverse drug reaction with regards to aspects such as the total number of drugs used by the patient on the day of reaction and preceding days, total number of new drugs used, and day when the reaction occurred. The concerns expressed by these and other authors pertained to what is an appropriate classification of drug adverse reactions, and the difficulty of ascertaining which drug caused a particular reaction.[30,31]

Another Canadian study of adverse reactions during hospitalization from the same period[31] was designed also to test the yield of different methods of reporting adverse reactions, and therefore included reports by nurses, interns, and residents. Interns and residents were instructed to report all adverse reactions by writing the patient's name, suspected drug or procedure, and type of reaction on a printed form placed on the patient's chart used for their daily bedside rounds. The nurses on each shift were instructed to list on specially provided forms the names of patients whose drug therapy was canceled or substituted, dose was reduced, or route of administration was changed. Nurses were also asked to record all diagnostic and therapeutic procedures administered to patients and any corresponding adverse effects.

In Ireland, Hurwitz and Wade[32] described an intensive monitoring study extending to seven wards in one hospital and another ward in a different hospital, compiling a large amount of information on the series of 1268 patients under surveillance. In addition to recording the name, sex, age, hospital number, ward, date of admission, and diagnosis, investigators interviewed patients regarding recent drug therapy, and any previous reactions to drugs, allergy, hay fever, or asthma. Ward notes about patients and their previous hospital records were examined. Information abstracted from each patient's daily prescription sheets included drugs administered, time and route of administration, dosage, and any changes in dosage or treatment. Also, the medical and nursing staffs were interviewed daily about suspected adverse reactions to drugs and reasons for any alterations in drug treatment or unusual disease courses. The authors noted the possibility that the direct questioning by the adverse reactions officer may have affected the reporting of subjective symptoms by introducing the notion of adverse drug reactions to patients.[32] On the positive side, however, they noted that in prior surveys of adverse reactions there had been no controlled observations of symptoms and signs of patients before administration of drugs.[32–34]

In an article on rational prescribing and drug usage, Philp[17] noted that physicians find it difficult to report adverse drug reactions, and argued that pharmacists should get involved in the wards. Several studies used clinical pharmacists as data collection monitors.[35,36] In particular, through monitoring drug order changes, the pharmacists would review with the physicians whether the reasons for changes in drug therapy were linked to possible adverse reactions. The pharmacist's role in surveying drug prescribing and usage was made more prominent by the requirement that hospitals needed to operate a drug utilization review plan as part of Medicare Conditions of Participation for hospitals (see below, and Chapter 29). In response to this requirement, the Shands Teaching Hospital in Gainesville, Florida, for example, undertook an extensive computerized review of drug utilization, using a pharmacist to collect numerator data and using an epidemiologist to collect denominator data, to estimate rates of adverse reactions to drugs.[37] As part of this program, the pharmacist generated a daily listing of all drugs discontinued or decreased in dosage in the previous 24-hour period, serving as an indicator of possible adverse reactions to drugs. Other uses of the drug monitoring program at the University of Florida included a bi-monthly report indicating the percentage of patients in the medical ward receiving a particular drug, thus identifying the usage of high-cost drugs. Another report detailed all adverse reactions on the medical ward during the prior reporting period, serving as a reminder to medical staff of the importance of rational drug prescribing. The program also made available the necessary data to select a particular diagnosis for analysis of the entire drug therapy during the patient stay, allowing for the assessment of rational prescribing and therapy cost for a particular disease.[37]

Ultimately, the most comprehensive intensive in-hospital drug surveillance program—started in 1966 and accumulating information on over 50 000 medical inpatients over a period of almost 20 years—was the Boston Collaborative Drug Surveillance Program (BCDSP). After initially monitoring the medical patients of a single Boston hospital, it was expanded to include multiple hospitals in several states in the US and abroad. Collection of new data from medical wards was discontinued in 1977, and collection of data from surgical wards (on about 5200 patients) was discontinued in 1984, but this old database remains available and has generated a considerable number of research papers about older drugs.[38–64] A similar intensive drug surveillance program was later launched by these investigators in pediatric wards at several teaching and community hospitals in several US states, accumulating data on 10 297 pediatric patients.[64]

Its early approach was similar to that at Johns Hopkins, that is continuously tracking and monitoring drug usage and adverse events of hospital patients. Later they added an inquiry about drug exposure in the three months before admission. Collaborative arrangements with multiple hospitals involved hiring local nurses at each site and training them to follow standardized procedures for collecting information from consecutive admissions to the hospital. In particular, detailed information was collected shortly after admission by structured patient interviews. Then, detailed information about drugs administered during hospitalization was obtained through chart reviews. In addition, the nurse monitors attended ward rounds and communicated with attending physicians to obtain their judgments about suspected adverse drug-related events. Further, in order not to miss associations that might

become the subject of later testing, a few selected major events (such as sudden death, jaundice, renal failure, gastrointestinal bleeding, and psychosis) were targeted for recording, regardless of whether they were thought to be drug related. All data collected were submitted to the Boston central research office to be subjected to tests for accuracy and completeness and to be processed and analyzed.

Because patient interviews focused on drugs used prior to hospitalization in relation to the causes of admission to the hospital, this database made it possible to examine and control for drug usage preceding hospitalization. Also, because medical record data in BCDSP were augmented with data from patient interviews that asked about alcohol and tobacco use, this database made it possible to control for these important confounders of drug effects. Another advantage of BCDSP was its large size, permitting the study of rare adverse medical events. Also, with multiple countries contributing data, study results could be evaluated for consistency cross-nationally. However, the major component of BCDSP data (for medical inpatients) is now almost 30 years old, and cannot support studies of the many important new drugs that have become available since the mid-1970s. Nonetheless, the BCDSP has supported a wide range of important studies since its inception.

Another initiative concurrent with the BCDSP was initiated in 1974 in Berne, Switzerland and is known as the Comprehensive Hospital Drug Monitoring Berne (CHDMB). Created by routine monitoring of all patients hospitalized in several medical wards in Berne, this has also served as a resource for published findings about drug-induced adverse reactions.[65] Other hospital monitoring efforts were reported in New Zealand[66] and Germany. A similarly intensive use of nurse monitors as described by Jick et al.[59] was described by other investigators.[24,67,68]

INPATIENT DATABASES

Multisite Databases

The Medimetrik and IHS databases were examples of early multisite hospital databases started as commercial enterprises. The Medimetrik database, for example, discontinued by 1988, could support research on rare drug events[69] because of its large size, as data were contributed from administrative, pharmacy, and discharge sites at 50 hospitals. However, it was not commercially viable, given the large costs of gathering such data.

Several noncommercial, large data collection systems in hospitals are described below.

The Health Evaluation through Logical Processing System (HELP)

The Health Evaluation through Logical Processing (HELP) database was developed at the LDS Hospital, a private community hospital, in Salt Lake City, Utah, and has been successfully operational since 1967. Intermountain Health Care (IHC), a large health care system that operates LDS Hospital, has installed HELP in a number of its other large hospitals, thereby permitting broader multi-hospital linkage. More recently, HELP was enhanced by the addition of pediatric data from the Primary Children's Medical Center.[70]

HELP is a computerized hospital information system that logs data for all inpatients from all hospital services (e.g., laboratory, pharmacy, radiology, pathology, operating rooms, intensive care units) and clinical information from the different reports found in medical records. All patient admissions, discharges, and transfers are processed electronically, as are bedside data entries by physicians, pharmacists, nurses, and therapists. HELP facilitates patient care as well as administrative and research functions by integrating this expansive inpatient information. Information relevant to the drugs administered to specific patients is linked by HELP with other therapies and procedures, and all other events developing in these patients. The database also incorporates algorithms that can identify adverse drug reactions by searching for signals that an adverse event has occurred and forwarding this information to a clinical pharmacist for investigation, thus serving a vital inpatient surveillance role. HELP is updated continually[71]. Therefore, these features of HELP make it a useful resource for pharmacoepidemiology studies.

Interestingly, despite its many useful features for supporting clinical and billing functions in the hospital, not all the member hospitals of IHC have accepted the sophisticated HELP system as it is in use at LDS Hospital. Among the barriers for more widespread use of the HELP system are the exorbitant initial investments in hardware and personnel training, the protracted period required for completing and implementing an integrated database, and the novelty of the belief that it is important to have an integrated and continuous medical record linking inpatient and outpatient data.[71]

As with earlier pharmacoepidemiology studies based on HELP data, recent studies have continued to focus on infectious diseases and antibiotic use. For example, one paper described a computer-assisted daily monitor of antibiotic use in hospitalized patients at the LDS Hospital for the purpose of identifying patients receiving excessive dosages of antibiotics.[72] This monitoring proved useful as it helped bring about a significant decrease in the number of patients administered excessive dosages of the study antibiotics, along with a

concomitant reduction in ADE incidence attributable to antibiotic use.[72] Another study[73] used HELP to assess the effectiveness of computer-assisted decision support programs for antimicrobial prescribing in intensive care units, demonstrating that this intervention promotes more selective prescribing patterns and overall reduction of antibiotic use. A similar recent example of the use of computerized inpatient medical data with HELP involved a study of a pediatric anti-infective monitor,[70] which helped reduce the rate of pharmacist intervention for erroneous drug orders.

Brigham and Women's Hospital

Brigham and Women's Hospital (BWH), a 720-bed medical center in Boston, has developed a computerized data collection and reporting capability called the Brigham Integrated Computing System (BICS) into which all orders for medications, laboratory tests, and other therapeutic interventions for all adult inpatients are entered. This database contains complete patient demographic information, discharge diagnoses, procedures, laboratory results, and pharmacy data from 1987, with less complete information available beginning in 1981.

As described by Teich et al., BICS provides Brigham and Women's Hospital with almost all of its clinical, administrative, and financial computing services. In particular, the BICS clinical information system includes a wide array of services such as test results review, longitudinal medical records, provider order entry, critical pathway management, critical-event detection and altering, automated inpatient summaries, operating-room scheduling, coverage lists, and an online reference library.[74]

Examples of the ways in which BICS is used to contribute to improved inpatient care and cost savings include a computerized physician order entry designed to display drug use guidelines, offer relevant alternatives, and suggest appropriate doses and frequencies whenever physicians enter drug orders for their patients;[75] a computer intervention designed to notify physicians when inpatients remain on expensive intravenous medications after they become able to take bioequivalent oral alternatives;[76] another computer intervention designed to provide physicians with electronic notification that certain clinical laboratory tests may be redundant;[77] a computer application to protect against errors in chemotherapy ordering and dosing and to coordinate the outpatient and inpatient chemotherapy services;[78] and a computer-based ADE monitor.[79]

The study by Teich et al.[75] showed that computerized guidelines prompted physicians to increase the use of recommended drugs and decrease the proportion of doses exceeding the recommended maximum. The study by Bates *et al.*[77] found that computerized alerts about potentially redundant clinical laboratory tests were effective, but limited because many tests were performed without the corresponding computer reminders, and many orders were not screened for redundancy. The study by Jha *et al.*[79] showed that using a computer-based ADE monitor resulted in identification of fewer ADEs than did chart review, leading them to conclude that different detection methods capture different events because of minimal overlap among the ADEs identified by the different methods. See Chapters 16 and 34 for examples of the use of BICS in pharmacoepidemiology.

Beth Israel Hospital

Also in Boston, the Beth Israel Hospital (BIH) developed an integrated clinical database with inpatient information (dating back to 1984) and outpatient information (dating back to 1977). The inpatient database includes demographic data, laboratory results, diagnostic tests, procedure codes, medications and blood products, admitting and discharge diagnosis codes, and hospital charges. The database can identify all patients with selected characteristics for purposes such as monitoring patient care, surveillance for ADEs, and other analyses of interest, including epidemiologic studies of stroke[80] and HIV.[81]

The Regenstrief Automated Medical Record System

The Regenstrief Medical Record System (RMRS) links 5 large hospitals and 44 outpatient clinics (most of which are associated with Indiana University), 13 homeless care sites, and the county and state health departments, all of which are located in and around Indianapolis. RMRS was developed over 20 years ago, and has been continuously updated and expanded. It was designed to store data on patient demographics, outpatient and inpatient diagnoses, laboratory test results, radiographic reports, prescriptions, and procedures, as well as information from physicians' notes, and emergency department data.[82,83] Because physicians enter their notes and prescription orders electronically, the likelihood of creating errors in transcribing physician handwriting from the medical record into the computer is reduced. The data system also creates global patient files that automatically link data from different patient care sites, allowing physicians to access patient data from one point of contact. Reports, such as encounter forms for outpatient clinic patient visits, information sheets for housestaff, discharge summaries, and chart abstracts, are generated by the RMRS. However, as described in Chapter 23, it suffers from incomplete ascertainment of outcomes, i.e., patients who go to other facilities in Indianapolis for some of their care will not have the associated care recorded. This means that key exposures or outcomes could be missed, as well as important confounders.

One recent epidemiologic study[84] identified in the database a cohort of 14 876 infants who were prescribed systemic erythromycin, or ophthalmic erythromycin ointment, or whose mothers were prescribed during pregnancy a macrolide antibiotic, to evaluate their risk for infantile hypertrophic pyloric stenosis. All the clinical data and information on inpatient and outpatient prescriptions for these medications were obtained from the database. Another study,[85] making use of the entire online information available for over 6000 patients admitted to a general medicine service over an 18-month period, evaluated whether computerized preventive care reminders to physicians influenced the rates at which several preventive therapies were ordered for these inpatients. Another study[86] evaluated if predictors for *Pneumocystis carinii* could be correctly determined from the available electronic data in the Regenstrief hospital records (along with other data not found in the Regenstrief database, such as vital signs and presenting symptoms obtained from emergency department records). The objective was to use available electronic data, rather than invasive diagnostic procedures, to identify patients with pneumocystis pneumonia. In another study, Clark *et al.*[87] interviewed patients admitted to a general medicine inpatient service about their health status at the time of admission, with the goal of using this information to predict length of stay. The Regenstrief Medical Record System was used to capture patient demographic and identification data to be entered electronically into the interview record and later to link also to clinical data. Other published studies involve informatics interventions[88] and the cost of inpatient care.[89]

US Department of Veterans Affairs

To buttress the VA health care system at the local and national levels, in 1995, the Department of Veterans Affairs (DVA) implemented a Decentralized Hospital Computer Program (DHCP). The comprehensive DHCP system covers medical management, as well as financial and clinical functions. In this system, all patient care events that occur in each of the local VA medical centers are registered in national databases within 1 to 7 days of their occurrence.[90]

The modular structure of DHCP is designed to gather data on admissions, discharges, transfers, clinic scheduling, and the whole gamut of information pertaining to patient care. Information from pharmacy, laboratory, radiology, surgery, dietetic, nursing, and administrative services is collected in some modules, while others capture data from progress notes, consults, mental health and psychological testing, dentistry, immunology case registries, oncology, social work, allergies and adverse reactions, and notifications and alerts. The system also includes order entry, results reporting, clinical measurements, medical images, X-rays, pathology slides, video views, electrocardiograms, and lesion images.[90] Data validation committees continuously scrutinize these data for quality and validity review. Information on services received from non-VA providers is also culled and incorporated into the Patient Treatment File. Inpatient and outpatient data are available at the patient- and physician-history levels, as well as aggregated by facility or systemwide.[90]

Application of the DHCP has been extended to the development of the VA Automated Tumor Registry for Oncology and the VA HIV Registry. The utility of these databases for epidemiologic research would appear to be formidable given the large, defined population base (i.e., veterans), but as yet has not been realized. In a 1996 paper, Graber *et al.*[91] noted that this database was difficult to use for epidemiologic analyses because it could be queried to retrieve data only about individual patients but not about a group of patients. In an attempt to address this problem, these authors performed a pilot project using a subset of the DHCP data to develop computer applications that can query information about groups of patients and their patterns of drug use.[91] Specifically, these applications were intended to screen for potential drug interactions and redundant drug therapies, identify polypharmacy, evaluate the use of potentially dangerous drug regimens, and verify appropriate monitoring of drug levels or laboratory tests.[91] These applications, however, were tested on a sample of all outpatient prescriptions during a limited time period and, as noted by the authors, implementation on the entire database would require considerable constant effort.[91]

Advantages and Limitations

There is merit and utility in the efforts of hospitals to establish comprehensive integrated automated data systems for enhancing the quality of patient care, reducing medical errors and adverse reactions to treatment, and supporting research. From the perspective of pharmacoepidemiologic research, however, it is unfortunate that these inpatient data systems are free-standing instead of integrated across institutions. The size and composition of patient populations in individual hospitals is likely to limit the ability to detect events of low incidence and produce generalizable results.

NEW HOSPITAL-BASED ADVERSE DRUG REACTION MONITORING AND DRUG USE EVALUATION PROGRAMS

A series of initiatives by the US Joint Commission on Accreditation of Healthcare Organizations (JCAHO)—the private nonprofit organization which must provide a hospital accreditation in order for it to qualify for payment by Medicare without separate inspections from the Federal government—have contributed significantly to the further development of hospital pharmacoepidemiology. These JCAHO initiatives began in 1986 with the "Agenda for Change," which placed emphasis on the quality of hospital performance.[92] This outlined the components of hospital drug use and associated requirements, specifically the development of adverse drug monitoring and reporting programs and drug usage evaluation programs. This was followed in 1989 by the "National Forum on Clinical Indicator Development," which encouraged the creation of expert panels and data-driven monitoring systems and outcome assessment.[93] In 1990, JCAHO established the "Medication Use Task Force,"[94] which developed specific, quantifiable indicators of good drug use with the intent that data on these indicators would be provided by all hospitals, and then a hospital would be provided data on where it stood versus other hospitals. These indicators were never implemented. The broad goals of these and related programs[95,96] were to improve the quality of patient care by improving the clinical use of medications and minimizing adverse drug reactions, to decrease hospital costs by eliminating inappropriate use of drugs or by offering acceptable low cost substitutions, and to decrease liability associated with the inappropriate use of high risk drugs.

As an example of a response by hospitals to the JCAHO initiatives, the Hospital of the University of Pennsylvania established the Drug Use and Effects Committee (DUEC), as a subcommittee of the Pharmacy and Therapeutics Committee, to provide guidance and oversight over these programs.[97]

To fulfill its mission, the *Adverse Drug Event (ADEs) Surveillance Program* in our hospital developed operational definitions of ADEs, publicized the program to nurses and physicians, arranged a mechanism for communicating spontaneous reports of ADEs, screened computerized discharge diagnoses for ADEs, targeted drugs, patients, and sites for intensive follow-up, triaged reports for in-depth investigation and reporting to the FDA, tabulated and analyzed the accumulated data on ADEs, reviewed these results on a continuous regular basis, and set up plans for any necessary follow-up. All of these activities have been routinized and are continuously ongoing. In addition, regular reports identify the top medications involved in ADEs, the severity of the reaction (mild or serious), whether they occur in the inpatient or outpatient setting, whether the event was dose-related, idiosyncratic, attributed to a new drug (defined as available on the market for three years) or multiple medications, and the source that reported the ADEs (e.g., admissions list, pharmacists, physicians, pharmacy students, tracer drugs, lab signals). Most of the tracer drugs are antidotes, and lab signals include all critical lab results reported in the hospital. The primary focus is on documenting severe, preventable, and rare ADEs, with secondary emphasis placed on documenting non-serious ADEs that are not dose-related.

As part of monitoring the program on adverse drug reactions, the DUEC also reviews monthly reports of *pharmacist interventions*. These can involve *preventive measures* (such as blocking an order for a prescription if the dose or regimen is considered inappropriate or because of potential drug–drug interactions) as well as *cost avoidance measures* (such as identifying unnecessary drug use when a physician orders two drugs when in fact one drug may be enough to achieve a therapeutic goal, suggesting that the regimen could be decreased, or suggesting a lower cost substitute drug). Along with these reviews, the DUEC's *Drug Usage Evaluation (DUE) Program* developed criteria for appropriate drug use, used the pharmacy computer to identify exposed patients, developed data entry forms for chart abstracting, performed medical chart reviews, organized and analyzed the collected data, reported the results to a review committee, and designed and implemented interventions to address any problems identified. Again, all these activities are now routinized and ongoing.

A DUE is defined as an authorized, structured, ongoing review of physician prescribing, pharmacist dispensing, and patient use of medication in the hospital. It involves a comprehensive review of patients' prescription and medication data before, during, and after dispensing, to ensure appropriate medication decision making and positive patient outcomes. Accordingly, the DUEC has targeted selected drugs for initial evaluation with the goal to document problems, identify the reasons for these problems, and make recommendations and/or design and implement some interventions to address the problems on an ongoing basis.

DUEC's *Cost Containment Program* was developed to identify potential problem areas based on ADEs, DUEs, and/or drugs generating the most expense, and to intercede to reduce costs, either through educational campaigns, formulary modifications, or other interventions.

The DUEC also monitors the monthly compilations of the lists of drug and vaccine shortages in the hospital pharmacy, caused either by national production shortages or recall by the manufacturer. As shortages are identified, the DUEC is notified of product changes to the hospital formulary, and of any dose strength differences between the products with limited supply and the substituted products. Appropriate clinical departments are, in turn, informed of these shortages and changes.

These combined activities constitute a criteria-based, ongoing, planned, systematic process to continuously improve the appropriate and effective use of drugs as well as the quality of care, while reducing both drug and non-drug expenditures.

In the years since its establishment in our hospital, the contributions of the DUEC to patient safety can be discerned from reviewing a few examples of its activities and outcomes. Table 35.1 and Figures 35.1 and 35.2 present some data from the DUEC ADE program. Included in the reports have been a number of previously unrecognized ADEs, which have led to changes in drug labels or manufacturing. As another example, the DUEC requested a DUE on allergy to determine compliance with the hospital's policies concerning the documentation of patient height, weight, and allergy information and the consistency of this information between sources. The findings from this DUE analysis triggered several recommendations by the DUEC, including: (i) developing a policy concerning which health care professional should be responsible for collecting and disseminating height, weight, and allergy information; (ii) incorporating height, weight, and allergy information into pharmacist medication histories; (iii) instituting data entry prompts for missing height, weight, and allergy information into both the computerized physician order entry system and the pharmacy computer system; (iv) educating health care professionals on the importance of recording reaction information on allergies; and (v) making patient allergy

Table 35.1. Medications involved in ADEs, Drug Use and Effects Committee, Hospital of the University of Pennsylvania, FY 2004

Medication	Total (%)
Warfarin	26.4
Heparin	17.4
Insulin	14.9
Acetaminophen	8.0
Amiodarone	7.0
Cefepime	5.5
Multiple Medications	5.5
Phenytoin	5.5
Vancomycin	4.5
Amphotericin B	3.0
Alemtuzumab	2.5

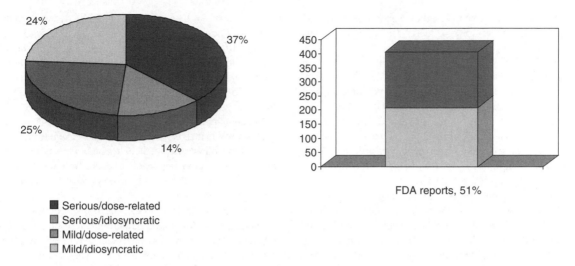

- ■ Serious/dose-related
- ■ Serious/idiosyncratic
- ■ Mild/dose-related
- □ Mild/idiosyncratic

Figure 35.1. Adverse drug events, 2003—Hospital of the University of Pennsylvania.

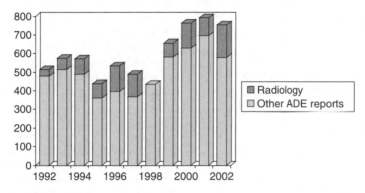

Figure 35.2. Adverse drug events, 1992–2002—Hospital of the University of Pennsylvania.

information a mandatory field prior to adding medication orders. Specific actions that were undertaken involved: (i) organizing a meeting with Admissions to discuss the policy and expectations of capturing the patient height, weight, and allergy history; (ii) investigating solutions with Information Systems regarding the capability of the Clinical Manager computer system to capture height, weight, and allergy information; and (iii) following up with Information Systems regarding pharmacist access to the computerized physician order entry system to add or change allergy information.

As another example, a request for DUE on heparin use was specifically designed to examine justification for use and appropriate use of bolus dosing and infusion dosing. Accordingly, this probe focused on whether there were a large

number of ADEs related to usage of the hospital guidelines, whether the hospital guidelines were being followed, and whether ADEs were possibly related to ordering within the computerized physician order entry system. This DUE also focused on monitoring to reveal the proportion of patients who, at 24 hours, had a therapeutic aPTT, a subtherapeutic aPTT, or a supratherapeutic aPTT, and whether there appeared to be a correlation between aPTT and incidence of bleeding. The findings from this DUE led to several recommendations, including: (i) educating the staff, (ii) adding American Health Association/American College of Cardiology recommendations for heparin dosing to our hospital's guidelines, (iii) entering patient weights into the computerized physician order entry system, (iv) decreasing the time patients are on heparin when possible, and (v) aiding appropriate prescribing through alerts and reminders, alerts for bed rest patients, alerts for dropping platelet counts below 150 or a 50% drop while on heparin, alert/warning and recommendations for dosing when PTTs get below 40, and order sets with lab orders. As with all DUEs, the ultimate outcome of such drug use evaluations is to enhance rational drug use.

The DUEC's oversight of the inpatient Cost Containment Program has targeted, for example, the antibiotic management program and anticoagulation management program. Some of these new initiatives involve including the daily cost information for antibiotic therapy on the Microbiology Laboratories Sensitivity report and including in the formulary the cost data for drug classes in table format to allow for easy reading by prescribers. Other examples to achieve cost savings were the restriction of high-dose hydromorphone PCA, removing zolpidem from the formulary due to a series of adverse drug events in ICU patients, developing guidelines for IVIG usage due to cost and safety issues, and favoring cimetidine as first-line H2 agonist and making famotidine available for use in certain patients (e.g., patients in intensive care units, transplant patients, or patients receiving drugs known to interact with cimetidine), but removing ranitidine from the formulary in order to force a change to another drug of that class. Obviously, as seen from the above examples, having a committee of experts regularly reviewing detailed information on drug use and ADEs in the hospital provides for continuous quality assurance and enhanced patient safety. However, in addition to these monitoring activities, the DUEC also designs and sponsors interventions.

THE FUTURE

In many ways, the history of pharmacoepidemiology started in the hospital, which was the easier place to conduct *ad hoc* studies, and then shifted to favor outpatient studies as the technology for outpatient databases emerged (see Part IIIb). Inpatient pharmacoepidemiology did not keep abreast, at least in part because the volume of data in hospitals made its automation, especially across many hospitals, infeasible. Yet, given the volume and toxicities of drugs used in the hospital, recent attention has turned back to hospitals.

According to all current indications, the trend toward more automated comprehensive inpatient data collection and storage is expected to continue in the future. This trend has been accelerated by requirements by JCAHO, the drive for improving patient safety, and the data indicating that the application of information technology may assist in achieving this goal (see Chapter 34). Nonetheless, further improvements in inpatient data are needed.

First, inpatient data systems need to be dynamic so as to change as new medical developments occur. For example, as new drugs are approved for use and genetic markers for diagnostic purposes are introduced, the data systems need to be expanded on an ongoing basis to include such developments. Likewise, data systems need to capture new ADEs as they emerge.

Second, inpatient data systems need to further develop and improve in their capability to extract free text from clinical notes throughout the medical record. This is needed to create a fully automated medical record for patient care and research purposes that can be linked to other elements in the data system such as drug use.

Third, inpatient data systems need to be developed and implemented in long-term care and nursing home facilities where a large proportion of drugs are used in elderly patients that are not currently well surveyed. The creation of such data systems will not only provide for improved patient care in these facilities, but will also make possible linking hospital and long-term care databases to permit tracing and follow-up of patients transferring between these types of inpatient care facilities.

Fourth, there still remains a need for the development of regional automated data systems that link inpatient data systems from multiple hospitals and link with outpatient data as well. For patient treatment, this will provide for more coordinated care as patients move between different providers and levels of care. For research purposes, regional data systems will provide a defined population, increased sample size, and longitudinal information for individual patients.

Fifth, a further need is to extend linkages of inpatient data systems across a nationally representative sample of hospitals to create a truly powerful resource for medical research.

Sixth, although there are these prospects for much improved inpatient data systems, privacy regulations (see Chapter 38) severely restrict access to these data for research purposes.

Thus, in conclusion, the future is likely to see a continuation of the increased interest in hospital pharmacoepidemiology that has emerged in the past few years, greatly accelerated by the increasing computerization of hospital care. In the process, we will hopefully be able to find out more, and faster, about those drugs we use primarily in hospitals.

REFERENCES

1. DeFrances CJ, Hall MJ. *2002 National Hospital Discharge Survey. Advanced Data from Vital and Health Statistics*, no. 343. Hyattsville, MD: National Center for Health Statistics, 2004.
2. Cowan C, Catlin A, Smith C, Sensenig A. National health expenditures, 2002. *Health Care Financ Rev* 2004; **25**: 143–66.

3. Standard & Poor Industry Surveys. Healthcare: Pharmaceuticals, June 24, 2004.

4. Birkmeyer JD, Siewers AE, Finlayson E, Stukel TA, Lucas Fl, Batista I et al. Hospital volume and surgical mortality in the United States. N Engl J Med 2002; **346**: 1128–37.

5. Person SD, Allison JJ, Kiefe CI, Weaver MT, Williams OD, Centor RM et al. Nurse staffing and mortality for Medicare patients with acute myocardial infarction. Med Care 2004; **42**: 4–12.

6. Allison JJ, Kiefe CI, Weissman NW, Person SD, Rousculp M, Canto JG et al. Relationship of hospital teaching status with quality of care and mortality for Medicare patients with acute MI. JAMA 2000; **284**: 1256–62.

7. National Center for Health Statistics, resident population data, http://www.cdc.gov/nchs/data/hus/tables/2003/03hus001.pdf.

8. Polanczyk CA, Marcantonio E, Goldman L, Rohde LE, Orav J, Mangione CM et al. Impact of age on perioperative complications and length of stay in patients undergoing non-cardiac surgery. Ann Intern Med 2001; **134**: 637–43.

9. AHRQ. Care of Women in U.S. Hospitals, 2000, HCUP fact book no. 3, AHRQ publication no. 02-0044. Rockville, MD: Agency for Healthcare Research and Quality, October 2002. Available at: http://www.ahrq.gov/data/hcup/factbk3/factbk3.htm.

10. Smith JW, Seidl LG, Cluff LE. Studies on the epidemiology of adverse drug reactions. V. Clinical factors influencing susceptibility. Ann Intern Med 1966; **65**: 629–40.

11. May FE, Stewart RB, Cluff LE. Drug interactions and multiple drug administration. Clin Pharmacol Ther 1977; **22**: 322–8.

12. Fattinger K, Roos M, Vergeres P, Holenstein C, Kind B, Masche U, Stocker DN et al. Epidemiology of drug exposure and adverse drug reactions in two Swiss departments of internal medicine. Br J Clin Pharmacol 2000; **49**: 158–67.

13. Onder G, Landi F, Cesari M, Gambassi G, Carbonin P, Bernabei R. Investigators of the GIFA Study. Inappropriate medication use among hospitalized older adults in Italy: results from the Italian Group of Pharmacoepidemiology in the Elderly. Eur J Clin Pharmacol 2003; **59**: 157–62.

14. Koh NY, Koo WH. Polypharmacy in palliative care: can it be reduced? Singapore Med J 2002; **43**: 279–83.

15. Kennedy JM, van Rij AM, Spears GF, Pettigrew RA, Tucker IG. Polypharmacy in a general surgical unit and consequences of drug withdrawal. Br J Clin Pharmacol 2000; **49**: 353–62.

16. Seidl LG, Thornton GF, Smith JW, Cluff LE. Studies on the epidemiology of adverse drug reactions. III. Reactions in patients on a general medical service. Bull Johns Hopkins Hosp 1966; **119**: 299–315.

17. Philp JR. Rational prescribing and drug usage. Am J Hosp Pharm 1970; **27**: 659–65.

18. Gouveia WA, Shane R, Clark T. Computerized prescriber order entry: power, not panacea (editorial). Am J Health Syst Pharm 2003; **60**: 1838.

19. Lau HS, Florax C, Porsius AJ, De Boer A. The completeness of medication histories in hospital medical records of patients admitted to general internal medicine wards. Br J Clin Pharmacol 2000; **49**: 597–603.

20. Lloyd SS, Rissing JP. Physician and coding errors in patient records. JAMA 1985; **254**: 1330–6.

21. Cluff LE. Adverse drug reactions: the need for detection and control. Am J Epidemiol 1971; **94**: 405–8.

22. Feinstein AR. Clinical biostatistics: the biostatistical problems of pharmaceutical surveillance. Clin Pharmacol Ther 1974; **16**: 110–23.

23. Edwards LD, Levin S, Lepper MH. A comprehensive surveillance system of infections and antimicrobials use at Presbytarian–St. Luke's Hospital, Chicago. Am J Hosp Pharm 1972; **94**: 1053–5.

24. Wang RI, Terry LC. Adverse drug reaction in a Veterans Administration hospital. J Clin Pharmacol 1971; **11**: 14–18.

25. Moser RH. Diseases of Medical Progress. Springfield, IL: Charles C. Thomas, 1959.

26. Finney DJ. The design and logic of a monitor of drug use. J Chronic Dis 1965; **18**: 77–98.

27. Cluff LE, Thornton GF, Seidl LG. Studies on the epidemiology of adverse drug reactions. I. Methods of surveillance. JAMA 1964; **188**: 976–83.

28. Seidl LG, Thornton GF, Cluff LE. Epidemiological studies of adverse drug reactions. Am J Public Health 1965; **55**: 1170–5.

29. Gardner P, Cluff LE. The epidemiology of adverse drug reactions. A review and perspective. Johns Hopkins Med J 1970; **126**: 77–87.

30. Hoddinott BC, Gowdey CW, Coulter WK, Parker JM. Drug reactions and errors in administration on a medical ward. Can Med Assoc J 1967; **97**: 1001–6.

31. Ogilvie RI, Ruedy J. Adverse reactions during hospitalization. Can Med Assoc J 1967; **97**: 1445–50.

32. Hurwitz N, Wade OL. Intensive hospital monitoring of adverse reactions to drugs. BMJ 1969; **1**: 531–6.

33. Reidenberg MM. Adverse drug reactions without drugs [letter]. Lancet 1967; **2**: 892.

34. Weston JK. The present status of adverse drug reaction reporting. JAMA 1968; **203**: 35–7.

35. Gardner P, Watson LJ. Adverse drug reactions: a pharmacy-based monitoring system. Clin Pharmacol Ther 1970; **11**: 802–7.

36. McKenzie MW, Stewart RB, Weiss CF, Cluff LE. A pharmacist-based study of the epidemiology of adverse drug reactions in pediatric medicine patients. Am J Hosp Pharmacy 1973; **30**: 898–903.

37. Lantos RL, Stewart RB. The hospital pharmacist's role in surveying drug prescribing and usage. Am J Hosp Pharm 1970; **27**: 666–70.

38. Stolley PD, Shapiro S, Slone D, Schinnar R. The cardiovascular effects of oral contraceptives. South Med J 1978; **71**: 821–4.

39. Rosenberg L, Shapiro S, Kaufman DW, Slone D, Miettinen OS, Stolley PD. Patterns and determinants of conjugated estrogen use. Am J Epidemiol 1979; **109**: 676–86.

40. Kaufman DW, Shapiro S, Rosenberg L, Monson RR, Miettinen OS, Stolley PD et al. Intrauterine contraceptive device use and pelvic inflammatory disease. Am J Obstet Gynecol 1980; **136**: 159–62.

41. Kaufman DW, Shapiro S, Slone D, Rosenberg L, Miettinen OS, Stolley PD et al. Decreased risk of endometrial cancer among oral contraceptive users. N Engl J Med 1980; **303**: 1045–7.

42. Levy M, Miller D, Kaufman D, Siskind V, Schwingl P, Rosenberg L et al. Major upper gastrointestinal bleeding and the use of aspirin and other nonnarcotic analgesics. *Arch Intern Med* 1988; **148**: 281–5.

43. Rosenberg L, Palmer JR, Kaufman DW, Strom BL, Schottenfeld D, Shapiro S. Breast cancer in relation to the occurrence and timing of induced and spontaneous abortion. *Am J Epidemiol* 1988; **127**: 981–9.

44. Kaufman DW, Kelly JP, Rosenberg L, Stolley PD, Warshauer ME, Shapiro S. Hydralazine use in relation to cancers of the lung, colon, and rectum. *Eur J Clin Pharmacol* 1989; **36**: 259–64.

45. Palmer JR, Rosenberg L, Rao RS, Strom BL, Warshauer ME, Harlap S et al. Oral contraceptive use and breast cancer risk among African-American women. *Cancer Causes Control* 1995; **6**: 321–31.

46. Rosenberg L, Palmer JR, Zauber AG, Warshauer ME, Strom BL, Harlap S et al. The relation of benzodiazepine use to the risk of selected cancers: breast, large bowel, malignant melanoma, lung, endometrium, ovary, non-Hodgkin's lymphoma, testis, Hodgkin's disease, thyroid, and liver *Am J Epidemiol* 1995; **141**: 1153–60.

47. Palmer JR, Rosenberg L, Kaufman DW, Warshauer ME, Stolley P, Shapiro S. Oral contraceptive use and liver cancer. *Am J Epidemiol* 1989; **130**: 878–82.

48. Rosenberg L, Werler MM, Palmer JR, Kaufman DW, Warshauer ME, Stolley PD et al. The risks of cancers of the colon and rectum in relation to coffee consumption. *Am J Epidemiol* 1989; **130**: 895–903.

49. Kaufman DW, Werler MM, Palmer JR, Rosenberg L, Stolley PD, Warshauer ME et al. Diazepam use in relation to breast cancer: results from two case–control studies. *Am J Epidemiol* 1990; **131**: 483–90.

50. Kaufman DW, Palmer JR, de Mouzon J, Rosenberg L, Stolley PD, Warshauer E et al. Estrogen replacement therapy and the risk of breast cancer: results from the case–control surveillance study. *Am J Epidemiol* 1991; **134**: 1375–85.

51. Lesko SM, Rosenberg L, Kaufman DW, Stolley PD, Warshauer ME, Lewis JL et al. Endometrial cancer and age at last delivery: evidence of an association. *Am J Epidemiol* 1991; **133**: 554–9.

52. Bigby M, Jick S, Jick H, Arndt K. Drug-induced cutaneous reactions. A report from the Boston Collaborative Drug Surveillance Program on 15,438 consecutive inpatients, 1975 to 1982. *JAMA* 1986; **256**: 3358–63.

53. Jick H. Effects of aspirin and acetaminophen in gastrointestinal hemorrhage. Results from the Boston Collaborative Drug Surveillance Program. *Arch Intern Med* 1981; **141**: 316–21.

54. Jick H, Porter J. Drug-induced gastrointestinal bleeding. Report from the Boston Collaborative Drug Surveillance Program, Boston University Medical Center. *Lancet* 1978; **2**: 87–9.

55. Levy M, Nir I, Superstine E, Birnbaum D, Eliakim M. Antimicrobial therapy in patients hospitalized in a medical ward. A report from the Boston Collaborative Drug Surveillance Program. *Isr J Med Sci* 1975; **11**: 322–34.

56. Miller RR. Hospital admissions due to adverse drug reactions. A report from the Boston Collaborative Drug Surveillance Program. *Arch Intern Med* 1974; **134**: 219–23.

57. Cohen MR. A compilation of abstracts and an index of articles published by the Boston Collaborative Drug Surveillance Program. *Hosp Pharm* 1977; **12**: 455–6, 458, 462 passim.

58. Borda IT, Slone D, Jick H. Assessment of adverse reactions within a drug surveillance program. *JAMA* 1968; **205**: 645–7.

59. Jick H, Miettinen OS, Shapiro S, Lewis GP, Siskind V, Slone D. Comprehensive drug surveillance. *JAMA* 1970; **213**: 1455–60.

60. Slone D, Gaetano LF, Lipworth L, Shapiro S, Lewis GP, Jick H. Computer analysis of epidemiologic data on effect of drugs on hospital patients. *Public Health Rep* 1969; **84**: 39–52.

61. Miller RR. Drug surveillance utilizing epidemiologic methods. A report from the Boston Collaborative Drug Surveillance Program. *Am J Hosp Pharm* 1973; **30**: 584–92.

62. Rosenberg L, Palmer JR, Rao RS, Zauber A, Strom BL, Warshauer ME et al. A case–control study of oral contraceptive use and risk of breast cancer. *Am J Epidemiol* 1996; **143**: 25–37.

63. Ory HW. Epidemiology of venous thromboembolic disease and OC use. *Dialogues Contracep* 1996; **5**: 4–7, 10.

64. Mitchell AA, Lacouture PG, Sheehan JE. Adverse drug reactions in children leading to hospital admission. *Pediatrics* 1988; **82**: 24–9.

65. Porter J, Jick H. Drug-related deaths among medical inpatients. *JAMA* 1977; **237**: 879–81.

66. Smidt NA, McQueen EG. Adverse reactions to drugs: a comprehensive hospital inpatient survey. *N Z Med J* 1972; **76**: 397–401.

67. Spino M, Sellers EM, Kaplan HL, Stapleton C, MacLeod SM. Adverse biochemical and clinical consequences of furosemide administration. *Can Med Assoc J* 1978; **118**: 1513–18.

68. Allen MD, Greenblatt DJ. Role of nurse and pharmacist monitors in the Boston Collaborative Drug Surveillance Program. *Drug Intell Clin Pharm* 1975; **9**: 648–54.

69. Jones JK, Staffa J. Estimation of the frequency of warfarin-associated necrosis in a large in-patient record-linked database. *Pharmacoepidemiol Drug Saf* 1993; **2**: 115–26.

70. Mullett CJ, Evans RS, Christenson JC, Dean JM. Development and impact of a computerized pediatric antiinfective decision support program. *Pediatrics* 2001; **108**: E75.

71. Gardner RM, Pryor TA, Warner HR. The HELP hospital information system: update 1998. *Int J Med Inform* 1999; **54**: 169–82.

72. Evans RS, Pestotnik SL, Classen DC, Burke JP. Evaluation of a computer-assisted antibiotic-dose monitor. *Ann Pharmacother* 1999; **33**: 1026–31.

73. Burke JP, Pestotnik SL. Antibiotic use and microbial resistance in intensive care units: impact of computer-assisted decision support. *J Chemother* 1999; **11**: 530–5.

74. Teich JM, Glaser JP, Beckley RF, Aranow M, Bates DW, Kuperman GJ et al. The Brigham integrated computing system (BICS): advanced clinical systems in an academic hospital environment. *Int J Med Inform* 1999; **54**: 197–208.

75. Teich JM, Merchia PR, Schmiz JL, Kuperman GJ, Spurr CD, Bates DW. Effects of computerized physician order entry on prescribing practices *Arch Intern Med* 2000; **160**: 2741–7.

76. Teich JM, Petronzio AM, Gerner JR, Seger DL, Shek C, Fanikos J. Partners HealthCare System, Boston, MA, USA. An information system to promote intravenous-to-oral medication conversion. *Proc AMIA Symp* 1999; 415–19.

77. Bates DW, Kuperman GJ, Rittenberg E, Teich JM, Fiskio J, Ma'luf N *et al*. A randomized trial of a computer-based intervention to reduce utilization of redundant laboratory tests. *Am J Med* 1999; **106**: 261–2.

78. Teich JM, Schmiz JL, O'Connell EM, Fanikos J, Marks PW, Shulman LN. An information system to improve the safety and efficiency of chemotherapy ordering. *Proc AMIA Annu Fall Symp* 1996; 498–502.

79. Jha AK, Kuperman GJ, Teich JM, Leape L, Shea B, Rittenberg E *et al*. Identifying adverse drug events: development of a computer-based monitor and comparison with chart review and stimulated voluntary report. *J Am Med Inform Assoc* 1998; **5**: 305–14.

80. Saposnik G, Caplan LR, Gonzalez LA, Baird A, Dashe J, Luraschi A *et al*. Differences in stroke subtypes among natives and caucasians in Boston and Buenos Aires. *Stroke* 2000; **31**: 2385–9.

81. Segal R, Poznansky MC, Connors L, Sands K, Barlam T. Changing patterns of presentations of patients with HIV-related disease at a tertiary referral centre and its implications for physician training. *Int J STD AIDS* 2001; **12**: 453–9.

82. McDonald CJ, Tierney WM, Overhage JM, Martin DK, Wilson GA. The Regenstrief Medical Record System: 20 years of experience in hospitals, clinics, and neighborhood health centers. *MD Comput* 1992, **9**: 206–17.

83. McDonald CJ, Overhage JM, Tierney WM, Dexter PR, Martin DK, Suico JG *et al*. The Regenstrief Medical Record System: a quarter century experience. *Int J Med Inform* 1999; **54**: 225–53.

84. Mahon BE, Rosenman MB, Kleiman MB. Maternal and infant use of erythromycin and other macrolide antibiotics as risk factors for infantile hypertrophic pyloric stenosis. *J Pediatr* 2001; **139**: 380–4.

85. Dexter PR, Perkins S, Overhage JM, Maharry K, Kohler RB, McDonald CJ. A computerized reminder system to increase the use of preventive care for hospitalized patients. *N Engl J Med* 2001; **345**: 965–70.

86. Diero L, Stiffler T, Einterz RM, Tierney WM. Can data from an electronic medical record identify which patients with pneumonia have *Pneumocystis carinii* infection? *Int J Med Inform* 2004; **73**: 743–50.

87. Clark DO, Kroenke K, Callahan CM, McDonald CJ. Validity and utility of patient-reported measures on hospital admission. *J Clin Epidemiol* 1999; **52**: 65–71.

88. Overhage JM, Tierney WM, McDonald CJ. Computer reminders to implement preventive care guidelines for hospitalized patients. *Arch Intern Med* 1996; **156**: 1551–6.

89. Tierney WM, Fitzgerald JF, Miller ME, James MK, McDonald CJ. Predicting inpatient costs with admitting clinical data. *Med Care* 1995; **33**: 1–14.

90. Lamoreaux J. The organizational structure for medical information management in the department of veterans affairs: an overview of major health care databases. *Med Care* 1996; **34**; 31–44.

91. Graber SE, Seneker JA, Stahl AA, Franklin KO, Neel TE, Miller RA. Development of a replicated database of DHCP data for evaluation of drug use. *J Am Med Inform Assoc* 1996; **3**: 149–56.

92. Joint Commission sets agenda for change. *JCAH Perspect* 1986; **6**: 6–8.

93. Marder RJ. Joint Commission plans for clinical indicator development for oncology. *Cancer* 1989; **64** (suppl 1): 310–6.

94. Medication Use Task Force refines components, processes. *Jt Comm Perspect* 1990; **10**: 5.

95. Nadzam DM, Turpin R, Hanold LS, White RE. Data-driven performance improvement in health care: the Joint Commission's Indicator Measurement System (IMSystem). *Jt Comm J Qual Improv* 1993; **19**: 492–500.

96. Joint Commission on Accreditation of Healthcare Organizations. ORYX. The next evolution in accreditation. *Nurs Manage* 1997; **28**: 49–52, 54.

97. Strom BL, Gibson GA. A systematic integrated approach to improvement of drug prescribing in an acute care hospital: a potential model for applied hospital pharmacoepidemiology. *Clin Pharmacol Ther* 1993; **54**: 126–33.

Part V

SELECTED SPECIAL METHODOLOGIC ISSUES IN PHARMACOEPIDEMIOLOGY

36

Determining Causation from Case Reports

JUDITH K. JONES

The Degge Group and Adjunct Faculty, Georgetown University, George Washington University School of Public Health,
Washington, DC, USA.

INTRODUCTION

A major component of the evaluation of reports of suspected adverse drug reactions in the clinical setting, or adverse events in a clinical trial, is a judgment about the degree to which any reported event is, in fact, causally associated with the suspected drug. In reality, a particular event is either associated or is not associated with a particular drug, but the current state of information almost never allows a definitive determination of this dichotomy. Accordingly, a number of approaches to the determination of the probability of a causal drug–event association have evolved over the past several years. This chapter will first discuss the historical development of these efforts, and several of the current approaches and uses. It will then review the evolving regulatory changes on this topic, including a brief consideration of the evaluation of single events in the clinical trial setting.

THE CLINICAL PROBLEM TO BE ADDRESSED BY PHARMACOEPIDEMIOLOGIC RESEARCH

The basic clinical problem to be addressed is illustrated in Figure 36.1. A clinical event occurs within the milieu of a number of possible causal factors. That event either occurred independently or in some way its occurrence was partially or totally linked to one or more of the potential causative agents. The primary task is to determine the degree to which the occurrence of the event is linked to one particular suspected causal agent, in this case a drug or other medicinal agent.

This task of evaluating causality in case reports shares some similarities with the problem of evaluating causality in chronic disease epidemiology, as discussed below and in more detail in Chapter 2. However, in the latter case, causality relates to events in populations and to the assessments of those events in one or more population studies. In individual case reports of suspected adverse reactions to a medicinal product that are submitted to the manufacturer or the regulatory agency, where data are often very incomplete, both the details of the exposure and sometimes the nature of the event make the determination of causality in case reports a major challenge. The evaluator of these cases makes, at the very least, an implicit judgment of causality. Because evaluation of these case reports is such a frequent activity in postmarketing surveillance, it would be optimal to have a coherent, consistent, and reliable method of determining the degree to which there may be a causal relationship

Pharmacoepidemiology, Fourth Edition   Edited by B.L. Strom

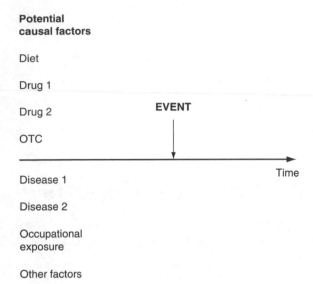

**Potential
causal factors**

Diet

Drug 1

Drug 2

OTC

Disease 1

Disease 2

Occupational
exposure

Other factors

Figure 36.1. The dilemma for determining causation of an event in a clinical setting. In reality a drug either did or did not cause or contribute to an event. However, given the multiple factors associated with the event, the actual truth can seldom be ascertained. Instead, some expression of probability that the drug was associated with the event is made. The method by which this expression is determined is the primary concern of those in adverse reaction causality research.

between given exposures and specific events. However, there are several attributes of single reports that represent obstacles to such assessments, specifically:

1. The usual focus of suspected adverse reaction assessment is an individual clinical event suspected of being associated with exposure to a drug or other medicinal product. The reporting of this event will typically be in the context of a suspicion by the reporter that the event is drug-induced, which will often bias the collection of data required to evaluate other possible causes.
2. The data available about a patient's drug exposure in the typical case report are often incomplete, usually missing precise information on duration, actual dose ingested, and/or concomitant drugs administered. Such information may be more often reported on events in the hospital setting.
3. The data available on the adverse event, including its onset, characteristics, and time course, are also typically incomplete, because the suspicion is usually retrospective and the desired data (e.g., baseline laboratory data) are often not available when the report is made.

4. Data on concomitant diseases and other confounding conditions, such as diet and habits, are typically not available, often because reports are made based upon the specific suspicion of a cause, rather than a differential diagnosis.

Since adverse reactions can be acute, subacute, or chronic, can be reversible or not (e.g., death and birth defects), can be rare or common, and can be pathologically unique or identical to known common diseases, the challenge has thus been to define general data elements and criteria for determining causality that will apply to most types of suspected adverse reactions. For example, for irreversible events such as birth defects or death, data on de-challenge (the result of discontinuing the drug) and re-challenge (the result of reintroducing the drug) are irrelevant.

Closely linked to the task of determining whether there is a causal relationship between a drug exposure and an event is the motivation for making that particular causality determination and the impact of that inference on any actions taken. If the determination is perceived to have little impact on future actions relating to either a patient in a clinical setting or to product labeling in the regulatory environment, the causality assessment might logically be less rigorous. Conversely, if, for example, continuation of a clinical trial hinges upon the assessment, the reliability of the method becomes more critical. With greater focus on the entire subject of adverse drug reactions and the introduction of concepts of causality assessment into more drug regulatory language, the need for consistent and reliable methods of causality determination[1] has become more important.

Specifically, with the appearance of US Food and Drug Administration (FDA) regulations for reporting in clinical trials of adverse events that are "reasonably" associated with a drug,[2] there is a growing need to describe the basis for defining an association within this setting. Although some of the above-listed uncertainties, such as details of exposure, are less likely to exist in clinical trials, there remain difficulties in assessing the likelihood of association for rare events, which will be considered below.

HISTORICAL PERSPECTIVES: DEVELOPMENT OF CONCEPTS OF CAUSALITY FOR ADVERSE REACTIONS

The development of thinking about the causality of adverse reactions has evolved in two disciplines: (i) in epidemiology, and (ii) in the study of individual case reports of adverse reactions. Consideration of both is important.

In the 1950s, epidemiologists grappled with the issue of causality, and Yerushalmy and Palmer, drawing upon the Bradford Hill epidemiologic criteria as well as the Koch–Henle postulates for establishing causation for infectious diseases, developed a set of proposed criteria for causality. These evolved, after considerable deliberation with other epidemiologists, into five criteria for the causal nature of an association.[3] These included determinations of:

1. the consistency of the association;
2. the strength of the association;
3. the specificity of the association;
4. the temporal relationship of the association;
5. the coherence, or biological plausibility, of the association.

These criteria continue to be generally used in chronic disease epidemiology, although they have also been actively discussed and criticized.[3] These criteria are most appropriately applied to population-based data in contrast to evaluation of individual cases or groups of cases from poorly defined populations. However, in some circumstances where large numbers of cases are considered, possibly along with population-based data on an adverse event, these criteria are invoked. For example, they form the basis for the World Health Organization's evaluation of collective data on vaccine adverse effects by the Global Advisory Committee on Vaccine Safety of the Immunization Safety Priority Project,[4] and more recently have been cited by Shakir and Layton[5] as useful for considering the overall data, including spontaneous reports, on an adverse event. The Bradford Hill criteria[6] are discussed in more detail in Chapter 2. Although seldom explicitly noted, the reasoning behind these criteria appeared at about the same time as did thinking about the causal assessment of individual reports of adverse reactions.

Prior to the past two or three decades in the adverse reactions field, the typical approach to case reports of suspected drug-associated clinical events submitted to regulatory agencies or for publication was to consider the events as possibly associated with the drug if there were a number of similar reports. Considerations of pharmacologic plausibility, dose–response, and timing factors were sometimes implicit, but seldom explicit. This approach continued until relatively recently, and in some cases is still used.

The more perplexing proposed drug–event associations were then typically referred to one or more experts, who generally approached the evaluation by what has been termed "global introspection." In this approach, the experts collect all the facts relevant to the problem at hand, compile them, and make unstructured judgments to decide the answer. In the causality assessment context, this answer has usually been expressed in terms of a qualitative probability scale, for example "definite" versus "probable" versus "possible" versus "doubtful" versus "unrelated".[7]

The recognized subjective nature of global reasoning as an approach led a number of investigators to develop more structured methods of causality assessment. Irey, in examining the details of cases of suspected reactions at the US Armed Forces Institute of Pathology, clearly demonstrated the discrepancy between cases initially reported as drug-associated and those found by careful detailed examination actually likely to be drug-associated.[8,9] Shortly thereafter, the clinical pharmacologists Karch and Lasagna also recognized the inadequacy of expert "global" evaluations of adverse reactions and developed a decision table, or algorithm, to segment the evaluation of a case into several components.[10] These two groups of investigators identified very similar basic data elements that they felt were necessary for a more standardized assessment:

1. the timing of the event, relative to the drug exposure;
2. the presence or absence of other factors which might also cause the event;
3. the result of withdrawing the drug ("de-challenge");
4. the result of reintroducing the drug ("re-challenge");
5. other data supporting an association, e.g., previous cases.

These criteria related to the special characteristics of suspected adverse drug reactions. The object for these causality assessments was either a single case or a group of cases from an ill-defined exposed population. Thus, there was only a vague resemblance to the criteria derived for chronic disease epidemiology. For example, in either a single report or even a series of cases, outside of a population context, there would be no way to evaluate the consistency, strength, or specificity of the association, although with some rare, drug-associated disorders, this might play some role. However, the temporal relationship does apply in both situations and in some cases the coherence or biological plausibility has been included in the criteria for single cases, as described in more detail below.

Following the introduction of these new methods for the assessment of suspected adverse drug reactions, a large number of other approaches were developed,[11–18] either as algorithms, decision tables, or, in at least one case, as a diagrammatic method.[18] These were reviewed and summarized in monographs from two conferences held in the early 1980s on the causality of adverse reactions, one in Morges, Switzerland,[19] and another in Crystal City, Virginia.[20]

The vast majority of these methods shared the basic elements originally suggested by Irey and Karch and Lasagna, but many added other details useful for the evaluation of special cases, such as injection site reactions or *in vitro* verification (e.g., Venulet *et al.*[17]). Some included extensive scoring systems linked to relatively extensive algorithms, such as the approach published by Kramer *et al.*[11] A summary of some of the major methods is presented in Table 36.1, and selected methods are discussed in detail in the next section of this chapter.

The 1981 Morges conference,[19] the 1983 Crystal City conference,[20] and a 1983 Paris meeting[21] were all convened to compare a number of these approaches and to consider whether a single "gold standard" method might be developed that could represent an international consensus that could be used by regulators and pharmaceutical sponsors alike. An international study group, the Associated Permanent Workshop of Imputologists (APWI) ("imputology" being the

French term for causality), was initiated at the Morges meeting and continued into the 1990s.[22,23] Although a consensus method was not established, the Crystal City conference had requested an outside observer (Dr David Lane, a theoretical statistician) to provide a critique of the deliberations.[24] His critique and subsequent participation in the Paris conference and APWI resulted in the development of a new approach for assessing the causality of adverse reactions based on Bayes probability theorem.[25] This approach considered the probability of an event occurring in the presence of a drug relative to its probability of occurring in the absence of the drug, considering all details of the case.[26–29] Although in use elsewhere in medicine, this approach had not been applied to analyses of suspected adverse effects. This method will be discussed in more detail in the next section of this chapter.

After this flux of activity in the mid-1980s, there was more limited activity in the area of adverse event causality, primarily marked by efforts in France in the mid-1990s, where causality assessment was required by the drug regulatory agency. This resulted in further elaboration of the Bayesian method by Begaud and colleagues in Bordeaux[30] and development of a further scoring method, RUCAM (Roussel Uclaf Causality Assessment Method), by Bénichou and Danan.[31] Since this time, although a standard method has not been adopted, causality assessment by varying methods has diffused into other regulatory requirements in the EU, Canada, and the US, into the requirement for publication of reports in at least one journal (*Annals of Pharmacotherapy*), and, sporadically, in analyses of both clinical trial data and spontaneous reports, as described below.

Table 36.1. A summary of the information categories in the method of Kramer *et al.*[11] for determining causality of adverse drug reactions

Axis[a]	Information category	Number of questions in the axis[b]	General content
I	Previous experience with drug	4	Literature or labeling information
II	Alternative etiologies	9	Character, frequency of event with disease versus drug
III	Timing of events	4	Timing consistent
IV	Drug levels, evidence of overdose	6	Blood levels, other dose-related events
V	De-challenge	23	All aspects of timing of de-challenge and results
VI	Re-challenge	10	All aspects of re-challenge—circumstances, timing, and results

[a] Axis in the published algorithmn. Although the visual format of the published algorithm appears complex, the axes correspond to the information considered in the majority of causality assessment methods. The authors then weight the answers to the questions to provide a score for each axis which, when summed, gives a numerical estimate of the probability of an association, ranging from 6 or 7 = definite to less than 0 = unlikely.
[b] Each question within an axis relates to a factor that might be considered to contribute to the causality assessment. However, not all questions are asked for any one problem.

ACTUAL AND POTENTIAL USES OF CAUSALITY ASSESSMENT

Despite the proliferation of methods and the great interest in adverse effects of drugs, the actual use of these methods for decision making has been infrequent, but may be increasing as interest in various methods of analysis of adverse events has burgeoned. However, causality assessment has been required in France for many years[32] and has been formally considered in a European Community Directive[33,34] (see also Chapter 10). This has resulted in a general consensus on the causality terms used by the European Union member states.[35] Further, since 1994, a formal method of causality assessment for reports of vaccine-associated adverse events has been instituted by Health Canada's Vaccine Safety Surveillance Section, Division of Immunization, Laboratory Center for Disease Control, which is conducted by the Advisory Committee on Causality Assessment.[36]

In fact, there are a variety of settings where standard assessments of causality could be useful, from the clinical trials activities in drug development by the pharmaceutical manufacturer, to evaluation and monitoring of postmarketing spontaneous reports by both sponsors and regulators, to the clinical setting, where suspected adverse reaction should be a common component of the differential diagnosis, and even possibly to the courtroom, and even the newsroom.[1]

Pharmaceutical Manufacturers

Manufacturers of pharmaceuticals must view causality assessment for events associated with their drugs from the standpoints of both regulatory requirements in different countries and product liability. Pharmaceutical manufacturers have not had to consider assessment of postmarketing report causality for FDA regulatory purposes. Regulations covering postmarketing event monitoring in the US required reporting of all events associated with the drug "whether or not thought to be associated with the drug" (earlier, US Code of Federal Regulations 21:310.300; now, 21:314.80) (see also Chapters 8 and 9), and causality assessment did not formally apply to events in clinical trials. However, with the revision of the FDA Investigational New Drug (IND) regulations (CFR 21:312.22) in the late 1980s, there was an implicit requirement for causality assessment to determine the need for reporting certain types of clinical events in clinical trials. This has come about by requiring the reporting of serious unexpected events associated with use of a drug where there is a reasonable possibility that the events may have been caused by the drug. A disclaimer is noted that such a report of a serious unexpected event does not constitute an admission that the drug caused the events. These regulations do not provide criteria or a suggested method; however, they do imply that such methods might be useful. In new proposed postmarketing regulations,[37] a similar concept alluding to causality has been introduced by designating adverse event reports as "suspected adverse drug reactions, or SADRs" defined as:

'A noxious and unintended response to any dose of a drug ("biological" for proposed § 600.80(a)) product for which there is a reasonable possibility that the product caused the response. In this definition, the phrase "a reasonable possibility" means that the relationship cannot be ruled out.'

This is further elaborated in the proposed regulations:

The phrase "the relationship cannot be ruled out" clarifies which individual cases would be reported to FDA. Classifying a case as "probably related," "possibly related," "remotely related," or "unlikely related" to the drug or biological product would signify that a causal relationship between the product and an adverse event could not be ruled out and, thus, the adverse event would be considered an SADR. For example, in some cases an adverse event may most probably have occurred as a result of a patient's underlying disease and not as a result of a drug or biological product the patient was taking, but it cannot usually be said with certainty that the product did not cause the adverse event. Therefore, such an adverse event would be classified as an SADR because there would be at least a "reasonable possibility" that the drug or biological product may have caused the adverse event. Of course, this classification would not establish causality (attributability) by itself, it would only indicate that causality could not be ruled out with certainty.

Independently, manufacturers faced with a serious event in drug development have also been motivated to explore formal evaluation methods for serious events that could be used to signal the need for discontinuation of drug development if causality is established.

Outside of the US, the requirements for manufacturers to consider causality have varied from country to country, but with promulgation of EU Directives on pharmacovigilance and related EU activities, the variation may decrease. Many regulatory agencies have requested or implied some type of evaluation to minimize the number of nonspecific events reported.[31] Given this environment, particularly in a growing international milieu, manufacturers have been actively interested in this area. In fact, several of the specific methods for causality assessment have been published by investigators based in the pharmaceutical industry.[14,17,18,38–41]

Causality definitely is an issue for pharmaceutical manufacturers in the arena of product liability, especially in the US. A number of years ago, Freilich considered many aspects of this,[42] concluding that a company must have a rigorous process for the review of any adverse event reports and "make causality assessments on an ongoing basis" for product liability purposes. This is necessary to comply with the duty to warn, which he summarizes as follows: "Information must be given of any risks of death or serious harm, no matter how rare, as well as information concerning side effects where there is a substantial probability of their occurrence, no matter how mild." Others in the legal arena dealing in product liability have considered causality issues and the notion of the "substantial factor" test for contributing to causation.[43,44]

Drug Regulators

The use by drug regulators of causality assessment of spontaneously reported postmarketing adverse reactions has varied considerably. Most countries' drug regulators have some method of approaching causality, but this method has been most well defined in France, Australia, and certain other countries[32,45,46] (also see Chapter 10).

In France—owing in part to the considerable original work and interest in adverse reaction causality by a regulator, J. Dangoumou, and his colleagues—all reports of suspected reactions must be evaluated by the "French method." This method combines symptom and chronologic criteria relating to the individual case to give a "global intrinsic score," and then adds bibliographic data relating to information on other cases and the known pharmacology and adverse effects of the drug from standardized sources to give an "extrinsic score".[13,47]

In the US (see also Chapter 9), although a data element for causality was incorporated into the initial file format for the computerized reports of suspected adverse reactions submitted to the FDA, no formal method for evaluating all reports was used until a simple algorithm was developed in the early 1980s, based on the Irey and Karch and Lasagna work.[15,16] This simple, basic method, based on only the timing, de- and re-challenge, and confounding factors criteria, very specifically excluded the consideration of previous literature reports as a basis for considering the strength of the association. It was reasoned that, in many cases, the FDA would be in the position of receiving the first reports of an association, and such a criterion would suppress a signal of a possibly new drug-associated event. The primary use of the assessment by the FDA was administrative, i.e., the causality assessment was a mechanism for identifying the best documented cases—those with a "probable" or "highly probable" association. The causality judgment was specifically deleted from publicly available files, which consistently carry the caveat, "a cause and effect relationship has not been established." Although the FDA algorithm existed for the reviewers of the reports, the frequency of its actual use was not determined, and this causality data element was removed from the computer file in 1986, but the caveat on all released adverse event information remains. The FDA does not now use formal causality assessment on a routine basis (see Chapters 8 and 9).

Publishers of Reports of Adverse Reactions

The medical literature containing case reports of suspected adverse reactions has largely avoided the issue of causality, although there are many published series of case reports that have applied the Naranjo scoring method that is described below and in Figure 36.2. In fact, the *Annals of Pharmacotherapy* now requires that this method be applied

and reported in all case reports published. The majority of single case reports, letters to the editor, or short publications do not provide an explicit judgment using any of the published algorithms. Further, many reports do not provide information on confounding drug therapy or medical conditions, data elements considered by most knowledgeable in adverse reaction assessment to be essential for considering causality. This issue was recognized as one of several problems relating to the publication of adverse reactions in the literature, and was discussed extensively during a conference on publication of adverse event reports in the medical literature in Morges, Switzerland in 1983. A number of editors of medical publications were present and discussed the quality of information in reported cases. They developed a list of the types of information that would be desirable for published reports, information that would permit the reader to assess independently the likelihood of the association.[48,49] In essence, the conclusion was that ideally publication of case reports should require at minimum the specifics of the five elements of the criteria for causality (e.g., details of timing, the nature of the reaction, discontinuation and re-introduction, and alternate causes based on prior history). The need for this publication requirement was underlined when Harambaru and her colleagues compared the value of 500 published reports with 500 spontaneous reports with respect to the availability of information needed in most standard causality assessments. Although analysis suggested the published reports contained significantly more information, the tabulation suggests very sparse data on both alternate causes/other diseases and other drugs in *both* types of reports.[50] Since at present, few journals appear to require specific types of information for publication of spontaneous reports, this has prompted another formal effort in 2004 by the International Society of Pharmacoepidemiology to address this issue.

METHODOLOGIC PROBLEMS TO BE ADDRESSED BY PHARMACOEPIDEMIOLOGIC RESEARCH

The problem to be solved in determining whether an event is caused by a drug is to find one or more methods that are reliable, consistent, accurate, and useful for determining the likelihood of association. This problem is compounded by the nature of drug-associated adverse events. They vary in their frequency, their manifestations, their timing relative to exposure, and their mechanism, and mimic almost the entire range of human pathology, as well as adding unique new pathologies (e.g., kidney stones consisting of drug crystals and the oculomucocutaneous syndrome caused by practolol). In addition, since drugs are used to treat illnesses, drug-associated events are always nested within other pathologies associated with the indication for the drug. Since drugs are used to produce a beneficial effect, known or expected adverse events are grudgingly accepted within the clinical risk/benefit equation. However, unknown or unexpected events are inconsistently recognized and described, and seldom are the desired baseline and other detailed measurements taken.

The nature of this task, and its context, has generated two divergent philosophies. One philosophy discounts the value or importance of causality assessment of individual reactions, deferring judgment to the results of formal epidemiologic studies or clinical trials.[51] The alternate view contends that the information in single reports can be evaluated to determine at least some degree of association, and that this can be useful, and sometimes critical, when discontinuation of a clinical trial or development of a drug, or drug withdrawal is a consideration.[52] This latter view has spurred the evolution of causal evaluation from expert consensual opinion based on global introspection to structured algorithms, and to elaborate probabilistic approaches, as described previously. Further, because of the nature of drug-associated effects, particularly those that are rare and serious, the question has been raised about whether epidemiologists need to consider using methods for causal evaluations of cases in their formal studies and in clinical trials, since the small numbers available may not be amenable to standard statistical analysis.[53]

CURRENTLY AVAILABLE SOLUTIONS

There are now a variety of methods for causality assessment of spontaneous reports. Four basic types will be described, chosen as illustrative examples and because they have been widely described in various publications.

UNSTRUCTURED CLINICAL JUDGMENT/ GLOBAL INTROSPECTION

Probably the most common approach to causality assessment is unstructured clinical judgment. An expert is asked to review the clinical information available and to make a judgment as to the likelihood that the adverse event resulted from drug exposure. However, it has been amply demonstrated that global introspection does not work well, for several reasons.[7]

First, cognitive psychologists have shown that the ability of the human brain to make unaided assessments of uncertainty in complicated situations is poor, especially when

assessing the probability of a cause given an effect, precisely the task of causality assessment.[54] This has been clearly demonstrated for the evaluation of suspected adverse reactions. Several studies have used "expert" clinical pharmacologists to review suspected reactions. Comparing their individual evaluations, these studies documented the extent of their disagreement and illustrated, thereby, how unreliable global introspection is as a causality assessment method.[14–16,55,56]

Second, global introspection is uncalibrated. One assessor's "possible" might mean the same thing as another assessor's "probable." This has been well demonstrated in a study of one pharmaceutical company's spontaneous report reviewers, who used both a verbal and numerical scale.[19]

These and other shortcomings of global introspection as a causality assessment method for adverse reactions are discussed in detail by Lane, Hutchinson, and Kramer.[7,27,28,57] Despite these concerns, global introspection for evaluation of adverse events continues to be used. Most notably, the Uppsala Sweden WHO Centre for Drug Monitoring that collects the spontaneous reports from national centers worldwide has published causality criteria ranging from "certain" to "unassessable/unclassifiable" that essentially represent six levels of global introspection, though they generally incorporate consideration of the more standard criteria for causality.[58] The Portuguese Nucleo de Farmacovigilancia do Centro central pharmacovigilance unit utilizes this WHO global introspection method, in part based upon a comparison of the results from an evaluation of 200 cases by both algorithm methods and the WHO global introspection method. They found a relatively moderate to high degree of correspondence of judgments for the reactions more likely associated.[59]

ALGORITHM/CRITERIAL METHOD WITH VERBAL JUDGMENTS

The subsequent attempts to address the limitations of global introspection have resulted in the proliferation of approaches (see Venulet et al.[19] and Herman[20] for reviews and examples of these methods, the appendix in Venulet[23] for a complete bibliography, and Herman and Fourrier[60] for a summary). These methods range from simple flow charts posing 10 or fewer questions to lengthy questionnaires containing up to 84 items. However, they share a common basic structure essentially based on the original Karch and Lasagna and Irey work—the timing of the adverse event in relation to administration of the drug, alternative etiological candidates, previous recognition of the event as a possible adverse reaction to the drug, the response when the drug is discontinued (de-challenge), and the response when the drug is subsequently readministered (re-challenge). Information relevant to each factor is elicited by a series of questions, the answers to which are restricted to "yes/no" (and, for some methods, "don't know").

These approaches have advantages when compared to global introspection,[57] since there is a great improvement in the consistency of ratings among reviewers. Since the consideration of each case is segmented into its components (e.g., timing, confounding diseases, etc.), this also allows for a better understanding of areas of disagreement. However, there is still considerable global introspection required to make judgments on the separate elements of the algorithms or decision tables. These judgments require, in some cases, "yes" or "no" answers where, in fact, a more quantitative estimate of uncertainty would be more appropriate. For example, the reviewer might have to consider whether the appearance of jaundice within one week represented a sufficient duration of drug exposure to be consistent with a drug–event association. Even adherents of some of the methods agree that their procedures for converting answers into probability ratings are arbitrary.

This type of approach, with various degrees of complexity, is used by some drug regulatory agencies, such as that of Australia.[45] The FDA algorithm, currently not in official use, was another example of this approach, inquiring sequentially about temporal sequence, de-challenge, re-challenge, and concomitant diseases which might have caused the event. Based on the Irey and Karch and Lasagna concepts, it was tailored to be amenable for rapid use by professionals with varied backgrounds for the administrative purpose of finding well-documented cases for regulatory signal evaluation. It was also considered useful and easily remembered by clinicians in initial differential diagnosis of a clinical event. However, this very simple approach is less useful for irreversible drug effects, since they have neither de-challenge nor re-challenge possibilities. To address this, an alternate algorithm for fatal outcome events was developed in the aftermath of the FDA algorithm.[16]

ALGORITHMS REQUIRING SCORING OF INDIVIDUAL JUDGMENTS

Many algorithms permit quantitative judgments by requiring the scoring of their criteria. The answers to the algorithms' questions are converted into a score for each factor, the factor scores are summed, and this overall score is converted into a value on a quantitative probability scale. These judgments range from the extensive, multiple question method of Venulet et al.,[17] which has now been translated for computer use, to the relatively simpler French method.[13]

The method developed by Kramer et al.[11] received considerable review and is representative of the scored methods. The authors categorized information needed into specific "axes" and each axis was composed of several questions about a case. Although it was presented in algorithm format with multiple steps, it can also be represented in tabular format, as shown here (see Table 36.1). One of the more practical methods of this type was developed by Naranjo et al.[12] This has been adopted in a number of clinical settings and by at least one publisher (Annals of Pharmacotherapy) and is shown in Figure 36.2. One of the more recent versions of this type of evaluation was developed by Bénichou and Danan,[31] called RUCAM, which, like the Naranjo method, has six criteria with three or four levels of scoring for each criterion to derive an overall score. This has recently been applied in evaluation of adverse events in HIV clinical trials,[61] and was more recently cited by Lee in review of methods of assessment of hepatic injury.[62]

These quantitative methods have found applications in a number of settings, ranging from evaluations of suspected adverse reactions by hospital committees (US hospitals are now required by the Joint Commission on Accreditation of Healthcare Organizations (JCAHO) to have programs of adverse reaction surveillance) to applications by some regulatory authorities, as in France. They are also used, although sometimes only in a research context, by some pharmaceutical manufacturers.[19,38] The specific manner in which they are used has not been well described in the literature.

PROBABILISTIC METHODS

Recognition of the various problems inherent in the previously existing methods set the stage for the development of an alternative approach based on the Bayesian probability approach to assessment of causality. This method has provided an opportunity for a fresh look at the issue of causality, and its initial apparent difficulty (due to its requirement for using all available information) raised some new issues about causality assessment of adverse reactions. It has also brought the area of adverse reactions evaluation into a larger discussion of the value of the Bayesian and probabilistic approaches to the analysis of medical and scientific data.[3]

First published as a method for adverse reaction assessment by Auriche,[41] who participated with Lane and others in a working group within the APWI organization, this method was first presented in extensive form in a workshop in 1985 (see Figure 36.3). Several examples were published in a monograph and subsequently in early papers.[28,29] The methods have been incorporated into automated versions by

**CAUSALITY ASSESSMENT
NARANJO SCORED ALGORITHM**

QUESTION	ANSWER			SCORE
	Yes	No	Unk	
Previous reports?	+1	0	0	_____
Event after drug?	+2	−1	0	_____
Event abate on drug removal?	+1	0	0	_____
+ Re-challenge?	+2	−1	0	_____
Alternative causes?	−1	+2	0	_____
Reaction with placebo?	−1	+1	0	_____
Drug blood level toxic?	+1	0	0	_____
Reaction dose-related?	+1	0	0	_____
Past history of similar event?	+1	0	0	_____
ADR confirmed objectively?	+1	0	0	_____
				_____
Total score				_____

Figure 36.2. A critical scored algorithm illustrated by the method of Naranjo *et al.*[12] in wide use. This particular method uses some of the basic data elements as well as more details of the history and characteristics of the case, and a score is designated for the response to each question.

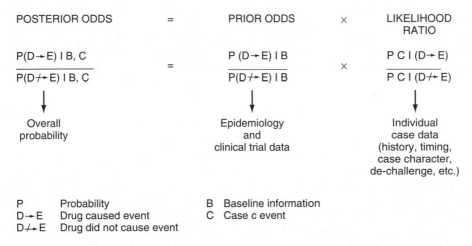

POSTERIOR ODDS	=	PRIOR ODDS	×	LIKELIHOOD RATIO

$$\frac{P(D{\rightarrow}E)\,|\,B,\,C}{P(D{\not\rightarrow}E)\,|\,B,\,C} = \frac{P(D{\rightarrow}E)\,|\,B}{P(D{\not\rightarrow}E)\,|\,B} \times \frac{P\,C\,|\,(D{\rightarrow}E)}{P\,C\,|\,(D{\not\rightarrow}E)}$$

Overall probability	Epidemiology and clinical trial data	Individual case data (history, timing, case character, de-challenge, etc.)

P	Probability	B	Baseline information
D→E	Drug caused event	C	Case c event
D↛E	Drug did not cause event		

Figure 36.3. The basic equations for the Bayesian analysis of suspected drug-associated events. These provide a structured yet flexible and explicit approach to estimating the probability that an event is associated with one, or more, drugs, as described in the text and extensive literature dating from Auriche,[41] Lane *et al.*,[28] and others. Since the prior probability estimate is dependent on explicit data from clinical trials and epidemiologic studies, this approach can provide a framework for specific event-related questions in these studies.

both Naranjo and Hutchinson, the latter developing a model using an expert system.[63,64] Naranjo and colleagues have implemented a practical spreadsheet/automated version called BARDI (Bayesian Adverse Reaction Diagnostic Instrument) and have now applied it to a number of practical adverse event problems.[54,65,66]

The Bayesian method determines the probability of an event occurring in the presence of a drug, relative to the probability of that event occurring in the absence of the drug, as illustrated in Figure 36.3. Estimation of this overall probability, the "posterior probability," is based on two components:

1. what is known prior to the event, the "prior probability" which is based on clinical trial and epidemiologic data;
2. what the likelihoods are, or are not, for drug causation of the components of the specific case, including its history, timing, characteristics, de-challenge and its timing components, re-challenge, and any other factors, such as multiple re-challenges.

The full application of this method requires knowledge of the clinical event, its epidemiology, and relatively specific information about the event's characteristics and kinetics over time. Examples have been published for several types of events, including Stevens–Johnson syndrome, renal toxicity, lithium dermatitis, and ampicillin-associated colitis, agranulocytosis, and Guillain–Barré syndrome.[24,54,65] Thus far, this approach appears to be useful for the analysis of the perplexing first events in new drug clinical trials, serious spontaneous adverse reaction reports, and possibly rare events discovered in both case–control and cohort pharmacoepidemiology studies, when standard methods of statistical analysis will not provide sufficient clues as to causality because of inadequate sample size.

With the logistic problem of the length of time required for the actual calculations minimized by automation, the major impediment to more general application of the Bayesian method is the frequent lack of the information required for robust analyses of events. There is no abundance of data on the incidence of most events and their occurrence in the presence and absence of most drugs (the required information for the prior probability). There are even fewer data available on the historical risk factors, the time course, and specific characteristics of the drug-associated conditions, as opposed to the naturally occurring conditions. Although this lack of information is a current limitation, it represents both an important challenge and a framework for structuring further understanding.

Bénichou and collaborators have delved further into a mapping process of reactions by type in an attempt to begin classifications of specific drug-associated disease, using acute liver disease as one model that incorporates qualitative clinical definitions of the disease into the judgment.[67,68]

For this reason, there appear to be several advantages of using this method for the analysis of suspected drug-associated events:

1. All judgments must be explicit and quantified, which permits better explanations of the degree of uncertainty about each component of information. Further, this approach makes maximum use of the available information and follows the basic rule of not discarding information.
2. Since each component is analyzed separately, a sensitivity analysis of each information component can estimate its overall contribution to the final posterior odds or probability estimate. This, in turn, can be used to determine which information is pivotal. For example, if a ten-fold difference in the estimate of the timing does not materially modify the overall posterior odds estimate, further efforts to determine the "best" estimate would not be worth while.
3. Because of the multistep approach to a judgment, combined with a lack of the prejudged weighting present in most other methods, this approach resists the tendency to achieve a result expected on an *a priori* global judgment. This is quite important in evaluating events with multiple causes.
4. This approach can provide an extensive summary of the information needed and areas needing further research and data compilation. Thus, the Bayesian approach ultimately provides a "map" to define the information most critical for understanding drug-induced disease and serves to help formulate the most critical questions to be researched. As disease natural histories and drug-induced diseases are now being described in large population databases, it will be essential to link these two types of analyses. An elegant example of the application of this Bayesian method, with an additional complimentary method developed by Begaud and colleagues using the Poisson method for estimating the probability of rare events in populations[30] has been published recently by Zapater *et al.*[69] These investigators have nicely demonstrated the feasibility of utilizing both clinical trial and population data to estimate the posterior probabilities of association in complex cases of ticlopidine-associated hepatitis.

COMPARISON AMONG THE DIFFERENT METHODS FOR CAUSALITY ASSESSMENT

Several efforts have been made to evaluate and compare these methods. The 1983 conference in Crystal City involved the application of several of the methods to a standardized case, illustrating a considerable lack of concordance for some methods.[21]

A much more elegant and detailed evaluation of six representative algorithmic methods has been carried out by Pere et al.,[70] who identified standard evaluation criteria and carried out an evaluation of 1134 adverse reactions using the various methods. Significantly, they found only moderate agreement between all pairs, and considerable disagreements on weightings of three of the major criteria—timing, de-challenge, and alternate etiologies—which tends to underline the lack of considerable information on the events and their characteristics.

Given the current state of affairs, where a number of published methods exist, the choice of a method for use in evaluating individual adverse effects will likely be determined by a number of practical factors. These include:

1. *How the evaluation will be used.* This refers to both its short-term use (e.g., a rating suggesting more-than-possible association may be needed to result in a "signal") and long-term use (e.g., will a single highly probable case in a file, not otherwise acted upon, be a source of liability for the evaluator?).
2. *The importance of the accuracy of the judgment.* If this evaluation will determine either a specific clinical outcome or, for example, the continuation of a clinical trial or the continued marketing of a drug, the accuracy of the judgment may be critical. Conversely, if little hinges upon the judgment, cruder estimates and methods, recognized as such, may suffice.
3. *The number of causality evaluations to be made.* The above considerations must also be weighed against the time required to make judgments on large numbers of reports. This is particularly a dilemma for regulatory agencies and manufacturers, where the need for accurate judgments is pitted against the volume of evaluations to be considered. One approach to this problem is suggested by the FDA's approach to identifying high priority problems according to their newness and seriousness (see Jones[1] and Chapter 8).
4. *The accrued value of thorough evaluations.* In some circumstances, the careful, rigorous evaluation of certain categories of drug-associated events will facilitate the more accurate evaluation of subsequent, related events.

For example, consider a case where a drug under development is anticipated to cause hepatic events. Detailed evaluations of hepatic events induced by other drugs may allow more satisfactory causality evaluation of reports received on the new drug.[71] In some cases this results from data collection being focused to a much greater degree, as has been initiated in France by Bénichou et al., where special reporting forms based on disease-specific criteria for events are being developed.[71,72] This is also clearly demonstrated in the efforts of Zapater et al. in the evaluation of ticlopidine-associated hepatic toxicity, where the evaluation and sensitivity analysis not only clarified the estimated probabilities for the cases, but also suggested that more careful examinations of relative values of hepatic enzymes might further understanding in the perplexing field of drug-associated hepatotoxicity.[69]

5. *Who will be carrying out the evaluation?* Although no specific studies have been carried out to evaluate the inter-rater differences among differently trained professionals, it is likely that the body of information held by each reviewer will have considerable impact on any of the methods used, including the Bayesian method.

THE FUTURE

The field of adverse reaction causality assessment has many unresolved issues, both methodological and practical, which have been described in the preceding sections. Although there was an original hope that there would be some basis for a consensus method,[21] the current state of the field would suggest that this is not likely to be the case, as again evidenced at the Third International APWI meeting in Paris (November 1992) and the ensuing absence of the emergence of a standard method. Several reasons can be suggested. First, a number of individuals and institutions have adopted one or sometimes a few methods and have committed to their use, often through their choice of data collecting systems or software.[17] Second, the practical aspects of the use of these methods have appeared to play a very real role. Although discussed with excitement as the possible "gold standard" for adverse reaction causality, the Bayesian method was not rapidly embraced, in part because of the difficulty of its use without automation. It was thought that with the lifting of this barrier, and with further use for practical applications, its potential would be realized, but this has generally not been the case. It is likely that the complex appearance of the Kramer et al. algorithm[11] likewise discourages its use in some sectors, although this has not been documented. Again, this is diminished with automation.

Third, the misuse of judgment terms or scores within the legal arena has generated concern,[42] particularly given the fact that there is not a gold standard method.

All of these factors suggest the need for considerable further work. This work would appear to fall into several areas:

1. Further definition of the *applications* of causality assessment, that is the "output" of the process, so as to better define the desired rigor, accuracy, and usability of the methods. It would appear that there will probably always be needs for simpler and rougher methods, as well as more complete and rigorous methods, when the determination has considerable impact.

2. Further definition of the *critical elements needed* for the evaluation of causality for different types of adverse reactions (e.g., hepatic, hematological, skin, etc.) so that this information may be collected at the time of reporting or publishing a spontaneous event. The need for this event-specific information has long been recognized[13,21,70] and is being implemented in some centers (e.g., Bordeaux, France, University of Toronto, as well as many pharmaceutical companies) that collect adverse events. Further work in this area can have a major impact on:

    a. the collection of better information on the different drug-associated events, using data collection instruments tailored to the event of interest, and

    b. the better definition of the dynamics and, ultimately, the pathophysiology and mechanisms of certain types of drug-induced conditions.

3. Gathering of data on these *critical elements* of the specific adverse events in the course of both clinical trials and epidemiologic studies. Risk factor, history, timing, characteristics, and resolution patterns of adverse events should be described in these studies and incorporated into general data resources on the characteristics of medical events and diseases.

4. Further work on *automation* of the causality evaluation process. Global introspection is still widely used because of the cumbersome nature of many of the more complete methods. Fortunately, several methods are now being automated, including the French method,[70] the Venulet method,[17] and the Bayesian BARDI method.[66] Convenient access to the proper questions, arrayed in logical order, as well as background data meeting quality criteria on the state of information to date, has the potential for considerably improving the state of adverse reaction causality evaluation.

5. Consideration of *new and different* methods for assessment. Although it is likely that further work will usually include use of the many available methods, it is of interest that other approaches have emerged. For example, as part of work on patient safety in the US (see also Chapter 34), "root cause analysis" is used to identify the important contributors to adverse events in clinical settings. This approach maps out functional maps of possible contributing factors to not only identify a cause but also determine methods of preventing it. Spath has provided one illustration of this approach.[73] Another approach described by investigators at the University of Toronto, although less generalizable, is the *N*-of-1 trial, which can evaluate the causality of adverse events in individuals, particularly those who have experienced multiple reactions to drugs[74] (see also Chapter 43).

In conclusion, the topic of causality of adverse reactions continues to represent a challenge. With increased awareness of the need to consider causality as part of the regulatory process, the need for consensus, possibly on more than one method depending on use, continues. One major result of the application of detailed causality assessment, particularly when it is viewed prospectively with collection of data in both pharmacovigilance centers and clinical studies, is that these data can ultimately contribute to the overall need to understand the details of the many drug-associated diseases.

REFERENCES

1. Jones JK. Uses of drug–event assessment. *Drug Inf J* 1984; **18**: 233–40.
2. Investigational New Drug Procedures, 21 CFR § 312.22, 1987.
3. Feinstein AR. Clinical biostatistics. XLVII. Scientific standards vs. statistical associations and biologic logic in the analysis of causation. *Clin Pharmacol Ther* 1979; **25**: 481–92.
4. Anonymous. Causality assessment of adverse events following immunization. *Wkly Epidemiol Rec* 2001; **76**: 85–9.
5. Shakir SAW, Layton D. Causal association in pharmacovigilance and Pharmacoepidemiology: thoughts on the application of the Austin Bradford Hill criteria. *Drug Saf* 2002; **25**: 467–71.
6. Hill AB. The environment and disease: association or causation? *Proc R Soc Med* 1965; **58**: 295–300.
7. Hutchinson TA, Lane DA. Assessing methods for causality assessment. *J Clin Epidemiol* 1989; **42**: 5–16.
8. Irey NS. Diagnostic problems in drug-induced diseases. In Meyler L, Peck HM, eds, *Drug-Induced Diseases*, vol. IV. Amsterdam: Elsevier Science, 1972; pp. 1–24.
9. Irey NS. Adverse drug reactions and death: a review of 827 cases. *JAMA* 1976; **236**: 575–8.
10. Karch FE, Lasagna L. Toward the operational identification of adverse drug reactions. *Clin Pharmacol Ther* 1977; **21**: 247–54.

11. Kramer MS, Leventhal JM, Hutchinson TA, Feinstein AR. An algorithm for the operational assessment of adverse drug reactions. I. Background, description, and instructions for use. *JAMA* 1979; **242**: 623–32.

12. Naranjo CA, Busto U, Sellers EM, Sandor P, Ruiz I, Roberts EA, Janecek E, Domecq C, Greenblatt DJ. A method for estimating the probability of adverse drug reactions. *Clin Pharmacol Ther* 1981; **30**: 239–45.

13. Begaud B, Evreux JC, Jouglard J, Lagier G. Unexpected or toxic drug reaction assessment (imputation). Actualization of the method used in France. *Therapie* 1985; **40**: 111–18.

14. Emanueli A, Sacchetti G. An algorithm for the classification of untoward events in large scale clinical trials. *Agents Actions* 1980; **7**: 318–22.

15. Jones JK. Adverse reactions in the community health setting: approaches to recognizing, counseling, and reporting. *Fam Community Health* 1985; **5**: 58–67.

16. Turner WM. The Food and Drug Administration algorithm. *Drug Inf J* 1984; **18**: 259–66.

17. Venulet J, Ciucci AG, Berneker GC. Updating of a method for causality assessment of adverse drug reactions. *Int J Clin Pharmacol Ther Toxicol* 1986; **24**: 559–68.

18. Castle WM. Assessment of causality in industrial settings. *Drug Inf J* 1984; **18**: 297–302.

19. Venulet J, Berneker GC, Ciucci AG, eds. *Assessing Causes of Adverse Drug Reactions*. London: Academic Press, 1982.

20. Herman RL, ed. *Drug–Event Associations: Perspectives, Methods, and Users*. Proceedings of Drug Information Association Workshop, Oct 30–Nov 2, 1983, Arlington, Virginia. *Drug Info J* 1984; **18**: 195–352.

21. Jones JK. Drug–event associations: a view of the current status [epilogue]. *Drug Inf J* 1984; **18**: 233–40.

22. Jones JK, Herman RL. Assessing adverse drug experiences [letter]. *Ann Intern Med* 1988; **108**: 160.

23. Venulet J. APWI: past and present. *Drug Inf J* 1991; **25**: 229–33.

24. Lane DA. A probabilist's view of causality assessment. *Drug Inf J* 1984; **18**: 323–30.

25. de Finetti B. *Theory of Probability*. New York: John Wiley & Sons, 1974.

26. Jones JK, Herman RL, guest eds. Introduction: the future of adverse drug reaction diagnosis: computers, clinical judgement and the logic of uncertainty. Proceedings of the Drug Information Association Workshop, Feb 1986, Arlington, VA. *Drug Inf J* 1986; **20**: 383.

27. Lane D. Causality assessment for adverse drug reactions: a probabilistic approach. In Berry D, ed., *Statistical Methodology in the Pharmaceutical Sciences*. New York: Marcel Dekker, 1990; pp. 475–507.

28. Lane DA, Kramer MS, Hutchinson TA, Naranjo C, Jones JK. The causality assessment of adverse drug reactions using a Bayesian approach. *Pharm Med* 1987; **2**: 265–83.

29. Jones JK. A Bayesian approach to causality assessment. *Psychopharm Bull* 1987; **23**: 395–9.

30. Begaud B, Moride Y, Tubert-Bitter P, Chaslerie A, Haramburu F. False-positives in spontaneous reporting: should we worry about them? *Br J Clin Pharmacol* 1994; **38**: 401–4.

31. Bénichou C, Danan G. A new method for drug causality assessment: RUCAM. In: Bénichou C, ed., *Adverse Drug Reactions. A Practical Guide to Diagnosis and Management*. New York: John Wiley & Sons, 1994; pp. 277–84.

32. Royer FJ. Adverse drug reaction monitoring: doing it the French way. *Lancet* 1985; **2**: 1056–8.

33. CPMP Working Party on Pharmacovigilance. *Procedure for Causality Classification in Pharmacovigilance in the European Community*. EC Document III/3445/91—EN, FINAL, July 1991.

34. Jones JK. Causality assessment of suspected adverse drug reactions: a transatlantic view. *Pharmacoepidemiol Drug Safety* 1992; **1**: 251–60.

35. Miremont G, Haramburu F, Begaud B, Pere JC, Dangoumou J. Adverse drug reactions: physicians' opinions versus a causality assessment method. *Eur J Clin Pharmacol* 1994; **46**: 285–9.

36. Collet J-P, MacDonald N, Cashman N, Pless R, Advisory Committee on Causality Assessment. Monitoring signals for vaccine safety: the assessment of individual adverse event reports by an expert advisory committee. *Bull World Health Organ* 2000; **78**: 178–85.

37. US Federal Register, vol. 68, no. 50, Friday, March 14, 2003, Proposed Rules.

38. Castle W, Baker A. Communication of ADR information: the viewpoint of a British company. *Drug Inf J* 1985; **19**: 375–80.

39. Stephens M. Assessment of causality in industrial settings. *Drug Inf J* 1984; **18**: 307–14.

40. Stephens M. *The Detection of New Adverse Drug Reactions*. London: Plenum Press, 1985.

41. Auriche M. Approache bayesienne de l'imputabilite des phenomenes indesirables aux medicaments. *Therapie* 1985; **40**: 301–6.

42. Freilich WB. Legal perspectives in causality assessment. *Drug Inf J* 1984; **18**: 211–17.

43. Margulies JB. Epidemiologic causation in the courtroom: square pegs in round holes? *Drug Inf J* 1991; **25**: 217–27.

44. Henderson TW. Legal aspects of disease clusters. Toxic tort litigation: medical and scientific principles in causation. *Am J Epidemiol* 1990; **132**: S69–78.

45. Mashford ML. The Australian method of drug–event assessment. *Drug Inf J* 1984; **18**: 271–3.

46. Wiholm BE. The Swedish drug–event assessment methods. *Drug Inf J* 1984; **18**: 267–9.

47. Dangoumau J, Begaud B, Boisseau A, Albin H.. Les effets indesirables des medicaments. *Presse Med* 1980; **9**: 1607–9.

48. Editorial. Improving reports of adverse drug reactions. *BMJ* 1984; **289**: 898–9.

49. Venulet J. Incomplete information as a limiting factor in causality assessment of adverse drug reactions and its practical consequences. *Drug Inf J* 1986; **20**: 423–31.

50. Haramburu F, Begaud, B, Pere JC. Comparison of 500 spontaneous and 500 published reports of adverse reactions. *Eur J Clin Pharmacol* 1990; **39**: 287–8.

51. Louik C, Lacouture PG, Mitchell AA, Kauffman R, Lovejoy FH, Yaffe SJ, Shapiro S.. A study of adverse reaction algorithms in a drug surveillance program. *Clin Pharmacol Ther* 1985; **38**: 183–7.

52. Naranjo CA, Lanctot KL, Lane DA. The Bayesian differential diagnosis of neutropenia and antiarrhythmic agents. *J Clin Pharmacol* 1990; **30**: 1120–7.

53. Jones JK. Epidemiologic perspective on causality assessment for drug associated events. *Drug Inf J* 1986; **20**: 413–22.

54. Kahneman D, Slovic P, Tversky A. *Judgement Under Uncertainty: Heuristics and Biases*. Cambridge, MA: Cambridge University Press, 1982.

55. Koch-Weser J, Sellers EM, Zacest R. The ambiguity of adverse drug reactions. *Eur J Clin Pharmacol* 1977; **11**: 75–8.

56. Karch FE, Smith CL, Kernzer B, MazulloJM, Weintraub M, Lasagna L. Adverse drug reactions—a matter of opinion. *Clin Pharmacol Ther* 1976; **19**: 489–92.

57. Kramer MS. Assessing causality of adverse reactions: global introspection and its limitations. *Drug Inf J* 1986; **20**: 433–7.

58. Uppsala Monitoring Centre, Definitions. Available at: http://www.who-umc.org/defs.html.

59. Macedo AF, Marques FB, Ribeiro CF, Texeira F. Causality assessment of adverse drug reactions: comparisons of the results obtained from published decisional algorithms and from the evaluations of an expert panel, according to different levels of imputability. *J Clin Pharm Ther* 2003; **28**: 137–43.

60. Herman RL, Fourrier A. List of References: Third International APWI Meeting. Paris, 1992.

61. Bonfanti P, Valsecchi L, Parazzini F, Carradori S, Purterla L, Fortuna P *et al.* Relazione di causalitá delle reaziioni averse a farmaci: un'esperienza nell'utilizzo degli inibitori della protease di HIV. *Clin Ter* 2000; **151**: 411–15.

62. Lee WM. Assessing causality in drug-induced liver injury. *J Hepatol* 2000; **33**: 1003–15.

63. Hutchinson TA, Dawid AP, Spiegelhalter DJ, Cowell RG, Roden S. Computerized aids for probabilistic assessment of drug safety I: A spreadsheet program. *Drug Inf J* 1991; **25**: 29–39.

64. Hutchinson TA, Dawid AP, Spiegelhalter DJ, Cowell RG, Roden, S. Computerized aids for probabilistic assessment of drug safety II: An expert system. *Drug Inf J* 1991; **25**: 41–8.

65. Lanctot KL, Naranjo, CA. Using microcomputers to simplify the Bayesian causality assessment of adverse drug reactions. *Pharm Med* 1990; **4**: 185–95.

66. Naranjo CA, Lanctot KL. Microcomputer assisted Bayesian differential diagnosis of severe adverse drug reactions to new drugs: a 4-year experience. *Drug Inf J* 1991; **25**: 243–50.

67. Bénichou C, Danan G, Flahault A. Causality assessment of adverse reactions to drugs—I. A novel method based on the conclusions of international consensus meetings: application to drug-induced liver injuries. *J Clin Epidemiol* 1993; **46**: 1323–30.

68. Bénichou C, Danan G, Flahault A. Causality assessment of adverse reactions to drugs—II. An original model for validation of drug causality assessment methods: case reports with positive rechallenge. *J Clin Epidemiol* 1993; **46**: 1331–6.

69. Zapater P, Such J, Perez-Mateo M, Horga JF. A new Poisson and Bayesian-based method to assign risk and causality in patients with suspected hepatic adverse drug reactions. *Drug Saf* 2002; **25**: 735–50.

70. Pere JC, Begaud B, Harambaru F, Albin H. Computerized comparison of six adverse drug reaction assessment procedures. *Clin Pharmacol Ther* 1986; **40**: 451–61.

71. Bénichou C. *Guide Practique de Pharmacovigilance*. Paris: Editions Pradel, 1992.

72. Bénichou C, Danon G. Experts' opinion in causality assessment: results of consensus meetings. *Drug Inf J* 1991; **25**: 251–5.

73. Spath P. Uncover root causes with E&CF charts: illustrate causal factors in accident sequence. *Hosp Peer Rev* 2000; **25**: 96–8.

74. Knowles AR, Uetrecht JP, Shear NH. Confirming false adverse reactions to drugs by performing individualized, randomized trials. *Can J Clin Pharmacol* 2002; **9**: 149–53.

37

Molecular Pharmacoepidemiology

STEPHEN E. KIMMEL[1], HUBERT G. LEUFKENS[2] and TIMOTHY R. REBBECK[1]

[1] University of Pennsylvania School of Medicine, Philadelphia, Pennsylvania, USA; [2] Utrecht Institute for Pharmaceutical Sciences, Utrecht, The Netherlands.

INTRODUCTION

One of the most challenging areas in clinical pharmacology and pharmacoepidemiology is to understand why individuals and groups of individuals respond differently to a specific drug therapy, both in terms of beneficial and adverse effects. Reidenberg observes that, while the prescriber has basically two decisions to make while treating patients (i.e., choosing the right drug and choosing the right dose), interpreting the inter-individual variability in outcomes of drug therapy includes a much wider spectrum of variables, including the patient's health profile, prognosis, disease severity, quality of drug prescribing and dispensing, adherence with prescribed drug regimen (see Chapter 46), and last, but not least, the genetic profile of the patient.[1]

Molecular pharmacoepidemiology is the study of the manner in which molecular biomarkers alter the clinical effects of medications in populations. Just as the basic science of pharmacoepidemiology is epidemiology, applied to the content area of clinical pharmacology, the basic science of molecular pharmacoepidemiology is epidemiology in general and molecular epidemiology specifically, also applied to the content area of clinical pharmacology. Thus, many of the

methods and techniques of epidemiology apply to molecular pharmacoepidemiologogy studies. However, there are several features of molecular pharmacoepidemiology that are somewhat unique to the field, as discussed later in this chapter. Most of the discussion will focus on studies related to genes, but the methodological considerations apply equally to studies of proteins and other biomarkers.

It has been suggested that, on average for each medication, about one out of three treated patients experience beneficial effects, one out of three do not show the intended beneficial effects, 10% experience only side effects, and the rest of the patient population is non-adherent so that the response to the drug is difficult to assess.[2] Although this is just a crude estimate, it highlights the challenge of individualizing therapy in order to produce a maximal beneficial response and minimize adverse effects. Although it is clear that many factors can influence medication efficacy and adverse effects, including age, drug interactions, and medication adherence, genetics can clearly be an important contributor in the response of an individual to a medication. Genetic variability can account for a large proportion (e.g., some estimates range from 20% to 95%[3]) of variability in drug disposition and medication effects.[3–7] In addition to altering dosing requirements, genetics can influence response to therapy by altering drug targets or the pathophysiology of the disease states that drugs are used to treat.[8–13]

GENETIC VARIABILITY IN DRUG RESPONSE: HISTORICAL PERSPECTIVE

Although molecular pharmacoepidemiology is a new subfield of a relatively new field, the idea that individuals have different susceptibility to medications is not new. Since the advent of modern drugs soon after the Second World War, physicians, pharmacists, and patients have been confronted with inter-individual variability in the effects of drug therapy. Some patients need higher than normal doses to achieve an optimum effect. In other patients, unwanted and adverse effects occur even in low doses, while some patients receive no apparent effect of the medication at all. History shows a number of cases where genetics or factors that may be correlated with genetic variability played a role in interpreting and predicting drug effects (Table 37 .1). One of the most well-known "classic" examples of genetic variance in drug response is the metabolic defect caused by glucose-6-phosphate dehydrogenase (G6PD) deficiency.[14] This X-linked disorder is present in about 10% of African men, and occurs at low expressed frequencies in some Mediterranean peoples. In carriers of this deficiency, hemolytic reaction occurs after exposure to oxidant drugs such as antimalarials (e.g., chloroquine), but is also seen in patients using drugs such as aspirin, probenecid, or vitamin K. Another early stimulus for pharmacogenetic thinking was the observation that, in the 1 in 3500 white subjects who are homozygous for the gene encoding an atypical form of butyrylcholinesterase, the inability to sufficiently hydrolyze the muscle relaxant drug succinylcholine could lead to prolonged, drug-induced muscle paralysis resulting in severe, frequently fatal, apnea.[15] A third pharmacogenetic antecedent is the example of drug-induced neuropathy in patients with genetically determined low active levels of the metabolic enzyme N-acetyltransferase.[16] This enzyme plays an important role

Table 37.1. Some examples of "old" clinically relevant gene–drug interactions

- Hemolysis in patients exposed to antimalarial therapy and G6PD deficiency[14]
- Prolonged action of suxamethonium due to plasma cholinesterase polymorphism[15]
- Neuropathy in patients exposed to isoniazide N-acetyltransferase polymorphism[16]
- Inefficacy of codeine as analgesic in poor metabolizers (CYP2D6)[17]

in Phase II pathways of drug metabolism, and genetic variance of the activity of this enzyme may lead to dramatic and clinically relevant differences in the plasma concentrations of drugs such as isoniazid, hydralazine, and procainamide. A final example is the metabolic variance caused by one of the many cytochrome P450 enzymes (CYP). Doctors treating patients with codeine as an analgesic have observed for decades that some patients do not respond at all to normal doses. These clinical observations were not well understood until it was discovered that a polymorphism of CYP2D6 (a subfamily of cytochrome P450) could result in suboptimal transformation of the inactive prodrug codeine into the active form, morphine.[17] The example of codeine points to inherited lack of efficacy. However, genetic polymorphisms of CYP2D6 also have consequences for drug safety, as discussed later in this chapter.

DEFINITIONS AND CONCEPTS

Genetic Variability

Building on the success of the various human genome initiatives, it is now estimated that there are approximately 30 000 regions of the human genome that are recognized as genes because they contain deoxyribonucleic acid (DNA) sequence elements including exons (sequences that encode proteins), introns (sequences between exons that do not directly encode amino acids), and regulatory regions (sequences that determine gene expression by regulating the transcription of DNA to RNA, and then the translation of RNA to protein). Some of these sequences have the ability to encode RNA (ribonucleic acid, the encoded messenger of a DNA sequence that mediates protein translation) and proteins (the amino acid sequence produced by the translation of RNA). We have also learned that there is a great deal of inter-individual variability in the human genome. The most common form of genomic variability is a single nucleotide polymorphism (SNP), which represents a substitution of one nucleotide (i.e., the basic building block of DNA, also referred to as a "base") for another, which is present in <1% of the population. Each person has inherited two copies of each gene (one from the paternal chromosome and one from the maternal chromosome). The term allele refers to the specific nucleotide sequence inherited either from the father or mother, and the combination of alleles in an individual is denoted a genotype. When the two alleles are identical (i.e., the same nucleotide sequence on both chromosomes), the genotype is referred to as "homozygous," and when the two alleles are different (i.e., different nucleotide sequences on each chromosome), the genotype is referred to as "heterozygous." Approximately 10 million SNPs are thought to exist in the human genome, with an estimated 2 common missense (i.e., amino acid changing) variants per gene (e.g., Cargill *et al.*[18]). It is likely that only a subset (perhaps 50 000–250 000) of the total number of SNPs in the human genome will actually confer small to moderate effects on phenotypes (the biochemical or physiological manifestation of gene expression) that are causally related to disease risk.[19] Finally, we also recognize that the genome is not simply a linear nucleotide sequence, but that population genomic structure exists in which regions as large as 100 kilobases (a kilobase being a thousand nucleotides, or bases) in length define units that remain intact over evolutionary time.[20] These regions define genomic block structure that may define haplotypes, which are sets of genetic variants that are transmitted as a unit across generations. Thus, the complexity of genome structure and genetic variability that influences response to medications provides unique challenges to molecular pharmacoepidemiology.

Pharmacogenetics and Pharmacogenomics

While the term *pharmacogenetics* is predominantly applied to the study of how genetic variability is responsible for differences in patients' responses to drug exposure, the term *pharmacogenomics*, along with including studies of genetic variability on drug response, also encompasses approaches simultaneously considering data about thousands of genotypes in drug discovery and development, as well as responses in gene expression to existing medications.[21,22] Although the term "pharmacogenetics" is sometimes used synonymously with pharmacogenomics, the former usually refers to a candidate-gene approach as opposed to a genome-wide approach in pharmacogenomics (both discussed later in this chapter).

THE INTERFACE OF PHARMACOGENETICS AND PHARMACOGENOMICS WITH MOLECULAR PHARMACOEPIDEMIOLOGY

Pharmacogenetic and pharmacogenomic studies usually are designed to examine intermediate endpoints between drugs and outcomes (such as drug levels, pharmacodynamic properties, or surrogate markers of drug effects) and often rely on detailed measurements of these surrogates in small groups of patients in highly controlled settings. Molecular pharmacoepidemiology focuses on the effects of genetics on clinical outcomes and uses larger observational and experimental methods to evaluate the effectiveness and safety of drug treatment in the population. Molecular pharmacoepidemiology uses similar methods as pharmacoepidemiology to answer questions related to the effects of genes on drug response. Thus, molecular pharmacoepidemiology answers questions related to:

1. the population prevalence of SNPs and other genetic variants;
2. evaluating how these SNPs alter disease outcomes;
3. assessing the impact of gene–drug and gene–gene interactions on disease risk;
4. evaluating the usefulness and impact of genetic tests in populations exposed, or to be exposed, to drugs.

There are, however, some aspects of molecular pharmacoepidemiology that differ from the rest of pharmacoepidemiology. These include the need to understand the complex relationship between medication response and the vast number of potential molecular and genetic influences on this response; a focus on interactions among these factors and interactions between genes and environment (including other medications) that raise issues of sample size has led to interest in novel designs; and the need to parse out the most likely associations between genes and drug response from among the massive number of potentially important genes identified through bioinformatics (the science of developing and utilizing computer databases and algorithms to accelerate and enhance biological research). As stated previously, the basic science of epidemiology underlies molecular pharmacoepidemiology just as it underlies all pharmacoepidemiology. What is different is the need for approaches that can deal with the vast number of potential genetic influences on outcomes; the possibility that "putative" genes associated with drug response may not be the actual causal genes, but rather a gene near the causal gene on the chromosome in the population studied (and that may not be similarly linked in other populations); the potential that multiple genes, each with a relatively small effect, work together to alter drug response; and the focus on complex interactions between and among genes, drugs, and environment. By discussing the potential approaches to these challenges in this chapter, it is hoped that both the similarities and differences between pharmacoepidemiology and molecular pharmacoepidemiology will be made clear.

CLINICAL PROBLEMS TO BE ADDRESSED BY PHARMACOEPIDEMIOLOGIC RESEARCH

Currently, there are relatively few examples of studies that have evaluated the association between genes and clinical outcomes.[23] The number of studies is likely to expand rapidly with our increasing understanding of the genome and improvements and developments in study design and statistical techniques. It is useful to conceptualize clinical problems in molecular pharmacoepidemiology by thinking about the mechanism by which genes can affect drug response.

THREE WAYS THAT GENES CAN AFFECT DRUG RESPONSE

The effect that a medication has on an individual can be affected at many points along the pathway of drug distribution and action. This includes absorption and distribution of medications to the site of action, interaction of the medication with its targets, metabolism of the drug, and drug excretion (see Chapter 4).[5,21,22,24] These mechanisms can be categorized into three general routes by which genes can affect a drug response: pharmacokinetic, pharmacodynamic, and gene–drug interactions in the causal pathway of disease. These will be discussed in turn below.

Pharmacokinetic Gene–Drug Interactions

Genes may influence the pharmacokinetics of a drug by altering its metabolism, absorption, or distribution. As discussed previously, the fact that different individuals might metabolize medications differently has been well known for decades (see also Chapter 4). Metabolism of medications can either inactivate their effect or convert an inactive prodrug into a therapeutically active compound. Drugs can be metabolized either through Phase I reactions (oxidation, reduction, and hydrolysis) or Phase II (conjugation) reactions (e.g., methylation).[25] The genes that are responsible for variable metabolism of medications are those that code for various enzyme systems, especially the cytochrome P450 enzymes.

The gene encoding CYP2D6 represents a good example of the various ways in which polymorphisms can alter drug response. Some of the genetic variants lead to low or no activity of the CYP2D6 enzyme whereas some individuals have multiple copies of the gene, leading to increased metabolism of drugs. A specific example is the clinically relevant association between polymorphism of CYP2D6 and the risk of antipsychotic-induced extrapyramidal syndromes, as measured by the need for antiparkinsonian medication. In a case–control study by Schillevoort *et al.* patients using the CYP2D6-dependent antipsychotic drugs (e.g., haloperidol) who were poor metabolizers were more than four times more likely to need antiparkinsonian

medication than the extensive metabolizers (odds ratio 4.4; 95% confidence interval (CI) 1.1–17.7).[26] An increased risk was not observed for patients using non-CYP2D6-dependent antipsychotic drugs (odds ratio 1.2; 95% CI 0.2–6.8). The decreased metabolic activity of CYP2D6 may also lead to lower drug efficacy, as illustrated previously for codeine, which is a prodrug that is metabolized to the active metabolite, morphine, by CYP2D6.[17,27] It has been estimated that approximately 6–10% of Caucasians have variants that result in CYP2D6 genotypes that encode dysfunctional or inactive CYP2D6 enzyme, in whom codeine is an ineffective analgesic.[9]

The genetic polymorphism of thiopurine methyltransferase (TPMT) is another example, and is one of the most developed examples of pharmacogenetics, with particular clinical relevance for treating cancer patients.[10,28,29] In its usual state, TPMT metabolizes thiopurine drugs, which would otherwise be toxic if not excreted. In approximately 90% of individuals TPMT activity is high and allows normal drug excretion. In 10% activity is intermediate due to the presence of a heterozygous variant in the TPMT gene. In 0.3% activity is so low (due to a homozygous variant in the TPMT gene) that patients using drugs such as azathioprine, mercaptopurine, or thioguanine accumulate excessive concentrations of the active thioguanine nucleotides, leading to severe hematological toxicity. Thus, TPMT genotyping can be determined prior to treatment with these agents to avoid potential toxicities.[30] Alternatively, as in usual clinical practice, individuals who experience treatment-related toxicities may be genotyped for TPMT and this may influence the course of further treatments.

In addition to metabolism, genes that alter the absorption and distribution of medications may also alter drug levels at tissue targets. These include, for example, genes that code for transporter proteins such as the ATP-binding cassette transporter proteins (ABCB, also known as the multidrug-resistance [MDR]-1 gene),[31] which has polymorphisms that have been associated with, for example, resistance to antiepileptic drugs.[32] It has been found that patients with drug-resistant epilepsy (approximately one of three patients with epilepsy is a nonresponder) are more likely to have the CC polymorphism of ABCB1, which is associated with increased expression of this transporter drug-efflux protein (odds ratio, 2.66; 95% CI 1.32–5.38).[32] Of note, and consistent with the complexities of molecular pharmacoepidemiologic research noted later, the ABCB1 polymorphism fell within an extensive block of linkage disequilibrium (LD). LD is defined by a region in which multiple genetic variants (e.g., SNPs) are correlated with one another due to population and evolutionary genetic history. As a result, an

SNP may be statistically associated with disease risk, but is also in LD with the true causative SNP. Therefore, the SNP under study may not itself be causal but simply linked to a true causal variant.[32] One of the major challenges in genetics research at this time is developing methods that can identify the true causal variant(s) that may reside in an LD block.

Pharmacodynamic Gene–Drug Interactions

Once a drug is absorbed and transported to its target site, its effect may be altered by differences in the response of drug targets. Therefore, polymorphisms in genes that code for drug targets may alter the response of an individual to a medication.

This is well illustrated by the polymorphisms of the $\beta(2)$-adrenergic receptor ($\beta(2)$-AR), known for their role in affecting response to β-agonists (e.g., albuterol) in asthma patients. In particular, the coding variants at position 16 within the $\beta(2)$-AR gene ($\beta(2)$-AR-16) have been shown to be important in determining patient response to albuterol treatment.[11] Israel et al. showed that the Arg-Arg genotype at $\beta(2)$-AR-16 was positively associated with clinical response to albuterol in patients who used this drug in an as-needed fashion.[11] However, patients with the same genotype showed a decrease in response after regular use of albuterol. The Gly-Gly genotype at $\beta(2)$-AR-16 was unaffected by regular use. This example shows that the clinical effects of genetic variants should be interpreted in the context of patterns of use of the drug regimen over time, in particular in cases where receptor kinetics (e.g., up- and downregulation of the receptor) play a critical role.

Pharmacodynamic gene–drug interactions may also result in mixed responses in terms of intended and non-intended effects. For example, the treatment of patients with schizophrenia is still unsatisfactory because of the highly variable and frequently poor response profiles of antipsychotic drugs.[33] It is thought that dopamine receptors play an important role in both achieving the wanted therapeutic benefits and the occurrence of side effects (e.g., drug-induced tardive dyskinesia and parkinsonism) with these drugs. It appears as though there is a complex interplay between available antipsychotics and an array of dopamine D2, D3, and D4 receptor actions. This example of pharmacodynamic drug–gene interactions illustrates that therapeutic responses are unlikely to be associated with a single polymorphism, in particular when the same receptor panel is responsible for both therapeutic and adverse responses.

Thus, pharmacodynamic gene–drug interactions may also affect the risk of adverse reactions. Another example is a polymorphism in the gene coding for the bradykinin B2 receptor that has been associated with an increased risk of angiotensin converting enzyme (ACE) inhibitor-induced cough.[34] Cough is one of the most frequently seen adverse drug reactions (ADRs) in ACE therapy and very often a reason for discontinuation of therapy. The TT genotype and T allele of the human bradykinin B(2) receptor gene are found to be significantly higher in subjects with cough and it may, therefore, be possible to predict in advance those who will cough on ACE inhibitors.[34]

Gene–Drug Interactions and the Causal Pathway of Disease

Along with altering the pharmacokinetic and pharmacodynamic properties of medications, genetic polymorphisms may also alter the disease state that is the target of drug therapy. As an example, hypertension is widely acknowledged to be a complex phenotype that involves many regulatory systems. These regulatory systems are associated with the responsiveness to different drug therapies. Medications that work by a particular mechanism, such as the increased sodium excretion of some antihypertensive medications, may have different effects depending on the susceptibility of the patient to the effects of the drug. One key polymorphism is in the α-adducin gene and its relation to treatment for hypertension. Cusi et al. found a significant association between the α-adducin locus (the site of the gene) and essential hypertension and greater sensitivity to changes in sodium balance among patients with the polymorphism of the gene.[35] These findings fueled various studies to evaluate whether the α-adducin polymorphism may also be useful to identify hypertensive patients who can optimally benefit from diuretic treatment. A case–control study has suggested that those with the α-adducin polymorphism may be more likely to benefit from diuretic therapy than those without the polymorphism.[8]

Genetic variability in disease states also can be critical for tailoring drug therapy to patients with a specific genotype related both to the disease and drug response. One example is the humanized monoclonal antibody trastuzumab (Herceptin®), which is used for the treatment of metastatic breast cancer patients with overexpression of the HER2 oncogene. The HER2 protein is thought to be a unique target for trastuzumab therapy in patients with this genetically associated overexpression, occurring in 10–34% of females with breast cancer.[12] The case of trastuzumab, together with another anti-cancer drug, imatinib, which is especially effective in patients with Philadelphia chromosome-positive leukemias, has pioneered successful genetically targeted therapy.[36]

Genetic polymorphisms that alter disease states can also play a role in drug safety. For example, factor V Leiden mutation, present in about one out of twenty Caucasians, is considered an important genetic risk factor for deep vein thrombosis and embolism.[37] A relative risk of about 30 in factor V carriers and users of oral contraceptives compared to non-carriers and non-oral-contraceptive users has been reported. This gene–drug interaction has recently also been linked to the differential thrombotic risk associated with third-generation oral contraceptives compared with second-generation oral contraceptives.[13] Despite this strong association, Vandenbroucke *et al.* have calculated that mass screening for factor V would result in denial of oral contraceptives for about 20 000 women positive for this mutation in order to prevent 1 death.[38] Therefore, they came to the conclusion that reviewing personal and family thrombosis history, and only if suitable, factor V testing before prescribing oral contraceptives, is the recommended approach to avoid this adverse gene–drug interaction.[38] This highlights another important role of molecular pharmacoepidemiology: determining the utility and cost-effectiveness of genetic screening to guide drug therapy.

The Interplay of Various Mechanisms

It is useful to conceptualize how the effects of genetic polymorphisms at different stages of drug disposition and response might influence an individual's response to a medication. As an example, an individual may have a genotype that alters the metabolism of the drug, the receptor for the drug, or both.[22] Depending on the combination of these genotypes, the individual might have a different response in terms of both efficacy and toxicity (see Table 37.2). In the simplified

Table 37.2. Hypothetical response to medications by genetic variants in metabolism and receptor genes

Gene affecting metabolism[a]	Gene affecting receptor response[a]	Drug response	
		Efficacy (%)	Toxicity (%)
Wild-type	Wild-type	70	2
Variant	Wild-type	85	20
Wild-type	Variant	20	2
Variant	Variant	35	20

[a] Wild-type associated with normal metabolism or receptor response and variants associated with reduced metabolism or receptor response.
Source: Modified from Evans and McLeod.[22]

example in Table 37.2, there is one genetic variant that alters drug metabolism and one genetic variant that alters receptor response to a medication of interest. In this example, among those who are homozygous for the alleles that encode normal drug metabolism and normal receptor response, there is relatively high efficacy and low toxicity. However, among those who have a variant that reduces drug metabolism, efficacy at a standard dose could actually be greater (assuming a linear dose–response relationship within the possible drug levels of the medication) but toxicity could be increased (if dose-related). Among those who have a variant that reduces receptor response, drug efficacy will be reduced while toxicity may not be different from those who carry genotypes that are not associated with impaired receptor response (assuming that toxicity is not related to the receptor responsible for efficacy). Among those who have variants for both genes, efficacy could be reduced because of the receptor variant (perhaps not as substantially as those with an isolated variant of the receptor gene because of the higher effective dose resulting from the metabolism gene variant), while toxicity could be increased because of the metabolism variant.

A summary of the specific examples cited earlier and their relationship with each of the three mechanisms of genetic variability in drug response is shown in Table 37.3.

SOME EXAMPLES OF THE PROGRESSION AND APPLICATION OF MOLECULAR PHARMACOEPIDEMIOLOGIC RESEARCH

Medications with a narrow therapeutic ratio are good targets for the use of molecular pharmacoepidemiology to improve the use and application of medications. One example is warfarin. This example illustrates both the logical progression of pharmacogenetics through molecular pharmacoepidemiology and the complexity of moving pharmacogenetic data into practice. The enzyme primarily responsible for the metabolism of warfarin to its inactive form is the cytochrome P450 2C9 variant (CYP2C9).[39–41] Pharmacogenetic studies identified polymorphisms in CYP2C9 that led to altered metabolism of warfarin.[42,43] One of the first molecular pharmacoepidemiology studies examining the clinical relevance of the CYP2C9 variants was a case–control study that reported that the odds ratio (OR) for a low warfarin dose requirement was 6.2 (95% CI 2.5, 15.6) among those having one or more CYP2C9 variant alleles compared with a control population with normal warfarin dose requirements.[44] The OR was elevated both in those with only one variant allele (i.e., heterozygotes: OR 2.7; 95% CI 1.2, 5.9) and in those with two variant alleles to an even greater extent (i.e., homozygotes:

Table 37.3. Pathways of gene–drug interactions and some relevant examples

Pharmacokinetic	Pharmacodynamic	In pathway of disease
CYP2D6 "poor metabolizer" type and antipsychotic-induced parkinsonism	β_2-adrenergic receptor (β2AR) and response to β_2 agonists	α-Adducin and salt-sensitive form (diuretic response) of hypertension
Thiopurine methyl-transferase defect and toxicity of cancer drugs (e.g., azathioprine)	Dopamine-4 receptor and response to antipsychotics	HER2-overexpression and response to Herceptin®
ABCB1 transporter gene and multidrug resistance in epilepsy (MDR1)	Bradykinin B(2) receptor gene and ACE induced cough	Factor V Leiden and VTE risk in OC users

OR 7.8; 95% CI 1.9, 32.1). Patients on low doses of warfarin also were more likely to have difficulty with anticoagulation control during the first week of therapy and more likely to have bleeding complications, based on unadjusted analyses. By design, this study selected subjects based on warfarin dose requirements, not genotype, and could only determine that lower doses of warfarin were more common among those with CYP2C9 variants. The other associations noted were between lower dose requirements and bleeding, not between genotype and bleeding. Certainly, there could be other factors related to lower dose requirements that increased the risk of bleeding, independent of genotype, but they were not examined. In addition, the study only examined anticoagulation control during the first week of warfarin therapy. A subsequent retrospective cohort study confirmed the lower dose requirement of patients with the genetic variant of CYP2C9, but did not examine clinical outcomes.[45] In order to address the clinically relevant question of bleeding, another retrospective cohort study was performed that demonstrated an increased risk of bleeding among patients followed in an anticoagulation clinic who had at least one variant of the CYP2C9 genotype.[46] The relatively small size of the study, retrospective nature, and selected population leave unanswered the question of whether there is an independent effect of CYP2C9 variants on the risk of clinical outcomes throughout the course of anticoagulation therapy, whether specific variants or combinations of variants (e.g., heterozygotes with only one variant allele versus homozygotes with two variant alleles) have different effects, and whether knowing that a patient carries a variant can alter therapy in a way that can reduce risk. Of note, there is still a large amount of inter-individual variability in response to warfarin within CYP2C9 genotypes, suggesting that other factors, both clinical and perhaps genetic, influence the response to the medication.[47] Another pharmacogenetic study, which identified other genes that might, in addition to CYP2C9, alter the response to warfarin, illustrates nicely the complexity of understanding the genetic variability of medication response

and the need for increasingly complex molecular pharmacoepidemiology studies.[48]

The ultimate question that molecular pharmacoepidemiology studies will have to answer is whether knowing that a patient carries a polymorphism or polymorphisms will lead to better outcomes. The recent development of an algorithm to predict a maintenance warfarin dose that combines clinical and genetic data suggests that improvements may be made by incorporating genetic data into dosing algorithms.[49] However, further pharmacoepidemiology studies, including prospective testing of genetic-based dosing algorithms, will be needed to determine if clinical outcomes can be improved by including genetic data when treating patients on warfarin.

Another pertinent example of how pharmacogenetics could lead to molecular pharmacoepidemiology studies that may guide decision makers in safe prescribing, and also fuel new drug development, is the HIV drug abacavir. Clinical trials have shown that severe hypersensitivity reaction to abacavir (HIV reverse transcriptase inhibitor) is seen in 4% of patients and results in switching to other HIV therapy.[50] These severe reactions could have resulted in cessation of development of the drug. However, the occurrence of hypersensitivity has been linked to the genetic variant HLA B5701 (data so far show that 55% of patients with the reaction are carriers of this SNP; 1% of patients without the reaction are carriers), raising the possibility that genetic screening could allow safe use of the drug.[51]

METHODOLOGIC PROBLEMS TO BE ADDRESSED BY PHARMACOEPIDEMIOLOGIC RESEARCH

As previously discussed, the basic science of molecular pharmacoepidemiology is the same basic science underlying pharmacoepidemiology. Therefore, the same methodological problems of pharmacoepidemiology must be addressed in molecular pharmacoepidemiology. These problems include those of chance and power, confounding, bias, and generalizability (see Chapters 2 and 3).

However, the complex relationship between medication response and molecular and genetic factors generates some unique challenges in molecular pharmacoepidemiology. Many of these challenges derive from the large number of potential genetic variants that can modify the response to a single drug, the possibility that there is a small individual effect of any one of these genes, the low prevalence of many genes, and the possibility that a presumptive gene–drug response relationship may be confounded by the racial and ethnic mixture of the population studied.[19,52] Thus, the methodological challenges of molecular pharmacoepidemiology are closely related to issues of statistical interactions, type I and type II errors, and confounding. First and foremost, however, molecular pharmacoepidemiology studies rely on proper identification of putative genes. In addition, in all research of this type, usage of appropriate laboratory methods, including the use of high-throughput genotyping technologies, is necessary. Similarly, appropriate quality control procedures must be considered to obtain meaningful data for research and clinical applications. This section will begin by highlighting the nature of gene discovery and then focus on the methodological challenges of studying interactions, minimizing type I and type II errors, and accounting for confounding, particularly by population admixture (defined below).

GENE DISCOVERY: GENOME-WIDE VERSUS CANDIDATE GENE APPROACHES

There are two primary, but not mutually exclusive, approaches for gene discovery: candidate gene association studies and genome-wide scans. In the former, genes are selected for study on the basis of their plausible biological relevance to drug response. In the latter, randomly selected DNA sequences are examined for associations with outcomes, initially irrespective of biological plausibility. Each approach has strengths and limitations. Candidate gene studies have the advantage of using knowledge of molecular biology, biochemistry, and physiology to elucidate biologically plausible associations of genotypes with outcomes of interest. However, it remains a challenge to choose appropriate candidate genes because the relevant biological information needed to choose candidates may not be available. A major challenge facing studies that measure the statistical relationship of a clinical outcome with candidate disease genes is to characterize the functional significance of genetic variants.

The amount of genomic information available vastly exceeds the information about the function of variants being applied in human disease studies. In contrast, genome-wide approaches avoid the need for biological plausibility in identifying genes for study, and instead use large-scale genetic or genomic information to search for genes with effects on phenotypes of interest. These approaches use the wealth of genomic information to scan the genome for important genes. However, the identification of these genes leads directly back to the need for biological information that explains the causal mechanism for the gene's association effect. Ultimately, genome-wide scans will identify genes that will become candidate genes, and will thus also require knowledge about gene function. A major limitation of genome-wide approaches is the limited ability to assess gene and variant function based on nucleotide sequence information alone. This is most likely to be true when variants do not alter an amino acid or disrupt a well-characterized motif that affects protein function or structure. It is likely that only a small subset of these variants will actually confer small to moderate effects on phenotypes that are causally related to disease risk.[19]

Some possible approaches to these challenges are discussed in the "Currently available solutions" section.

INTERACTIONS

Along with examining the direct effect of genes and other biomarkers on outcomes, molecular pharmacoepidemiology studies must often be designed to examine effect modification between medication use and the genes or biomarkers of interest. That is, the primary measure of interest is often the role of biomarker information on the effect of a medication. For purposes of simplicity, this discussion will use genetic variability as the measure of interest.

Effect modification is present if there is a difference in the effect of the medication depending on the presence or absence of the genetic variant. This difference can be either on the multiplicative or additive scale. On the multiplicative scale, interaction is present if the effect of the combination of the genotype and medication exposure relative to neither is greater than the product of the measure of effect of each (genotype alone or medication alone) relative to neither. On the additive scale, interaction is present if the effect of the combination of the genotype and medication exposure is greater than the sum of the measures of effect of each alone, again all relative to neither.[53]

For studies examining a dichotomous medication exposure (e.g., medication use versus nonuse), a dichotomous genetic exposure (e.g., presence versus absence of a genetic variant), and a dichotomous outcome (e.g., myocardial infarction occurrence versus none), there are two ways to consider presenting and analyzing interactions.[54] The first is as a stratified analysis, comparing the effect of medication exposure versus non-exposure on the outcome in two strata: those with the genetic variant and those without (e.g., see Table 37.4). The second is to present a 2×4 table (also shown in Table 37.4). In the first example (stratified analyses), one compares the effect of the medication among those with the genetic variant to the effect of the medication among those without the genetic variant. In the second example (the 2×4 table), the effect of each combination of exposure (i.e., with both genetic variant and medication; with genetic variant minus medication; with medication minus genetic variant) is determined relative to the lack of exposure to either. The advantage of the 2×4 table is that it presents separately the effect of the drug, the gene, and both relative to those without the genetic variant and without medication exposure. In addition, presentation of the data as a 2×4 table allows one to directly compute both multiplicative and additive interactions.[54] In the example given in Table 37.4, multiplicative interaction would be assessed by comparing the odds ratio for the combination of genotype and medication exposure to the product of the odds ratios for medication alone and genotype alone. Multiplicative interaction would be considered present if the odds ratios for the combination of medication and genotype (A in Table 37.4) was greater than the product of the odds ratios for either alone (B $\times$ C). Additive interaction would be considered present if the odds ratio for the combination of genotype and medication use (A) was greater than the sum of the odds ratios for medication use alone and genotype alone (B + C). The 2×4 table also allows the direct assessment of the number of subjects in

each group along with the respective confidence interval for the measured effect in each of the groups, making it possible to directly observe the precision of the estimates in each of the groups and therefore better understand the power of the study. Furthermore, attributable fractions can be computed separately for each of the exposures alone and for the combination of exposures. In general, we believe that presenting the data in both manners is optimal because it allows the reader to understand the effect of each of the exposures (2×4 table) as well as the effect of the medication in the presence or absence of the genotypic variant (stratified table).

TYPE I ERROR

The chance of type I error (concluding there is an association when in fact one does not exist) increases with the number of statistical tests performed on any one data set (see also Chapter 3).[55] It is easy to appreciate the potential for type I error in a molecular pharmacoepidemiology study that examines, simultaneously, the effects of multiple genetic factors, the effects of multiple nongenetic factors, and the interaction between and among these factors.[55–57] One of the reasons cited for nonreplication of study findings in molecular pharmacoepidemiology is type I error.[58] Limiting the number of associations examined to those of specific candidate genetic variants that are suspected of being associated with the outcome is a "standard" method to limit type I error in pharmacoepidemiology.[59] However, with increasing emphasis in molecular pharmacoepidemiology studies on identifying all variants within a gene and examining multiple interactions, this method of limiting type I error may not be

Table 37.4. Two ways to present effect modification in molecular pharmacoepidemiologic studies using case–control study as a model

Genotype	Medication	Cases	Controls	Odds ratio	Information provided
Stratified analysis					
+	+	a	b	ad/bc	Effect of medication versus no medication among
	–	c	d		those with the genotype
–	+	e	f	eh/fg	Effect of medication versus no medication among
	–	g	h		those without the genotype
2 × 4 Table					
+	+	a	b	ah/bg = A	Joint genotype and medication versus neither
+	–	c	d	ch/dg = B	Genotype alone versus neither
–	+	e	f	eh/fg = C	Medication alone versus neither
–	–	g	h	Reference	Reference group

Source: Modified from Botto *et al.*[54]

desirable.[60] Some other currently available solutions are discussed in the next section.

TYPE II ERROR

Because it has been hypothesized that much of the genetic variability leading to phenotypic expression of complex diseases results from the relatively small effects of many relatively low prevalence genetic variants,[61] the ability to detect a gene–response relationship is likely to require relatively large sample sizes to avoid type II error (concluding there is no association when in fact one does exist).[62] The sample size requirements for studies that examine the direct effect of genes on medication response will be the same as the requirements for examining direct effects of individual risk factors on outcomes. With relatively low prevalences of polymorphisms and often low incidence of outcomes (particularly in studies of adverse drug reactions), large sample sizes are typically required to detect even modest associations. For such studies, the case–control design has become a particularly favored approach for molecular pharmacoepidemiology studies because of its ability to select participants based on the outcome of interest (and its ability to study the effects of multiple potential genotypes in the same study).

Studies that are designed to examine the interaction between a genetic polymorphism and a medication will require even larger sample sizes.[63] This is because such studies need to be powered to compare those with both the genetic polymorphism and the medication exposure with those who have neither. As an example, the previously mentioned case–control study of the α-adducin gene and diuretic therapy in patients with treated hypertension examined the effects of the genetic polymorphism, the diuretic therapy, and both in combination.[8] There were a total of 1038 participants in the study. When comparing the effect of diuretic use with no use and comparing the effect of the genetic variant with the nonvariant allele, all 1038 participants were available for comparison (Table 37.5). However, when examining the effect of diuretic therapy versus nonuse among those with the genetic variant, only 385 participants contributed to the analyses. Of note, this study presented the data for interaction in the two ways presented in Table 37.4.

In order to minimize false negative findings, further efforts must be made to ensure adequate sample sizes, both for pharmacology studies as well as for molecular pharmacoepidemiology studies. Because of the complex nature of medication response, and the likelihood that at least several genes are responsible for the variability in drug response, studies designed to test for multiple gene–gene and

Table 37.5. Gene-exposure interaction analysis in a case–control study

Diuretic use	Adducin variant	Cases	Controls	Odds ratio (OR) for stroke or myocardial infarction
0	0	A_{00} 103	B_{00} 248	1.0
0	1	A_{01} 85	B_{01} 131	1.56
1	0	A_{10} 94	B_{10} 208	1.09
1	1	A_{11} 41	B_{11} 128	0.77

Case control OR for diuretic use in variant carriers: $OR_{variant} = A_{11}B_{01}/A_{01}B_{11} = 41 \times 131/85 \times 128 = 0.49$
Case control OR for diuretic use in wild-type carriers: $OR_{wild\text{-}type} = A_{10}B_{00}/A_{00}B_{10} = 94 \times 248/103 \times 208 = 1.09$
Synergy index $= OR_{variant}/OR_{wild\text{-}type} = 0.45$
Case-only OR $= A_{11}A_{00}/A_{10}A_{01} = 41 \times 103/94 \times 85 = 0.53$
Source: Adapted from Psaty et al.[8]

gene–environment interactions (including other medications, environmental factors, adherence to medications, and clinical factors) will, similarly, require large sample sizes.

CONFOUNDING BY POPULATION ADMIXTURE

When there is evidence that baseline disease risks and genotype frequencies differ among ethnicities, the conditions for population stratification (i.e., population admixture or confounding by ethnicity) may be met.[64] Population admixture is simply a manifestation of confounding by ethnicity, which can occur if both baseline disease risks and genotype frequency vary across ethnicity. The African American population is an admixture of at least three major ethnicities (African, European Caucasian, and Native American). Wacholder et al.[64] demonstrated that the larger the number of ethnicities involved in an admixed population, the less likely that population stratification can be the explanation for an observation. Millikan[65] and Wang et al.[66] also reported that a minimal bias in point estimates is likely in African American populations, suggesting that point estimates of association will not usually be influenced by population stratification in studies that involve African American populations under most usual circumstances. Ardlie et al.[67] used empirical data to show that carefully matched, moderate-sized case–control samples in Caucasian populations are unlikely to contain levels of population admixture that would result in significantly inflated numbers of false-positive associations. They did observe the potential for population structure to exist in African American populations, but this structure was eliminated by removing recent African or Caribbean immigrants, and limiting study samples to resident African Americans. Furthermore, Cardon and Palmer[68] argued that poor study design may be more important than population stratification in conferring bias to association studies. Thus, based on the current literature that evaluates the effects of confounding by ethnicity overall, and specifically in African Americans, there is little evidence that population stratification is a likely explanation for bias in point estimates or incorrect inferences.[64] Nonetheless, population admixture must be considered in designing and analyzing molecular pharmacoepidemiology studies to ensure that adequate adjustment can be made for this potential confounder. New approaches to addressing population admixture are presented in the following section.

CURRENTLY AVAILABLE SOLUTIONS

GENE DISCOVERY: GENOME-WIDE VERSUS CANDIDATE GENE APPROACHES

As discussed in the "Methodologic problems" section, there are two primary approaches for gene discovery: candidate gene association studies and genome-wide screens. The latter approach relies on linkage disequilibrium (LD), defined above as the correlation between alleles at two loci. The genome-wide association approach uses DNA sequence variation (e.g., SNPs) found throughout the genome, and does not rely on *a priori* functional knowledge of gene function. Therefore, this approach can be used to identify new candidate genes or regions. These approaches rely on the potential for truly causative gene effects to be detected using genetic variants that may not have a functional effect. A number of factors influence the success of these studies. Appropriate epidemiological study designs and adequate statistical power remain essential. Thorough characterization of LD is essential for replication of genome-wide association studies: the haplotype mapping (HapMap) consortium and other groups have shown that the extent of LD varies by ethnicity, which may affect the ability to replicate findings in subsequent studies.[61] Particularly informative SNPs that best characterize a genomic region can be used to limit the amount of laboratory and analytical work in haplotype-based studies.[69] It has been hypothesized that studies that consider LD involving multiple SNPs in a genomic region (i.e., a haplotype) can increase power to detect associations by 15–50% compared with analyses involving only individual SNPs.[70] Finally, even if genome-wide scans may identify

markers associated with the trait of interest, a challenge will be to identify the causative SNPs.

Clearly, candidate gene and genome-wide approaches are not mutually exclusive. It has been suggested that gene discovery should focus on SNPs or haplotypes based on: (i) strong prior information about biological pathways or linkage data; (ii) information about the functional significance of an SNP or haplotype; and/or (iii) studies that start with a "simple" haplotype involving a small number of SNPs that can be expanded to increase the number of SNPs that constitute haplotypes in a specific region of the genome.[61] Figure 37.1 presents a simple paradigm for considering SNPs and haplotypes. On the one hand, investigators can begin by studying simple haplotypes, and then move to more complete haplotype characterization. Similarly, investigators can study candidate genes, then move to characterization of haplotypes in the candidate region to better understand the spectrum of genetic variability that may be associated with the trait of interest. Ultimately, both individual SNPs with known functional significance as well as haplotype data may be required to fully understand the basis of human pharmacogenetics. Haplotypes will capture information about the total genetic variability in a genomic region, but knowledge about etiologically significant functional genetic changes will still be required to understand the biological basis of phenotypically relevant associations.

INTERACTIONS

Along with traditional case–control and cohort studies, the case-only study can be used for molecular pharmacoepidemiology studies designed to examine interactions between genes and medications.[71,72] In this design, cases, representing those with the outcome or phenotype of interest, are selected for study, and the association between genetic variants and

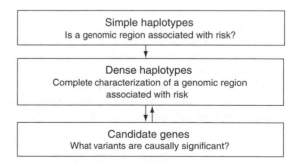

Figure 37.1. Paradigm for candidate gene and haplotype-based association studies.

medication use is determined among these cases. Under the assumption that there is no association between the gene and medication exposure among those without the disease (i.e., controls), the odds ratio for the association between genetic variants and medication use in the cases is equivalent to the synergy index on a multiplicative scale for a case–control study.[71] (The synergy index is the odds ratio for medication use versus the outcome of interest in those with the variant alleles divided by the odds ratio for medication use versus the outcome in those without the variant alleles—see Table 37.5 footnote.) In other words, assuming that the use of the medication is unrelated to the genotype, the case-only study provides a valid measure of the interaction of the genotype and the medication on the risk of the outcome.

One strength of the case-only study design is that it eliminates the need to identify controls, which is often a major methodological and logistical challenge in case–control studies. In addition, the case-only study can result in greater precision in estimating interactions compared with case–control analyses.[71,72] It also is possible to use the case-only approach to estimate interactions between genes and medications in large-scale registries of people with diseases or disease outcomes (e.g., cancer registries with genotypes and medication information available).[54]

There are several limitations of the case-only design.[71] As stated above, the design relies on the assumption of independence between exposure (medication use) and genotype. Although this assumption may be valid (in the absence of performing genotyping, it may be reasonable to assume that the use of the medication is not related to patients' genotypes), it is certainly possible that the genotype, by altering response to medications targeted at a specific disease, could affect the medications being prescribed to patients. For example, the use of a particular antihypertensive medication may be related to prior success with other medications. Patients carrying genotypic variants that diminish the response to one class of antihypertensive medication may be more likely to be on other classes of antihypertensive medications. Thus, there would be an association between the genotype and the medication exposure. One way to minimize this possibility is to include only first-time prescriptions for hypertensive medications.

Another limitation of the case-only design is that it does not allow assessment of the independent effects of medication use or genotype on outcome. Further, the assessment of interaction can only be interpreted on a multiplicative scale.

TYPE I ERROR AND REPLICATION

Given concerns of type I error (along with other methodological concerns such as uncontrolled confounding, publication bias, and linkage disequilibrium), a key issue in molecular epidemiology is the ability to replicate association study findings. Replication of association studies is required not only to identify biologically plausible causative associations, but also to conclude that a candidate gene has a meaningful etiological effect. Lohmueller et al.[58] observed that many associations are not replicated. This lack of replication can be explained by false positive reports (e.g., spurious associations), by false negative reports (e.g., studies that are insufficiently powerful to identify the association), or by actual population differences (e.g., the true associations are different because of differences in genetic background, exposures, etc.). Given the perceived lack of consistency in association studies, what level of confidence can we have in associations reported to date?

Lohmueller et al.[58] addressed these issues by undertaking a meta-analysis of 25 inconsistent associations and 301 "replication" studies (i.e., by ignoring the initial positive report). Most initial associations were not replicated, but an excess (20%) of replicated associations were seen, while only 5% were expected under the null hypothesis. This replication is not solely due to publication bias, since one would have to hypothesize 40–80 negative studies were not reported rather than the average of 12 reported studies per association. Lohmueller et al. also concluded that it was unlikely that these replications represented false positives due to ethnic stratification. Different linkage disequilibrium patterns or other population patterns or population-specific modifiers (genes and/or environments) could also explain lack of replication, but this was unlikely to be a significant source of study inconsistency. The first positive reports also tended to be unreliable estimates for subsequently reported ORs,[73] perhaps due to the "winner's curse" phenomenon which predicts that the initial positive report overestimates the "true" value.[74] Indeed, 23 of 25 associations studied showed evidence for a "winner's curse." An additional consequence of this phenomenon is that replication studies may therefore require larger sample sizes since the actual replication effects may be smaller than suggested by the initial report. Despite these limitations, these data indicate that associations are replicable more often than expected by chance, and may therefore represent truly causative effects on disease.

In order to achieve believable, replicable association results, investigators must consider factors that influence the design, analysis, and interpretation of these studies. These include, as discussed above, adequate sample size, proper study design, and characterization of the study population, particularly when replication studies themselves are not comparable in terms of ethnicity or other confounding factors.

One approach to assessing for possible type I error is the use of "genomic controls." This approach uses the distribution of test statistics obtained for unlinked markers (genotypes at loci that lie in regions other than the location of the gene of interest) to adjust the usual chi square test for the association of interest. For example, if 20 unlinked markers are studied in addition to the candidate gene of interest, none of these 20 should be associated with disease if they are truly random markers with no biological effect. If one or more of these unlinked markers is associated with disease, this implies that the association represents a type I error because associations of these unlinked markers cannot be causally associated with disease, and therefore can only represent false positive associations. Therefore, the observation of associations with the unlinked markers is a measure of the potential for type I error. This approach is also useful for assessing for possible population admixture, as discussed below.

association studies, a number of analytical approaches exist to either circumvent problems imposed by population genetic structure, or that use this structure in gene identification.[79,80] The "structured association" approach identifies a set of individuals who are drawing their alleles from different background populations or ethnicities. This approach uses information about genotypes at loci that lie in regions other than the location of the gene of interest (i.e., "unlinked markers") to infer their ancestry and learn about population structure. It further uses the data derived from these unlinked markers to adjust the association test statistic. Using a similar conceptual model, the "genomic control," discussed above in "Type I Error and Replication," uses a similar conceptual model. If unlinked markers are associated with disease, one possible explanation is the presence of population admixture.

TYPE II ERROR

Reducing type II error essentially involves a logistical need to ensure adequate sample size (see also Chapter 3). One approach to increasing the sample size of molecular pharmacoepidemiology studies is to perform large, multicenter collaborative studies. Another is to assemble large, relatively homogenous populations for multiple studies, such as the deCode project.[75,76] This project has established a cohort of almost 100 000 inhabitants of Iceland with available genetic data that can be used for both population- and genome-wide linkage studies. This represents half of the total adult population of Iceland and includes more than 90% of people over the age of 65.[77] This project has also generated debate about the process of informed consent.[78]

Another potential solution to minimizing type II error is through meta-analysis, whereby smaller studies, which are, individually, not powered to detect specific associations (such as interactions) are combined in order to improve the ability to detect such associations (see Chapter 44). One particularly intriguing approach is the concept of prospective meta-analysis in which studies are planned or identified in advance of performing a meta-analysis so that important elements of study design complement each other across studies and important potential sources of bias that hamper the interpretation of retrospective meta-analyses can be avoided (see Chapter 44).

POPULATION ADMIXTURE

As presented above, although population stratification is unlikely to be a significant source of bias in epidemiological

THE FUTURE

Ultimately, the ability of genes and other biomarkers to improve patient care and outcomes will need to be tested in properly controlled studies, including randomized controlled trials. The positive and negative predictive value of carrying a genetic variant will be important determinants of the ability of the variant to improve outcomes. Those genetic variants with good test characteristics will still need to be evaluated in properly controlled trials. Such studies could examine several ways to incorporate genetic testing into clinical practice, including the use of genetic variants in dosing algorithms,[30,49] in selection of a specific therapeutic class of drug to treat a disease,[8] and in avoidance of using specific medications in those at high risk for adverse drug reactions.[34] Somewhat relatedly, the measurement of genotypes in randomized trials of medications is a powerful way to assess the effect of genetic variation on medication response in a relatively unbiased fashion.

The cost-effectiveness of such approaches is also of great interest because the addition of genetic testing adds cost to clinical care (see also Chapter 41). Veenstra and colleagues have developed a set of criteria for evaluating the potential clinical and economic benefits of pharmacogenetic testing.[23] These criteria include the severity of the outcome avoided, the availability of other means to monitor drug response without the need for additional pharmacogenetics testing, the strength of association between the genetic variants and clinically relevant outcomes, the availability of a rapid and relatively inexpensive assay, and the frequency of the variant alleles. In essence, these criteria could be applied to any new diagnostic test. Clearly, additional research will be needed to determine the cost-effectiveness of new biomarker and genetic tests as they are developed.

Just as for all research, the ethical, legal, and social implications of genetic testing must be considered and addressed.[5,81–83] (See also Chapter 38.) Pharmacogenetic testing raises issues of privacy concerns, access to health care services, and informed consent. For example, concern has been raised that the use of genetic testing could lead to targeting of therapies to only specific groups (ethnic or racial) of patients, ignoring others, and to loss of insurance coverage for certain groups of individuals.[83] There also is a concern that medicines will be developed only for the most common, commercially attractive, genotypes, leading to "orphan genotypes".[83,84] The previously mentioned cases of idiosyncratic side effects in susceptible patients based on genotyping also point to the question of whether it would be feasible to develop alternative drugs targeted to these nonresponders (e.g., carriers of HLA B5701 in the example of abacavir). For sure these would be "orphan drugs," according to current epidemiologic data on HIV and associated drug-induced side effects in the US and Europe. Would it then be economically realistic for the pharmaceutical industry to invest in such drugs? Subsetting of patients according to response to therapy based on gene–drug interactions may have a plethora of consequences for the pharmaceutical marketplace; some will be predictable and others will not. Although beyond the scope of discussion for this chapter, it is important to note that ethical, legal, and social implications of genetic testing in general are critically important issues that will need to be addressed along with the methodological challenges of molecular pharmacoepidemiologic research.[81]

Finally, it is important to recognize that genetic and other biomarkers are unlikely to fully explain the variability in drug response.[85,86] Continued efforts at characterizing other causes of drug failures and adverse reactions and understanding how these causes interact with genetic polymorphisms are critical to fully characterize the variability of drug response and to ultimately improve patient outcomes.

REFERENCES

1. Reidenberg MM. Evolving ways that drug therapy is individualized. *Clin Pharmacol Ther* 2003; **74**: 197–202.
2. Maitland-van der Zee AH, de Boer A, Leufkens HG. The interface between pharmacoepidemiology and pharmacogenetics. *Eur J Pharmacol* 2000; **410**: 121–30.
3. Kalow W, Tang BK, Endrenyi L. Hypothesis: comparisons of inter- and intra-individual variations can substitute for twin studies in drug research. *Pharmacogenetics* 1998; **8**: 283–9.
4. Phillips KA, Veenstra DL, Oren E, Lee JK, Sadee W. Potential role of pharmacogenomics in reducing adverse drug reactions: a systematic review. *JAMA* 2001; **286**: 2270–9.
5. Johnson JA. Pharmacogenetics: potential for individualized drug therapy through genetics. *Trends Genet* 2003; **19**: 660–6.
6. Roden DM. Cardiovascular pharmacogenomics. *Circulation* 2003; **108**: 3071–4.
7. Roden DM, George AL, Jr. The genetic basis of variability in drug responses. *Nat Rev Drug Discov* 2002; **1**: 37–44.
8. Psaty BM, Smith NL, Heckbert SR, Vos HL, Lemaitre RN, Reiner AP *et al.* Diuretic therapy, the alpha-adducin gene variant, and the risk of myocardial infarction or stroke in persons with treated hypertension. *JAMA* 2002; **287**: 1680–9.
9. Rogers JF, Nafziger AN, Bertino JS, Jr. Pharmacogenetics affects dosing, efficacy, and toxicity of cytochrome P450-metabolized drugs. *Am J Med* 2002; **113**: 746–50.
10. Krynetski E, Evans WE. Drug methylation in cancer therapy: lessons from the TPMT polymorphism. *Oncogene* 2003; **22**: 7403–13.
11. Israel E, Drazen JM, Liggett SB, Boushey HA, Cherniack RM, Chinchilli VM *et al.* The effect of polymorphisms of the beta(2)-adrenergic receptor on the response to regular use of albuterol in asthma. *Am J Respir Crit Care Med* 2000; **162**: 75–80.
12. Slamon DJ, Leyland-Jones B, Shak S, Fuchs H, Paton V, Bajamonde A *et al.* Use of chemotherapy plus a monoclonal antibody against HER2 for metastatic breast cancer that overexpresses HER2. *N Engl J Med* 2001; **344**: 783–792.
13. Kemmeren JM, Algra A, Meijers JC, Tans G, Bouma BN, Curvers J *et al.* Effect of second- and third-generation oral contraceptives on the protein C system in the absence or presence of the factor V Leiden mutation: a randomized trial. *Blood* 2004; **103**: 927–33.
14. Alving AS, Carson PE, Flanagan CL, Ickes CE. Enzymatic deficiency in primaquine-sensitive erythrocytes. *Science* 1956; **124**: 484–5.
15. Kalow W. Familial incidence of low pseudocholinesterase level. *Lancet* 1956; **268**: 576–7.
16. Evans DA, Manley KA, McKusick VA. Genetic control of isoniazid metabolism in man. *BMJ* 1960; **5197**: 485–91.
17. Sindrup SH, Brosen K. The pharmacogenetics of codeine hypoalgesia. *Pharmacogenetics* 1995; **5**: 335–46.
18. Cargill M, Altshuler D, Ireland J, Sklar P, Ardlie K, Patil N *et al.* Characterization of single-nucleotide polymorphisms in coding regions of human genes. *Nat Genet* 1999; **22**: 231–8.
19. Chanock S. Candidate genes and single nucleotide polymorphisms (SNPs) in the study of human disease. *Dis Markers* 2001; **17**: 89–98.
20. Reich DE, Cargill M, Bolk S, Ireland J, Sabeti PC, Richter DJ *et al.* Linkage disequilibrium in the human genome. *Nature* 2001; **411**: 199–204.
21. Evans WE, Relling MV. Pharmacogenomics: translating functional genomics into rational therapeutics. *Science* 1999; **286**: 487–91.
22. Evans WE, McLeod LJ. Pharmacogenomics—drug disposition, drug targets, and side effects. *N Engl J Med* 2003; **348**: 528–49.

23. Veenstra DL. The interface between epidemiology and pharmacogenomics. In: Khoury MJ, Little J, Burke W, eds, *Human Genome Epidemiology*. New York: Oxford University Press, 2004; pp. 234–46.

24. Weinshilboum R. Inheritance and drug response. *N Engl J Med* 2003; **348**: 529–37.

25. Benet LZ, Kroetz DL, Sheiner LB. Pharmacokinetics: the dynamics of drug absorption, distribution, and elimination. In: Hardman JG, Limbird LE, Molinoff PB, Ruddon RW, Goodman Gilman A, eds, *The Pharmacological Basis of Therapeutics*. New York: McGraw-Hill, 2004; pp. 3–27.

26. Schillevoort I, de Boer A, van der WJ, Steijns LS, Roos RA, Jansen PA *et al.* Antipsychotic-induced extrapyramidal syndromes and cytochrome P450 2D6 genotype: a case–control study. *Pharmacogenetics* 2002; **12**: 235–40.

27. Poulsen L, Brosen K, Arendt-Nielsen L, Gram LF, Elbaek K, Sindrup SH. Codeine and morphine in extensive and poor metabolizers of sparteine: pharmacokinetics, analgesic effect and side effects. *Eur J Clin Pharmacol* 1996; **51**: 289–95.

28. McLeod HL, Krynetski EY, Relling MV, Evans WE. Genetic polymorphism of thiopurine methyltransferase and its clinical relevance for childhood acute lymphoblastic leukemia. *Leukemia* 2000; **14**: 567–72.

29. Krynetski EY, Schuetz JD, Galpin AJ, Pui CH, Relling MV, Evans WE. A single point mutation leading to loss of catalytic activity in human thiopurine S-methyltransferase. *Proc Natl Acad Sci U S A* 1995; **92**: 949 53.

30. Marsh S, McLeod HL. Cancer pharmacogenetics. *Br J Cancer* 2004; **90**: 8–11.

31. Hoffmeyer S, Burk O, von Richter O, Arnold HP, Brockmoller J, Johne A *et al.* Functional polymorphisms of the human multidrug-resistance gene: multiple sequence variations and correlation of one allele with P-glycoprotein expression and activity in vivo. *Proc Natl Acad Sci U S A* 2000; **97**: 3473–8.

32. Siddiqui A, Kerb R, Weale ME, Brinkmann U, Smith A, Goldstein DB *et al.* Association of multidrug resistance in epilepsy with a polymorphism in the drug-transporter gene ABCB1. *N Engl J Med* 2003; **348**: 1442–8.

33. Schafer M, Rujescu D, Giegling I, Guntermann A, Erfurth A, Bondy B *et al.* Association of short-term response to haloperidol treatment with a polymorphism in the dopamine D(2) receptor gene. *Am J Psychiatry* 2001; **158**: 802–4.

34. Mukae S, Aoki S, Itoh S, Iwata T, Ueda H, Katagiri T. Bradykinin B(2) receptor gene polymorphism is associated with angiotensin-converting enzyme inhibitor-related cough. *Hypertension* 2000; **36**: 127–31.

35. Cusi D, Barlassina C, Azzani T, Casari G, Citterio L, Devoto M *et al.* Polymorphisms of alpha-adducin and salt sensitivity in patients with essential hypertension. *Lancet* 1997; **349**: 1353–7.

36. Kurzrock R, Kantarjian HM, Druker BJ, Talpaz M. Philadelphia chromosome-positive leukemias: from basic mechanisms to molecular therapeutics. *Ann Intern Med* 2003; **138**: 819–30.

37. Vandenbroucke JP, Koster T, Briet E, Reitsma PH, Bertina RM, Rosendaal FR. Increased risk of venous thrombosis in oral-contraceptive users who are carriers of factor V Leiden mutation. *Lancet* 1994; **344**: 1453–7.

38. Vandenbroucke JP, van der Meer FJ, Helmerhorst FM, Rosendaal FR. Factor V Leiden: should we screen oral contraceptive users and pregnant women? *BMJ* 1996; **313**: 1127–30.

39. Kaminsky LS, Zhang ZY. Human P450 metabolism of warfarin. *Pharmacol Ther* 1997; **73**: 67–74.

40. Hirsh J, Dalen JE, Deykin D, Poller L, Bussey H. Oral anticoagulants. Mechanism of action, clinical effectiveness, and optimal therapeutic range. *Chest* 1995; **108**(suppl 4): 231S–46S.

41. Majerus PW, Broze GJ Jr., Miletich JP, Tollefsen DM. Anticoagulant, thrombolytic, and antiplatelet drugs. In: Hardman JG, Limbird LE, Molinoff PB, Ruddon RW, Goodman Gilman A, eds, *Goodman and Gilman's The Pharmacological Basis of Therapeutics*. New York: McGraw-Hill, 1996; pp. 1341–59.

42. Takahashi H, Kashima T, Nomoto S, Iwade K, Tainaka H, Shimizu T *et al.* Comparisons between in-vitro and in-vivo metabolism of (S)-warfarin: catalytic activities of cDNA-expressed CYP2C9, its Leu359 variant and their mixture versus unbound clearance in patients with the corresponding CYP2C9 genotypes. *Pharmacogenetics* 1998; **8**: 365–73.

43. Steward DJ, Haining RL, Henne KR, Davis G, Rushmore TH, Trager WF *et al.* Genetic association between sensitivity to warfarin and expression of CYP2C9*3. *Pharmacogenetics* 1997; **7**: 361–7.

44. Aithal GP, Day CP, Kesteven PJ, Daly AK. Association of polymorphisms in the cytochrome P450 CYP2C9 with warfarin dose requirement and risk of bleeding complications. *Lancet* 1999; **353**: 717–19.

45. Taube J, Halsall D, Baglin T. Influence of cytochrome P-450 CYP2C9 polymorphisms on warfarin sensitivity and risk of over-anticoagulation in patients on long-term treatment. *Blood* 2000; **96**: 1816–19.

46. Higashi MK, Veenstra DL, Kondo LM, Wittkowsky AK, Srinouanprachanh SL, Farin FM *et al.* Association between CYP2C9 genetic variants and anticoagulation-related outcomes during warfarin therapy. *JAMA* 2002; **287**: 1690–8.

47. Daly AK, King BP. Pharmacogenetics of oral anticoagulants. *Pharmacogenetics* 2003; **13**: 247–52.

48. Wadelius M, Sorlin K, Wallerman O, Karlsson J, Yue QY, Magnusson PK *et al.* Warfarin sensitivity related to CYP2C9, CYP3A5, ABCB1 (MDR1) and other factors. *Pharmacogenomics J* 2004; **4** :40–8.

49. Gage BF, Eby C, Milligan PE, Banet GA, Duncan JR, McLeod HL. Use of pharmacogenetics and clinical factors to predict the maintenance dose of warfarin. *Thromb Haemost* 2004; **91**: 87–94.

50. Hetherington S, Hughes AR, Mosteller M, Shortino D, Baker KL, Spreen W *et al.* Genetic variations in HLA-B region and hypersensitivity reactions to abacavir. *Lancet* 2002; **359**: 1121–2.

51. Mallal S, Nolan D, Witt C, Masel G, Martin AM, Moore C *et al.* Association between presence of HLA-B*5701, HLA-DR7, and HLA-DQ3 and hypersensitivity to HIV-1 reverse-transcriptase inhibitor abacavir. *Lancet* 2002; **359**: 727–32.

52. Nebert DW, Jorge-Nebert L, Vesell ES. Pharmacogenomics and "individualized drug therapy": high expectations and disappointing achievements. *Am J Pharmacogenomics* 2003; **3**: 361–70.

53. Kleinbaum DG, Kupper LL, Morgenstern H. Interaction, effect modification, and synergism. In: Kleinbaum DG, Kupper LL, Morgenstern H, eds, *Epidemiologic Research. Principles and Quantitive Methods*. New York: Van Nostrand Reinhold, 1982; pp. 403–18.

54. Botto LD, Khoury MJ. Facing the challenge of complex genotypes and gene–environment interaction: the basic epidemiologic units in case–control and case-only designs. In: Khoury MJ, Little J, Burke W, eds, *Human Genome Epidemiology*. New York: Oxford University Press, 2004; pp. 111–26.

55. Kraft P. Multiple comparisons in studies of gene × gene and gene × environment interaction. *Am J Hum Genet* 2004; **74**: 582–4.

56. Cardon LR, Bell JI. Association study designs for complex diseases. *Nat Rev Genet* 2001; **2**: 91–9.

57. Rao DC. Genetic dissection of complex traits: an overview. *Adv Genet* 2001; **42**: 13–34.

58. Lohmueller KE, Pearce CL, Pike M, Lander ES, Hirschhorn JN. Meta-analysis of genetic association studies supports a contribution of common variants to susceptibility to common disease. *Nat Genet* 2003; **33**: 177–82.

59. Kelada SN, Eaton DL, Wang SS, Rothman NR, Khoury MJ. Applications of human genome epidemiology to environmental health. In: Khoury MJ, Little J, Burke W, eds, *Human Genome Epidemiology*. New York: Oxford University Press, 2004; pp. 145–67.

60. Kerwin RW. A perspective on progress in pharmacogenomics. *Am J Pharmacogenomics* 2003; **3**: 371–3.

61. Rebbeck TR, Ambrosone CB, Bell D, Chanock S, Hayes R, Kadlubar F, Thomas DC. SNPs haplotypes and cancer: applications in molecular epidemiology. *Cancer Epidemiol Biomarkers Prev* 2004; **13**: 681–7.

62. Dupont WD, Plummer WD Jr. Power and sample size calculations. A review and computer program. *Control Clin Trials* 1990; **11**: 116–28.

63. Lachenbruch PA. A note on sample size computation for testing interactions. *Stat Med* 1988; **7**: 467–9.

64. Wacholder S, Rothman N, Caporaso N. Population stratification in epidemiologic studies of common genetic variants and cancer: quantification of bias. *J Natl Cancer Inst* 2000; **92**: 1151–8.

65. Millikan RC. Re: Population stratification in epidemiologic studies of common genetic variants and cancer: quantification of bias. *J Natl Cancer Inst* 2001; **93**: 156–8.

66. Wang Y, Localio R, Rebbeck TR. Evaluating bias due to population stratification in case–control association studies of admixed populations. *Genet Epidemiol* 2004; **27**: 14–20.

67. Ardlie KG, Lunetta KL, Seielstad M. Testing for population subdivision and association in four case–control studies. *Am J Hum Genet* 2002; **71**: 304–11.

68. Cardon LR, Palmer LJ. Population stratification and spurious allelic association. *Lancet* 2003; **361**: 598–604.

69. Thompson D, Stram D, Goldgar D, Witte JS. Haplotype tagging single nucleotide polymorphisms and association studies. *Hum Hered* 2003; **56**: 48–55.

70. Gabriel SB, Schaffner SF, Nguyen H, Moore JM, Roy J, Blumenstiel B *et al*. The structure of haplotype blocks in the human genome. *Science* 2002; **296**: 2225–9.

71. Khoury MJ, Flanders WD. Nontraditional epidemiologic approaches in the analysis of gene–environment interaction: case–control studies with no controls! *Am J Epidemiol* 1996; **144**: 207–13.

72. Piegorsch WW, Weinberg CR, Taylor JA. Non-hierarchical logistic models and case-only designs for assessing susceptibility in population-based case–control studies. *Stat Med* 1994; **13**: 153–62.

73. Ioannidis JP, Rosenberg PS, Goedert JJ, O'Brien TR, International meta-analysis of HIV host genetics. Commentary: meta-analysis of individual participants' data in genetic epidemiology. *Am J Epidemiol* 2002; **156**: 204–10.

74. Capen EC, Clapp RV, Campbell WM. Competitive bidding in high risk situations. *J Petroleum Technol* 1971; **23**: 641–53.

75. Hakonarson H, Gulcher JR, Stefansson K. deCODE genetics, Inc. *Pharmacogenomics* 2003; **4**: 209–15.

76. Stefansson H, Sigurdsson E, Steinthorsdottir V, Bjornsdottir S, Sigmundsson T, Ghosh S *et al*. Neuregulin 1 and susceptibility to schizophrenia. *Am J Hum Genet* 2002; **71**: 877–92.

77. deCode Genetics, nrg1-Markers. Available at: http://www.decode.com/nrg1/markers/. Accessed: February 12, 2004.

78. Merz JF, McGee GE, Sankar P. "Iceland Inc."?: On the ethics of commercial population genomics. *Soc Sci Med* 2004; **58**: 1201–9.

79. Pritchard JK, Rosenberg NA. Use of unlinked genetic markers to detect population stratification in association studies. *Am J Hum Genet* 1999; **65**: 220–8.

80. Devlin B, Roeder K. Genomic control for association studies. *Biometrics* 1999; **55**: 997–1004.

81. Nuffield Council on Bioethics. Available at: http://www.nuffieldbioethics.org/home/. Accessed: July 12, 2004.

82. Thomas DC. Genetic epidemiology with a capital "E". *Genet Epidemiol* 2000; **19**: 289–300.

83. Williams-Jones B, Corrigan OP. Rhetoric and hype: where's the "ethics" in pharmacogenomics? *Am J Pharmacogenomics* 2003; **3**: 375–83.

84. Serono VP. Genomics raising disease redefinition, other orphan issues. *The Pink Sheet* April 10, 2000, pp. 20–1. Available at: http://www.thepinksheet.com/. Accessed: July 12, 2004.

85. Vesell ES. Therapeutic lessons from pharmacogenetics. *Ann Intern Med* 1997; **126**: 653–5.

86. Vesell ES. Pharmacogenetics: multiple interactions between genes and environment as determinants of drug response. *Am J Med* 1979; **66**: 183–7.

38

Bioethical Issues in Pharmacoepidemiologic Research

DAVID CASARETT[1], JASON KARLAWISH[1], ELIZABETH ANDREWS[2]
and ARTHUR CAPLAN[3]

[1] University of Pennsylvania, Department of Medicine, Division of Geriatrics, Philadelphia, Pennsylvania, USA;
[2] Research Triangle Institute Health Solutions, Research Triangle Park, North Carolina, USA; [3] University of Pennsylvania,
Department of Medicine, Center for Bioethics, Philadelphia, Pennsylvania, USA.

INTRODUCTION

In the past 50 years as medical research has evolved rapidly, the discipline of research ethics has assumed a largely protectionist posture, largely because of a series of unfortunate scandals and the public outcry that ensued.[1-3] As a result, research ethics has focused primarily on protecting human subjects from the risks of research. The goal has been to minimize risks to subjects, rather than minimizing the risks and maximizing the potential benefits for both subjects and society.[4] Themes that run through many of these scandals are scientists' failure to adequately review and disclose research risks and potential benefits, and their failure to obtain explicit permission from research subjects. As a result of these events, review by an institutional review board (IRB) and full informed consent have become the cornerstones of the protection of human subjects from research risks.

Research ethics and research practice have become separate and even, sometimes, antagonistic enterprises. The role society expects of ethics is to regulate science. Scientific practice reflects this fact. IRB review and the practice of informed consent have become as integral to the design of a clinical research as sample size calculations, the accurate measurement of endpoints, or robust statistical analysis.

These and other requirements have been remarkably effective in defining the limits of ethical research, and have made it much less likely that the most egregious ethical errors of the past will be repeated. Overall, they should be viewed as welcome additions to the practice of clinical research. However, serious scientific and ethical problems may arise when the requirements that were developed to guide clinical research are applied to other kinds of research. In particular, standard protections in clinical research are not easily exported and applied to the very different challenges of epidemiologic research. Therefore, as these rules have

---

been applied to pharmacoepidemiologic research, the result has been the parallel development of modifications to the ethical guidelines and principles, on one hand, and increasing consternation and confusion, on the other, about how these modifications should be applied.

The central problem has been that, while the ethics of human subjects research has been built upon the protection of human subjects, the human subjects involved in pharmacoepidemiologic research are quite different. Indeed, it may be difficult to see how the analysis of a data set makes the patients whose information contributes to that data set "human subjects" and why this research requires review by an ethics review board. The idea that a patient can become a subject without his or her knowledge, and without any direct contact with an investigator, is not intuitively clear. Moreover, the risks to the subjects of epidemiology research are not the usual health risks of research that can be balanced against the potential health benefits of research. Harm is not the issue in pharmacoepidemiologic research. It is almost always what in law and philosophy is referred to as "wrong," that is, a violation of a person's rights. The chief risk is the violation of confidentiality. While investigators and ethics review boards may be able to balance medical risks against medical benefits, they may find balancing these different currencies to be challenging.

In an effort to deal with these problems, investigators, governments, and professional associations have developed regulations and guidelines to provide ethical structure to the growing field of epidemiology.[5–7] Most of these guidelines apply equally well to pharmacoepidemiologic research, although this field has begun to develop its own principles.[7] These guidelines and regulations have made it clear that the protection of subjects in epidemiology research represents only one part of the ethical obligations of epidemiology investigators. Guidelines have addressed four broad categories of ethical issues in epidemiology research: obligations to society, obligations to funders and employers, obligations to colleagues, and obligations to subjects.[5–7]

Although these guidelines acknowledge a range of ethical obligations, one of these, the investigators' obligations to subjects, has clearly proven to be the most challenging. This is because the procedures of ethical research, like ethics board review and informed consent, may be overly protectionistic or prohibitively difficult in epidemiologic research. Ethical concerns about pharmacoepidemiologic research, and more broadly about epidemiology research, have therefore focused on the kinds of research that require ethics board review and the kinds of research that require the subject's informed consent.

The answers to these questions define the ethical procedures that allow researchers to have access to information gathered for clinical and administrative purposes. Therefore, investigators face a considerable challenge. They must protect patients' privacy and confidentiality in a way that accomplishes research goals accurately and efficiently. This challenge lies at the heart of the ethics of pharmacoepidemiologic research.

National and international organizations have created principles that provide a backdrop to the research framework, the most well established being those adopted by the Organization for Economic Cooperation and Development (OECD) in 1980.[8] These recommendations suggest that limits to the collection of data should be sought, that the quality of data is important, that data use should be specified in advance, and that investigators should adhere to specified uses. Finally, the OECD suggests a requirement of "openness"— that is, a requirement that goals, uses, and access to data should be a matter of public record, and that individuals should be able to determine whether and how data about them are being used. Despite general agreement about these and other principles, the international community has failed to achieve a consensus about the proper balance of protections and research progress.

The goal of this chapter is to present an overview of this balance and specifically of the challenges that arise when the principles of research ethics are applied to issues surrounding privacy and confidentiality. In order to accomplish this goal, this chapter will tend to emphasize regulations in the United States. This is not because these regulations can or should be generalized to other countries, but simply because at the current time international guidelines vary widely and are often contradictory.[9,10] Therefore, although the experience of the United States is not universal, these regulations provide a frame of reference for comparison. Where instructive, however, experience from other countries is discussed as well.

This chapter begins by defining the terms that describe the procedures and requirements of ethical research. These are the normative boundaries in which pharmacoepidemiology must operate in order to maintain the public's trust. If research is to move forward, pharmacoepidemiologists must develop procedures that permit them to balance a need for scientific rigor, on one hand, with respect for ethical requirements, on the other. This chapter will discuss three such strategies and the challenges that investigators face in applying them: delinking subject identifiers from their information, modifications to bioethics review board review, and modifications to subject informed consent requirements. This chapter concludes with a critical consideration of some of the available guidelines and regulations, and recommendations for future regulatory efforts.

CLINICAL PROBLEMS TO BE ADDRESSED BY PHARMACOEPIDEMIOLOGIC RESEARCH

The birth and subsequent development of research and scholarship in research ethics, like any field of specialized knowledge, has constructed a language that is particularly its own. This language provides a taxonomy of ethical issues in research and is essential to this discussion because it forms the foundation of any communication and discourse between the fields of ethics and epidemiology. These terms also offer an excellent vantage point from which to examine critically the current emphasis on human subjects protection and its applicability to pharmacoepidemiologic research.

RESEARCH

Any productive analysis of the ethics of pharmacoepidemiologic research is critically dependent on a clear and precise understanding of the term "research." Given the frequency with which this term is used by ethicists, investigators, and the public, a definition would seem to be a simple matter. Unfortunately, this has been far from the truth.[11] Yet, perhaps the most well established definition is also the oldest. In its summary statement (the Belmont Report), the US National Commission for the Protection of Human Subjects defined "research" as any activity designed to "develop or contribute to generalizable knowledge."[12] This is a definition that has been embraced by other scholars, and has become the standard by which a proposed project is assessed.[13]

Unfortunately, this definition creates a challenge for pharmacoepidemiologic researchers and ethics review boards, because it is not always easy to characterize the intent of the person who generates the knowledge. For instance, data may be gathered as part of a health care organization's drug surveillance program, the intent of which is define the patterns of medication use in a local population. It is not clear, given the definition based on "generalizable knowledge," whether this project should be construed as research, clinical care, or even as a quality improvement activity. These distinctions are important because once a project is identified as "research," investigators must meet a series of requirements designed to protect the patients, who are now human subjects.

This definition is particularly problematic in pharmacoepidemiologic research, because it is hard to distinguish the routine practice of epidemiology from research. The

extremes are evident. The paradigmatic *practice* of epidemiology is public health case finding and surveillance for adverse drug reactions. This is a social good that we do not, generally, consider to be research, although the activities are conducted for the purpose of creating generalizable knowledge upon which to base public health decisions. Analogous would be the quality assurance activities of health plans or hospitals, seeking to improve the use of medications in their settings. These sorts of investigations proceed, and sometimes even produce publishable data, without review by ethics review boards. These activities differ from more "research oriented" epidemiology designed to test hypotheses about drug adverse event associations, interactions, compliance, or efficacy. These investigations may be identified as research, and they may be required to undergo ethics review board review. However, the difference between these two types of activity can be difficult to demarcate.

HUMAN SUBJECTS

Although it is important that any discussion of research and research ethics be clear about the definition of a research subject, this definition is as elusive as the definition of research, on which it depends. Broadly, though, a useful definition comes from the United States "Common Rule," the set of Federal regulations first promulgated in 1981 that govern research ethics.[14] The Common Rule defines a "research subject" as "a living individual, about whom an investigator (whether professional or student) conducting research obtains either: 1) data through intervention or interaction with the individual, or 2) identifiable private information"[14] (US Code of Federal Regulations 46.102f). For pharmacoepidemiologists, the key issue here is that the use of information that can be linked to an individual constitutes a contact between an investigator and a human subject. This is true even if the information was gathered in the past and no contact occurs between the investigator and the person. A key issue, then, becomes whether information can be linked to an individual.

This may not be a universally accepted definition. However, the Common Rule applies, at a minimum, to all research carried out by US investigators using Federal funds. In addition, its influence is far greater because the vast majority of institutions that accept these Federal funds have signed an agreement, called a Federalwide Assurance (FWA), to abide by the Common Rule requirements in all research, regardless of the source of funding.[14] Therefore, the Common Rule serves as *de facto* law governing research at the most productive research institutions in the US and offers a reasonable working definition. Further, even when research is performed outside the United States, if it is done with US Federal support or at an institution with an FWA then it must conform to American regulations governing research ethics.

ETHICS REVIEW BOARDS

In many countries over the past 30 years, ethics review boards have become central to the practice of research. In the US context, these are committees with at least one "community representative," appointed by institutions that receive Federal monies to conduct research. In other nations, there are regional or national committees that are appointed by professional organizations or government agencies.

This requirement reflects the consensus that scientists, and science, could benefit from independent review of research protocols. This idea first appeared in the World Medical Association's Declaration of Helsinki in 1964, which requires that an independent committee review all protocols. The Declaration recommends that this committee be responsible for "consideration, comment and guidance," but does not define further the committee's authority to approve or reject protocols that it finds unacceptable.[10] These recommendations have been taken up rapidly, and review boards have become widespread. Their authority has been clarified as well, and these committees typically have the power to review and reject all research that takes place in their institution or in which their institution's investigators are involved.

In the US, while some states have enacted legislation governing human subjects research, the formal system of review has evolved primarily in a manner that links Federal authority and funding. A committee, referred to as an Institutional Review Board (IRB), is required to review all research that is funded by all Federal government branches that have signed on to the "Common Rule."[14] Examples of Federal agencies that abide by the Common Rule are the National Institutes of Health (NIH), the Food and Drug Administration (FDA), and the Agency for Healthcare Research and Quality (AHRQ). Further, as noted above, institutions that have filed an FWA have agreed to abide by the Common Rule requirements in all research, regardless of the source of funding. In most other countries, research regulations are not limited by provisions regarding funding but, instead, apply to all research conducted in that country.

The composition of these review boards varies widely across international boundaries. However, a consistent feature is the need for inclusion of expertise from outside the scientific community. For instance, the US regulations mandate the inclusion of at least one member who is not affiliated with the institution, and one member who may be affiliated but who represents law, ethics, or another non-science discipline[14] (Code of Federal Regulations (CFR) 46.107). Australian regulations mandate a committee's composition by requiring a mix of genders, and by extending the inclusion of non-science representatives.[10] The purpose of these requirements is to introduce accountability to society and minimize conflicts of interest between scientists who act as research reviewers and researchers.

Although review boards have become a commonplace feature on the research landscape, even under US Federal guidelines, not all research requires review. Certain kinds of research can receive expedited review, that is, review by the IRB chair or a designated member of the IRB instead of the full committee, and some may be exempt. This is a means to assure that the research risks are truly minor and the research fulfills basic subject protections without expending unnecessary IRB resources. Research that does not require ethics board review is any project that does not involve human subjects[14] (CFR 46.101). For example, when investigators use data in which nothing would permit the investigator to identify the individual from whom the data came, ethics board review is not required. In addition, according to the Common Rule, research may be eligible for expedited review if it poses no more than minimal risk (see below for definition) and the research involves "existing data," which means a retrospective analysis of records that exist as of the date the research is proposed[12] (CFR 46.110). Most European nations have similar provisions for expediting the review of research that poses no more than minimal risks to subjects. Internationally, there is some disagreement about whether pharmacoepidemiologic research should require review. For instance, while the Royal College of Physicians would not require review,[15] the Council for International Organizations of Medical Sciences (CIOMS) recommends ethics board review for all research.[16]

PRIVACY AND CONFIDENTIALITY

In pharmacoepidemiologic research, these terms are of paramount concern. Although they are often discussed together, they are distinct concepts. It is useful to distinguish them, and to describe individually the ethical basis for requirements of each. Of these, privacy is the most basic and confidentiality is in a sense derivative.

Privacy, in the setting of research, refers to each individual's right to be free from unwanted inspection of, access to, or physical manipulation of records and documents containing personal information. In the case of epidemiology research in particular, privacy refers to each individual's right to prevent access to his or her medical records. The right to privacy, and others' corresponding obligation to respect privacy, is justified in part by each individual's right to be left alone.[17] This is a legal way of considering a right to privacy, but privacy has an important social function as well. Viewed in this light, a right to privacy is a precondition for social interaction and cooperation because it allows and requires a degree of trust.[18]

Confidentiality is a derivative right that is based upon the right to privacy. When individuals choose to allow a health care provider access to personal medical information, they have chosen to waive their right to privacy.[6] Individuals may choose to exercise this right with the expectation, either implicit or explicit, that no one else will have access to that information without the patient's permission. This right to limit the transfer of information, to control the secondary use of information by others, is the right to confidentiality.

Like the right to privacy, the right to confidentiality is also based on a basic right to a freedom from interference, in the sense that a right to confidentiality is not possible unless there is an underlying right to privacy. However, the right to confidentiality also engenders a responsibility on the part of the person who has information about another person. The expectation that someone will not disclose the information to a third party creates a fiduciary relationship. That is, it creates an agreement based on a mutually understood set of goals and understandings. This means that confidentiality may be more highly specified by arrangements that may be made at the time that an individual initially grants access to information. For instance, patients may have specific concerns or expectations about ways in which the information they divulge may be used. These expectations may include transfer to a third party in either identifiable or unidentifiable form, or access to particular kinds of information within a medical record, or limits as to the period of time information may be available to others.

The fundamental issue is whether information that was gathered in a clinical setting, where rules of confidentiality apply, can be used for reasons, such as research, that were not part of the conditions of that relationship. Both the law and research regulations are ambiguous over what constitutes a substantive violation of confidentiality. Does the use of records without prior authorization constitute a violation of confidentiality? Or does it constitute a risk of a violation that depends on how those records are used, and on what is done with the information?

In general, society has not articulated clear answers to these questions, in large part because the questions engage well-formed but conflicting political and philosophical views about how society should organize the exchange of information. For example, proponents of communitarianism (the perspective of a community created by voluntary association) argue that the good of the individual is inextricably tied to the public good.[19] Thus, ethical dichotomies that pit individuals against society (such as the unauthorized use of a person's clinical information for research) must be resolved with attention to both personal and public goods.

However, proponents of liberalism, or a rights-based individualism, disagree. From this perspective, what is right exists prior to what is good. This means that any unauthorized use of a person's information threatens to violate a fundamental right to privacy and the potential good derived from that use is not a proper condition to balance against that violation.

In most states in the US, these conflicting views exist in a perhaps deliberately unresolved tension. Laws (or the absence of laws) generally allow procedures that attempt to circumscribe the extremes of either view. Laws are silent on whether medical records can be used for research without the prior authorization of the patient, although a few states have laws that records can be used for research after IRB review.[17] Many European nations have very strict protections of individual rights to privacy and confidentiality. For example, Iceland and Sweden have very strict requirements for individual informed consent for the use of identifiable information such as requirements for individual consent. Other nations lean toward a more communitarian perspective with respect to epidemiologic research and allow waivers of consent for many studies.

However, US research regulations do provide a set of conditions that permit the use of records regardless of whether the patient authorized their use for research. The key features of these conditions are that the research risks are minimal and the potential violation does not adversely affect subjects' rights and welfare[12] (CFR 46.116). The following sections will discuss both of these key arguments.

MINIMAL RISK

Although the general goal of research is to produce knowledge that will benefit society, investigators must also minimize the risks to subjects. It is axiomatic that, as risks to subjects increase, the degree of subject protections, such as ethics review and informed consent, increases as well. The concept of minimal risk attempts to operationalize a risk threshold, above which protections should be stricter. Conversely, subject protections are relaxed if a research protocol does not exceed the level of minimal risk. Although the concept of minimal risk is relatively straightforward, and would apply to most pharmacoepidemiology protocols, its definition is problematic.

According to US regulations stated in the Common Rule, research risks are "minimal" if "the probability and magnitude of harm or discomfort are not greater in and of themselves than those ordinarily encountered in daily life or during the performance of routine physical or psychological examinations or tests"[14] (CFR 46.102.i) In most situations, this concept is difficult to operationalize.[20] This is in large part because the definition lacks a clear standard against which to compare the research risks: the daily lives of healthy or "normal" persons, or the daily lives of persons who might be subjects of the research. In pharmacoepidemiologic research, where the risk is a potential violation of confidentiality, there is the additional problem of deciding whether any such violation is ordinarily encountered during daily life, such that a violation in the course of research is "minimal risk."

INFORMED CONSENT

Perhaps the most disturbing feature of many of the research scandals in recent history has been the total disregard for informed consent. Every nation which has addressed the subject, as reflected in international codes of ethics and professional society statements about research ethics, recognizes that subjects, or for incompetent patients, their surrogates, are to be told about the nature of research and alternatives to participation, and to have the chance to volunteer to participate. It is not surprising, therefore, that research ethics guidelines, recommendations, and regulations have stressed the procedural requirement of a subject's informed consent. In order for a subject's consent to be informed, he or she must understand the research and must agree to participate voluntarily, without inducement or coercion.[21]

The regulations governing research informed consent in the US, while not universal, are illustrative of these features[14] (CFR 46.116). The US regulations convey the feature of understanding by requiring that the investigator explain the research risks, benefits, and alternatives of research participation; the confidentiality of any information obtained; and the procedures for compensation and for contacting a person responsible for the research. Voluntariness is expressed by the requirement that investigators tell subjects that participation in the research study is voluntary, and that subjects have the right to discontinue participation at any time. In some situations, informed consent may be modified to be verbal instead of written, or even may not

need to be obtained at all. Whether informed consent must always be obtained, and in what form consent should be documented, have been the subject of vigorous debate.[22,23]

Again, while the US guidelines are not universal, they offer a helpful perspective on the complexities that this issue raises. The Common Rule requires that written informed consent be obtained in most research situations[14] (CFR 46.116). However, it makes two notable exceptions. First, written documentation of informed consent is not required if the principal risk of the research is a breach of confidentiality and if the written record is the only link between personal data and the subject's identity[14] (CFR 46.117.c). In this case, whether or not a written informed consent document is used depends on each subject's preferences regarding whether he/she wishes to sign a consent document that could be used to link data with identifiable information. Second, informed consent can be entirely waived if the research meets four conditions[14] (CFR 46.116):

1. the research involves no more than minimal risk to the subjects;
2. the waiver or alteration will not adversely affect the rights and welfare of the subjects;
3. the research could not practicably be carried out without the waiver or alteration;
4. whenever appropriate, the subjects will be provided with additional pertinent information after participation.

These criteria are often applied to pharmacoepidemiologic research and other forms of research that rely on the use of pre-existing records. The controversial conditions here are whether the research risks are minimal and whether a waiver of informed consent will adversely affect the subjects' rights and welfare. These are controversial, because in research that involves the use of medical records, the principal risk is the violation of the subjects' confidentiality. A consensus about the proper application of these conditions requires a consensus about whether access to the patient's medical record without the patient's permission is a violation of confidentiality that is greater than minimal risk and violates the subject's rights and welfare.

There are two competing answers to this question. The first relies upon a strict adherence to the principle of respect for autonomy. Accordingly, any unauthorized use of records violates confidentiality, presents more than minimal risk, and adversely affects subjects' rights and welfare. Hence, in all human subjects research, the subject's informed consent could be perceived as an absolute requirement. Although this view follows from strict adherence to some research ethics codes,[24] this is not the view held by most contemporary researchers and ethicists.

Instead, a second interpretation allows for flexibility in the priority of the principle of respect for autonomy. Accordingly, some potential or even actual violations of confidentiality do not adversely affect the subject's rights and welfare or present more than minimal risk. This interpretation requires that we be able to determine to which kinds of information, if any, most people would be willing to grant access. For instance, at one extreme, research using information about patients' sexual activity or certain genetic characteristics might well be perceived as posing a greater than minimal risk. In such a study, obtaining that information without patients' consent might well have an adverse impact upon patients' rights and welfare, depending on the use of the information and the safeguards in place to protect access by third parties. In contrast, information about patients' age and blood pressure might seem to pose only minimal risks, even though blood pressure information could be more predictive of future disability status than the results of a genetic test. Obtaining information without patients' consent must be considered in the appropriate context in a rapidly changing environment, because the potential impact on an individual is heavily dependent on social, economic, and medical factors.

In between these extremes, reasonable people can and do disagree about the magnitude of harm and impact upon rights caused by unauthorized use of information. There are two useful ways to settle this. The first is to assure that the ethics board review is truly multidisciplinary so that a variety of reasonable views are heard. The second is to require that researchers take steps to minimize the risks and adverse effect upon rights if patient confidentiality is violated. These methods are addressed in the next section.

METHODOLOGIC PROBLEMS TO BE ADDRESSED BY PHARMACOEPIDEMIOLOGIC RESEARCH

There are several procedures available that can protect patient confidentiality. These methods allow patients to control who has access to information. At the time that clinical data are gathered, such as upon enrollment in a health system, a patient can provide a "universal consent" to determine whether his or her medical record can be used for research. This term should not be construed to mean an informed consent to participate in research, because the patient is simply consenting to the generic use of his or her records and not whether to participate in actual protocols.

A variation on this method is that patients can shield some aspects of their medical records from use in research. This is possible in some electronic record management systems. For example, patients could place into an electronic "black box," records of certain medications, such as antidepressants. Finally, at the time of the research, patients can be contacted to provide informed consent for the use of their archived records. However, there are two problems in applying these methods to pharmacoepidemiologic research. First, they may not really protect privacy to the degree that investigators and ethics review boards would hope. Second, they may erode the validity of the research findings (as will be further discussed below), and therefore generalizability to the population that stands to benefit from the research.

First, there is reason for skepticism about whether these interventions actually foster patient confidentiality. For instance, if individuals must be contacted each time their records may be used in a particular study, the individual may consider such contact intrusive. Furthermore, individuals might consider that their confidentiality has been violated if researchers access research information and contact them directly in order to obtain consent for the use of otherwise de-identified records. Individuals may also refuse participation if contacted for a study they consider irrelevant to their health. An individual may also become alarmed if asked to consent for records to be used in such a study of a disease for which she has not been diagnosed (e.g., a case–control study of patients with and without breast cancer). Although these concerns cover very different ground, they all provide grounds for concern that a variety of procedures for protecting privacy may not be ideal.

Validity is a necessary precondition for all ethical research,[25] and research should not be done if it cannot answer the hypothesis it claims to test. In pharmacoepidemiology studies that use archival records, methods that allow patients to control who has access to data can severely limit the validity of the research to be done. For instance, consider the procedure of universal consent, in which each patient is given the opportunity to remove his or her electronic medical records (such as Medicaid data) from use for research. It is certain that at least some patients will opt out. The problem is that willingness to provide consent is generally not random, and varies in ways that may bias study results, as demonstrated in a study of consent bias in the Rochester Epidemiology Project.[26] In an ethics review board-approved study at the Mayo Clinic, patients were mailed an educational brochure and a request for authorization to allow use of medical records for research. Characteristics of patients who did and did not provide written authorization were compared. Among persons returning the form, the refusal rate was low (3.2%), but the persons declining consent varied from the study population by age, gender, residence, and prior diagnoses, suggesting that the ability to opt out of databases creates a potential bias in the data.

Selective consent by patients may prohibit the evaluation of a key medication-adverse event association if the shielded information is in the pathway between the medication exposure and outcome of interest. For example, the results of a study of a drug–outcome association may be misleading if there is a large increased risk due only to an interaction between the study medication and the confounder drug. The overall study results may show a low-level association between the study drug and the outcome. No interaction could be analyzed. Further, if all patients treated with antidepressants chose to withhold their medical records from any research, the drug–outcome study would show no association, since no data on patients experiencing the reaction would be included in the research data file.

When researchers attempt to contact all patients in a database to seek informed consent, some patients may be unavailable to provide consent because they have died, moved, or changed health plans. Those patients are likely to be distributed in a nonrandom fashion. The potential bias was demonstrated using data from the Mayo Clinic Rochester Epidemiology Project.[27] Data available from all patients over a 50-year period showed a decrease in the population incidence of hip fracture. Data from only those patients known to be alive and able to give consent would produce results showing an increasing risk of hip fracture over time. This consent issue poses particular challenges in studies requiring long periods of exposure or follow-up, studies evaluating events of long latency, and the evaluation of intergenerational effects of medications.

The number of studies using archival records will likely increase with the growing availability of electronic records and increasing interest in answering important drug safety questions. However, as the number of studies increases, there will undoubtedly be a decreasing consent rate if all studies require consent. Jacobsen et al. showed a high consent rate among persons who returned consent forms, but only 79.3% of persons contacted returned the consent forms.[26] This return rate should be considered optimal, given the high credibility of the Mayo Clinic within Minnesota. Another study of consent, a drug safety study within a population of members of a Minnesota health plan, showed much poorer participation. In this study, with more representative results, only 19% of individuals contacted provided consent, and only 52% provided any response.[28]

An additional problem is encountered in the conduct of large, multi-institutional case–control studies in which access to a large amount of data must be reviewed in order to identify the cases and controls prior to contacting the appropriate patients for consent. Ethics review boards typically waive the requirement for consent in the initial case-finding review of records, and evaluate the consent used when patients are invited to participate in the study. Applying the current Common Rule framework to these studies requires separate review by ethics review boards from each participating institution of the same protocol. Issues raised by these ethics review boards and encountered in the review process may relate less to true local differences in the research environment than to the administrative differences of each institution's ethics review board process. Absent a more streamlined approach to the current ethics review board process, the time and cost of seeking multiple approvals discourage the conduct of these studies that may have important public health implications.

CURRENTLY AVAILABLE SOLUTIONS

These methodological challenges pose considerable obstacles to the conduct of pharmacoepidemiologic research. For records-based studies using data not directly identifying subjects, investigators have relied on the confidentiality policies governing the use of information in the individual institution. For studies using identifiable records, investigators receive guidance and direction, if they receive it at all, through a process of negotiation with local ethics review boards, whose task is to balance the requirements of the research design with the rights and welfare of prospective subjects. Because the tension between ethics requirements and the exigencies of pharmacoepidemiologic research require this balancing process, in a very real sense the ethics of pharmacoepidemiologic research is a negotiated agreement between investigators and one or more review boards. The available solutions to the methodological challenges outlined in the previous section, therefore, depend upon two factors. First, they depend upon the steps investigators can take in gathering and handling data. Second, they depend upon the degree to which review boards can and should be involved in research, and on their ability to review research in a manner that is both competent and efficient. We examine each of these in turn.

The past several years have seen a rapid movement toward legislative protections for data privacy both in the US and internationally. These legislative approaches to protect the confidentiality of medical data provide potentially strong protections and safeguards on the creation and reuse of confidential information. For instance, the European Union (EU) Directive that went into effect October, 1998 covers all information that is either directly identifiable or information from which identity could be inferred.[29] EU member states are currently bringing their laws into conformity with the Directive and tailoring these laws to the individual concerns and circumstances of their countries. The EU Directive requires first, consent for all uses of information beyond that for which the information was originally collected. Safeguards on the use and transfer of information are required as well. Each institution must have a data controller/data privacy officer, who is accountable for appropriate procedures and use of data within the institution. In addition, data cannot be transferred from a member state of the EU to another country outside the EU unless that country has safeguards at least as stringent as those of the EU. Notably, however, member states may grant deviations from some provisions of the Directive for activities of substantial public interest. Interestingly, there is no mention of ethics review boards in the Directive. All research would presumably: (i) be conducted with explicit consent, (ii) be conducted only with delinked records, or (iii) be exempted by a specific member state as a type of activity of substantial public interest.

For pharmacoepidemiology, a number of implications of the Directive are of concern. For example, pharmacovigilance activities currently must be conducted using identifiable data. A requirement for patient consent would stifle the collection of a substantial proportion of cases and therefore hinder the ability to identify signals of drug safety problems. Furthermore, analysis of secondary information (from clinical trials or administrative databases) for research questions not anticipated at the time patients signed consent would not be possible without additional consent. Very little research could be conducted using secondary files from which direct patient identifiers have been deleted. This restriction is due to the broad definition in the Directive of identifiable and "indirectly identifiable" data.

In the US, the Health Insurance Portability and Accountability Act (HIPAA) of 1996 called for Congress to pass legislation on medical data privacy, and for the Department of Health and Human Services to promulgate regulations if Congress failed to act. While Congress considered numerous bills that promised stricter scrutiny of research and tighter protections, none was passed. Therefore, the Privacy Rule (Standard for Privacy of Individually Identifiable Health Information, in Title 45 of the Code of Federal Regulation, Part 160 and Subparts A and E of Part 164) was developed, and went into effect April 14, 2003

(see www.hhs.gov/ocr/hipaa). The Privacy Rule offers greater protections of privacy, restrictions on the uses to which existing data can be put, and requirements that individuals must be able to determine who and why others may have access to their personal data in many cases outside of standard medical practice. The rule applies to "covered entities" or organizations that generate and manage personally identifiable health data. While some researchers may not be directly covered by the rule, they generally must obtain access to information from organizations considered covered entities.

Of specific interest for pharmacoepidemiologists are the strategies for protecting confidentiality and enabling researchers to access existing data sets. Under the new rule, data sets that are de-identified can be disclosed and used freely. The Privacy Rule defines de-identified data as: (i) a data set from which 18 specified items that could be considered identifiers have been removed, and (ii) a data set which the covered entity knows will not be used alone or with other data for the purpose of subsequently identifying individuals. The covered entity can alternatively use a satisfactory statistical method to de-identify the data set while maintaining some of the 18 elements.

However, epidemiologists would rarely find a data set stripped of these 18 elements appropriate for research because the elements include some items that are essential for research. For example, any specific date field would have to be removed. Specific dates are usually required to evaluate sequence and timing of drug exposures and adverse events.

There are several methods researchers can use to gain access to a data set that has not been completely de-identified. First, patient authorization can be obtained. Second, the requirement for patient authorization can be waived by either an IRB or a Privacy Board (which is defined in the rule) if certain conditions are met, such as limits on access to the data, and assurances that the research could not be conducted without the waiver. Third, a "limited data set," that contains some of the 18 elements considered identifiers (e.g., dates and geocodes) can be provided to a researcher if a "data use agreement" has been signed by the researcher assuring the appropriate use and disclosure of the information for research.

There are two additional features of the Privacy Rule that are important in protecting research. A data set can be considered to be de-identified even though a covered entity maintains a code by which the de-identified database can be relinked to personally identifiable data. The code itself cannot be disclosed. In some early drafts of legislation and rules, retention of these codes would not have been allowed. The ability to relink a data set to original data in order to supplement a de-identified data set with information on risk factors, outcomes, or extended follow-up time can be critically important in pharmacoepidemiology studies. In addition, the Privacy Rule has preserved access by researchers to patient information in certain circumstances for activities "preparatory for research." A preliminary review of medical records is often important to identify patients potentially eligible for a study prior to approaching a patient for consent. Researchers may have access under the Privacy Rule only if the identifiable data are necessary for the preparatory work, and the identifiable information may not be removed from the covered entity as it is reviewed. However, early implementation of the Privacy Rule suggests that the intended balance between protecting patient confidentiality and promoting careful research has not yet been realized, as some covered entities are reluctant to permit research access to data even when all aspects of the Privacy Rule are honored.

There are also opportunities to improve the ethics board review process. Ethics review varies widely from country to country, and there may even be differences within one country. In existing guidelines there is general agreement that protocol review by ethics review boards is valuable in principle. However, there is considerably less agreement about what kinds of pharmacoepidemiologic research require this review.

For instance, as noted above, the Royal College of Physicians position statement on ethics board review suggests that ethics board review is not necessary, even for linked studies, as long as investigators take appropriate precautions to safeguard the confidentiality of information.[15] On the other hand, the Council for International Organizations of Medical Sciences recommends ethics board review for all epidemiology research, whether or not they involve identifiable data.[16] In the middle are the recommendations of the International Society for Pharmacoepidemiology (ISPE)[7] and the Common Rule[14] (CFR 101.b4), which require ethics board review only when subjects are identifiable through linked data.

In some cases, it is not even the features of the research, but the source of funding that determines whether ethics board review is necessary. For example, as noted above, the Common Rule regulations apply only to research that is conducted using Federal funds or research that is conducted in institutions that have agreed to follow these regulations voluntarily. The result is that while some researchers are required to apply for ethics review board approval, other researchers whose research presents the same kinds of research risks are not. Although this distinction on the basis of funding source respects the limits of Federal authority in intrastate activities, it lacks moral force.

As examples of efficient protection of human subjects, the Common Rule and ISPE positions seem the most sensible. This means that investigators and ethics review boards will at times need to negotiate the kinds of research that achieve standards such as "existing data" and minimal risk. However, this negotiation is a far better system to assure adequate subject protection for research than a system in which decisions are either entirely left in the hands of the investigators or made by others.

Nevertheless, this system of research oversight, and its heavy dependence on ethics board review, means that oversight can vary widely among institutions. This variability creates enormous administrative challenges for pharmacoepidemiology investigators, challenges that may be magnified in the case of multicenter research that crosses international borders. Certainly, sensitivity to local issues may be a desirable feature for the ethical review of research, particularly if institutions have special populations or circumstances that warrant special scrutiny of protocols. However, this variability may also be the result of variability in the quality of the ethics review board's skills and resources.

The ability of ethics review boards to review research in a manner that is both competent and efficient addresses issues of the training and certification of membership and resources for handling the volume of new and renewing research protocols. In general, the requirements for the skills and knowledge needed for ethics review board membership are handled by the local ethics review board. No certification exists to assure that ethics review board members possess adequate understanding of research ethics and regulation. Finally, ethics review boards are funded through indirect means, such as the general pool of indirect funds generated from grants. Potential ways to improve the quality and efficiency of ethics board review include training and certification of board members, reduction in the amount of paperwork for routine monitoring of protocols, and explicit funding that is proportionate to an ethics review board's workload.

THE FUTURE

The variability and quality of ethics board review pose significant challenges for pharmacoepidemiology investigators. These should be the focus of future efforts to harmonize research regulations and set minimum standards for ethics review board competency and funding. However, these solutions do not adequately address a larger problem. Although ethics review boards may offer a reasonable procedural solution to ethics review, it is less clear how ethics review boards should make the sorts of decisions that are required of them. Specifically, it is not clear how ethics review boards and investigators should balance ethical and methodological requirements. Without a careful consideration of this balancing process, any efforts at regulation, and particularly efforts to standardize ethics board review and boost their resources, will achieve only limited success.

The idea of balancing is not new. Traditional approaches to balancing the ethical and methodological requirements of research typically use as their guide the research risks. In most guidelines, and the Common Rule is an excellent case in point, increasing risks to subjects requires increasing attention to full ethics board review and the informed consent process, including written documentation of informed consent.[14] Seen in this light, there is a simple proportional relationship between research risks and subject protections such as informed consent. This relationship describes the degree of subject protections solely in terms of the balance of the risks and potential benefits to the subjects of the proposed research.

The problem, though, is that this relationship is too simple for the situation of pharmacoepidemiologic research. The ethical requirements of traditional biomedical research do not fit entirely with the practice of pharmacoepidemiologic research. The risks to the subjects of epidemiology research are not the usual health risks of research that can be balanced against the potential health benefits of research. They are instead largely risks of another kind. The chief risk is the violation of confidentiality, which is really a civil, rather than a medical, risk.

We suggest that investigators and ethics review boards should consider an additional factor in this relationship: the value of the knowledge to be gained[14] (CFR 46.111a). An ethical justification for this position begins, first, with the example of social services research. United States research regulations currently include an exception for studies designed to evaluate social programs[14] (CFR 46.101). The implicit argument for this exception is that these social programs offer clear and evident value. They contribute in an important way to the social good. Studies designed to evaluate them, even if these studies bear all of the markings of "research," are considered to be exempt from the requirements of ethics board review and subject to informed consent that govern the ethical conduct of research. In a sense, the requirements of ethical research are suspended for studies that offer significant and generally agreed upon value.

This is an extreme case of balancing value against research risks. Indeed, it effectively removes research involving social programs from the purview of ethics oversight. This example is informative not only because it is so extreme, but also because studies of social programs have a great deal in common with pharmacoepidemiologic research. Pharmacoepidemiology's goals of studying medication use and identifying adverse drug reactions are directed as much toward the preservation of the public's health as they are toward the production of generalizable knowledge. The value of pharmacoepidemiologic research is therefore as clear and as readily evident as it is in studies designed to evaluate social programs. On these grounds alone, a compelling argument might be made that some kinds of pharmacoepi- demiology projects, like projects to evaluate important social programs, should be exempt from research review.

Of course, this argument may not be equally cogent and convincing for all pharmacoepidemiologic research because pharmacoepidemiologic research, like any research, spans a continuum. Certainly studies of adverse drug reactions resemble closely the example of social program research. This is one standard, perhaps the highest standard, for a study's potential to produce valuable knowledge. Phrased somewhat differently, the knowledge must be immediately relevant and applicable to the subjects who are being studied. In pharmacoepidemiologic research, one example might be a study of adverse drug reactions among individuals taking a certain medication. Results of this research would have immediate consequences for the health of the patients, or "subjects," for whom data is gathered.

Other studies may be done for private companies or organizations following vigorous methodological standards but where the findings would not be made public or shared with anyone outside the sponsoring organization. It is difficult to know how to balance concerns for privacy against the desire of private entities to obtain pharmacoepidemiology data. Studies like these should arguably be held to a different ethical standard because they do not hold the immediate possibility of clinically relevant knowledge that could be applicable to the people involved. The problem is that no public and national body exists to decide what kinds of research achieve this level of value.

The central ethical issue in pharmacoepidemiologic research is deciding what kinds of projects will generate generalizable knowledge that is widely available and highly valued, and do this in a manner that protects individuals' right to privacy and confidentiality. The problem is that these two ends differ in kind. The knowledge generated by pharmacoepidemiology is health-related knowledge about such things as the risks and benefits of medicines. In contrast, individuals' right to privacy is a matter of civil law. Although the two are frequently cast as in need of balancing, it may not be possible to weigh a certain amount of knowledge to be gained against a certain amount of confidentiality to be lost.

Instead, perhaps the most productive approach will be to determine what kinds of procedures and practices warrant crossing thresholds of confidentiality in the pursuit of valuable knowledge. Such a discussion should include research, but should not by any means be limited to it. For example, society allows journalists wide access to gather and disseminate information, provided the journalist adheres to standards of practice (such as preserving the confidentiality of sources) and journalism is still viewed as a valuable instrument for preserving a democratic society.

Therefore, if the ethical requirement of informed consent is absolute and inviolable, then any balancing would be indefensible. However, this is not a tenable solution, nor is it a solution that would be consistent with the way that society responds to a need for valuable information in other settings. Further public discussion is needed to identify ways in which the policies and procedures for the protection of privacy and the maintenance of confidentiality are fair and consistent with the requirements imposed on other sectors of society.

REFERENCES

1. Advisory Committee on Human Radiation Experiments. Final Report, no. 00000848-9, vol. 061. Washington, DC: Government Printing Office, 1995.
2. Caplan AL. Twenty years after. The legacy of the Tuskegee Syphilis Study. When evil intrudes. *Hastings Cent Rep* 1992; **22**: 29–32.
3. Beecher HK. Ethics and clinical research. *N Engl J Med* 1966; **274**: 1354–60.
4. Kahn JP, Mastroianni AC, Sugarman J. *Beyond Consent. Seeking Justice in Research*. New York: Oxford University Press, 1998.
5. Last JM. Guidelines on ethics for epidemiologists. *Int J Epidemiol* 1990; **16**: 226–9.
6. Beauchamp TL, Cook RR, Fayerweather WE, Raabe GK, Thar WE, Cowles SR, Spivey GH. Ethical guidelines for epidemiologists. *J Clin Epid* 1991; **44**: 151S–69S.
7. Andrews E. Data privacy, medical record confidentiality, and research in the interest of the public health. *Pharmacoepidemiol Drug Saf* 1999; **8**: 247–60.
8. Organization for Economic Cooperation and Development. Guidelines on the Protection of Privacy and Transborder Flow of Personal Data. Recommendation of the OECD Council, September 1980.
9. Mann RD, Bertelsmann A. The issue of data privacy and confidentiality in Europe—1998. *Pharmacoepidemiology Drug Saf* 1999; **8**: 261–4.
10. Brody BA. *The Ethics of Biomedical Research: An International Perspective*. New York: Oxford University Press, 1998.
11. Lynn J, Johnson J, Levine RJ. The ethical conduct of health services research: a case study of 55 institutions' applications to the SUPPORT project. *Clin Res* 1994; **42**: 3–10.
12. National Commission for the Protection of Human Subjects of Biomedical and Behavioral Research. The Belmont Report. *Ethical Principles and Guidelines for the Protection of Human Subjects of Research*. Washington, DC: US Government Printing Office, 1979.
13. Levine RJ. *Ethics and Regulation of Clinical Research*, 2nd edn. Baltimore, MD: Urban and Schwartzenberg, 1986.
14. Department of Health and Human Services, Protection of Human Subjects. Title 45 Part 46: Revised. Code of Federal Regulation; June 18, 1991.
15. Royal College of Physicians. Research involving patients. Reprinted in: Brody, H. *The Ethics of Biomedical Research. An International Perspective*. New York: Oxford University Press, 1990; pp. 315–20.
16. Council for International Organizations of Medical Sciences. International Guidelines for ethical review of epidemiological studies. Reprinted in: Brody, H. *The Ethics of Biomedical Research. An International Perspective*. New York: Oxford University Press, 1998; pp. 225–32.
17. Warren S, Brandeis L. The right to privacy. *Harv Law Rev* 1890; **4**: 193–220.
18. Fried C. Privacy: a rational context. *Yale Law J* 1968; **77**: 475–93.
19. Avineri S, de-Shalit A. *Individualism and Communitarianism*. New York: Oxford University Press, 1992.
20. Freedman B, Fuks A, Weijer C. In loco parentis. Minimal risk as the ethical threshhold for research upon children. *Hastings Cent Rep* 1993; **23**: 13–19.
21. Grisso T, Appelbaum PS. *Assessing Competence to Consent to Treatment*. New York: Oxford University Press, 1998.
22. Brett A, Grodin M. Ethical aspects of human experimentation in health services research. *JAMA* 1991; **265**: 1854–7.
23. Truog RD, Robinson W, Randolph A. Is informed consent always necessary for randomized, controlled trials? *N Engl J Med* 1999; **340**: 804–7.
24. The Nuremberg Code. Reprinted in: Brody, H. T*he Ethics of Biomedical Research. An International Perspective*. New York: Oxford University Press, 1998; p. 213.
25. Freedman B. Scientific value and validity as ethical requirements for research: a proposed explication. *IRB* 1987; **9**: 7–10.
26. Jacobsen SJ, Xia Z, Campion ME, Darby CH, Plevak MF, Seltman KD, Melton LJ 3rd. Potential effect of authorization bias on medical record research. *Mayo Clin Proc* 1999; **74**: 330–8.
27. Melton LJ. The threat to medical-records research. *N Engl J Med* 1997; **337**: 1466–70.
28. McCarthy DB, Shatin D, Drinkard CR. Medical records and privacy: empirical effects of legislation. *Health Serv Res*; **34**: 417–25.
29. Olsen J, Breart G, Feskens E, Grabauskas V, Noah N, Olsen J, Porta M, Saracci R. Directive of the European Parliament and of the Council on the protection of individuals with regard to the processing of personal data and on the free movement of such data. *Int J Epidemiol* 1995; **24**: 462–3.

39

The Use of Randomized Controlled Trials for Pharmacoepidemiology Studies

SAMUEL M. LESKO and ALLEN A. MITCHELL
Slone Epidemiology Center, Boston University, Boston, Massachusetts, USA.

INTRODUCTION

When properly conducted, randomized controlled trials (RCTs) are considered the gold standard for demonstrating the effectiveness of a new medication because they provide unbiased estimates of effect (see Chapter 2). While RCTs are generally used to evaluate beneficial drug effects (see also Chapter 40), too often pharmacoepidemiologists overlook the fact that the advantages of this study design also make it ideal for obtaining an unbiased estimate of the risk of adverse outcomes.

During the premarketing phases of drug development, RCTs involve highly selected subjects and in the aggregate include at most a few thousand patients. These studies are designed to be sufficiently large to provide evidence of a beneficial clinical effect and to exclude large increases in risk of common adverse clinical events. However, premarketing trials are rarely large enough to detect small differences in the risk of common adverse events or to estimate reliably the risk of rare events, whether serious or trivial. Identification and quantification of these potentially important risks require large studies, which typically are conducted after a drug has been marketed. Because of design complexity and costs, large controlled trials have not generally been considered in the pharmacoepidemiologist's armamentarium for the postmarketing evaluation of drugs. Until recently, the authors also did not consider this approach for our postmarketing studies. However, our search for the best method to assess the risk of serious but rare adverse reactions to pediatric ibuprofen caused us to expand our view.[1] The experience that led to that change serves as the basis for this chapter and may prompt others to consider randomized trials for the postmarketing assessment of drug safety.

CLINICAL PROBLEMS TO BE ADDRESSED BY PHARMACOEPIDEMIOLOGIC RESEARCH

Pharmacoepidemiologic methods are used to quantify risks and benefits of medications that could not be adequately evaluated in studies performed during the premarketing phase of drug testing. In this chapter, we will consider the role of postmarketing randomized trials in assessing only the risks of medications; however, the same principles can

Pharmacoepidemiology, Fourth Edition   Edited by B.L. Strom
© 2005 John Wiley & Sons, Ltd

be applied to the postmarketing evaluation of the benefits of medications (see also Chapter 40).

As noted above, premarketing studies are typically too small to detect modest differences in the incidence rates (e.g., relative risks of 2.0 or less) for common adverse events or even large differences in the incidence rates for rare events, such as those that affect 1 per 1000 treated patients. Modest differences in risk of non-life-threatening adverse events can be of substantial public health importance, particularly if the medication is likely to be used by large numbers of patients. For example, following the introduction of angiotensin converting enzyme (ACE) inhibitor use in patients with congestive heart failure, case reports of severe hypotension began to appear in the literature. Although similar events were noted after initial use of other medications (e.g., vasodilators) in congestive heart failure patients, reliable estimates of the risk for different classes of medications were not available. Because of the high prevalence of the indication, differences in risk too small to be detected by conventional RCTs were judged to be clinically important, and a large RCT was conducted to resolve the question.[2]

Modest risks are especially relevant for nutritional supplements or drugs being considered for over-the-counter (OTC) sale, because these agents are likely to be very commonly used and are widely viewed by the public as safe. If there are questions about the safety of a drug after it has been licensed, large observational studies are typically used to satisfy the sample sizes needed to identify (or rule out) the relevant risks. The respective strengths and weaknesses of these designs are discussed elsewhere in this volume (see Chapter 2). However, potential confounding is a major concern for virtually every observational study, and uncontrolled or incompletely controlled confounding can easily account for modest associations between a drug and an adverse clinical event (see Chapters 2 and 47). For example, in the relation between phenylpropanolamine and cerebrovascular disease, obesity increases both the likelihood of exposure to the drug and the risk of a cerebrovascular accident; thus, body weight must be controlled in any analysis of this association. The challenge to the pharmacoepidemiologist is to recognize those factors that represent potential confounders and then control for their effects. To do so requires the relevant information to be included in the data to be analyzed, but information on important confounding factors is frequently incomplete or unavailable. Although surrogate variables are often used (e.g., years of education to reflect socioeconomic status), these may be poor measures of the underlying confounding factor, and their control therefore may not eliminate confounding.

An investigator observing a crude (i.e., unadjusted) association between a drug and an effect attempts to control for confounding by adjusting for one or more factors. If a crude odds ratio (or relative risk) of 5.0 (for example) remains essentially unchanged after all known confounders have been controlled, residual confounding is usually not considered an important concern; although the true (unconfounded) odds ratio may be somewhat smaller than the unadjusted estimate, it is generally assumed to be of similar magnitude. On the other hand, in the same example, if the adjusted odds ratio (or relative risk) is closer to the null value of 1.0, there is empirical evidence of confounding in the data, and the adjusted odds ratio is usually considered the "best" (least biased) measure of the association. However, it is not possible to determine whether there remains any residual confounding in this best estimate, which if *completely* controlled might reveal that the true association is still weaker or even nonexistent.

The authors have direct experience with this concern. Infants treated in newborn intensive care units often receive medications and intravenous fluids through indwelling catheters, and low doses of heparin are periodically infused to help maintain the patency of these catheters. In 1986, we published the results of a case–control study of the use of intravenous heparin in relation to the risk of intraventricular hemorrhage (IVH) in low-birth-weight infants.[3] We compared 66 infants with IVH (cases) to 254 infants with no evidence of IVH (controls), matched on study hospital and duration of observation. Compared to no heparin exposure, the matched odds ratio for heparin exposure on the day prior to detection of IVH was 14 (95% confidence interval [CI] 5.4–34). As additional potential confounders were taken into account, the magnitude of the association became progressively smaller (Table 39.1). Adjustment by logistic regression for the matching factors, birth weight, volume of

Table 39.1. Effect of potential confounding factors on the relation between heparin exposure and intraventricular hemorrhage in 320 premature infants

Model	Potential confounders included	Odds ratio[a]	95% CI
1	Hospital and duration of observation	14.0	5.4–34
2	Model 1 + birth weight	7.5	2.8–20
3	Model 2 + IV fluids	4.4	1.6–12
4	Model 3 + pneumothorax	3.9	1.4–11

[a] Calculated by logistic regression controlling for the potential confounders listed.
Source: Adapted from Lesko *et al.*[3]

parenteral fluids administered, and the presence of pneumo-thorax reduced the odds ratio to 3.9 (95% CI 1.4–11), which did not change further when other potential confounding factors were added to the multivariate model. Although we described an observation that was statistically significant, biologically plausible, and clinically important, we concluded that control of confounding may have been incomplete and that "the association could have been partly, or even wholly, due to the severity of the infants' underlying conditions rather than to the use of heparin." We suggested that the question could only be answered by a randomized trial. A second observational study also found an increased risk (odds ratio 1.96) among infants who received doses of heparin above the lowest quartile of exposure.[4] Uncertainty about the association persisted until 1997, when results were published from a randomized, double blind trial of heparin added to umbilical catheters used to treat premature infants.[5] In this study involving 113 infants, Chang et al. found no difference in the incidence of intraventricular hemorrhage between the heparin treated and control groups ($p = 0.6$). Although the odds ratios from the earlier obser-vational studies were moderately large (3.9 and 1.96) and statistically significant, these "best" estimates of risk were likely due to confounding by one or more factors not completely controlled in the analyses.

Another, perhaps more familiar, example is the purported cardioprotective effect of estrogens. Because women have a lower incidence of heart disease than men, and incidence increases substantially after menopause, it has been hypothe-sized that estrogens reduce the risk of heart disease. Although not all published observational studies have confirmed this association,[6,7] numerous studies, including at least one large prospective cohort study, have reported significantly lower risks of cardiovascular events among women using postmenopausal hormone replacement therapy.[8–10] The Women's Health Initiative (WHI) is a large, complex clinical investigation of several strategies intended to prevent cardiovascular disease and cancer in postmenopausal women.[11] The study included a placebo-controlled, randomized clinical trial of hormone replacement therapy and the risk of coronary heart disease. This compon-ent of the WHI was closed early when a planned interim analysis indicated that the risk of coronary heart disease was significantly elevated among women randomized to hormone replacement therapy (hazard ratio 1.29; 95% CI 1.02–1.63).[12] Further, hazard ratios were also elevated for breast cancer (1.26; 95% CI 1.00–1.59), stroke (1.41; 95% CI 1.07–1.85), and pulmonary embolism (2.13; 95% CI 1.39–3.25). It seems likely that incomplete control of confounding in the observational studies obscured these associations. As these examples demonstrate, when residual confounding is a pos-sible explanation for an apparent association, additional research is needed to determine the true unbiased relationship.

Weak associations deserve particular attention. Although there are important exceptions, the general view is that the stronger the association, the more likely the observed rela-tionship is causal. This is not to say that a weak association (e.g., a relative risk ≤1.5) can never be causal; rather, it is more difficult to be certain of it because such associations, even if statistically significant, can easily be an artifact of confounding. As an example, consider an analysis where socioeconomic status is a potential confounder and education is used as a surrogate for this factor. Because the relation between years of education completed (the surrogate) and socioeconomic status (the potential confounder) is, at best, imperfect, analyses controlling for years of education can only partially control for confounding. This leads to the familiar caveat in reports of observational studies, "residual confounding may account for the observed association." This qualification is no more appropriate than for studies reporting weak associations. As a consequence, even after rigorous efforts have been made to control for confounding, seasoned epidemiologists consider small relative risk estimates to be most compatible with no association, regardless of the confidence interval (or p value). Whether or not one subscribes to this view, it is advisable to use extreme caution in making causal inferences from small relative risks derived from observational studies.

When there is concern about residual confounding prior to embarking on an observational study, one may wish to consider using a non-observational study design. We faced just this situation when we considered how to best assess the safety of pediatric ibuprofen. Ibuprofen is a nonsteroidal anti-inflammatory drug (NSAID) that has become widely used among adults in the US, first by prescription and then as an OTC drug. In 1989, ibuprofen suspension was licensed as a prescription product for fever control in children. It was approved based on premarketing studies in children, which established that it was effective and safe for use under a physician's supervision. Events known to occur in adults using ibuprofen, such as acute gastrointestinal bleeding, acute renal failure, and anaphylaxis, were either not observed at all during the premarketing trials in children or occurred so infrequently that it was not possible to obtain reliable estimates of the risk. In addition, it was at least theoretically possible that Reye's syndrome (a toxic encephalopathy in children associated with another NSAID, aspirin) might be associated with ibuprofen use in children. Other events, possibly unique to children, might also be associated with this drug. Thus, premarketing studies were unable to exclude even a substantially increased risk of important rare but serious adverse reactions.

Once available OTC, pediatric ibuprofen would likely be widely used for the treatment of fever, which is typically a minor and self-limited condition. (We will not discuss whether and when it is appropriate to treat fever in children.) Given the generally benign nature of this indication, it is reasonable to require greater assurance of safety than may be expected for a drug used to treat a life-threatening illness. Further, an effective antipyretic with an excellent record of safety in children, acetaminophen, had been available OTC in the US for more than 20 years. For these reasons, the US Food and Drug Administration required additional data concerning the risk of rare but serious adverse events before it would approve pediatric ibuprofen for OTC sale.

What approach would best provide this information? Observational postmarketing studies, especially case–control studies, are one source of data for very rare conditions. However, the circumstances surrounding ibuprofen use in 1989–90 raised serious concern about whether observational studies could adequately control confounding. Specifically, prior to the availability of pediatric ibuprofen, febrile children in the US received no antipyretic or were given acetaminophen, which was generally considered safe by both physicians and parents. On the other hand, because ibuprofen was available only by prescription, treatment with this drug required contact with a physician. In addition, for fever less than 102.5 °F, the recommended dose of prescription ibuprofen was 5 mg/kg, whereas for fever of 102.5 °F or greater, the dose was 10 mg/kg. Both its status as a prescription medication and the two-tier dosing schedule predicted that ibuprofen would be used for more severe illness than acetaminophen. This prediction was supported by a survey of 108 physicians (61 pediatricians, 47 family practitioners) conducted in 1992.[1] More than half of the physicians in the study reported that they treated children with ibuprofen after acetaminophen failed, but none reported using acetaminophen only when ibuprofen was not effective. Further, both the minimum age and temperature at which the physicians recommended using these drugs were higher for ibuprofen than acetaminophen. It seemed clear that pediatric ibuprofen would be most commonly used among children whose illness was relatively severe, or whose fever was particularly high or unresponsive to acetaminophen. Because of the greater severity of illness (and potential exposure to antibiotics or other medications), there was a reasonable basis to believe that ibuprofen users would experience relatively high rates of adverse clinical events, *unrelated to the ibuprofen itself*. It was apparent, then, that to provide a valid assessment of the risks of pediatric ibuprofen, a study must be able to distinguish the risks of the drug from the risks associated with the illness for which ibuprofen was given.

METHODOLOGIC PROBLEMS TO BE SOLVED BY PHARMACOEPIDEMIOLOGIC RESEARCH

The phenomenon described above for pediatric ibuprofen is known as confounding by indication (also referred to as indication bias, channeling, confounding by severity, or contraindication bias). According to Slone *et al.* confounding by indication exists when "patients who receive different treatments . . . differ in their risk of adverse outcomes, independent of the treatment received."[13] In general, confounding by indication occurs when an observed association between a drug and an outcome is due to the underlying illness (or its severity) and not to any effect of the drug. Put another way, confounding by indication occurs when the risk of an adverse event is related to the *indication* for medication use but not the use of medication itself. As with any other form of confounding, one can, in theory, control for its effects if one can reliably measure the severity of the underlying illness. In practice, however, this is not easily done.

Confounding by indication is a particular concern in a number of settings (see Chapters 40 and 47). When there is a single therapy for an illness, and all patients receive the therapy (i.e., are "channeled" to the treatment), it is not possible to control for confounding in an observational study simply because no patients are left untreated to serve as controls. For example, it is standard practice to administer artificial surfactant to premature infants at risk for respiratory distress syndrome of the newborn. If any infants are not treated, they are likely to differ from treated infants in that they may have a very mild form of the illness, or they may have a major congenital malformation and not be expected to survive. Thus, they are also likely to have different risks for many clinical outcomes. While it may be rare for all patients with a given illness to be treated in exactly the same way, this situation is not unusual for subgroups of patients. For example, all patients with diabetes are not treated with insulin, but patients with type I (insulin-dependent) diabetes are. In general, observational studies are most informative when patients receiving different medications are similar with respect to their risks of adverse events. Cohort studies will be compromised if there is no reasonable alternative to the study treatment, including no treatment, to serve as a control. Case–control studies may be infeasible if one cannot identify controls that, aside from any effect of the exposure, are equally at risk of having the outcome diagnosed as the cases.

When there is at least one alternate treatment option and it is possible to control for obvious confounding, observational studies can contribute to our understanding of a medication's risks, particularly where the adjusted relative risk is large. However, as discussed above, a small relative risk (e.g., 1.3) can easily be an artifact of confounding by an unknown factor or by incomplete control of a recognized confounder.

When confronted with the task of assessing the safety of a marketed drug product, the pharmacoepidemiologist must evaluate the specific hypothesis to be tested and estimate the magnitude of the hypothesized association and determine whether confounding by indication is possible. If incomplete control of confounding is likely, it is important to recognize the limitations of observational research designs and consider conducting an RCT. There is nothing inherent in an RCT that precludes a pharmacoepidemiologist from designing and carrying out these studies. To the contrary, the special skills of a pharmacoepidemiologist can be very useful in performing large-scale RCTs after a drug is marketed.

OVERVIEW OF CLASSIC RCTs

As noted above, RCTs are most commonly used during the premarketing phases of drug development to demonstrate a drug's efficacy (and to gather general information concerning safety). By randomization, one hopes to make the distributions of confounding factors (both known and unknown) equal in all groups. If the study is sufficiently large, the assigned treatment is the most likely explanation for any observed differences in the clinical outcomes (improvement in the illness or the occurrence of adverse clinical events) between the treatment groups. By definition, participants in observational studies are not assigned treatment at random. As we have seen, the choice of treatment may be determined by the stage or severity of the illness or by the patient's poor response to or adverse experience with alternative therapies, which can introduce bias.

Sample Size

In homogeneous populations, balanced treatment groups can be achieved with relatively small study sizes. In heterogeneous populations (e.g., children less than 12 years of age), a large sample size may be required to insure the equal distribution of uncommon confounders between study groups (e.g., infants versus toddlers versus school-age children). Study size is determined by the need to assure balance between treatment groups and the magnitude of the effect to be detected. Large randomized studies minimize the chance

that the treatment groups are different with respect to potential confounders and permit the detection of small differences in clinical outcomes.

Blinding

Blinding is used to minimize detection bias, and is particularly important where the outcome is at all subjective. Reporting of subjective symptoms by study participants and the detection of even objectively defined outcome events may be influenced by knowledge of the medications the patient is using. For example, if a patient complains of abdominal pain, a physician may be more likely to perform a test for occult blood in the stool if that patient was being treated with ibuprofen rather than acetaminophen. Thus, follow-up data collection will only be unbiased if both parties (patients and investigators) are unaware of the treatment assigned. Blinding may not be possible for non-drug treatments such as diet, exercise, and surgery, and double blinding may be difficult to achieve and maintain in drug studies as well, particularly if either the study or control medication produces specific symptoms (i.e., side effects) or easily observable physiologic effects (e.g., change in pulse rate or blood pressure).

Choice of Control Treatment

The hypothesis being tested determines the choice of control treatment. Placebo controls are most useful for making comparisons with untreated disease but may not represent standard of care and have been challenged as unethical.[14] Further, it may be difficult to maintain blinding in placebo-controlled studies, as noted above. Studies employing an active control typically utilize common drug treatments, which frequently represent the standard of care. Although often considered more ethical and easier to keep blinded because the illness and symptoms are not left untreated, these studies do not permit comparison with the natural history of the illness.

Data Collection

Data collection in a premarketing clinical trial is generally resource intensive. Detailed descriptive and clinical data are collected at enrollment, and extensive clinical and laboratory data are collected at regular and often frequent intervals during follow-up. In addition to the data needed to test the hypothesis of a clinical benefit, premarketing trials of medications must also assess safety and therefore must collect extensive data on symptoms, physical signs, and laboratory evaluations. Such data collection contributes substantially to the high cost of these trials.

Data Analysis

In observational studies, data analyses may be quite complex because of the need to adjust for potential confounders. In contrast, analysis of the primary hypothesis in many clinical trials is straightforward and involves a comparison of some measure of the outcome event (which may be either a continuous or categorical variable) in different groups. Analyses involving repeated measures, subgroups of study subjects, or adjustment to control for incomplete or ineffective randomization may be performed, but they add complexity.

Methodologic strengths notwithstanding, there are several features of the classic RCT that limit its use as a postmarketing study design. First, the complexity and cost of traditional premarket RCTs, with their detailed observations and resource-intensive follow-up, make very large studies of this type generally infeasible. Second, it may be unethical to conduct a study in which patients are randomly assigned a potentially harmful treatment. For example, an RCT to test the hypothesis that cigarette smoking increases the risk of heart disease would not be acceptable. However, if the study can be simplified and use the epidemiologist's tools to track patients and collect follow-up data, it may be possible to both control costs and make a large study feasible. The ethical dilemma can be resolved by studying only questions that are truly important to the public's health and for which the answers are not known.

Generalizability of Results

The usual clinical trial conducted during the premarketing evaluation of a drug almost always involves highly selected patients; as a consequence, the results of the trial may not be generalizable to the large numbers of patients who may use the medication after licensing. Traditionally, pharmacoepidemiologists may be more attracted to observational studies because they can reflect the real-world experience of medication use and clinical outcomes, and because their modest costs permit studies involving large numbers of patients.

CURRENTLY AVAILABLE SOLUTIONS

LARGE SIMPLE TRIALS

Large, simple trials (LSTs) may be the best solution when it is not possible to completely control confounding by means other than randomization. If the volume and complexity of data collection can be kept to a minimum, there is no reason that large trials cannot be conducted. Indeed, the US Salk vaccine trial of the early 1950s is an example of a very large trial.[15] More recently, large randomized trials have been used to test the efficacy of therapeutic interventions, especially in cardiology,[16–23] or to evaluate dietary supplements or pharmaceuticals for primary prevention of cardiovascular disease and cancer.[24–33] This approach has also been used successfully to evaluate the risk of adverse drug effects when the more common observational designs have been judged inadequate.[2,34] LSTs are really just very large randomized trials made simple by reducing data collection to the minimum needed to test only a single hypothesis (or at most a few hypotheses). Randomization of treatment assignment is the key feature of the design, which controls for confounding by known and unknown factors. The large study size provides the power needed to evaluate small risks, either absolute or relative.

How Simple Is Simple?

Yusuf *et al.* have suggested that very large randomized studies of treatment-related mortality need collect only data concerning the vital status of participants at the conclusion of the study.[35] Because the question of drug safety frequently concerns outcomes less severe than mortality, these ultra simple trials may not be sufficient. Hasford has suggested a somewhat less restrictive approach to data collection, in which "large trials with lean protocols" include only *relevant* baseline, follow-up, and outcome data.[36] Collecting far less data than is common in the usual RCT is the key feature of both approaches. With simplified protocols that take advantage of epidemiologic follow-up methods, very large trials can be conducted to test hypotheses of interest to pharmacoepidemiologists.

Power/Sample Size

Study power is not simply a function of the number of subjects enrolled. It is related to the number of events observed during the course of the study, which in turn is a function of the incidence rate for the event, the sample size, and the duration of observation (or follow-up). Power requirements can be satisfied by studying a population at high risk, enrolling a large sample size, or conducting follow-up for a prolonged period. The appropriate approach will be determined by considering the goal of the study and the hypothesis to be tested. Allergic or idiosyncratic events may require a very large study population, and events with long latency periods may be best studied with long duration follow-up. While an elderly population may be at high risk for gastrointestinal bleeding or cardiovascular events, a study limited to this group may lack generalizability and would be inappropriate to assess the risk of these events in younger adults or children.

Data Elements

The data collection process can be kept simple by restricting the study to a few primary endpoints that satisfy the study hypothesis, are objective, are easily identified, and are verifiable. Epidemiologists may need to overcome their predisposition to comprehensive data collection when it comes to secondary outcomes (i.e., those that do not directly relate to the study hypothesis), as these must be ignored to eliminate unnecessary effort. Because confounding is controlled by randomization, data on all potential confounders need not be collected. Rather, a few basic demographic variables can be collected at enrollment in order to characterize the population studied and allow the investigators to confirm that effective randomization was achieved.

Data Collection

The data collection process itself can be streamlined to keep the study simple. Follow-up data can be collected by mailed questionnaires or telephone interviews conducted directly with the study participants. Because the study will be limited to clear and objective outcomes (see below) which can be confirmed by medical record review or other means, self-report by the study participants can be an appropriate source of follow-up data. Other sources of follow-up data could include electronic medical records (e.g., for studies conducted among subscribers of a large health maintenance organization) or vital status records for fatal outcomes (e.g., the US National Death Index).

The primary advantage of this simplicity is that it allows very large groups of study participants to be followed at reasonable cost. The trade-off, of course, is that a simple trial cannot answer all possible questions about the safety of a drug but must be limited to testing, at most, a few related hypotheses.

WHEN IS A LARGE SIMPLE RANDOMIZED TRIAL APPROPRIATE?

LSTs are appropriate when all of the conditions in Table 39.2 apply.

Table 39.2. Conditions appropriate for the conduct of a large randomized trial

(1)	The research question is important.
(2)	Genuine uncertainty exists about the likely results.
(3a)	The absolute risk is small and confounding by indication is likely or
(3b)	The relative risk is small, regardless of the absolute risk.
(4)	Important effect modification (interaction) is unlikely.

Important Research Question

Although a simple trial will cost less per subject than a traditional clinical trial, the total cost of a large study (in money and human resources) will still be substantial. The cost will usually be justified only when there is a clear need for a reliable answer to a question concerning the risk of a serious outcome. A minor medication side effect such as headache or nausea may not be trivial for the individual patient but may not warrant the expense of a large study. On the other hand, if the question involves the risk of premature death, permanent disability, hospitalization, or other serious events, the cost may well be justified.

Uncertainty Must Exist

An additional condition has been referred to as the "uncertainty principle." This was originally described by Gray et al. as a simple criterion to assess subject eligibility in LSTs.[37] It states that "both patient and doctor should be *substantially uncertain* about the appropriateness, for this particular patient, of each of the trial treatments. If the patient and doctor are *reasonably certain* that one or other treatment is inappropriate then it would not be ethical for the patient's treatment to be chosen at random" (italic in the original). We support this principle and would extend its use to evaluate when it is appropriate to conduct an LST to test a given hypothesis related to the risk of an adverse clinical event. Very large randomized trials are justified only when there is true uncertainty about the risk of the treatment in the population. Apart from considerations of benefit, it would not be ethical to subject large numbers of patients to a treatment that was reasonably believed to place them at increased risk, however small, of a potentially serious or permanent adverse clinical event. The concept of uncertainty can thus be extended to include a global assessment of the combined risks and benefits of the treatments being compared. One treatment may be known to provide therapeutic benefits that are superior to an alternative, but it may be unknown whether the risks of important side effects outweigh the therapeutic advantage. For example, the antiestrogen tamoxifen may improve breast cancer survival, but may do so only at the cost of an increased risk of endometrial cancer. Appropriately, a randomized trial was undertaken to resolve uncertainty in this situation.[25]

Power and Confounding

LSTs will only be needed if (i) the *absolute* risk of the study outcome is small and there are concerns about confounding by indication, *or* (ii) the *relative* risk is small (in which case, there are inherent concerns about residual confounding from any source).[23] By contrast, LSTs would not be necessary if the *absolute* risk were large, because premarket or other conventional RCTs should be adequate, or where confounding by indication is not an issue, because observational studies would suffice; also, if the *relative* risk were large (and confounding by indication is not a concern), observational studies would be appropriate.

No Interaction between Treatment and Outcome

An additional requirement for LSTs is that important interactions between the treatment and patient characteristics (effect modification) are unlikely.[23] In other words, the available evidence should suggest that the association will be qualitatively similar in all patient subgroups. Variation in the strength of the association is acceptable among subgroups, but there should be no suggestion that the effect would be completely reversed in one or more subgroups. Because of the limited data available in a truly simple trial, it may not be possible to test whether an interaction has occurred, and the data collected may not be sufficient to identify relevant subgroups. Because randomization only controls confounding for comparisons made between the groups that were randomized, subsets of these groups may not be strictly comparable with respect to one or more confounding factors. Thus, if clinically important interaction is considered likely, additional steps must be taken to permit the appropriate analyses (e.g., stratified randomization). This added complexity may result in a study that is no longer a truly simple trial.

WHEN IS AN LST FEASIBLE?

LSTs are feasible when all of the conditions in Table 39.3 are met.

Table 39.3. Conditions which make a large, simple randomized trial feasible

---

(1) The study question can be expressed as a simple testable hypothesis.
(2) The treatment to be tested is simple (uncomplicated).
(3) The outcome is objectively defined (e.g., hospitalization, death).
(4) Epidemiologic follow-up methods are appropriate.
(5) A cooperative and motivated population is available for study.

Simple Hypothesis

LSTs are best suited to answer focused and relatively uncomplicated questions. For example, an LST can be designed to test the hypothesis that the risk of hospitalization for any reason, or for acute gastrointestinal bleeding, is increased in children treated with ibuprofen. However, it may not be possible for a single LST to answer the much more general question, "Is ibuprofen safe with respect to all possible outcomes in children?"

Simple Treatments

Simple therapies (e.g., a single drug at a fixed dose for a short duration) are most amenable to study with LSTs. They are likely to be commonly used, so that it will be easy to enroll large numbers of patients, and the results will be applicable to a large segment of the population. Complex therapeutic protocols are difficult to manage, reduce patient compliance, and by their very nature may not be compatible with the simple trial design.

Objective and Easily Measured Outcomes

The outcomes to be studied should be objective, easy to define ("simple"), and easy to recall. An example might include hospitalization for acute gastrointestinal bleeding. Study participants may not correctly recall the details of a hospital admission, or even the specific reason for admission, but they likely will recall the fact that they were admitted, the name of the hospital, and at least the approximate date of admission. Medical records can be obtained to document the details of the clinical events that occurred. Events of this type can be reliably recorded using epidemiologic follow-up methods (e.g., questionnaires, telephone interviews, or linkage with public vital status records). On the other hand, clinical outcomes which can be reliably detected only by detailed in-person interviews, physical examinations, or extensive physiologic testing are not as amenable for study in simple trials.

Cooperative Population

Particularly in LSTs, a cooperative and motivated study population will greatly increase the probability of success. Striking examples are the large populations in the Physicians' and Women's Health Studies; the success of these studies is at least partly due to the willingness of large numbers of knowledgeable health professionals to participate.[38,39] Because of the participants' knowledge of medical conditions and symptoms and participation in the US health care system, relatively sophisticated information could be obtained using mailed questionnaires, and even biologic samples could be collected. Success of the Boston University Fever Study was also largely due to parents whose motivation and cooperation were encouraged by their private physicians who had invited them to participate in the study.[34]

LOGISTICS OF CONDUCTING AN LST

An LST may be appropriate and feasible, but it will only succeed if all logistical aspects of the study are kept simple as well. In general, LSTs are "multicenter" studies involving a group of primary investigators who are responsible for the scientific conduct of the study, a central data coordinating facility, and a network of enrollment sites (possibly the offices of collaborating physicians or other health care providers). Health care professionals (e.g., physicians, nurse practitioners, and pharmacists in private practice or members of large health care organizations) can participate by recruiting eligible patients and obtaining informed consent. Alternative methods to identify and enroll eligible subjects (e.g., direct mailings to professional groups or print ads) may be appropriate for some studies. Because success depends on the cooperation of multiple health care providers and a large number of patients, it may be best to limit the demands placed on each practitioner (or his/her clinical practice).

To facilitate patient recruitment and to maximize generalizability of the results, minimal restrictions should be placed on patient eligibility. As Gray *et al.* have said, "Any obstacle to simplicity is an obstacle to large size, and the wider the range of the patients studied, the wider the generalizability of the results will be."[37] Patients with a medical contraindication or known sensitivity to either the study or control drug should not, of course, be enrolled, but other restrictions should be kept to a minimum and should ideally reflect only restrictions that would apply in a typical clinical setting.

Simple informed consent and registration documents should be completed in triplicate with one copy kept on file by the enrolling collaborator, one given to the study participant, and one forwarded to the data coordinating center by mail or facsimile. Registration of study subjects can also be accomplished online using a secure Internet (or dialup) connection to the coordinating center, which allows for immediate confirmation of eligibility and randomization.[40] Substantial bias can be introduced if either physician or patient can choose not to participate after learning (or guessing) which treatment the patient has been assigned. Therefore, patients should be randomized only after eligibility has been confirmed and the enrollment process completed.

Particularly in studies requiring a long duration of medication use, validity may be seriously compromised by poor compliance with the treatment regimen. A run-in period prior to randomization can be used to identify patients who are unable or unwilling to adhere to a chronic treatment regimen and are likely to drop out of the study. During the run-in period, eligible subjects are given a "test" medication and their compliance with the protocol is assessed. Patients who cannot comply with the protocol are withdrawn from the trial. Patients who remain in the study are likely to be highly compliant, so that relatively few will drop out after randomization. Depending on the characteristics of drugs under study, either the active drug or the control may be preferable for the run-in period. In the Physicians' Health Study, for example, the study drug aspirin was used for the run-in period to identify subjects who could not tolerate the gastrointestinal side effects of the drug.[38] As a consequence, however, the data cannot be used to assess the risk of gastrointestinal bleeding following aspirin use.

Importance of Complete Follow-Up

Because dropouts and losses to follow-up may not be random but rather may be related to adverse treatment effects, it is important to make every effort to obtain follow-up data on all enrolled subjects. For example, a study that has follow-up data on even tens of thousands of patients may not be able to provide a valid answer to the primary study question if this number represents only half of those randomized. The duration of the follow-up period can affect the completeness of follow-up data collection. If the duration of follow-up is too short, important outcomes may be missed (i.e., they may not be diagnosed until after the end of the follow-up period). On the other hand, as the length of the follow-up period increases, the number lost to follow-up or exposed to the alternate treatment (contaminated exposure) increases. In the extreme, a randomized trial becomes a cohort study because of selective dropouts in either or both of the treatment arms. Beyond choosing a motivated and interested study population, the investigators can minimize losses to follow-up by maintaining regular contact with all study participants.

Regular mailings of supplies of medication, a study newsletter, or email reminders can be helpful, and memory aids such as medication calendar packs or other devices may help maintain compliance with chronic treatment schedules. In addition, follow-up data collection itself can help maintain contact with study participants.

Follow-Up Data Collection

An important element of a successful LST is that follow-up data collection is the responsibility of the central study staff. Busy health care providers frequently cannot commit the time required to consistently obtain even minimal but specific follow-up data from large numbers of subjects. However, the clinician who originally enrolled the subject may be able to provide limited follow-up data (e.g., vital status) or a current address or telephone number for the occasional patient who would otherwise be lost to follow-up. A questionnaire delivered by mail, supplemented by telephone interviews when needed, has been shown to work quite well.[34] The response rate will likely be greatest if the questions are both simple and direct and the time required to complete the questionnaire is limited. Medical records can be reviewed to verify important outcomes, such as rare adverse events, and the work needed to obtain and abstract the relevant records should be manageable. If there is a need to confirm a diagnosis or evaluate symptoms, a limited number of participants can be referred to their enrolling health care provider for examination or to have blood or other studies performed. In addition, a search of public records (e.g., the National Death Index in the US) can identify study subjects who have died during follow-up.

ANALYSIS

Primary Analysis

Analyses of the primary outcomes are usually straightforward and involve a simple comparison of incidence rates between the treatment and control groups. Under the assumption that confounding has been controlled by the randomization procedure, complex multivariate analyses are not necessary (and may not be possible because only limited data on potential confounders are available). Descriptive data collected at enrollment should be analyzed by treatment group to test the randomization procedure; any material differences between treatment groups suggest an imbalance despite randomization. As noted above, it is assumed that there is no material interaction between patient characteristics and medication effects, thus eliminating the need for complex statistical analyses to test for effect modification.

Subgroup Analyses

It is important to remember that confounding factors will be distributed evenly only among groups that were randomized; subgroups which are not random samples of the original randomization groups may not have similar distributions of confounding factors. For example, participants who have remained in the study (i.e., have not dropped out or been lost to follow-up) may not be fully representative of the original randomization groups and may not be comparable with respect to confounders. Despite all efforts, complete follow-up is rarely achieved, and because only the original randomization groups can be assumed to be free of confounding, at least one analysis involving all enrolled study subjects (i.e., an intention-to-treat analysis) should be performed. Also, unless a stratified randomization scheme was used, one cannot be certain that unmeasured confounding variables will be evenly distributed in subgroups of participants, and the smaller the subgroup, the greater the potential for imbalance. Therefore, subgroup analyses will be subject to the same limitations as observational studies (i.e., the potential for uncontrolled confounding).

Data Monitoring/Interim Analyses

Because of the substantial commitment of resources and large number of patients potentially at risk for adverse outcomes, it is often appropriate to monitor the accumulating data over the course of the study. The study may sometimes be ended prematurely if participants experience unacceptable risks, if the hypothesis can be satisfactorily tested earlier than anticipated, or if it becomes clear that a statistically significant result cannot be achieved, even if the study were to be completed as planned. A data monitoring committee, independent of the study investigators, can conduct periodic reviews of the data using an appropriate group sequential analysis procedure to preserve the study's overall type I error rate.[41,42]

THE FUTURE

With accelerated approval of new medications and rapid increases in their use, we may see a greater need for large postmarketing studies capable of randomizing exposures in order to assess small differences in risk. This is particularly the case for drugs that are being considered for OTC switch, because the risks of rare and unknown events that would be acceptable under prescription status might be unacceptable when the drug is self-administered and likely used by much larger and diverse populations. In the absence of techniques that reliably control for confounding by indication in observational studies, there may be a growing need for LSTs to evaluate larger relative risks. Improvements in the efficiency with which such trials can be carried out may lead to their increased use.

One possible approach that may improve efficiency in large studies would be to conduct trials involving patients who receive care from very large health delivery systems with automated medical records. If reliable data concerning relevant outcomes (e.g., hospitalization for gastrointestinal bleeding) were available in automated medical records for all study participants, it would be theoretically possible to eliminate the need to contact patients to collect follow-up data. It would still be necessary to identify eligible subjects, obtain consent, and randomize treatment. In addition, assurance would have to be provided that events were not being missed by patients presenting to out-of-plan providers. In theory, it may be possible to conduct such a "hybrid trial," but to our knowledge, such a trial has not been attempted.

In settings where there is no appropriate control treatment and it is not ethical to randomize between active drug and placebo, an alternative to an LST might be to enroll and follow a single cohort of perhaps the first 10 000 users of a study medication. However, the absence of a comparison group would make it impossible to determine whether the observed risks were due to the drug, the disease, or other factors, although it would at least be possible to accurately estimate the absolute risk of important events, whatever their cause, among exposed subjects. An alternative and perhaps preferable approach would be to randomize to different doses, when possible, and search for a dose–response relationship.

It is clear that very large simple controlled trials of drug safety can be successfully carried out.[2,34] It is less clear, however, how frequently the factors that indicate the need for a very large trial (Table 39.2) will converge with those that permit such a trial to be carried out (Table 39.3). As pharmacoepidemiologists become more comfortable with LSTs, we may see more of them being conducted, and new methods of subject recruitment and more efficient sources of follow-up data are likely to be developed.

REFERENCES

1. Mitchell AA, Lesko SM. When a randomized controlled trial is needed to assess drug safety: the case of pediatric ibuprofen. *Drug Saf* 1995; **13**: 15–24.

2. Hasford J, Bussmann W-D, Delius W, Koepcke W, Lehmann K, Weber E. First dose hypotension with enalapril and prazosin in congestive heart failure. *Int J Cardiol* 1991; **31**: 287–94.

3. Lesko S, Mitchell AA, Epstein MF, Louik C, Giacoia GP, Shapiro S. Heparin use as a risk factor for intraventricular hemorrhage in low-birth-weight infants. *N Engl J Med* 1986; **314**: 1156–60.

4. Malloy MH, Cutter GR. The association of heparin exposure with intraventricular hemorrhage among very low birth weight infants. *J Perinatol* 1995; **15**: 185–91.

5. Chang GY, Leuder FL, DiMichele DM, Radkowski MA, McWilliams LJ, Jansen RD. Heparin and the risk of intraventricular hemorrhage in premature infants. *J Pediatr* 1997; **131**: 362–6.

6. Rosenberg L, Armstrong B, Jick H. Myocardial infarction and estrogen therapy in post-menopausal women. *N Engl J Med* 1976; **294**: 1256–9.

7. Wilson PW, Garrison RJ, Castelli WP. Postmenopausal estrogen use, cigarette smoking, and cardiovascular morbidity in women over 50. The Framingham Study. *N Engl J Med* 1985; **313**: 1038–43.

8. Byrd BF, Burch JC, Vaughn WK. The impact of long term estrogen support after hysterectomy. A report of 1016 cases. *Ann Surg* 1977; **185**: 574–80.

9. Ross RK, Paganini-Hill A, Mack TM, Arthur M, Henderson BE. Menopausal oestrogen therapy and protection from death from ischaemic heart disease. *Lancet* 1981; **1**: 858–60.

10. Stampfer MJ, Willett WC, Colditz GA, Rosner B, Speizer FE, Hennekens CH. A prospective study of postmenopausal estrogen therapy and coronary heart disease. *N Engl J Med* 1985; **313**: 1044–9.

11. Women's Health Initiative (WHI) Study Group. Design of the Women's Health Initiative clinical trial and observational study. *Control Clin Trials* 1998; **19**: 61–109.

12. Rossouw JE, Anderson GL, Prentice RL, LaCroix AZ, Kooperberg C, Stefanick ML *et al*. Writing Group for the Women's Health Initiative Investigators. Risks and benefits of estrogen plus progestin in healthy postmenopausal women: principal results from the Women's Health Initiative randomized controlled trial. *JAMA* 2002; **288**: 321–33.

13. Slone D, Shapiro S, Miettinen OS, Finkle WD, Stolley PD. Drug evaluation after marketing. A policy perspective. *Ann Intern Med* 1979; **90**: 257–61.

14. Rothman KJ, Michels KB. The continuing unethical use of placebo controls. *N Engl J Med* 1994; **331**: 394–8.

15. Francis T Jr, Korns R, Voight R, Boisen M, Hemphill F, Napier J *et al*. An evaluation of the 1954 poliomyelitis vaccine trials: summary report. *Am J Public Health* 1955; **45** (suppl): 1–50.

16. Gruppo Italiano per lo Studio della Streptochinasi nell'infarto miocardico (GISSI). Effectiveness of intravenous thrombolytic treatment in acute myocardial infarction. *Lancet* 1986; **i**: 397–402.

17. Gruppo Italiano per lo Studio della Streptochinasi nell'infarto miocardico (GISSI). GISSI-2: a factorial randomized trial of alteplase versus streptokinase and heparin versus no heparin

among 12 490 patients with acute myocardial infarction. *Lancet* 1990; **336**: 65–71.

18. GUSTO investigators. An international randomized trial comparing four thrombolytic strategies for acute myocardial infarction. *N Engl J Med* 1993; **329**: 673–82.

19. ISIS-1 (First International Study of Infarct Survival) Collaborative Group. Randomised trial of intravenous atenolol among 16,027 cases of suspected acute myocardial infarction: ISIS-1. *Lancet* 1986; **ii**: 57–66.

20. ISIS-2 (Second International Study of Infarct Survival) Collaborative Group. Randomised trial of intravenous streptokinase, oral aspirin, both, or neither among 17,187 cases of suspected acute myocardial infarction: ISIS-2. *Lancet* 1988; **ii**: 349–60.

21. ISIS-3 (Third International Study of Infarct Survival) Collaborative Group. A randomised trial of streptokinase *vs* tissue plasminogen activator *vs* anistreplase and of aspirin plus heparin *vs* aspirin alone among 41,299 cases of suspected acute myocardial infarction. *Lancet* 1992; **399**: 753–70.

22. ISIS-4 Collaborative Group Fourth International Study of Infarct Survival: Protocol for a large, simple study of the effects of oral mononitrate, of oral captopril, and of intravenous magnesium. *Am J Cardiol* 1991; **68**: 87D–100D.

23. Yusuf S. Reduced mortality and morbidity with the use of angiotensin-converting enzyme inhibitors in patients with left ventricular dysfunction and congestive heart failure. *Herz* 1993; **18**(suppl): 444–8.

24. Alpha-Tocopherol, Beta Carotene Cancer Prevention Study Group. The effect of vitamin E and beta carotene on the incidence of lung cancer and other cancer in male smokers. *N Engl J Med* 1994; **330**: 1029–35.

25. Fisher B, Costantion JP, Wickerham DL, Redmond CK, Kavannah M, Cronin WM *et al*. Tamoxifen for prevention of breast cancer: report of the National Surgical Adjuvant Breast and Bowel Project P-1 Study. *J Natl Cancer Inst* 1998; **90**: 1371–88.

26. Gerstein HC, Bosch J, Pogue J, Taylor DW, Zinman B, Yusuf S. Rationale and design of a large study to evaluate the renal and cardiovascular effects of an ACE inhibitor and vitamin E in high-risk patients with diabetes. The MICRO-HOPE Study. Microalbuminuria, cardiovascular, and renal outcomes. Heart Outcomes Prevention Evaluation. *Diabetes Care* 1996; **19**: 1225–8.

27. GISSI Prevenzione Investigators. Dietary supplementation with n-3 polyunsaturated fatty acids and vitamin E after myocardial infarction: results of the GISSI Prevenzione trial. *Lancet* 1999; **354**: 447–55.

28. Heart Outcomes Prevention Evaluation (HOPE) Study Investigators. Vitamin E supplementation and cardiovascular events in high risk patients. *N Engl J Med* 2000; **342**: 154–60.

29. Hennekens CH, Buring JE, Manson JE, Stampfer M, Rosner B, Cook NR *et al*. Lack of effect of long-term supplementation with beta carotene on the incidence of malignant neoplasms and cardiovascular disease. *N Engl J Med* 1996; **334**: 1145–9.

30. Klein EA, Lippman SM, Thompson IM, Goodman PJ, Albanes D, Taylor PR, Coltman C. The selenim and vitamin E cancer prevention trial. *World J Urol* 2003; **21**: 21–7.

31. Omenn GS, Goodman GE, Thornquist MD, Balmes J, Cullen MR, Glass A *et al*. Effects of combination of beta carotene and vitamin A on lung cancer and cardiovascular disease. *N Engl J Med* 1996; **334**: 1150–5.

32. Steering Committee of the Physicians' Health Study Research Group. Final report on the aspirin component of the ongoing Physicians' Health Study. *N Engl J Med* 1989; **321**: 129–35.

33. Thompson IM, Goodman PJ, Tangen CM, Lucia MS, Miller GJ, Ford LG *et al*. The influence of finasteride on the development of prostate cancer. *N Engl J Med* 2003; **349**: 215–24.

34. Lesko SM, Mitchell AA. An assessment of the safety of pediatric ibuprofen: a practitioner-based randomized clinical trial. *JAMA* 1995; **273**: 929–33.

35. Yusuf S, Collins R, Peto R. Why do we need some large, simple randomized trials? *Stat Med* 1984; **3**: 409–20.

36. Hasford J. Drug risk assessment: a case for large trials with lean protocols. *Pharmacoepidemiol Drug Saf* 1994; **3**: 321–7.

37. Gray R, Clarke M, Collins R, Peto R Making randomized trials larger: a simple solution? *Eur J Surg Oncol* 1995; **2**: 137–9.

38. Hennekens CH, Buring JE. Methodologic considerations in the design and conduct of randomized trials: the U.S. Physicians' Health Study. *Control Clin Trials* 1989; **10**: 142S–50S.

39. Lee IM, Cook NR, Manson JE, Buring JE, Hennekens CH. Beta-carotene supplementation and incidence of cancer and cardiovascular disease: the Women's Health Study. *J Natl Cancer Inst*. 1999; **91**(24): 2102–6.

40. Santoro E, Nicolis E, Grazia Franzosi M. Telecommunications technology for the management of large scale clinical trials: the GISSI experience. *Comput Methods Programs Biomed* 1999; **60**: 215–23.

41. O'Brien PC. Data and safety monitoring. In: Armitage P, Colton T, eds, *Encyclopedia of Biostatistics*. Chichester: John Wiley & Sons, 1998; pp. 1058–66.

42. DeMets DL. Data and safety monitoring boards. In: Armitage P, Colton T, eds, *Encyclopedia of Biostatistics*. Chichester: John Wiley & Sons, 1998; pp. 1067–71.

40

The Use of Pharmacoepidemiology to Study Beneficial Drug Effects

BRIAN L. STROM[1] and the late KENNETH L. MELMON[2]

[1] University of Pennsylvania School of Medicine, Philadelphia, Pennsylvania, USA; [2] Stanford University School of Medicine, Stanford, California, USA.

INTRODUCTION

In order to be approved for marketing in the United States, drugs must be proven to be safe and effective using "adequate and well-controlled investigations." Earlier chapters in this book have shown that this premarketing information often is insufficient to provide some of the information about drug toxicity which is clinically most important. The same applies to information about drug efficacy.

In this chapter we will begin by clarifying the different definitions of various types of beneficial drug effects. Then we will discuss the need for *postmarketing studies of drug effectiveness*. Next, we will present the unique methodologic problems raised by studies of beneficial drug effects, as well as potential solutions to these problems. Finally we will evaluate the frequency with which these proposed solutions might be successful. Specific examples of approaches to the study of efficacy also will be presented.

DEFINITIONS

There are at least four different types of measurable drug effects of interest to a prescriber. *Unanticipated harmful effects* are the unwanted effects of drugs that could not have been predicted on the basis of their preclinical pharmacologic profile or the results of premarketing clinical studies. These effects are most often Type B adverse reactions, as defined in Chapter 1. For example, chloramphenicol was not known to cause aplastic anemia at the time it was marketed,[1] nor was the skeletal muscle pain associated with use of HMG-CoA reductase inhibitors known. A major research challenge is to discover medically important unanticipated harmful effects as soon as possible after drug marketing. Quantitation of the incidence of these effects is medically useful as well.

Anticipated harmful effects are unwanted effects of drugs that could have been predicted on the basis of preclinical and premarketing studies. They can be either Type A reactions or Type B reactions (see Chapter 1). One example is the syncope that sometimes occurs after patients take their first dose of prazosin.[2] Although this effect was known to occur at the time of marketing, a major question remaining to be answered was how often the event occurred. The dominant research challenge that this type of drug effect presents is establishing its incidence.

Unanticipated beneficial effects are desirable effects of drugs that were not anticipated at the time of drug marketing. Although these effects may be medically useful, they are nevertheless side effects, if they are not the purpose for which the drug was given. An example of an unanticipated beneficial effect is aspirin's ability to decrease the probability of a subsequent myocardial infarction in patients who were given the drug for its analgesic or anti-inflammatory action.[3] Only recently, relative to how long aspirin has been around, has this been confirmed as a valid new indication for the use of aspirin. A major research challenge is to discover this type of drug effect. For example, it currently remains an open question whether non-aspirin nonsteroidal anti-inflammatory drugs have the same beneficial effects, although data are accumulating to that effect.[4] Secondarily, it is useful to quantitate the frequency of the event.

Anticipated beneficial effects are the desirable effects that are known to be caused by the drug. They represent the reason for prescribing the drug. The study of anticipated beneficial effects has three aspects. A study of drug *efficacy* investigates whether a drug *has the ability* to bring about the intended effect. In an *ideal* world, with perfect compliance, no interactions with other drugs or other diseases, etc., *could* the drug achieve its intended effects? Drug efficacy usually is studied using a randomized clinical trial.

In contrast, a study of drug *effectiveness* investigates whether, in the *real* world, a drug *in fact* achieves its desired effect. For example, a drug given in experimental conditions might be able to lower blood pressure but if it causes such severe sedation that patients refuse to ingest it, it will not be effective. Thus an efficacious drug may lack effectiveness. Studies of drug effectiveness usually are performed after a drug's efficacy has been established. In contrast, if a drug is demonstrated to be effective, it also is obviously efficacious. Studies of drug effectiveness generally would best be conducted using nonexperimental study designs. However, these raise special methodologic problems, which are discussed below.

Lastly, a study of *efficiency* investigates whether a drug can bring about a desired effect at an acceptable cost. This type of assessment falls in the province of health economics, and is discussed in Chapter 41.

Note that the outcome variable for any of these studies can be of multiple different types. They can be clinical outcomes (diseased/undiseased), or so-called "outcomes research," as defined by health services researchers (see Chapter 45 for a discussion of the validity issues involved in measuring such outcomes); they can be measures of quality-of-life (see Chapter 42), often referred to in the pharmaceutical industry as "outcomes research"; they can be measures of utility, i.e., global measures of the desirability of certain clinical outcomes (see Chapters 41 and 42); they can be economic outcomes (see Chapter 41); etc. Regardless, the same methodologic issues apply to each.

CLINICAL PROBLEMS TO BE ADDRESSED BY PHARMACOEPIDEMIOLOGIC RESEARCH

In order to make optimal clinical decisions about whether to use a drug, a prescriber needs to know whether, and to what degree, the drug actually is able to produce the intended effect (see Table 40.1).[5] Premarketing randomized clinical trials generally provide information on whether a drug can produce at least one beneficial effect. Specifically, premarketing studies generally investigate the efficacy of drug relative to a placebo, when both are used to treat a particular illness. These premarketing studies of efficacy tend to be conducted in very atypical clinical settings, compared to those in which the drug ultimately will be used. Patient compliance (now more often called adherence) during these studies is assured, and the patients included are similar to each other in age and sex, do not have other diseases, and

Table 40.1. Clinically important information about intended beneficial effects of drugs

---

(1) Can the drug have the desired effect?
(2) Does the drug actually achieve the desired effects when used in practice?
(3) Can and does the drug have other beneficial effects, including long-term effects for the same indication?
(4) Can the drug achieve these desired effects better than other alternative drugs available for the same indication?
(5) For each of the above, what is the magnitude of the effect in light of the many different factors in medical practice that might modify the effect, including:
    (a) variations in drug regimen: dose per unit time, distribution of dose over time, duration of regimen;
    (b) Characteristics of the indication: severity, subcategories of the illness, changes over time;
    (c) Characteristics of the patient: age, sex, race, genetics, geographic location, diet, nutritional status, compliance, other illnesses, drugs taken for this or other illness (including tobacco and alcohol), etc.

Source: Modified from Strom *et al.*[5]

are not taking other drugs. Such restrictions maximize the ability of premarketing studies to demonstrate a drug's efficacy, if the drug actually is efficacious. Additional information may then be needed on whether, in the world of daily medical practice, the drug actually achieves the same beneficial effects and whether the drug can and does have other beneficial effects. In addition, at the time of marketing there may be little data on a drug's efficacy relative to other medical or surgical alternatives available for the same indication. Finally, a number of factors that are encountered in the practice of medicine can modify a drug's ability to achieve its beneficial effects. Included are variations in the drug regimen, characteristics of the indication for the drug, and characteristics of the patient receiving the drug, including demographic factors, nutritional status, the presence of concomitant illnesses, the ingestion of drugs, and so on. Many, if not most, of these factors that can influence the effects of drugs are not fully explored prior to marketing.

In order to quantitate the need for postmarketing studies of the beneficial effects of drugs, a comparison was made of the 100 most common drug uses in 1978 (drug–indication pairs) to the information available to the Food and Drug Administration (FDA) at the time of its regulatory decisions about the marketing and labeling of the drugs involved in these uses.[5] The comparison was restricted to drugs approved after 1962, when the Kefauver–Harris Amendments first introduced a requirement for the submission of data about drug efficacy prior to approval of a drug for marketing.

Of the 100 common drug uses, 31 had not been approved by the FDA at the time of initial marketing, and 18 still had not been approved at the time of the comparison; 8 of the 18 unapproved uses were probably medically and therapeutically inappropriate. For example, the use of antibiotics is not justified for the treatment of viral infections, but such use was common. Other unapproved drug–indication pairs could well have been quite appropriate, but the regulatory process does not need to and did not reflect the current medical practice.

Of the 100 common drug uses, 8 were based on the assumption that a drug had a particular long-term effect, but only an intermediate effect had been studied prior to marketing. For example, antihypertensive drugs are used for their presumed ability to prevent long-term cardiovascular complications, but are approved for marketing on the basis of their ability to lower blood pressure. Of the 100 common drug uses, 5 may have been for either the intermediate effect or the long-term effect of the drugs, but only the intermediate effect was studied prior to marketing. For example, hypoglycemic agents may be used to control the symptoms of diabetes or to prevent the vascular complications of diabetes, but only the former was studied before drug marketing.

Drugs other than those in the list of 100 common uses were sometimes prescribed as treatment for each of the 52 indications included in those 100 uses. Yet, eight of the uses involved drugs whose effects relative to alternative drugs had not been studied prior to marketing.

The 100 common drug uses also included a number of examples of clinical factors that are able to modify the effects of the drug, but these were not discovered until after drug marketing. Some are listed in Table 40.2.[6–19] In addition, additional prescriptions accompanied 62% of the prescriptions studied, and 41% of the prescriptions were for patients who had illnesses other than just the one that the drug was being used to treat. Of the 100 common drug uses, the mean number of concomitantly administered drugs ranged from 0.04 to 2.1. The mean number of concomitant diagnoses ranged from 0.1 to 1.2. Yet, for none of the uses was the potential for modification of the drug effect by concomitant drugs or concomitant diagnoses fully explored before marketing.

The proportion of prescriptions which were for patients less than age 20 ranged from 0.0%, for 43 of the uses, to 97%. Yet, many of these uses had not been tested in children prior to marketing. Analogously, only three of the drugs were approved for use in pregnant patients, yet we know that drug use in pregnancy was common, even then.[20–22]

Thus, this study revealed considerable gaps in the information about beneficial drug effects at the time of drug marketing. These deficiencies in the available information should not be surprising, nor should they be considered inadequacies that ought to prevent the release of the drug to the marketplace. The data needed for clinical decisions are frequently and understandably different from those needed for regulatory decisions. Studies performed prior to marketing per force are focused predominantly on meeting appropriate regulatory requirements, and only secondarily on providing a basis for optimal therapeutic decisions. The physician also should keep in mind that the FDA is not allowed to regulate physicians but, rather, pharmaceutical manufacturers. This regulation is not aimed at telling a physician precisely how an agent should be used. In addition, the FDA does not initiate its own studies of drug effects, but generally evaluates those submitted to it by manufacturers. Finally, there are reasonable logistical limitations on what can be expected prior to marketing, without undue cost in time and resources, as well as delaying the availability of a chemical entity with a proven potential for efficacy. Thus, it seems that more studies of beneficial drug effects are needed, perhaps as a routine part of postmarketing drug surveillance.

Table 40.2. Examples of factors determining drug efficacy that were demonstrated after marketing, selected from the 100 most common drug uses of 1978

Factors	Drug	Indication	Comments	Reference
Regimen				
Dose per unit time	Ibuprofen	Rheumatoid arthritis, osteoarthritis	Daily dosage initially approved proved to be suboptimal	6
Distribution of dose over time	Furosemide	Congestive heart failure	Efficacy improved by more frequent, smaller doses	7
Duration	Clonidine	Hypertension	Tolerance develops in the absence of a diuretic	8
	Hypoglycemics (e.g., acetohexamide and tolazamide)	Diabetes mellitus	Tolerance develops in many patients	9
Indication				
Severity	Metaproterenol	Asthma	Patients with severe illness do not have a response without additional, supplementary therapy	10
Subcategories	Desipramine	Depression	May vary with endogenous versus exogenous depression	11
Changes over time	Ampicillin	Otitis media	No longer the drug of choice in some geographic areas due to bacterial resistance	12, 13
Patient				
Age	Diazepam	Anxiety	A given regimen is more effective in the aged than in the young	14
			Metabolism varies markedly from premature infants (half-life 54 hours), to full-term infants, to older children (half-life 18 hours); young children can have paradoxic reactions	15
Other illness	Gentamicin	Infection	Lower doses required in renal failure	16
Other				
Drugs	Lithium	Manic-depressive illness	Clearance impaired by diuretics, e.g., furosemide	17
	Acetohexamide	Diabetes mellitus	Many drugs interfere, by causing hyperglycemia (e.g., diuretics), displacing drug from binding sites (e.g., nonsteroidal anti-inflammatory drugs), etc.	18
Diet	Diuretics (e.g., metolazone, furosemide)	Hypertension	A decrease in sodium intake can improve efficacy	19
	Lithium	Manic-depressive illness	Significant sodium depletion or excess can modify renal excretion	17

Source: Strom BL *et al.*[5]

METHODOLOGIC PROBLEMS TO BE ADDRESSED BY PHARMACOEPIDEMIOLOGIC RESEARCH

Chapter 2 introduced the concept of a confounding variable, that is a variable other than the risk factor and outcome variable under study which is related independently to each of the other two and, thereby, can create an apparent association or mask a real one. This is discussed in more depth in Chapter 47. Studies of intended drug effects present a special methodologic problem of confounding by the indication for therapy.[23,24] In this case, the risk factor under study is the

drug being evaluated and the outcome variable under study is the clinical condition that the drug is supposed to change (cure, ameliorate, or prevent). In clinical practice, one would expect treated patients to differ from untreated patients, as the former have an indication for the treatment. To the extent that the indication is related to the outcome variable as well, the indication can function as a confounding variable.

For example, if one wanted to evaluate the effectiveness of a β-blocker used after a myocardial infarction in preventing a recurrent myocardial infarction, one might conduct a cohort study comparing patients who were treated with the β-blocker as part of their usual post-myocardial infarction medical care to patients who were not treated, measuring the incidence of subsequent myocardial infarction in both groups. However, patients with angina, arrhythmias, and hypertension, all indications for β-blocker therapy, are at increased risk of subsequent myocardial infarction. As such, one might well observe an increase in the risk of myocardial infarction, rather than the expected decrease. Thus, even if use of the drug was beneficial, it might appear to be harmful!

Confounding by the indication for the treatment generally is not a problem if a study is focusing on unexpected drug effects, or side effects, whether they are harmful or beneficial. In this situation, the indication for treatment is not usually related to the outcome variable under study. For example, in a study of gastrointestinal bleeding from nonsteroidal anti-inflammatory drugs, the possible indications for treatment, such as arthritis, dysmenorrhea, and acute pain, have little or no relationship in and of themselves to the risk of gastrointestinal bleeding.[25] Nevertheless, sometimes the problem of confounding by indication can emerge even in studies of unexpected drug effects (beneficial or harmful). For instance, in a study of hypersensitivity reactions associated with the use of nonsteroidal anti-inflammatory drugs, the increased risk of hypersensitivity reactions evident in patients taking nonsteroidal anti-inflammatory drugs was higher in those using the drugs for acute pain than in those using the drugs for osteoarthritis and other chronic conditions. This probably was because of the intermittent ingestion of the drug by those receiving it for acute pain.[26]

Although confounding by the indication is a less common problem for studies of side effects, this is not the case for studies of anticipated beneficial effects. In these studies one would expect the indication to be more closely related to the outcome variable. In fact, the problem presented by confounding by the indication has been thought by some to invalidate nonexperimental approaches to studies of the beneficial effects of drugs. Some have felt that questions of beneficial drug effects can be addressed only by using randomized clinical trials.[27] Yet, although postmarketing randomized clinical trials certainly can be very useful, they are vexed by many of the same logistical problems, ethical restrictions, and artificial medical settings found in premarketing clinical trials.

CURRENTLY AVAILABLE SOLUTIONS

Not all studies of beneficial drug effects need be randomized clinical trials (see Table 40.3).[23] First, some questions do not require any comparative (analytic) research for their answer. For these, simple clinical observations, as reported in a case report or case series, can be sufficient. For example, the efficacy and effectiveness of naloxone, used as a narcotic antagonist, is demonstrable simply through the observation of a single patient. Consider a patient comatose from an overdose of methadone. An injection of naloxone results in his prompt awakening. However, 30 minutes later, as the effects of the narcotic antagonist wear off, the patient returns to coma. Another injection of the naloxone results in awakening once more, and then later the coma returns again. This sequence of events represents a convincing demonstration of the drug's ability to have its desired effect. No elaborate studies are needed to make this point. The same would be true for a case series of patients treated with penicillin to treat pneumococcal pneumonia.

However, in applying this simple approach of clinical observations based on a case report or case series, the course of a patient's disease must be sufficiently predictable that one can differentiate a true drug effect from spontaneous improvement. In particular, one must be able to exclude *regression to the mean* as the mechanism of the observed change: individuals selected to participate in a study based upon the severity of their disease spontaneously and usually will tend to improve. One example would be a patient with recurrent headaches. The patient would most likely seek medical attention when the headaches are most severe or most frequent. A spontaneous return to the baseline pattern of headaches generally could be expected. However, if the patient were treated in the interim, then the treating physician likely would view the return to normality as evidence of successful therapy, no matter what treatment was used or whether it contributed anything to the recovery.

Second, some questions about beneficial drug effects can be answered using formal nonexperimental studies, because there is no confounding by the indication. If the decision about whether to treat is not based on a formal indication, but on some other factor that may not be related to the outcome variable under study, such as the limited availability of the drug in question, then there is no opportunity for confounding by the indication. This situation occurs most commonly in studies of primary prevention. The use of measles vaccine, routinely administered to healthy infants, is one example.

Third, there are several settings in which confounding by the indication may exist but theoretically can be controlled. When the indication can be measured sufficiently well, then traditional epidemiologic techniques of exclusion, matching, stratification, and mathematical modeling can be applied. The indication clearly can be sufficiently measured if it is dichotomous or binary. In this situation, the indication

Table 40.3. Classification of research questions according to their problems of confounding by the indication for therapy

Situation	Example
(1) Comparative studies unnecessary	
(a) Drug effect obvious in the individual patient, or	Naloxone used for methadone overdose
(b) Drug effect obvious in a series of patients	Penicillin used for pneumococcal pneumonia
(2) Confounding by the indication nonexistent: there is no indication	Measles vaccine given routinely to healthy infants
(3) Confounding by the indication exists but is controllable	
(a) The indication is dichotomous	
(i) Gradations in the indication do not exist, or	Anti-Rh (D) immune globulin given to Rh (D) negative mothers who deliver Rh (D) positive newborns to prevent future erythroblastosis fetalis
(ii) Gradations in the indication are unrelated to the choice of treatment, or	Penicillin used for endocarditis prophylaxis in patients with congenital aortic stenosis who are undergoing tooth extraction
(iii) Gradations in the indication are unrelated to expected outcome, or	Penicillin used to prevent tertiary syphilis, given to patients with an asymptomatic positive serologic test for syphilis
(iv) Special clinical settings	Anticoagulants used after myocardial infarctions to prevent death
(b) The indication is sufficiently characterizable	Isoniazid used for tuberculosis prophylaxis in a patient with an asymptomatic positive PPD
(i) Complete characterization of the indication as it relates to choice of therapy or as it relates to expected outcome, and	
(ii) Characterization must continue after initiation of therapy	
(4) Confounding by the indication exists and is not controllable	Ampicillin used to treat urinary tract infection

Source: Strom et al.[23]

either is present or absent, but has no gradations in severity. The indication also can be sufficiently measured if any gradations in severity either are unrelated to the choice of whether or not to treat or are unrelated to the expected outcome. Alternatively, sometimes one can find special clinical settings in which the gradations are not related to the choice of therapy. For example, if the availability of drugs is limited or there are consistent philosophical differences among prescribers for using or not using the drug, then gradations in the indication will not be related to the choice of therapy.

Finally, if an indication is graded but can be sufficiently precisely measured, it can be controlled by mathematical modeling using, for example, multiple regression. Then confounding by the indication can be controlled and ruled out as the cause for an observed beneficial effect of the drug.

Recently, researchers have begun to use *propensity scores* towards this end.[28,29] This is an approach that uses mathematical modeling to predict *exposure*, rather than the traditional approach of predicting *outcome*.[30] This is, essentially, a direct measure of indication. One can then use the propensity score to create categories of probability of exposure, and control for those categories in the analysis. While this approach has many attractive features, especially as a direct way to control for confounding by indication, it is important to point out that it is still dependent on identifying and measuring those variables which are the true predictors of therapeutic choice. Further, based on very recent data,[31] propensity score only has advantages when there are seven or fewer outcome events per confounder. When there are at least eight outcome events per confounder, logistic regression represents a preferable approach.[31]

When questions of intended drug effects do not fall into any of the preceding categories, *confounding by the indication cannot be controlled*. Nonexperimental study designs cannot then be used, or they can only be used to demonstrate qualitatively some degree of beneficial effect. Specifically, if confounding by the indication is such that treated patients would have a worse clinical outcome than untreated patients, yet the outcome observed in treated patients is better than that observed in untreated patients, some degree of confidence that the drug has a beneficial effect can be built. As an example, patients treated with corticosteroids for status asthmaticus would be expected to be sicker than those not so treated. If patients receiving corticosteroids stop wheezing sooner than those not receiving corticosteroids, corticosteroids would indeed seem to have a beneficial effect. However, if the patients receiving corticosteroids do not stop wheezing sooner than those not receiving corticosteroids, the results of the study are uninterpretable. It is possible that the corticosteroids in fact have no beneficial effect. However, it is also possible that a beneficial effect was present but was being masked by the difference in severity between the two treatment groups.

The qualitative approach illustrated above must be used with caution. First, the effect of the confounding by indication must be opposite in direction to the expected effect of the drug. Second, the effect of the confounding by indication must be absolutely predictable in its direction. Third, the effect of the confounding by indication must be sufficiently large so as to exclude regression to the mean as an explanation for the results. Even if all of these conditions are met, the results must be interpreted only qualitatively, not quantitatively.

Examples of each of these situations are presented in Table 40.3 and discussed further in Strom et al.[23]

APPLICABILITY OF THE PROPOSED APPROACHES

How commonly are the nonexperimental approaches we have described applicable for the study of beneficial drug effects? A list of the 100 most recently approved new molecular entities as of December 1978 was studied to determine what types of nonexperimental study designs, if any, could be used to evaluate drug effectiveness.[32] After excluding from this list seven entities that were used in contact lenses, the remaining 93 drugs were examined for all potential indications and clinical outcomes that could be used to evaluate intended drug effects. Ultimately we assessed 131 drug uses, that is 131 drug–indication pairs. Each drug use was categorized as to whether a study evaluating the effectiveness of that drug for that indication would present the problem of confounding by the indication and, if so, whether one of the approaches described above would be adequate to address it. Of these drug uses, 89 (67.9%) could have been evaluated using simple clinical observations, without formal comparative research. A very few of these drugs were, in fact, approved by FDA on the basis of such studies, e.g., nitroprusside (approved for malignant hypertension) and bretylium (approved for life-threatening arrhythmias, in patients refractory to all other antiarrhythmics). The remaining 42 drug uses required comparative research for their evaluation, because they all presented the problem of confounding by the indication. In 7 of the 42 (5.3% of the total), this confounding was not an obstacle to valid nonexperimental research. Most often the validity of

the approach rested on the observation that any given physician usually used the drug to treat either all or none of his patients with the indication.

In the remaining 35 of the 42 uses (26.7% of the total), confounding by the indication was judged to be uncontrollable using currently available nonexperimental techniques.

To place these findings in perspective, of the 42 drug uses that required comparative research to evaluate their effectiveness, 30 could not ethically be addressed using a randomized clinical trial and a placebo control. Most of these 30 involved the use of drugs to treat infections or malignancies. In these situations, patients could not ethically be left "untreated," that is assigned to the placebo group.

Studies of the effects of one drug relative to another active drug, of course, gave different results. Formal comparative research was necessary for all 131 drug uses. Nonexperimental studies theoretically could be conducted validly for 94 of the 131 drug uses (71.8%). Experimental studies would be ethical for all of them.

Of course, judging theoretically that a question of effectiveness is "studiable" by a given technique is not the same as proving that a valid outcome would emerge from such a study. There are many particular details in the actual conduct of such studies that must be addressed on a case-by-case basis. It is, therefore, instructive to examine some specific examples of nonexperimental research into beneficial drug effects.

SPECIFIC EXAMPLES

Estrogens for Prevention of Osteoporotic Fractures

One of the first series of studies of drug effectiveness using rigorous nonexperimental study designs examined whether exogenous estrogens could prevent fractures in postmenopausal women with osteoporosis.[33] Biochemical studies had documented that the menopause resulted in a negative calcium and phosphorus balance, and that the balance returned toward normal with the ingestion of exogenous estrogens.[34] Studies of bone density documented that exogenous estrogens prevented the loss of bone density that was associated with the menopause,[35] for as long as the estrogens were continued.[36] It seemed plausible that the use of estrogens might prevent fractures from osteoporosis, but no data directly addressed that question. On the other hand, postmenopausal estrogens had been shown to cause endometrial cancer.[37,38]

A randomized clinical trial would have been the ideal way to address the effect of estrogen on fractures. However, such a study was impractical for many reasons. This is prophylactic therapy. Although postmenopausal fractures are common, they are experienced by a sufficiently small proportion of the population during any defined time period that an extremely large sample size would be needed. Also, the study would need to be carried on for many years before a beneficial effect could begin to be seen.

Instead of a randomized clinical trial, a series of nonexperimental studies were performed. Both case–control and cohort designs were used.[39–56] In general, these studies were rigorous and well done. Unfortunately, however, the question of confounding by the indication was not addressed in most of the studies.[33] In particular, most of the studies failed to address why some of the women received the postmenopausal exogenous estrogens and others did not. Given the data already available on the effects of estrogens on bone density and endometrial cancer, it is reasonable to assume that some physicians might preferentially routinely use the drugs and others might routinely avoid them. In such a setting, nonexperimental techniques could yield valid results, unaffected by confounding by the indication (category (3)(a)(iv) in Table 40.3). However, many physicians might try to selectively prescribe the drugs for patients who have undergone hysterectomy, because these patients are at no risk of endometrial cancer. Alternatively, some physicians may try to use the drugs only on patients who they feel are at high risk of fractures or are at high risk of complications from fractures. These situations would represent uncontrollable confounding by the indication—category (4) in Table 40.3. Finally, one might expect that the direction of the confounding by indication might be opposite to that of the drug effect, allowing one to use these data to make at least qualitative conclusions. This assumes, however, that physicians can accurately predict who is at high risk of fracture. Such a presumption was not borne out by the available data.[50]

In fact, the three studies that closely examined the comparability of the study groups were able to document that they were not comparable.[39,50,52] Specifically, one study was a case–control study within an orthopedic service, and documented that cases with fractures of the hip or radius weighed less than controls matched for age and race, had a later menopause, and more frequently were alcoholics.[39] A second was a cohort study of patients with known estrogen deficiency. In this study, those who were treated with estrogens differed from those who were not in age, age of menopause, duration of follow-up, height, weight, blood pressure, marital status, race, economic status, and gravidity, as well as in the frequency of the following diagnoses: atrophic vaginitis, bilateral oophorectomy, premature ovarian failure,

hypopituitarism, gonadal dysgenesis, endocrine disease, hypertension, and osteoporosis.[50]

A third study used a case–control design to investigate patients admitted to surgical services.[52] It compared cases with hip fractures to a control group of surgical patients, divided into those with trauma and those without trauma. Cases were noted to be older, taller, and to have a lower body weight than the controls. The cases more frequently had undergone ovariectomy, breastfed fewer times and for fewer months, and were hypothyroid less frequently than the controls. When these factors were controlled for as confounding variables, the effect of estrogens was still apparent. However, as in the other studies, there was no information on how or why the decision was made to treat with or withhold estrogens.

A number of other nonexperimental studies published since then showed similar results.[57–62] Since then, the finding that estrogens have a beneficial effect on hip fractures has been confirmed in a massive clinical trial, i.e., the Women's Health Initiative.[63]

Anticoagulants for Prevention of Recurrent Venous Thromboembolism

The use of intravenous anticoagulants reduces the risk of recurrent venous thromboembolism,[64] and the addition of oral anticoagulants to intravenous anticoagulants probably reduces the risk even further.[65] However, how long oral anticoagulant treatment should be continued had not been well studied. Most explicit advice from experts on the optimal duration of anticoagulation therapy was based on anecdotal experience.[66,67] Most of the data available that were used to suggest the appropriate duration of therapy are derived from clinical observations in a single medical center.[65,68–70] They represent an accumulating case series. Over time, gradually patients' treatment has been prolonged. Thus, changes in the duration of treatment are intermingled with other changes in medical care over decades. In addition, the studies do not compare patients receiving treatments of different length, but simply observe when most recurrences tend to occur. The investigators have assumed that treatment should be prolonged sufficiently to include that time when recurrences can be expected. Problems with these studies have been detailed.[66,67]

As with the question of the effect of estrogens on bone fractures from osteoporosis, a randomized clinical trial would be the ideal design to address the question of the optimal duration of anticoagulation after venous thromboembolism, but such a study is impractical. After patients have been anticoagulated in the hospital and followed for a short time as outpatients, the risk of recurrence is sufficiently small that an enormous population would be needed to detect a difference in outcome due to differences in therapy. Until recently, the only randomized clinical trial in the literature that addressed this question compared six weeks of outpatient treatment to six months of treatment. No difference in recurrence rate between these two groups of patients was observed.[71] However, only 186 subjects were included, yielding a total of only 7 recurrences. In addition, over half the study subjects had some known short-term risk factors for venous thromboembolism. These included pregnancy, use of oral contraceptives, and recent surgery. Patients with these transient underlying risk factors might be expected to be less likely to benefit from longer-term anticoagulant therapy than patients with idiopathic disease.

The question of the optimal duration of anticoagulation was addressed in a cohort study using data from the Northern California Kaiser Permanente Medical Program.[72] The study required the use of ten years of data from this population of 1.6 million, or a total of 16 million patient-years of experience. There were a total of 3384 individuals identified as being hospitalized for venous thromboembolism. Of these, 2473 suffered from idiopathic venous thromboembolism. Their clinical outcomes were evaluated, according to how long they had been treated with oral anticoagulants. Using those treated with six weeks of therapy or less as a control group, prolongation of therapy beyond that point was found to increase the risk of major bleeding dramatically, but to have no effect on recurrence rates.

The feature of this study that allowed the investigators to overcome the problem of confounding by indication was that physician behavior regarding how long therapy was continued was essentially random (category (3)(a)(ii) in Table 40.3). The choice of how long to treat became random, because there was no prior information on how long one should treat. In fact, the duration of treatment was relatively uniformly distributed across the years of follow-up, and the results were no different when one restricted the analysis to those who had their anticoagulation stopped because of hemorrhage, rather than at the option of their physician.

More recently, a randomized trial was published which showed that long-term low-dose warfarin therapy was effective in decreasing the subsequent risk of recurrence of idiopathic venous thromboembolism.[73] However, this was in patients who had already received full dose warfarin for a median of 6.5 months.

Lidocaine for Prevention of Death from Myocardial Infarction

In another study, the efficacy of lidocaine in preventing death from myocardial infarction was studied using a case–control design.[74] Among patients admitted to a coronary or intensive care unit for acute myocardial infarction, those who died were compared to an equal number of patients who survived. The controls were matched to the cases for age, gender, race, and date of hospitalization. Overall, lidocaine did not protect against death. Lidocaine was effective only when deaths attributable to ventricular arrhythmia were analyzed separately.

In this careful study, the investigators obviously were well aware of the risk of confounding by indication. They attempted to control for this confounding by using the epidemiologic technique of stratification, that is classifying patients according to their risk of dying from myocardial infarction, in order to control for this inequality of risk as a confounding variable. Thus, they treated the study as a category (3)(b) question in Table 40.3. Unfortunately, however, it is doubtful that one can accurately and fully measure the basis for physicians' judgments about who they think is at high risk of death from myocardial infarction. Similarly, it is unlikely that each individual's risk of dying from a myocardial infarction can be predicted, especially death by ventricular arrhythmia. Certainly a classification according to just the presence or absence of congestive heart failure, as was used, is overly simplistic. In fact, the rates of death attributed to ventricular arrhythmia were virtually identical in those patients with and without congestive heart failure. Nevertheless the results do coincide with those of a randomized clinical trial evaluating the efficacy of lidocaine in preventing primary ventricular fibrillation.[75] However, while the drug prevented the arrhythmia in that randomized clinical trial, it did not alter mortality. Since then, there have been more than 20 randomized trials and 4 meta-analyses, indicating that lidocaine reduces ventricular fibrillation but increases mortality in acute myocardial infarction.[76] This was not confirmed in a subsequent paper, which re-analyzed the data from the 43 704 patients enrolled in GUSTO-I or GUSTO-IIb.[77]

Anticoagulants for Prevention of Death from Myocardial Infarction

Whether anticoagulants can prevent death from myocardial infarction had been addressed using randomized clinical trials.[78] However, the results had been inconsistent and inconclusive, possibly because of problems of sample size.

Thus, this question would appear to be a good candidate for a case–control study. Such a study was done,[79] with the investigators treating this research question as if it were a category (3)(b) question in Table 40.3. However, as with the study of the effects of lidocaine on myocardial infarction, it is doubtful whether one can measure and quantitate precisely the risk of dying from a myocardial infarction at the time of the acute episode. This study might have been more convincing if the investigators had identified the patients of practitioners who always used anticoagulants for their patients with myocardial infarctions, and then compared them to a control group of patients of practitioners who never used anticoagulants for their patients with myocardial infarctions. Inasmuch as the choice of therapy in these patients would not have been made on the basis of any perceived difference among the patients in their risk of dying from myocardial infarction, confounding by the indication would not be a problem. Of course, if the investigators had designed the study as we suggest, they then would have had to consider whether the physicians themselves were somehow a predictor of outcome, and whether this was consistently related to their philosophy of using anticoagulants, across multiple physicians. Thus, randomized trials are really needed to provide the answer to this question, and of course in recent years, with the advent of low molecular weight heparin and thrombolytic therapy, many have been forthcoming.

Generic versus Brand Name Drugs

Another potential use of nonexperimental study designs to study the beneficial effects of drugs arose with the passage of the 1984 Waxman–Hatch Act in the US. Generic drugs can now be marketed after simple demonstration of bioequivalence, i.e., equivalent bioavailability, in 18 to 24 normal adults.[80] However, it is not clear whether bioequivalence assures clinical equivalence, that is equivalent efficacy and toxicity.[81] *Clinical inequivalence is more likely to be evident as a difference in beneficial effects than as a difference in adverse effects.* In developing a drug, dosages are sought which optimize drug efficacy. Toxicity, other than idiosyncratic or allergic reactions, usually occurs at higher doses and concentrations than needed for efficacy. Modest variations in the plasma concentration on the active drug, created by receiving the same dose in different preparations, are most likely, therefore, to be a problem for drug efficacy than for drug toxicity. Variations in plasma concentration are even more likely to be a problem for drug effectiveness and cost-effectiveness. Even a simple change in the physical appearance of the drug could conceivably lead to a decrease in compliance and, thereby, effectiveness.

Studies designed to evaluate differences in efficacy among different preparations of the same drug require enormous sample sizes, as one would be searching for relatively small differences. However, such sample sizes can be achieved relatively easily and efficiently as part of nonexperimental pharmacoepidemiology studies. Thus, the suggestion has been made that studies of clinical equivalence could possibly be carried out as postmarketing surveillance studies.[81] Confounding by the indication is unlikely to be a problem because, as far as the physician is concerned, he or she is dealing with different products of the same drug, products that are theoretically interchangeable. The choice among the alternative therapies is not being made by the prescriber on the basis of patient characteristics, but by the pharmacist on the basis of product availability—category (3)(a)(ii) in Table 40.3.

A few pharmacoepidemiology studies (unpublished) on the relative effectiveness of different preparations used for the same purpose have been performed by Strom, using the COMPASS® database. These studies compared patients who were started on a brand name product and were switched to a generic product when it became available, and patients who remained on the brand name product. The drugs studied were thioridazine, chlorpropamide, and slow-absorption theophylline. These studies naturally raise concerns about the ability to identify the actual product dispensed. Very few of the pharmacoepidemiology approaches described in Part III of the book are able to identify the specific product dispensed. Often the approach does not even distinguish whether it is a brand name product or a generic product that is being used. Even when the distinction is made—for example most Medicaid data sets use the National Drug Code to identify specifically the drug, the manufacturer, the dosage form, and the dose—one is inevitably left with questions about whether a brand name is being billed for, while a generic drug is dispensed. In addition, such studies raise concerns about how to define the clinical outcome variable. For example, how is drug efficacy reflected in a claims database? The studies described above used proxy outcomes such as number of physician visits, number of hospitalizations, and use of adjunctive therapy to obtain an estimate of drug efficacy.

Using these outcomes, the investigators first analyzed the baseline data, comparing the experience, prior to switching, of those who ultimately switched to generic products to the experience of those who did not later switch to a generic product. In each of the three studies, the future switchers were different from the future non-switchers, prior to the switch. Thus, it appears that patients who were to be switched to generic products were different from patients who stayed on the brand name products: confounding by indication was indeed operating. Because of this, no analyses of efficacy after the switch were performed. Parenthetically, because of this, and questions about the uncertain interpretability of the clinical outcomes, it was elected not to publish the results of these papers.

Cost-Effectiveness Studies

An important new category of studies of beneficial drug effects includes studies of their cost-effectiveness. These studies measure the resources necessary to achieve a particular beneficial outcome, and thus have two main study variables—one that is clinical and one that is economic. For example, one could perform a cohort study comparing treated patients to untreated patients, and determine whether the clinical outcomes they experience and the cost of the medical care they subsequently receive is different. In such a study, one would need to consider the possibility of confounding by the indication for both the clinical outcome and the cost variables. It should be noted that the indication may have different effects on the clinical outcomes and the costs. Thus, while performing the clinical outcome assessment, one needs to consider and, potentially, quantify the implications of the indication for the treatment on the clinical outcome variable. In contrast, while performing the cost assessment, one needs to consider and, potentially, quantify the cost implications of the indication on both the clinical outcomes and the costs. The subject of health economics as applied to drug use is discussed in more detail in Chapter 41.

Vaccines

In the past several years, nonexperimental study designs have been widely used to evaluate the efficacy of vaccines. Specifically, case–control studies have been used to explore the efficacy of pneumococcal vaccine,[82,83] rubella vaccine,[84,85] measles vaccine,[86–90] *Hemophilus influenzae* type b polysaccharide vaccine,[91–100] oral poliovirus vaccine,[101,102] meningococcus vaccine,[103–105] Japanese encephalitis vaccine,[106] and BCG vaccine in protecting against tuberculosis,[107–114] diphtheria toxoid vaccine,[115] and leprosy.[116,117] Cohort studies have been used to explore the efficacy of *Hemophilus influenzae* type b polysaccharide vaccine,[93] measles vaccine,[118,119] and pertussis vaccine.[120,121] Again, studies like these should ideally be conducted as randomized clinical trials. However, the relative infrequency of the diseases that the above vaccines are designed to prevent, particularly in populations which are partly vaccinated, make use of this design difficult, although not impossible. In fact, in one

situation, a new Japanese encephalitis vaccine manufactured in China was studied for efficacy using a case–control design,[107] while a study of its safety, conducted by the same authors, used a randomized clinical trial design.[122] In considering the applicability of nonexperimental study designs, the relatively indiscriminate use of such vaccines places the study in category (2) of Table 40.3. Patients who receive these vaccines differ from those who do not in their socioeconomic status, their access to medical care, and their physicians' attitudes towards vaccines. However, for most vaccines, an individual physician is not likely to give only some of his eligible patients the vaccine, withholding it from other eligible patients. Thus, patients receiving vaccines are not likely to differ from those who do not get the vaccine, at least in their physicians' perceptions about the patients' risk of contracting these diseases. Nonexperimental studies of such questions should produce valid results, therefore. Indeed, as is evident from the large number of examples, this is becoming a standard and accepted approach. We refer the interested reader to some methodologic papers on the subtleties of designing nonexperimental studies of vaccine efficacy.[123–129]

Cancer Screening

Another more recent and frequent use of nonexperimental study designs is to evaluate the efficacy of cancer screening programs. Although this does not directly relate to drugs, the methodological implications are the same, and have been better enunciated than in the pharmacoepidemiology literature. The use of nonexperimental study designs to evaluate the efficacy of cancer screening programs will be briefly discussed here, therefore.

Once again, ideally questions about the value of screening would be addressed using randomized clinical trials. However, most diseases that are screened for are relatively uncommon. Only a very small fraction of participants in a broad screening program could be expected to benefit from the screening program. Thus, randomized clinical trials of screening can be expensive and may require years to complete. Even more importantly, once a screening procedure is widely accepted, even without data documenting its efficacy, recruiting patients into a randomized clinical trial can be impractical and possibly truly unethical.

Instead, investigators have used nonexperimental designs. Screening procedures that have been evaluated repeatedly in this fashion include the value of "Pap" smears for cervical cancer[130–145] and mammography and self-examination for breast cancer.[146–163] Other studies investigated screening measures for lung cancer[164,165] and gastric cancer.[166] All of these were case–control studies. Many more have been published since. Again, they raise similar methodologic considerations of confounding by indication. Specifically, why do some women choose to have the screening procedure and others do not? One randomized clinical trial documented that women who attended screening sessions were at higher risk of developing breast cancer than women who were offered screening but did not attend.[167] In addition, case–control studies of screening present additional thorny methodologic problems regarding how to define cases, how to define controls, the time period to choose for the study, etc.[168–183]

Other Examples

Other analogous work using case–control study designs has explored the effectiveness of bicycle safety helmets in preventing face injuries,[184] antibiotic prophylaxis in preventing post-dental infective endocarditis,[185] β-blockers in preventing mortality in patients with acute myocardial infarction,[186] β-blockers and incident coronary artery events,[187] etc.

THE FUTURE

Clinicians have long recognized the value of clinical observations and nonexperimental research. Much of our current knowledge about the usefulness of medical interventions is based on information that is nonexperimental. Yet the data and conclusions from the information are useful and valid. However, the information that observational techniques generate cannot be accepted uncritically. Perhaps in reaction to the limitations of nonexperimental studies, some scientists have insisted that "the randomized clinical trial (RCT) is the only scientifically reliable method for assessment of the efficacy (and risks) of most clinical treatments."[27] Sackett *et al.* argue: "to keep up with the clinical literature…discard at once all articles on therapy that are not randomized trials."[188] In light of the analysis presented above, this posture seems too simplistic and far reaching. If overbearing, it results in clinically necessary and potentially available information being uncollected and unused. The proper balance in attitude about the value of these approaches probably lies somewhere between the two extremes. To quote Sir Austin Bradford Hill, one of the developers of the randomized trial: "Any belief that the controlled trial is the only way [to study therapeutic efficacy] would mean not only that the pendulum had swung too far but that it had come right off its hook."[189] Many investigators are now applying nonexperimental designs to studies of beneficial drug effects. However, careful attention

needs to be paid to the possibility of confounding by the indication. Some approaches to this problem are now available, and hopefully more will be available in the future. However, when confounding by indication can be addressed, clinical observations and nonexperimental research can be used. The results of nonexperimental research are unlikely to be as powerful or as convincing as those of experimental research. We are not suggesting that nonexperimental research, and certainly we are not suggesting that nonexperimental studies, be used as replacements for experimental studies. However, when an experimental study is deemed to be unnecessary, unethical, infeasible, or too costly relative to the expected benefits, there frequently is a good alternative.

REFERENCES

1. Wallerstein RO, Condit PK, Kasper CK, Brown JW, Morrison FR. Statewide study of chloramphenicol therapy and fatal aplastic anemia. *JAMA* 1969; **208**: 2045–50.
2. Graham RM, Thornell IR, Gain JM, Bagnoli C, Oates HF, Stokes GS. Prazosin: the first dose phenomenon. *BMJ* 1976; **2**: 1293–4.
3. Boston Collaborative Drug Surveillance Group. Regular aspirin intake and acute myocardial infarction. *BMJ* 1974; **1**: 440–3.
4. Kimmel SE, Berlin JA, Reilly M, Jaskowiak J, Kishel L, Chittams J, Strom BL. The effects of nonselective non-aspirin non-steroidal anti-inflammatory medications on the risk of nonfatal myocardial infarction and their interaction with aspirin. *J Am Coll Cardiol* 2004; **43**: 985–90.
5. Strom BL, Melmon KL, Miettinen OS. Post-marketing studies of drug efficacy: why? *Am J Med* 1985; **78**: 475–80.
6. Anonymous. Ibuprofen (Motrin)—a new drug for arthritis. *Med Lett Drugs Ther* 1974; **16**: 109–10.
7. Wilson TW, Falk KJ, Labelle JL, Nguyen KB. Effect of dosage regimen on natriuretic response to furosemide. *Clin Pharmacol Ther* 1975; **18**: 165–9.
8. Anonymous. Clonidine (Catapres) for hypertension. *Med Lett Drugs Ther* 1975; **17**: 45–6.
9. Shen SW, Bressler R. Clinical pharmacology of oral antidiabetic agents. *N Engl J Med* 1977; **296**: 787–93.
10. Webb-Johnson DC, Andrews JL. Bronchodilator therapy. *N Engl J Med* 1977; **297**: 758–64.
11. Hollister LE. Tricyclic antidepressants. *N Engl J Med* 1978; **299**: 1106–9.
12. Syriopoulou V, Scheifele D, Howie V, Ploussard J, Sloyer J, Smith AL. Incidence of ampicillin-resistant *Hemophilus influenzae* in otitis media. *J Pediatr* 1976; **89**: 839–41.
13. Schwartz R, Rodriquez W, Khan W, Ross S. The increasing incidence of ampicillin-resistant *Hemophilus influenzae*. *JAMA* 1978; **239**: 320–3.
14. Vestal RE. Drug use in the elderly: a review of problems and special considerations. *Drugs* 1978; **16**: 358–82.

15. Morselli PL, Principi N, Tognoni G, Reali E, Belvedere G, Standen SM *et al.* Diazepam elimination in premature and full term infants, and children. *J Perinat Med* 1973; **1**: 133–41.

16. Chan RA, Bennes EJ, Hoeprich PD. Gentamicin therapy in renal failure: a nomogram for dosage. *Ann Intern Med* 1972; **76**: 773–8.

17. Hansten PD. *Drug Interactions*, 4th edn. Philadelphia, PA: Lea & Febiger, 1979.

18. *Physicians' Desk Reference*, 33rd edn. Oradell, NJ: Medical Economics, 1979.

19. Parijs J, Joossens JV, Van der Linden L, Verstreken G, Amery AK Moderate sodium restriction and diuretics in the treatment of hypertension. *Am Heart J* 1973; **85**: 22–34.

20. Doering PL, Stewart RB. The extent and character of drug consumption during pregnancy. *JAMA* 1978; **239**: 843–6.

21. Boethius G. Recording of drug prescriptions in the county of Jämtland, Sweden. II. Drug exposure of pregnant women in relation to course and outcome of pregnancy. *Eur J Clin Pharmacol* 1977; **12**: 37–43.

22. Degenhardt KH, Kerken H, Knörr K. Drug usage and fetal development: preliminary evaluations of a prospective investigation. *Adv Exp Med Biol* 1972; **27**: 467–79.

23. Strom BL, Miettinen OS, Melmon KL. Postmarketing studies of drug efficacy: when must they be randomized? *Clin Pharmacol Ther* 1983; **34**: 1–7.

24. Psaty BM, Koepsell TD, Siscovick D, Wahl P, Logerfo JP, Inui TS, Wagner EH. An approach to several problems in using large databases for population-based case–control studies of the therapeutic efficacy and safety of anti-hypertensive medicines. *Stat Med* 1991; **10**: 653–62.

25. Carson JL, Strom BL, Soper KA, West SL, Morse ML. The association of nonsteroidal anti-inflammatory drugs with upper gastrointestinal tract bleeding. *Arch Int Med* 1987; **147**: 85–8.

26. Strom BL, Carson JL, Morse ML, West SL, Soper KA. The effect of indication on hypersensitivity reactions associated with zomepirac sodium and other nonsteroidal antiinflammatory drugs. *Arthritis Rheum* 1987; **30**: 1142–8.

27. Juhl E, Christensen E, Tygstrup N. The epidemiology of the gastrointestinal randomized clinical trial. *N Engl J Med* 1977; **296**: 20–2.

28. Rosenbaum PR. *Observational Studies*, Springer series in statistics. New York: Springer-Verlag, 1995; pp. 200–24.

29. D'Agostino RB Jr. Propensity score methods for bias reduction in the comparison of a treatment to a non-randomized control group. *Stat Med* 1998; **17**: 2265–81.

30. Paul R, Rosenbaum PR, Rubin DB. The central role of the propensity score in observational studies for causal effects. *Biometrika* 1983; **70**: 41–55.

31. Cepeda MS, Boston R, Farrar JT, Strom BL. Comparison of logistic regression versus propensity score when the number of events is low and there are multiple confounders. *Am J Epidemiol* 2003; **158**: 280–7.

32. Strom BL, Miettinen OS, Melmon KL. Post-marketing studies of drug efficacy: how? *Am J Med* 1984; **77**: 703–8.

33. Strom BL. Are estrogens effective in preventing fractures from post-menopausal osteoporosis? In: Melmon KL, ed., *Drug Therapeutics: Concepts for Physicians*. New York: Elsevier-North Holland, 1982; pp. 67–80.

34. Lagrelius A. Treatment with oral estrone sulphate in the female climacteric. III. Effects on bone density and on certain biochemical parameters. *Acta Obstet Gynecol Scand* 1981; **60**: 481–8.

35. Lindsay R, Hart DM, Aitken JM, MacDonald EB, Anderson JB, Clarke AC. Long-term prevention of postmenopausal osteoporosis by oestrogen. Evidence for an increased bone mass after delayed onset of oestrogen treatment. *Lancet* 1976; **1**: 1038–41.

36. Lindsay R, Hart DM, MacLean A, Clark AC, Kraszewski A. Bone response to termination of oestrogen treatment. *Lancet* 1978; **1**: 1325–7.

37. Ziel HK, Finkle WD. Increased risk of endometrial cancer among users of conjugated estrogens. *N Engl J Med* 1975; **293**: 1167–70.

38. Antunes CM, Strolley PD, Rosenshein NB, Davies JL, Tonascia JA, Brown C *et al.* Endometrial cancer and estrogen use. Report of a large case–control study. *N Engl J Med* 1979; **300**: 9–13.

39. Hutchinson TA, Polansky SM, Feinstein AR. Post-menopausal oestrogens protect against fractures of hip and distal radius. *Lancet* 1979; **2**: 705–9.

40. Weiss NS, Ure CL, Ballard JH, Williams AR, Daling JR. Decreased risk of fractures of the hip and lower forearm with postmenopausal use of estrogen. *N Engl J Med* 1980; **303**: 1195–8.

41. Johnson RE, Specht EE. The risk of hip fracture in postmenopausal females with and without estrogen drug exposure. *Am J Public Health* 1981; **71**: 138–44.

42. Wallach S, Henneman PH. Prolonged estrogen therapy in post-menopausal women. *JAMA* 1959; **171**: 1637–42.

43. Gordon GS, Picchi J, Roof BS. Antifracture efficacy of long-term estrogens for osteoporosis. *Trans Assoc Am Phys* 1973; **86**: 326–32.

44. Burch JC, Byrd BF, Vaughn WK. The effects of long-term estrogen on hysterectomized women. *Am J Obstet Gynecol* 1974; **118**: 778–82.

45. Burch JC, Byrd BF, Vaughn WK. The effects of long-term estrogen administration to women following hysterectomy. *Front Horm Res* 1975; **3**: 208–14.

46. Nachtigall LE, Nachtigall RH, Nachtigall RD, Beckman EM. Estrogen replacement therapy I. A 10-year prospective study in the relationship to osteoporosis. *Obstet Gynecol* 1979; **53**: 277–81.

47. Nachtigall LE, Nachtigall RH, Nachtigall RD, Beckman EM. Estrogen replacement therapy II. A prospective study in the relationship to carcinoma and cardiovascular and metabolic problems. *Obstet Gynecol* 1979; **54**: 74–9.

48. Nordin BE, Horsman A, Crilly RG, Marshall DH, Simpson M. Treatment of spinal osteoporosis in postmenopausal women. *BMJ* 1980; **280**: 451–5.

49. Paganini-Hill A, Ross RK, Gerkins VR, Henderson BE, Arthur M, Mack TM. Menopausal estrogen therapy and hip fractures. *Ann Intern Med* 1981; **95**: 28–31.

50. Hammond CB, Jelovsek FR, Lee KL, Creasman WT, Parker RT. Effects of long-term estrogen replacement therapy I. Metabolic effects. *Am J Obstet Gynecol* 1979; **133**: 525–36.

51. Riggs BL, Seeman E, Hodgson SF, Taves DR, O'Fallon WM. Effect of the fluoride/calcium regimen on vertebral fracture occurrence in postmenopausal osteoporosis. Comparison with conventional therapy. *N Engl J Med* 1982; **306**: 446–50.

52. Krieger N, Kelsey JL, Holford TR, O'Connor T. An epidemiologic study of hip fracture in postmenopausal women. *Am J Epidemiol* 1982; **116**: 141–8.

53. Hooyman JR, Melton LJ, Nelson AM, O'Fallon WM, Riggs BL. Fractures after rheumatoid arthritis. *Arthritis Rheum* 1984; **27**: 1353–61.

54. Ettinger B, Genant HK, Cann CE. Long-term estrogen replacement therapy prevents bone loss and fractures. *Ann Intern Med* 1985; **102**: 319–24.

55. Wasnich RD, Ross PD, Heilbrun LK, Vogel JM, Yano K, Benfante RJ. Differential effects of thiazide and estrogen upon bone mineral content and fracture prevalence. *Obstet Gynecol* 1986; **67**: 457–62.

56. Michaelsson K, Baron JA, Farahmand BY, Johnell O, Magnusson C, Persson PG *et al*. Hormone replacement therapy and risk of hip fracture: population based case–control study. The Swedish Hip Fracture Study Group. *BMJ* 1998; **316**: 1858–63.

57. Nelson HD, Rizzo J, Harris E, Cauley J, Ensrud K, Bauer DC *et al*. Osteoporosis and fractures in postmenopausal women using estrogen. *Arch Intern Med* 2002; **162**: 2278–84.

58. Randell KM, Honkanen RJ, Kroger H, Saarikoski S. Does hormone-replacement therapy prevent fractures in early postmenopausal women? *J Bone Miner Res* 2002; **17**: 528–33.

59. Cauley JA, Zmuda JM, Ensrud KE, Bauer DC, Ettinger B. Timing of estrogen replacement therapy for optimal osteoporosis prevention. *J Clin Endocrinol Metab* 2002; **86**: 5700–5.

60. Mosekilde L, Beck-Nielsen H, Sorensen OH, Nielsen SP, Vestergaard P, Hermann AP *et al*. Hormonal replacement therapy reduces forearm fracture incidence in recent postmenopausal women—results of the Danish Osteoporosis Prevention Study. *Maturitas* 2000; **36**: 181–93.

61. Honkanen RJ, Honkanen K, Kroger H, Alhava E, Tuppurainen M, Saarikoski S. Risk factors for perimenopausal distal forearm fracture. *Osteoporos Int* 2000; **11**: 265–70.

62. Grodstein F, Stampfer MJ, Falkeborn M, Naessen T, Persson I. Postmenopausal hormone therapy and risk of cardiovascular disease and hip fracture in a cohort of Swedish women. *Epidemiology* 1999; **10**: 476–80.

63. Rossouw JE, Anderson GL, Prentice RL, LaCroix AZ, Kooperberg C, Stefanick ML. Risks and benefits of estrogen plus progestin in healthy postmenopausal women: principal results from the Women's Health Initiative randomized controlled trial. *JAMA* 2002; **288**: 321–33.

64. Barritt DW, Jordan SC. Anticoagulant drugs in the treatment of pulmonary embolism. *Lancet* 1960; **1**: 1309–12.

65. Coon WW, Willis PW. Recurrence of venous thromboembolism. *Surgery* 1973; **73**: 823–7.

66. Acheson L, Speizer FE, Tager I. Venous thrombosis: duration of anticoagulant therapy [letter]. *N Engl J Med* 1975; **293**: 879.

67. Salzman EW. Venous thrombosis. *West J Med* 1976; **125**: 220–2.

68. Coon WW, Mackenzie JW, Hodgson PE. A critical evaluation of anticoagulant therapy in peripheral venous thrombosis and pulmonary embolism. *Surg Gynecol Obstet* 1958; **106**: 129–36.

69. Coon WW, Willis PW, Symons MJ. Assessment of anticoagulant treatment of venous thromboembolism. *Ann Surg* 1969; **170**: 559–68.

70. Coon WW, Willis PW. Thromboembolic complications during anticoagulant therapy. *Arch Surg* 1972; **105**: 209–12.

71. O'Sullivan EF. Duration of anticoagulant therapy in venous thrombo-embolism. *Med J Aust* 1972; **2**: 1104–7.

72. Petitti DB, Strom BL, Melmon KL. Duration of warfarin anticoagulant therapy and the probabilities of recurrent thromboembolism and hemorrhage. *Am J Med* 1986; **81**: 255–9.

73. Ridker PM, Goldhaber SZ, Danielson E, Rosenberg Y, Eby CS, Deitcher SR *et al*. Long-term, low-intensity warfarin therapy for the prevention of recurrent venous thromboembolism. *N Engl J Med* 2003; **348**: 1425–34.

74. Horwitz RI, Feinstein AR. Improved observational method for studying therapeutic efficacy. Suggestive evidence that lidocaine prophylaxis prevents death in acute myocardial infarction. *JAMA* 1981; **246**: 2455–9.

75. Lie KI, Wellens HJ, van Capelle FJ, Durrer D. Lidocaine in the prevention of primary ventricular fibrillation. A double-blind, randomized study of 212 consecutive patients. *N Engl J Med* 1974; **291**: 1324–6.

76. Sadowski ZP, Alexander JH, Skrabucha B, Dyduszynski A, Kuch J, Nartowicz E *et al*. Multicenter randomized trial and a systematic overview of lidocaine in acute myocardial infarction. *Am Heart J* 1999; **137**: 792–8.

77. Alexander JH, Granger CB, Sadowski Z, Aylward PE, White HD, Thompson TD *et al*. Prophylactic lidocaine use in acute myocardial infarction: incidence and outcomes from two international trials. The GUSTO-I and GUSTO-IIb Investigators. *Am Heart J* 1999; **137**: 799–805.

78. Hirsh J. Effectiveness of anticoagulants. *Semin Thromb Hemost* 1986; **12**: 21–37.

79. Horwitz RI, Feinstein AR. The application of therapeutic-trial principles to improve the design of epidemiologic research: a case–control study suggesting that anticoagulants reduce mortality in patients with myocardial infarction. *J Chronic Dis* 1981; **34**: 575–83.

80. Mattison N. Pharmaceutical innovation and generic drug competition in the USA: effects of the Drug Price Competition and Patent Term Restoration Act of 1984. *Pharmaceut Med* 1986; **1**: 177–85.

81. Strom BL. Generic drug substitution—revisited. *N Engl J Med* 1987; **316**: 1456–62.

82. Shapiro ED, Clemens JD. A controlled evaluation of the protective efficacy of pneumococcal vaccine for patients at high risk of serious pneumococcal infections. *Ann Intern Med* 1984; **101**: 325–30.

83. Mills OF, Rhoads GG. The contribution of the case–control approach to vaccine evaluation: pneumococcal and *Haemophilus influenzae* type B PRP vaccines. *J Clin Epidemiol* 1996; **49**: 631–6.

84. Greaves WL, Orenstein WA, Hinman AR, Nersesian WS. Clinical efficacy of rubella vaccine. *Pediatr Infect Dis* 1983; **2**: 284–6.

85. Strassburg MA, Greenland S, Stephenson TG, Weiss BP, Auerbach D, Habel LA *et al*. Clinical effectiveness of rubella vaccine in a college population. *Vaccine* 1985; **3**: 109–12.

86. Killewo J, Makwaya C, Munubhi E, Mpembeni R. The protective effect of measles vaccine under rountine vaccination conditions in Dar Es Salaam, Tanzania: a case–control study. *Int J Epidemiol* 1991; **20**: 508–14.

87. Mahomva AI, Moyo IM, Mbengeranwa LO. Evaluation of a measles vaccine efficacy during a measles outbreak in Mbare, City of Harare Zimbabwe. *Cent Afr J Med* 1997; **43**: 254–6.

88. Mudzamiri WS, Peterson DE, Marufu T, Biellik RJ, L'Herminez M. Measles vaccine efficacy in Masvingo district, Zimbabwe. *Cent Afr J Med* 1996; **42**: 195–7.

89. Kabir Z, Long J, Reddaiah VP, Kevany J, Kapoor SK. Non-specific effect of measles vaccination on overall child mortality in an area of rural India with high vaccination coverage: a population-based case–control study. *Bull World Health Organ* 2003; **81**: 244–50.

90. Akramuzzaman SM, Cutts FT, Hossain MJ, Wahedi OK, Nahar N, Islam D, Shaha NC, Mahalanabis D. Measles vaccine effectiveness and risk factors for measles in Dhaka, Bangladesh. *Bull World Health Organ* 2002; **80**: 776–82.

91. Wenger JD, Pierce R, Deaver KA, Plikaytis BD, Facklam RR, Broome CV and the *Haemophilus influenzae* Vaccine Efficacy Study Group. Efficacy of *Haemophilus influenzae* type b polysaccharide–diphtheria toxoid conjugate vaccine in US children aged 18–59 months. *Lancet* 1991; **338**: 395–8.

92. Greenberg DP, Vadheim CM, Bordenave N, Ziontz L, Christenson P, Waterman SH, Ward JI. Protective efficacy of *Haemophilus influenzae* type b polysaccharide and conjugate vaccines in children 18 months of age and older. *JAMA* 1991; **265**: 987–92.

93. Black SB, Shinefield HR, Hiatt RA, Fireman BH, and the Kaiser Permanente Pediatric Vaccine Study Group. Efficacy of *Haemophilus influenzae* type b capsular polysaccharide vaccine. *Pediatr Infect Dis J* 1988; **7**: 149–56.

94. Harrison LH, Broome CV, Hightower AW, Hoppe CC, Makintubee S, Sitze SL *et al*. A day care-based study of the efficacy of Haemophilus b polysaccharide vaccine. *JAMA* 1988; **260**: 1413–18.

95. Shapiro ED, Murphy TV, Wald ER, Brady CA. The protective efficacy of Haemophilus b polysaccharide vaccine. *JAMA* 1988; **260**: 1419–22.

96. Osterholm MT, Rambeck JH, White KE, Jacobs JL, Pierson LM, Neaton JD, Hedberg CW, MacDonald KL, Granoff DM. Lack of efficacy of Haemophilus b polysaccharide vaccine in Minnesota. *JAMA* 1988; **260**: 1423–8.

97. Bower C, Condon R, Payne J, Burton P, Watson C, Wild B. Measuring the impact of conjugate vaccines on invasive *Haemophilus influenzae* type b infection in Western Australia. *Aust N Z J Public Health* 1998; **22**: 67–72.

98. Muhlemann K, Alexander ER, Weiss NS, Pepe M, Schopfer K. Risk factors for invasive *Haemophilus influenzae* disease among children 2–16 years of age in the vaccine era, Switzerland 1991–1993. The Swiss H. Influenzae Study Group. *Int J Epidemiol* 1996; **25**: 1280–5.

99. McVernon J, Andrews N, Slack MP, Ramsay ME. Risk of vaccine failure after *Haemophilus influenzae* type b (Hib) combination vaccine with acellular pertussis. *Lancet* 2003; **361**: 1521–3.

100. McVernon J, Johnson PD, Pollard AJ, Slack MP, Moxon ER. Immunologic memory in *Haemophilus influenzae* type b conjugate vaccine failure. *Arch Dis Child* 2003; **88**: 379–83.

101. Balraj V, John TJ, Thomas M, Mukundan S. Efficacy of oral poliovirus vaccine in rural communities of North District, India. *Int J Epidemiol* 1990; **19**: 711–4.

102. Deming MS, Jaiteh KO, Otten MW Jr, Flagg EW, Jallow M, Cham M *et al*. Epidemic poliomyelitis in The Gambia following the control of poliomyelitis as an endemic disease. II. Clinical efficacy of trivalent oral polio vaccine. *Am J Epidemiol* 1992; **135**: 393–408.

103. Rheingold AL, Broome CV, Hightower AW, Ajello GW, Bolan GA, Adamsbaum C *et al*. Age-specific differences in duration of clinical protection after vaccination with meningococcal polysaccharide A vaccine. *Lancet* 1985; **2**: 114–21.

104. Rosenstein N, Levine O, Taylor JP, Evans D, Plikaytis BD, Wenger JD, Perkins BA. Efficacy of meningococcal vaccine and barriers to vaccination. *JAMA* 1998; **279**: 435–9.

105. Bose A, Coen P, Tully J, Viner R, Booy R. Effectiveness of meningococcal C conjugate vaccine in teenagers in England. *Lancet* 2003; **361**: 675–6.

106. Hennessy S, Lui Z, Tsai TF, Strom BL, Wan CM, Liu HL *et al*. Effectiveness of live-attenuated Japanese encephalitis vaccine (SA14-14-2): a case–control study. *Lancet* 1996; **347**: 1583–6.

107. Miceli I, Colaiacovo D, Kantor IN, Peluffo G. Evaluation of the effectiveness of BCG vaccination using the case–control method. *Dev Biol Stand* 1986; **58**: 293–6.

108. Shapiro C, Cook N, Evans D, Willett W, Fajardo I, Koch-Weser D *et al*. A case–control study of BCG and childhood tuberculosis in Cali, Colombia. *Int J Epidemiol* 1985; **14**: 441–6.

109. Young TK, Hershfield ES. A case–control study to evaluate the effectiveness of mass BCG vaccination among Canadian Indians. *Am J Public Health* 1986; **76**: 783–6.

110. Houston S, Fanning A, Soskolne CL, Fraser N. The effectiveness of bacillus Calmette-guérin (BCG) vaccination against

tuberculosis: a case–control study in Treaty Indians, Alberta, Canada. *Am J Epidemiol* 1990; **131**: 340–8.

111. Filho VW, de Castilho EA, Rodrigues LC, Huttly SRA. Effectiveness of BCG vaccination against tuberculous meningitis: a case–control study in Sao Paulo, Brazil. *Bull World Health Organ* 1990; **68**: 69–74.

112. Patel A, Schofield F, Siskind V, Abrahams E, Parker J. Case–control evaluation of a school-age BCG vaccination programme in subtropical Australia. *Bull World Health Organ* 1991; **69**: 425–33.

113. Sirinavin S, Chotpitayasunondh T, Suwanjutha S, Sunakorn P, Chantarojanasiri T. Protective efficacy of neonatal Bacillus Calmette-Guérin vaccination against tuberculosis. *Pediatr Infect Dis J* 1991; **10**: 359–65.

114. Sharma RS, Srivastava DK, Singh AA, Kumaraswamy RK, Mullick DN, Rungsung N *et al*. Epidemiological evaluation of BCG vaccine efficacy in Delhi—1989. *J Commun Dis* 1989; **21**: 200–6.

115. Bisgard KM, Rhodes P, Hardy IR, Litkina IL, Filatov NN, Monisov AA *et al*. Diphtheria toxoid vaccine effectiveness: a case–control study in Russia. *J Infect Dis* 2000; **181**(suppl 1): 84–7.

116. Fine PEM, Ponninghaus JM, Maine N, Clarkson JA, Bliss L. Protective efficacy of BCG against leprosy in Northern Malawi. *Lancet* 1986; **2**: 499–502.

117. Muliyil J, Nelson KE, Diamond EL. Effect of BCG on the risk of leprosy in an endemic area: a case control study. *Int J Lepr* 1991; **59**: 229–36.

118. Sutcliffe PA, Rea E. Outbreak of measles in a highly vaccinated secondary school population. *Can Med Assoc J* 1996; **155**: 1407–13.

119. Ramsay ME, Moffatt D, O'Connor M. Measles vaccine: a 27-year follow-up. *Epidemiol Infect* 1994; **112**: 409–12.

120. Isomura S. Clinical studies on efficacy and safety of an acellular pertussis vaccine in Aichi prefecture, Japan. *Dev Biol Stand* 1991; **73**: 37–42.

121. Report from the PHLS Epidemiological Research Laboratory and 21 area health authorities. Efficacy of pertussis vaccination in England. *BMJ* 1982; **285**: 357–9.

122. Liu ZL, Hennessy S, Strom BL, Tsai TF, Wan CM, Tang SC *et al*. Short-term safety of live-attenuated Japanese encephalitis vaccine (SA14–14–2): results of a 26,239-subject randomized clinical trial. *J Infect Dis* 1997; **176**: 1366–9.

123. Smith PG. Retrospective assessment of the effectiveness of BCG vaccination against tuberculosis using the case–control method. *Tubercle* 1982; **63**: 23–35.

124. Smith PG, Rodrigues LC, Fine PEM. Assessment of the protective efficacy of vaccines against common diseases using case–control and cohort studies. *Int J Epidemiol* 1984; **13**: 87–93.

125. Clemens JD, Shapiro ED. Resolving the pneumococcal vaccine controversy: are there alternatives to clinical trials? *Rev Inf Dis* 1984; **6**: 589–600.

126. Orenstein WA, Bernier RH, Dondero TJ, Hinman AR, Marks JS, Bart KJ *et al*. Field evaluation of vaccine efficacy. *Bull World Health Organ* 1985; **63**: 1055–68.

127. Smith PG. Evaluating interventions against tropical diseases. *Int J Epidemiol* 1987; **16**: 159–66.

128. Farrington CP. Quantifying misclassification bias in cohort studies of vaccine efficacy. *Stat Med* 1990; **9**: 1327–37.

129. Joseph KS. A potential bias in the estimation of vaccine efficacy through observational study designs [letter]. *Int J Epidemiol* 1989; **18**: 729–31.

130. Clarke EA, Anderson TW. Does screening by "Pap" smears help prevent cervical cancer? *Lancet* 1979; **2**: 1–4.

131. Aristizabal N, Cuello C, Correa P, Collazos T, Haenszel W. The impact of vaginal cytology on cervical cancer risks in Cali, Colombia. *Int J Cancer* 1984; **34**: 5–9.

132. LaVecchia C, Franceschi S, Decarli A, Fasoli M, Gentile A, Tognoni G. "Pap" smear and the risk of cervical neoplasia: quantitative estimates from a case–control study. *Lancet* 1984; **2**: 779–82.

133. MacGregor E, Moss SM, Parkin DM, Day NE. A case–control study of cervical cancer screening in north east Scotland. *BMJ* 1985; **290**: 1543–6.

134. van der Graaf Y, Zielhuis GA, Peer PG, Vooijs PG. The effectiveness of cervical screening: a population-based case–control study. *J Clin Epidemiol* 1988; **41**: 21–6.

135. Clarke EA, Hilditch S, Anderson TW. Optimal frequency of screening for cervical cancer: a Toronto case–control study. *IARC Sci Publ* 1986; **76**: 125–31.

136. Raymond L, Obradovic M, Riotton G. Additional results on relative protection of cervical cancer screening according to stage of tumour from the Geneva case–control study. *IARC Sci Publ* 1986; **76**: 107–10.

137. Geirsson G, Kristiansdottir R, Sigurdsson K, Moss S, Tulinius H. Cervical cancer screening in Iceland: a case–control study. *IARC Sci Publ* 1986; **76**: 37–41.

138. Berrino F, Gatta G, d'Alto M, Crosignani P, Riboli E. Efficacy of screening in preventing invasive cervical cancer: a case–control study in Milan, Italy. *IARC Sci Publ* 1986; **76**: 111–23.

139. Miller MG, Sung HY, Sawaya GF, Kearney KA, Kinney W, Hiatt RA. Screening interval and risk of invasive squamous cell cervical cancer. *Obstet Gynecol* 2003; **101**: 29–37.

140. Herrero R, Brinton LA, Reeves WC, Brenes MM, de Britton RC, Gaitan E *et al*. Screening for cervical cancer in Latin America: a case–control study. *Int J Epidemiol* 1992; **21**: 1050–6.

141. Sato S, Makino H, Yajima A, Fukao A. Cervical cancer screening in Japan. A case–control study. *Acta Cytol* 1997; **41**: 1103–6.

142. Celentano DD, Klassen AC, Weisman CS, Rosenshein NB. Cervical cancer screening practices among older women: results from the Maryland cervical cancer case–control study. *J Clin Epidemiol* 1988; **41**: 531–41.

143. Celentano DD, Klassen AC, Weisman CS, Rosenshein NB. Duration of relative protection of screening for cervical cancer. *Prev Med* 1989; **18**: 411–22.

144. Zhang ZF, Parkin DM, Yu SZ, Esteve J, Yang XZ, Day NE. Cervical screening attendance and its effectiveness in a rural population in China. *Canc Detect Prev* 1989; **13**: 337–42.

145. Sobue T, Suzuki T, Fujimoto I, Yokoi N, Naruke T. Population-based case–control study on cancer screening. *Environ Health Perspect* 1990; **87**: 57–62.

146. McCarthy EP, Burns RB, Freund KM, Ash AS, Shwartz M, Marwill SL *et al.* Mammography use, breast cancer stage at diagnosis, and survival among older women. *J Am Geriatr Soc* 2000; **48**: 1226–33.

147. Wojcik BE, Spinks MK, Stein CR. Effects of screening mammography on the comparative survival rates of African American, white, and Hispanic beneficiaries of a comprehensive health care system. *Breast J* 2003; **9**: 175–83.

148. Collette JHA, Day NE, Rombach JJ, de Waard F. Evaluation of screening for breast cancer in a non-randomized study (the DOM project) by means of a case–control study. *Lancet* 1984; **1**: 1224–6.

149. Verbeek ALM, Hendriks JHCL, Holland R, Mravunac M, Sturmans F, Day NE. Reduction of breast cancer mortality through mass screening with modern mammography. First results of the Nijmegen project, 1975–1981. *Lancet* 1984; **1**: 1222–4.

150. Foster RS Jr, Costanza MC. Breast self-examination practices and breast cancer survival. *Cancer* 1984; **53**: 999–1005.

151. Greenwald P, Nasca PC, Lawrence CE, Horton J, McGarrah RP, Gabriele T *et al.* Estimated effect of breast self-examination and routine physician examinations on breast cancer mortality. *N Engl J Med* 1978; **299**: 271–3.

152. Smith EM, Francis AM, Polissar L. The effect of breast self-exam practices and physical examination on extent of disease at diagnosis. *Prev Med* 1980; **9**: 409–17.

153. Huquely CM, Brown RL. The value of breast self-examination. *Cancer* 1981; **47**: 989–95.

154. Senie RT, Rosen PP, Lesser ML, Kinne DW. Breast self-examination and medical examination related to breast cancer stage. *Am J Public Health* 1981; **71**: 583–90.

155. Feldman JG, Carter AC, Nicastri AD, Hosat ST. Breast self-examination, relationship to stage of breast cancer at diagnosis. *Cancer* 1981; **47**: 2740–5.

156. Dubin N, Pasternack BS. Breast cancer screening data in case–control studies. *Am J Epidemiol* 1984; **120**: 8–16.

157. Dubin N, Friedman DR, Toniolo PG, Pasternack BS. Breast cancer detection centers and case–control studies of the efficacy of screening. *J Chronic Dis* 1987; **40**: 1041–50.

158. Collette HJA, Rombach JJ, Day NE, de Waard F. *Lancet* 1984; **1**: 1224–6.

159. Hunt KA, Rosen EL, Sickles EA. Outcome analysis for women undergoing annual versus biennial screening mammography: a review of 24,211 examinations. *Am J Roentgenol* 1999; **173**: 285–9.

160. Palli D, Del Turco MR, Buiatti E, Carli S, Ciatto S, Toscani L *et al.* A case–control study of the efficacy of a non-randomized breast cancer screening program in Florence (Italy). *Int J Cancer* 1986; **38**: 501–4.

161. Palli D, Del Turco MR, Buiatti E, Ciatto S, Crocetti E, Paci E. Time interval since last test in a breast cancer screening programme: a case–control study in Italy. *J Epidemiol Community Health* 1989; **43**: 241–8.

162. Friedman DR, Dubin N. Case–control evaluation of breast cancer screening efficacy. *Am J Epidemiol* 1991; **133**: 974–84.

163. Randolph WM, Goodwin JS, Mahnken JD, Freeman JL. Regular mammography use is associated with elimination of age-related disparities in size and stage of breast cancer at diagnosis. *Ann Intern Med* 2002; **137**: 783–90.

164. Ebeling K, Nischan P. Screening for lung cancer—results from a case–control study. *Int J Cancer* 1987; **40**: 141–4.

165. Sobue T, Suzuki T, Naruke T, and the Japanese Lung-Cancer-Screening Research Group. A case–control study for evaluating lung-cancer screening in Japan. *Int J Cancer* 1992; **50**: 230–7.

166. Oshima A, Hirata N, Ubukata T, Umeda K, Fujimoto I. Evaluation of a mass screening program for stomach cancer with a case–control study design. *Int J Cancer* 1986; **38**: 829–33.

167. Shapiro S, Venet W, Strax P, Venet L, Roeser R. Selection, follow-up, and analysis in the Health Insurance Plan Study: a randomized trial with breast cancer screening. *Natl Cancer Inst Monogr* 1985; **67**: 65–74.

168. Connor RJ, Prorok PC, Weed DL. The case–control design and the assessment of the efficacy of cancer screening. *J Clin Epidemiol* 1991; **44**: 1215–21.

169. Morrison AS. Case definition in case–control studies of the efficacy of screening. *Am J Epidemiol* 1982; **115**: 6–8.

170. Weiss NS. Control definition in case–control studies of the efficacy of screening and diagnostic testing. *Am J Epidemiol* 1983; **118**: 457–60.

171. Sasco AJ, Day NE, Walter SD. Case–control studies for the evaluation of screening. *J Chronic Dis* 1986; **39**: 399–405.

172. Frommer DJ. Case–control studies of screening. *J Clin Epidemiol* 1988; **41**: 101.

173. Sasco AJ. Lead time and length bias in case–control studies for the evaluation of screening. *J Clin Epidemiol* 1988; **41**: 103–4.

174. Cole P, Morrison AS. Basic issues in population screening for cancer. *J Natl Cancer Inst* 1980; **64**: 1263–72.

175. Morrison AS. Case definition in case–control studies of the efficacy of screening. *Am J Epidemiol* 1982; **115**: 6–8.

176. Baum M, MacRae KD. Screening for breast cancer. *Lancet* 1984; **2**: 462.

177. Flanders WD, Longini IM Jr. Estimating benefits of screening from observational cohort studies. *Stat Med* 1990; **9**: 969–80.

178. Weiss NS, McKnight B, Stevens NG. Approaches to the analysis of case–control studies of the efficacy of screening for cancer. *Am J Epidemiol* 1992; **135**: 817–23.

179. Knox G. Case–control studies of screening procedures. *Public Health* 1991; **105**: 55–61.

180. Weiss NS. Case–control studies of the efficacy of screening tests designed to prevent the incidence of cancer. *Am J Epidemiol* 1999; **149**: 1–4.

181. Weiss NS. Analysis of case–control studies of the efficacy of screening for cancer: how should we deal with tests done in persons with symptoms? *Am J Epidemiol* 1998; **147**: 1099–102.

182. Cronin KA, Weed DL, Connor RJ, Prorok PC. Case–control studies of cancer screening: theory and practice. *J Natl Cancer Inst* 1998; **90**: 498–504.

183. Weiss NS, Lazovich D. Case–control studies of screening efficacy: the use of persons newly diagnosed with cancer who later sustain an unfavorable outcome. *Am J Epidemiol* 1996; **143**: 319–22.

184. Thompson DC, Thompson RS, Rivara FP, Wolf ME. A case–control study of the effectiveness of bicycle safety helmets in preventing facial injury. *Am J Public Health* 1990; **80**: 1471–4.

185. Imperiale TF, Horwitz RI. Does prophylaxis prevent postdental infective endocarditis? A controlled evaluation of protective efficacy. *Am J Med* 1990; **88**: 131–6.

186. Horwitz RI, Viscoli CM, Clemens JD, Sadock RT. Developing improved observational methods for evaluating therapeutic effectiveness. *Am J Med* 1990; **89**: 630–8.

187. Psaty BM, Koepsell TD, LoGerfo JP, Wagner EH, Inui TS. Beta-blockers and primary prevention of coronary heart disease in patients with high blood pressure. *JAMA* 1989; **261**: 2087–94.

188. Sackett DL, Haynes RB, Tugwell PT. *Clinical Epidemiology. A Basic Science for Clinical Medicine*. Boston, MA: Little, Brown and Co., 1985.

189. Hill AB. Reflections on the controlled trial. *Ann Rheum Dis* 1966; **25**: 107–13.

41

Pharmacoeconomics: Economic Evaluation of Pharmaceuticals

KEVIN A. SCHULMAN[1], HENRY A. GLICK[2] and DANIEL POLSKY[2]

[1] Center for Clinical and Genetic Economics, Duke Clinical Research Institute, Duke University Medical Center, Durham, North Carolina, USA; [2] Leonard Davis Institute of Health Economics, University of Pennsylvania School of Medicine, Philadelphia, Pennsylvania, USA.

INTRODUCTION

Conventional evaluation of new medical technologies such as pharmaceutical products includes consideration of efficacy, effectiveness, and safety. Other chapters of this book describe in detail how such evaluations are carried out. The methodology is well developed, and Federal regulation requires studies of safety and efficacy to be performed prior to drug marketing. More recently, health care researchers from a variety of disciplines have developed techniques for the evaluation of the economic effects of clinical care and new medical technologies. Clinicians, pharmacists, economists, epidemiologists, operations researchers, and others have contributed to the field of "clinical economics," an evolving discipline dedicated to the study of how different approaches to patient care and treatment influence the resources consumed in clinical medicine.[1-14]

The growth of clinical economics has proceeded rapidly as health policy makers have faced a continuing series of decisions about funding new clinical therapies in an era of increasingly constrained health care resources. Assessments of new therapies include the resources required for the new therapy, the extent of the substitution of the new resources for existing resources, if any, and the health outcomes that result from therapeutic intervention. Thus, clinical economics includes not just an assessment of the cost of a new therapy, but an assessment of its overall economic and clinical effects.

This chapter discusses the need for applying economic concepts to the study of pharmaceuticals, introduces the concepts of clinical economics and the application of these concepts to pharmaceutical research, reviews some of the methodologic issues addressed by investigators studying the economics of pharmaceuticals, and finally offers examples of this type of research.

Pharmacoepidemiology, Fourth Edition   Edited by B.L. Strom
© 2005 John Wiley & Sons, Ltd

CLINICAL PROBLEMS TO BE ADDRESSED BY PHARMACOEPIDEMIOLOGIC RESEARCH

There is ongoing concern about the cost of medical care, which has caused both purchasers and producers of pharmaceuticals to realize that the cost of drugs is not limited to their purchase price. The accompanying costs of preparation, administration, monitoring for and treating side effects, and the economic consequences of successful disease treatment are all influenced by the clinical and pharmacologic characteristics of pharmaceuticals. Thus, in addition to differences in efficacy and safety, differences in efficiency (or the effectiveness of the agent in actual clinical practice compared to its cost) distinguish drugs from one another.

Concerns about the cost of medical care in general and pharmaceuticals specifically are being felt in nearly all developed nations. Several national governments now require or are in the process of implementing requirements for the presentation of pharmacoeconomic data at the time of product registration for pharmaceuticals to qualify for reimbursement through the national health insurance systems.[15–21] Clinical economics research is being used increasingly by managed care organizations in the United States to inform funding decisions for new therapies. At the local level, hospital administrators and other providers of health care are seeking ways of delivering high-quality care within the constraints of limited budgets or reduced fee schedules. These decision makers increasingly are interested in guidance regarding the cost-effectiveness of new medical technologies such as pharmaceuticals. This guidance can be provided by clinical economic analyses.

TRENDS IN PHARMACOECONOMIC RESEARCH

The biotechnology revolution in medical research has added another challenge to pharmacoeconomic research. Pharmacoeconomics is increasingly being used to help determine the effect on patients of new classes of therapies before they are brought to the marketplace and to help determine appropriate clinical and economic outcomes for the clinical development program. The challenge is twofold: (i) understanding the potential effect of a therapy (e.g., whether a new antisepsis agent is a new type of antibiotic compound, where a short-term evaluation, efficacy at 14 days, is the appropriate clinical endpoint for analysis, or a life supporting therapy, where a longer-term evaluation, efficacy at 6 or 12 months, is the appropriate clinical endpoint for efficacy assessment), and (ii) understanding the transition from efficacy to efficiency in clinical practice.[22,23] These challenges span the clinical development spectrum. As we learn more about the potential effect and use of a new product, these

issues can be re-addressed in an iterative process. Finally, more and more firms are beginning to use economic models to help guide the business planning process and the new product development process to address the economic issues surrounding new therapies at the beginning of the product development cycle.

Pharmacoeconomic studies are designed to meet the different information needs of health care purchasers and regulatory authorities. Economic data from Phase III studies are used to support initial pricing of new therapies and are used in professional educational activities by pharmaceutical firms. Postmarketing economic studies are used to compare new therapies with existing therapies and increasingly to confirm the initial Phase III economic assessments of the product.

No single study can possibly provide all interested audiences with complete economic information on a new therapy. Thus, specific studies are undertaken to address economic concerns from specific perspectives, such as a postmarketing study of a new therapy from the perspective of a health maintenance organization (HMO). They may also be undertaken to assess the effect of therapy on specific cost categories, such as an assessment of the productivity costs of treatment to provide data to federal governments in Europe, since these governments fund both the health insurance system and the disability system.

ECONOMIC EVALUATION AND THE DRUG DEVELOPMENT PROCESS

New pharmaceuticals are developed in a series of well-defined stages due to the regulatory process of drug approval. After a compound is identified and thought to be clinically useful, four distinct sets of evaluations—referred to as Phase I through IV studies—are mandated by the US Food and Drug Administration (FDA) and most other equivalent regulatory bodies. Phase I studies represent the first introduction of a new compound into (usually undiseased) humans, principally for the evaluation of safety and dosage. In Phase II studies, the drug is introduced into a patient population with the disease of interest, again principally for the evaluation of safety and dosing. Phase III studies are randomized trials evaluating the safety and efficacy of new drugs, compared either with placebo or with a therapy that the new drug might replace (in the US, the appropriate comparator often is the subject of negotiations between the developer of the drug and the FDA). In addition to these three types of studies, drugs often are evaluated after they are marketed in what are referred to as Phase IV or postmarketing studies. The drug development process allows for timely collection of data that can be used to evaluate the costs and effects of pharmaceuticals early in their product life, with an opportunity for further data collection and evaluation once the product has been approved and marketed.

Clinical economics has been integrated throughout the development process, with goals that parallel the clinical development stages. Phase I and II studies are used to develop pilot economic data, such as estimates of the mean and variance estimates for costs, quality-of-life, and utilities for patients with a specific clinical syndrome. These studies are also used to perform pilot tests of data collection tools, including economic case report forms that prospectively capture resources used by patients who will be entered into the Phase III and postmarketing clinical trials. From these data, issues such as sample size and power for pharmacoeconomic studies can be assessed.

One of the fastest growing areas in the economic assessment of new drugs is the incorporation of economic analyses as part of Phase III clinical trials. Phase III studies can include economic assessments of new therapies as a primary or secondary endpoint (i.e., an assessment of changes in the use of specific resource categories resulting from treatment, such as changes in length of hospital stay or changes in hospitalization rates).[24-29]

Lastly, a wide variety of postmarketing economic studies can be performed. These include efficiency trials (also known as "pragmatic" or "practical" trials) in which comparisons between products are made in more realistic settings with less restrictive protocols than those designed for Phase III safety and efficacy trials.[30] These postmarketing studies may include assessments of the new therapy compared with "usual care" or compared with specific therapeutic agents. Again, the economic analysis can serve as a primary or secondary endpoint of the study.

Developing economic data as an endpoint in a clinical trial requires integrating pharmacoeconomics into the clinical development process. While there recently has been an increase in the number of trials that collect economic data, the challenge remains to ensure that pharmacoeconomic endpoints are considered sufficiently early in the clinical development process so that designing the economic protocol does not impede the process of designing the clinical trial. Economic analysis requires the establishment of a set of economic endpoints for study (e.g., direct, productivity, and intangible cost to patients and caregivers, as well as quality-of-life or preference measures for patients and caregivers), review of the clinical protocol to ensure that there are no economic biases in the design of the clinical trial—such as requirements for differential resource use between the treatment arms of the study—and the development of the economic protocol. Ideally, the economic study will be integrated into the clinical protocol and the economic data will be collected as part of a unified case report form for both clinical and economic variables.

In the following sections, we briefly review the research methods of pharmacoeconomics, discuss some methodologic issues that have confronted researchers investigating the economics of pharmaceuticals, and review several studies that illustrate the usefulness of pharmacoeconomic research.

METHODOLOGIC PROBLEMS TO BE ADDRESSED BY PHARMACOEPIDEMIOLOGIC RESEARCH

TECHNIQUES OF CLINICAL ECONOMICS

Economists emphasize that costs are more than just transactions of currency. Cost represents the consumption of a resource that could otherwise be used for another purpose. The value of the resource is that of its next best use, which no longer is possible once the resource has been used. This value is called the resource's "opportunity cost." For example, the time it takes to read this chapter is a cost for the reader, because it is time that cannot be used again; the opportunity to use it for another purpose has been forgone. Good investments are made when the benefits of the investment (e.g., what you learn) are greater than or equal to the value of the opportunities you have forgone (e.g., what you would be doing if you were not reading this chapter).

In addition to the fact that not all costs involve a transaction of money, it is important to remember that, at least from the perspective of society as a whole, not all transactions of money should be considered costs. For example, monetary transactions that do not represent the consumption of resources (e.g., social security payments, disability payments, or other retirement benefits) are not costs by this definition. They simply transfer the right to consume the resources represented by the money from one individual to another.

In considering economic analysis of medical care, there are three dimensions of analysis, (represented by the three axes of the cube in Figure 41.1) with which readers should become familiar.[1] Along the X axis are three types of economic analysis—cost identification, cost-effectiveness, and cost–benefit. Along the Y axis are four points of view, or perspectives, that one may take in carrying out an analysis. One may take the point of view of society in assessing the costs and benefits of a new medical therapy. Alternatively, one may take the point of view of the patient, the payer, or the provider. Along the third axis, the Z axis, are the types of costs and benefits that can be included in economic analysis of medical care. These costs and benefits, which will be defined

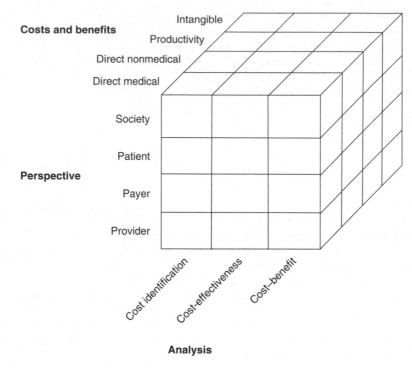

Figure 41.1. The three dimensions of economic evaluation of clinical care.
Source: Bombardier and Eisenberg.[1]

below, include direct costs and benefits, productivity costs and benefits, and intangible costs and benefits.

Types of Analysis

Cost–Benefit Analysis

Cost–benefit analysis of medical care compares the cost of a medical intervention to its benefit. Both costs and benefits are measured in the same (usually monetary) units (e.g., dollars). These measurements are used to determine either the ratio of dollars spent to dollars saved or the net saving (if benefits are greater than costs) or net cost. All else equal, an investment should be undertaken when its benefits exceed its costs.

The methods of cost–benefit analysis may be applied to evaluate the total costs and benefits of the interventions that are being compared by analyzing their cost–benefit ratios or their net benefits. Furthermore, the additional or "incremental" cost of an intervention (i.e., the difference in cost between a new therapy and conventional medical care) may be compared with its additional or "incremental" benefit. Incremental analysis is generally preferred to comparisons

of totals because it allows the analyst to focus on the differences between any two treatment modalities.

One potential difficulty of cost–benefit analysis is that it requires researchers to express an intervention's costs and outcomes in the same units. Thus, monetary values must be associated with years of life lost and morbidity due to disease and with years of life gained and morbidity avoided due to intervention. Expressing costs in this way is obviously difficult in health care analyses. Outcomes (treatment benefits) may be difficult to measure in units of currency. Translating disease and treatment outcomes into monetary measures may be more difficult than translating them into clinical outcome measures, such as years of life saved or years of life saved adjusted for quality.

Cost-Effectiveness Analysis

Cost-effectiveness analysis provides an approach to the dilemma of assessing the monetary value of health outcomes as part of the evaluation. While cost generally is still calculated only in terms of dollars spent, effectiveness is determined independently and may be measured only in clinical terms, using any meaningful clinical unit. For example, one might measure clinical outcomes in terms of number of lives saved, complications prevented, or diseases cured. Alternatively, health outcomes can be reported in terms of a change in an intermediate clinical outcome, such as cost per percent change in blood cholesterol level. These results generally are reported as a ratio of costs to clinical benefits, with costs measured in monetary terms but with benefits measured in the units of the relevant outcome measure (for example, dollars per year of life saved).

When several outcomes result from a medical intervention (e.g., the prevention of both death and disability), cost-effectiveness analysis may consider these two outcomes together only if a common measure of outcome can be developed. Frequently, analysts combine different categories of clinical outcomes according to their desirability, assigning a weighted utility, or value, to the overall treatment outcome.[3] A utility weight is a measure of the patient's preferences for his/her health state or for the outcome of an intervention. The comparison of costs and utilities sometimes is referred to as cost–utility analysis, with the denominator expressed as quality-adjusted life-years (QALYs).

As with cost–benefit analysis, cost-effectiveness analysis can compare a treatment's total costs and total effectiveness, or it can assess only the treatment's incremental costs and incremental effectiveness. In the former, the cost effectiveness ratio of each intervention is calculated and the two ratios are compared (e.g., the cost per life saved using each intervention). In the latter approach, which assesses incremental costs and benefits, the incremental cost of the innovation is calculated, as is the incremental effectiveness, and the analyst can calculate the additional effect (e.g., lives saved) per additional treatment dollar spent. Programs that cost less and demonstrate improved or equivalent treatment outcomes are said to be dominant and should always be adopted. Programs that cost more and are more effective should be adopted if both their cost-effectiveness and incremental cost-effectiveness ratios fall within an acceptable range and the budget for the program is acceptable. Programs that cost more and have worse clinical outcomes are said to be dominated and should never be adopted. Programs that cost less and have reduced clinical outcomes may be adopted depending upon the magnitude of the changes in cost and outcome.

As with the translation of clinical outcomes into monetary measures, there also are difficulties associated with combining different outcomes into a common measure in cost-effectiveness analysis. However, it generally is considered more difficult to translate all health benefits into monetary units for the purposes of cost–benefit analysis than to combine clinical outcomes measures. Thus, cost-effectiveness

analysis is used more frequently than cost–benefit analysis in the medical care literature.

Cost Identification Analysis

An even less complex approach than cost–benefit or cost-effectiveness analysis would be simply to enumerate the costs involved in medical care and to ignore the outcomes that result from that care. This approach is known as cost identification analysis. By performing cost identification analysis, the researcher can determine alternative ways of providing a service. The analysis might be expressed in terms of the cost per unit of service provided. For example, a cost identification study might measure the cost of a course of antibiotic treatment, but it would not calculate the clinical outcomes (cost-effectiveness analysis) or the value of the outcomes in units of currency (cost–benefit analysis). Cost identification studies, which include comparisons among different treatments based upon their costs alone, are appropriate only if treatment outcomes or benefits are equivalent for the therapies being evaluated.

Sensitivity Analysis

Most cost–benefit and cost-effectiveness studies require large amounts of data that may vary in reliability, validity, or the effect on the overall results of the study. This is especially the case when models are developed for the economic analysis using secondary data sources, when data collection is performed retrospectively, or when critical data elements are unmeasured or unknown. Sensitivity analysis is a set of procedures in which the results of a study are recalculated using alternate values for some of the study's variables in order to test the sensitivity of the conclusions to these altered specifications. Such an analysis can yield several important results by demonstrating the independence or dependence of a result on particular assumptions, establishing the minimum or maximum values of a variable that would be required to affect a recommendation to adopt or reject a program, and identifying clinical or economic uncertainties that require additional research. In general, sensitivity analyses are performed on variables that have a significant effect on the study's conclusions but for which values are uncertain.

Types of Costs

Another dimension of economic analysis of clinical practice illustrated by Figure 41.1 is the evaluation of costs of a therapy. Economists consider three types of costs: direct, productivity, and intangible.

Direct Medical Costs

The direct medical costs of care usually are associated with monetary transactions and represent costs that are incurred during the provision of care. Examples of direct medical costs include payments for purchasing a pharmaceutical product, payments for physicians' fees, salaries of allied health professionals, or purchases of diagnostic tests. Because the charge for medical care may not accurately reflect the resources consumed, accounting or statistical techniques may be needed to determine direct costs.[7,31–35]

Direct Nonmedical Costs

Monetary transactions undertaken as a result of illness or health care to detect, prevent, or treat disease are not limited to direct medical costs. There is another type of cost that often is overlooked: direct nonmedical costs. These costs are incurred because of illness or the need to seek medical care. They include the cost of transportation to the hospital or physician's office, the cost of special clothing needed because of the illness, the cost of hotel stays for receiving medical treatment at a distant medical facility, and the cost of special housing (e.g., the cost of modification of a home to accommodate an ill individual). Direct nonmedical costs, which are generally paid out of pocket by patients and their families, are just as much direct medical costs as are expenses that are more usually covered by third-party insurance plans.

Direct costs can be further classified to help determine the potential effect of a therapy in terms of the ability to change patterns of resource consumption by patients. If these costs increase with increasing volume of activity, they are described as variable costs. However, if the same costs are incurred regardless of the volume of activity, they are described as fixed costs. For example, the paper used in an electrocardiogram machine is a variable cost, since a strip of paper is used for every tracing. However, the machine itself is a fixed cost since it must be purchased whether one tracing is needed or many are performed. Of course, fixed costs are fixed only within certain bounds. A very large increase in activity will require the purchase of another piece of equipment. Even the fixed cost of a hospital's building is only fixed within certain limits of activity and a certain time frame. If enough increase in activity occurs, a new building might be needed. Alternatively, if patient care is transferred from an inpatient to an outpatient setting, a part of the building may be closed and the staff size decreased. Still, for the purposes of most decisions in clinical practice, costs can be considered to be fixed or variable.

Productivity Costs

In contrast to direct costs, productivity costs do not stem from transactions for goods or services. Instead, they represent the cost of morbidity (e.g., time lost from work) or mortality (e.g., premature death leading to removal from the work force). They are costs because they represent the loss of opportunities to use a valuable resource, a life, in alternative ways. A variety of techniques are used to estimate productivity costs of illness or health care.[36–40] Sometimes, as with patients infected with human immunodeficiency virus,[41] the productivity costs of an illness are substantially greater than the direct costs of the illness.

Intangible Costs

Intangible costs are those of pain, suffering, and grief. These costs result from medical illness itself and from the services used to treat the illness. They are difficult to measure as part of a pharmacoeconomic study, though they are clearly considered by clinicians and patients in considering potential alternative treatments. Although investigators are developing ways to measure intangible costs—such as willingness-to-pay analysis whereby patients are asked to place monetary values on intangible costs[3]—at present these costs are often omitted in clinical economics research.

Perspective of Analysis

The third axis in Figure 41.1 is that of the perspective of an economic analysis of medical care. Costs and benefits can be calculated with respect to society's, the patient's, the payer's, and the provider's points of view. A study's perspective determines how costs and benefits are measured, and the economist's strict definition of costs (the consumption of a resource that could otherwise be used for another purpose) no longer may be appropriate when perspectives different from that of society as a whole are used. For example, a hospital's cost of providing a service may be less than its charge. From the hospital's perspective, then, the charge could be an overstatement of the resources consumed for some services. However, if the patient has to pay the full charge, it is an accurate reflection of the cost of the service to the patient. Alternatively, if the hospital decreases its costs by discharging patients early, the hospital's costs may decrease, but patients' costs may increase because of the need for increased outpatient expenses that are not covered by their health insurance plan.

Because costs will differ depending on the perspective, the economic impact of an intervention will be different from different perspectives. To make comparisons of the economic impact across different interventions, it is important for all economic analyses to adopt a similar perspective. It has been recommended that, as a base case, all analyses adopt a societal perspective. The cost to society is the opportunity cost, the value of the opportunities forgone because of the resource having been consumed. Society's perspective usually is taken by measuring the consumption of real resources, including the loss of potentially productive human lives. As already noted, this cost does not count transfer payments, such as social security benefits. (From the point of view of the Social Security Administration, however, these payments would be a cost, because the perspective of the Social Security Administration is not the perspective of society.) If an intervention is not good value for money from the societal perspective, it would not be a worthwhile intervention for society, even if the intervention may have economic advantages for other stakeholders.

Nevertheless, conducting the economic analysis from other perspectives, in addition to the societal perspective, is important. This is because the costs of medical care may not be borne solely by the same parties who stand to benefit from it. Economic analysis of medical care often raises vexing ethical problems related to equity, distribution of resources, and responsibility for the health of society's members.[42,43] Economic analyses from multiple perspectives shed light on the equity issues associated with new interventions.

In summary, economic analysis of medical technology or medical care evaluates a medical service by comparing its dollar cost with its dollar benefit (cost–benefit), by measuring its dollar cost in relation to its outcomes (cost-effectiveness), or simply by tabulating the costs involved (cost identification). Direct costs are generated as services are provided. In addition, productivity costs should be considered, especially in determining the benefit of a service that decreases morbidity or mortality. Finally, the perspective of the study determines the costs and benefits that will be quantified in the analysis, and sensitivity analyses test the effects of changes in variable specifications for estimated measures on the results of the study.

METHODOLOGIC ISSUES IN THE PHARMACOECONOMIC ASSESSMENT OF THERAPIES

The basic approach for performing economic assessments of pharmaceutical products, as discussed above, has been adapted from the general methodology for cost-effectiveness and cost–benefit analysis. These methods have been well developed in medical technology assessment as well as in other fields of economic research. However, there remain a number of methodological issues that confront investigators in economic evaluations of pharmaceutical therapies. This section reviews some of these issues as they arise in the design, analysis, and interpretation of pharmacoeconomic evaluations.

Clinical Trials versus Common Practice

One of the most vexing of these issues is how to assess the cost implications of products during clinical trials. Ascertaining whether or not a product's costs are adequately offset by its effects or benefits presents a number of issues for consideration.[44,45] We shall discuss some of these issues related to the case of the pharmacoeconomic assessment of a new prophylactic therapy for thromboembolic disease.

The Problem

As has been pointed out in other chapters of this volume, clinical trials are useful for determining the efficacy of therapeutic agents. However, their focus on efficacy rather than effectiveness and their use of protocols for testing and treating patients pose problems for cost-effectiveness analysis. One difficulty in assessing the economic impact of a drug as an endpoint in a clinical trial is the performance of routine testing to determine the presence or absence of a study outcome. For example, in a study of prophylaxis against thromboembolic events, the protocol may specify testing of all patients for deep vein thromboses (DVT) (e.g., fibrinogen scanning, venograms, or Doppler testing), whether or not the patients show clinical signs of these events. While this diagnostic strategy may be appropriate, it is not necessarily common practice. Yet, it can have wide-ranging effects on the calculated costs and outcomes of care.

First, the protocol may induce the detection of extra cases—cases that would have gone undetected if no protocol were used in the usual care of patients. These cases may be detected earlier than they would have been in usual care. In the prophylaxis example above, repeated testing of all patients is likely to increase the number of DVTs that are detected, especially if, in usual care, patients are only tested when they develop clinical symptoms or signs of DVT. This extra or early detection may also reduce the average costs for each case detected, because subclinical cases or those detected early may be less costly to treat than clinically detected cases. However, because these two potential biases—more cases, each of which may cost less—work in opposite directions, the total costs of care for the patients in the trial may or may not exceed those that would occur in usual care.

Second, protocol-induced testing may lead to the detection of adverse drug effects that would otherwise have gone undetected. As above, the average costs of each may be less because the adverse effects would be milder. However, their frequency would obviously be higher, and they could result in additional testing and treatment.

Third, protocol-induced testing also may lead to the occurrence of fewer adverse events from the pharmaceutical product than would occur in usual care. The extra tests done in compliance with the protocol may provide information that otherwise would not have been available to clinicians, allowing them to take steps to prevent adverse events and their resulting costs. For example, an antibiotic protocol may call for more frequent testing of creatinine levels than would be conducted in usual care. These tests may warn physicians of impending renal problems, allowing them to change the drug dosage or the antibiotic. Thus, cases of nephrotoxicity that would have occurred in usual care may be avoided. This potential bias of reducing the costs of side effects and adverse events would tend to lower the overall costs of care observed in the trial compared to usual care.

Fourth, due to ethical obligations that arise when patients are enrolled in trials, outcomes detected in trials may be treated more aggressively than they would be in usual care. In trials, it is likely that physicians will treat all detected treatable clinical outcomes. In usual care, physicians may treat only those outcomes that in their judgment are clinically relevant. This potential bias would tend to increase the costs of care observed in the trial compared to usual care.

Fifth, protocol-induced testing to determine the efficacy of a product or to monitor the occurrence of all side effects, whether clinically detectable or not, generally will increase the costs of diagnostic testing in the trial, because many of these tests likely would be omitted in usual care. Alternatively, the protocol may reduce these costs in environments where there is overuse of testing. In teaching settings, for example, some residents may normally order more tests than are needed, and this excess testing may be limited by the protocol's testing prescriptions.

Sixth, clinical protocols may offer patients additional resources that are not routinely available in clinical practice. These additional resources may provide health benefits to patients. For example, protocols offering extensive home care services may affect the observed benefits of a therapy if the nursing intervention improves the management of the patient's illness. This could result in a bias in the study design if there are differences in the amount of home care services provided to patients in the treatment and control arms of a trial, or may result in additional health benefits to all study patients.

Seventh, patients in trials often are carefully selected. If a study sample has a mean patient age of 45 years, the result of the trial may not be readily generalizable to substantially older or younger populations. Similarly, exclusion criteria in clinical protocols may rule out patients with specific clinical syndromes (e.g., diabetes mellitus), women of childbearing potential, or patients of advanced age. These patients may require additional resources or may receive less benefit from therapy because their life span is shorter. These exclusions further limit the generalizability of the findings of efficacy studies.

A related issue in pharmacoeconomics trials is the generalizability of the health care delivery system of the patients in the study. A pharmacoeconomic study conducted through an HMO using its members as subjects may observe fewer referrals to specialist physicians than would the same clinical study in a different practice setting. This effect may be even more pronounced in multinational clinical trials, where health care systems, physician education, and patients' expectations for treatment differ by country.

Other difficulties in projecting the results of clinical trials to usual care arise because the patients in clinical trials generally comply more completely with their treatment than do patients in usual care, because they receive prescribed patterns of care, and because trials often have a placebo arm. If there is an actual placebo effect, this last factor may tend to understate the effectiveness the agent will have when it is utilized in usual care.

Routinely appending economic evaluations to clinical trials will likely yield "cost-efficacy" analyses, the results of which may be substantially different from the result of cost-effectiveness analyses conducted in the usual care setting. The problem of generalizability is similar to that found in clinical epidemiology research. However, clinical economics explicitly recognizes the added complexity of having different resource-induced costs and benefits derived from clinical protocols and from observing patients in different health care systems in multicenter clinical trials.

Pharmacogenomic strategies offer opportunities to segment populations of patients according to clinical benefit or risk.[46] (See also Chapter 37.) Application of these new tools to the clinical development program will allow for tailoring of therapies in ways that could alter economic evaluations of therapies.[23]

Possible Solutions

One possible solution to this problem will be illustrated by examining the impact of a "usual care" arm appended as a third arm of a clinical trial. In such a three-arm study, patients randomized to the usual care arm of the study would be treated as they would be outside of the trial, rather than as mandated by the study protocol, and economic and outcomes data from usual care could thus be collected. These data would make it possible to quantify the number of outcomes that likely would be detected in usual care and the costs of these outcomes.

One drawback to this method is that physicians in the trial may treat all patients similarly, whether they are in the protocol-driven arm or the usual care arm of the study. This contamination can be partially overcome by randomizing physicians to the protocol or usual care arms, and can be overcome more completely by randomizing the sites of care (e.g., different hospitals for different arms of the study). However, these options require large numbers of physicians and/or sites of care and, thus, are very costly to implement. Moreover, such a strategy may result in nonrandom assignment of patients to treatment arms.

A second method that has been used to overcome these problems[7] is to collect data from patients who are not in the trial but who would have met its entry criteria, using these data to estimate the likely costs and outcomes in usual care. These patients could have received their care prior to the trial (historical comparison group) or concurrent with it (concurrent comparison group). In either case, some of the data available in the trial may not be available for patients in the comparison groups. Thus, investigators must insure comparability between the data for usual care patients and trial patients.

Two problems arise when using a concurrent comparison group to project the results of a trial to usual care. First, as with the randomization scheme above, the use of a protocol in the trial may affect the care delivered to patients who are not in the trial. If so, usual care patients may not receive the same care they would have received if the trial had not been performed. Thus, the results of the trial may lose generalizability to other settings. Second, the trial may enroll a particular type of patient (e.g., investigators may "cream-skim" by enrolling the healthiest patients with the fewest complications), possibly leaving a biased sample (e.g., of sicker and more complicated patients) for inclusion in the concurrent comparison group. This potential bias would tend to affect the estimate of the treatment costs that would be experienced in usual care.

Adoption of a historical comparison group would offset the issue of contamination. Because the trial was not ongoing when these patients received their care, it could not affect how they were treated. A historical comparison group would also tend to offset the selection bias: the subset of patients who would have been included in the trial if it had been carried out in the historic period will be candidates for the comparison group. However, use of a historic comparison group is unlikely to offset this bias entirely. Because

this group is identified retrospectively, its attributes likely will reflect those of the average patients eligible for the trial, rather than those of the subset of patients that would have been enrolled in the trial (e.g., if cream-skimming had occurred).

However, differences between the care provided to patients in the trial and that provided to patients in this group may be due as much to secular trends in the provision of medical care as they are to the adoption of a study protocol. For example, length of stay in the United States has decreased since the early 1980s, due in part to the implementation of the Medicare Prospective Payment System. Thus, historical cohorts from earlier periods may have had longer lengths of stay as inpatients than is currently seen in clinical practice. These data may suggest a protocol-induced decrease in length of stay when one really does not exist.

To avoid these difficulties, the usual care comparison group may include both historic and concurrent comparison groups. In this case, multivariable methods such as multiple regression analysis or other analytic techniques must be used to control for differences among the historic and concurrent comparison groups as well as between the comparison groups and the patients in the trial. For example, in a regression analysis of length of stay in the trial and in usual care, variables representing each of the groups will indicate the magnitude of the secular trends, the selection bias, and the protocol effects of the trial.

A number of methods currently are being investigated to help overcome the potential biases of resource-induced costs and benefits in clinical trials. These approaches include the development of "large and simple clinical trials" (see Chapter 39), increased attention to the generalizability of patient selection criteria in study design, and conducting the trial in different health systems simultaneously to assess the impact of the therapy in different delivery settings (e.g., using a large HMO as a clinical testing site).

Issues in the Design of Prospective Pharmacoeconomic Studies

We have already addressed some of the general issues in the design and interpretation of pharmacoeconomic studies. Yet, prospective pharmacoeconomic studies, especially within Phase III clinical trials, are often our only opportunity to collect and analyze information on new therapeutic products before decisions are made concerning insurance reimbursement and formulary inclusion for these agents. We now address issues that arise in the design of these studies.

Sample Size

The size required of the sample to identify a meaningful economic difference is frequently problematic. Often those setting up clinical trials focus on the primary clinical question when developing sample-size estimates. They fail to consider the fact that the sample required to address the economic questions posed in the trial may differ from that needed for the primary clinical question. In some cases, the sample size required for the economic analysis is smaller than that required to address the clinical question. More often, however, the opposite is true, in that the variances in cost and patient preference data are larger than those for clinical data. Then one needs to confront the question of whether it is either ethical or practical to prolong the study for longer than need be to establish the drug's clinical effects. Furthermore, in many cases the variances for the pharmacoeconomic data are unknown. Power calculations can be performed, however, to determine the detectable differences between the arms of the study given a fixed patient population and various standard deviations around cost and patient preference data (see Table 41.1). Methods for calculating sample size in economic evaluations have been described elsewhere.[47,48]

Participation Of Patients

Those planning Phase III clinical trials usually are more focused on the clinical results of the trial than they are on the economic results; they would usually like to keep the number of centers needed to complete the trial to a minimum; and they would rather finish the trial sooner than later. Thus, they have a concern that patients might agree to participate in the clinical trial, but not be willing to participate in the economic portion of the trial. In such a case, the investigators often argue that patients should be allowed to participate in the clinical portion of the trial but be excluded from the economic portion of the trial. While self-selection always poses difficulties for trials, it should be clear that this suggestion is particularly worrisome. The economic assessment would end up comparing an estimate of effects from the entire sample with an estimate of costs from a non-random subset of the entire sample, thus allowing substantial bias to enter the analysis. Protocols should allow prospective collection of resource consumption and patient preference data, while sometimes incorporating a second consent to allow access to patients' financial information. This second consent would be important if the primary concern was the possibility of patient selection bias in the analysis of clinical endpoints. However, given the low rates of refusal to the release of financial information, a single consent form

Table 41.1. Study differences detectable given a fixed sample size

Standard deviation (LOS/$)	Detectable difference R^2 for covariables			
	0.0	0.1	0.2	0.3
n = 150/group				
5	2	2	1	1
10	3	3	3	3
20	6	6	6	6
30	10	9	9	8
40	13	12	12	11
50	16	15	14	14
100	32	31	29	27
500	162	153	145	135
1000	324	307	289	271
2500	809	767	723	677
5000	1618	1535	1447	1354
n = 300/group				
5	1	1	1	1
10	2	2	2	2
20	4	4	4	4
30	7	7	6	6
40	9	9	8	8
50	11	11	10	10
100	23	22	20	19
500	114	109	102	96
1000	229	217	205	191
2500	572	543	512	479
5000	1144	1085	1024	957
n = 450/group				
5	1	1	1	1
10	2	2	2	2
20	4	4	3	3
30	6	5	5	5
40	7	7	7	6
50	9	9	8	8
100	19	18	17	16
500	93	89	84	78
1000	187	177	167	156
2500	467	443	418	391
5000	934	886	836	782

Note: Values represent minimum detectable differences between trial arms given the standard deviation reported for the row in the table, and a fixed sample size for each arm of the trial.

should be considered for all trial data. The single consent would avoid the possibility of selection bias in the economic endpoints relative to the clinical endpoints.

Data Collection

In many cases, by the time clinical investigators think to include economic assessments in their trials, they generally have asked for the collection of so much clinical data that it is nearly impossible to ask the data collectors to collect any economic data. Collection of resource consumption data from primary or secondary sources is essential for a prospective economic evaluation of a pharmaceutical therapy. Some data elements, such as patient preference assessments, can only be collected on a prospective basis. Other data elements, such as outpatient physician treatment records for a linked inpatient and outpatient economic evaluation of a therapy, or patient resource consumption information for many European hospitals without centralized billing systems, must be collected prospectively to simplify the data collection process for the study.

While some prospective data collection is required for almost all pharmacoeconomic studies, the amount of data to be collected for the pharmacoeconomic evaluation is still the subject of much debate. There is no definitive means of addressing this issue at present. Phase II studies can be used to develop data that will help determine which resource consumption items are essential for the economic evaluation. Without this opportunity for prior data collection, however, we have to rely upon expert opinion to suggest major resource consumption items that should be monitored within the study. Duplicate data collection strategies (prospective evaluation of resource consumption within the study's case report form with retrospective assessment of resource consumption from hospital bills) can be used to ensure that data collection strategies do not miss critical data elements.

Resources are divided into specific categories for assessment for prospective data collection: inpatient resource use, outpatient resource use, and non-acute-care resource use. Within each of these categories, data can be subdivided into several categories: professional services (physicians, nurses, allied health professionals), hospital setting (intensive care unit, step-down unit, general medical floor), major diagnostic tests, (radiologic tests, laboratory tests, nuclear medicine studies), major surgical procedures (operations and non-operating room procedures), and medications. Sample data collection forms for inpatient and outpatient resource consumption are presented as Figures 41.2 and 41.3. Issues related to data collection for economic studies have been reviewed elsewhere.[49]

Appropriate Comparators

Selection of appropriate treatment alternatives in a clinical study is essential for a useful economic evaluation of a pharmaceutical therapy. This issue is both a clinical and an economic one. Comparators can be the most common alternative therapies for a condition, or the lowest possible cost alternatives, even when not frequently used. However, in pharmacoeconomic studies, treatment comparators may be inappropriately selected as much for their relatively high price as they are for their likely effectiveness. Phase III studies have special limitations in this regard, because agents will be compared against the placebo to assess efficacy rather than against alternative treatments to assess the relative effectiveness of the agent.

Multicenter Evaluations

The primary result of economic evaluations usually is a comparison of average, or pooled, differences in costs and differences in effects among patients who received the therapies under study. It is an open question, however, whether pooled results are representative of the results that would be observed in the individual centers or countries that participated in the study.[29] In some, the therapy may provide good value for the cost, while in others it may provide poor value. Three reasons commonly cited for these differences are differences in practice patterns (i.e., medical service use), differences in absolute and relative prices for medical service use (i.e., unit costs), and differences in underlying morbidity/mortality patterns in different centers and countries.[50–53]

There is a growing literature that addresses the transferability of a study's pooled results to subgroups.[29,50,52] Approaches include evaluation of the homogeneity of different centers' and countries' results,[54,55] use of random effects models to borrow information from the pooled results when deriving center-specific or country-specific estimates, direct statistical inference by use of net monetary benefit regression,[56] and use of decision analysis.

Factors Affecting Resource Consumption

Pharmacoeconomic research holds as a basic assumption the proposition that clinical severity of disease is the sole determinant of resource use by patients. Studies of regional variation, such as those by Perrin *et al.*,[57] highlight the shortcomings of this assumption. This creates a significant challenge for health services research, and for pharmacoeconomics in particular. For example, when a new therapy is introduced to reduce severity of disease as a substitute for physician services that similarly reduce the severity of disease, if physicians either continue to provide the service to maintain their clinical practice or change the characteristics of the patients to whom they provide services (i.e., operate on less severely ill patients), we will not achieve the potential economic advantage afforded by the new therapy.

Economic Data

Analysts generally have access to resource utilization data such as length of stay, monitoring tests performed, and pharmaceutical agents received. When evaluating a therapy

HOSPITAL DISCHARGE FORM		Patient No. __ __ __ __
Principal Investigator _____	Study Hospital _____	Date of Admission _____
		Date of Discharge _____
Source of Admission [ ] Emergency room [ ] Transfer (from _____) [ ] Elective	Discharge Diagnosis 1._____ 2._____	

Unit Type	Number of Days
Intensive Care Unit	
Intensive Care Unit with Mechanical Ventilator	
Bone Marrow Transplant Unit	
Step-Down/Intermediate Care Unit	
General Medical or Surgical Floor	

Pharmacologic Therapy	Total Dose
[ ] Study Drug _____	
[ ] Control _____	
Continuous IV Medication _____	

Types of Procedures	Date

Diagnostic Tests	Number of Tests
MRI	
CT Scan	
Bone Scan	

Figure 41.2. Inpatient resource assessment. This is a sample case report form for prospective assessment of inpatient resource consumption in a pharmacoeconomic study.

from a perspective that requires cost data rather than charge data, however, it may be difficult to translate these resources into costs. For example, does a technology that frees up nursing time reduce costs, or are nursing costs fixed in the sense that the technology is likely to have little or no effect on the hospital payroll? Economists taking the social perspective would argue that real resource consumption has decreased and thus nursing is a variable cost.

OUTPATIENT VISIT RECORD	Patient No. __ __ __ __					
	Duration (in minutes)					
Name of Physician and Location of Visit (e.g., Emergency Room, Outpatient Clinic, Day Surgery, Home, Office)	date ____	date ____	date ____	date ____	date ____	
1.						
2.						
3.						
Name of Nurse Clinician and Location of Visit (e.g., Emergency Room, Outpatient Clinic, Day Surgery, Home, Office)	date ____	date ____	date ____	date ____	date ____	
1.						
2.						

Type of Procedure	Date
1.	
2.	
3.	

Diagnostic Tests	Number of Tests
MRI	
CT Scan	
Bone Scan	
Other	

Other Therapy (medications, etc.)	Date
1.	
2.	
3.	

Figure 41.3. Outpatient resource assessment. This is a sample case report form for prospective assessment of outpatient resource consumption in a pharmacoeconomic study.

Accountants or others taking the hospital perspective might argue that, unless the change affects overall staffing or the need for overtime, it is not a saving. This issue depends in part on the temporal perspective taken by the analyst. In the short term, it is unlikely that nursing savings are recouped; in the long term, however, there probably will be a redirection of services. This analysis may also be confounded by the potential increase in the quality of care that nurses with more time may be able to provide to their patients. In countries that have a shortage of hospital beds, hospital administrators often do not recognize staffing savings from early discharge programs, because the bed will be occupied by a new patient as soon as the old patient is discharged.

Perspective

When perspectives other than the societal perspective are adopted, it is unclear what benefits or outcomes should be counted in the analysis. For example, if a governmental agency's perspective is adopted, in which transfer payments such as pensions are counted as costs, quick deaths at age 65 may be valued more than long, costly deaths at age 75. Independent of whether we should condone this perspective, we must determine whether health status is an independent goal to be included in the analysis.

In summary, due to their focus on efficacy and their use of clinical protocols, economic assessments of pharmaceutical products based upon Phase III clinical trials are not without their problems. However, these issues can be developed in pharmacoeconomic analysis plans and addressed prospectively or through supplemental data collection activities conducted concurrently with the clinical trial.

Measurement and Modeling in Clinical Trials

Previously, we have discussed the development of pharmacoeconomic data throughout the drug development process. However, the types of data available at the end of the trial will depend upon the trial's sample size, duration, and clinical endpoint.

There are two categories of clinical endpoints considered in pharmacoeconomic analysis: intermediate endpoints and final endpoints. An intermediate endpoint is a clinical parameter, such as systolic blood pressure, which varies as a result of therapy. A final endpoint is an outcome variable, such as change in survival, or quality-adjusted survival, that is common to several economic trials, which allows for comparisons of economic data across clinical studies and is of relevance to policy makers.

The use of intermediate endpoints to demonstrate clinical efficacy is common in clinical trials, because it reduces both the cost of the clinical development process and the time needed to demonstrate the efficacy of the therapy. Intermediate endpoints are most appropriate in clinical research if they have been shown to be related to the clinical outcome of interest, as in the following:

- the use of changes in blood cholesterol levels to demonstrate the efficacy of new lipid lowering agents (intermediate endpoint: changes in low-density and high-density lipoprotein levels; final endpoint: changes in myocardial infarction rate and survival; demonstration of the relationship between intermediate and final endpoints: Framingham Heart Study[58]);
- the use of change in blood pressure to demonstrate the efficacy of new antihypertensive agents (intermediate endpoint: changes in systolic and diastolic blood pressure; final endpoint: changes in stroke rates and survival; demonstration of the relationship between intermediate and final endpoints: Framingham Heart Study[59]).

Ideally, a clinical trial would be designed to follow patients throughout their lives, assessing both clinical and economic variables, to allow an incremental assessment of the full impact of the therapy on patients over their lifetimes. Of course, this type of study is almost never performed. Instead, most clinical trials assess patients over a relatively short period of time. Thus, some pharmacoeconomic assessments must utilize data collected from within the clinical trial in combination with an epidemiologic model to project the clinical and economic trial results over an appropriate period of a patient's lifetime.

The importance of this effort is illustrated in the following hypothetical example. A new therapy is under development that reduces the absolute risk of dying from a chronic disease by 50% as measured in a one-year trial. However, this therapy is not curative. A four-year trial was initiated at the same time as the one-year trial. The first-year results were the same in both the four-year trial and the one-year trial. However, there was an increased risk of death for treatment patients in the second and third year of the four-year trial, and by the end of the third year of the trial the survival rate was identical in the treatment and control arms of the four-year trial. While there was a clear benefit to the new therapy in terms of postponing events from the first year of treatment to later years, the economic assessment of the therapy would suggest a greatly reduced treatment benefit from the four-year trial as compared with the one-year trial.

In projecting results of short-term trials over patients' lifetimes, it is typical to present at least two of the many potential projections of lifetime treatment benefit.[60] A one-time effect model assumes that the clinical benefit observed in the trial is the only clinical benefit received by patients. Under this model, after the trial has ended, the conditional probability of disease progression for patients is the same in both arms of the trial. Given that it is unlikely that a therapy will lose all benefits as soon as one stops measuring them, this projection method generally is pessimistic compared to the actual outcome. A continuous-benefit effect model assumes that the clinical benefit observed in the trial is continued throughout the patients' lifetimes. Under this model, the conditional probability of disease progression for treatment and control patients continues at the same rate as that measured in the clinical trial. In contrast to the one-time model, this projection of treatment benefit most likely is optimistic compared to the treatment outcome.

While we and others have developed models as secondary analyses of new therapies,[22,23,60–63] a number of clinical trials have included collection of primary economic data.[25,27,28,64–69] This change has resulted from an increasing awareness of the need for reliable economic data about new therapies at the time when the therapies are being introduced to the market. This impetus has also resulted from issues related to the complexity and cost of developing appropriate economic data for a secondary analysis of a new therapy, and issues related to the potential for bias in the design of economic studies conducted from analysis of secondary data sources.[15,16,70–72] However, as illustrated above, even primary data collection in clinical trials does not eliminate the need for treatment models in the economic analysis of new therapies.

Analysis Plan for Cost Data

Analysis of cost data shares many features with analysis of clinical data. One of the most important is the need to develop an analysis plan before performing the analysis. Table 41.2 identifies a set of tasks that should be addressed in such a plan. The analysis plan should describe the study design (e.g., report on whether the trial is randomized and double-blind; identify the randomization groups; outline the recruitment strategy; describe the criteria for patient evaluation) and any implications the design has for the analysis of costs (e.g., how one will account for recruiting strategies such as rolling admission and a fixed stopping date).

Table 41.2. Steps in an economic analysis plan

 (1) Study design/summary
 (2) Study hypothesis/objectives
 (3) Definition of endpoints
 (4) Covariates
 (5) Prespecification of time periods of interest
 (6) Statistical methods
 (7) Types of analyses
 (8) Hypothesis tests
 (9) Interim analyses
(10) Multiple testing issues
(11) Subgroup analyses
(12) Power/sample size calculations

The analysis plan should also specify the hypothesis and objectives of the study, define the primary and secondary endpoints, and describe how the endpoints will be constructed (e.g., multiplying resource counts measured in the trial times a set of unit costs measured outside the trial). In addition, the analysis plan should identify the potential covariables that will be used in the analysis and specify the time periods of interest (e.g., costs and clinical outcomes at 6 months might be the primary outcome, while costs and clinical outcomes at 12 months might be a secondary outcome).

Also, the analysis plan should identify the statistical methods that will be used and how hypotheses will be tested (e.g., a p-value cutoff or a confidence interval for the difference that excludes 0). Further, the plan should prespecify whether interim analyses are planned, indicate how issues of multiple testing will be addressed, and predefine any subgroup analyses that will be conducted. Finally, the analysis plan should include the results of power and sample size calculations.

If there are separate analysis plans for the clinical and economic evaluations, efforts should be made to make them as consistent as possible (e.g., shared use of an intention-to-treat analysis, shared use of statistical tests for variables used commonly by both analyses, etc.). At the same time, the outcomes of the clinical and economic studies can differ (e.g., the primary outcome of the clinical evaluation might focus on event-free survival while the primary outcome of the economic evaluation might focus on quality-adjusted survival). Thus, the two plans need not be identical.

The analysis plan should also indicate the level of blinding that will be imposed on the analyst. Most, if not all, analytic decisions should be made while the analyst is blinded to the treatment groups (i.e., fully blinded rather than being simply blinded to treatment A versus treatment B). Blinding is particularly important when investigators have not precisely specified the models that will be estimated, but instead rely on the structure of the data to help make decisions about these issues.

Methods for Analysis of Costs

When one analyzes cost data derived from randomized trials, one should report means of costs for the groups under study as well as the difference in the means, measures of variability and precision, such as the standard deviation and quantiles of costs (particularly if the data are skewed), and an indication of whether or not the costs are likely to be meaningfully different from each other in economic terms.

Traditionally, the determination of a difference in costs between the groups has been made using Student's t-tests or analysis of variance (ANOVA) (univariate analysis) and ordinary least squares regression (multivariable analysis). The recent proposal of the generalized linear model promises to improve the predictive power of multivariable analyses.

Univariate Analysis A basic assumption underlying t-tests and ANOVA (which are parametric tests) is that cost data are normally distributed. Given that the distribution of these data often violates this assumption, a number of analysts have begun using nonparametric tests, such as the Wilcoxon rank-sum test (a test of median costs) and the Kolmogorov–Smirnov test (a test for differences in cost distributions), which make no assumptions about the underlying distribution of costs. The principal problem with these nonparametric approaches is that statistical conclusions about the mean need not translate into statistical conclusions about the median (e.g., the means could differ yet the medians could be identical), nor do conclusions about the median necessarily translate into conclusions about the mean. Similar difficulties arise when—to avoid the problems of nonnormal distribution—one analyzes cost data that have been transformed to be more normal in their distribution (e.g., the log transformation of the square root of costs). Rather, if one is concerned about nonnormal distribution, one should use statistical procedures that do not depend on the assumption of normal distribution of costs (e.g., nonparametric tests of means).

Table 41.3 shows the results of the univariate analysis of hospital costs measured among men receiving vehicle and an investigational medication for the treatment of aneurysmal subarachnoid hemorrhage.[73] The mean cost for patients receiving vehicle was $20 287 (SD, $22 542); the mean cost for patients receiving the investigational medication was $25 185 (SD, $22 619). The distribution (as seen from the quantiles reported in Table 41.3, which shows the distribution of costs for the two groups) is skewed. For example, the difference between the 25th and 50th percentiles is approximately $4500 for the two treatment groups, but is approximately $10 000 between the 50th and 75th percentiles. Of note, from the 5th to the 75th percentile, there was approximately a $5000 difference between the two treatment groups. By the 95th percentile, the costs in the two groups were similar. These distributions provide evidence that the costs differ between the two treatment groups.

The parametric and nonparametric statistical tests, however, yielded conflicting conclusions about whether or not the cost differences were statistically different from one another. The t-test comparing mean costs between the groups indicated a nonsignificant difference ($p=0.15$), whereas the t-test comparing the mean log of costs and both of the nonparametric statistical tests indicated they differed ($p<0.02$). In this case, one might conclude that the difference in the medians between groups is statistically significant, whereas the difference in the means between groups is not. Similarly conflicting conclusions about the statistical significance of observed differences in costs have been reported in other studies.[74] Although each of these statistical tests is informative, given that the important outcome for the analysis of the value for the cost of the new therapy (e.g., the cost-effectiveness ratio) is the difference in mean costs, the statistical test of differences in means (e.g., t-test) should be used for inferences about this outcome. Measuring the correct parameter should take precedence over threats to the efficiency of the way that parameter is measured.

Multivariable Analysis Regression analysis often is used to assess differences in costs, in part because the sample size needed to detect economic differences may be larger than the sample needed to detect clinical differences (i.e., to overcome power problems). Traditionally, ordinary least squares regression has been used to predict costs (or their log) as a function of the treatment group while controlling for covariables such as disease severity, costs prior to randomization, etc. However, use of the log of costs as the outcome variable simply to avoid statistical problems posed by untransformed costs leaves one with the problem that we are not interested in this outcome itself; rather we are interested in the difference in untransformed costs. In addition, the retransformation of the predicted difference in the log of costs into an estimate of the predicted difference in costs is not trivial.[75,76] A generalized linear model framework has been proposed to maintain the log distribution and overcome issues related to retransformation.[77]

Table 41.3. Hospital costs of tirilazad mesylate for subarachnoid hemorrhage in men

Variable	Vehicle	Tirilazad, 6 mg/kg per day
Cost ($)	20 287	25 185
Standard deviation	(22 542)	(22 619)
Distribution		
5%	4 506	10 490
25%	9 691	13 765
50%	13 773	18 834
75%	23 044	31 069
95%	53 728	51 771
Comparison of differences		
t-test	0.15	
t-test (log of costs)	0.02	
Wilcoxon rank-sum	0.001	
Kolmogorov–Smirnov	0.001	

While univariate t-tests and ANOVAs assume the normal distribution of cost data, ordinary least squares regression assumes that the error terms from the prediction of costs are normally distributed. Because of the potential violation of this assumption, however, a number of alternative multivariable methods have recently been proposed for analyzing costs. In addition to the generalized linear model mentioned above, these methods include nonparametric hazards models,[78–82] parametric failure-time models,[78] Cox semiparametric regression,[83] and joint distributions of survival and cost.[84] The relative merits of several of these methods have been compared by Lipscomb and colleagues[85] and by Manning and Mullahy;[86] however, there is little conclusive evidence regarding which model is best in a given analytic circumstance.

Table 41.4 shows selected results of an ordinary least squares regression predicting hospital costs measured among men receiving vehicle and the investigational medication for the treatment of aneurysmal subarachnoid hemorrhage. On average, costs among those receiving the investigational medication were $6058 higher than costs among patients receiving vehicle ($p = 0.03$). Increasing levels in the neurograde of subarachnoid hemorrhage upon entry to the study (grades of subarachnoid hemorrhage range from I to V, with V being the most severe) were generally associated with increasing costs; the reduction in costs among those in grade V was due principally to the large number of patients in this category who died in the hospital. Other predictors of hospital costs included the additional days between onset of subarachnoid hemorrhage and

Table 41.4 Selected coefficients and p values for the hospital cost regressions for men receiving tirilazad for subarachnoid hemorrhage

	Coefficient	p
Intercept	1747	0.90
Randomization group[a]		0.05
6 mg/kg per day	6058	
2 mg/kg per day	−100	
0.6 mg/kg per day	−247	
Neurograde of subarachnoid hemorrhage		0.0001
Grade II	3950	
Grade III	3904	
Grade IV	9132	
Grade V	5406	

[a] 6 mg/kg/day versus vehicle, 2 mg/kg/day, and 0.6 mg/kg/day, $p = 0.03$, 0.03, and 0.02, respectively; no other comparisons statistically significant.

randomization into the trial (+), age (+), and country (+/−) (data not shown).[73]

Uncertainty in Economic Assessment

There are a number of sources of uncertainty surrounding the results of economic assessments. One source relates to sampling error (stochastic uncertainty). The point estimates are the result of a single sample from a population. If we ran the experiment many times, we would expect the point estimates to vary. One approach to addressing this uncertainty is to construct confidence intervals both for the separate estimates of costs and effects as well as for the resulting cost-effectiveness ratio. A substantial literature has developed related to construction of confidence intervals for cost-effectiveness ratios.[87–90]

One of the most dependably accurate methods for deriving 95% confidence intervals for cost-effectiveness ratios is the nonparametric bootstrap method.[91] In this method, one re-samples from the study sample and computes cost-effectiveness ratios in each of the multiple samples. To do so, one (i) draws a sample of size n with replacement from the empiric distribution and uses it to compute a cost-effectiveness ratio; (ii) repeats this sampling and calculation of the ratio (by convention, at least 1000 times for confidence intervals); (iii) orders the repeated estimates of the ratio from lowest (best) to highest (worst); and (iv) identifies a 95% confidence interval from this rank-ordered distribution. The percentile method is one of the simplest means of identifying a confidence interval, but it may not be as accurate as other methods. When using 1000 repeated estimates, the percentile method uses the 26th and 975th ranked cost-effectiveness ratios to define the confidence interval.[92]

In the multivariable regression analysis above, we estimated that therapy with the investigational medication added $6058 to the cost of hospitalization (95% CI, $693 to $11 423). The results of a logistic regression predicting death indicated that the investigational medication yielded a difference in the predicted probability of death of 0.225.[73] The cost per death averted was $26 924 ($6058/0.225). The results of the bootstrap analysis indicated that the 95% CI for the cost-effectiveness ratio ranged from $4300 to $54 600.[76] Interpreting the results of the bootstrap in a Bayesian sense, evaluating stochastic uncertainty alone, there is a 96% chance that the ratio is below $50 000 per death averted.

In addition to addressing stochastic uncertainty, one may want to address uncertainty related to parameters measured without variation (e.g., unit cost estimates, discount rates, etc.), whether or not the results are generalizable to settings other than those studied in the trial, and, for chronic therapies, whether the cost-effectiveness ratio observed within the trial is likely to be representative of the ratio that would have been observed if the trial had been conducted for a longer period. These sources of uncertainty are often addressed using sensitivity analysis.

CURRENTLY AVAILABLE SOLUTIONS

The previous sections of this chapter dealt with the principles of clinical economics and methodological issues surrounding the economic analysis of pharmaceutical products. This section presents a set of case studies that illustrate the practical application of these methods to the evaluation of pharmaceuticals. The following cases illustrate cost-effectiveness analyses of valsartan for patients with chronic heart failure, tirilazad mesylate for aneurysmal subarachnoid hemorrhage, and high-dose chemotherapy plus autologous stem cell transplantation for patients with metastatic breast cancer.

MULTINATIONAL ECONOMIC EVALUATION OF VALSARTAN IN PATIENTS WITH CHRONIC HEART FAILURE

In this study, data on resource use and direct medical costs were analyzed to assess the economic impact of an angiotensin receptor blocker, valsartan, in combination with prescribed therapy for patients with New York Heart Association class II to IV heart failure.[27,93] Patients who enrolled in this clinical trial were receiving a standard regimen of medication for heart failure (e.g., angiotensin-converting enzyme (ACE) inhibitors) and were randomized to receive 160 mg of valsartan or placebo twice daily. A total of 5010 patients in 16 countries were enrolled in the trial. The clinical investigators found no differences in mortality; however, the valsartan group had a lower risk of experiencing the combined mortality–morbidity endpoint (i.e., death, hospitalization for heart failure, cardiac arrest with resuscitation, or receipt of intravenous inotropic or vasodilator drugs). Most of the difference was attributable to a lower risk of first hospitalization for heart failure among patients receiving valsartan. Economic data were collected prospectively as part of the clinical trial.

Resource use data were collected in a case report form at regular trial visits every 2 weeks for 2 months, at 4 months and 6 months, and then every 3 months. Unit costs were collected for each of the resource categories assessed (hospitalizations, outpatient visits, and medications). For US patients, the cost estimates for hospital resources and outpatient visits were based on 1999 Medicare reimbursement

rates. Unit costs for medications for all countries were derived from an international drug pricing database. For patients in countries outside of the United States, local health economists in each country provided mean cost estimates of outpatient and hospital care for discharge diagnoses, including heart failure, acute myocardial infarction, and several others. In most cases, these unit cost estimates were based on national fee schedules or hospital accounting systems. Cost estimates were converted to US dollars using purchasing power parties from the Organization for Economic Cooperation and Development. Costs were reported in 1999 US dollars.

To assign costs to hospitalizations for which the diagnosis was not included in the cost survey, unit costs for individual countries were imputed using diagnosis related group (DRG) weights from the US Centers for Medicare and Medicaid Services and the cost estimates provided for hospitalizations due to heart failure. At that point, country-level costs were assigned to individual hospital events and adjusted for differences in length of stay. Daily medication costs were assigned to patients based on a mean daily dose indicated for patients with heart failure and on the duration for which the patient was on the medication.

The results of the resource use analysis indicate that half of the patients in each group were hospitalized at least once during the trial; however, patients in the valsartan group were 13.9% less likely than patients in the placebo group to have a heart failure hospitalization. In addition, patients in the valsartan group spent less time in hospital than did patients in the placebo group.

The results of the cost analysis indicate that the mean cost of a hospitalization for heart failure was $423 less for patients in the valsartan group, compared to patients in the placebo group. However, much of the savings was offset by higher costs for non-heart-failure hospitalizations among patients in the valsartan group, yielding a nonsignificant decrease in inpatient costs of $193 for patients in the valsartan group. The difference in outpatient costs also was nonsignificant. Overall within-trial costs, including the cost of valsartan, were $545 higher for patients in the valsartan group.

In exploratory subgroup analyses, the investigators found that costs were higher for patients aged 65 years and older, and the difference in costs between treatment groups was greater among older patients. Also, costs varied according to the heart failure medications patients were taking at baseline. Patients receiving valsartan and who were not taking an ACE inhibitor at baseline had lower morbidity and mortality and $929 lower costs compared to their counterparts receiving placebo, even after including the cost of valsartan. Thus, valsartan was the dominant strategy in this subgroup of patients. However, patients receiving valsartan and who had both an ACE inhibitor and a β-blocker at baseline had lower survival and higher costs. Thus, valsartan was the dominated strategy in this subgroup. Analysis of the subgroup of patients receiving valsartan and who had an ACE inhibitor at baseline was inconclusive.

The authors conclude that patients receiving valsartan experienced clinical benefit at a mean incremental cost of $285 per year. In patients who were not taking an ACE inhibitor at baseline, valsartan was the dominant strategy.

ECONOMIC ANALYSIS OF TIRILAZAD MESYLATE FOR ANEURYSMAL SUBARACHNOID HEMORRHAGE

The investigators undertook a cost-effectiveness analysis on the use of tirilazad mesylate, a potential free-radical scavenger and lipid peroxidation inhibitor, for the treatment of aneurysmal subarachnoid hemorrhage in a randomized, double-blind, placebo-controlled Phase III clinical trial.[73] A sample of 1023 patients from nine European countries, Australia, and New Zealand were randomized to receive one of four treatments: vehicle or tirilazad 0.6, 2.0, or 6 mg/kg of body weight per day for eight to ten days. All treatments were administered within 48 hours of the occurrence of a subarachnoid hemorrhage and ceased ten days after the initial hemorrhagic event. All patients received nimodipine treatment concomitantly.

Clinical and economic outcomes at three months and hospital costs were estimated using data from 1019 of the 1023 patients enrolled in the study. Death during the three months after randomization was the clinical outcome. The primary clinical outcome was occurrence of vasospasm, and the secondary outcome was Glasgow Outcome Scale (GOS) score and mortality. The authors evaluated the costs of hospitalizations during the trial as well as patients' residence and employment status three months after randomization. Cost estimates were based on resource use and unit costs for resources used.

Data on the length of stay, number of imaging studies, number and types of surgical procedures, and medication use were collected prospectively. Information on the site of care in the hospital was obtained retrospectively but was collected before the study results were known and while the investigators were blinded to the treatment groups. Patient status at three months was evaluated prospectively by assessing daily residence costs at three months for patients living at home with supervision or dependent on others as well as for those in minimal care, skilled care, or long-term rehabilitation institutions. The daily employment value at

three months was also assessed for homemakers and for full- and part-time workers.

Local health economists from six countries collected unit costs of inpatient resource utilization. The averages of the unit costs from the six countries were used for the five other countries. The $137.50 cost per 150 mg of tirilazad was based on a price set by the manufacturer. The authors determined values for employment using wage and salary data from the participating countries. The unit costs from other countries were converted into 1993 US dollars. The authors state that during the sensitivity analysis, deaths averted were translated into gains in life expectancy both with and without adjustments for quality-of-life.

The results of the study indicate that patients were similar in all groups except in the proportions having right-to-left and left-to-right shifts of the midline structures and those having generalized, as opposed to localized, brain swelling. Total length of hospital stay, number of days between the onset of subarachnoid hemorrhage and randomization, number of days the patient was intubated, characteristics of the hemorrhage, the country in which patients received care, and mortality of the patients were all predictors of stay by unit type.

Results of the economic analysis showed that the average hospital cost was $20 341 (SD, ±$17 239) for the whole sample. The average hospital cost for women ($19 569 ± $15 156) was less than the cost among men ($21 835 ± $20 743). The results also indicated that the majority of the cost was attributable to the length of stay and the greatest difference in cost was due to the costs of tirilazad. The cost analysis at three months showed that the largest difference in employment value was observed between men who received tirilazad 6 mg/kg per day and those who received vehicle ($9.20 additional earnings per day). In addition, the results showed that the largest difference in residence cost was also between these two groups ($15.80 additional residence cost per day for the 6 mg/kg group). However, none of these differences was statistically significant. One significant finding of this study was that those who received tirilazad 6 mg/kg per day had a significant reduction in the probability of death in the whole sample ($p = 0.002$) and in men ($p = 0.0001$). There was no significant difference in the probability of death among women between the group who received tirilazad 6 mg/kg per day and those who received vehicle. When costs and outcomes were compared, the results showed that in both the entire sample and in men, tirilazad 6 mg/kg per day was associated with improved survival compared to vehicle, but also with increased hospital costs. The cost per death averted was $29 615 for the sample as a whole and $26 924 for men. There were no significant differences in costs or probability of survival of women in either the tirilazad 6 mg/kg per day or vehicle group.

The results were subjected to a sensitivity analysis, showing that the cost-effectiveness ratio (95% confidence interval) between those in the entire sample who received tirilazad 6 mg/kg per day and vehicle was $9189 per death averted due to tirilazad, adding hospital costs and mortality. The cost-effectiveness ratios among men (95% CI) ranged from $4300 to $54 600 per death averted. The sensitivity analysis also showed that in 68.8% of women, 6 mg/kg per day of tirilazad resulted in an increase in hospital costs and survival. Five percent experienced decreased costs and survival, 11.6% had decreased costs and increased survival, and 14.3% had increased costs and decreased survival. Another finding was that in the entire sample, the ratios of cost per year of life saved and cost per quality-adjusted year of life saved fell below $50 000 if survivors live on average 0.6 and 0.8 years respectively. For men, these ratios fell below $50 000 if survivors at the end of the trial live an average of 1.1 and 2.4 years. Among men, the ratio of cost per year of life saved did not fall below $27 500. Also, the ratio of the cost per quality-adjusted year of life saved did not fall under $36 400.

The economic analysis of this study showed that treatment with tirilazad mesylate is associated with a significant increase in survival and increase in the cost of care. The results also showed that the ratios of cost per death averted, cost per year of life saved, and cost per quality-adjusted year of life saved are favorable when compared to other interventions.

ECONOMIC EVALUATION OF HIGH-DOSE CHEMOTHERAPY PLUS AUTOLOGOUS STEM CELL TRANSPLANTATION FOR METASTATIC BREAST CANCER

The Philadelphia Bone Marrow Transplant Group conducted a clinical trial to compare survival associated with high-dose chemotherapy plus autologous hematopoietic stem cell transplantation versus conventional-dose chemotherapy in women with metastatic breast cancer. Data on resource use and costs were collected as secondary endpoints of the study. Because the clinical trial found no significant differences in survival between the two treatment groups, the economic evaluation[94] would provide important additional information about the two therapies.

Because resource use data were not captured explicitly in the clinical case report form, the investigators abstracted the clinical trial records and oncology department flow sheets retrospectively to document the resources used by each patient. The abstraction process captured information about

hospitalizations, medical procedures, medications, tests, and inpatient and outpatient physician services for each patient from the time of randomization through death or end of follow-up. Each patient's course of treatment and resource use was analyzed in four phases—randomization, treatment, progression, and remission. (The treatment phase for patients in the transplantation group was further divided into an inpatient phase and postdischarge phase.) Based on these clinical phases, the investigators grouped the patients into one of three clinical "trajectories." Patients in trajectory 1 went through all four clinical phases before the end of the study. Patients in trajectory 2 went through randomization, treatment, and immediately to progression. Patients in trajectory 3 went through randomization, treatment, and immediately to remission until the end of the study.

Daily costs for inpatient care in both treatment groups were assigned according to each patient's length of stay. They were estimated using data from the cost accounting system of an academic medical center. Cost estimates for transplantation hospitalizations were based on the mean daily cost of hospitalization for stem cell transplantation. Cost estimates for other hospitalizations were based on the mean daily cost of a hospitalization for neutropenic fever. The investigators used Medicare reimbursement rates to estimate costs for inpatient and outpatient laboratory tests and physician fees. They estimated medication costs by referring to each drug's average wholesale price. The study medication cost estimates were added to the estimate of inpatient costs for patients undergoing transplantation, and they were added to the estimate of outpatient costs for patients in the conventional-dose chemotherapy group. When a patient was missing costs for any month in the study, the investigators imputed the costs using median costs for each clinical phase, clinical trajectory, and treatment group.

The results of the economic analysis showed that patients in the transplantation group had significantly more inpatient days (28.6 versus 17.8; $p = 0.004$) and significantly greater mean length of stay per hospitalization (21.9 days versus 15.2 days; $p = 0.02$) than did patients in the conventional-dose chemotherapy group. Patients in the transplantation group also had more procedures per outpatient visit. Mean total costs were higher for patients in the transplantation group ($84 055 versus $28 169), for a mean cost difference of $55 886 (95% CI, $47 298 to $63 666). Most of the difference was attributable to the $52 448 difference in inpatient care. The investigators also found differences by clinical trajectory, and these differences were not consistent between treatment strategies. For example, outpatient costs for patients in trajectory 3 who were randomized to conventional-dose chemotherapy were much higher than outpatient costs for patients in trajectories 1 and 2. Because patients in trajectory 3 completed more cycles of treatment, they spent more time in the treatment phase and accrued greater costs associated with administering therapy.

In sensitivity analysis, the investigators confirmed the robustness of their findings by varying the discount rate, the hospital costs, and the number of cycles of paclitaxel and docetaxel that patients were assumed to have received. Varying the discount rate had little effect on the mean difference in cost between treatment groups. Increasing and decreasing the hospital costs by 50% yielded mean differences in total costs ranging from $36 528 to $75 531. Increasing the number of cycles of paclitaxel and docetaxel caused a greater increase in costs for patients in the conventional-dose chemotherapy group, because more patients in this group were treated with these drugs.

The authors concluded that high-dose chemotherapy plus stem-cell transplantation for women with metastatic breast cancer was more costly and resulted in greater morbidity with no improvement in survival. By studying resource use and estimating costs, the authors were able to quantify the economic burden associated with the two treatments and to provide information about the clinical trajectories of patients with metastatic breast cancer.

THE FUTURE

The emergence of cost as a criterion for the evaluation of pharmaceutical products requires the continued development and application of research methods to guide decision makers. Patients, and physicians acting on their behalf, are principally concerned about the effectiveness and safety of drugs. However, as patients, payers, and society become more concerned about the cost of medical care, the clinical contribution of pharmaceutical agents will be weighed against their costs and compared with the next best alternative. As third-party payers increasingly cover drug costs, they will be concerned with their expenditures on pharmaceuticals and the value obtained for the money spent. Hospitals and other providers of care, operating under increasingly constrained budgets, will increase their assessments of pharmaceutical expenditures.

The naive decision maker might weigh drugs according to their purchase price alone. This paradigm ignores two essential elements in choosing pharmaceuticals. First, in identifying a drug's cost, its purchase price is only part of its real economic impact. The costs of preparation and delivery, as well as the cost of monitoring for and treating adverse events and side effects, are unavoidable elements of the cost of treating patients.

Second, a full analysis should go beyond the identification of cost. Only if the safety and effectiveness of two pharmaceutical agents are equivalent will cost alone determine the choice of therapy. Cost-effectiveness analysis requires that cost be weighed against effectiveness and that when two or more alternatives are being compared, the additional cost per additional unit of effectiveness be measured. Beyond these considerations of cost identification and cost-effectiveness, a full economic analysis will also assess the net value, or utility, of the drug's clinical contribution.

This is a challenging period for the field of clinical economics. Many of the earlier methodologic challenges of the field have been addressed, and researchers have gained experience in implementing economic evaluations in a multitude of settings. This experience has raised new questions for those interested in the development of new clinical therapies and in the application of economic data to the decision making process.

With the increasing importance of multinational clinical trials in the clinical development process, many of the problems facing researchers today involve the conduct of economic evaluations in multinational settings. Foremost among these is the problem of generalizability.[29] There is little consensus among experts as to whether the findings of multinational clinical trials are more generalizable than findings from trials conducted in single countries. This question is even more problematic for multinational economic evaluations, because the findings of economic evaluations reflect complex interactions between biology, epidemiology, practice patterns, and costs that differ from country to country.

As physicians are asked simultaneously to represent their patients' interests while being asked to deliver clinical services with parsimony, and as reimbursement for medical services becomes more centralized in the United States and other countries, decision makers must turn for assistance to collaborative efforts of epidemiologists and economists in the assessment of new therapeutic agents. Through a merger of epidemiology and economics,[95] better information can be provided to the greatest number of decision makers, and limited resources can be used most effectively for the health of the public.

ACKNOWLEDGMENTS

The authors dedicate this chapter to John M. Eisenberg, MD (1946–2002), mentor, friend, and fellow author in previous editions of this work.

The authors also acknowledge Harris Koffer, Pharm D, vice president of Quest Diagnostics, Inc., and Shelby D. Reed, PhD, assistant research professor of medicine at Duke University, for their contributions to this chapter.

REFERENCES

1. Bombardier C, Eisenberg J. Looking into the crystal ball: can we estimate the lifetime cost of rheumatoid arthritis? *J Rheumatol* 1985; **12**: 201–4.

2. Drummond MF. *Principles of Economic Appraisal in Health Care*. New York: Oxford University Press, 1980.

3. Drummond MF, Stoddart GL, Torrance GW. *Methods for the Evaluation of Health Care Programs*. New York: Oxford Medical Publications, 1987.

4. Drummond MF, Davies L. Economic analysis alongside clinical trials: revisiting the methodological issues. *Int J Technol Assess Health Care* 1991; **7**: 561–73.

5. Detsky AS, Naglie IG. A clinician's guide to cost effectiveness analysis. *Ann Intern Med* 1990; **113**: 147–54.

6. Eddy DM. Cost-effectiveness analysis: is it up to the task? *JAMA* 1992; **267**: 3342–8.

7. Eisenberg JM, Koffer H, Finkler SA. Economic analysis of a new drug: potential savings in hospital operating costs from the use of a once-daily regimen of a parenteral cephalosporin. *Rev Infect Dis* 1984; **6**: S909.

8. Eisenberg JM, Koffer H, Glick HA, Connell ML, Loss LE, Talbot GH *et al*. What is the cost of nephrotoxicity associated with aminoglycosides? *Ann Intern Med* 1987; **107**: 900–9.

9. Eisenberg JM. Clinical economics: a guide to the economic analysis of clinical practices. *JAMA* 1989; **262**: 2879–86.

10. Glick HA, Connell ML, Koffer H, Eisenberg JM, Kelley MA. The economic impact of prophylaxis against venous thromboembolism in patients undergoing total hip replacement. *Clin Res* 1988; **36**: A337.

11. Warner KE, Luce BR. *Cost Benefit and Cost Effectiveness Analysis in Health Care: Principles, Practice and Potential*. Ann Arbor, MI: Health Administration Press, 1982.

12. Weinstein MC. Economic assessments of medical practices and technologies. *Med Decis Making* 1981; **1**: 309.

13. Weinstein MC, Stason WB. Cost-effectiveness of coronary artery bypass surgery. *Circulation* 1982; **66**: 56–68.

14. Weinstein MC. Principles of cost-effective resource allocation in health care organizations. *Int J Technol Assess Health Care* 1990; **6**: 93–103.

15. Glennie JL, Torrance GW, Baladi JF, Berka C, Hubbard E, Menon D *et al*. The revised Canadian Guidelines for the Economic Evaluation of Pharmaceuticals. *Pharmacoeconomics* 1999; **15**: 459–68.

16. Commonwealth Department of Human Services and Health. *Guidelines for the Pharmaceutical Industry on Preparation of Submissions to the Pharmaceutical Benefits Advisory Committee Including Major Submission Involving Economic Analyses*. Canberra, Australia: Australian Government Publishing Service, 1995.

17. Drummond MF. The use of health economic information by reimbursement authorities. *Rheumatology* 2003; **42**(suppl 3): iii60–iii3.

18. Nishimura S, Torrance GW, Ikegami N, Fukuhara S, Drummond M, Schubert F. Information barriers to the implementation of economic evaluations in Japan. *Pharmacoeconomics* 2002; **20**(suppl 2): 9–15.

19. National Institute for Clinical Guidance. *Guidance for Manufacturers and Sponsors*, Technology Appraisals Process Series no. 5. London: National Institute for Clinical Excellence, 2001.

20. Pharmaceutical Management Agency Ltd (PHARMAC). *A Prescription for Pharmacoeconomic Analysis*, version 1, September 24, 1999.

21. Elsinga E, Rutten FF. Economic evaluation in support of national health policy: the case of The Netherlands. *Soc Sci Med* 1997; **45**: 605–20.

22. Schulman KA, Kinosian BP, Jacobson TA, Glick HA, Willian MK, Koffer H *et al*. Reducing high blood cholesterol level with drugs: cost effectiveness of pharmacologic management. *JAMA* 1990; **264**: 3025–33.

23. Schulman KA, Glick HA, Rubin H, Eisenberg JM. Cost effectiveness of HA-1A monoclonal antibody for gram-negative sepsis: prospective economic assessment of a new therapeutic agent. *JAMA* 1991; **226**: 3466–71.

24. Mark DB, Hlatky MA, Califf RM, Naylor CD, Lee KL, Armstrong PW *et al*. Cost effectiveness of thrombolytic therapy with tissue plasminogen activator as compared with streptokinase for acute myocardial infarction. *N Engl J Med* 1995; **332**: 1418–24.

25. Reed SD, Radeva JI, Glendenning GA, Saad F, Schulman KA. Cost-effectiveness of zoledronic acid for the prevention of skeletal complications in patients with prostate cancer. *J Urol* 2004; **171**: 1537–42.

26. Reed SD, Anstrom KJ, Ludmer JA, Glendenning GA, Schulman KA. Cost-effectiveness of imatinib versus interferon-alpha plus low-dose cytarabine for patients with newly diagnosed chronic-phase chronic myeloid leukemia. *Cancer* 2004; **101**: 2574–83.

27. Reed SD, Friedman JY, Velazquez EJ, Gnanasakthy A, Califf RM, Schulman KA. Multinational economic evaluation of valsartan in patients with chronic heart failure: results from the Valsartan Heart Failure Trial (Val-HeFT). *Am Heart J* 2004; **148**: 122–8.

28. Reed SD, Radeva JI, Weinfurt KP, McMurray JJV, Pfeffer MA, Velazquez EJ *et al*. Resource use, costs, and quality of life among patients in the multinational Valsartan in Acute Myocardial Infarction Trial. *Am Heart J* in press.

29. Reed SD, Anstrom KJ, Bakhai A, Briggs AH, Califf RM, Cohen DJ *et al*. Conducting economic evaluations alongside multinational clinical trials: toward a research consensus. *Am Heart J* 2005; **149**: 434–43.

30. Tunis SR, Stryer DB, Clancy CM. Practical clinical trials: increasing the value of clinical research for decision making in clinical and health policy. *JAMA* 2003; **290**: 1624–32.

31. Finkler SA. The distinction between cost and charges. *Ann Intern Med* 1982; **96**: 102–9.

32. Bridges JM, Jacobs P. Obtaining estimates of marginal cost by DRG. *Healthc Financ Manage* 1986; **40**: 40–6.

33. Hsiao WC, Braun P, Becker ER, Becker ER, Yntema D, Verrilli DK *et al*. An overview of the development and refinement of the resource-based relative value scale: the foundation for reform of U.S. physician payment. *Med Care* 1992; **30** (suppl): NS1–12.

34. Granneman TW, Brown RS, Pauly MV. Estimating hospital costs. *J Health Econ* 1986; **5**: 107–27.

35. Reed SD, Friedman JY, Gnanasakthy A, Schulman KA. Comparison of hospital costing methods in an economic evaluation of a multinational clinical trial. *Int J Technol Assess Health Care* 2003; **19**: 396–406.

36. Landefeld JS, Seskin EP. The economic value of life: linking theory to practice. *Am J Public Health* 1982; **72**: 555–65.

37. Rice DP, Hodgson TA. The value of human life revisited. *Am J Public Health* 1982; **72**: 536–8.

38. Thompson MS, Read JL, Liang M. Feasibility of willingness-to-pay measurement in chronic arthritis. *Med Decis Making* 1984; **4**: 195–215.

39. Mishan EJ. *Cost–Benefit Analysis*, 3rd edn. London: George Allen & Unwin, 1992.

40. Shelling TC, Chase SB, eds, The life you save may be your own. In: *Problems in Public Expenditure Analysis*. Washington, DC: The Brookings Institution, 1968.

41. Lynn LA, Schulman KA, Eisenberg JM. The pharmacoeconomics of HIV disease. *Pharmacoeconomics* 1992; **1**: 161–74.

42. Strosberg MA, Wiener JM, Baker R, Fein IA, eds, *Rationing America's Medical Care: The Oregon Plan and Beyond*. Washington, DC: The Brookings Institution, 1992.

43. Sulmasy DP. Physicians, cost-control, and ethics. *Ann Intern Med* 1992; **116**: 920–6.

44. Drummond MF, Stoddart GL. Economic analysis and clinical trials. *Control Clin Trials* 1984; **5**: 115–28.

45. Weinstein MC. Methodologic considerations in planning clinical trials of cost effectiveness of magnetic resonance imaging. *Int J Technol Assess* 1985; **1**: 567–81.

46. Evans WE, McLeod HL. Pharmacogenomics—drug disposition, drug targets, and side effects. *N Engl J Med* 2003; **348**: 538–49.

47. Laska EM, Meisner M, Seigel C. Power and sample size in cost-effectiveness analysis. *Med Decis Making* 1999; **19**: 339–43.

48. Willan AR. Analysis, sample size, and power for estimating incremental net health benefit from clinical trial data. *Control Clin Trials* 2001; **22**: 228–37.

49. Brown M, Glick HA, Harrell F, Herndon J, McCabe M, Moinpour C *et al*. Integrating economic analysis into cancer clinical trials: the National Cancer Institute–American Society of Clinical Oncology Economics workbook. *J Natl Cancer Inst Monogr* 1998; **24**: 1–28.

50. Cook JR, Drummond M, Glick H, Heyse JF. Assessing the appropriateness of combining economic data from multinational clinical trials. *Stat Med* 2003; **22**: 1955–76.

51. Drummond M, Pang F. Transferability of economic evaluation results. In: Drummond M, McGuire A, eds, *Economic Evaluation in Health Care. Merging Theory with Practice*. Oxford: Oxford University Press, 2001; pp. 254–76.

52. Willke RJ, Glick HA, Polsky D, Schulman K. Estimating country-specific cost-effectiveness from multinational clinical trials. *Health Econ* 1998; **7**: 481–93.

53. O'Brien BS. A tale of two (or more) cities: geographic transferability of pharmacoeconomic data. *Am J Manag Care* 1997; **3**: S33–40.

54. Willan AR, Pinto EM, O'Brien BJ *et al*. Country specific cost comparisons from multinational clinical trials using empirical Bayesian shrinkage estimation: the Canadian ASSENT-3 economic analysis. *Health Econ* 2005; **14**: 327–38.

55. Pinto EM, Willan AR, O'Brien BJ. Cost-effectiveness analysis for multinational clinical trials. *Stat Med* 2005, April 1 (online).

56. Hoch JS, Briggs AH, Willan AR. Something old, something new, something borrowed, something blue: a framework for the marriage of health econometrics and cost-effectiveness analysis. *Health Econ* 2002; **11**: 415–30.

57. Perrin JM, Homer CJ, Berwick DM, Woolf AD, Freeman JL, Wennberg JE. Variations in rates of hospitalizations of children in three urban communities. *N Engl J Med* 1989; **320**: 1183–7.

58. Anderson KM, Odell PM, Wilson PW, Kunnel WB. Cardiovascular disease risk profiles. *Am Heart J* 1991; **121**: 293–8.

59. Stokes J 3rd, Kannel WB, Wolf PA, Dagostino RB, Lupples LA. Blood pressure as a risk factor for cardiovascular disease. The Framingham Study—30 years of follow-up. *Hypertension* 1989; **13**(suppl): I13–18.

60. Schulman KA, Lynn LA, Glick HA, Eisenberg JM. Cost effectiveness of low-dose zidovudine therapy for asymptomatic patients with human immunodeficiency virus (HIV) infection. *Ann Intern Med* 1991; **114**: 798–802.

61. Glick H, Heyse JF, Thompson D, Epstein RS, Smith ME, Oster G. A model for evaluating the cost-effectiveness of cholesterol-lowering treatment. *Int J Technol Assess Health Care* 1992; **8**: 719–34.

62. Goldman L, Weinstein MC, Goldman PA, Williams LW. Cost-effectiveness of HMG-CoA reductase inhibition for primary and secondary prevention of coronary heart disease. *JAMA* 1991; **265**: 1145–51.

63. Grover SA, Abrahamowicz M, Joseph L, Brewer C, Coupal L, Suissa S. The benefits of treating hyperlipidemia to prevent coronary heart disease: expected changes in life expectancy and morbidity. *JAMA* 1992; **267**: 816–22.

64. Mark DB, Talley JD, Topol EJ, Bowman L, Lam LC, Anderson KM *et al*. Economic assessment of platelet glycoprotein IIb/IIIa inhibition for prevention of ischemic complications of high-risk coronary angioplasty. EPIC Investigators. *Circulation* 1996; **94**: 629–35.

65. Lincoff AM, Mark DB, Tcheng JE, Califf RM, Bala MV, Anderson KM *et al*. Economic assessment of platelet glycoprotein IIb/IIIa receptor blockade with abciximab and low-dose heparin during percutaneous coronary revascularization: results from the EPILOG randomized trial. Evaluation in PTCA to improve long-term outcome with abciximab GP IIb/IIIa blockade. *Circulation* 2000; **102**: 2923–9.

66. Topol EJ, Mark DB, Lincoff AM, Cohen E, Burton J, Kleiman N *et al*. Outcomes at 1 year and economic implications of platelet glycoprotein IIb/IIIa blockade in patients undergoing coronary stenting: results from a multicentre randomised trial. EPIST-ENT Investigators. Evaluation of platelet IIb/IIIa inhibitor for stenting. *Lancet* 1999; **354**: 2019–24.

67. Drummond MF, Becker DL, Hux M, Chancellor JV, Duprat-Lomon I, Kubin R *et al*. An economic evaluation of sequential i.v./ po moxifloxacin therapy compared to i.v./ po co-amoxiclav with or without clarithromycin in the treatment of community-acquired pneumonia. *Chest* 2003; **124**: 526–35.

68. Lorber MI, Fastenau J, Wilson D, DiCesare J, Hall ML. A prospective economic evaluation of basiliximab (Simulect) therapy following renal transplantation. *Clin Transplant* 2000; **14**: 479–85.

69. Ramsey SD, Moinpour CM, Lovato LC, Crowley JJ, Grevstad P, Presant CA *et al*. Economic analysis of vinorelbine plus cisplatin versus paclitaxel plus carboplatin for advanced non-small-cell lung cancer. *J Natl Cancer Inst* 2002; **94**: 291–7.

70. Adams ME, McCall NT, Gray DT, Orza MJ, Chalmers TC. Economic analysis in randomized control trials. *Med Care* 1992; **30**: 2–243.

71. Hillman AL, Eisenberg JM, Pauly MV, Bloom BS, Glick H, Kinosian B *et al*. Avoiding bias in the conduct and reporting of cost-effectiveness research sponsored by pharmaceutical companies. *N Engl J Med* 1991; **324**: 1362–5.

72. Udvarhelyi IS, Colditz GA, Ri A, Epstein AM. Cost-effectiveness and cost–benefit analyses in the medical literature: are the methods being used correctly? *Ann Intern Med* 1992; **116**: 238–44.

73. Glick H, Willke R, Polsky D, Llana T, Alves WM, Kassell N *et al*. Economic analysis of tirilazad mesylate for aneurysmal subarachnoid hemorrhage: economic evaluation of a phase III clinical trial in Europe and Australia. *Int J Technol Assess Health Care* 1998; **14**: 145–60.

74. Zhou X-H, Melfi CA, Hui SL. Methods for comparison of cost data. *Ann Intern Med* 1997; **127**: 752–6.

75. Manning WG. The logged dependent variable, heteroscedasticity, and the retransformation problem. *J Health Econ* 1998; **17**: 283–95.

76. Duan N. Smearing estimate: a nonparametric retransformation method. *J Am Stat Assoc* 1983; **78**: 605–10.

77. Blough DK, Madden CW, Hornbrook MC. Modeling risk using generalized linear models. *J Health Econ* 1999; **18**: 153–71.

78. Dudley RA, Harrell FE, Smith LR, Mark DB, Califf RM, Pryor DB *et al*. Comparison of analytic models for estimating the effect of clinical factors on the cost of coronary artery bypass graft surgery. *J Clin Epidemiol* 1993; **46**: 261–71.

79. Lin DY, Feuer EJ, Etzioni R, Wax Y. Estimating medical costs from incomplete follow-up data. *Biometrics* 1997; **53**: 113–28.

80. Fenn P, McGuire A, Phillips V, Backhouse M, Jones D. The analysis of censored treatment cost data in economic evaluation. *Med Care* 1995; **33**: 851–61.

81. Fenn P, Mcguire A, Backhouse M, Jones D. Modeling programme costs in economic evaluation. *J Health Economics* 1996; **15**: 115–25.

82. Schulman KA, Buxton M, Glick H, Sculpher M, Guzman G, Kong J *et al*. Results of the economic evaluation of the FIRST study. *Int J Technol Assess Health Care* 1996; **12**: 698–713.

83. Harrell F, Lee K, Mark D. Multivariable prognostic models: issues in developing models, evaluating assumptions and adequacy, and measuring and reducing errors. *Stat Med* 1996; **15**: 361–87.

84. Lancaster T, Intrator O. *Panel data with survival: hospitalization of HIV patients*, Brown University Department of Economics, Working Paper Series, #95–36, 1995.

85. Lipscomb J, Ancukiewicz M, Parmigiani G, Hasselblad V, Samsa G, Matchar DBJ. Predicting the cost of illness: a comparison of alternative models applied to stroke. *Med Decis Making* 1998; **18**: S39–56.

86. Manning WG, Mullahy J. Estimating log models: to transform or not to transform. *J Health Econ* 2000; **20**: 461–94.

87. Heyse J, Cook J. *A New Measure of Cost Effectiveness in Comparative Clinical Economic Trials*. Boston, MA: American Statistical Association, 1992.

88. O'Brien BJ, Drummond MF, Labelle RJ, Willan A. In search of power and significance: issues in the design and analysis of stochastic cost effectiveness studies in health care. *Med Care* 1994; **32**: 150–63.

89. Willan AR, O'Brien BJ. Confidence intervals for cost-effectiveness ratios: an application of Fieller's theorem. *Health Econ* 1996; **5**: 297–305.

90. Chaudhary MA, Stearns SC. Estimating confidence intervals for cost-effectiveness ratios: an example from a randomized trial. *Stat Med* 1996; **15**: 1447–58.

91. Polsky DP, Glick HA, Willke R, Schulman K. Confidence intervals for cost-effectiveness ratios: a comparison of four methods. *Health Econ* 1997; **6**: 243–52.

92. Efron B, Tibshirani RJ. *An Introduction to the Bootstrap*. New York: Chapman & Hall, 1993.

93. Cohn JN, Tognoni G, Valsartan Heart Failure Trial Investigators. A randomized trial of the angiotensin-receptor blocker valsartan in chronic heart failure. *N Engl J Med* 2001; **345**: 1667–75.

94. Schulman KA, Stadtmauer EA, Reed SD, Glick HA, Goldstein LJ, Pines JM *et al*. Economic analysis of conventional-dose chemotherapy compared with high-dose chemotherapy plus autologous hematopoietic stem-cell transplantation for metastatic breast cancer. *Bone Marrow Transplant* 2003; **31**: 205–10.

95. Eisenberg JM. From clinical epidemiology to clinical economics. *J Gen Intern Med* 1988; **3**: 299–300.

42

Using Quality-of-Life Measurements in Pharmacoepidemiologic Research

HOLGER SCHÜNEMANN[1], GORDON H. GUYATT[2,3] and ROMAN JAESCHKE[3]

[1] Department of Medicine, University at Buffalo, State University of New York, USA, Department of Clinical Epidemiology and Biostatistics, McMaster University, Hamilton, Ontario, Canada and Division of Clinical Research Development and Information Translation/INFORMA, Italian National Cancer Institute, Rome, Italy; [2] Department of Medicine and Department of Clinical Epidemiology and Biostatistics, McMaster University, Hamilton, Ontario, Canada; [3] Department of Medicine, St. Joseph's Hospital, and Department of Medicine, McMaster University, Hamilton, Ontario, Canada.

INTRODUCTION

One may judge the impact of drug interventions by examining a variety of outcomes. In some situations, the most compelling evidence of drug efficacy may be found as a reduction in mortality (β-blockers after myocardial infarction), rate of hospitalization (neuroleptic agents for schizophrenia), rate of disease occurrence (antihypertensives for strokes), or rate of disease recurrence (chemotherapy after surgical cancer treatment). Alternatively, clinicians frequently rely on direct physiological or biochemical measures of the severity of a disease process and the way drugs influence these measures—for example, left ventricular ejection fraction in congestive heart failure, spirometry in chronic airflow limitation, or glycosylated hemoglobin level in diabetes mellitus.

However, clinical investigators have recognized that there are other important aspects of the usefulness of the interventions which these epidemiologic, physiologic, or biochemical outcomes do not address, and are typically patient-reported outcomes. These areas encompass the ability to function normally; to be free of pain and physical, psychological, and social limitations or dysfunction; and to be free from iatrogenic problems associated with treatment. On occasion, the conclusions reached when evaluating different outcomes may differ: physiologic measurements may change without people feeling better,[1,2] a drug may ameliorate symptoms without a measurable change in physiologic function, or life prolongation may be achieved at the expense of unacceptable pain and suffering.[3] The recognition of these patient-important (versus disease-oriented) and patient-reported areas of well-being led to the introduction of a technical term: health-related quality-of-life (HRQL).

The term "quality-of-life," as it is often used, lacks focus and precision and, because it is an abstract concept, its

Pharmacoepidemiology, Fourth Edition   Edited by B.L. Strom

definition has led to much debate. Since the patient's subjective well-being is influenced by many factors unrelated to the disease process or treatment (e.g., education, income, quality of the environment, etc.), investigators have adopted the narrower term, HRQL. Some definitions of HRQL reflect the evaluation of patients' overall well-being, several broad domains (physiologic, functional, psychological, and social status), and subcomponents of each domain—for example, pain, sleep, activities of daily living, and sexual function within physical and functional domains.

It follows that HRQL is a multifactorial concept that, from the patient's perspective, represents the final common pathway of all the physiological, psychological, and social influences of the therapeutic process.[4] It follows also that, when assessing the impact of a drug on a patient's HRQL, one may be interested in describing the patient's status (or changes in the patient status) on a whole variety of domains, and that different strategies and instruments are required to explore separate domains.

Definitions of HRQL, both theoretical and practical, remain controversial. Most HRQL measurement instruments focus largely on how patients are functioning, e.g., their ability to care for themselves and carry out their usual roles in life. While this pragmatic view of HRQL has gained ascendancy, there remain those who argue that, unless you are tapping into individual patients' own values and preferences of health states, you may be measuring health status but you are not measuring HRQL.[5] Consider, for instance, a woman with quadriplegia who, despite her limitations, is very happy and fulfilled and values her life highly (more, for instance, than most people, or more than she did before she suffered quadriplegia). On most domains of most HRQL instruments, this woman's results would suggest a poor HRQL, despite the high value she places on her health state. Investigators and those interpreting the results of HRQL measure should be aware of the varying emphasis put on individual patient values and preferences in the different types of instruments.[6]

CLINICAL PROBLEMS TO BE ADDRESSED BY PHARMACOEPIDEMIOLOGIC RESEARCH

HRQL effects may be pertinent in investigating and documenting both beneficial as well as harmful aspects of drug action. The knowledge of these drug effects may be important, not only to the regulatory agencies and physicians prescribing the drugs, but to the people who agree to take the medication and live with both its beneficial actions and detrimental side effects. Investigators must therefore recognize the clinical situations where a drug may have an important effect on HRQL. This requires careful examination of data available from earlier phases of drug testing and, until now, has usually been performed in the latter stages of Phase III testing. For example, Croog and colleagues studied the effect of three established antihypertensive drugs—captopril, methyldopa, and propranolol—on quality-of-life, long after their introduction in clinical practice.[7] Their report, which showed an advantage of captopril in several HRQL domains, had a major impact on drug prescription patterns at the time of its publication. The earlier in the process of drug development potential effects on quality-of-life are recognized, the sooner appropriate data may be collected and analyzed.

METHODOLOGIC PROBLEMS TO BE ADDRESSED BY PHARMACOEPIDEMIOLOGIC RESEARCH

Researchers willing to accept the notion of the importance of measuring HRQL in pharmacoepidemiologic research and ready to use HRQL instruments in postmarketing (or, in some cases, premarketing) trials, face a considerable number of challenges. These challenges start with the realization that, as we have noted, there is no universal agreement on what the concept of quality-of-life actually entails. Thus, investigators must define as precisely as possible the aspects of HRQL in which they are interested.

Having identified the purpose for which an investigator wishes to use an HRQL instrument, one must be aware of the measurement properties required for it to fulfill its purpose. An additional problem occurs at this stage if researchers developed the original instrument in a different language, because one cannot assume the adequate performance of an instrument after its translation. At the next step, the investigator must choose from many available HRQL measurement instruments. When one has dealt satisfactorily with all these problems, the investigator has to ensure—as in any measurement—the rigorous fashion (standardized, reproducible, unbiased) with which to obtain the measurements (interviews or self- or computer-administered questionnaires). Finally, one is left with the chore of interpreting the data and translating the results into clinically meaningful terms.[8,9]

CURRENTLY AVAILABLE SOLUTIONS

QUALITY-OF-LIFE MEASUREMENT INSTRUMENTS IN INVESTIGATING NEW DRUGS: POTENTIAL USE AND NECESSARY ATTRIBUTES

In theory, any HRQL instrument could be used either to discriminate among patients (either according to current function or according to future prognosis), or to evaluate changes occurring in the health status (including HRQL) over time.[10,11] In most clinical trials, the primary objective of quality-of-life instruments is the evaluation of the effects of therapy, expressing treatment effects as a change in the score of the instrument over time. Occasionally, the intended use of instruments is to discriminate among patients. An example would be a study evaluating the effect of drug treatment on functional status in patients after myocardial infarction, where the investigators may wish to divide potential patients into those with moderate versus poor function (with a view toward intervening in the latter group).

The purpose for which investigators use an instrument dictates, to some degree, its necessary attributes. Each HRQL measurement instrument, regardless of its particular use, should be valid. The *validity* of an instrument refers to its ability to measure what it is intended to measure. This attribute of a measurement instrument is difficult to establish when there is no gold standard, as is the case with evaluation of HRQL. In such situations, where so-called *criterion validity* cannot be established, the validity of an instrument is frequently established in a step-wise process including examination of *face validity* (or sensibility)[12] and *construct validity*.

Sensibility relies on an intuitive assessment of the extent to which an instrument meets a number of criteria, including applicability, clarity and simplicity, likelihood of bias, comprehensiveness, and whether redundant items have been included. *Construct validity* refers to the extent to which results from a given instrument relate to other measures in a manner consistent with theoretical hypotheses. It is useful to distinguish between *cross-sectional construct validity* and *longitudinal construct validity*. To explain the former one could hypothesize that scores on one HRQL instrument should correlate with scores on another HRQL instrument or a physiological measure when measured at one point in time. For example, for identification of patients with chronic airflow limitation who have moderate to severe functional status impairment, an instrument measuring patient-reported dyspnea should show correlation with spirometry. In contrast, one would anticipate that spirometry would discriminate less well between those with worse and better emotional

function than it does between those with worse and better physical function. To exemplify longitudinal construct validity one could hypothesize that *changes* in spirometry related to a use of a new drug in patients with chronic airflow limitation should bear a close correlation with *changes* in functional status of the patient and a weaker correlation with *changes* in their emotional status.

The second attribute of an HRQL instrument is its ability to detect the "signal," over and above the "noise" which is introduced in the measurement process. For *discriminative instruments*, those that measure differences among people at a single point in time, this "signal" comes from differences between patients in HRQL. In this context, the way of quantifying the signal-to-noise ratio is called *reliability*. If the variability in scores between subjects (the signal) is much greater than the variability within subjects (the noise), an instrument will be deemed reliable. Reliable instruments will generally demonstrate that stable subjects show more or less the same results on repeated administration. The reliability coefficient (in general most appropriately an intraclass correlation coefficient) measuring the ratio of between-subject variance to total variance (which includes both between- and within-subject variance) is the statistic most frequently used to measure signal-to-noise ratio for discriminative instruments.

For *evaluative instruments*, those designed to measure changes within individuals over time, the "signal" comes from the differences in HRQL within patients associated with the intervention. The way of determining the signal-to-noise ratio is called *responsiveness* and refers to an instrument's ability to detect change. If a treatment results in an important difference in HRQL, investigators wish to be confident they will detect that difference, even if it is small. The responsiveness of an instrument is directly related to: (i) the magnitude of the difference in score in patients who have improved or deteriorated (the capacity to measure this signal can be called *changeability*), and (ii) the extent to which patients who have not changed obtain more or less the same scores (the capacity to minimize this noise can be called *reproducibility*). It follows that, to be of use, the ability of an instrument to show change when such change occurs has to be combined with its stability under unchanged conditions.

An example of an index of responsiveness is the ratio of the magnitude of change that corresponds to the minimally important difference (MID), to the variability in score in stable subjects.[13] Alternatively, the minimally important difference can be related to the variability associated with measuring differences in subjects who are changing. Investigators have suggested other measurements of responsiveness, but they all rely on some way of relating signal to noise.[13–17]

Another essential measurement property of an instrument is the extent to which one can understand the magnitude of any differences between treatments that a study demonstrates—the instrument's *interpretability*. If a treatment improves HRQL score by 3 points relative to control, what are we to conclude? Is the treatment effect very large, warranting widespread dissemination, or is it trivial, suggesting the new treatment should be abandoned? This question highlights the importance of being able to interpret the results of our HRQL questionnaire scores.

While our capacity to interpret results remains limited, investigators are adducing more and more information to enhance instrument interpretability.[8,9] Researchers have developed a number of strategies to address this difficult issue. Successful strategies have three things in common. First, they require an independent standard of comparison. Second, this independent standard must itself be interpretable. Third, there must be at least a moderate relationship between changes in questionnaire score and changes in the independent standard. The authors of this chapter have found that a correlation of 0.5 approximates the boundary between an acceptable and unacceptable relationship for establishing interpretability.

In our own work, we have often used global ratings of change (patients classifying themselves as unchanged, or experiencing small, medium, and large improvements or deteriorations) as the independent standard. We construct our disease-specific instruments using 7-point scales with an associated verbal descriptor for each level on the scale. For each questionnaire domain, we divide the total score by the number of items so that domain scores can range from 1 to 7. Using this approach to framing response options, we have found that the smallest difference that patients consider important is often approximately 0.5 per question.[16,18] A moderate difference corresponds to a change of approximately 1.0 per question, and changes of greater than 1.5 can be considered large. So, for example, in a domain with four items, patients will consider a one point change in two or more items as important. This finding seems to apply across different areas of function, including dyspnea, fatigue, and emotional function in patients with chronic airflow limitation;[16] symptoms, emotional function, and activity limitations in both adult[18] and child[19] asthma patients, and parents of child asthma patients;[20] and symptoms, emotional function, and activity limitations in adults with rhinoconjunctivitis.[21] Similar observations may be derived from reports of other investigators.[22]

The approach that we have just described relies on within-patient comparisons as the independent standard. An alternative is between-patient comparisons. In one example of this approach, we formed groups of seven patients with chronic airflow limitation participating in a respiratory rehabilitation program.[23] Each patient completed the Chronic Respiratory Questionnaire (CRQ). The patients conversed with one another long enough to make judgments about their relative experience of fatigue in daily life. While there was a bias in their assessment (patients generally considered themselves better off than one another), their relative ratings allow estimates of what differences in CRQ score constitute small, medium, and large differences. The results were largely congruent with the findings from the within-patient rating studies.[23]

Another anchor-based approach uses HRQL instruments for which investigators have established the minimal important difference (MID). Investigators can apply regression or other statistical methods to compute the changes on a new instrument that correspond to those of the instrument with the established MID. For example, using the established MID of the CRQ we computed the MID for two other instruments that measure HRQL in patients with chronic airflow limitation, the feeling thermometer and the St George's Respiratory Questionnaire.[24] Similar to the anchor-based approach using transition ratings, investigators should ensure that the strength of the correlation between the change scores of these instruments exceeds a minimum (for example, a correlation coefficient of 0.5).

Yet another approach to estimate the MID involves enrolling panels of experts or patients and using qualitative research methods, such as Delphi techniques. Using a panel-based approach, Wyrwich *et al.* enrolled pulmonary physicians to determine the MID of the CRQ.[25] All panel members were familiar with the CRQ, received information about the instrument, and received materials about the previously established MID for the instrument. The experts came to a consensus on what constitutes the MID of the CRQ. The results for the MID were similar to those obtained with the anchor-based approach described above (a change of 0.5 on the 7-point scale).

Investigators proposed distribution-based methods to determine interpretability of HRQL instruments. Distribution-based methods differ from anchor-based methods in that they interpret results in terms of the relation between the magnitude of effect and some measure or measures of variability in results.[9] The magnitude of effect can be the difference in an individual patient's score before and after treatment, a single group's score before and after treatment, or the difference in score between treatment and control groups.

As a measure of variability, investigators may choose between-patient variability (the standard deviation of patients at baseline, for instance) or within-patient variability (the standard deviation of change that patients experienced during a study).

If an investigator used the distribution-based approach, the clinician would see a treatment effect reported as, for instance, 0.3 standard deviation units. The great advantage of distribution-based methods is that the values are easy to generate for almost any HRQL instrument because there will always be one or more measures of variability available. This contrasts with the work needed to generate an anchor-based interpretation, evident from the prior discussion. The problem related to this methodology is that the units do not have intuitive meaning to clinicians. It is possible, however, that clinicians could gain experience with standard deviation units in the same way they learn to understand other HRQL scores.

Cohen addressed this problem in a seminal work by suggesting that changes in the range of 0.2 standard deviation units represent small changes, those in the range of 0.5 standard deviation units represent moderate changes, and those in the range of 0.8 standard deviation units represent large changes.[26] Thus, one would tell a clinician that if trial results show a 0.3 standard deviation difference between treatment and control, then the patient can anticipate a small improvement in HRQL with treatment. The problem with this approach is the arbitrariness. Do 0.2, 0.5, and 0.8 standard deviation units consistently represent small, medium, and large effects?

In response to this problem, investigators have attempted to provide empirical evidence about the relationship between distribution-based and anchor-based results. These studies address the question, "What is the appropriate interpretation of a particular magnitude of effect in distribution-based units, as judged by the results of anchor-based studies?" For example, we described the MID for the CRQ based on Cohen's effects size in patients completing a respiratory rehabilitation program.[24] The CRQ scores that corresponded to 0.2, 0.5, and 0.8 standard deviation units were as follows: CRQ dyspnea 0.24, 0.61, and 0.98; CRQ fatigue 0.27, 0.67, and 1.08; CRQ emotional function 0.24, 0.60, and 0.96; and CRQ mastery 0.24, 0.60, and 0.96. Thus, this work indicates the MID to be in the range of 0.2 to 0.5 standard deviation units.

The standard error of measurement (SEM) presents another distribution-based method. It is defined as the variability between an individual's observed score and the true score, and is computed as the baseline standard deviation multiplied by the square root of 1 minus the reliability of the QOL measure. In theory, a QOL measure's standard error of measurement is sample independent, whereas its component statistics, the standard deviation and the reliability estimate, are sample dependent and vary around the standard error of measurement.[27] When the between-person variability in the population increases, the standard deviation will increase (tending to raise the standard error of measurement), but the reliability will also increase (tending to lower the standard error of measurement). Thus, the standard error of measurement largely reflects within-person variability over time. Wyrwich and colleagues provide an example of using the SEM approach in their study following 471 outpatients with COPD. The authors used the SEM to correlate this distribution-based method with the MID.[28] They found that the SEM method consistently suggested an MID of the CRQ of approximately 0.5. In addition, the research revealed that this methodology shows consistent estimates for the MID across a wide range of HRQL scores on the CRQ.

Investigators can also use as independent standards measures that clinicians, through long experience, already know well. For example, scores on a generic measure of HRQL, the Sickness Impact Profile (SIP), range from an average of 8.2 in patients with American Rheumatism Association arthritis class I, to 25.8 in class IV.[29] Another standard would be obtained by administering questionnaires to patients before and after an intervention of known effectiveness with which clinicians are familiar, so that they can see the change in score associated with response to treatment. For example, patients shortly after hip replacement have scores of 30 on the SIP, scores which decrease to less than 5 after full convalescence.[30] Relationships between HRQL and a variety of marker states can also be useful: SIP scores in patients with chronic airflow limitation severe enough to require home oxygen are approximately 24;[31] scores in patients with chronic, stable angina are approximately 11.5.[32]

Clinicians and investigators tend to assume that, if the mean difference between a treatment and a control is appreciably less than the smallest change that is important, then the treatment has a trivial effect. This may not be so. Let us assume that a randomized clinical trial (RCT) shows a mean difference of 0.25 in a questionnaire with an MID of 0.5. One may conclude that the difference is unimportant, and the result does not support administration of the treatment. This interpretation assumes that every patient given treatment scored 0.25 better than they would have, had they received the control. However, it ignores possible heterogeneity of the treatment effect. Depending on the true distribution of results, the appropriate interpretation may be different.

Consider a situation where 25% of the treated patients improved by a magnitude of 1.0, while the other 75% did not improve at all (mean change of 0). This would indicate that the 25% of treated patients obtained moderate benefit from the intervention. Using the number needed to treat (NNT), a methodology developed for interpreting the magnitude of treatment effects, investigators have found that clinicians commonly treat 25 to 50 patients, and often as many as 100, to prevent a single adverse event.[33] Thus, the hypothetical treatment with a mean difference of 0.25 and an NNT of 4 proves to have a powerful effect.

We have shown that this issue is much more than hypothetical.[34] In a crossover randomized trial in asthmatic patients comparing the short-acting inhaled β-agonist salbutamol to the long-acting inhaled β-agonist salmeterol, we found a mean difference of 0.3 between groups in the activity dimension of the Asthma Quality-of-Life Questionnaire (AQLQ). This mean difference represents slightly more than half the minimal important difference in an individual patient. Knowing that the minimal important difference is 0.5 allows us to calculate the proportion of patients who achieved benefit from salmeterol—that is, the proportion who had an important improvement (greater than 0.5 in one of the HRQL domains) while receiving salmeterol relative to salbutamol. For the activity domain of the AQLQ, this proportion proved to be 0.22 (22%). The NNT is simply the inverse of the proportion who benefit, in this case 4.5. Thus, clinicians need to treat fewer than five patients with salmeterol to ensure that one patient obtains an important improvement in their ability to undertake activities of daily living.

In another randomized trial examining the effect of a respiratory rehabilitation program in patients with chronic lung disease, we found a mean difference between rehabilitation patients and the community controls of 0.40 in the emotions domain of the CRQ.[35] This difference is less than the value of 0.5 that represents the minimal important difference in an individual patient. However, the data from the trial allow us to calculate the proportion of patients who were ≥0.5 better in their emotional function while receiving rehabilitation than would have been the case had they been in the community control group. This turned out to be 0.30, which translates into an NNT of 4 (or exactly 3.3) patients.

This discussion emphasizes that, to interpret the results of HRQL measurement in pharmacoepidemiology studies requires clinicians to be aware of the changes in score that constitute trivial, small, medium, and large differences in HRQL. Further, looking at mean differences between groups can be misleading. The distribution of differences is critical, and can be summarized in an informative manner using the NNT.

QUALITY-OF-LIFE MEASUREMENT INSTRUMENTS: TAXONOMY AND POTENTIAL USE

Clinical journals have published trials in which HRQL instruments are the primary outcome measures. With the expanding importance of HRQL in evaluating new therapeutic interventions, investigators (and readers) are faced with a large array of instruments. Researchers have proposed different ways of categorizing these instruments, according to the purpose of their use, into instruments designed for screening, providing health profiles, measuring preference, and making clinical decisions,[36] or into discriminative and evaluative instruments (as above).

We have also suggested a taxonomy based on the domains of HRQL which an instrument attempts to cover.[37] According to this taxonomy, an HRQL instrument may be categorized, in a broad sense, as generic or specific. *Generic instruments* cover (or at least aim to cover) the complete spectrum of function, disability, and distress of the patient, and are applicable to a variety of populations and conditions. Within the framework of generic instruments, health profiles and utility measures provide two distinct approaches to measurement of global quality-of-life. *Specific instruments* are focused on disease or treatment issues particularly relevant to the disease or condition of interest.

GENERIC INSTRUMENTS

Health Profiles

Health profiles are single instruments that measure multiple different aspects of quality-of-life. They usually provide a scoring system that allows aggregation of the results into a small number of scores and sometimes into a single score (in which case, it may be referred to as an index). As generic measures, they are designed for use in a wide variety of conditions. For example, one health profile, the SIP contains twelve "categories" which can be aggregated into two dimensions and five independent categories, and also into a single overall score.[30] The SIP has been used in studies of cardiac rehabilitation,[38] total hip joint arthroplasty,[39] and treatment of back pain.[40] In addition to the SIP, there are a number of other health profiles available: the Nottingham Health Profile,[41] the Duke–UNC Health Profile,[42] and the McMaster Health Index Questionnaire.[43] Increasingly, a collection of related instruments from the Medical Outcomes Study[44] have become the most popular and widely used generic instruments. Particularly popular is one version that includes 36 items, the SF-36.[45–47] The SF-36 is available in over 40 languages, and normal values for the general population in many countries are available.

While each health profile attempts to measure all important aspects of HRQL, they may slice the HRQL pie quite differently. For example, the McMaster Health Index Questionnaire follows the World Health Organization approach and identifies three dimensions: physical, emotional, and social. The SIP includes a physical dimension (with categories of ambulation, mobility, body care, and movement), a psychosocial dimension (with categories including social interaction and emotional behavior), and five independent categories including eating, work, home management, sleep and rest, and recreations and pastimes.

General health profiles offer a number of advantages to the clinical investigator. Their reproducibility and validity have been established, often in a variety of populations. When using them for discriminative purposes, one can examine and establish areas of dysfunction affecting a particular population. Identification of these areas of dysfunction may guide investigators who are constructing disease-specific instruments to potentially target areas with the greatest impact on the quality-of-life. Health profiles, used as evaluative instruments, allow determination of the effects of an intervention on different aspects of quality-of-life, without necessitating the use of multiple instruments (which may save both the investigator's and the patient's time). Because health profiles are designed for a wide variety of conditions, one can potentially compare the effects on HRQL of different interventions in different diseases. Profiles that allow computation of a single score can be used in a cost-effectiveness analysis, in which the cost of an intervention in dollars is related to its outcome in natural units (see Chapter 41).

The main limitation of health profiles is that they may not focus adequately on the aspects of quality-of-life specifically influenced by a particular intervention. This may result in an inability of the instrument to detect a real effect in the area of importance (i.e., lack of responsiveness). In fact, disease-specific instruments offer greater responsiveness compared with generic instruments.[48,49] We will return to this issue when we discuss the alternative approach, specific instruments.

Utility Measurement

Economic and decision theory provides the underlying basis for *utility measures* (see Chapter 41). The key elements of a utility instrument are, first, that it is preference-based, and second, that scores are tied to death as an outcome. Typically, HRQL can be measured as a utility measure using a single number along a continuum from dead (0.0) to full health (1.0). The use of utility measures in clinical studies requires serial measurement of the utility of the patient's quality-of-life throughout the study.

There are two fundamental approaches to utility measurement in clinical studies. One is to ask patients a number of questions about their function and well-being. Based on their responses, patients are classified into one of a number of categories. Each category has a utility value associated with it, the utility having been established in previous ratings by another group (ideally a random sample of the general population). This approach is typified by three widely used instruments: the Quality of Well-Being Scale,[50–52] the Health Utilities Index,[53] and the Euroqol (EQ5).[54]

The second approach is to ask patients to make a single rating that takes into account all aspects of their quality-of-life.[55] This rating can be made many ways. The "standard gamble" asks patients to choose between their own health state and a gamble in which they may die immediately or achieve full health for the remainder of their lives. Using the standard gamble, patients' utility or HRQL is determined by the choices they make, as the probabilities of immediate death or full health are varied. Another technique is the "time trade-off," in which subjects are asked about the number of years in their present health state they would be willing to trade-off for a shorter life span in full health. A third technique is the use of a simple visual analogue scale presented as a thermometer, the "feeling thermometer."[56] When completing the feeling thermometer, patients choose the score on the thermometer that represents the value they place on their health state. The best state is full health (equal to a score of 100) and the worst state is dead (a score of 0).

A major advantage of utility measurement is its amenability to cost–utility analysis (see Chapter 41). In cost–utility analysis, the cost of an intervention is related to the number of quality-adjusted life-years (QALYs) gained through application of the intervention.[57] Cost per QALY may be compared and provides a basis for allocation of scarce resources among different health care programs. Results from the utility approach may thus be of particular interest to program evaluators and health policy decision makers.

However, utility measurement also has limitations. Utilities can vary depending on how they are obtained, raising questions of the validity of any single measurement.[58,59] Utility measurement does not allow the investigator to determine which aspects of HRQL are responsible for changes in utility. Finally, utilities potentially share the disadvantage of health profiles, in that they may not be responsive to small but still clinically important changes.

SPECIFIC INSTRUMENTS

An alternative approach to HRQL measurement is to focus on aspects of health status that are specific to the area of primary interest. The rationale for this approach lies in the increased responsiveness that may result from including only those aspects of HRQL that are relevant and important in a particular disease process or even in a particular patient situation. One could also focus an instrument only on the areas that are likely to be affected by a particular drug. This latter approach is advanced in the design and conduct of randomized controlled trials with individual patients— N-of-1 Randomized Clinical Trials[60] (see Chapter 43).

In other situations, the instrument may be specific to the disease (e.g., for chronic lung disease, for rheumatoid arthritis, for cardiovascular diseases, for endocrine problems); specific to a population of patients (e.g., the frail elderly, who are afflicted with a wide variety of different diseases); specific to a certain function (e.g., emotional or sexual function); or specific to a given condition or problem (e.g., pain), which can be caused by a variety of underlying pathologies. Within a single condition, the instrument may differ depending on the intervention. For example, while success of a disease modifying agent in rheumatoid arthritis should result in improved HRQL by enabling a patient to increase performance of physically stressful activities of daily living, occupational therapy may achieve improved HRQL by encouraging family members to take over activities formerly accomplished with difficulty by the patient. Appropriate disease-specific HRQL outcome measures should reflect this difference.

Specific instruments can be constructed to reflect the "single state" ("How tired have you been: very tired, somewhat tired, full of energy?") or a "transition" ("How has your tiredness been: better, the same, worse?").[61] Theoretically, the same could be said of generic instruments, although none of the available generic instruments has used the transition approach. Specific measures can integrate aspects of morbidity, including events such as recurrent myocardial infarction.[62]

Like generic instruments, disease-specific instruments may be used for discriminative purposes. They may aid, for example, in evaluating the extent to which a primary symptom (for example dyspnea) is related to the magnitude of physiological abnormality (for example exercise capacity).[63] Disease-specific instruments can be applied for evaluative purposes to establish the impact of an intervention on a specific area of dysfunction, and hence aid in elucidating the mechanisms of drug action.[64] Guidelines provide structured approaches for constructing specific measures.[65]

Whatever approaches one takes to the construction of disease-specific measures, a number of head-to-head comparisons between generic and specific instruments suggest that the latter approach will fulfill its promise of enhancing responsiveness.[22,66–70]

In addition to the improved responsiveness, specific measures have the advantage of relating closely to areas routinely explored by the physician. For example, a disease-specific measure of quality-of-life in chronic lung disease focuses on dyspnea during day-to-day activities, fatigue, and areas of emotional dysfunction, including frustration and impatience.[13] Specific measures may therefore appear clinically sensible to the clinician.

The disadvantages of specific measures are that they are (deliberately) not comprehensive, and cannot be used to compare across conditions or, at times, even across programs. This suggests that there is no one group of instruments that will achieve all the potential goals of HRQL measurement. Thus, investigators may choose to use multiple instruments, an issue we will deal with in the next section.

USE OF MULTIPLE QUALITY-OF-LIFE MEASURES IN CLINICAL STUDIES

Clinical investigators are not restricted to using a single instrument in their studies, and investigators will often conclude that a single instrument cannot yield all the relevant information. For example, utility and disease-specific measures contribute quite different sorts of data, and an investigator may want to use one of each.

Another, somewhat different way of using multiple instruments is to administer a battery of specific instruments. An example of such an approach was a blinded, randomized trial of three antihypertensive agents in primary hypertension.[7] The investigators identified five dimensions of health they were measuring: the sense of well-being and satisfaction with life, the physical state, the emotional state, intellectual functioning, and the ability to perform in social roles and the degree of satisfaction from those roles. Even within these five dimensions, additional components were present. For example, separate measurements of sleep and sexual function existed. Patients taking one of the three drugs under investigation, captopril, scored better on measures of general well-being, work performance, and life satisfaction. The lesson for the clinician is clearly important: one can have an impact on not only the length, but also the quality of the patient's life according to choice of antihypertensive agent.

The approach of using multiple instruments, although comprehensive, has limitations. First, investigators must find a valid, responsive instrument for every attribute they wish to measure. Second, it is possible (indeed likely) that only some of the instruments chosen will show differences between the treatments under investigation. Unless one of the instruments has been designated as the primary measure of outcome before the study started, different results in different measures may make interpretation difficult. The greater the number of instruments used, the greater the probability that one or more instruments will favor one treatment or the other, even if the treatments' true effectiveness is identical. Thus, the alpha error (the probability of finding an apparent difference between treatments when in fact their outcomes do not differ) increases with each new instrument used. Although this problem may be dealt with through statistical adjustment for the number of instruments used, such adjustment is often not made.[71]

Another problem occurs if only a small proportion of the instruments used favor an intervention (or if some instruments favor one treatment and other instruments favor the other). In these situations, the clinician may be unsure how to interpret the results. The use of multiple instruments opens the door to such potential controversy.

A final limitation of using a battery of instruments is that it gives no indication of the relative importance of various areas of dysfunction to the patient. For example, had Croog *et al.*[7] found that one antihypertensive agent disturbed sleep, while another had an adverse impact on sexual function, their approach would not have allowed determination of which drug had a greater net adverse impact on patients' lives.

THE FUTURE

The considerations we have raised suggest a step-by-step approach to addressing issues of HRQL in pharmacoepidemiology studies.[72–74] Clinicians must begin by asking themselves if investigators have addressed all the important effects of treatment on patients' quantity and quality-of-life. If they have not, clinicians may have more difficulty applying the results to their patients.

If the study has addressed HRQL issues, have investigators chosen the appropriate instruments? In particular, does evidence suggest the measures used are valid measures of HRQL? If so, and the study failed to demonstrate differences between groups, is there good reason to believe the instrument is responsive in this context? If not, the results may be a false negative, failing to show the true underlying difference in HRQL.

Whatever the differences between groups, the clinician must be able to interpret their magnitude. Knowledge of the difference in score that represents small, medium, and large differences in HRQL will be very helpful in making this interpretation. Clinicians must still look beyond mean differences between groups, and consider the distribution of differences. The NNT for a single patient to achieve an important benefit in HRQL offers one way of expressing results that clinicians are likely to find meaningful.

REFERENCES

1. Franciosa J, Jordan R, Wilen M. Minoxidil in patients with chronic left heart failure: contrasting hemodynamic and clinical effects in a controlled trial. *Circulation* 1984; **70**: 63–8.
2. Packer M. How should we judge the efficacy of drug therapy in patients with chronic congestive heart failure? The insight of the six blind men. *J Am Coll Cardiol* 1987; **9**: 433–8.
3. Danis M, Gerrity M, Southerland L, Patrick D. A comparison of patient, family, and physician assessment of the value of medical intensive care. *Crit Care Med* 1988; **16**: 594–600.
4. Schipper H, Clinch J, Powell V. Definitions and conceptual issues. In: Spilker B, ed., *Quality-of-Life Assessment in Clinical Trials*. New York: Raven Press, 1990; pp. 11–24.
5. Gill T, Feinstein A. A critical appraisal of the quality of quality-of-life measurements. *JAMA* 1994; **272**: 619–26.
6. Guyatt G, Cook D. Health status, quality-of-life, and the individual patient. A commentary on: Gill TM, Feinstein AR. A critical appraisal of quality-of-life measurements. *JAMA* 1994; **272**: 630–1.
7. Croog S, Levine S, Testa M. The effects of antihypertensive therapy on the quality-of-life. *N Engl J Med* 1986; **314**: 1657–64.
8. Guyatt GH. Making sense of quality-of-life data. *Med Care* 2000; **38**(suppl II): 175–9.
9. Guyatt GH, Osoba D, Wu AW, Wyrwich KW, Norman GR, Clinical Significance Consensus Meeting G. Methods to explain the clinical significance of health status measures. *Mayo Clin Proc* 2002; **77**: 371–83.
10. Kirshner B, Guyatt G. A methodologic framework for assessing health care indices. *J Chronic Dis* 1985; **38**: 27–36.
11. Guyatt G, Kirshner B, Jaeschke R. Measuring health status: what are the necessary measurement properties? *J Clin Epidemiol* 1992; **45**: 1341–5.
12. Feinstein A. The theory and evaluation of sensibility. In: Feinstein A, ed. *Clinimetrics*. New Haven, CT: Yale University Press, 1987; pp. 141–65.
13. Guyatt G, Walter S, Norman G. Measuring change over time: assessing the usefulness of evaluative instruments. *J Chronic Dis* 1987; **40**: 171–8.

14. Levine M. Incorporation of quality-of-life assessment into clinical trials. In: Osoba D, ed., *Effect of Cancer on Quality-of-Life*. Boston, MA: CRC Press, 1991; pp. 105–111.

15. Guyatt G, Feeny D, Patrick D. Measuring health-related quality-of-life: basic sciences review. *Ann Intern Med* 1993; **70**: 225–30.

16. Jaeschke R, Guyatt G, Keller J, Singer J. Measurement of health status: ascertaining the meaning of a change in quality-of-life questionnaire score. *Control Clin Trials* 1989; **10**: 407–15.

17. Husted JA, Cook RJ, Farewell VT, Gladman DD. Methods for assessing responsiveness: a critical review and recommendations. *J Clin Epidemiol* 2000; **53**: 459–68.

18. Juniper E, Guyatt G, Willan A, Griffth L. Determining a minimal important change in a disease-specific quality-of-life questionnaire. *J Clin Epidemiol* 1994; **47**: 81–7.

19. Juniper E, Guyatt G, Feeny D, Ferrie PJ, Griffith LE, Townsend M. Measuring quality-of-life in children with asthma. *Qual Life Res* 1996; **5**: 35–46.

20. Juniper E, Guyatt G, Feeny D, Ferrie P, Griffith L, Townsend M. Measuring quality-of-life in the parents of children with asthma. *Qual Life Res* 1996; **5**: 27–34.

21. Juniper EF, Guyatt GH, Griffith LE, Ferrie PJ. Interpretation of rhinoconjunctivitis quality-of-life questionnaire data. *J Allergy Clin Immunol* 1996; **98**: 843–5.

22. Laupacis A, Wong C, Churchill D. The use of generic and specific quality-of-life measures in hemodialysis patients treated with erythropoietin. *Control Clin Trials* 1991; **12**: 168S–79S.

23. Redelmeier D, Guyatt G, Goldstein R. Assessing the minimal important difference in symptoms: a comparison of two techniques. *J Clin Epidemiol* 1996; **49**: 1215–19.

24. Schünemann H, Griffith L, Jaeschke R, Stubbing D, Goldstein R, Guyatt GH. Evaluation of the minimal important difference for the feeling thermometer and St. George's Respiratory Questionnaire in patients with chronic airflow limitation. *J Clin Epidemiol* 2003; **56**: 1170–6.

25. Wyrwich KW, Fihn SD, Tierney WM, Kroenke K, Babu AN, Wolinsky FD. Clinically important changes in health-related quality-of-life for patients with chronic obstructive pulmonary disease. An expert consensus panel report. *J Gen Intern Med* 2003; **18**: 196–202.

26. Cohen J. *Statistical Power Analysis for the Behavioral Sciences*, 2nd edn. Hillsdale, NJ: Lawrence Erlbaum Associates, 1988.

27. Wyrwich KW, Nienaber NA, Tierney WM, Wolinsky FD. Linking clinical relevance and statistical significance in evaluating intra-individual changes in health-related quality-of-life. *Med Care* 1999; **37**: 469–78.

28. Wyrwich KW, Tierney WM, Wolinsky FD. Further evidence supporting an SEM-based criterion for identifying meaningful intra-individual changes in health-related quality-of-life. *J Clin Epidemiol* 1999; **52**: 861–73.

29. Deyo R, Inui T, Leininger J, Overman S. Measuring functional outcomes in chronic disease: a comparison of traditional scales and a self-administered health status questionnaire in patients with rheumatoid arthritis. *Med Care* 1983; **21**: 180–92.

30. Bergner M, Bobbitt R, Carter W, Gilson B. The Sickness Impact Profile: development and final revision of a health status measure. *Med Care* 1981; **19**: 787–805.

31. McSweeney A, Grant I, Heaton R, Adams KM, Timms RM. Life quality of patients with chronic obstructive pulmonary disease. *Arch Intern Med* 1982; **142**: 473–478.

32. Fletcher A, McLoone P, Bulpitt C. quality-of-life on angina therapy: a randomised controlled trial of transdermal glyceryl trinitrate against placebo. *Lancet* 1988; **2**: 4–7.

33. Laupacis A, Sackett D, Roberts R. An assessment of clinically useful measures of the consequences of treatment. *N Engl J Med* 1988; **318**: 1728–33.

34. Guyatt G, Juniper E, Walter S, Griffith L, Goldstein R. Interpreting treatment effects in randomized trials. *BMJ* 1998; **316**: 690–3.

35. Guyatt GH, Berman LB, Townsend M, Pugsley SO, Chambers LW. A measure of quality-of-life for clinical trials in chronic lung disease. *Thorax* 1987; **42**(10): 773–8.

36. Osoba D. *Effect of Cancer on Quality-of-Life*. Boston, MA: CRC Press, 1991.

37. Guyatt G, Zanten SVV, Feeny D, Patrick D. Measuring quality-of-life in clinical trials: a taxonomy and review. *Can Med Assoc J* 1989; **140**: 1441–7.

38. Ott C, Sivarajan E, Newton K, Almes MJ, Bruce RA, Bergner M, Gilson BS. A controlled randomized study of early cardiac rehabilitation: the sickness impact profile as an assessment tool. *Heart Lung* 1983; **12**: 162–70.

39. Liang M, Larson M, Cullen K, Schwartz J. Comparative measurement efficiency and sensitivity of five health status instruments for arthritis research. *Arthritis Rheum* 1985; **28**: 542–7.

40. Deyo R, Diehl A, Rosenthal M. How many days of bed rest for acute low back pain? A randomized clinical trial. *N Engl J Med* 1986; **315**: 1064–70.

41. Hunt S, McKenna S, McEwen J, Backett E, Williams J, Papp E. A quantitative approach to perceived health status: a validation study. *J Epidemiol Community Health* 1980; **34**: 281–6.

42. Parkerson G, Gehlback S, Wagner E, Sherman A, Clapp N, Muhlbaier L. The Duke–UNC Health Profile: an adult health status instrument for primary care. *Med Care* 1981; **19**: 806–28.

43. Sackett D, Chambers L, MacPherson A, Goldsmith C, McAuley R. The development and application of indices of health: general methods and a summary of results. *Am J Public Health* 1977; **67**: 423–8.

44. Tarlov A, Ware J, Greenfield S, Nelson E, Perrin E, Zubkoff M. The Medical Outcomes Study. *JAMA* 1989; **262**: 925–30.

45. Brook R, Ware J, Davies-Avery A, Stewart A, Donald C, Rogers WH, Williams KN, Johnston SA. Overview of adult health status measures fielded in Rand's health insurance study. *Med Care* 1979; **17**(suppl 7): 1–131.

46. Ware J, Sherbourne C. The MOS 36-item short-form health survey (SF-36). *Med Care* 1992; **30**: 473–83.

47. Ware J, Kozinski M, Bayliss M, McHorney CA, Rogers WH, Raczek A. Comparison of methods for the scoring and statistical

analysis of SF-36 health profile and summary measures: summary of results of the Medical Outcomes Study. *Med Care* 1995; **33**: AS264–79.

48. Guyatt G, King DR, Feeny DH, Stubbing D, Goldstein RS.. Generic and specific measurement of health-related quality-of-life in a clinical trial of respiratory rehabilitation. *J Clin Epidemiol* 1999; **52**: 187–192.

49. Wiebe S, Guyatt G, Weaver B, Matijevic S, Sidwell C. Comparative responsiveness of generic and specific quality-of-life instruments. *J Clin Epidemiol* 2003; **56**: 52–60.

50. Kaplan R, Anderson J, Wu A, Mathews W, Kozin F, Orenstein D. The quality of well-being scale: applications in AIDS, cystic fibrosis, and arthritis. *Med Care* 1989; **27**(suppl): S27–43.

51. Kaplan R, Bush J, Berry C. Health status: types of validity and the index of well-being. *Health Serv Res* 1976; **11**: 478–507.

52. Kaplan R, Bush J. Health-related quality-of-life measurement for evaluation research and policy analysis. *Health Psychol* 1982; **1**: 61–80.

53. Feeny D, Furlong W, Boyle M, Torrance G. Multi-attribute health status classification systems: health utilities index. *Pharmacoeconomics* 1995; **7**: 490–502.

54. Anonymous. EuroQol—a new facility for the measurement of health-related quality-of-life. The EuroQol Group. *Health Policy* 1990; **16**: 199–208.

55. Torrance G. Measurement of health state utilities for economic appraisal: a review. *J Health Econ* 1986; **5**: 1–30.

56. Bennett K. Measuring health state preferences and utilities: rating scale, time trade-off, and standard gamble techniques. In: Spilker B, ed., *quality-of-life and Pharmacoeconomics in Clinical Trials*. Philadelphia, PA: Lippincott-Raven, 1996; p. 259.

57. Mehrez A, Gafni A. Quality-adjusted life years, utility theory, and healthy-years equivalents. *Med Decis Making* 1989; **9**: 142–9.

58. Sutherland H, Dunn V, Boyd N. Measurement of values for states of health with linear analog scales. *Med Decis Making* 1983; **3**: 477–87.

59. Llewellyn-Thomas H, Sutherland HJ, Tibshirani R, Ciampi A, Till JE, Boyd NF. The measurement of patients' values in medicine. *Med Decis Making* 1982; **3**: 477–87.

60. Guyatt G, Keller J, Jaeschke R, Rosenbloom D, Adachi J, Newhouse M. The *N*-of-1 randomized controlled trials: clinical usefulness. Three year experience. *Ann Intern Med* 1990; **112**: 293–9.

61. MacKenzie M, Charlson M. Standards for the use of ordinal scales in clinical trials. *BMJ* 1986; **292**: 40–43.

62. Olsson G, Lubsen J, VanEs G, Rehnqvist N. Quality-of-life after myocardial infarction: effect of long term metoprolol on mortality and morbidity. *BMJ* 1986; **292**: 1491–3.

63. Mahler D, Rosiello R, Harver A, Lentine T, McGovern J, Daubenspeck J. Comparison of clinical dyspnea ratings and psychophysical measurements of respiratory sensation in obstructive airway disease. *Am Rev Respir Dis* 1987; **135**: 1229–33.

64. Jaeschke R, Singer J, Guyatt G. Using quality-of-life measures to elucidate mechanism of action. *Can Med Assoc J* 1991; **144**: 35–39.

65. Guyatt G, Bombardier C, Tugwell P. Measuring disease-specific quality-of-life in clinical trials. *Can Med Assoc J* 1986; **134**: 889–95.

66. Tandon P, Stander H, Schwarz RP Jr. Analysis of quality-of-life data from a randomized, placebo controlled heart-failure trial. *J Clin Epidemiol* 1989; **42**: 955–62.

67. Smith D, Baker G, Davies G, Dewey M, Chadwick. D. Outcomes of add-on treatment with Lamotrigine in partial epilepsy. *Epilepsia* 1993; **34**: 312–22.

68. Chang S, Fine R, Siegel D, Chesney M, Black D, Hulley S. The impact of diuretic therapy on reported sexual function. *Arch Intern Med* 1991; **151**: 2402–8.

69. Tugwell P, Bombardier C, Buchanan W, Goldsmith C, Grace E, Bennett K *et al.* Methotrexate in rheumatoid arthritis. Impact on quality-of-life assessed by traditional standard-item and individualized patient preference health status questionnaires. *Arch Intern Med* 1990; **150**: 59–62.

70. Goldstein R, Gort E, Guyatt G, Stubbing D, Avendano M. Prospective randomized controlled trial of respiratory rehabilitation. *Lancet* 1994; **344**: 1394–7.

71. Pocock S, Hughes M, Lee R. Statistical problems in the reporting of clinical trials. *N Engl J Med* 1987; **317**: 426–432.

72. Guyatt G, Naylor C, Juniper EF, Heyland D, Jaeschke R, Cook DJ. Therapy and understanding the results: quality-of-life. In: Guyatt G, Rennie D, eds, *Users' Guides to the Medical Literature: A Manual for Evidence-Based Clinical Practice*. Chicago, IL: American Medical Association Press, 2002; pp. 49–100.

73. Guyatt G. Therapy and harm: an introduction. In: Guyatt G, Renne D, eds, *Users' Guides to the Medical Literature: A Manual for Evidence-Based Clinical Practice*. Chicago, IL: American Medical Association Press, 2002; pp. 49–100.

74. Guyatt G, Naylor C, Juniper E, Keyland D, Jaeschke R, Cook D. Users' guides to the medical literature: XII. How to use articles about health-related quality-of-life. *JAMA* 1997; **277**: 1232–7.

75. Dans A, Dans L, Guyatt G, Richardson S. For the Evidence-based Medicine Working Group. User's guides to the medical literature: XIV. How to decide on the applicability of clinical trial results to your patient. *JAMA* 1998; **279**: 545–9.

43

N-of-1 Randomized Clinical Trials in Pharmacoepidemiology

GORDON H. GUYATT[1], ROMAN JAESCHKE[2] and ROBIN ROBERTS[3]

[1] Department of Medicine and Department of Clinical Epidemiology and Biostatistics, McMaster University, Hamilton, Ontario, Canada; [2] Department of Medicine, McMaster University, Hamilton, Ontario, Canada, and Polish Institute of EBM, Krakow, Poland; [3] Department of Clinical Epidemiology and Biostatistics, McMaster University, Hamilton, Ontario, Canada.

INTRODUCTION

Clinicians are used to, and comfortable with, making initial clinical recommendations for their patients on the basis of medical research consisting of formal randomized clinical trials of groups of patients (see Chapter 2). However, individual patients may not behave the same way as the group. Responding to this heterogeneity of treatment effect, psychological research has long taken advantage of experimental studies of single subjects. In this chapter, we describe how clinicians can use an experimental approach that focuses on the individual to facilitate clinical research and, especially, to enhance the clinical care of their patients. We believe the approaches we describe are highly relevant to pharmacoepidemiology because they apply fundamental epidemiological principles to the selection of drugs for individual patients, and to the drug development process.

CLINICAL PROBLEMS TO BE ADDRESSED BY PHARMACOEPIDEMIOLOGIC RESEARCH

Traditionally, important questions that patients, and clinicians caring for them, consider include: does treatment have the potential to eradicate the disease? What is the probability of prolonging the life of the patient? What is the chance of delaying the progression of a disease? What is the frequency and impact of a drug's side effects? Randomized controlled trials (RCTs) address these questions, and are usually necessary to establish valid evidence of drug efficacy[1] (see also Chapters 1, 2, 39, and 40). When deciding which therapy is more beneficial for an individual patient, however, clinicians often cannot rely on the results of RCTs. For example, an RCT addressing the issue may not be available; some conditions are so rare that even multicenter collaborative trials may not be feasible. Further, even when a relevant RCT generated a clear answer, its

Pharmacoepidemiology, Fourth Edition   Edited by B.L. Strom
© 2005 John Wiley & Sons, Ltd

result may not apply to an individual patient. First, if the patient does not meet the eligibility criteria, extrapolation may not be appropriate.[2] Second, regardless of the overall trial results, some patients may benefit from a given therapy while others do not.

Under these circumstances, clinicians typically conduct the time-honored "trial of therapy," in which the patient is given a treatment and the subsequent clinical course determines whether the treatment is judged effective and continued. However, many factors may mislead physicians conducting conventional therapeutic trials. They include the placebo effect, the natural history of the illness, the expectations that the clinician and patient have about the treatment effect, and the desire of the patient and the clinician not to disappoint one another. To avoid these pitfalls, clinicians must conduct trials of therapy with safeguards that keep both patients and themselves "blind" to the treatment being administered. Investigators routinely use such safeguards in large-scale RCTs involving dozens or hundreds of patients. To implement these safeguards in a clinically sensible manner while investigating drug effects in the individual patient constitutes a considerable challenge.

METHODOLOGIC PROBLEMS TO BE ADDRESSED BY PHARMACOEPIDEMIOLOGIC RESEARCH

To maintain the methodological safeguards provided by RCTs and to avoid the disadvantages of large sample multicenter studies, we built on the work of experimental psychologists to develop a corresponding methodology for examination of an intervention's effect in individual patients in clinical practice.[3] Any person conducting an RCT in an individual patient (N-of-1 RCT) faces several formidable methodological challenges. The first one is to identify a clinical situation in which an N-of-1 RCT may potentially provide useful information. The second is to assess properly the patient's (and clinician's) willingness to undergo the time and effort consuming process of the N-of-1 RCT. The third is to choose appropriate treatment targets to monitor the effects of therapy (both beneficial and potentially harmful). Once these elements are in place, the clinician–patient team has to design, execute, and analyze the results of the trial. The clinician must carefully think through each of these elements before commencing an N-of-1 RCT.

CURRENTLY AVAILABLE SOLUTIONS

THE GENERAL CASE

The methodology of experimental studies of single patients is known as "single case" or "single subject" research, $N = 1$, or, as we call it, N-of-1 RCTs.[4,5] We have previously described how N-of-1 RCTs may be used in medical practice to determine the optimum treatment of an individual patient, described an "N-of-1 service" designed to assist clinicians who wish to conduct such a trial, provided detailed guidelines for clinicians interested in conducting their own N-of-1 RCTs, and reviewed our own three years' experience in conducting such studies.[6,7] In each of two conditions (chronic airflow limitation and fibromyalgia) we conducted over 20 N-of-1 RCTs, and described our experience with these patients in two separate reports.[8,9]

In general terms, the N-of-1 RCT design is based on pairs of active/placebo, high dose/low dose, or first drug/alternate drug combinations, the order of administration within each pair determined by random allocation (see Figure 43.1). Treatment targets (directed specifically at the patient's complaints) are monitored in a double-blind fashion on a regular, predetermined schedule. The trial continues as long as the clinician and patient agree that they need more information to get a definite answer regarding the efficacy, superiority, or side effects of the treatment, or until the patient or clinician decides for any other reason to end the trial. Experience drawn from conducting numerous N-of-1 RCTs[6–9] indicates that each individual patient trial should usually include at least three treatment pairs. It is unusual to obtain a clear answer from a smaller number of pairs, and three pairs is the minimum for any statistical analysis. Even three pairs will likely limit the strength of inference, and certainly limits the power of any statistical analysis, and if a very short duration of treatment periods is feasible, the number of pairs could be greater.

Several criteria must be satisfied before clinicians begin an N-of-1 RCT. In addition to the effectiveness or harmful side effects of treatment being in doubt, the disorder should be relatively chronic and stable. The treatment, if effective, should be continued relatively long term, and the patient should be eager to collaborate in designing and carrying out the N-of-1 RCT. The treatment(s) must have a rapid onset and termination of action, and the clinician should be aware of the optimal treatment duration, which must be practical. Last but not least, the clinician must secure the cooperation of a pharmacy in the preparation of blinded medication.

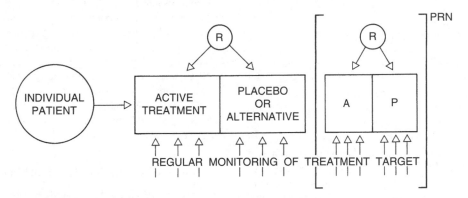

Figure 43.1. *N*-of-1 study design.

CHOOSING APPROPRIATE OUTCOME MEASURES

The choice of the target to be monitored during *N*-of-1 RCTs depends on the clinical context. While one may choose physiological variables as treatment targets (say forced expired volume in one second in an RCT of a bronchodilator, or postural blood pressure change in a trial of amitriptyline in symptomatic postural hypotension), we have little experience in the use of physiological endpoints. When investigators have experimented with use of *N*-of-1 RCTs to sort out physiological responses such as blood pressure they have found intra-individual variability too great. In our experience, *N*-of-1 RCTs are uniquely suitable in sorting out the effects of a given drug on different aspects of health-related quality of life (HRQL; see Chapter 42).

Let us assume that the problem with which the clinician is faced is new onset of pain associated with walking (intermittent claudication) in a patient with peripheral vascular disease. This patient was recently diagnosed with portal hypertension and esophageal varices secondary to liver cirrhosis, and subsequently began taking β-blockers to prevent bleeding from esophageal varices. Now the clinician reads the insert to the β-blocker and confirms what she remembers from medical school: β-blockers may exacerbate the symptoms of peripheral vascular disease. She then finds a meta-analysis that concludes that β-blockers do not have this effect.[10] A clinical dilemma ensues—should the patient (free of symptoms of claudication before being put on the β-blocker) stay on the medication or should it be discontinued? This situation fulfills all the requirements necessary for conduct of an *N*-of-1 RCT: the condition is chronic; the

potential effect of the β-blocker on peripheral vasculature should have rapid onset and termination of action; and the drug, if proven not to cause the troublesome symptoms, will be continued long term.

The clinician should establish the treatment targets most important for the patient before the trial, tailoring the choice to the individual case. The patient may be concerned about his ability to walk a dog, visiting a family who lives on the fourth floor of a building with no elevator, the severity of his discomfort when playing golf, or embarrassment due to other people noticing problems with walking. The clinician must monitor whatever symptoms the patient judges as sufficiently important and troublesome that getting rid of them may be worth about 10% absolute increase in the risk of bleeding during the next 1–2 years that this patient with esophageal varices might expect if the β-blocker is discontinued.

The simplest outcome measure could be the preference for β-blocker or placebo in a pair of treatment periods. If one would like to quantify the degree of symptoms and explore the reasons behind the patient's preference, the response options depend on the nature of the treatment target. We have found seven-point scales an optimal method for recording the severity of symptoms because of their ability to detect small degrees of change, patients' ease in understanding them, and their ease of interpretation.[11] Using a seven-point scale response, for example, one may ask:

Please indicate how much leg discomfort you have been experiencing while playing golf last week by choosing one of the options from the scale below:

1. Extreme discomfort
2. Severe discomfort

3. Quite a lot of discomfort
4. Moderate discomfort
5. Mild discomfort
6. A little discomfort
7. No discomfort at all

Using the taxonomy introduced in the chapter on quality of life studies, we call a set of such questions a disease- and patient-specific questionnaire (see Chapter 42). Other options for monitoring treatment targets include other disease-specific or general quality of life questionnaires.

To summarize our hypothetical example, one could conduct an N-of-1 RCT consisting of three treatment pairs, with each treatment pair including a two-week treatment period on β-blocker and a two-week period on placebo with a 2–4 day transition period of gradually decreasing doses. The patient could complete the outcome measures (a disease- and patient-specific three- to five-item symptom questionnaire) twice during the second week of each treatment period (second week only as the results during the first week could be influenced by the medication taken during the preceding treatment period).

STATISTICAL INTERPRETATION OF THE RESULTS

An Example Trial

To illustrate issues in the interpretation of data from N-of-1 trials, we will use an example of an N-of-1 RCT in which we tested the effectiveness of ipratropium bromide in a dose of four inhalations four times a day (each inhalation 20 micrograms of the drug) in a patient with chronic airflow limitation. Each day, the patient rated the severity of a number of

symptoms, judged by him as important in his daily life. The symptoms included shortness of breath while walking upstairs, playing a musical instrument, drying the dishes, and overall shortness of breath. Each symptom was rated on a seven-point scale in which a higher score represented better function (i.e., "1" = extremely short of breath, . . . , "7" = not at all short of breath). The treatment periods were seven days in length (with measurements obtained during the last five days of each period), and the trial included four pairs of treatment periods. Table 43.1 presents the mean scores for each of the 8 weeks of the study.

Interpreting the Results: Visual Inspection

One way of evaluating these data is by visual inspection. Visual inspection of the data is based on a graphical display of outcome assessments over time and in relation to the treatment being received. A conclusion that the treatment is effective would be supported to the extent that there is minimal variability within periods, that the difference between active and placebo periods is large relative to the within-period variability that is seen, and to the extent that the magnitude of the difference between active and placebo periods is consistent. Using the visual inspection of data one tries to draw conclusions intuitively about the direction, magnitude, and consistency of response to experimental treatment. We invite readers to make conclusions on the basis of the data presented in Table 43.1 and Figure 43.2 before considering a more formal analysis.

Visual inspection is appealing in that it makes intuitive sense to both patient and clinician. Yet, visual inspection is

Table 43.1. Results of an N-of-1 RCT: ipratropium, symptom score (data represent mean score on four questions)

Pair	Treatment	Day 1	Day 2	Day 3	Day 4	Day 5	Treatment mean
1	Placebo	3.25	3.25	3.00	3.00	3.00	3.10
	Active	5.00	5.25	4.75	5.25	5.25	5.10
	Difference						+2.00
2	Placebo	3.75	3.25	3.25	2.75	2.75	3.15
	Active	4.50	4.50	4.75	4.50	4.70	4.59
	Difference						+1.44
3	Placebo	2.75	2.75	3.00	2.25	3.25	2.80
	Active	2.50	3.25	3.25	2.75	3.00	3.15
	Difference						+0.35
4	Placebo	3.00	3.00	2.75	2.75	2.75	2.85
	Active	4.50	4.50	5.00	5.25	—	4.81
	Difference						+1.96
All pairs	Placebo						2.975
	Active						4.413
	Difference						+1.438

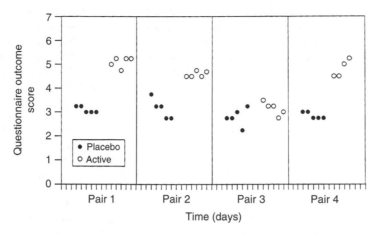

Figure 43.2. Results of an N-of-1 RCT: a visual display of mean daily symptom scores in a trial of ipratropium bromide versus placebo.

subjective and thus may allow inconsistency in the evaluation of intervention effects. Use of the criteria presented above will help reduce subjectivity and thus increase the likelihood of consistent interpretation. However, even experts in visual analysis often disagree about particular data patterns and whether the effects are reliable.[12]

Interpreting the Results: Nonparametric Tests

An alternative approach to analysis of data from N-of-1 RCTs is to utilize a statistical test of significance, and a number of tests are possible candidates. These tests fall into two main classes: nonparametric and parametric tests. The major problematic issue in the interpretation of the results of N-of-1 RCTs is that the errors associated with each data point may be correlated with the errors associated with other data points. This is called "autocorrelation" or "serial dependency," related to the fact that the outcomes are all measures in the same person, and we will address the issue in detail later in the discussion.

Like most statistical comparisons, nonparametric tests start from the hypothesis that treatment has no effect. An apparent effect of treatment observed in an N-of-1 RCT may well be due to a quirk of the order in which treatments were allocated within pairs. To evaluate this possibility, one considers the apparent treatment effects that would result from all other randomized treatment orders that could have occurred. The proportion of randomizations that produce apparent treatment effects as or more extreme than that actually observed is the p-value of the test.

In its simplest form, a randomization test would be based on the direction (i.e., sign) of the observed treatment difference in each pair. One can compute the p-value for the sign test which is appropriate for this form of randomization test from the binomial distribution or it can be obtained from published tables.[13] Using this approach for the analysis of the results of the ipratropium study described above, the first step is to calculate the mean score for each treatment period (presented in the last column of Table 43.1). In each pair of periods, the mean score favored the active treatment. Using the binomial theorem, the probability of this result occurring by chance if the treatment was ineffective is $1/2 \times 1/2 \times 1/2 \times 1/2 = 1/16$ (or 0.0625 for a one-sided test). If one chose to adopt a threshold approach to interpretation (ipratropium works or does not work), one would not reject the null hypothesis that the treatment works if one's threshold were less than 0.0625, and one would reject the null hypothesis if one's threshold were greater than 0.0625.

Two other nonparametric tests that incorporate the size of the outcome score differences are also commonly used. The Wilcoxon signed rank test[14] uses the ranks of score differences. The absolute differences within pairs are first ordered from smallest to largest and ranks given to the difference, then if the two treatments are equivalent we would expect that the sum of ranks for positive differences should equal the sum of negative ranks.

One can utilize a third option, a "pure" quantitative randomization test,[15] by building up the empirical distribution of the difference in mean treatment outcome over all possible randomizations of the observed data. Under the null hypothesis of no systematic difference, the distribution of treatment mean difference would be centered on zero, but particular random treatment orderings would have led to variability in mean difference in both the positive and negative directions. The p-value of the test is again simply the proportion of randomizations that would have led to treatment differences as, or more extreme than, the one actually observed in the trial itself. This randomization test takes into account not only the direction of the difference (as the sign test does) and its relative size (as the signed rank test does), but also its numerical size.

If one uses randomization tests to obtain conventional one-tailed statistical significance one must complete at least five pairs and hope to obtain the most extreme result, because $1/2^5 = 1/32 = 0.0313$, while $1/2^4 = 1/16 = 0.0625$. The advantage of tests that quantify the size of the paired treatment differences rather than just their sign is manifest when one does not observe this extreme result. Whereas the sign test immediately drops to a p-value of 6/32 (0.1875) if only four of five pairs favor active treatment, the signed rank and, particularly, the pure randomization test can yield lower p-values (perhaps as low as 2/32) if the one pair favoring placebo does so only marginally. Thus, the expected p-values associated with an efficacious treatment tend to decrease from the sign test through the signed rank test to the randomization test, as each one is using more information. Tables for the Wilcoxon signed rank test are available,[14] but the randomization test approach depends upon the actual data observed and must be calculated anew (either by hand or with a computer program) for each application.

Interpreting the Data: Parametric Tests

While nonparametric tests are very appealing in the context of an N-of-1 trial, their avoidance of strong distributional assumptions about the data make them relatively conservative compared to tests which make such assumptions. More powerful techniques for normally distributed outcomes, which we will refer to generally as analysis of variance, include analysis of variance itself and, as a special case, the Student's t-test (either in the paired or unpaired forms).

In the ipratropium trial, there were four pairs of treatment periods and five symptom scores per period. If one assumes that the day-to-day fluctuation in outcome within treatment period is simply inherent random variation in the disease process one would call this, in the parlance of analysis of variance, a balanced two-factor crossed design with replication. The factor of interest is treatment, but we must also

allow for possible shifts in mean from one pair of periods to another and thus period pair represents the second factor. Less obvious to the statistical layperson is the need to allow for the possibility of interaction between treatment and period pair. In this situation, the interaction measures the tendency of the treatment effect to vary in size from one period pair to another.

Table 43.2 presents the results of the analysis of variance with the imputed missing value for the final observation of the active treatment period during the fourth pair. The mean square for between pairs measures the variation in mean symptom score between period pairs, the mean square for between treatments reflects consistent differences in mean between active and placebo periods, and the mean square for interaction reflects the variation in active–placebo mean difference over period pairs. It is crucial to realize that period pair is a random factor in this design; in other words, that the four pairs of periods in which the study was run can be thought of as a sample from a much larger population of time periods that could have been used. Because of this, the appropriate test of treatment compares the average difference between active and placebo means to the variability in active–placebo differences over treatment pairs, in the ratio of the mean square treatment to mean square interaction. The resulting F test ($F1$, $3 = 13.99$, $p = 0.033$) is identical to the square of the paired

Table 43.2. Analysis of variance: ipratropium trial symptom scores

Source	Degrees of freedom	Sum of squares	Mean square	F value
Between pairs	3	7.32	2.44	$\frac{2.44}{0.88} = 31.33$ ($p \leq 0.0001$)
Between treatments	1	20.68	20.68	$\frac{20.68}{1.48} = 13.99$ ($p = 0.033$)
Interaction treatment × pairs	3	4.44	1.48	$\frac{1.48}{0.08} = 19.03$ ($p < 0.0001$)
Error	31	2.41	0.08	
Total	38	34.84		
Paired t approach				
Mean	Active–placebo difference		=	1.438
SD	Active–placebo difference)		=	0.7686
t3	= 1.438/(0.7686/4)		=	3.74
[NB	t3 = 14.00]			

Student's *t*-test conducted on the four pairs of treatment means.

One might reasonably question why one should use ANOVA here when the result is identical to the simple and more familiar paired *t*-test. The answer lies in the second test provided by the ANOVA, namely the test of interaction, which is computed as the ratio of the mean square interaction to the mean square error ($F3, 31 = 19.03$, $p < 0.0001$). This formally asks the question, "Is there evidence of extra variation in treatment effect from period pair to period pair over and above what we would expect from the inherent day-to-day variation in symptom score?" If evidence for this extra variation were very weak, we would gain great advantage statistically by comparing the mean square treatments to the mean square error (or even the pooled error incorporating the interaction). Although the numerical size of the *F* would not change much, the gain in degrees of freedom could have an appreciable effect on the *p*-value. In essence, the switch from using the yardstick of the interaction mean square to the error mean square in testing the treatment effect allows us to use the variation in all forty individual observations, rather than only the treatment mean differences in the four pairs of periods.

The ipratropium trial shows relatively strong evidence of extra variation through the test of interaction ($F3, 31 = 19.03$, $p < 0.0001$). Thus, in this particular case, one could have used the simple paired *t*-test. However, we have used this approach in sixteen *N*-of-1 trials to look at serial dependency. We found clear evidence of extra variation in treatment effect over period pairs in about 50% of trials. The additional variation could be a reflection of the long-term ebb and flow of the disease. Alternatively, isolated, short-term, truly random changes in symptom severity could also be responsible. In any case, the presence of the interaction dictates that in the majority of situations, the simple paired ANOVA is not an appropriate approach.

Given that the test of interaction may be of limited power in the context of an *N*-of-1 trial, because of the relatively small number of period pairs, one should err on the side of caution and in general use the more conservative paired *t*-test. However, in those situations where there is no evidence of extra variation (say when the mean square interaction is less than or equal to the mean square error), then one should consider the comparison based upon the pooled error. We acknowledge that many statisticians may be reluctant to accept our position regarding the appropriateness of use of any parametric methods, including the paired *t*-test. More conservative practitioners,

therefore, will restrict themselves to use of nonparametric methods.

Interpreting the Data: Autocorrelation

Large group studies are usually so designed that, within the constraints of the design, the responses of the different patients are statistically independent. On the other hand, data for successive treatment periods for one and the same patient are of the nature of a "time series" and may be serially dependent or "autocorrelated." That is, any individual observation is to some extent a function of the previous observation. Thus, an individual observation may bear a closer relation to an adjacent observation than to an observation much earlier or later in the series. Serial dependency can occur for instance when there is a natural ebb and flow of the severity of the underlying disease process. The lack of independence of individual outcome assessments over time, if present, is important to recognize since it constitutes a serious threat to the valid application of either parametric or nonparametric methods to *N*-of-1 RCTs.

While one can postulate all kinds of biologic reasons why symptom scores could be expected to be correlated from day to day, it is necessary to formally examine many *N*-of-1 trials in similar disease processes to demonstrate empirically the level of dependence. One such investigation has already been reported by Huitema.[16] He reviewed the results of almost 500 *N*-of-1 trials in the behavioral area, and concluded there was very little evidence of important serial dependence. He refers to the widely held belief that autocorrelation is a problem in *N*-of-1 studies as a "myth."

We have conducted a similar analysis in 16 *N*-of-1 trials in patients with a spectrum of medical conditions. The 16 *N*-of-1 RCTs involved repeated outcome assessments during each treatment period, and between three and six pairs of treatment periods. Autocorrelations were estimated from data that have firstly been "detrended" by subtraction of the period mean to produce residual variation. Serial correlation coefficients can be calculated for pairs of residuals that are one time unit apart (i.e., adjacent in time), two units apart, etc. Even if there is no real correlation between successive raw observations, the subtraction of period means will create slight negative correlation among pairs of residuals within a period. This correlation, equal to $1/(k - 1)$ (where k is the number of observations per period), is created by the fact that the sum of residuals within a period must add to zero. One must take this feature into account when examining observed residuals for autocorrelation.

In practice, only the first few autocorrelations need to be investigated. Since one might expect that serial dependency, if present in this type of data, would be in the form of a first order autoregressive process (highest correlation between adjacent observations), one should be sensitive to the appearance of the characteristic exponentially decaying pattern of autocorrelations. We found almost no evidence of autocorrelation of individual assessments over time and reasonable normality for a variety of composite symptom scores and physiologic outcomes (Table 43.3). Although 22 of 64 of the autocorrelations shown in Table 43.3 are greater than 0.2, only 5 of these are statistically significant and only 2 of these are first order correlations. The pattern of autocorrelation is little different from that which would be expected by chance if there were no underlying autocorrelation at all.

While the power of the tests for autocorrelation is limited, the data nevertheless suggest that autocorrelation is the exception rather than the rule. Autocorrelations of 0.2 and higher can alter p-values, so that the true p-value will be greater than the p-value that one observes when one conducts the statistical test.[17] An autocorrelation of 0.2 for instance, will result in a true p-value of 0.089 being associated with an observed p-value of 0.05. However, even if such autocorrelations were present in the individual data, the autocorrelation of the mean scores from each treatment period (which we advocate using in the paired t-test described above) would be substantially lower and unlikely to significantly distort observed p-values.

If one wishes to be reasonably secure in the use of parametric or nonparametric methods that assume no serial dependence in an individual N-of-1 RCT, one can begin by testing for the presence of autocorrelation of the residuals.

In our trial of ipratropium, for instance, the first and second order autocorrelations ($\pm$ standard error) for the symptom data were 0.10 (± 0.11) and -0.06 (± 0.10) respectively. The corresponding figures for the peak flow data were 0.07 (± 0.16) and -0.24 (± 0.16). These autocorrelations are not statistically significant and their magnitude is small. The results therefore support application of standard parametric or nonparametric analysis to the data. Had significant autocorrelation been found, we could have turned to an analytic method applicable for dealing with autocorrelated data from N-of-1 RCTs.[18]

A summary of our viewpoint regarding autocorrelation is as follows. First, in 16 N-of-1 studies we found consistently small magnitudes of autocorrelation. The pattern of the serial dependence observed suggests that most of the autocorrelation was due to the play of chance, rather than a true finding. Although this is a small sample, the results suggest that autocorrelation of large magnitude may be unusual in N-of-1 RCTs. Second, Huitema's study of almost 500 single case studies supports the hypothesis that important correlation is unusual in these experiments. Third, the impact of any autocorrelation would be minimized by using mean scores from each period and by the paired design. Fourth, if concern regarding autocorrelation remains, the data from an individual study should be tested to determine the extent of autocorrelation.

CLINICAL INTERPRETATION OF THE RESULTS

We have touched on the problem of interpreting the results of studies using HRQL measurements in assessing the effectiveness of therapeutic interventions in the quality of life chapter in this book (see Chapter 42). In that chapter we noted that, while conducting classical (multi-subject) RCTs and measuring symptoms on a seven-point scale, we have noted that a difference of 0.5 points per question approximates the smallest important difference. This observation was made when the minimal important difference was defined as the smallest difference in score in the domain of interest which patients perceive as a change and which would mandate, in the absence of troublesome side effects and excessive cost, modification in the patient's management. While the clinician would participate in the decision regarding modification of management, the definition otherwise focuses on the patient's experience. This follows from a conceptual or philosophical perspective that sees quality of life as part of an individual's subjective experience.

Conducting N-of-1 RCTs provides an opportunity to define the size of the minimally important difference and

Table 43.3. Number of N-of-1 RCTs showing varying magnitude of autocorrelation

Degree of separation	Magnitude of autocorrelation				
	≤0.1	>0.1–≤0.2	>0.2–≤0.3	>0.3–≤0.4	>0.4
+1	7/16	3/16	2/16	2/16[a]	2/16[a]
+2	5/16	7/16	2/16	2/16	0/16
+3	4/16	8/16	3/16	1/16	0/16
+4	5/16	3/16	4/16	3/16[b]	1/16[a]

No correlations reach conventional levels of statistical significance unless otherwise stated.
[a] One of these correlations reached conventional levels of statistical significance ($p < 0.05$).
[b] Two of these correlations reached conventional levels of statistical significance ($p < 0.05$).

other effect sizes. The strategy that we have used in the N-of-1 RCTs performed to date could be summarized as follows.[19]

All these N-of-1 RCTs were designed to examine the efficacy of specific interventions in ameliorating symptoms due to a variety of conditions. The primary outcome measure in each N-of-1 RCT was an HRQL questionnaire measuring the severity of symptoms identified by patients as related to their disease and important in their day-to-day life. The operational definition of the minimal important difference that we used was the smallest difference that was important enough that patients would choose to continue indefinitely with the intervention.

We conducted each trial according to the principles outlined in the previous sections. To assess drug efficacy and side effects, we constructed an individualized questionnaire examining the severity of symptoms identified by patients as part of their disease and as being important in their day-to-day life. We identified the symptoms to be measured from detailed patient interviews in which we elicited patients' experience of the illness or the drug, and what bothered them most. The questionnaires that followed consisted of four to seven items (symptoms), with severity of symptoms measured on a seven-point scale (see previously presented response option example). We calculated the difference in the mean score per question between treatment periods for each treatment pair.

To directly assess the patient's perception of the drug's effect, we asked the following questions after each pair of treatment periods:

Overall, in which of the two periods did you feel better?

1. First period
2. Second period
3. No difference.

If the patient expressed a preference on the above question we then asked:

Would you continue drug A indefinitely if it was actually drug A that made you feel better?

1. Yes
2. No.

When the patient answered *yes* to the above question we asked her/him to provide us with the magnitude of the drug effect by asking the following question (global rating):

If it turns out that you felt better during the period in which you were on drug A, we would like you to rate how important the difference between the two periods is to you:

1. Not important
2. Slight importance
3. Some importance, consistent benefit
4. Moderate importance, consistent benefit
5. Much importance, good deal of benefit
6. Very important
7. Great importance.

A global rating score of 0 was assigned if the patient indicated that there was no difference between periods, or if the observed difference was not sufficient to make him or her take the drug indefinitely.

We subsequently examined the relation between patients' subjective assessment of drug efficacy (global rating) and differences in the quality of life questionnaire score in every pair of every N-of-1 RCT in which data were available. As different questionnaires included from four to seven questions, the difference in the HRQL score was expressed as the total difference in score divided by the number of questions in a particular questionnaire. The minimal important difference was defined as the difference in the questionnaire score corresponding to a small degree of importance (answers 1 to 3 on the global rating), moderate benefit as differences corresponding to answers 4 or 5, and large benefit as differences corresponding to answers 6 or 7.

To help understand the significance of different changes in questionnaire score, we calculated the mean differences on the HRQL questionnaire score in patients who told us they had experienced small, moderate, and large changes using the global rating. A mean difference of 0.29 points per question in HRQL questionnaire score corresponded to a global rating of a small degree of change—the minimal important difference. Differences of approximately 0.66 points per question corresponded to the moderate difference by the global rating; differences of about 1.09 points per question represented a marked difference.[19] We have found similar results in the setting of quality of life measurement in conventional multi-patient studies using a variety of interventions, though the difference corresponding to a minimal important difference has tended to be somewhat higher (around 0.5).[20–23]

While analyzing the size of minimal important difference in the setting of N-of-1 RCTs, we observed large between-patient variability in the changes in symptom questionnaire score, corresponding to varying estimates of drug efficacy. Some portion of this variability is certainly due to the less than perfect validity of the independent standard (in this case, the global rating of drug efficacy). However, it is likely that patients have different standards about the changes in symptoms that they view as important or trivial.

Physiological measures also display the same variability in the clinical significance of a particular change in score or value. On the other hand, establishing the range of changes in score that correspond to small, medium, and large effects across a group of patients undergoing N-of-1 RCTs and confirming that these changes conform to the previous estimates[20] provided us with information allowing meaningful interpretation of study results and was useful in the planning of future studies.

PRACTICAL ASPECTS

Collaboration with a Pharmacy

Conducting an N-of-1 RCT that incorporates the appropriate safeguards against bias and misinterpretation can be challenging. Usually, the clinician requires collaboration with a pharmacist or pharmacy service. Preparation of placebos identical to the active medication in appearance, taste, and texture is required. Occasionally, pharmaceutical firms can supply such placebos. More often, however, clinicians must collaborate with a local pharmacist to repackage the active medication; if it comes in pill form, it can be crushed and repackaged in capsule form. Identical appearing placebo capsules can be filled with lactose. While somewhat time consuming, preparation of placebos is not technically difficult. Our own average cost for preparing medication for N-of-1 studies in which placebos have not been available from the drug's manufacturer has been $125. The pharmacist is also generally charged with preparing the randomization schedule (which requires nothing more than a "coin toss" for each pair of treatment periods). This allows the clinician, along with the patient, to remain blind to allocation.

The pharmacist may also be helpful in planning the design of the trial through knowledge of the drug's action and the washout period needed, thus helping with decisions about the duration of study periods. The pharmacist can also help monitor compliance and drug absorption. Both pill counts and the drawing of serum drug levels at the end of each treatment period can help establish that the patient is taking the study medication conscientiously throughout the trial.

Ethics of an N-of-1 RCT

Is the conduct of an N-of-1 RCT a clinical or a research undertaking? If the former, is it the sort of clinical procedure, analogous to an invasive diagnostic test, that requires written informed consent? We would argue that the N-of-1 RCT

could, and should, be a part of routine clinical practice. Irrespective of one's point of view on this matter, a number of ethical issues are important. We believe that patients should be fully informed of the nature of the study in which they are participating, and there should be no element of deception in the use of placebos as part of the study. Clinicians should obtain consent, which can be verbal and documented in the clinical medical record. This may be perfectly adequate, though we prefer to obtain written informed consent for all N-of-1 RCTs (the consent form we use is presented in the Appendix). The consent in the Appendix will not be acceptable for research purposes, and may be too complex for some patients—we provide it only as an example that we have used with considerable success. Patients should be aware that they could terminate the trial at any time without jeopardizing their care or their relationship with their physician. Finally, follow-up should be close enough to prevent any important deleterious consequences of initiation or withdrawal of therapy.

All these considerations suggest that setting up an N-of-1 trial can involve a substantial amount of effort. One must explain the endeavor fully to the patient, obtain informed consent, construct the outcome questionnaire, negotiate with the pharmacist regarding preparation of medication, carry out the study, and conduct the analysis. These challenges may seem formidable to the busy clinician. Nevertheless, with effort, they can be managed.[24–26]

If an N-of-1 RCT is undertaken as part of a research endeavor, Institutional Review Board (IRB) approval is necessary. Whatever definition of research one uses, one could mount arguments for or against a particular N-of-1 RCT constituting a piece of research. As a result, a safe approach would be to take each individual N-of-1 RCT before one's local IRB. The IRB may then, as ours did at McMaster, grant blanket approval for all N-of-1 RCTs that follow specified procedures and principles. If an IRB decides an N-of-1 RCT is a research undertaking then clinicians subject to HIPAA must follow HIPAA requirements.

EXPLORING NEW DRUG USE

The Conventional Approach

In the preceding sections, we described the application of N-of-1 RCTs in deciding about optimal therapy in individual patients. The concept of N-of-1 RCTs, however, could also be used to draw more general conclusions regarding drug efficacy. The main role for this methodology is likely in the early, premarketing stages of drug development (Phase II),[27] but the same principles may apply in the postmarketing phase while exploring new areas of possible drug utilization—using different doses, examining the effects in different populations, or investigating previously unrecognized beneficial actions or side effects.

Let us use as an example the hypothetical observation that a long-used antidepressant medication (drug A) improves itching associated with renal failure. Although this example is hypothetical, it is not inconceivable; recall amantadine's use in Parkinson's disease, β-blockers in familial tremor, or amitriptyline in fibrositis, chronic pain, or diabetic neuropathy. Now, the investigators wish to compare drug A with currently used modes of therapy. In large sample parallel group trials, patients are assigned at random to drug A or an alternative drug (say, an antihistamine). The treatment groups are followed and the treatment target monitored. These trials are the standard approach to establishing drug efficacy, and to persuading regulatory agencies that a new medication should be placed on the market or a new indication for an old medication accepted.

There are three major hurdles that need to be overcome before such large sample parallel group studies of the efficacy and safety of a drug can be undertaken. First, investigators must determine whether the drug shows sufficient promise to justify the initiation of a large clinical research program. Second, they must define the patient population to be studied. Third, they must establish the dose regimen to be used in the major trials.

These decisions are generally based on findings from early clinical safety, tolerance, pharmacology, and drug disposition studies in healthy volunteers and patients, augmented by information gained from initial small-scale efficacy studies. These efficacy studies are often open, and use baseline status or a historical reference group as a control. Such studies tend to yield anecdotal information of questionable validity. Investigators may use classical double blind randomized parallel group studies in the early exploration of drug properties, but their small sample size results in findings that leave considerable uncertainty about the answers to the three key questions described above.

Thus, when designing the first large-sample efficacy study, investigators face difficult decisions concerning both dose regimen and sample selection. They may gamble on a single dose (with a possibility of suboptimal efficacy with too small a dose or excessive side effects with too large a dose), or take a safer approach that includes two or more different regimens for comparison. At the same time, they may hazard a guess at a suitable homogeneous target population of patients, or take a more conservative approach that includes a heterogeneous (possibly stratified) population.

If the investigators decide to gamble or guess and turn out to be wrong, the large-sample efficacy study misfires. Nevertheless, the choice for gambling and guessing is frequently made. The reason is that, even with a well-defined, homogeneous patient population, a parallel group study of a single dose of a new drug often requires large numbers of patients for adequate statistical power. The extra numbers required for a heterogeneous patient population and/or several different dosage regimens might well be considered prohibitive.

Even if, through good luck or sound judgment, the first large-sample efficacy study is successful and the study population is clearly shown to benefit from the selected dosage of the new drug, important questions are likely to remain. Would an equivalent benefit have been obtained at lower doses, or would there be additional benefit with higher doses? Will the use of lower dose allow preservation of drug benefit with reduced side effects? Are there subgroups of patients who are particularly responsive or resistant to the new drug?

Several successive rounds of large-sample parallel group studies may well fail to provide clear-cut answers. One reason is that in such studies, there is usually much uncontrolled variation among patients. The result of this variation is that the determination of the profiles of responsive and drug resistant subpopulations of patients is hindered and at times rendered impossible.

The Role of *N*-of-1 RCTs

N-of-1 trials share many features in common with the traditional crossover trials used in drug evaluation. The fundamental difference between the *N*-of-1 approach and traditional crossover trials is their primary purpose: *N*-of-1 trials attempt to establish effects in an individual, whereas crossover trials attempt to establish effects in a group. As a secondary goal, one may use a crossover trial to examine individual responses. Similarly, one may analyze a series of *N*-of-1 trials with a similar design as a multiple crossover trial. However, the *N*-of-1 trial will be designed so that individual effects can be reliably detected; the crossover trial will be designed so that individual estimates of response are imprecisely estimated but the magnitude of the average group effect can be efficiently determined.

In some therapeutic indications (including our hypothetical example of itch), the problems faced by investigators involved in drug development may be overcome by including in the program a short series of carefully designed N-of-1 RCTs. These studies will permit the reliable identification of responders and non-responders to the new treatment and an estimate of the proportion of patients in each category. They may also make it possible to determine the optimal dosage regimen for individual patients. The availability of this type of information makes the design of large-scale parallel group studies less problematic.

In relating the foregoing example to the general use of N-of-1 RCTs in drug development, we will deal in turn with the following seven issues: (i) the role of an open run-in period, (ii) determining the rapidity of onset of drug action, (iii) optimizing dose, (iv) measuring outcome, (v) assessing potential drug impact, (vi) predicting response, and (vii) confirming side effects.

The Role of an Open Run-In Period

To increase the efficiency of generating data in drug development (or in the exploration of a new indication), one could argue for first conducting formal N-of-1 RCTs only among patients who showed an apparent benefit during an open run-in period. Then, only responders in N-of-1 trials would be included in subsequent large-sample parallel group studies. In open therapeutic trials—that is, trials of medication when both patient and clinician are aware that the patient is taking active medication—potential biases are likely to favor a false positive conclusion. These biases include patient and physician expectations and the benefit that patients sometimes experience when they believe that they are taking a beneficial intervention—the so-called placebo effect. Thus, a false positive conclusion (concluding the drug works better when actually it does not) may be more likely than a false negative conclusion (concluding the drug does not work when in fact it does).

Accordingly, it would be reasonable to conduct formal N-of-1 studies only on the subgroup of patients with apparent benefit from a new drug in open trials. Investigators used this approach in evaluating oral ketamine in patients with chronic pain.[28] In this study, only 9 out of 21 patients proceeded to formal N-of-1 trial, with the remaining 12 having either no response or intolerable side effects during an open run-in period. Obviously, any estimates of the degree to which patients prefer drug A over drug B then have to take into account that only potential respondents were included in the formal evaluation. While one may question the ethics

of including someone with a positive response in the open trial in a subsequent N-of-1, the high frequency of negative N-of-1 trials under these circumstances leaves us uncomfortable with assuming that anything other than the largest and most compelling responses in an open trial are biological responses to the intervention.

Determining the Rapidity of Onset and Termination of Action

Conducting visual and statistical analyses of the data generated while obtaining numerous measurements during each treatment period in an N-of-1 RCT may help in determining the rapidity of the onset and termination of the treatment effect.[29] One may incorporate this knowledge into the design of subsequent N-of-1 RCTs and large-sample parallel group studies may then incorporate this knowledge. Precise information about the rapidity of action may also add to the understanding of the drug's mechanism of action—a drug exerting its action within minutes of administration and another drug starting to act only after days of use are likely to have different biological modes of action.

Optimizing Dose

When one does not know the optimal dose of a drug, one option is to allow open, unblinded dose titration to obtain a response in the individual patient. One of many alternative approaches would be to conduct an N-of-1 RCT, beginning with the lowest plausible effective dose of the new drug. If the first pair or set of pairs showed superiority of drug B (the accepted method of treatment), a higher dose of drug A could be used in the next pair. The process could continue until side effects appeared, the highest acceptable dose of drug A was reached, or a difference in favor of drug A emerged. This last observation could be confirmed by conducting additional pairs of treatment in the same patient on the apparently favorable dose of drug A. This approach would not only help determine the optimal dose, but would reveal whether this optimal dose differed among different patients, an issue that would be very difficult to elucidate using parallel group studies. In addition, it would be possible to modify the doses used after only a few N-of-1 trials, if a high incidence of toxicity (use lower doses) or a low incidence of response (use higher doses) were found.

Measurement of Outcome

In the initial study of a drug in a new setting, investigators may be uncertain about the outcomes upon which to focus.

This is particularly true if the primary outcomes relate to patients' symptoms, and if the condition being treated (or the treatment) results in a spectrum of problems. For example, an antidepressant used for itchiness may have differential impact on the primary complaint, mood, and a number of possible side effects, including problems with vision, dry mouth, and constipation (some of which may be idiosyncratic to people with renal failure). These differences may become apparent in the initial positive *N*-of-1 RCTs, giving the investigator an opportunity to shift the focus of outcome measurement to the areas most likely to show benefit or to important side effects.

Assessing Potential Drug Impact

Once a number of *N*-of-1 trials have been conducted, one is in a position to evaluate the potential impact of the medication. If only 1 out of 20 patients has an *N*-of-1 RCT that shows drug A relatively superior, the drug may not be worth further development; if 15 out of 20 patients favor a new drug, one clearly has an important new treatment. Between such extremes, the decision concerning further study of the drug will depend on factors such as the prevalence of the condition being treated, its associated morbidity, the expense and toxicity of the treatment, and the availability of other effective treatments. If a condition is of major importance to a relatively large population of patients, and if the drug (at the doses used) is inexpensive and nontoxic (both of which would be true for the use of amitriptyline in renal failure-induced itchiness), a 25% response rate likely suggests an important role for the medication. In a condition that results in severe morbidity and for which there is no other treatment, the use of an inexpensive and nontoxic drug might be worth exploring and using even if only a small proportion of patients gained a clinically important benefit.

If initial *N*-of-1 RCTs suggest further study is warranted, the results can help in planning subsequent investigations. For example, sample size for a parallel groups study can be informed by prior *N*-of-1 RCTs which provide accurate information concerning both within-person variability over time and heterogeneity of treatment response. The lower the response rate in preceding *N*-of-1 RCTs, the larger the sample size required in subsequent parallel group designs to detect the desired clinically important difference.

Predicting Response

N-of-1 RCTs can also help determine eligibility criteria for subsequent studies. The precise identification of responders and non-responders to therapy allows powerful examination of predictors of response. If there is very little overlap between responders and non-responders (for example, if virtually all people on peritoneal dialysis respond and all those on hemodialysis do not), a small number of *N*-of-1 RCTs will allow identification of variables associated with response. If a larger number of *N*-of-1 RCTs have been completed, weaker predictors may also be identified.

Identifying variables associated with response is important for clinicians in deciding when to use a drug. In addition, the ability of *N*-of-1 RCTs to define responders precisely may provide a solution to one of the major dilemmas facing those exploring the use of a drug in a new situation: choosing the population for the first large-sample parallel groups RCT.

Confirming Side Effects

Clinicians from a Drug Safety Clinic in Toronto, Ontario have described the use of *N*-of-1 RCTs to confirm or reject the causal role of medications in producing side effects. These investigators found blinding and randomization helpful in the management of patients with nonspecific symptomatology potentially attributable to drug ingestion.[30]

In summary, *N*-of-1 RCTs have a potentially important role to play in the development of new drugs or in explorations of the use of an old drug in a new clinical situation. Information regarding rapidity of onset and termination of drug action, the optimal dose, the outcomes on which to focus, and predictors of response may be obtained most efficiently using *N*-of-1 RCTs. The ultimate impact of a medication can be thus assessed early in the process of clinical testing.

THE FUTURE

We have previously reported our experience with the use of *N*-of-1 methodology and found that the method is able to aid in resolution of difficult clinical dilemmas; that, based on the results of *N*-of-1 trials, treatment frequently changes; and that, with long-term follow-up, physicians continue to follow the conclusions based on the *N*-of-1 RCT results.[7] In addition to Larson's work, which we have already cited, other clinical groups have reported on their experience with *N*-of-1 RCTs, generally confirming the feasibility and usefulness of the approach.[31–43] Some of these studies have reinforced the potential for a series of *N*-of-1 RCTs to simultaneously provide information about individuals, and about the effectiveness of particular agents in groups of individuals.[39] Patients who undergo *N*-of-1 RCTs are better off than those whose treatment regimen is determined by conventional methods. The most rigorous test of the usefulness of *N*-of-1 RCTs would be a randomized trial. Three such trials, in which investigators randomized patients to conventional care or to undergo *N*-of-1 RCTs, have addressed the impact of *N*-of-1 RCTs.[44–46] The same group of investigators conducted two of these studies; both examined the use of theophylline in patients with chronic airflow limitation. The investigators found that, while using *N*-of-1 RCTs did not affect patients' quality of life or functional status, of patients initially on theophylline, fewer in the *N*-of-1 RCT groups ended up receiving the drug in the long term. Thus, *N*-of-1 RCTs saved patients the expense, inconvenience, and potential toxicity of long-term theophylline therapy of no use to them.

The third trial randomized 27 patients with osteoarthritis who were uncertain of the additional benefit of a nonsteroidal anti-inflammatory in alleviating their pain to conventional management, and another 24 similar patients to undergo an *N*-of-1 randomized trial comparing diclofenac and misoprostol (the latter agent to avoid gastrointestinal side effects) to placebo.[46] The results showed few differences between groups (similar proportion of patients ended up taking diclofenac, similar quality of life) though all quality of life measures showed trends in favor of the *N*-of-1 arm. Costs were higher in the *N*-of-1 arm. These results suggest that *N*-of-1 RCTs are unlikely to be uniformly superior to conventional trials. If we are ever to understand when *N*-of-1 RCTs will benefit patients, considerable further study will be required.

While confirming the potential of *N*-of-1 RCTs, groups with extensive experience with *N*-of-1 RCTs have noted the time and effort required. It is unlikely that full implementation of *N*-of-1 RCTs will become a major part of clinical practice. Clinicians can, however, incorporate many of the key principles of *N*-of-1 RCTs into their practice without adopting the full rigor of the approach presented here. Medication can be repeatedly withdrawn and reintroduced in an open or unmasked fashion. Symptoms and physical findings can be carefully quantified. However, without the additional feature of double blinding, both the placebo effect and physician and patient expectations can still bias the results.

In summary, the *N*-of-1 approach clearly has potential for improving the quality of medical care and the judicious use of expensive and potentially toxic medication in patients with chronic disease. Using the guidelines offered here, we believe that clinicians will find the conduct of *N*-of-1 RCTs feasible, highly informative, and stimulating.

APPENDIX: CONSENT FORM FOR *N*-OF-1 RANDOMIZED TRIALS

Often, doctors and patients try to decide what treatment is best by starting a particular drug and seeing if it makes the patient feel better. Unfortunately, the results of such "therapeutic trials," as we call them, are often misleading. The patient may have gotten better anyway, even without any medication. Or, the doctor and the patient may be so optimistic that they may misinterpret the results of the therapeutic trial. Finally, people often feel better when they are taking new medication even when it doesn't have any specific activity against their illness (the placebo effect), and this may also lead to a misleading interpretation of the value of the new treatment.

We believe we have developed a better way of conducting therapeutic trials. In this new approach, the patient alternates between taking active drug and placebo. The placebo is a medication that looks identical, but doesn't contain the active ingredient. While taking the active and placebo medication the patient keeps careful track of how he or she is feeling. Neither the doctor nor the patient knows when the patient is taking the active drug and when the patient is taking the placebo. After several periods on both active and placebo medication the "code" is broken and the patient and the doctor then look at the results. Together, they decide whether the drug is of any benefit and should be continued.

We think that it would help you to take part in one of these therapeutic trials of [NAME OF DRUG] —————. We will conduct a number of pairs of periods. Each period will be [DURATION OF PERIOD] —————. During one period of each pair you will be taking the active treatment, and during the other you will be using the placebo. If at any time during the study you are feeling worse we can consider that treatment period at an end and can go on to the next treatment. Therefore, if you begin to feel worse, just call my office at [INSERT NUMBER] and I will get in touch with you.

If you don't think this new way of conducting a therapeutic trial is a good idea for you, we will try the new drug in the usual way. Your decision will not interfere with your treatment in any way. You can decide to stop the trial any time along the way, and this will not interfere with your treatment either. All information we collect during the trial will remain confidential.

PATIENT SIGNATURE —————

WITNESS SIGNATURE —————

PHYSICIAN SIGNATURE —————

DATE —————

REFERENCES

1. Guyatt G, Cook D, Devereaux PJ, Meade M, Straus S. Therapy. In: Guyatt G, Rennie D, eds, *The Users' Guides to the Medical Literature: A Manual for Evidence-Based Clinical Practice.* Chicago, IL: AMA, 2002.

2. Dans A, McAlister F, Dans L, Richardson WS, Straus S, Guyatt G. Applying results to individual patients. In: Guyatt G, Rennie D, eds, *The Users' Guides to the Medical Literature: A Manual for Evidence-Based Clinical Practice.* Chicago, IL: AMA, 2002.

3. Guyatt GH, Sackett D, Taylor DW, Chong J, Roberts R, Pugsley S. Determining optimal therapy: randomized trials in individual patients. *N Engl J Med* 1986; **314**: 889–92.

4. Kratchwill TR. *Single Subject Research: Strategies for Evaluating Change.* Orlando, FL: Academic Press, 1978.

5. Kazdin AE. *Single-Case Research Designs: Methods for Clinical and Applied Settings.* New York: Oxford University Press, 1982.

6. Guyatt GH, Sackett DL, Adachi JD, Roberts RS, Chong J, Rosenbloom D *et al.* A clinician's guide for conducting randomized trials in individual patients. *Can Med Assoc J* 1988; **139**: 497–503.

7. Guyatt GH, Keller JL, Jaeschke R, Rosenbloom R, Adachi JD, Newhouse MT. Clinical usefulness of the N of 1 randomized control trials: three year experience. *Ann Intern Med* 1990; **112**: 293–9.

8. Jaeschke R, Adachi JD, Guyatt GH, Keller JL, Wong B. Clinical usefulness of amitryptiline in fibromyalgia: the results of 23 randomized controlled trials. *J Rheumatol* 1991; **18**: 226S–33S.

9. Patel A, Jaeschke R, Guyatt G, Newhouse MT, Keller J. Clinical usefulness of N-of-1 RCTs in patients with chronic airflow limitation. *Am Rev Respir Dis* 1991; **144**: 962–4.

10. Radack K, Deck C. Beta-adrenergic blocker therapy does not worsen intermittent claudication in subjects with peripheral arterial disease. A meta-analysis of randomized controlled trials. *Arch Intern Med* 1991; **151**: 1769–76.

11. Jaeschke R, Singer J, Guyatt GH. A comparison of 7 point and visual analogue scales: data from a randomized trial. *Control Clin Trials* 1990; **11**: 43–51.

12. DeProspero A, Cohen S. Inconsistent visual analysis of intrasubject data. *J Appl Behav Anal* 1979; **12**: 573–9.

13. Beyer WH, ed., *CRC Handbook of Tables for Probability and Statistics,* 2nd edn. Cleveland, OH: Chemical Research Co., 1968.

14. Conover WJ. *Practical Nonparametric Statistics.* New York: John Wiley & Sons, 1971; pp. 206–15.

15. Edgington ES. *Randomization Tests,* 2nd edn. New York: Marcel Dekker, 1987.

16. Huitema BE. Autocorrelation in applied behavior analysis: a myth. *Behav Assess* 1985; **7**: 107–18.

17. Gastwirth JL, Bubin H. Effect of dependence on level of significance of a one sample test. *J Am Stat Assoc* 1971; **66**: 816–20.

18. Rochon J. A statistical model for the "N-of-1" study. *J Clin Epidemiol* 1990; **43**: 499–508.

19. Jaeschke R, Guyatt GH, Keller J, Singer J. Interpreting changes in quality-of-life score in *N* of 1 randomized trials. *Control Clin Trials* 1991; **12** (suppl): 226S–33S.

20. Jaeschke R, Guyatt G, Keller J, Singer J. Measurement of health status: ascertaining the meaning of a change in quality-of-life questionnaire score. *Control Clin Trials* 1989; **10**: 407–15.

21. Juniper EF, Guyatt GH, Willan A, Griffith LE. Determining a minimal important change in a disease-specific quality-of-life questionnaire. *J Clin Epidemiol* 1994; **47**: 81–7.

22. Juniper EF, Guyatt GH, Griffith LE, Ferrie PJ. Interpretation of rhinoconjunctivitis quality-of-life questionnaire data. *J Allergy Clin Immunol* 1996; **98**: 843–5.

23. Juniper EF, Guyatt GH, Feeny DH, Ferrie PJ, Griffith LE, Townsend M. Measuring quality-of-life in children with asthma. *Qual Life Res* 1996; **5**: 35–46.

24. Keller JL, Guyatt GH, Roberts RS, Adachi JD, Rosenbloom D. An *N*-of-1 service: applying the scientific method in clinical practice. *Scand J Gastroenterol* 1988; **23**: 22–9.

25. Larson EB. *N*-of-1 clinical trials. A technique for improving medical therapeutics. *West J Med* 1990; **152**: 52–6.

26. Larson EB, Ellsworth AJ, Oas J. Randomized clinical trials in single patients during a two-year period. *JAMA* 1993; **270**: 2708–12.

27. Guyatt GH, Heyting A, Jaeschke R, Keller J, Adachi JD, Roberts RS. *N*-of-1 trials for investigating new drugs. *Control Clin Trials* 1990; **11**: 88–100.

28. Haines DR, Gaines SP. *N* of 1 randomised controlled trials of oral ketamine in patients with chronic pain. *Pain* 1999; **83**: 283–7.

29. Chatellier G, Day M, Bobrie G, Menard J. Feasibility study of *N*-of-1 trials with blood pressure self-monitoring in hypertension. *Hypertension* 1995; **25**: 294–301.

30. Knowles SR, Uetrecht JP, Shear NH. Confirming false adverse reactions to drug by performing individualized, randomized trials. *Can J Clin Pharmacol* 2002; **9**: 149–53.

31. Menard J, Serrurier D, Bautier P, Plouin PF, Corvol P. Crossover design to test antihypertensive drugs with self-recorded blood pressure. *Hypertension* 1988; **11**: 153–9.

32. Johannessen T. Controlled trials in single subjects. 1. Value in clinical medicine. *BMJ* 1991; **303**: 173–4.

33. Nikles CJ, Glasziou PP, Del Mar CB, Duggan CM, Mitchell G. *N* of 1 trials. Practical tools for medication management. *Aust Fam Physician* 2000; **29**: 1108–12.

34. Notcutt W, Price M, Miller R, Newport S, Phillips C, Simmons S, Sansom C. Initial experiences with medicinal extracts of cannabis for chronic pain: results from 34 '*N* of 1' studies. *Anaesthesia* 2004; **59**: 440–52.

35. Wegman AC, van der Windt DA, de Haan M, Deville WL, Fo CT, de Vries TP. Switching from NSAIDs to paracetamol: a series of *n* of 1 trials for individual patients with osteoarthritis. *Ann RheumDis* 2003; **62**: 1156–61.

36. Price JD, Grimley Evans J. An *N*-of-1 randomized controlled trial ('*N*-of-1 trial') of donepezil in the treatment of non-progressive amnestic syndrome. *Age Ageing* 2002; **31**: 307–9.

37. Jansen IH, Olde Rikkert MG, Hulsbos HA, Hoefnagels WH. Toward individualized evidence-based medicine: five "*N* of 1" trials of methylphenidate in geriatric patients. *J Am Geriatr Soc* 2001; **49**: 474–6.

38. Duggan CM, Mitchell G, Nikles CJ, Glasziou PP, Del Mar CB, Clavarino A. Managing ADHD in general practice. *N* of 1 trials can help! *Aust Fam Physician* 2002; **29**: 1205–9.

39. Coxeter PD, Schluter PJ, Eastwood HL, Nikles CJ, Glasziou PP. Valerian does not appear to reduce symptoms for patients with chronic insomnia in general practice using a series of randomised *n*-of-1 trials. *Complement Ther Med* 2003; **11**: 215–22.

40. Hart A, Sutton CJ. *N*-of-1 trials and their combination: suitable approaches for CAM research? *Complement Ther Med* 2003; **11**: 213–14.

41. Peloso PM. Are individual patient trials (*n*-of-1 trials) in rheumatology worth the extra effort? *J Rheumatol* 2004; **31**: 8–11.

42. Price JD, Grimley Evans J. *N*-of-1 randomized controlled trials ('*N*-of-1 trials'): singularly useful in geriatric medicine. *Age Ageing* 2002; **31**: 227–32.

43. Karnon J, Qizilbash N. Economic evaluation alongside *n*-of-1 trials: getting closer to the margin. *Health Econ* 2001; **10**: 79–82.

44. Mahon J, Laupacis A, Donner A, Wood T. Randomised study of n of 1 trials versus standard practice. *BMJ* 1996; **312**: 1069–74.

45. Mahon J, Laupacis A, Hodder RV, McKim DA, Paterson NA, Wood TE *et al.* Theophylline for irreversible chronic airflow limitation: a randomized study comparing *n* of 1 trials to standard practice. *Chest* 1999; **115**: 38–48.

46. Pope JE, Prashker M, Anderson J. The efficacy and cost effectiveness of *N* of 1 studies with diclofenac compared to standard treatment with nonsteroidal anti-inflammatory drugs in osteoarthritis. *J Rheumatol* 2004; **31**: 140–9.

44

The Use of Meta-analysis in Pharmacoepidemiology

JESSE A. BERLIN and CARIN J. KIM

University of Pennsylvania School of Medicine, Philadelphia, Pennsylvania, USA.

INTRODUCTION

DEFINITIONS

Meta-analysis has been defined as "the statistical analysis of a collection of analytic results for the purpose of integrating the findings."[1] Other definitions have included qualitative, as well as quantitative, analyses.[2] Meta-analysis is used to identify sources of variation among study findings and, when appropriate, to provide an overall measure of effect as a summary of those findings.[3] While epidemiologists have been cautious about adopting meta-analysis, because of the inherent biases in the component studies and the great diversity in study designs and populations,[4–6] the need to make the most efficient and intelligent use of existing data prior to (or instead of) embarking on a large, primary data collection effort has dictated a progressively more accepting approach.[6–12] Meta-analysis of randomized clinical trials has found such wide acceptance that an entire international organization, the Cochrane Collaboration, has been built around the performance and updating of meta-analyses of trials.[13] Cochrane Reviews are maintained in a publicly available electronic library. More information is available on the Cochrane web site (http://www.cochrane.org). A similar structure has developed in the social sciences, in the form of the Campbell Collaboration.[14]

Meta-analysis may be regarded as a "state-of-the-art" literature review, employing statistical methods in conjunction with a thorough and systematic qualitative review.[15] The distinguishing feature of meta-analysis, as opposed to the usual qualitative literature review, is its systematic, structured, and presumably objective presentation and analysis of available data. The traditional review has been increasingly recognized as being subjective.[15–18] With the support of leading scientists[19] and journal editors,[20] there has been growing acceptance of the concept that the literature review can be approached as a more rigorous scientific endeavor, specifically, an observational study with the same requirements for planning, prespecification of definitions, use of eligibility definitions, etc., as any other observational study. In recent years, the terms "research synthesis" and "systematic review" have been used to describe the structured review process in general, while "meta-analysis" has been

Pharmacoepidemiology, Fourth Edition   Edited by B.L. Strom
© 2005 John Wiley & Sons, Ltd

reserved for the quantitative aspects of the process. For the purposes of this chapter, we shall use "meta-analysis" in the more general sense. Meta-analysis provides the conceptual and quantitative framework for such rigorous literature reviews; similar measures from comparable studies are tabulated systematically and the effect measures are combined when appropriate.

Several activities may be included under the above definition of meta-analysis. Perhaps the most popular conception of meta-analysis, for most clinically oriented researchers, is the summary of a group of randomized clinical trials dealing with a particular therapy for a particular disease. An example of this approach would be a study that examined the effects of aspirin following myocardial infarction. Typically, this type of meta-analysis would present an overall measure of the efficacy of treatment, e.g., a summary odds ratio. Summary measures may be presented for different subsets of trials involving specific types of patients, e.g., studies restricted to men versus studies that include both men and women. More sophisticated meta-analyses also examine the variability of results among trials and, when results have been conflicting, attempt to uncover the sources of the disagreements.[21]

More recently, meta-analyses of nonexperimental epidemiologic studies have been performed[22–31] and articles have been written describing the methodologic considerations specific to those meta-analyses.[3,6,11,15,32–42] In general, both the meta-analyses of nonexperimental studies and the associated methodologic articles tend to focus more on the exploration of reasons for disagreement among the results of prior studies, including the possibility of bias. Given the greater diversity of designs of nonexperimental studies, it is logical to find more disagreement among nonexperimental studies than among randomized trials.

This chapter summarizes many of the major conceptual and methodologic issues surrounding meta-analysis and offers the views of one meta-analyst about possible avenues for future research in this field.

CLINICAL PROBLEMS TO BE ADDRESSED BY PHARMACOEPIDEMIOLOGIC RESEARCH

There are a number of reasons why a pharmacoepidemiologist might be interested in conducting a meta-analysis. These include the study of uncommon adverse outcomes of therapies free of the confounding and bias of non-experimental studies, the exploration of reasons for inconsistencies of results across previous studies, the exploration of subgroups of patients in whom therapy

may be more or less effective, the combination of studies involved in the approval process for new therapies, and the study of positive effects of therapies, as in the investigation of new indications for existing therapies, particularly when the outcomes being studied are uncommon or the past studies have been small.

The investigation of adverse effects has been a recurring theme throughout this book, as it is a major focus of pharmacoepidemiology. It is most often, but not always, pursued through nonexperimental studies. The difficulties in studying these events have also been detailed throughout this book. One major challenge involves obtaining information on adverse reactions that is unconfounded by indication (see Chapter 40). These adverse events often occur only rarely, making their evaluation still more difficult. The results of nonexperimental studies of whether such events are associated with a particular drug may be conflicting, leaving a confusing picture for the practicing clinician and the policy makers to interpret. Meta-analysis, by combining results from many randomized studies, can address the problem of rare events and rectify the associated lack of adequate statistical power in a setting free of the confounding and bias of nonexperimental studies. For example, Chalmers and colleagues used meta-analysis of randomized clinical trials to explore possible gastrointestinal side effects of nonsteroidal anti-inflammatory drugs (NSAIDs).[43] These studies individually had almost no power to detect any association between NSAIDs and adverse gastrointestinal outcomes, but collectively the number of subjects was adequate both to show some important associations and to show the rarity of most complications. The details of this NSAID meta-analysis will be presented later in this chapter. MacLean and colleagues[44] also studied randomized trials of NSAIDs, as part of a similar effort regarding adverse gastrointestinal events.

When reports of several investigations of a specific adverse drug reaction disagree, whether randomized or nonexperimental in design, meta-analysis can also be used to help resolve these disagreements. These disagreements among studies may arise from differences in the choice of endpoints, the exact definition of exposure, the eligibility criteria for study subjects, the methods of obtaining information, other differences in protocols, or a host of other reasons possibly related to the quality of the studies. While it is not possible to produce a definitive answer to every research question, the exploration of the reasons for heterogeneity among studies' results may at least provide valuable guidance concerning the design of future studies.

The exploration of subgroups of patients in whom therapy may be more or less effective is a controversial question in individual randomized trials. Most trials are not designed with sample sizes adequate to address efficacy in subgroups. The finding of statistically significant differences between the effects of therapy in different subgroups, particularly when those groups were not defined *a priori*, raises the question of whether those are spurious findings. Conversely, the lack of statistical significance for clinically important differences between prospectively defined subgroups can often be attributed to a lack of statistical power. Such clinically meaningful but statistically nonsignificant findings are difficult to interpret. Meta-analysis can be used to explore these questions with improved statistical power.

The use of meta-analysis in the approval process for new drugs represents another potential application, although experience in this area is as yet rather limited. However, many of the methodologic issues arising in the context of new drug approval also arise in the investigation of new indications for pharmaceutical products that have previously been approved for other purposes. For some therapies, such as streptokinase in the treatment of myocardial infarction, meta-analysis could have been used to summarize evidence prior to embarking on a very large-scale, multicenter, randomized trial.[45]

METHODOLOGIC PROBLEMS TO BE ADDRESSED BY PHARMACOEPIDEMIOLOGIC RESEARCH

As the skeptical reader might imagine, many methodologic issues can arise in the context of performing a meta-analysis. Many, but not all, of these problems relate to the process of combining studies that are often diverse with respect to specific aspects of design or protocol, some of which may be of questionable quality.

QUALITY OF THE ORIGINAL STUDIES

Meta-analysis seems particularly prone to the "garbage in = garbage out" phenomenon. Combining a group of poorly done studies can produce a precise summary result built on a very weak foundation. This apparent precision may lend undue credibility to a result that truly should not be used as a basis for formulating clinical or policy strategies.[5] However, if the quality judgment is subtly influenced by the direction or magnitude of the findings of the study, excluding studies based on such a subjective judgment about their quality could open the meta-analytic process to a serious form of bias.

COMBINABILITY OF STUDIES

Clearly, no one would suggest combining studies that are so diverse that a summary would be nonsensical. For example, one would not combine studies of hormone replacement therapy in relation to risk of breast cancer with studies of hormone replacement therapy in relation to risk of coronary heart disease. Beyond obvious examples like this, however, the choices may not be so clear. Should studies with different patient populations be combined? How different can those populations be before it becomes unacceptable to combine the studies? Should nonrandomized studies be combined with randomized studies? Should nonrandomized studies ever be used in a meta-analysis? These are questions that cannot be answered without generating some controversy.

PUBLICATION BIAS

Unpublished material cannot be retrieved by literature searches and is likely to be difficult to find referenced in published articles. *Publication bias* occurs when study results are not published, or their publication is delayed, because of the results.[46–56] The usual pattern is that statistically significant results are published more easily than nonsignificant results, although this bias may not be as severe for randomized studies as it is for nonrandomized studies.[48,57,58] While one could simply decide not to include unpublished studies in a meta-analysis, since those data have often not been peer-reviewed,[59] unpublished data can represent a large proportion of all available data.[60] If the results of unpublished studies are systematically different from those of published studies, particularly with respect to the magnitude and/or direction of the findings, their omission from a meta-analysis would yield a biased summary estimate (assuming that the quality of the unpublished studies is at least equal to the quality of the published studies).

Publication bias is a potentially serious limitation to any meta-analysis. For example, Sutton and colleagues[61] found that in 4 of 48 meta-analyses they examined, there was evidence that the statistical inferences would have changed after the overall effect estimate was adjusted for publication bias. The retrospective identification of completed unpublished trials is clearly possible[60] in some instances, but generally is not practical. One study[62] used a survey of investigators to attempt to identify unpublished studies. The authors surveyed 42 000 obstetricians and pediatricians, asking whether they had participated in any unpublished trials completed more than two years previously, i.e., during the period prior to the end of 1984. They identified only

18 such studies, despite an overall response rate of 94% to their survey.

Other forms of bias, related to publication bias, have also been identified.[49] These include reference bias, i.e., preferential citation of significant findings,[63] language bias, i.e., exclusion of studies in languages other than English,[64,65] and bias related to source of funding.[48,50,66–68] These related biases have been termed "dissemination bias" by Sutton and colleagues, who found that the threat of such biases is more severe in nonrandomized studies of an intervention.[58]

BIAS IN THE ABSTRACTION OF DATA

Meta-analysis, by virtue of being conducted after the data are available, is a form of retrospective research and is thus subject to the potential biases inherent in such research.[69] In the meta-analysis of gastrointestinal side effects of NSAIDs mentioned above[43] and described more fully below, Chalmers and colleagues examined over 500 randomized studies. They measured the agreement of different individuals when reading the "methods" sections of papers that had been masked as to their source and the results. There were disagreements on 10–20% of items, which had to be resolved in conference with a third person. These disagreements arose from errors on the part of the reader and from lack of clarity of the presentation of material in the original articles. Whatever its source, when such variability exists, the opportunity for observer bias may exist as well.[69]

In a number of instances, more than one meta-analysis has been performed in the same general area of disease and treatment. A review of 20 of these instances[59] showed that, for almost all disease/treatment areas, there were differences between two meta-analyses of the same topic in the acceptance and rejection of papers to be included. While there was only one case (out of the 20) of extreme disagreement regarding efficacy, there were several cases in which one or more analyses showed a statistically significant result while the other(s) showed only a trend. These disagreements were not easily explainable. For example, differences between meta-analyses of the same topic in the acceptance and rejection of papers did not always lead to differences in conclusions.

More generally, the acceptance or rejection of different sets of studies can drastically change conclusions. This is illustrated by several meta-analyses of whether or not corticosteroid drugs cause peptic ulcer. The first published paper argued that corticosteroids did not cause peptic ulcer, because the p-value for the meta-analysis was only 0.07.[70] Five years later, a second analysis, by a second set of authors, included a larger number of studies and found

evidence for an association with a p-value of less than 0.001.[71] Re-analysis of the data from the second meta-analysis by the authors of the first meta-analysis, with the addition of several more studies, gave a p-value of 0.40.[72] Another meta-analysis done by the second team gave a revised p-value of 0.01.[73] Despite efforts to make meta-analysis an objective, reproducible activity, there is evidently some judgment involved.

In a separate commentary, DerSimonian[74] re-analyzed data from one meta-analysis and one clinical review of parenteral nutrition with branched-chain amino acids in hepatic encephalopathy. She pointed to differences in the data extracted by the two sets of authors[75,76] for the same endpoints from the same original papers. When combined statistically, the data extracted by the two sets of authors led to substantively different conclusions about the efficacy of therapy.

CURRENTLY AVAILABLE SOLUTIONS

This section will first present the general principles of meta-analysis and a general framework for the methods typically employed in a meta-analysis. Much of this material has been presented in review articles in major clinical journals,[7,9,10] so only the most important points will be highlighted here. In the second part of this section, specific solutions to the methodologic issues raised in the previous section are presented. Finally, case studies of applications that should be of interest to pharmacoepidemiologists will be presented, illustrating approaches to some of the clinical and methodologic problems raised earlier.

STEPS INVOLVED IN PERFORMING A META-ANALYSIS (TABLE 44.1)

Define the Purpose

While this is an obvious component of any research, it is particularly important to define precisely the primary and secondary objectives of a meta-analysis. The important

Table 44.1. General steps involved in conducting a meta-analysis

(1) Define the purpose
(2) Perform the literature search
(3) Establish inclusion/exclusion criteria
(4) Collect the data
(5) Perform statistical analyses
(6) Formulate conclusions and recommendations

primary question might be "Are NSAIDs associated with an increased risk of gastrointestinal side effects?" Another might be "Are corticosteroids effective in the treatment of alcoholic hepatitis?" Secondary objectives might include the identification of subgroups in which a treatment appears to be uniquely more or less effective. For NSAIDs, estimating the absolute risk difference (and, thus, the public health implications) as well as the relative risk (and, thus, the etiologic implications) might be a secondary objective.

Perform the Literature Search

While computerized searches of the literature can facilitate the retrieval of all relevant published studies, these searches are not always reliable. Several studies have examined problems with the use of electronic searches.[77-79] Use of search terms that are too nonspecific can result in large numbers of mostly irrelevant citations that need to be reviewed to determine relevance. Use of too many restrictions can result in missing a substantial number of relevant publications. For example, in preparing for meta-analyses of neonatal hyperbilirubinemia, MEDLINE was searched for relevant clinical trials.[77] A search by a trained librarian identified only 29% of known trials in the Oxford Database of Perinatal Trials.[80] It is generally suggested that a professional librarian with training and experience in searches of clinical topics be consulted, although, as just cited, even a trained librarian may not perform perfectly. Other methods of searching, such as review of the reference sections of retrieved publications found to be relevant, and hand searches of relevant journals, are also recommended.

Establish Inclusion/Exclusion Criteria

A set of rules for including and excluding studies from the meta-analysis should be defined during the planning stage of the meta-analysis and should be based on the specific hypotheses being tested in the analysis. One might, for example, wish to limit consideration to randomized studies with more than some minimum number of patients. In a meta-analysis of epidemiologic studies, one might wish to include studies of incident cases only, excluding studies of prevalent cases, assuming that the relationship between exposure and outcome could be different in the two types of study. Practical considerations may, of course, force changes in the inclusion criteria. For example, one might find no randomized studies of a particular new indication for an existing therapeutic agent, thus forcing consideration of nonrandomized studies.

In establishing inclusion/exclusion criteria, one is also necessarily defining the question being addressed by the meta-analysis. If broad inclusion criteria are established, then a broad, and perhaps more generalizable, hypothesis may be tested. The use of broad entry criteria also permits the examination of the effects of research design on outcome (e.g., do randomized and nonrandomized studies tend to show different effects of therapy?) or the exploration of subgroup effects. As an example, in a meta-analysis of aspirin administered following myocardial infarction, restriction of the meta-analysis to studies using more than a certain dose of aspirin would not permit an exploratory, cross-study comparison of dose–response effects, which might prove illuminating.

A key point is that exclusion criteria should be based on *a priori* considerations of design of the original studies and completeness of the reports and specifically not on the results of the studies. To exclude studies solely on the basis of results that contradict the majority of the other studies will clearly introduce bias into the process.[11] While that may seem obvious, the temptation to try to justify such exclusions on a *post hoc* basis may be strong, particularly when a clinically plausible basis for the exclusion can be found. Such exclusions made after having seen the data, and the effect of individual studies on the pooled result, may form the basis for legitimate sensitivity analyses (comparing pooled results with and without that particular study included), but should not be viewed as primary exclusion criteria.

Another important note is that studies may often generate more than one published paper. For example, later reports might update analyses previously published, or might report on outcomes not addressed in earlier papers. It is essential, for two reasons, that only one report on the same patients be accepted into the meta-analysis. First, the validity of the statistical methods depends on the assumption that the different studies represent different groups of individuals. Second, the inclusion of a study more than once would assign undue weight to that study in the summary measure. A caution is that it is not always obvious that the same patients have been described in two different publications. Contacting the authors may be of some help in determining if there is duplication, although some authors may perceive the inquiry as questioning their academic integrity. It is also not always obvious what the right choice of report should be for a given study. Certain aspects of the methods may only be reported in earlier publications, which necessitates at least referring to those papers. Methods of analysis may change from paper to paper, or degree of control of confounding, or inclusion or exclusion of certain subpopulations. Thus, there is no general rule we can recommend in such situations, other than trying to exercise good judgment and reporting clearly the reasons for choosing one publication over others. The issue of multiple publications based on the same study has been addressed in more detail by Huston and Moher.[81]

Collect the Data

When the relevant studies have been identified and retrieved, the important information regarding study design and outcome needs to be extracted. Typically, data abstraction forms are developed, pilot tested on a few articles, and revised as needed. As in any research, it is necessary to strike a balance between the completeness of the information abstracted and the amount of time needed to extract that information. Careful specification in the protocol for the meta-analysis of the design features and patient characteristics that will be of clinical or academic interest may help avoid over- or under-collecting information. It is generally advisable, when possible, to collect raw data on outcome measures, e.g., numbers treated and number of events in each group, rather than derived measures such as odds ratios, which may not be the outcome measures of interest in the meta-analysis or may have been calculated incorrectly by the original authors.

Many articles on "how to do a meta-analysis" (e.g., Sacks *et al.*,[9] L'Abbe *et al.*[10]) recommend that the meta-analyst assess the quality of the studies being considered in a meta-analysis. One might wish to use a measure of study quality as part of the weight assigned to each study in the analysis, as an exclusion criterion (e.g., excluding studies with quality scores below some arbitrary threshold), or as a stratification factor allowing the separate estimation of effects for good quality and poor quality studies.[82,83] Chalmers and colleagues have developed a quality assessment scoring system for randomized trials.[84] Several groups have opted for other, far shorter and simpler, systems.[85–88] Issues related to quality scoring have been discussed more generally by Moher and colleagues,[89] and an annotated checklist of quality scoring systems is available.[90] Most of these systems were proposed as very general systems that could be applied to clinical trials covering a wide range of therapies and endpoints. Scoring systems designed for epidemiologic studies have been developed as well, in the context of evaluating studies of specific exposure–disease relationships (e.g., Longnecker *et al.*[22]).

The argument has been made, however, that general scoring systems are arbitrary in their assignment of weights to particular aspects of study design, and that such systems risk losing information, and can even be misleading.[41,91,92]

Jüni and colleagues, for example, examined studies comparing low molecular weight heparin with standard heparin with respect to prevention of postoperative thrombosis. They used 25 different quality assessment scales to identify high quality trials. For six scales, the studies identified as being of high quality showed little to no benefit of low molecular weight heparin, while for seven scales, the "high quality" studies showed a significant advantage of low molecular weight heparin. This apparent contradiction raises questions about the validity of such scales as methods for stratifying studies. One reason the contradiction arises, the authors argue, is that the quality scores tend to measure a combination of completeness of reporting and factors that might relate to the potential for bias. They recommend, instead, a focus on particular aspects of study design as potential predictors of study outcome, e.g., whether or not the assessment of outcome is blinded to treatment status.

Thus, in a given meta-analysis, one might wish to examine *specific* aspects of study design that are unique to that clinical or statistical situation.[41,91–93] For example, Schulz and colleagues[93] found that trials in which the concealment of randomized allocation was inadequate, on average produced larger estimates of treatment effects, compared with trials in which allocation was adequately concealed. This specific finding was not detected when these same authors looked for an overall association between quality score and treatment effect. In the analysis of low molecular weight heparin, Jüni and colleagues[92] found that studies with unmasked outcome assessment showed larger, and presumably biased, benefits of low molecular weight heparin than studies using masked assessment of outcome. Such explorations clearly need to be guided by common sense. As Jüni and colleagues point out, for studies with total mortality as an outcome, masking of outcome assessment would not be expected to impact directly on study findings.

Other authors have suggested essentially similar approaches to that recommended by Jüni and colleagues. For example, Greenland and O'Rourke[94] suggest the use of statistical models to investigate the association between specific design factors and study findings. This approach, known as "response–surface estimation," can be used to derive the predicted outcome for a study with specified (and presumably desirable) characteristics, while at the same time borrowing strength from all of the available studies. Once again, caution is needed in performing such analyses, with respect to such issues as extrapolation beyond the range of the data. (What if there are *no* studies of sufficient quality on a given dimension included in the model? Is it valid to extrapolate to such studies based on trends observed for lower quality studies?) This is a specific example of the more general issue of modeling heterogeneity in results across studies, in which the heterogeneity is thought to stem from study design issues, rather than from true biological or clinical variability in response to therapy. Models for heterogeneity are discussed in greater detail later in this chapter.

Two procedural recommendations have been made regarding the actual techniques for data extraction. One is that studies should be read independently by two readers. The justification for this comes from meta-analyses in which modest but important inter-reader variability has been demonstrated.[43,69] A second recommendation is that readers be masked to certain information in studies, such as the identity of the authors and the institutions at which a study was conducted, and masked to the specific treatment assignments.[59] While masking has a high degree of intuitive appeal, the effectiveness of masking in avoiding bias has not been demonstrated. Only one randomized trial examines the issue of the effect of masking on the results of meta-analyses.[95] This study compared the results of the same meta-analyses performed independently by separate teams of meta-analysts, with one team masked and the other unmasked. The masked and unmasked teams produced nearly identical results on a series of five meta-analyses, lending little support to the need for masking.

Perform Statistical Analyses

In most situations, the statistical methods for the actual combination of results across studies are fairly straightforward, although a great deal of literature in recent years has focused on the use of increasingly sophisticated methods. If one is interested in combining odds ratios or other estimates of relative risk across studies, for example, some form of weighted average of within-study results is appropriate, and several of these exist.[96] A popular example of this is the Mantel–Haenszel procedure, in which odds ratios are combined across studies with weights proportional to the inverse of the variance of the within-study odds ratio.[34,35,96] Other approaches include inverse-variance weighted averages of study-specific estimates of multivariate-adjusted relative risks[35,96] and exact stratified odds ratios.[97] One popular method, sometimes called the "one-step" method, which is similar to the Mantel–Haenszel method,[98] has been shown to be biased under some circumstances. Since this method offers no clear advantage over the Mantel–Haenszel method, which is more robust, the Mantel–Haenszel method may be preferable in many circumstances.[34]

Bias in statistical methods is also discussed by Tang,[99] who shows that inverse-variance methods may introduce bias in meta-analyses of binary outcomes. Essentially, the problem with those approaches is that the inverse-variance weights depend not only on study size, but on the event rates themselves. For example, consider an analysis of 10 trials that all have sample sizes of 500 in both the treated and control groups. Suppose nine studies have event rates of 28% in the treated groups compared with 30% in the control groups. In this same analysis, a single study has event rates of 3% in the treated group versus 1% in controls. For an inverse-variance weighted analysis of risk differences, which are −2% in the nine studies and +2% in the single study, the single study with the low event rates would get 54% of the weight in the meta-analysis, compared with 5.1% of the weight for each of the other nine studies. For an analysis of (log) relative risks, the single study would get 0.4% of the weight, compared with 11.1% of the weight for each of the other nine studies. Appropriate use of weights is also addressed by Chang and colleagues.[100]

Choices are never simple, however. In a simulation study, Deeks and colleagues[101] showed, at an international meeting, that in situations where there are rare events, and consequently frequent zero cells in contingency tables, the one-step method tended to perform better than other alternatives, including Mantel–Haenszel and exact methods.

One basic principle in many analytic approaches is that the comparisons between treated (exposed) and untreated (unexposed) patients are typically made within a study prior to combination across studies. In the combination of randomized trial results, this amounts to preserving the randomization within each study prior to combination. In all of the procedures developed for stratified data, "study" plays the role of the stratifying variable. In general, more weight is assigned to large studies than to small studies because of the increased precision of larger studies.

A second basic principle to note is that some of these methods assume that the studies are all estimating a single, common effect, e.g., a common odds ratio. In other words, the underlying treatment effect (whether beneficial or harmful) that all studies are estimating is assumed to be the same for all studies. Any variability among study results is assumed to be random and is ignored in producing a summary estimate of the effect.[102,103]

In any meta-analysis, however, the possible existence of heterogeneity among study designs and results should be examined, and may warrant a set of exploratory analyses designed to investigate the sources of that heterogeneity. Methods for detecting and describing heterogeneity are described in more detail below. Depending on the results of such exploratory analyses, one may wish to use methods for combining studies that do not make the assumption of a common treatment effect across all studies. These are the so-called "random-effects" models, which allow for the possibility that the underlying true treatment effect, which each study is estimating, may not be the same for all studies, even when examining studies with similar designs, protocols, and patient populations. Hidden or unmeasured sources of among-study variability of results are taken into account by these random-effects models through the incorporation of such variability into the weighting scheme when computing a weighted average summary estimate. Random effects models are described in much greater detail in several recent papers.[104–108] The similarity of meta-analytic methods to methods for multicenter trials is discussed by Senn.[107]

The practical consequence of the random-effects models is to produce wider confidence intervals than would otherwise be produced by the traditional methods.[102,103] This approach is considered particularly useful when there is heterogeneity among study results, and exploratory analyses have failed to uncover any known sources of observed heterogeneity. However, random-effects models should not be viewed as a panacea for unexplained heterogeneity. One danger is that a summary measure of heterogeneous studies may not really apply to any particular study population or study design, i.e., they lose information by averaging over potentially important study and population characteristics.[41]

A second practical effect of random-effects models, which is only apparent from examining the mathematics involved, is that they tend to assign relatively higher weights to small studies than the traditional methods would assign.[102] This equalization of weights may have unwanted consequences in some circumstances, and can lead to counterintuitive results, with very small studies making contributions to the summary equal to those of very large studies. A thorough discussion of the interpretation and application of fixed- versus random-effects models is presented by Hedges and Vevea.[109] Villar and colleagues[110] compare results of fixed- and random-effects models on an empirical basis. As expected, in the presence of heterogeneity, they found that the random-effects models gave wider confidence intervals. Interestingly, these random-effects models also showed larger treatment effects than the corresponding fixed-effects models applied to the same data. Explanations for this phenomenon are considered in the section on publication bias, below.

Bayesian statistical methods are also being proposed with increasing frequency in the statistical literature.[111–119] These methods can incorporate into the analysis the investigator's prior beliefs about the size of an effect or about the factors biasing the observed effects. When the investigator has no

prior beliefs about the effect, the results of the observed studies are sometimes used to estimate the components of the "prior" distribution. Thus, the final answers reflect the observed data very closely. In practice, when the investigator does not specify prior beliefs, the summary results are similar to those from standard methods, especially the random effects models described above, except that generally speaking, confidence intervals produced by Bayesian methods will be still wider than those produced by other methods.

Another approach within a Bayesian framework[120] is based on summing the statistical evidence provided by each study for each value of the effect measure (e.g., the odds ratio). The value of the odds ratio with the maximum evidence (the maximum likelihood estimate) has usually proved the same as the pooled estimate produced by other methods, in the situations where this method has been used.[120] By providing a mathematical and graphical picture of what is occurring at other values of the effect estimate, this method also provides information on the contribution of each study to the total.

A number of somewhat specialized statistical issues have been addressed in recent years. These include how to include both parallel and crossover trials in a single meta-analysis,[121–124] the inclusion of trials in which some form of group (e.g., medical practice or hospital) is the unit of randomization (so-called "cluster randomized" trials) in meta-analyses,[125] converting odds ratios to effect sizes so that studies with dichotomous outcomes may be combined directly with studies having continuous outcome measures,[126] and the analysis of single patient (N-of-1) trials to estimate population treatment effects and to evaluate individual responses to treatment.[127] These N-of-1 designs are also discussed elsewhere in this volume (see Chapter 43). Nam and colleagues[128] discuss the analysis of studies with multiple, correlated outcomes. Recently published work of particular interest to epidemiologists includes the analysis of dose–response data from epidemiologic data,[129,130] a method for combining disparate designs (case–control, comparative cohort, and uncontrolled cohort studies),[131] and exact methods for case–control and follow-up studies.[132] Of note, a paper by Shi and Copas, on trend estimation, presents a method that allows for aggregated dose data that does not rely on the usual approach of trying to assign a single exposure value to an exposure category. Their approach relies on making distributional assumptions about the doses within categories (e.g., a lognormal distribution for alcohol consumption across all subjects in a series of case–control studies).[130]

One should probably assume, when undertaking a meta-analysis, that heterogeneity of findings across studies will be present, whether or not a formal statistical test is able to detect it. Thus, an important part of performing the subsequent analyses will involve somehow quantifying the degree of heterogeneity and understanding the potential sources of heterogeneity. An important word of caution is that statistical tests of heterogeneity, i.e., formal statistical tests of the variability among the studies, suffer from a notorious lack of statistical power.[133,134] Thus, a finding of significant heterogeneity may safely be interpreted as meaning the studies are not all estimating the same parameter. A lack of statistical significance, however, may not mean that heterogeneity is not important in a data set or that sources of variability should not be explored.

Higgins and Thompson propose alternative measures of heterogeneity.[135–137] They argue that one problem with tests of heterogeneity is that they are sensitive to the number of trials included in the meta-analysis. Current approaches to statistical quantification of the among-study variability are sensitive to the "metric" on which the outcome is measured, e.g., continuous versus dichotomous outcomes. They propose several alternative measures of heterogeneity, which they call H, R, and I^2. These are measures quantifying the impact of heterogeneity on summary estimates, rather than quantifying the extent of heterogeneity *per se*. R is the ratio of the standard error of the underlying mean from a random effects meta-analysis to the standard error of a fixed effect meta-analytic estimate. Both H and I^2 relate to the proportion of variability in point estimates due to heterogeneity rather than sampling error. The advantages of the three methods are in the fact that the comparisons can be made across meta-analyses of different sizes and with different outcome measures. In particular, these authors recommend I^2 because:

- it focuses attention on the effect of any heterogeneity on the meta-analytic result;
- its interpretation is intuitive, i.e., the percentage of total variation across studies due to heterogeneity;
- it can be accompanied by an uncertainty interval;
- it is simple to calculate and can usually be derived from published meta-analyses;
- it does not inherently depend on the number of studies in the meta-analysis;
- it may be interpreted similarly irrespective of the type of outcome data (e.g., time to event, quantitative, or dichotomous) and choice of effect measure (e.g., OR or hazard ratio).

With respect to how one should approach the search for sources of heterogeneity, a number of options are available. One might stratify the studies according to patient characteristics or study design features and investigate heterogeneity within and across strata. To the extent that the stratification explains the heterogeneity, the combined results would differ between or among strata and the heterogeneity within the strata would be reduced compared to the overall result. In addition to stratification, regression methods such as weighted least squares linear regression could be used to explore sources of heterogeneity.[3,35,138–141] These might be important when various components of study design are correlated with each other, acting as potential confounders. Graphical methods for meta-analysis have also been proposed, that focus on issues related to heterogeneity.[142,143]

In recent years, increasingly sophisticated (and complex) approaches to the statistical modeling of heterogeneity have been proposed. Thompson and Sharp,[144] for example, compared different forms of weighted normal errors regression and random effects logistic regression. Hardy and Thompson reviewed regression methods to investigate heterogeneity.[138]

A topic of recurring interest in the meta-analysis literature has been the investigation of risk in the control group as a predictor of treatment benefit. The question generally being addressed is whether high-risk patients benefit more from therapy than low-risk patients. However, the question is analyzed using the estimated risk in the control group as an indicator of risk in the *population* under study, making this strictly a meta-analytic exercise. Importantly, risk estimates for individual patients are generally not available in such analyses.[114,145–147] One exception to the lack of patient-level risk estimates is a paper by Trikalinos and Ioannidis,[148] who present methods for modeling study findings as a function of the risk in the control group, using individual patient data. Sharp and Thompson[145] present a Bayesian approach to this problem, based only on group-level data. They recommend a method relying on the underlying binomial distribution of the binary outcomes. That is, this method is analogous to a logistic regression, in which the *risk* is modeled as a function of treatment status and a study-level summary of patient characteristics. This differs from other approaches based on modeling the treatment effects.[114,149]

Helpful overviews of statistical methods for meta-analysis are provided in a number of sources, including a recent text[150] and several review articles.[107,117,151,152] Tutorials on basic[117] and more advanced[153] meta-regression methods are also available.

Formulate Conclusions and Recommendations

As with all research, the conclusions of a meta-analysis should be clearly summarized, with appropriate interpretation of the strengths and weaknesses of the meta-analysis. Authors should clearly state how generalizable the result is and how definitive it is and should outline the areas that need future research. Any hypotheses generated by the meta-analysis should be stated as such, and not as conclusions.

APPROACHES TO SELECTED METHODOLOGIC PROBLEMS IN META-ANALYSIS

Combinability of Results from Diverse Studies: Heterogeneity is Your Friend

The underlying question in any meta-analysis is whether it is clinically and statistically reasonable to estimate an average effect of therapy, either positive or negative. If one errs on the side of being too inclusive, and the studies differ too greatly, there is the possibility that the average effect may not apply to any particular subgroup of patients.[35,154] Conversely, diversity of designs and results may provide an opportunity to understand the factors that modify the effectiveness (or toxicity) of a drug. Glasziou and Sanders[155] nicely summarize issues related to potential sources of heterogeneity. They highlight an important distinction between artifacts that might be related to either the choice of summary measure or to study design features, and real biological or clinical variation in treatment effect. The former would include issues such as whether relative risk or risk difference is the more appropriate measure of treatment effect, and design issues mentioned above in the context of study quality, such as use of blinding in the evaluation of endpoints within a study. Such features are modifiable aspects of the conduct and analysis of studies. Variation due to clinical factors, in contrast, represents the potential to target therapy to the appropriate patient populations.

It has been argued that because of the potential for bias in observational epidemiologic studies, exploring heterogeneity should be the main point of meta-analyses of such studies, rather than producing a single summary measure.[6,41,156]

The generality of the question posed will clearly influence the generalizability of the result, but also may affect whether the primary studies involved are viewed as combinable or not. Because the set of available studies is likely to be heterogeneous with respect to design features, the choice of a more general question may be preferred to a very specific one. For example, Dickersin and Berlin[15] suggest that a more general question might be "Is taking aspirin associated with decreased mortality in patients who have already had a myocardial infarction?" rather than "Is administration of 325 milligrams of aspirin per day, started within seven days

of a first documented myocardial infarction and taken for at least six months, in the absence of other preventive treatments, in patients followed for at least one year, associated with a decrease in subsequent cardiovascular mortality?" If addressing the second question, the meta-analyst may quickly find him or herself with only one available study. Diversity of study designs, on the other hand, can provide a more generalizable result than restriction to a very narrowly-defined group of studies. Issues of study design, such as dose or duration of therapy, and how study design relates to study results, could be addressed through a series of exploratory analyses.[15]

As an example of the type of analysis that could be used to investigate study design issues, Hennessy and colleagues[31] performed a meta-analysis of nonexperimental studies comparing third generation oral contraceptives (those containing gestodene and desogestrel) to second generation pills (those containing levenorgestrel) with respect to the risk of venous thromboembolic events. A major issue in these studies has been the possibility of depletion of susceptibles. Specifically, the concern is that users of the newer drugs might tend to be new users of *any* oral contraceptives, whereas users of the older, second generation drugs, would tend to be established users. The risk of venous events tends to be highest for new users, who have events soon after beginning pill use. These susceptible individuals, the argument goes, would be depleted from the ranks of users of second generation pills, but not from among the third generation pill users, thereby leaving a more susceptible population of third generation pill users. The authors found several studies that had performed subgroup analyses of new users in their first year of use. When combined, these subgroups still demonstrated an increased risk from third generation pills. The power to look within subgroups was only available within the context of the meta-analysis, not within any of the individual studies.

The example just presented was motivated by a specific concern about a hypothesized source of bias in studies. It is sometimes instructive to perform more exploratory analyses of meta-analytic data as well. These may provide valuable insights into the biology of the problem and/or may generate hypotheses for future confirmation. Morgenstern and colleagues[30] found that the association between neuroleptic medication and tardive dyskinesia was stronger in studies conducted in the United States than in studies conducted elsewhere. They used regression methods to show that this association was not simply the product of confounding by other study design features. The authors suggest that the US study samples may have had a higher baseline frequency of unmeasured factors (e.g., affective disorders such as schizophrenia) than the exposed groups in other countries. As with any exploratory analysis, due caution must be exercised in the interpretation of such *a posteriori* hypotheses, even though they may be based on very sound biological reasoning.

Publication Bias

As discussed above, when the primary source of data for a meta-analysis is published data, there is usually a danger that the published studies represent a biased subset of all the studies that have been done. In general, it is more likely that studies with statistically significant findings will be published than studies with no significant findings. A practical technique for determining the potential for publication bias is the "funnel plot," first proposed by Light and Pillemer.[157] The method involves plotting the effect size (e.g., the risk difference) against a measure of study size, such as the sample size, or the inverse of the variance of the individual effect sizes. If there is no publication bias, the points should produce a kind of funnel shape, with a scatter of points centered around the true value of the effect size, and with the degree of scatter narrowing as the variances decrease. If publication bias is a problem, the funnel would look as though a bite had been taken out, with very few (if any) points around the point indicating no effect (e.g., odds ratio of 1.0) for studies with large variances. This method requires a sufficient number of studies to permit the visualization of a funnel shape to the data. If the funnel plot does indicate the existence of publication bias, then one or more of the correction methods described below should be considered. In the presence of publication bias, the responsible meta-analyst should also evaluate the ethics of presenting a summary result that is likely to represent an overestimate of the effect in question.

Two examples of funnel plots are given in Figures 44.1 and 44.2. These plots represent studies of psychoeducational programs for surgical patients.[157,158] In the first plot, only the published studies are represented. The funnel appears to have a "bite" taken out of it where the small studies showing no effect of these programs should be. In the second plot, the unpublished studies, including doctoral dissertations, are included, and the former "bite" is now filled with these unpublished studies.

Sterne and Egger[159] provide guidelines for the choice of axes in funnel plots of studies with dichotomous outcomes, recommending that the standard error of the treatment effect (e.g., the standard error of the log odds ratio) be used as the measure of study size and that relative measures (relative risk, as opposed to risk difference) be used as the treatment

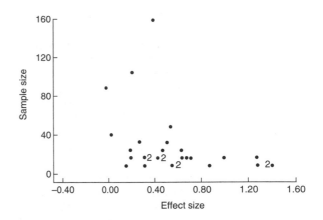

Figure 44.1. Funnel plot for published studies only: analysis of data from Devine and Cook's[158] review of psychoeducational programs for surgical patients. Reprinted by permission of the publishers from *Summing Up: The Science of Reviewing Research* by Richard J. Light and David B. Pillemer, Cambridge MA: Harvard University Press. Copyright 1984 by the President and Fellows of Harvard College.

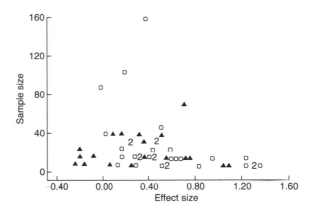

Figure 44.2. Funnel plot for published (open boxes) and unpublished (closed triangles) combined: analysis of data from Devine and Cook's[158] review of psychoeducational programs for surgical patients. Reprinted by permission of the publishers from *Summing Up: The Science of Reviewing Research* by Richard J. Light and David B. Pillemer, Cambridge, MA: Harvard University Press. Copyright 1984 by the President and Fellows of Harvard College.

effect measures. These same authors and a colleague point out that publication bias is only one possible explanation for funnel plot asymmetry, so that the funnel plot should be seen as estimating "small study effects," rather than necessarily publication bias.[160] A similar point is made by Terrin and colleagues.[161]

Several mathematical approaches to the problem of publication bias have been proposed. An early method, first described by Rosenthal,[162] is the calculation of a "fail-safe N" when the result of the meta-analysis is a statistically significant rejection of the null hypothesis. This method, in a kind of sensitivity analysis, uses the Z-statistics from the individual studies included in a meta-analysis to calculate the number of *unpublished* studies with a Z-statistic of exactly 0 that would be required to exist, in order for the combined Z-score (published + unpublished studies) to become nonsignificant. Because this method focuses only on Z-statistics, and ignores the estimation of effects (e.g., odds ratios), it is of limited utility. That is, the fail-safe N approach focuses only on the statistical significance of the combined result and does not help provide an overall estimate of the effect that is "adjusted" for publication bias.

A number of related methods to deal with potential unpublished studies have been developed in recent years. These include other methods for estimating the number of unpublished studies,[163,164] formal methods to test for the presence of publication bias,[165–167] and methods to adjust summary estimates to account for unpublished studies,[109,163,168–171] but several of those methods make some fairly strong assumptions about the specific mechanism producing the publication bias. A method called "trim-and-fill" has a fair amount of intuitive appeal,[172] although it, too, relies on assumptions about the missing studies. It is based on the funnel plot, focusing on the studies that lead to the appearance of funnel plot asymmetry. Under this approach, a mirror image of the studies producing the asymmetry is imputed, using a carefully defined statistical algorithm to determine which studies to mirror, and the impact of adding those mirror image studies to the pooled analysis is assessed.

An additional methodologic caution generated by publication bias relates to the use of random-effects models for combining results. When the results of the studies being analyzed are heterogeneous and a random-effects model is being used to combine those results, one of the properties of the model, described above, is to assign relatively higher weights to small studies than would otherwise be assigned by more traditional methods of combining data. If publication bias is a problem in a particular data set, one consequence implied by the funnel plot is that small studies would tend to show larger effects than large studies. Thus, if publication bias is present, one of the reasons for heterogeneity of study results is that the small studies show systematically larger effects than the large studies. The

assignment of higher relative weights to the small studies could, when publication bias is present, lead to a biased summary result. In fact, this appears to be exactly the situation presented by Poole and Greenland in an examination of studies of water chlorination and cancer.[38] Random-effects summary estimates of the relative risk for various cancers were larger than corresponding fixed-effects summaries. This was apparently due to the assignment of higher relative weights to small studies which, in this case, showed relatively larger effects, that may not be representative of the findings of all small studies. Data presented by Villar and colleagues[110] found a similar phenomenon in studies in perinatal medicine.

A proposed solution to the problem of publication bias is the use of prospective registration of studies at their inception, prior to the availability of results.[49,173–180] Others have suggested obtaining unpublished data from the Food and Drug Administration (FDA), but one case study of such an approach found only a very small advantage to inclusion of data from the FDA. Going one step further, several prospective meta-analyses are either being planned or have been conducted.[181–184] These are meta-analyses that are planned, with complete protocols, including proposed tests of subgroup effects, prior to having knowledge of the results of any of the component studies. More on the topic of prospective meta-analysis is presented below.

CASE STUDIES OF APPLICATIONS OF META-ANALYSIS

Investigation of Adverse Effects

As mentioned earlier, the investigation of adverse or unwanted effects of existing therapies is an important application of meta-analysis. As discussed in Chapters 1 and 3, adverse events associated with pharmaceutical products are often so uncommon as to be difficult to study. In particular, the usual premarketing randomized studies frequently have too few patients to provide any useful information on the incidence of uncommon adverse events. By the same token, individual studies may have low statistical power to address particular questions. Meta-analysis provides the benefit of vastly increased statistical power to investigate adverse events. In fact, since 1982, the safety evaluation of drugs in the US has included pooled analyses.[185]

The assessment of the excess risk of gastrointestinal side effects associated with NSAIDs provides an excellent example of a situation in which meta-analysis has been helpful. Four different meta-analytic approaches to this problem will be reviewed here.

Chalmers and colleagues examined data from randomized trials of NSAIDs.[43] They argued that the typical epidemiologic approaches to investigating NSAIDs as risk factors for gastrointestinal side effects, i.e., cohort or case–control studies, are subject to too many potential biases. Randomized trials, on the other hand, would provide internally valid comparisons of NSAID users to nonusers. Presumably, although not stated explicitly, the combination of results from numerous studies, with varied entry and exclusion criteria, would alleviate the problem of the potential lack of generalizability from patients enrolled in a particular trial. The pooling of results from numerous studies would permit the assessment of rare events.

The authors performed a meta-analysis of randomized trials, excluding trials involving topical usage of NSAIDs, those that examined pharmacological endpoints only, studies of newborns, trials involving fewer than four days of treatment, trials in which patients were taking NSAIDs within the three days before randomization, and trials of drugs for dysmenorrhea (because of the short duration of the drug regimen and the confounding gastrointestinal symptoms from the dysmenorrhea). The meta-analysis was limited to those trials in which the anti-inflammatory drug was compared with a placebo, no drug, or a drug with no anti-inflammatory property. Photocopies of the "Methods" sections of 525 potentially relevant studies (blinded as to author, journal, and time and place of study, as well as all allusions to results) were read by two independent observers who determined inclusion suitability according to the above criteria.

Data were extracted for the following endpoints: nausea, indigestion or dyspepsia, gross gastrointestinal bleeding, suspected ulcer only, proven ulcer, gastric side effects, and unspecified gastric side effects. Factors that might be related to the incidence of these endpoints were also extracted from the studies: disease under study, drug ingested, dose and duration of drug, age of patients, sex of patients, and date of publication. The data were analyzed by crude pooling (i.e., ignoring the stratification by study and simply collapsing over studies), by unweighted averaging of the within-study risk differences, and by a weighted average of the risk differences. Additional analyses were performed to determine whether any factors seemed to be associated with a study showing a harmful effect of NSAIDs.

As a methodologic aside, the authors examined inter-reader disagreements. Overall, a disagreement rate of 19% was observed for the final decision on inclusion or exclusion of studies. These disagreements were resolved in conference.

There were 100 randomized trials of non-aspirin NSAIDs included in the final analysis, containing 123 comparisons

with a no-treatment control group, which usually received a placebo. A total of 12 853 patients were included in these trials, with a mean duration of treatment of about 67 days (median 21 days) and a mean age of 46 years. For the sake of brevity, the aspirin trials will not be discussed here. The data revealed a generally low risk of gastrointestinal side effects. For example, only two patients were reported with proven ulcers out of 6460 treated patients, with none in the controls. In the 10 studies explicitly mentioning gross upper-gastrointestinal hemorrhage, the risk was 8/1103 (0.73%) in the control patients and 24/1157 (2.1%) in treated patients, giving a crude relative risk of 2.8. The length of follow-up for these 10 studies was not specifically mentioned by the authors of the meta-analysis. However, the analysis of duration of therapy showed that duration was longer for studies showing a harmful effect of NSAIDs (geometric mean = 81 days) than for studies showing no effect of NSAIDs (geometric mean = 25 days) for the gross hemorrhage endpoint, consistent with a duration–response effect.

This meta-analysis was faced with some interesting statistical and other methodologic questions. There were numerous studies that did not explicitly mention side effects in general or did not mention particular side effects, even though others were mentioned. The authors chose to do a kind of sensitivity analysis by analyzing all studies, assuming that the risk of an unreported side effect was zero, and separately analyzing results from only those studies explicitly mentioning a particular side effect.

Another issue was the extensive number of studies with no occurrences of a particular endpoint in either the treated or the control group. The usual pooling procedures, e.g., the Mantel–Haenszel procedure,[96] essentially ignore such studies, since they contribute no information, under one interpretation, concerning the common odds ratio. On the other hand, if over 90 of 100 separate trials report no proven ulcers in either the treated or the control groups, then another interpretation of those results is that the risk of an ulcer is fairly low. Chalmers and colleagues chose to work with risk differences to address this issue, allowing studies with no events in either group to enter the calculations. This is the type of situation considered by Deeks and colleagues,[101] whose results suggest that the one-step method would have been the most appropriate for these studies with frequent occurrence of zero cells.

The use of randomized trials to study uncommon adverse effects of NSAIDs was also the strategy adopted by the Southern California Evidence-Based Practice Center. Their work is cited elsewhere in this chapter in the context of publication bias, but they also present results on relative risks.[44]

Another meta-analytic approach to the problem of side effects of NSAIDs was used by Gabriel and colleagues,[186] who examined the results of 16 nonexperimental studies (9 case–control and 7 cohort) of serious gastrointestinal complications related to use of NSAIDs. The studies had to have a comparison group and provide an estimate of risk for serious gastrointestinal complications (defined as bleeding, perforation, or other adverse gastrointestinal events resulting in hospitalization or death) in NSAID users compared with nonusers, regardless of underlying disease. They excluded studies if the primary goal was to assess effectiveness.

The odds ratio found by these authors for gastrointestinal bleeding, based on 9 studies reporting this endpoint, was 2.39 (CI 2.11, 2.70). The authors performed separate analyses for case–control and cohort studies. Although these separate summaries are only reported graphically and the exact values are difficult to read, the summary odds ratio from the cohort studies is clearly closer to unity than the result from the case–control studies. These authors also found that the size of the odds ratio was related to the duration of NSAID use. Interestingly, though, the highest odds ratios were obtained from studies in which the duration of NSAID consumption was less than 1 month. (Note: Gabriel, *et al.* only presented this finding without adjustment for study design, case–control versus cohort. Although they performed a multiple regression to examine inter-study heterogeneity, the findings of that model with respect to the individual potential sources of heterogeneity were not presented. It is possible that the studies with under one month of NSAID use were also predominantly case–control studies, but that cannot be determined from their paper, leaving the underlying source of heterogeneity somewhat ambiguous.)

The consistency of results for gastrointestinal bleeding between the two meta-analyses is of interest and lends some support to a causal association. Several points are important in considering the above results. In a cohort study of gastrointestinal bleeding and NSAIDs, Carson and colleagues[187] found a quadratic duration–response relation. They argue that this is compatible with an increasing risk with increasing duration of NSAID use, as suggested by Chalmers *et al.*,[43] until many of those patients who would develop gastrointestinal bleeding from NSAIDs were removed from the cohort and then the risk declined. This reasoning may explain the apparently anomalous finding by Gabriel *et al.*[186] of highest odds ratios for studies with less than one month of NSAID use.

Bollini and colleagues[188] also examined epidemiologic studies that investigated the association between NSAIDs and severe upper gastrointestinal tract disease, including hematemesis, melena, peptic ulcer, ulcer perforation, and death attributable to these outcomes. The studies had to compare groups exposed and unexposed to NSAIDs. Of the 34 studies they examined, 7 were cohort, 8 case–control with community controls, and 19 case–control with hospital controls. The type of study design was associated with varying estimates of the relative risk. Case–control studies with hospital controls had the highest average relative risk (4.4 CI 3.3, 6.0) and the cohort studies had the lowest (2.0 CI 1.2, 3.2). They found that studies with satisfactory methods yielded on average a lower relative risk (2.6 CI 1.8, 3.9) as compared with studies whose methods were unsatisfactory (4.2 CI 3.1, 5.6).

In perhaps the most comprehensive and clinically useful of the systematic reviews in the area of NSAIDs side effects, Henry and colleagues[189] addressed the issue of *comparative* relative risks of serious gastrointestinal complications with individual NSAIDs. Their stated motivation for this approach was that one strategy for reducing NSAID toxicity in populations would be to choose, as first line therapy, a drug and dose with a comparatively low risk of gastrointestinal side effects.

The authors used meta-analytic methods to examine the range of relative risks for particular NSAIDs and explore the extent to which differences in toxicity could be related to different doses, or to different susceptibility among patients receiving the various drugs. To do this, they identified case–control or cohort studies of relationships between use of specific NSAIDs in the community and development of serious peptic ulcer complications requiring hospital admission. In estimating pooled relative risks, analyses were restricted to studies that compared another drug with ibuprofen as the reference. They used unadjusted relative risks based on 2×2 tables in the pooling.

The authors found 12 studies examining 14 NSAIDs, including two unpublished reports. Eleven of the studies were case–control studies. The estimated relative risks for specific drugs versus ibuprofen ranged from 1.6 (CI 1.0, 2.5) for fenoprofen, to 9.2 (CI 4.0, 21) for azapropazone. All of the relative risks were significantly greater than 1.0. Using a weighted ranking system, which incorporated study size into the weights, the authors found that ibuprofen had the lowest rank (least toxicity), followed by diclofenac. Aspirin and naproxen had intermediate risks, while azapropazone, tolmetin, and ketoprofen had the highest risks. High dose ibuprofen (i.e., greater than 1600 mg daily) was also associated with an elevated relative risk.

It is important to keep in mind that the conclusions reached by Henry *et al.* were based on indirect comparisons of the various drugs with ibuprofen. They claimed to find little evidence that the relative rankings were due to confounding by patient susceptibility. Despite any shortcomings of their approach, as the authors point out, clinical and regulatory decisions have to be made on some type of scientific basis, and these are the only data available. Risks need to be weighed against benefit, and the authors highlight the known variability across patients in clinical response to particular drugs. Thus, it seems that this systematic review provided useful information for clinical decision making.

In qualitative reviews of the literature on the gastrointestinal side effects of NSAIDs, Taragin *et al.*[190] and Carson and Strom[191] point out differences in study designs that could lead to differences in results. For example, bleeding could be defined as all bleeding, fatal bleeding, bleeding requiring hospitalization, bleeding requiring transfusions, or bleeding requiring surgery. Several procedures exist for the detection of gastrointestinal bleeding. The clinical relevance of the different methods is sometimes unclear. Case–control studies may show higher odds ratios because of the likelihood of recall bias; patients with bleeding requiring hospitalization might be more likely to recall NSAID use than controls, particularly if probing by interviewers, or by health care providers prior to interview, is more extensive for cases than for controls. This possibility is supported by the data from the Gabriel *et al.* meta-analysis. Cohort studies based on claims data, such as that conducted by Carson and colleagues[187] described above, sometimes use unvalidated outcomes. To the extent that false events may be documented for both the exposed and unexposed cohorts, the relative risk observed in such studies would show less of an effect of exposure. Of course, these cohort studies may exaggerate the apparent effect of exposure if spurious diagnoses of gastrointestinal events are more likely to occur when a patient has a history of NSAID use. Further variability may be generated among study results by the inclusion of many different kinds of NSAIDs, some of which may have more potential to cause gastrointestinal side effects than others.

Thus, another benefit of meta-analysis is the ability to examine findings according to study characteristics and study design, leading to hypotheses about subgroups or particular therapies of special interest and suggestions for the design of subsequent studies. Meta-analysis can quantify differences related to study design that the traditional review can only observe in qualitative terms.

There are numerous other examples of the application of meta-analysis to the evaluation of adverse effects of pharmaceutical therapies. These include:

1. Two meta-analyses have been published on the effects of prophylactic lidocaine in acute myocardial infarction.[192–194] These studies showed that, although lidocaine effectively prevented ventricular fibrillation,[194] there seemed to be an excess in mortality among those patients randomly allocated to lidocaine compared with those allocated to placebo. In a related paper, using meta-analytic regression methods, Antman and Berlin[195] calculated that, given the low baseline incidence of ventricular fibrillation in the current coronary care unit environment, 400 patients would require treatment with lidocaine to prevent a single episode of ventricular fibrillation. Considering this estimate in addition to the possibly increased risk of mortality, the authors suggest that prophylactic lidocaine should not be given routinely.

2. In a meta-analysis of randomized trials regarding the efficacy and safety of quinidine therapy for the maintenance of sinus rhythm after cardioversion,[196] the authors showed that quinidine is, indeed, effective at maintaining sinus rhythm, but that mortality seems to be elevated in quinidine patients (mortality odds ratio = 2.98, CI 1.1, 8.3, based on 12 deaths among patients randomized to quinidine versus only 3 among patients randomized to placebo). In a subsequent paper, the authors examined the relationship between study design and outcome.[197] The nonrandomized studies tended to show less benefit of quinidine with respect to maintenance of sinus rhythm compared with the randomized studies. The odds ratios for mortality also varied according to study design, although there were few deaths overall: OR = 3.5 (CI 1.0, 12.4) for randomized studies; OR = 9.9 (CI 0.8, 123.2) for nonrandomized studies. The overall mortality risk was 2.0% (34/1709) for quinidine-treated patients and 0.6% (4/681) for all control patients.

3. A third example is the meta-analysis of nonexperimental studies of oral contraceptives and the risk of breast cancer discussed above.[23] An association between increasing odds ratio and increasing duration of oral contraceptive use was found in case–control studies in which the cases were mostly premenopausal (defined as age limit of 45 years old or less). In a subsequent methodologic paper, Berlin and colleagues[3] used these same data to show that the magnitude of the odds ratio depends not only on the menopausal status of the cases but on the calendar years during which cases were accrued, presumably because of the changing formulations of oral contraceptives.

New Indications for Existing Therapies

Meta-analysis has also been used to assess the effectiveness of existing therapies for new indications. As an example, the efficacy of antilymphocyte antibodies in the perioperative period of cadaveric kidney transplantation (induction therapy) had not, until recently, been conclusively demonstrated. Individual studies, both randomized and nonexperimental, had failed individually to show a significant benefit of induction therapy with respect to allograft survival. Szczech and colleagues performed a meta-analysis of the published data from the randomized trials of induction therapy[198] in adults receiving cadaveric renal transplants. That analysis, using survival analytic methods on the group-level (published) data, showed a statistically significant 31% lower rate of allograft failure at two years in patients receiving induction therapy.

In a subsequent analysis of the individual patient data from five of the seven randomized trials of induction therapy, Szczech and colleagues examined the effect of induction therapy beyond two years and in subgroups of patients with risk factors for early allograft failure.[199] The subgroup analyses are examined in the next section. The five studies included in the individual patient analyses yielded results for the two-year analysis virtually identical to those obtained from the full set of seven studies using the published data, i.e., a relative rate of 0.69 favoring induction therapy. When extended to five years, the rate of allograft survival was 69.0% in patients receiving induction therapy and 64.4% in those not receiving induction therapy ($p = 0.13$). Thus, the overall benefit demonstrated at two years was smaller and no longer significant at five years.

Differential Effects among Subgroups of Patients

In the analysis of individual patient data by Szczech and colleagues,[199] the authors were able to examine the specific effects of induction therapy in subgroups of patients at high risk for allograft failure. Before proceeding to analyses *within* particular subgroups, the authors tested statistical interactions between each of the relevant patient characteristics and induction therapy. One of the patient characteristics of interest was the panel reactive antibody level (PRA), an indicator of immune system presensitization. Patients with PRA levels less than 20% were considered unsensitized, while those with PRA of 20% or higher were considered presensitized. At two years, the effect of induction therapy differed in presensitized and unsensitized patients ($p = 0.03$ for interaction). The rate ratio at two years was

0.12 (CI 0.03 to 0.44, $p = 0.002$) in presensitized patients (85 patients with 15 failures) and 0.74 (CI 0.50 to 1.09, $p = 0.13$) in unsensitized patients (511 patients with 100 failures). This interaction was still significant at five years ($p = 0.009$ for interaction), with a rate ratio of 0.20 (CI 0.09 to 0.47, $p < 0.001$) in presensitized patients (85 patients with 33 failures) and 0.97 (CI 0.71 to 1.32, $p > 0.2$) in unsensitized patients (510 patients with 163 failures). The authors found no other significant interactions between induction therapy and any other variable.[199]

Several advantages of meta-analysis, and particularly individual-patient analyses, are demonstrated by this example. The improved precision provided by large numbers of patients is an important benefit. Having individual-level data allowed an analysis that could go beyond the simple, unadjusted analyses to which most meta-analyses of published data are limited. The availability of patient characteristics permitted not only *adjustment* for those characteristics, but also examination of subgroup effects in larger numbers of patients than would typically be included in a single trial. Although one might wish to confirm these subgroup results in an independent data set, the patient-level analyses strongly suggest that induction therapy is effective in the 14% of patients who are presensitized. If confirmed, these results could mean that induction therapy could be targeted to the group in which it is highly effective, while avoiding needless treatment and potential toxicity in other patients.

Selection from among Several Alternative Therapies

In a meta-analysis of therapies for the prevention of supraventricular arrhythmias after coronary bypass surgery, Andrews *et al.*[47] looked separately at verapamil, digoxin, and β-adrenoceptor blockers as prophylactic agents. Only randomized trials were included. Neither digoxin nor verapamil reduced the risk of supraventricular arrhythmias after coronary artery bypass surgery (digoxin: OR = 0.97, CI = 0.62, 1.49; verapamil: OR = 0.91, CI = 0.57, 1.46). The risk of a supraventricular arrhythmia in patients treated with β-blockers was dramatically reduced (OR = 0.28, CI = 0.21, 0.36), although significant heterogeneity among the study results was present. The authors explored this heterogeneity by examining separately studies of different β-blockers, and by summarizing separately preoperative and postoperative treatment. While these separate summaries suggested varying degrees of heterogeneity within subgroups of studies, all of the summaries showed statistically significant benefits of β-blockers. The authors drew no firm conclusions from the subgroup analyses other than to suggest directions for future research.

As another example, for several decades, heparin has been used as the primary antithrombotic drug for the initial treatment of venous thromboembolism. There has been some controversy over the optimal mode of administration of heparin: intermittent intravenous, continuous intravenous, or subcutaneous injection. While continuous infusion has been shown to be safer than intermittent injection, and equally effective, continuous infusion has disadvantages, such as the need for hospitalization for most patients, possibly prolonged immobilization, enhanced risk for sepsis related to the infusion cannula, and possible increased cost.[200] Hommes and colleagues performed a meta-analysis of randomized trials of intravenous versus subcutaneous heparin administration in the initial treatment of deep vein thrombosis.[200] They found eight studies meeting their inclusion criteria. The overall summary relative risk for efficacy was 0.62 (CI 0.39, 0.98), indicating a benefit from the use of subcutaneous compared with intravenous administration. The analysis of safety (i.e., risk of major hemorrhage) also showed a modest benefit of subcutaneous injection (relative risk=0.79; CI 0.42, 1.46). In the analysis of efficacy, as in others described above, there was highly significant among-study heterogeneity. The source of this heterogeneity was apparently a single study showing a significant benefit from intravenous administration.[201] The authors of the meta-analysis speculated that the particular study failed to achieve therapeutic levels of heparin in the subcutaneous group.

A somewhat different approach to subgroup analyses has emerged in recent years. This strategy views the risk of events in the control group of a trial (baseline risk) as a general indicator of severity of disease in the treated population. The relationship between treatment benefit and baseline risk can then be estimated, i.e., examining whether there is an interaction between treatment and baseline risk.[111–114,147] A number of statistical issues arise in such analyses, including the inherent association induced by regressing treatment benefit (e.g., the log relative risk, which is calculated using the baseline risk) on baseline risk, and the fact that the baseline risk, except in very large studies, is affected by sampling variability. These approaches all use group-level (published) data, examining whether the risk in the *population* is associated with the magnitude of treatment benefit. This may not necessarily yield the same result as looking at the interaction on an *individual patient* basis between treatment and *individual-level* estimates of risk. It is also clearly different clinically from examining specific patient characteristics, as opposed to calculating estimates of risk that depend on several characteristics. Information may be lost by using multivariable risk estimates,

as opposed to potentially biologically specific patient characteristics.

Saving Time and Money if You Believe a Meta-analysis

One of the potential benefits of meta-analysis is the potential to shorten the time between a medical research finding and the clinical implementation of a new therapy. This is a concern not only for the development of new drugs, but for the exploration of new indications for existing therapies. As a simple but elegant example of the use of meta-analysis in the approval context, Webber and colleagues[202] report the use of meta-analysis of ECG data from several clinical pharmacology studies for two submissions. They calculated a pooled estimate for the difference between active doses and placebo in a continuous measure of QT prolongation. This approach allowed the sponsor to avoid having to perform a new safety study to address the question of QT prolongation.

One prominent group has advocated the routine use of what they have termed "cumulative meta-analysis," i.e., performing a new meta-analysis each time the results of a new clinical trial are published.[45,203] Antman et al.[45] applied this technique in combination with a classification scheme of the treatment recommendations for myocardial infarction found in review articles and textbook chapters. They found many discrepancies between the evidence contained in the published randomized trials and the timeliness of the recommendations.

As an example, Antman and colleagues analyzed data from 17 trials of β-blockers for the prevention of death in the years following a myocardial infarction.[45] In the left-hand side of Figure 44.3, reproduced from their paper, the data are presented as a traditional meta-analysis, with individual study results presented along with the summary odds ratio arbitrarily estimated after 17 trials had been completed. In the right-hand side of Figure 44.3, the same data are presented as a cumulative meta-analysis, with an updated summary estimate calculated after the completion of each new trial. The cumulative meta-analysis clearly shows that the updated pooled estimate became statistically significant in 1977 and has remained so ever since.

The process of cumulative meta-analysis was applied by these authors to eight therapies for acute myocardial infarction. In five of the six instances in which the cumulative meta-analyses revealed the therapies to be of statistically significant benefit in reducing in-hospital mortality, it was several years before experts recommended the therapy with any consistency. An important example was thrombolytic therapy, which did not begin to be recommended by more

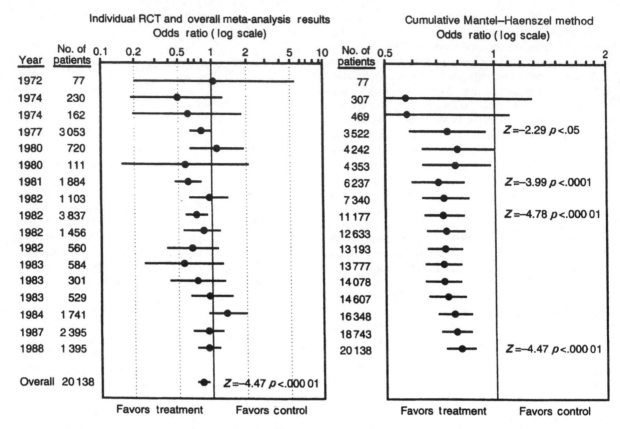

Figure 44.3. Results of 17 randomized control trials of the effects of oral β-blockers for secondary prevention of mortality in patients surviving a myocardial infarction presented as two types of meta-analyses. On the left is the traditional one, revealing many trials with nonsignificant results but a highly significant estimate of the pooled results on the bottom of the panel. On the right, the same data are presented as cumulative meta-analyses, illustrating that the updated pooled estimate became statistically significant in 1977 and has remained so up to the present. Note that the scale is changed on the right graph to improve clarity of the confidence intervals. Reprinted with permission from: Antman *et al*, *JAMA* 1992; **268**: 240–8. Copyright 1992. American Medical Association. All rights reserved.

than half the experts, even for specific indications, until 13 years after the cumulative meta-analysis would have shown therapy to be effective. Six years passed between the publication, in a major journal,[45,204] of the first meta-analysis showing an impressive reduction in mortality by thrombolytic therapy and the year in which the majority of the experts, whose opinions were studied by the authors, recommended it for routine or specific use. In 1985, a 20% reduction in mortality was established at the $p < 0.001$ level (OR = 0.78; CI 0.69, 0.90). A total of 14 reviews after 1985 did not mention the treatment or felt that it was still experimental. The authors concluded that identifying and interpreting the therapeutic trials in a given field is extremely difficult, so that clinical experts need access to better

databases and new statistical techniques (like cumulative meta-analysis).

Some caution may be advised in interpreting cumulative meta-analyses. The issue of multiple statistical tests, for example, is considered by some to be an important consideration. The problem is that testing and estimation procedures may need to make adjustments for the increased probability of a spurious positive finding (type I, or α, error) introduced by the use of repeated statistical tests.[112,205] At the least, one might wish to consider using a more stringent criterion for statistical significance than the traditional $p < 0.05$ cutoff. A recent paper proposes a correction to p-values in the context of cumulative meta-analysis.[206] Another consideration is that estimates of treatment effect may not be stable over time, perhaps due to changing clinical environments. In the β-blocker example, there is an apparent "drift" of the effect estimate back toward the null in more recent years, i.e., treatment appears to be less effective in the most recent studies. Thus, it may be important to re-evaluate therapies as other treatment strategies evolve for the same conditions.

A final caution with regard to interpreting cumulative meta-analyses relates to the continuing need for well-designed randomized controlled trials. New indications for existing therapies, for example, are often suggested by nonexperimental studies, including cohort and case–control studies and nonrandomized Phase II clinical trials. The results of these studies are not always confirmed by subsequent, properly designed randomized trials. For example, consider the case of β-carotene in the prevention of cancer. A series of observational studies (see Ziegler et al.[207] for a review) examined the relation between dietary intake of foods rich in β-carotene and the risk of lung cancer. Overall, they showed a relatively consistent association between diets rich in β-carotene and reduced risk of lung cancer. Subsequent randomized trials of this specific nutrient as a supplement have failed to confirm a protective effect against lung cancer.[208,209] A similar, and much publicized, situation arose with respect to combination estrogen plus progestin as hormone replacement therapy. A series of nonexperimental studies had shown a protective effect against cardiovascular disease. The Women's Health Initiative combination therapy arm[210] was terminated early, partly because of increased risk of cardiovascular disease.

THE FUTURE

The examples above have raised several important issues that will need to be addressed in the future. A set of issues not fully addressed above relates to the availability of individual-level data. From the above examples, it becomes increasingly apparent that the pursuit of questions about subgroups of patients is often an informative and important element of a well-conducted meta-analysis, at least for certain therapies. One should certainly exercise due caution in the interpretation of subgroup effects, emphasizing those that are specified *a priori* with biological justification. By assembling large numbers of patients, meta-analysis can at least begin to address the problems related to statistical instability of subgroup effects. It is too often the case, however, that results are not reported separately for subgroups of patients. Typically, some trials will exclude particular patients while others will not exclude them. At the level of grouped data from published

reports, one is faced with analyzing the two groups of studies separately as the only way of addressing the subgroup question, or using meta-regression techniques on what amounts to ecological data. As a trivial hypothetical example, suppose one wanted to perform separate analyses of the effect of treatment X in men and women. Among the existing randomized trials, six exclude women and four do not, but the four also include men. Ideally, one would like to obtain information on the effect in men alone from all of the 10 trials, since all include men. Similarly, one could obtain a separate estimate of the effect of treatment in women from the four studies including women. It is possible to use the group-level data only to show, for example, that studies that include women tend to show different effects than studies excluding women, but one cannot perform a separate analysis of women. One might alternatively regress the treatment effect measure (e.g., log relative risk) against the percentage male (or female), but that is still less satisfactory than obtaining patient-level data. For further practical discussions of the use of individual patient data, see Stewart and Clarke,[211] Stewart and Parmar,[212] Duchateau et al.,[213] and Schmid et al.[214] Mechanisms for the sharing of person-level data need to be promoted.

In practice, an important question is whether results for subgroups obtained using group-level data are consistent with what one would find using patient-level data. Increasing evidence is accumulating that such consistency is not the rule. In a methodologic paper extending the work on induction therapy described above, Berlin and colleagues[215] found that the conclusion that induction therapy in renal transplant patients is limited to those with elevated PRA was not found consistently in the group-level data. Lambert and colleagues, in a simulation study, point out that the group-level analyses often have low statistical power, even in the absence of systematic bias in the group-level comparisons. Thus, it seems there is a trade-off between the resource-intensive individual patient analysis against the less expensive but potentially invalid group-level analysis. Again, the need to facilitate availability of individual patient data is apparent and has been recognized by the US government. The National Institutes of Health (NIH) in the US have developed a policy on data sharing of final research data from NIH-supported studies for use by other researchers. Investigators submitting an NIH application will be required to include a plan for data sharing or to state why data sharing is not possible. NIH will support such sharing, financially, either in project budgets or through administrative supplements to grants. (For more details, see http://grants2.nih.gov/grants/guide/notice-files/NOT-OD-03-032.html.)

In the development of cumulative meta-analysis, some of the most important issues will be philosophical ones. Some of the same issues apply to the approval process for new drugs. How much evidence is required before a therapy can be accepted as efficacious? Should we require the existence of a certain minimum number of trials showing a statistically significant benefit of a therapy? Suppose 10 studies all show a 20% (or thereabouts) reduction in mortality in patients treated with drug X compared to placebo, but none of the individual studies shows a statistically significant effect. If the combined analysis shows a highly statistically significant 20% reduction in mortality due to treatment X, and 20% is considered clinically significant, should the combined analysis be sufficient evidence for the acceptance of drug X as beneficial? What would an additional, large clinical trial contribute?

In this context, it is worth noting that several empirical studies have examined discrepancies between large trials and meta-analyses of the same therapies.[216–221] The assumption made by some of the authors of these studies, that larger studies are necessarily better studies, may not be valid. Replication of a finding by independent studies must certainly be a key element to establishing efficacy, as compared with a single trial. Large trials may also be poorly designed. For example, for BCG vaccine, a huge trial using passive follow-up, and therefore missing (by the authors' own admission) at least 50% of all cases of tuberculosis, failed to show the protective effect found in a number of other studies with more complete follow-up.[222,223] Another paper[224] points out that one can also find discrepancies between large trials of the same therapy. They found that in approximately 27% of pairs of large studies identified from the Cochrane Library, the two studies had findings that were statistically significantly different from each other. This is identical to the proportion of discrepant comparisons in a highly visible paper by LeLorier et al.,[216] in which comparisons between meta-analyses and subsequent large trials were made.

When there is little or no heterogeneity of results among trials, and the likelihood of serious publication bias is minimal, one might be willing to accept meta-analytic evidence as helping to establish effectiveness. It is less obvious what to do with the results of a meta-analysis when there is substantial heterogeneity. If the heterogeneity is adequately explained in the analysis in terms of subgroup effects, or trial quality, meta-analysis might still be an acceptable part of demonstrating effectiveness, but such a conclusion might be conditional on the type of patient or other factors.

Similarly, the technique of cumulative meta-analysis could be applied to the analysis of adverse events. As nonexperimental studies of adverse effects are completed, the same approach could be applied. The likelihood seems to be, however, that such meta-analyses would be faced with much more serious issues of heterogeneity of findings than meta-analyses of randomized studies typically have to confront. The acceptance of meta-analytic results in this context might be extremely slow. (Consider the slow pace, demonstrated by Antman et al.,[45] with which new therapies are accepted even when the evidence is provided by randomized trials.) Even if a meta-analysis of, for example, oral contraceptive use and breast cancer risk were to show a convincing, consistent duration–response relationship, the issue of what to do with that information is complex. If the relative risk for 10 years of use is 1.5, is that sufficient to warrant removal of oral contraceptives from the market? Would 2.5 be a sufficiently high relative risk? What other factors, e.g., family history, etc., need to be considered when prescribing oral contraceptives? While these are clearly more general issues, not restricted to the interpretation of meta-analyses, the additional precision provided by meta-analyses makes their interpretation all the more difficult.

There has been growing attention paid to the potential for indirect comparisons to contribute evidence regarding the efficacy and safety of therapies. Alternative treatments for the same indication are often available, but have not always been evaluated in head-to-head randomized comparisons. Even when there are direct comparisons available, these may constitute a small portion of the available evidence. Several papers have presented statistical methods for performing indirect comparisons.[225–227] The basic principle of these methods is most clearly discussed by Bucher and colleagues.[225] If drug A is compared to placebo in one randomized trial using an odds ratio for a dichotomous outcome, and drug B is similarly compared to placebo in another randomized trial, the comparison of A to B is achieved essentially by dividing the odds ratios, in effect "subtracting out" the placebo. The assumption needed for these indirect comparisons to be valid is that there is no modification of the treatment effect by patient characteristics that may differ in their distribution between the two trials (even if that factor is balanced within each trial). So, for example, if treatments A and B in the hypothetical trials above were both effective in men but not in women, the trial of drug A had 20% men in each of the active and placebo arms, and the trial of drug B had 50% men in each arm, drug B could appear to more effective than drug A, even if the two drugs were truly equally effective, simply because of the imbalance *between* the trials in the sex distribution of the patients. Psaty and colleagues[228] used both direct and indirect comparisons of drugs for hypertension. Song and colleagues[229] reviewed 44 published meta-analyses in which both direct and indirect comparisons had been made, and found that adjusted indirect comparisons often, but not always, agree with the corresponding direct comparisons. In 3 of the 44 comparisons, a significant discrepancy between the adjusted indirect and the direct comparisons was found.

The concept of prospective meta-analysis also merits further attention. Along with registration of trials, this closely related strategy has been advocated as a means of avoiding publication bias.[181–184] It may be possible, however, to go beyond simply planning the logistics of multiple trials and the collection of common data elements to allow pooling of results upon the completion of all trials. It may be possible to go further toward planning the scientific questions to be addressed. As a simple example, by regulation, sex and age (adult versus pediatric) would need to be addressed for a new analgesic. In addition, it would be important to consider indication (emergency department, postoperative, etc.) and dose (cumulative dose, daily dose, need for a loading dose, etc.). How best to design the *series* of studies to address all of these questions, either simultaneously or sequentially, needs further consideration (see Berlin and Colditz[32] for a more complete discussion of this issue).

While there are no easy answers to many of these questions, it is clear that meta-analysis will play an increasingly important role in the formulation of treatment and policy recommendations. Thus, the quality of the meta-analyses performed is of the utmost importance and needs to be reviewed by the scientific community in an open, published forum. Meta-analyses, if they are carefully interpreted in view of their strengths and weaknesses, should prove to be extremely helpful in pharmacoepidemiologic research.

REFERENCES

1. DerSimonian R, Laird N. Meta-analysis in clinical trials. *Controlled Clin Trials* 1986; **7**: 177–88.
2. Last JM. *A Dictionary of Epidemiology*, 2nd edn. New York: Oxford University Press, 1988.
3. Berlin JA, Longnecker MP, Greenland S. Meta-analysis of epidemiologic dose–response data. *Epidemiology* 1993; **4**: 218–28.
4. Feinstein AR. Para-analysis, faute de mieux, and the perils of riding on a data barge. *J Clin Epidemiol* 1989; **42**: 929–35.
5. Shapiro S. Is meta-analysis a valid approach to the evaluation of small effects in observational studies? *J Clin Epidemiol* 1997; **50**: 223–9.
6. Egger M, Schneider M, Davey Smith G. Spurious precision? Meta-analysis of observational studies. *BMJ* 1998; **316**: 140–4.
7. Thacker SB. Meta-analysis. A quantitative approach to research integration. *JAMA* 1988; **259**: 1685–9.
8. Buffler PA. The evaluation of negative epidemiologic studies: the importance of all available evidence in risk characterization. *Regul Toxicol Pharmacol* 1989; **9**: 34–43.
9. Sacks HS, Berrier J, Reitman D, Ancona-Berk VA, Chalmers TC. Meta-analyses of randomized controlled trials. *N Engl J Med* 1987; **316**: 450–5.
10. L'Abbe KA, Detsky AS, O'Rourke K. Meta-analysis in clinical research. *Ann Intern Med* 1987; **107**: 224–33.
11. Colditz GA, Burdick E, Mosteller F. Heterogeneity in meta-analysis of data from epidemiologic studies: a commentary. *Am J Epidemiol* 1995; **142**: 371–82.
12. Berlin JA. Invited commentary: benefits of heterogeneity in meta-analysis of data from epidemiologic studies. *Am J Epidemiol* 1995; **142**: 383–7.
13. Bero LA, Rennie D. The Cochrane Collaboration—preparing, maintaining, and disseminating systematic reviews of the effects of health care. *JAMA* 1995; **274**: 1935–38.
14. Davies P, Boruch R. The Campbell Collaboration does for public policy what Cochrane does for health. *BMJ* 2001; **323**: 294–5.
15. Dickersin K, Berlin JA. Meta-analysis: state-of-the-science. *Epidemiol Rev* 1992; **14**: 154–76.
16. Mulrow CD. The medical review article: state of the science. *Ann Intern Med* 1987; **106**: 485–8.
17. Oxman AD, Guyatt GH. Guidelines for reading literature reviews. *Can Med Assoc J* 1988; **138**: 697–703.
18. Chalmers I. Improving the quality and dissemination of clinical research. In: Lock S, ed., *The Future of Medical Journals: In Commemoration of 150 Years of the British Medical Journal*. London: British Medical Society, 1991; pp. 127–46.
19. Kass EH. Reviewing reviews. In: Warren KS, ed., *Coping with the Biomedical Literature: A Primer for the Scientist and the Clinician*. New York: Praeger, 1981; pp. 71–91.
20. Huth EJ. Needed: review articles with more scientific rigor. *Ann Intern Med* 1987; **106**: 470–1.
21. Canner PL. An overview of six clinical trials of aspirin in coronary heart disease. *Stat Med* 1987; **6**: 255–67.
22. Longnecker MP, Berlin JA, Orza MJ, Chalmers TC. A meta-analysis of alcohol consumption in relation to risk of breast cancer. *JAMA* 1988; **260**: 652–6.
23. Romieu I, Berlin JA, Colditz G. Oral contraceptives and breast cancer. Review and meta-analysis. *Cancer* 1990; **66**: 2253–63.
24. Frumkin H, Berlin J. Asbestos exposure and gastrointestinal malignancy: review and meta-analysis. *Am J Ind Med* 1988; **14**: 79–95 (published erratum appears in *Am J Ind Med* 1988; **14**: 493).
25. Berlin JA, Colditz GA. A meta-analysis of physical activity in the prevention of coronary heart disease. *Am J Epidemiol* 1990; **132**: 612–28.
26. Gray A, Berlin JA, McKinlay JB, Longcope C. An examination of research design effects on the association of testosterone and male aging: results of a meta-analysis. *J Clin Epidemiol* 1991; **44**: 671–84.

27. Longnecker MP, Orza MJ, Adams ME, Vioque J, Chalmers TC. A meta-analysis of alcoholic beverage consumption in relation to risk of colorectal cancer. *Cancer Causes Control* 1990; **1**: 59–68.

28. Wong O, Raabe GK. Critical review of cancer epidemiology in petroleum industry employees, with a quantitative meta-analysis by cancer site. *Am J Ind Med* 1989; **15**: 283–310.

29. Booth-Kewley S, Friedman HS. Psychological predictors of heart disease: a quantitative review. *Psychol Bull* 1987; **101**: 343–62.

30. Morgenstern H, Glazer WM, Niedzwiecki D, Nourjah P. The impact of neuroleptic medication on tardive dyskinesia: a meta-analysis of published studies. *Am J Pub Health* 1987; **77**: 717–24.

31. Hennessy S, Berlin J, Kinman JL, Margolis DJ, Marcus SM, Strom BL. Risk of venous thromboembolism from oral contraceptives containing gestodene and desogestrel versus levonorgestrel: a meta-analysis and formal sensitivity analysis. *Contraception* 2001; **64**: 125–33.

32. Berlin JA, Colditz GA. The role of meta-analysis in the regulatory process for foods, drugs, and devices. *JAMA* 1999; **281**: 830–4.

33. Greenland S, Longnecker MP. Methods for trend estimation from summarized dose–response data, with applications to meta-analysis. *Am J Epidemiol* 1992; **135**: 1301–9.

34. Greenland S, Salvan A. Bias in the one-step method for pooling study results. *Stat Med* 1990; **9**: 247–52.

35. Greenland S. Quantitative methods in the review of epidemiologic literature. *Epidemiol Rev* 1987; **9**: 1–30.

36. Fleiss JL, Gross AJ. Meta-analysis in epidemiology, with special reference to studies of the association between exposure to environmental tobacco smoke and lung cancer: a critique. *J Clin Epidemiol* 1991; **44**: 127–39.

37. O'Neill RT, Anello C. Does research synthesis have a place in drug regulatory policy? Synopsis of issues: assessment of efficacy and drug approval. *Clin Res Reg Aff* 1996; **13**: 23–9.

38. Poole C, Greenland S. Random-effects meta-analyses are not always conservative. *Am J Epidemiol* 1999; **150**: 469–75.

39. Jones DR. Meta-analysis of observational epidemiological studies: a review. *J R Soc Med* 1992; **85**: 165–8.

40. Einarson TR, Leeder JS, Koren G. A method for meta-analysis of epidemiological studies. *Drug Intell Clin Pharm* 1988; **22**: 813–24.

41. Greenland S. Invited commentary: a critical look at some popular meta-analytic methods. *Am J Epidemiol* 1994; **140**: 290–6.

42. Stroup D, Berlin J, Morton S, Olkin I, Williamson G, Rennie D *et al.* Meta-analysis of observational studies in epidemiology—a proposal for reporting. *JAMA* 2000; **283**: 2008–12.

43. Chalmers TC, Berrier J, Hewitt P, Berlin J, Reitman D, Nagalingam R *et al.* Meta-analysis of randomized controlled trials as a method of estimating rare complications of non-steroidal anti-inflammatory drug therapy. *Aliment Pharmacol Ther* 1988; **2** (suppl 25): 9–26.

44. MacLean CH, Morton SC, Ofman JJ, Roth EA, Shekelle PG. How useful are unpublished data from the Food and Drug Administration in meta-analysis? *J Clin Epidemiol* 2003; **56**: 44–51.

45. Antman EM, Lau J, Kupelnick B, Mosteller F, Chalmers TC. A comparison of results of meta-analyses of randomized control trials and recommendations of clinical experts. Treatments for myocardial infarction. *JAMA* 1992; **268**: 240–8.

46. Begg CB, Berlin JA. Publication bias and dissemination of clinical research. *J Natl Cancer Inst* 1989; **81**: 107–15.

47. Andrews TC, Reimold SC, Berlin JA, Antman EM. Prevention of supraventricular arrhythmias after coronary artery bypass surgery. A meta-analysis of randomized control trials. *Circulation* 1991; **84** (suppl 5): 236–44.

48. Easterbrook PJ, Berlin JA, Gopalan R, Matthews DR. Publication bias in clinical research. *Lancet* 1991; **337**: 867–72.

49. Moher D, Berlin J. Improving the reporting of randomised controlled trials. In: Maynard A, Chalmers I, eds, *Non-Random Reflections on Health Services Research*. London: BMJ Publishing Group, 1997; pp. 250–71.

50. Dickersin K, Min YI, Meinert CL. Factors influencing publication of research results. Follow-up of applications submitted to two institutional review boards. *JAMA* 1992; **267**: 374–8.

51. Dickersin K. The existence of publication bias and risk factors for its occurrence. *JAMA* 1990; **263**: 1385–9.

52. Dickersin K, Min YI. NIH clinical trials and publication bias. *Online J Curr Clin Trials* 1993; doc. no. 50.

53. Chalmers I. Underreporting research is scientific misconduct. *JAMA* 1990; **263**: 1405–8.

54. Chalmers TC, Frank CS, Reitman D. Minimizing the three stages of publication bias. *JAMA* 1990; **263**: 1392–5.

55. Stern JM, Simes RJ. Publication bias: evidence of delayed publication in a cohort study of clinical research projects. *BMJ* 1997; **315**: 640–5.

56. Ioannidis JP. Effect of the statistical significance of results on the time to completion and publication of randomized efficacy trials. *JAMA* 1998; **279**: 281–6.

57. Berlin JA, Begg CB, Louis TA. An assessment of publication bias using a sample of published clinical trials. *J Am Stat Assoc* 1989; **84**: 381–92.

58. Sutton AJ, Abrams KR, Jones DR. Generalized synthesis of evidence and the threat of dissemination bias: the example of electronic fetal heart rate monitoring (EFM). *J Clin Epidemiol* 2002; **55**: 1013–24.

59. Chalmers TC, Berrier J, Sacks HS, Levin H, Reitman D, Nagalingam R. Meta-analysis of clinical trials as a scientific discipline. II: Replicate variability and comparison of studies that agree and disagree. *Stat Med* 1987; **6**: 733–44.

60. Early Breast Cancer Trialists' Collaborative Group. *Treatment of Early Breast Cancer*, vol. I: *Worldwide Evidence*. New York: Oxford University Press, 1990.

61. Sutton AJ, Duval S, Tweedie R, Abrams KR, Jones DR. Empirical assessment of effect of publication bias on meta-analyses. *BMJ* 2000; **320**: 1574–7.

62. Hetherington J, Dickersin K, Chalmers I, Meinert CL. Retrospective and prospective identification of unpublished

controlled trials: lessons from a survey of obstetricians and pediatricians. *Pediatrics* 1989; **84**: 374–80.

63. Gotzsche PC. Reference bias in reports of drug trials. *BMJ (Clin Res Ed)* 1987; **295**: 654–6.

64. Egger M, Zellweger-Zahner T, Schneider M, Junker C, Lengeler C, Antes G. Language bias in randomised controlled trials published in English and German. *Lancet* 1997; **350**: 326–9.

65. Moher D, Fortin P, Jadad AR, Juni P, Klassen T, Le Lorier J *et al.* Completeness of reporting of trials published in languages other than English: implications for conduct and reporting of systematic reviews. *Lancet* 1996; **347**: 363–6.

66. Davidson RA. Source of funding and outcome of clinical trials. *J Gen Intern Med* 1986; **1**: 155–8.

67. Hemminki E. Study of information submitted by drug companies to licensing authorities. *BMJ* 1980; **280**: 833–6.

68. Cho MK, Bero LA. The quality of drug studies published in symposium proceedings. *Ann Intern Med* 1996; **124**: 485–9.

69. Chalmers TC. Problems induced by meta-analyses. *Stat Med* 1991; **10**: 971–9.

70. Conn HO, Blitzer BL. Nonassociation of adrenocorticosteroid therapy and peptic ulcer. *N Engl J Med* 1976; **294**: 473–9.

71. Messer J, Reitman D, Sacks HS, Smith H, Jr, Chalmers TC. Association of adrenocorticosteroid therapy and peptic-ulcer disease. *N Engl J Med* 1983; **309**: 21–4.

72. Conn HO, Poynard T. Adrenocorticosteroid administration and peptic ulcer: a critical analysis. *J Chronic Dis* 1985; **38**: 457–68.

73. Chalmers TC. Meta-analysis in clinical medicine. *Trans Am Clin Climatol Assoc* 1987; **99**: 144–50.

74. DerSimonian R. Parenteral nutrition with branched-chain amino acids in hepatic encephalopathy: meta-analysis. *Hepatology* 1990; **11**: 1083–4.

75. Erikkson LS, Conn HO. Branched-chain amino acids in hepatic encephalopathy. *Gastroenterology* 1990; **99**: 604–7 (published erratum appears in *Gastroenterology* 1990; **99**: 1547).

76. Naylor CD, O'Rourke K, Detsky AS, Baker JP. Parenteral nutrition with branched-chain amino acids in hepatic encephalopathy. A meta-analysis. *Gastroenterology* 1989; **97**: 1033–42.

77. Dickersin K, Hewitt P, Mutch L, Chalmers I, Chalmers TC. Perusing the literature: comparison of MEDLINE searching with a perinatal trials database. *Control Clin Trials* 1985; **6**: 306–17.

78. Poynard T, Conn HO. The retrieval of randomized clinical trials in liver disease from the medical literature. A comparison of MEDLARS and manual methods. *Control Clin Trials* 1985; **6**: 271–9.

79. Bernstein F. The retrieval of randomized clinical trials in liver diseases from the medical literature: manual versus MEDLARS searches. *Control Clin Trials* 1988; **9**: 23–31.

80. Chalmers I. *Oxford Database of Perinatal Trials*. Oxford: Oxford University Press, 1988.

81. Huston P, Moher D. Redundancy, disaggregation, and the integrity of medical research. *Lancet* 1996; **347**: 1024–6.

82. Detsky AS, Naylor CD, O'Rourke K, McGeer AJ, L'Abbe KA. Incorporating variations in the quality of individual randomized trials into meta-analysis. *J Clin Epidemiol* 1992; **45**: 255–65.

83. Berard A, Bravo G. Combining studies using effect sizes and quality scores: application to bone loss in postmenopausal women. *J Clin Epidemiol* 1998; **51**: 801–7.

84. Chalmers TC, Smith H, Jr, Blackburn B, Silverman B, Schroeder B, Reitman D *et al.* A method for assessing the quality of a randomized control trial. *Control Clin Trials* 1981; **2**: 31–49.

85. Imperiale TF, McCullough AJ. Do corticosteroids reduce mortality from alcoholic hepatitis? A meta-analysis of the randomized trials. *Ann Intern Med* 1990; **113**: 299–307.

86. Prendiville W, Elbourne D, Chalmers I. The effects of routine oxytocic administration in the management of the third stage of labour: an overview of the evidence from controlled trials. *Br J Obstet Gynaecol* 1988; **95**: 3–16.

87. Mahon WA, Daniel EE. A method for the assessment of reports of drug trials. *Can Med Assoc J* 1964; **90**: 565–9.

88. Verhagen AP, de Vet HCW, de Bie RA, Kessels AGH, Boers M, Bouter LM *et al.* The Delphi list: a criteria list for quality assessment of randomized clinical trials for conducting systematic reviews developed by Delphi consensus. *J Clin Epidemiol* 1998; **51**: 1235–41.

89. Moher D, Jadad AR, Tugwell P. Assessing the quality of randomized controlled trials. Current issues and future directions. *Int J Technol Assess Health Care* 1996; **12**: 195–208.

90. Moher D, Jadad AR, Nichol G, Penman M, Tugwell P, Walsh S. Assessing the quality of randomized controlled trials: an annotated bibliography of scales and checklists. *Control Clin Trials* 1995; **16**: 62–73.

91. Greenland S. Quality scores are useless and potentially misleading. *Am J Epidemiol* 1994; **140**: 300–1.

92. Jüni P, Witschi A, Block R, Egger M. The hazards of scoring the quality of clinical trials for meta-analysis. *JAMA* 1999; **282**: 1054–60.

93. Schulz KF, Chalmers I, Hayes RJ, Altman DG. Empirical evidence of bias. Dimensions of methodological quality associated with estimates of treatment effects in controlled trials. *JAMA* 1995; **273**: 408–12.

94. Greenland S, O'Rourke K. On the bias produced by quality scores in meta-analysis, and a hierarchical view of proposed solutions. *Biostatistics* 2001; **2**: 463–71.

95. Berlin JA, Miles CG, Cirigliano MD, Conill AM, Goldmann DR, Horowitz DA *et al.* Does blinding of readers affect the results of metaanalyses? Results of a randomized trial. *Online J Curr Clin Trials* 1997; doc. no. 205.

96. Kleinbaum DG, Kupper LL, Morgenstern H. *Epidemiologic Research: Principles and Quantitative Methods*. New York: Van Nostrand Reinhold, 1982.

97. Rothman KJ, Greenland S. *Modern Epidemiology*, 2nd edn. Philadelphia, PA: Lippincott, Williams and Wilkins, 1998.

98. Yusuf S, Peto R, Lewis J, Collins R, Sleight P. Beta blockade during and after myocardial infarction: an overview of the randomized trials. *Prog Cardiovasc Dis* 1985; **27**: 335–71.

99. Tang J-L. Weighting bias in meta-analysis of binary outcomes. *J Clin Epidemiol* 2000; **53**: 1130–6.

100. Chang B-H, Waternaux C, Lipsitz S. Meta-analysis of binary data: which within study variance estimate to use? *Stat Med* 2001; **20**: 1947–56.
101. Deeks J, Bradburn M, Localio R, Berlin J. Much ado about nothing: statistical models for meta-analysis with rare events. 6th International Cochrane Colloquium, Baltimore, MD, 1998.
102. Berlin JA, Laird NM, Sacks HS, Chalmers TC. A comparison of statistical methods for combining event rates from clinical trials. *Stat Med* 1989; **8**: 141–51.
103. Fleiss JL. The statistical basis of meta-analysis. *Stat Methods Med Res* 1993; **2**: 121–45.
104. Follmann DA, Proschan MA. Valid inference in random effects meta-analysis. *Biometrics* 1999; **55**: 732–7.
105. Aitkin M. Meta-analysis by random effect modelling in generalized linear models. *Stat Med* 1999; **18**: 2343–51.
106. Frost C, Clarke R, Beacon H. Use of hierarchical models for meta-analysis: experience in the metabolic ward studies of diet and blood cholesterol. *Stat Med* 1999; **18**: 1657–76.
107. Senn SJ. The many modes of META. *Drug Inf J* 2000; **34**: 535–49.
108. Sidek K, Jonkman J. A simple confidence interval for meta-analysis. *Stat Med* 2002; **21**: 3153–9.
109. Hedges LV, Vevea JL. Fixed- and random-effects models in meta-analysis. *Psychol Meth* 1998; **3**: 486–504.
110. Villar J, Mackey ME, Carroli G, Donner A. Meta-analyses in systematic reviews of randomized controlled trials in perinatal medicine; comparison of fixed and random effects models. *Stat Med* 2001; **20**: 3635–47.
111. Carlin JB. Meta-analysis for 2×2 tables: a Bayesian approach. *Stat Med* 1992; **11**: 141–58.
112. Whitehead A, Whitehead J. A general parametric approach to the meta-analysis of randomized clinical trials. *Stat Med* 1991; **10**: 1665–77.
113. Thompson SG, Smith TC, Sharp SJ. Investigating underlying risk as a source of heterogeneity in meta-analysis. *Stat Med* 1997; **16**: 2741–58.
114. McIntosh MW. The population risk as an explanatory variable in research synthesis of clinical trials. *Stat Med* 1996; **15**: 1713–28.
115. Larose DT, Dey DK. Grouped random effects models for Bayesian meta-analysis. *Stat Med* 1997; **16**: 1817–29.
116. Smith TC, Spiegelhalter DJ, Thomas A. Bayesian approaches to random-effects meta-analysis: a comparative study. *Stat Med* 1995; **14**: 2685–99.
117. Normand S-LT. Tutorial in biostatistics. Meta-analysis: formulating, evaluating, combining, and reporting. *Stat Med* 1999; **18**: 321–59.
118. Eddy DM, Hasselblad V, Shachter R. *Meta-Analysis by the Confidence Profile Method: The Statistical Synthesis of Evidence*. Boston, MA: Academic Press, 1990.
119. Eddy DM, Hasselblad V, Shachter R. An introduction to a Bayesian method for meta-analysis: the confidence profile method. *Med Decis Making* 1990; **10**: 15–23.
120. Goodman SN. Meta-analysis and evidence. *Control Clin Trials* 1989; **10**: 188–204 (published erratum appears in *Control Clin Trials* 1989; **10**: 435).
121. Curtin F, Altman DG, Elbourne D. Meta-analysis combining parallel and cross-over clinical trials. I: Continuous outcomes. *Stat Med* 2002; **21**: 2131–44.
122. Curtin F, Elbourne D, Altman DG. Meta-analysis combining parallel and cross-over clinical trials, II: Binary outcomes. *Stat Med* 2002; **21**: 2145–59.
123. Curtin F, Elbourne D, Altman DG. Meta-analysis combining parallel and cross-over clinical trials. III: The issue of carry-over. *Stat Med* 2002; **21**: 2161–73.
124. Elbourne D, Altman DG, Higgins J, Curtin F, Worthington H, Vail A. Meta-analysis involving cross-over trials: methodological issues. *Int J Epidemiol* 2002; **31**: 140–9.
125. Donner A, Klar N. Issues in the meta-analysis of cluster randomized trials. *Stat Med* 2002; **21**: 2971–80.
126. Chinn S. A simple method for converting an odds ratio to effect size for use in meta-analysis. *Stat Med* 2000; **19**: 3127–31.
127. Zucker D, Schmid CH, McIntosh MW, D'Agostino RB, Selker HP, Lau J. Combining single patient (*N*-of-1) trials to estimate population treatment effects and to evaluate individual patient responses to treatment. *J Clin Epidemiol* 1997; **50**: 401–10.
128. Nam I-S, Mengersen KL, Garthwaite P. Multivariate meta-analysis. *Stat Med* 2003; **22**: 2309–33.
129. Cook R, Brumback BA, Wigg M, Ryan L. Synthesis of evidence from epidemiological studies with interval-censored exposure due to grouping. *Biometrics* 2001; **57**: 671–80.
130. Shi J, Copas J. Meta-analysis for trend estimation. *Stat Med* 2004; **23**: 3–19.
131. Brumback BA, Holmes LB, Ryan LM. Adverse effects of chorionic villus sampling: a meta-analysis. *Stat Med* 1999; **18**: 2163–75.
132. Martin DO, Austin H. An exact method for meta-analysis of case–control and follow-up studies. *Epidemiology* 2000; **11**: 255–60.
133. Fleiss JL. Analysis of data from multiclinic trials. *Control Clin Trials* 1986; **7**: 267–75.
134. Takkouche B, Cadarso-Suarez C, Spiegelman D. Evaluation of old and new tests of heterogeneity in epidemiologic meta-analysis. *Am J Epidemiol* 1999; **150**: 206–15.
135. Higgins J, Thompson SG. Quantifying heterogeneity in a meta-analysis. *Stat Med* 2002; **21**: 1539–58.
136. Higgins J, Thompson SG, Deeks J, Altman DG. Measuring inconsistency in meta-analysis. *BMJ* 2003; **327**: 557–60.
137. Higgins J, Thompson SG, Deeks J, Altman DG. Statistical heterogeneity in systematic reviews of clinical trials: a critical appraisal of guidelines and practice. *J Health Serv Res Policy* 2002; **7**: 51–61.
138. Hardy RJ, Thompson SG. Detecting and describing heterogeneity in meta-analysis. *Stat Med* 1998; **17**: 841–56.
139. Berlin JA, Antman EM. Advantages and limitations of metaanalytic regressions of clinical trials data. *Online J Curr Clin Trials* 1994; doc. no. 134.
140. Berkey CS, Hoaglin DC, Mosteller F, Colditz GA. A random-effects regression model for meta-analysis. *Stat Med* 1995; **14**: 395–411.

141. Vanhonacker WR. Meta-analysis and response surface extrapolation: a least squares approach. *Amer Stat* 1996; **50**: 294–9.

142. Walker AM, Martin-Moreno JM, Artalejo FR. Odd man out: a graphical approach to meta-analysis. *Am J Pub Health* 1988; **78**: 961–6.

143. Song F. Exploring heterogeneity in meta-analysis: is the L'Abbe plot useful? *J Clin Epidemiol* 1999; **52**: 725–30.

144. Thompson SG, Sharp SJ. Explaining heterogeneity in meta-analysis: a comparison of methods. *Stat Med* 1999; **18**: 2693–708.

145. Sharp SJ, Thompson SG. Analysing the relationship between treatment effect and underlying risk in meta-analysis: comparison and development of approaches. *Stat Med* 2000; **19**: 3251–74.

146. Schmid C, Lau J, McIntosh M, Cappelleri J. An empirical study of the effect of the control rate as a predictor of treatment efficacy in meta-analysis of clinical trials. *Stat Med* 1998; **17**: 1924–42.

147. Cook RJ, Walter SD. A logistic model for trend in $2 \times 2 \times$ kappa tables with applications to meta-analyses. *Biometrics* 1997; **53**: 352–7.

148. Trikalinos T, Ioannidis JP. Predictive modeling and heterogeneity of baseline risk in meta-analysis of individual patient data. *J Clin Epidemiol* 2001; **54**: 245–52.

149. Schmid CH. Exploring heterogeneity in randomized trials via meta-analysis. *Drug Inf J* 1999; **33**: 211–24.

150. Sutton AJ, Abrams KR, Jones DR, Sheldon TA, Song F. *Methods for Meta-Analysis in Medical Research*. Chichester: John Wiley & Sons, 2000.

151. Brockwell S, Gordon I. A comparison of statistical methods for mcta-analysis. *Stat Med* 2001; **20**: 825–40.

152. Sterne JAC, Juni P, Schulz KF, Altman DG, Bartlett C, Egger M. Statistical methods for assessing the influence of study characteristics on treatment effects in "meta-epidemiological" research. *Stat Med* 2002; **21**: 1513–24.

153. Van Houwelingen HC, Arends LR, Stijnen T. Tutorial in biostatistics—advanced methods in meta-analysis: multivariate approach and meta-regression. *Stat Med* 2002; **21**: 589–624.

154. Simon R. Overviews of randomized clinical trials. *Cancer Treat Rep* 1987; **71**: 3–5.

155. Glasziou PP, Sanders SL. Investigating causes of heterogeneity in systematic reviews. *Stat Med* 2002; **21**: 1503–11.

156. Davey Smith G, Egger M, Phillips AN. Meta-analysis. Beyond the grand mean? *BMJ* 1997; **315**: 1610–14.

157. Light RJ, Pillemer DB. *Summing Up: The Science of Reviewing Research*. Cambridge, MA: Harvard University Press, 1984.

158. Devine EC, Cook TD. Effects of psycho-educational interventions on length of hospital stay: a meta-analytic review of 34 studies. In: Light RJ, ed., *Evaluation Studies Review Annual,* vol. 8. Beverly Hills, CA: Sage, 1983.

159. Sterne JAC, Egger M. Funnel plots for detecting bias in meta-analysis: guidelines on choice of axis. *J Clin Epidemiol* 2001; **54**: 1046–55.

160. Sterne JAC, Egger M, Smith GD. Investigating and dealing with publication and other biases in meta-analysis. *BMJ* 2001; **323**: 101–5.

161. Terrin N, Schmid CH, Lau J, Olkin I. Adjusting for publication bias in the presence of heterogeneity. *Stat Med* 2003; **22**: 2113–26.

162. Rosenthal R. The file drawer problem and tolerance for null results. *Psychol Bull* 1979; **86**: 638–41.

163. Iyengar S, Greenhouse JB. Selection models and the file-drawer problem. *Stat Sci* 1988; **3**: 109–17.

164. Gleser LJ, Olkin I. Models for estimating the number of unpublished studies. *Stat Med* 1996; **15**: 2493–507.

165. Egger M, Davey Smith G, Schneider M, Minder C. Bias in meta-analysis detected by a simple, graphical test. *BMJ* 1997; **315**: 629–34.

166. Begg CB, Mazumdar M. Operating characteristics of a rank correlation test for publication bias. *Biometrics* 1994; **50**: 1088–101.

167. Dear KBG, Begg CB. An approach for assessing publication bias prior to performing a meta-analysis. *Stat Sci* 1992; **7**: 237–45.

168. Hedges LV, Olkin I. *Statistical Methods for Meta-Analysis*. Orlando, FL: Academic Press, 1985.

169. Hedges LV, Vevea JL. Estimating effect size under publication bias: small sample properties and robustness of a random effects selection model. *J Educational Behavioral Stat* 1996; **21**: 299–332.

170. Vevea JL, Hedges LV. A general linear model for estimating effect size in the presence of publication bias. *Psychometrika* 1995; **60**: 419–35.

171. Givens GH, Smith DD, Tweedie RL. Publication bias in meta-analysis: a Bayesian data-augmentation approach to account for issues exemplified in the passive smoking debate. *Stat Sci* 1997; **12**: 221–50.

172. Duval S, Tweedie R. Trim and fill: a simple funnel-plot-based method of testing and adjusting for publication bias in meta-analysis. *Biometrics* 2000; **56**: 455–63.

173. Meinert CL. Toward prospective registration of clinical trials. *Control Clin Trials* 1988; **9**: 1–5.

174. Simes RJ. Publication bias: the case for an international registry of clinical trials. *J Clin Oncol* 1986; **4**: 1529–41.

175. Chalmers I, Dickersin K, Chalmers TC. Getting to grips with Archie Cochrane's agenda. *BMJ* 1992; **305**: 786–8.

176. Dickersin K. Why register clinical trials?—Revisited. *Control Clin Trials* 1992; **13**: 170–7.

177. Dickersin K. Report from the panel on the case for registers of clinical trials at the Eighth Annual Meeting of the Society for Clinical Trials. *Control Clin Trials* 1988; **9**: 76–81.

178. Savulescu J, Chalmers I, Blunt J. Are research ethics committees behaving unethically? Some suggestions for improving performance and accountability. *BMJ* 1996; **313**: 1390–3.

179. Anonymous. Making clinical trials register. *Lancet* 1992; **338**: 244–5.

180. Dickersin K, Rennie D. Registering clinical trials. *JAMA* 2003; **290**: 516–23.

181. Valsecchi MG, Masera G. A new challenge in clinical research in childhood ALL: the prospective meta-analysis strategy for intergroup collaboration. *Ann Oncol* 1996; **7**: 1005–8.

182. Margitic SE, Morgan TM, Sager MA, Furberg CD. Lessons learned from a prospective meta-analysis. *J Am Geriatr Soc* 1995; **43**: 435–9.

183. Simes RJ. Prospective meta-analysis of cholesterol-lowering studies: the Prospective Pravastatin Pooling (PPP) project and the cholesterol Treatment Trialists (CTT) collaboration. *Am J Cardiol* 1995; **76**: 122C–6C.

184. Whitehead A. A prospectively planned cumulative meta-analysis applied to a series of concurrent clinical trials. *Stat Med* 1997; **16**: 2901–13.

185. Temple RJ. The regulatory evolution of the integrated safety summary. *Drug Inf J* 1991; **25**: 485–92.

186. Gabriel SE, Jaakkimainen L, Bombardier C. Risk for serious gastrointestinal complications related to use of nonsteroidal anti-inflammatory drugs. A meta-analysis. *Ann Intern Med* 1991; **115**: 787–96.

187. Carson JL, Strom BL, Soper KA, West SL, Morse ML. The association of nonsteroidal anti-inflammatory drugs with upper gastrointestinal tract bleeding. *Arch Intern Med* 1987; **147**: 85–8.

188. Bollini P, Garcia Rodriguez L, Perez Gutthann S, Walker AM. The impact of research quality and study design on epidemiologic estimates of the effect of nonsteroidal anti-inflammatory drugs on upper gastrointestinal tract disease. *Arch Intern Med* 1992; **152**: 1289–95.

189. Henry D, Lim LL, Garcia Rodriguez LA, Perez GS, Carson JL, Griffin M et al. Variability in risk of gastrointestinal complications with individual non-steroidal anti-inflammatory drugs: results of a collaborative meta-analysis [see comments]. *BMJ* 1996; **312**: 1563–6.

190. Taragin MI, Carson JL, Strom BL. Gastrointestinal side effects of the nonsteroidal anti-inflammatory drugs. *Dig Dis* 1990; **8**: 269–80.

191. Carson JL, Strom BL. The gastrointestinal toxicity of the non-steroidal anti-inflammatory drugs. In: Rainsford KD, Velo GP, eds, *Side-effects of Anti-inflammatory Drugs 3*. Boston, MA: Kluwer, 1992; pp. 1–8.

192. Hine LK, Laird N, Hewitt P, Chalmers TC. Meta-analytic evidence against prophylactic use of lidocaine in acute myocardial infarction. *Arch Intern Med* 1989; **149**: 2694–8.

193. Hine LK, Laird NM, Hewitt P, Chalmers TC. Meta-analysis of empirical long-term antiarrhythmic therapy after myocardial infarction. *JAMA* 1989; **262**: 3037–40.

194. MacMahon S, Collins R, Peto R, Koster RW, Yusuf S. Effects of prophylactic lidocaine in suspected acute myocardial infarction. An overview of results from the randomized, controlled trials. *JAMA* 1988; **260**: 1910–16.

195. Antman EM, Berlin JA. Declining incidence of ventricular fibrillation in myocardial infarction. Implications for the prophylactic use of lidocaine. *Circulation* 1992; **86**: 764–73.

196. Coplen SE, Antman EM, Berlin JA, Hewitt P, Chalmers TC. Efficacy and safety of quinidine therapy for maintenance of sinus rhythm after cardioversion. A meta-analysis of randomized control trials. *Circulation* 1990; **82**: 1106–16. (published erratum appears in *Circulation* 1991; **83**: 714).

197. Reimold SC, Chalmers TC, Berlin JA, Antman EM. Assessment of the efficacy and safety of antiarrhythmic therapy for chronic atrial fibrillation: observations on the role of trial design and implications of drug-related mortality. *Am Heart J* 1992; **124**: 924–32.

198. Szczech LA, Berlin JA, Aradhye S, Grossman RA, Feldman HI. Effect of anti-lymphocyte induction therapy on renal allograft survival: a meta-analysis. *J Am Soc Nephrol* 1997; **8**: 1771–7.

199. Szczech LA, Berlin JA, Feldman HI. The effect of anti-lymphocyte induction therapy on renal allograft survival. A meta-analysis of individual patient-level data. Anti-Lymphocyte Antibody Induction Therapy Study Group. *Ann Intern Med* 1998; **128**: 817–26.

200. Hommes DW, Bura A, Mazzolai L, Buller HR, ten Cate JW. Subcutaneous heparin compared with continuous intravenous heparin administration in the initial treatment of deep vein thrombosis. A meta-analysis. *Ann Intern Med* 1992; **116**: 279–84.

201. Hull RD, Raskob GE, Hirsh J, Jay RM, Leclerc JR, Geerts WH et al. Continuous intravenous heparin compared with intermittent subcutaneous heparin in the initial treatment of proximal-vein thrombosis. *N Engl J Med* 1986; **315**: 1109–14.

202. Webber DM, Montague TH, Bird NP. Meta-analysis of QTc interval-pooling data from heterogeneous trials. *Pharmaceut Stat* 2002; **1**: 17–23.

203. Lau J, Antman EM, Jimenez-Silva J, Kupelnick B, Mosteller F, Chalmers TC. Cumulative meta-analysis of therapeutic trials for myocardial infarction. *N Engl J Med* 1992; **327**: 248–54.

204. Stampfer MJ, Goldhaber SZ, Yusuf S, Peto R, Hennekens CH. Effect of intravenous streptokinase on acute myocardial infarction: pooled results from randomized trials. *N Engl J Med* 1982; **307**: 1180–2.

205. Berkey CS, Mosteller F, Lau J, Antman EM. Uncertainty of the time of first significance in random effects cumulative meta-analysis. *Control Clin Trials* 1996; **17**: 357–71.

206. Lan KKG, Hu M, Cappelleri JC. Applying the law of iterated logarithm to cumulative meta-analysis of a continuous endpoint. *Statistica Sinica* 2003; **13**: 1135–45.

207. Ziegler RG, Mayne ST, Swanson CA. Nutrition and lung cancer. *Cancer Causes Control* 1996; **7**: 157–77.

208. Hennekens CH, Buring JE, Manson JE, Stampfer M, Rosner B, Cook NR et al. Lack of effect of long-term supplementation with beta carotene on the incidence of malignant neoplasms and cardiovascular disease. *N Engl J Med* 1996; **334**: 1145–9.

209. Omenn GS, Goodman GE, Thornquist MD, Balmes J, Cullen MR, Glass A et al. Effects of a combination of beta carotene and vitamin A on lung cancer and cardiovascular disease. *N Engl J Med* 1996; **334**: 1150–5.

210. Rossouw JE, Anderson GL. Risks and benefits of estrogen plus progestin in healthy postmenopausal women: principal results from the Women's Health Initiative randomized controlled trial. *JAMA* 2002; **288**: 321–33.

211. Stewart LA, Clarke MJ. Practical methodology of meta-analyses (overviews) using updated individual patient data. *Stat Med* 1995; **14**: 2057–79.

212. Stewart LA, Parmar MK. Meta-analysis of the literature or of individual patient data: is there a difference? *Lancet* 1993; **341**: 418–22.

213. Duchateau L, Pignon JP, Bijnens L, Bertin S, Bourhis J, Sylvester R. Individual patient- versus literature-based meta-analysis of survival data: time to event and event rate at a particular time can make a difference, an example based on head and neck cancer. *Control Clin Trials* 2001; **22**: 538–47.

214. Schmid CH, Landa M, Jafar TH, Giatras I, Karim T, Reddy M *et al.* Constructing a database of individual clinical trials for longitudinal analysis. *Control Clin Trials* 2003; **24**: 324–40.

215. Berlin J, Santanna J, Schmid CH, Szczech LA, Feldman H. Individual patient- versus group-level data meta-regressions for the investigation of treatment effect modifiers: ecological bias rears its ugly head. *Stat Med* 2002; **21**: 371–87.

216. LeLorier J, Gregoire G, Benhaddad A, Lapierre J, Derderian F. Discrepancies between meta-analyses and subsequent large randomized, controlled trials. *N Engl J Med* 1997; **337**: 536–42.

217. Ioannidis JP, Cappelleri JC, Lau J. Issues in comparisons between meta-analyses and large trials. *JAMA* 1998; **279**: 1089–93.

218. Cappelleri JC, Ioannidis JP, Schmid CH, de Ferranti SD, Aubert M, Chalmers TC *et al.* Large trials vs meta-analysis of smaller trials: how do their results compare? *JAMA* 1996; **276**: 1332–8.

219. Peto R, Collins R, Gray R. Large-scale randomized evidence: large, simple trials and overviews of trials. *J Clin Epidemiol* 1995; **48**: 23–40.

220. Villar J, Piaggio G, Carroli G, Donner A. Factors affecting the comparability of meta-analyses and largest trials results in perinatology. *J Clin Epidemiol* 1997; **50**: 997–1002.

221. Borzak S, Ridker PM. Discordance between meta-analyses and large-scale randomized, controlled trials. Examples from the management of acute myocardial infarction. *Ann Intern Med* 1995; **123**: 873–7.

222. Colditz GA, Brewer TF, Berkey CS, Wilson ME, Burdick E, Fineberg HV *et al.* The efficacy of bacillus Calmette-Guerin vaccination in the prevention of tuberculosis: meta-analysis of the published literature. *JAMA* 1994; **271**: 698–702.

223. Colditz GA, Berkey CS, Mosteller F, Brewer TF, Wilson ME, Burdick E *et al.* The efficacy of bacillus Calmette-Guerin vaccination of newborns and infants in the prevention of tuberculosis: meta-analyses of the published literature. *Pediatrics* 1995; **96**: 29–35.

224. Furukawa T, Streiner D, Hori S. Discrepancies among megatrials. *J Clin Epidemiol* 2001; **53**: 1193–9.

225. Bucher HC, Guyatt GH, Griffith LE, Walter SD. The results of direct and indirect treatment comparisons in meta-analysis of randomized controlled trials. *J Clin Epidemiol* 1997; **50**: 683–91.

226. Lumley T. Network meta-analysis for indirect treatment comparisons. *Stat Med* 2002; **21**: 2313–24.

227. Ades AE. A chain of evidence with mixed comparisons: models for multi-parameter synthesis and consistency of evidence. *Stat Med* 2003; **22**: 2995–3016.

228. Psaty BM, Lumley T, Furberg CD, Schellenbaum G, Pahor M, Alderman MH *et al.* Health outcomes associated with various antihypertensive therapies used as first-line agents: a network meta-analysis. *JAMA* 2003; **289**: 2534–44.

229. Song F, Glenny AM, Altman DG. Indirect comparison in evaluating relative efficacy illustrated by antimicrobial prophylaxis in colorectal surgery. *Control Clin Trials* 2000; **21**: 488–97.

45

Validity of Pharmacoepidemiologic Drug and Diagnosis Data

SUZANNE L. WEST[1], BRIAN L. STROM[2] and CHARLES POOLE[1]

[1] School of Public Health, University of North Carolina at Chapel Hill, North Carolina, USA;
[2] University of Pennsylvania School of Medicine, Philadelphia, Pennsylvania, USA.

INTRODUCTION

In discussing the quality of data for research, Gordis remarked that epidemiologists have become so enamored with statistical analysis of the data that they have paid too little attention to the validity of the raw data being analyzed with these sophisticated techniques.[1] Although this statement referred to questionnaire data, it applies equally to data generated by abstracting medical records or data from automated databases. Whatever the source of the data, the veracity of a study's conclusions rests on the validity of its data.

We begin this chapter by discussing the validity of the drug and diagnosis information used by clinicians in the management of patients' care. Next, the methodologic problems involved in validity assessment are presented, with some background on measurement error and the most recent information on the cognitive theories of memory systems, including semantic and episodic memory. Most of the chapter presents a literature review of the studies that have evaluated the validity of drug, diagnosis, and hospitalization data and the factors that influence the accuracy of these data. This information will be presented for the two primary information sources available for pharmacoepidemiology studies: questionnaires and administrative databases. The chapter concludes with a summary of our current knowledge in the field as well as directions for future research.

CLINICAL PROBLEMS TO BE ADDRESSED BY PHARMACOEPIDEMIOLOGIC RESEARCH

Physicians rely on patient-supplied information on past drug use and illness to assist with the diagnosis of current disease. Proper diagnosis and treatment of current illnesses may be compromised by poor recall of past illnesses and drugs. This problem is particularly relevant in the clinical situation, where a patient may be treated concurrently or sequentially by several different physicians. In circumstances such as these, the physician may not have a complete past history recorded in the chart and may need to rely on the patient to provide this information, especially for drugs that were not efficacious or that resulted in an adverse drug reaction. Because patients have difficulty recalling their medications, physicians may request that patients bring their medications or a comprehensive listing of their medications to their medical visits. A recent survey of 774 patients attending a university cardiology clinic found that 15% of patients attended with their medications, 19% brought a comprehensive medication list, 9% brought a list of the medication names only, 40% were confident that they knew their medication regimens but did not bring their medications with them, and 17% were unsure of the medications they were on.[2] The 17% who were unsure of what they were taking dropped to 2% once appointment cards indicated that the patients should bring their medications to their clinic visits. This very practical study is important for two reasons. First, it shows that a good number of patients cannot communicate their medication regimens to the clinician, which can impede their care. More importantly, a simple reminder stamped on the appointment card can provide physicians with knowledge that will improve the care of their patients.

Patients' recall abilities compromise a physician's ability to diagnose and/or prescribe successfully and may play a role in the success of drug therapy. The patient needs to recall the physician's instructions for most efficacious drug use. Brody[3] found that 55 (53%) of 104 patients interviewed immediately after seeing their physician made one or more errors in recalling their therapeutic regimens. Patient recall may be even poorer for illnesses and medication use that occurred many years previously.

Of particular concern to the subject of this book is the validity of data on drug exposure and disease occurrence because the typical focus of pharmacoepidemiologic research is often the association between a medication and an adverse drug event. Further, many potential confounders of importance in pharmacoepidemiologic research (although certainly not all) are either drugs or diseases. As noted, clinicians recognize that patients very often do not know the names of the drugs they are taking currently. Thus, it is a given that patients have difficulty recalling past drug use accurately, at least absent any aids to this recall. Superficially at least, patients cannot be considered reliable sources of diagnosis information either; in some instances they may not even have been told the correct diagnosis, still less recall it. Yet, these data elements are crucial to pharmacoepidemiology

studies that ascertain data using questionnaires. Special approaches have been developed by pharmacoepidemiologists to obtain such data more accurately, from patients and other sources, but the success of these approaches needs to be considered in detail.

METHODOLOGIC PROBLEMS TO BE ADDRESSED BY PHARMACOEPIDEMIOLOGIC RESEARCH

COGNITIVE THEORY OF AUTOBIOGRAPHICAL MEMORY

Epidemiologic research often relies on asking study subjects to recall events or exposures that occurred at some time in the past, with recall intervals spanning from days to several years. To appreciate the accuracy of data derived by recollection, it is important to understand the response process in general and the organization of memory, a key element of the response process.

Measurement error for survey data depends on the adequacy of the response process, which is made up of four key respondent tasks: (i) question comprehension and interpretation; (ii) search for and retrieval of information to construct an answer to the question; (iii) judgment to discern the completeness and relevance of memory for formulating a response; and (iv) development of the response based on retrieved memories.[4–7] Often, too little attention is paid to the first two key tasks when developing survey instruments, the result of which is questions that are too vague or complex for respondents to marshal retrieval processes appropriately. Thus, understanding memory organization and retrieval are critical components for developing questionnaires for collecting accurate health-related data on drug use or events such as doctor visits.

Based on current memory theory, autobiographical memory is used to store events, most of which are catalogued for retrieval in a more general fashion and are sequenced based on important personal milestones.[7] Thus, when respondents are asked to recall a visit to a doctor that may have occurred at a particular point in time, researchers believe that the respondents use scripts (a generic mental representation of the event) to help retrieval. For example, the respondent first contemplates a doctor visit in general and then supplements this script with details relevant to the particular visit that requires contemplation for specific criteria (e.g., diagnosis) and timing (e.g., a particular year).

Autobiographical memory appears to contain generic events that are somehow linked to details for individual events that occurred during specific points in a person's lifetime. How autobiographical memory is organized is still being debated by memory theorists. Conway suggests that autobiographical memory is based on three levels, where the highest level relates to periods defined by personal life events such as one's first job, first child, first year of college, etc.[7] This period organization has both a temporal and thematic structure so that subsequent events can be catalogued appropriately. The next level stores general knowledge and script-type generic information whereas the third level contains detailed information to distinguish among events. This third level, which is more sensory and perceptual, is thought to be similar to episodic memory, described below.

Other memory researchers suggest that autobiographical events are stored in three types of hypothetical memory systems: semantic, episodic, and procedural (related to a learned motor skill which is not usually of concern in the acquisition of data via questionnaires),[8,9] where the semantic memory system is used for retaining general knowledge, including facts and concepts. In the autobiographical context as related to responses to a questionnaire, this would be the recall of one's birth date, height, or educational attainment. Whereas semantic memory retains factual information, the episodic memory system is believed to maintain detailed sensory–perceptual knowledge of very recent experiences (in the past 24–48 hours).[10] Episodic memories have a temporal structure but a very short retention span (on the order of minutes or hours), with the implication that for episodic memories to be retained, the specific events must be organized thematically or temporally within the hierarchy of autobiographical memory. The key differentiating factor between semantic and episodic memories is the temporal nature of episodic memories. Once incorporated into autobiographical memory, episodic memories can be recollected when necessary. This "mental time travel" allows an individual to re-experience previous events cognitively,[11] and it is this recollection of episodic memories that facilitates responses to questionnaires. Those who theorize a semantic and episodic hierarchy have shown that semantic memory shows little deterioration with age but there may be age-related effects for the encoding (or establishment) of memories.[12,13] Unlike semantic memory, age has a much greater influence on episodic memory because information encoding, storage, and retrieval are adversely affected by age. In addition, episodic memory is more vulnerable to neuronal dysfunction than the other memory systems.[11,13]

There are four types of temporal questions often included in questionnaires.[7] They include:

- time of occurrence, which requires respondents to provide a date when an event occurred such as when were they diagnosed with a particular condition;
- duration questions such as "How long did you take drug A?";
- elapsed time, which asks how long it has been since an event occurred, including questions such as "How many months has it been since you last took drug A?";
- temporal frequency questions that ask respondents to report the number of events that occurred over a specific time period, such as "How many visits did you make to your primary care practitioner in the past 6 months?".

The cognitive processes the respondent uses to answer temporal questions will determine the accuracy of the response, and respondents use many different recall processes in combination to develop a response. Memory researchers believe that, although the recall process is individualistic, the types of information used and its integration typically include four concepts, namely recalling the exact date, temporal sequencing, correlating with other events, and determining adequacy of response.[7] For landmark events such as marriage or the birth of a child, respondents are capable of recalling the exact date for the event; less significant events are not stored with their date of occurrence. When events are less significant, relative ordering of events within a time period may enhance recall. For example, a respondent may remember that the event being queried occurred during his or her employment with company X, which occurred between July 1998 and February 2000. Landmark events also provide useful indicators to sequence events of interest, i.e., a diagnosis made after a child's birth. Being able to recall some details about the event may provide useful clues to the date in which it occurred, such as being hospitalized during the summer months when the weather was so sunny. Finally, after respondents derive an answer based on several cognitive processes, they judge the adequacy of their recall with regard to the timing of other events that occurred during the same temporal period.

An example best illustrates the theory of Tourangeau and colleagues[7] on how respondents use a cyclic process of recalling details about a particular event. As new information is recalled, this new information helps shape the memory and adds details to describe the event in question: "When was your major depression first diagnosed?" The respondent may use the following process to provide the correct date, namely January 1998.

The recall process begins with the respondent being uncertain whether the depression was diagnosed in 1997 or 1998. To work towards identifying the correct year, the respondent recalls that the depression was the result of his losing his job. The job loss was particularly traumatic because he and his wife just purchased their first home a few months previously and now, with the loss of his income, they were at risk of losing the house. The home purchase was a landmark event for this respondent and he remembers that it occurred in mid-1997, just as their children finished the school year. So, it was 1997 when he lost his job, toward the end of the year because the holiday season was particularly grim. His remembers that his depression was diagnosed after the holidays, but was it January or February of 1998? It was January 1998 because he was already taking antidepressants by Valentine's Day, when he went out to dinner with his wife and he could not drink wine with his meal. This is diagrammed in Figure 45.1.

Landmark events such as marriage and childrearing probably serve as the primary organizational units of autobiographical knowledge and as such, provide an anchor for information retrieval.[9] In particular, the example shows how the respondent used landmark and other notable events, relationships among datable events, and general knowledge (holiday period and children finishing the school year) to reconstruct when his major depression was first diagnosed. An important caveat is that the respondent described above was willing to expend considerable effort to search his memory to determine when his depression was diagnosed—this may not be the situation for all respondents.

Understanding the complexity of memory and making use of our current knowledge of how memory is organized will enhance our ability to collect data using questionnaires. With regard to pharmacoepidemiologic surveys, ascertaining the timing of events and exposures is the most difficult and requires flexibility in question design and sufficient cognitive testing and pretesting to enhance response accuracy.

As will be evident in the studies described below, researchers have been employing most of the findings from cognitive research to pharmacoepidemiology studies. The continued and innovative application of these findings can only further improve the methodology for collecting health-related data via questionnaire. Tourangeau and colleagues[7] provide an enlightening discussion of their theory of survey response along with the possible memory processes underlying retrieval and questionnaire response.

THE INFLUENCE OF MEASUREMENT ERROR ON PHARMACOEPIDEMIOLOGIC RESEARCH

Epidemiologic assessments of the effects of a drug on disease incidence depend upon an accurate assessment of both drug exposure and disease occurrence. Measurement error for either factor, whether due to inaccurate recall or poorly acquired data, may identify a risk factor in the study which does not exist in the population or, conversely, may fail to detect a risk factor when one truly exists.

In an epidemiologic study, the measure of association is often based on the number of subjects categorized by

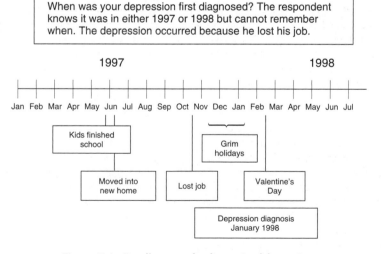

Figure 45.1. Recall process for diagnosis of depression.

the cross-classification of presence or absence of disease and exposure. In a study of the association between drug A and disease B, if some study participants forgot their past exposure to drug A, they would be incorrectly classified as nonexposed. This misclassification is a measurement error. Although the measurement process usually involves some error, if this measurement error is of sufficient magnitude, the validity of the study's findings is diminished.

There are two types of measurement error or misclassification: nondifferential and differential.[14] The difference between these errors relates to the variables under study. In particular, differential misclassification is said to occur when the misclassification of one variable (e.g., drug usage) varies according to the level of another variable (e.g., disease status), so that the direction of the bias can be toward or away from the null. For example, in a case–control study of oral contraceptives (OC) and breast cancer, there would be concern that those with breast cancer would recall past OC use differently from those without breast cancer. Cases might ponder the origins of their illness and recall and report OC use they otherwise would have forgotten or failed to report. Alternatively, cases might be distracted by their illness during the interview and forget their past OC use, fail to report it to get the interview over more quickly, or because of psychological denial in favor of something else that they may feel is more likely as an explanation for that disease (e.g., pesticide exposure). The state of mind of the respondent and of the interviewer at the time of the interviews are crucial determinants of the overall accuracy of the interview or questionnaire information and of the degree to which the accuracy might differ by respondent characteristics (e.g., case or control status). Patients who learn they have serious diseases, and parents who learn the same about their children, often go through phases or stages in questioning how these illnesses might have come about. In earlier stages, attention is often directed inward toward self-blame. As the time passes, external explanations are often sought. The time course of the psychological state of seriously ill patients and their close family members is highly variable, but potentially of great importance to the validity of interview and questionnaire data obtained from them. The traditional assumptions that cases remember true exposures better than non-cases (i.e., that exposure classification has higher sensitivity among cases than among controls) and that cases intentionally or unintentionally report more false-positive exposures than non-cases (i.e., that exposure classification has lower specificity among cases than among non-cases) are undoubtedly too simplistic for general reliance.

A difference in the accuracy of recall between cases and non-cases could influence the determination of OC exposure and the resulting measure of association. In case–control studies, differential misclassification of exposure can result from recall bias.[15] It is commonly thought that the potential for recall bias can be minimized if the study is designed to obtain complete exposure data, i.e., information on the names and usage dates for every drug used in the time period of interest.[16]

Nondifferential misclassification of exposure occurs when the misclassification of one variable does not vary by the level of another variable and may occur if both cases and controls simply forget their exposures to the same degree. The measure of association is affected by nondifferential misclassification of exposure as well; it is usually biased toward the null. Exceptions can occur when classification errors are not independent of each other,[17,18] as when participants who are particularly reluctant to report health outcomes that they have experienced are especially unwilling to report medications they have taken as well. Other exceptions to the rule about bias toward the null from nondifferential misclassification can occur when there are more than two categories of exposure.[19] Rothman and Greenland give a simple hypothetical example to illustrate the potential for bias away from the null from independent, nondifferential misclassification of an exposure with more than two categories of exposure.[20] Consider a case–control study of an exposure with three categories—low, medium, and high—and suppose the correctly classified case and control counts are 100/100, 200/100, and 600/100, respectively. With low exposure as the referent, the odds ratios are 2.0 for medium exposure and 6.0 for high exposure. Now suppose that 40% of the cases and controls in the high exposure group are misclassified into the medium exposure group. The odds ratio for high exposure is unbiased, (360/60) / (100/100) = 6.0, and the odds ratio for medium exposure is biased upward to (440/140) / (100/100) = 3.1. Finally, there is no bias from independent, nondifferential misclassification of a binary outcome measure under some circumstances.[21,22] For instance, if there are no false-positive cases, the expected risk ratio will be the risk ratio given correct disease classification multiplied by the ratio of the sensitivity in the exposed group to the sensitivity in the unexposed group. If the sensitivity is independent and nondifferential, this ratio equals unity and the risk ratio is unbiased. In addition, it is important to keep in mind that when an expected bias is toward the null, this is the direction of the bias on average. The actual bias in any given study may be away from the null even when the misclassification probabilities are nondifferential.[23,24]

QUANTITATIVE INDICES OF MEASUREMENT ERROR

Three kinds of comparisons may be drawn between two (or more) methods of data collection or sources of information on exposure or outcome. Many different terms have been used to describe each of them, resulting in a certain amount of confusion.

When the same data collection method or source of information is used more than once for the same information on the same individual, comparisons of the results measure the reliability of the method or information source. An example of a reliability study would be a comparison of responses in repeat interviews using the same interview instrument. Reliability is not validity, though the term is sometimes used as such.

When different data collection methods or different sources of information are compared (e.g., comparing prescription dispensation records with interview responses), and neither of them can be considered distinctly superior to the other, the comparisons measure mere agreement. Agreement between two sources or methods does not imply that either is valid or reliable.

Only when one of the methods or sources is clearly superior to the other can the comparison be said to measure validity, a synonym for which is accuracy. The superior method or source is often called a "gold standard." In recognition that a method or source can be superior to another method or source without being perfect, the term "alloyed gold standard" has been used.[25]

For a binary exposure or outcome measure, such as ever versus never use of a particular drug, there are two measures of validity. Sensitivity (also called completeness) measures the degree to which the inferior source or method correctly identifies individuals who, according to the superior method or source, possess the characteristic of interest (i.e., ever used the drug). Specificity measures the degree to which the inferior source or method correctly identifies individuals who, according to the superior method or source, lack the characteristic of interest (i.e., never used the drug).

Sensitivity and specificity are the two sides of the validity coin for a dichotomous exposure or outcome variable. In general, sources or methods that have high sensitivity tend to have low specificity, and methods with high specificity tend to have low sensitivity. In these situations, which are very common, neither of the two sources or methods being compared can be said to have superior overall validity to the other. Depending on particulars of the study setting, either

sensitivity or specificity may be the more "important" validity measure. Moreover, absolute values of these measures can be deceiving. For instance, if the true prevalence of ever use of a drug is 5%, then an exposure classification method or information source with 95% specificity (and perfect sensitivity) will double the measured prevalence to 10%. The ultimate criterion of importance of a given combination of sensitivity and specificity is the degree of bias exerted on a measure of effect such as an estimated relative risk. Because the degree of bias depends on such study-specific conditions as the true prevalence of exposure, no general guidelines can be given. Each study situation must be evaluated on its own merits. For example, suppose in a case–control study that the true odds ratio is OR = 3.0, the sensitivity of an exposure measure is higher among cases (90%) than among controls (80%), the specificity is lower among cases (95%) than among controls (99%), and, for simplification, that the outcome is measured perfectly and there is no control-selection bias. The exposure misclassification will bias the expected effect estimate upward to OR = 3.6 if the true exposure prevalence in the source population is 10%, downward to OR = 2.6 if the true exposure prevalence is 90%, and leave it unbiased at OR = 3.0 if the true exposure prevalence is 70%.[26]

As measures of validity, sensitivity and specificity have "truth" (i.e., the classification according to a gold standard or an alloyed gold standard) in their denominators. Investigators should take care not to confuse these measures with the predictive values of positive and negative classifications, which have the classification according to the inferior measure in their denominators. We distinguish here between the persons who actually do or do not have an exposure or outcome and those who are classified as having it or not having it. The proportion of persons classified as having the exposure or outcome who are correctly classified is the positive predictive value. The proportion of persons classified as lacking the exposure or outcome who are correctly classified is the negative predictive value. Predictive values are measures of performance of a classification method or information source, not measures of validity. Predictive values depend not only on the sensitivity and specificity (i.e., on validity), but on the true prevalence of the exposure or outcome as well. Thus, if a method or information source for classifying persons with respect to outcome or exposure has the same validity (i.e., the same sensitivity and specificity) in two populations, but those populations differ in their outcome or exposure prevalence, the source or method will have different predictive values in the two populations.

In many "validation" studies, the "confirmation" or "verification" rates are not measures of validity, but merely measures of agreement. In other such investigations, one method or source may be used as a gold standard or as an alloyed gold standard to assess another method or source with respect to only one side of the validity coin. Studies that focus on the "completeness" of one source, such as studies in which interview responses are compared with prescription dispensation records to identify drug exposures that were forgotten or otherwise not reported by the respondents, may measure (more or less accurately) the sensitivity of the interview data. However, such studies are silent on the specificity without strong assumptions (e.g., that the respondent could not have obtained the drug in any way that would not be recorded in the prescription dispensation records).

In general, it is all too common for studies that measure mere agreement to be interpreted as though they measured validity or accuracy. The term "reliability" tends to be used far too broadly, to refer variously not only to reliability itself, but to agreement or validity as well. A widespread increase in the care with which such terms are used would be very helpful.

Figure 45.2 illustrates the calculation of sensitivity and specificity. For a drug exposure, a true gold standard would be a list of all drugs the study participant has taken, including dose, duration, and dates of exposure. This drug list might be a diary of prescriptions kept by the study participants or, perhaps more readily available, a computerized database of filled prescriptions, although neither of these data sources might be a genuine gold standard. Prescription diaries cannot be assumed to be kept in perfect accuracy. For instance, there may be a tendency to record that drug use was more regular and complete than it actually was, or that it was used according to the typical prescribed regimen. Similarly, there may be substantial gaps between when a prescription is filled and when it is ingested.

There are two methods to quantify the validity of continuously distributed variables, such as duration of drug usage. The mean and standard error of the differences between the data in question and the valid reference measurement are typically used when the measurement error is constant across the range of true values (i.e., when measurement error is independent of where an individual's true exposure falls on the exposure distribution in the study population).[27] Realizing that it is only generalizable to populations with similar exposure distributions, the product–moment correlation coefficient may also be used. However, high correlation between two measures does not necessarily mean high agreement. For instance, the correlation coefficient could be very high (i.e., close to 1), even though one of the variables systematically overestimates or underestimates values of the other variable. The high correlation means that the over- or underestimation is systematic and very consistent. When the two measures being compared are plotted against one another and they have the same scale, full agreement occurs only when the points fall on the line of equality, which is 45° from either axis.[28] However, one is said to have perfect correlation when the points lie along any straight line parallel to the line of equality. It is difficult to tell from the value of a correlation coefficient how much bias will be produced by using an inaccurate measure of disease exposure.

Quantitative Measurement of Reliability

To evaluate reliability for categorical variables, the percentage agreement between two or more sources and related (κ) coefficient are used. They are used only when two imperfect classification schemes are being compared, not when there is one classification method that may be considered *a priori* superior to the other.[14,27] The κ statistic is the percentage agreement corrected for chance.[27] Agreement is conventionally considered poor for a κ statistic less than zero, slight for κ between zero and 0.20, fair for a κ of 0.21–0.40, moderate for a κ of 0.41–0.60, substantial for a κ of 0.61–0.80, and almost perfect for a κ of 0.81–1.00.[29] Figure 45.3

		Gold standard		
		Exposed	Not exposed	
Questionnaire data	Exposed	A true positive	B false positive	m_1
	Not exposed	C false negative	D true negative	m_2
		n_1	n_2	N

Sensitivity $= A/A + C$

Specificity $= D/B + D$

Figure 45.2. Formulas for calculating sensitivity and specificity.

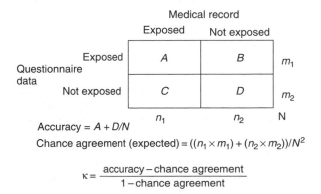

Accuracy $= A + D/N$

Chance agreement (expected) $= ((n_1 \times m_1) + (n_2 \times m_2))/N^2$

$$\kappa = \frac{\text{accuracy} - \text{chance agreement}}{1 - \text{chance agreement}}$$

Figure 45.3. Formulas for calculating the percent agreement and κ.

illustrates the percentage agreement and κ calculations for a reliability assessment between questionnaire data and medical record information.

The intraclass correlation coefficient is used to evaluate the reliability of continuous variables.[14] It reflects both the average differences in mean values as well as the correlation between measurements. The intraclass correlation coefficient indicates how much of the total measurement variation is due to the differences between the subjects being evaluated and to differences in measurement for one individual. When the data from two sets of measurements are identical, the intraclass correlation coefficient equals 1.0. Under certain conditions, the intraclass correlation coefficient is exactly equivalent to Cohen's weighted κ.[27] It is impossible to translate values of measures of agreement, such as κ, into expected degrees of bias in exposure or disease associations.

EFFECTS OF MEASUREMENT ERROR ON THE POINT ESTIMATE OF ASSOCIATION

Copeland *et al.* evaluated misclassification in epidemiologic studies using a series of computer-generated graphs. They showed that the bias—i.e., discrepancy between the point estimate and the true value of the measure of association— was a function of the disease frequency, exposure frequency, sensitivity, and specificity of the classification.[30] It is instructive to note that Copeland *et al.* were not able to describe bias as a function of the product-moment correlation coefficient, the intraclass correlation coefficient, percentage agreement, or κ. This means that higher or lower values of these measures, even when one of the measurement methods is a gold standard, should not be interpreted as evidence of greater or lesser degrees of bias. When nondifferential misclassification occurred, the point estimate was biased toward the null. Their results for nondifferential misclassification also indicated that the rarer the disease, the more the potential for bias in cohort studies. Likewise, the less prevalent the exposure, the more the potential for bias increases in case–control studies. For differential misclassification, the point estimate could be biased toward or away from the null. This presents a problem for *ad hoc* case–control studies, where recall bias is always a concern.

Copeland *et al.*'s simulations were all done on binary disease and exposure variables. Dosemeci *et al.* presented additional simulations to show that nondifferential misclassification of exposure may bias the point estimate toward or away from the null, or may cause the point estimate to change direction when polychotomous exposure variables (i.e., variables with more than two categories) are considered.[19] A typical example of a polychotomous variable would be never, some, or frequent use of a drug. For a continuous variable, nondifferential misclassification may not produce a bias towards the null if there is perfect correlation between the variable as measured and the true value.[14] For example, if both cases and controls in a case–control study underestimate duration of drug use by an equal percentage, then there would not be a bias towards the null.

CORRECTING MEASURES OF ASSOCIATION FOR MEASUREMENT ERROR

To correct effect estimates for measurement error, estimates of sensitivity and specificity are required.[30] These estimates can be derived from previous research or from a subsample within the study being analyzed. However, estimates of sensitivity and specificity of exposure classification from previous research are rarely available. Should these estimates be available, they may not prove to be useful since the classification methods need to be similar in both the correctly classified and misclassified data.[31] The classification probabilities will vary according to the questionnaire design, study population, and time period of administration. In addition, the correction methods most familiar to epidemiologists are appropriate for bivariate, not multivariate, data.[32]

For differential misclassification of exposure by disease status (recall bias), Raphael[33] contends that it is the researcher's responsibility to either present a strong case that recall bias did not threaten the study's validity or to control for it statistically. One extremely important way to help make the case for which Raphael has called is to conduct a sensitivity analysis.[34] Sensitivity analysis is the last line of defense against biases after every effort has been made to eliminate, reduce, or control them in study design, data collection, and data analysis. As used in this context, the meaning of the term "sensitivity" differs from its other epidemiologic meaning as the counterpart to specificity as a measure of classification validity. In a sensitivity analysis, one alters key assumptions or methods reasonably to see how sensitive the results of a study are to those variations. One key assumption, usually implicit, is that the exposure and the outcome in a study have been measured accurately. With estimates from previous research or "guesstimates" from expert experience and judgment, one can modify this assumption and use analytic methods ranging from the very simple[26] to the highly complex[35] to "back calculate" what the results might have looked like if more accurate methods had been used to classify participants with respect to outcome, exposure, or both. Sometimes it may be found that wildly implausible degrees of inaccuracy would have to have been present to produce observed associations. Other times it may be found that the overall study results would be appreciably biased by values of sensitivity and specificity that, if viewed in isolation and out of the context of the particulars of the study in question, might seem high enough or close enough to being nondifferential to be reassuring.

For many years, this kind of assessment has been conducted informally and qualitatively. However, the net result is controversy, with investigators judging the bias small and critics judging it large. Further, intuitive judgments, even those of the most highly trained and widely experienced investigators, can be poorly calibrated in such matters. Formal sensitivity analysis makes the assessment of residual bias transparent and quantitative, and forces the investigator (and other critics) to defend criticisms that in earlier times would have remained qualitative and unsubstantiated. An important and well-known historical example is the bias from nondifferential misclassification of disease proposed by Horwitz and Feinstein[36] to explain associations between early exogenous estrogen preparations and endometrial cancer. When proper sensitivity analyses were conducted of this bias, it was found to be capable of explaining only a negligible proportion of those associations.[36–38]

Epidemiologic applications of quantitative methods with long history in the decision sciences have become accessible for quantifying uncertainties about multiple sources of systematic error in a probabilistic manner.[35,39–41] These methods permit the incorporation of available validation data as well as expert judgment about measurement error, uncontrolled confounding, and selection bias along with conventional sampling error, and prior probability distributions for effect measures themselves, to form uncertainty distributions. These approaches have been used practically in pharmacoepidemiology in the assessment of selection bias in a study of topical coal tar therapy and skin cancer among severe psoriasis patients,[39] exposure misclassification and selection bias in a study of propanolamine use and stroke,[40] and selection bias, confounder misclassification, and unmeasured confounding in a study of less than definitive therapy and breast cancer mortality,[35] as well as in other clinical and nonclinical applications.[41–43] Pharmacoepidemiologists would be well advised to continue setting good examples in the application of these methods. Sometimes biases can be shown to be of more concern and sometimes of less concern than intuition or simple sensitivity analysis might suggest. Almost always the probabilistic uncertainty

about these sources of systematic error dwarfs the uncertainty reflected by conventional confidence intervals. By the use of these methods, the assessment of systematic error can move from a qualitative discussion of "study limitations," beyond sensitivity analyses of one scenario at a time for one source of error at a time, to a comprehensive analysis of all sources of error simultaneously. The resulting uncertainty distributions not only supplement, but supplant, conventional likelihood and p-value functions, which reflect only random sampling error. As a result, much more realistic, probabilistic assessments of total uncertainty attending to effect measure estimates are in the offing.

CURRENTLY AVAILABLE SOLUTIONS

OVERVIEW OF APPROACHES USED TO EVALUATE THE ACCURACY OF PHARMACOEPIDEMIOLOGIC DATA SOURCES

The accuracy of drug exposure and diagnostic data has been measured in pharmacoepidemiology studies, sometimes as a validation effort in etiologic studies and elsewhere as separate methodologic evaluations.

Medical Record Validation for Etiologic Studies

In etiologic studies, where drug exposure and disease occurrence are typically derived from questionnaires, "validation" is often done by comparison with medical records. Although the literature uses the term "validation study" or "verification" to describe the agreement between two sources of information, "concordance" or "agreement" might be a more appropriate term to describe the comparison between questionnaire data and medical records, because the medical record itself is not a true "gold standard" for several reasons.

First, retrieval of medical records depends not only on a person's ability to remember and report who prescribed the drug or diagnosed the condition in question, but on the health care provider's attention in recording the information, and on the availability of the medical record for review. If the medical record cannot be retrieved because the health care provider could not be identified, had retired, or the record was destroyed or lost, the events cannot be verified.

In addition, even if the medical record is available, it may not list all diagnoses and medications prescribed. Kirking and colleagues[44] found that prescriptions were poorly documented in the medical record when compared with a pharmacy claims database. Based on the number of prescriptions dispensed, only 39% of prescriptions were documented in the prescriber visit notes of the chart. This varied from 34% for persons with 12 or more dispensings in a six-month period to 56% for those with fewer than 12 prescriptions in the same time period.

Monson and Bond used individual pharmacy folders that contained all prescription drug orders as the gold standard for evaluating outpatient medical record completeness.[45] Virtually all outpatient medications were obtained from the hospital pharmacy. The medical records for 89% of all persons who received drugs from the pharmacy had documentation that any prescription had been written. Of the 1326 individual prescriptions issued for the 355 persons, 26% were not recorded in the chart, and for only 38% of the 1326 prescriptions did the medical record contain the name, dose, strength, and directions as they appeared on the prescription form. Documentation of therapy was inversely correlated with the number of drugs dispensed, a similar result to that of Kirking and colleagues.

Using a different study design that looked at documentation of a single drug, West *et al.* reported that 89% of the outpatient medical records of persons who were dispensed one fill of one NSAID prescription contained documentation of that prescription.[46] Age, gender, and whether the NSAID was used for an acute or chronic condition did not influence the likelihood that the drug was documented on the chart. Similarly, Christensen and colleagues reported that 92–95% of antihypertensive medications were noted in the medical record, using a database of drug dispensations for comparison.[47] Thus, study design appears to influence the findings of medical record documentation, with better results noted for those studies that evaluated only one drug[46] or one therapeutic class[47] compared to those that looked for documentation of all prescriptions in a given period of time.[44,45,48]

The therapeutic class may also affect medical record completeness, with psychotropic medications being poorly documented. Buchsbaum *et al.* reported that the names of benzodiazepines were more often omitted from the chart than the names of non-benzodiazepine medications (95% versus 81%, respectively, $p < 0.01$), as were the indications for use (95% versus 57%, respectively, $p < 0.0001$), with 15% of benzodiazepine and only 2% of non-benzodiazepine prescriptions missing from the chart entirely.[48]

Three studies have used pharmacy dispensings to evaluate the completeness of drug documentation in the inpatient medical record. Lau and colleagues used a structured interview conducted during the two-day hospital stay and dispensings from a community pharmacy to determine the completeness of recording current medication use in hospital medical records for patients admitted to a general medicine ward.[49] Three types of errors were evaluated for the 1606 medications evaluated in the study. An omission error was defined as medication use according to the structured interview and pharmacy records but there was no entry of the medication in the hospital chart ($n = 406$, 26% of all errors). Less than 3% of medications were listed in the hospital medical record without corroboration by the patient's structured interview. Finally, of the 1606 medications used by the patients, 97.6% of them had been dispensed according to the pharmacy records.

In a similar study evaluating the completeness of the inpatient medical record for admissions due to Stevens–Johnson syndrome, Strom *et al.* focused specifically on drugs commonly suspected of causing the syndrome.[50] The persons' inpatient medical records recorded only 50% of the 234 prescriptions for these drugs known to be dispensed to these individuals in the 30 days prior to hospitalization, according to computerized Medicaid pharmacy claims files. These data indicate that drugs prescribed during an outpatient visit often are not documented in a subsequent inpatient chart, even when the drugs may have caused the disease resulting in the hospitalization. Guess *et al.* reported similarly poor completeness comparing discharge and autopsy reports to the computerized drug file from the Saskatchewan Health Plan.[51] In their study of persons with fatal upper gastrointestinal hemorrhage or perforation, NSAID use was mentioned in the discharge or autopsy report for only 31% of cases identified as exposed according to the drug file.

In another inpatient medical record study, Lloyd and Rissing reported that the average inpatient medical record contains approximately 2.3 physician errors, such as failure to list treatments or diagnoses that were either treated or affected length of stay.[52] They also noted that procedures performed in locations other than the operating room were often omitted from the chart.

In summary, the medical record does not document all medications prescribed for individuals. Record completeness is likely to vary by type of drug, type of chart (outpatient versus inpatient), and the number of drugs prescribed in a given period. This diminishes the usefulness of medical records for verifying self-reported drug exposure.

Methodologic Studies

Exposure confirmation performed as part of etiologic studies is often only partial verification, for two reasons. First, the comparison data source may be an alloyed gold standard, where the rate calculated is a measure of agreement, not a measure of validity. More commonly, verification studies using a gold or an alloyed gold standard, can assess only one of the two validity measures, either sensitivity or specificity.

Methodologic studies that use alternative data sources such as prospectively collected data or databases of dispensed drugs can measure both the sensitivity and specificity, if one assumes that the prescription database is a gold standard. Lower sensitivity is often more of a concern than is lower specificity, depending on the data source used for the study. Drug exposures or diseases that are underreported on questionnaires or are missing due to incompleteness of claims processing in a record-linked database, i.e., data sources with low sensitivity, cannot be evaluated as risk factors for the association under investigation. Alternatively, low specificity is often less of a problem in pharmacoepidemiology unless the characteristic with low specificity also has very low prevalence in the population being studied. In situations where the factor has low prevalence and low sensitivity, a small degree of misclassification can have a dramatic effect on measures of association. Because the incidence of Stevens–Johnson syndrome is rare, a small degree of misclassification when using administrative claims data where the case definition uses the ICD-9-CM code 695.1 will include several skin problems other than Stevens–Johnson (i.e., the false-positive rate would be high).

Besides the need for completeness on the individual level, it is also critical that information from all persons who are covered by the health plan from which the database is generated appear in the database. Systematic omissions of specific population groups, such as certain ethnic or racial groups, diminish the quality of the database.

In the remainder of the chapter, we will examine the available data on the validity and reliability of data obtained from *ad hoc* questionnaires and automated databases containing person-level data. In each case, we will examine the information available regarding drug exposure data and medical diagnoses separately. We will then end with some conclusions, as well as recommendations for related areas requiring research in the future.

SELF-REPORTED DRUG DATA FROM *AD HOC* QUESTIONNAIRE STUDIES

Accuracy

Concern for the validity of medication data obtained from subjects prompted the conduct of several studies, the first of which was published in 1967.[53] This study evaluated whether recall of medication use during pregnancy was influenced by the outcome of the birth. Since then, numerous

studies have evaluated self-reported medication use for oral contraceptives, for postmenopausal estrogens, and for exposures during pregnancy. Recall accuracy for each of these different types of exposures will be discussed in this section, as well as information from the few studies that report on medications other than hormones or pregnancy-related exposures.

Oral Contraceptive Use

Most of the studies concerned with the accuracy of interview data have evaluated how well women remember past use of oral contraceptives (OC)[54–60] (Table 45.1) and hormone replacement therapy[61–65] (Table 45.2). Accuracy of self-reported OC and hormone replacement therapy has been assessed as part of etiologic studies by verifying exposure using medical records[56–60,62–65] or as separate, methodologic studies.[53,54,61,66,67] The latter have compared self-reported data to prospectively collected information ascertained as part of cohort studies[53,54,66] or from drug dispensation records and files.[61,67]

First examining the OC studies (Table 45.1), the time between when the exposure occurred and when it was queried (period of recall or recall length) varied from 0 (i.e., current use) to 17 or more years between use and questionnaire date. Two[54,66] of the five methodologic studies[53,54,61,66,67] were of OC recall. The methodologic study by Coulter *et al.*[66] employed memory prompts whereas that by Bean *et al.*[54] did not. The former study employed two different types of memory aids, one which listed the different OC brands available (Memory Aid A) and the second that used both pictures of OCs and a calendar to record life events (Memory Aid B).

Overall, the available studies indicate that women accurately remember when they first began using OCs, although the brand names and duration of use are not remembered as well (see Table 45.1). We will present the available data on the accuracy of the date or age of initiation of OC use, duration of use, and brand name in turn.

The two methodologic studies reported that approximately 90% of women were able to recall the age (±1 year) that they began using OCs, regardless of whether a memory aid was used or the type of memory aid used.[54,66] Of the studies which verified OC questionnaire data using medical records,[56–60] the results indicate that women's recall of the exact month and year when they began or stopped OC use was poorly recalled (Table 45.1). The difference in the rates between studies may be attributed to the recall length, which was estimated at up to 10 years for the Stolley *et al.* study and up to 20 years for the Nischan *et al.* study.

Table 45.1. Studies of self-reported prior oral contraceptive use by period of recall and type of questionnaire administration

Author	Recall period	Questionnaire and sample size	Memory aids	Comparison data source	Findings
Glass et al., 1974[57]	3–17 years, median: 5	Personal interview $n=75$	No	Medical records	Percentage agreement: First brand used: 74 Most recent used: 79 Current use: 100
Stolley et al., 1978[60]	2+ years	Personal interview $n=246$	List of brand names	Medical records	Percentage agreement: Most recent OC: 89, $\kappa=0.93$ Previous OC: 63, $\kappa=0.57$ Start date of most recent ±1 month: 52 Stop date of most recent ±1 month: 74 Total duration ±1 month: 36 Total duration ±1 year: 77
Bean et al., 1979[54]	9.1 years	Personal interview $n=160$	No	Menstrual and Reproductive History Cohort	Percentage agreement: First use, exact age: 55 Age ±1 year: 88
Adam et al., 1981[56]	Unknown	Self-administered $n=676$	No	Medical records	25% exposed by questionnaire 32% exposed by medical charts
Rosenberg et al., 1983[59]	4–16 years	Personal interview $n=130$	Calendar and photos	Medical records	Month specific agreement as a percentage: Duration: 90 Duration and brand: 62 Duration, brand and dose: 54
Coulter et al., 1986[66]	10–15 years	Personal interview $n=99$	A: Brand names listed only B: Calendar and photos	Oxford Family Planning Association Cohort	Percentage agreement: (All ±1 yr) Aid A Aid B Duration 57 69 First use 90 90 Last use 63 79 First brand 69 69 Recent brand 53 63
Nischan et al., 1993[58]	≤20 years	Personal interview $n=758$	Calendar and samples	Medical records	Percentage agreement: Cases Controls First brand used: 77 78 Last brand used: 70 66 First use (± 1 year): 72 ($r=0.83$) 68 ($r=0.88$) Last use (±1 year): 70 ($r=0.89$) 69 ($r=0.88$) Total duration (±1 month): 24 17 Total duration (±1 year): 65 ($r=0.83$) 59 ($r=0.91$)

The accuracy of self-reported data on the exact months of use varied from a high of 90% in the study by Rosenberg et al.,[59] which used picture memory aids but measured agreement differently from other authors, to a low of 17% reported by Nischan et al., which provided the respondents with both a calendar and samples of OCs.[58]

Recall accuracy for OC brand names depended on the order of their use. The first brand used was recalled with reasonable accuracy.[57,58,66] There were far greater discrepancies among the studies for the accuracy of the most recent OC brand used, but this may be due to how accuracy was defined, by name[57,60] or by name and dose.[58,66] It was very difficult for respondents to recall all OC brands with their correct dosages. Coulter et al. found that only 33% of those provided Memory Aid A and 48% of those given Memory Aid B could recall all OCs used for six months or longer.[66] Rosenberg et al. reported similarly poor results for the recall accuracy of OC duration, brand, and dose.[59] In the Nischan et al. study,[58] agreement on duration of brand-specific OC use ranged from 31.4% to 100% ($r=0.21$–0.96). Agreement was best for the most recently introduced product and lowest for the OCs that had similar brand names.

Table 45.2. Studies of self-reported prior estrogen use by period of recall and type of questionnaire administration

Author	Recall period	Questionnaire and sample size	Memory aids	Comparison data source	Findings	κ/correlation
Horwitz et al., 1980[63]	Unknown	Telephone interviews n = 324	None	Medical records	Percentage agreement: Ever use: Conventional controls: 80 Alternative controls: 86	κ = 0.58 κ = 0.71
Spengler et al., 1981[65]	Unknown	Personal interview n = 153	Samples of estrogens	Medical records	Ever use, pooled cases and controls (percentage agreement): Versus private MD's records: 82 Versus hospital records: 80	κ = 0.63 κ = 0.59
Paganini-Hill and Ross, 1982[64]	Unknown	Personal interview n = 334	None	Medical and pharmacy records	Percentage agreement: Ever use (versus medical record): 75 Dose (versus medical record): 80 Total duration (by month)[a]	κ = 0.51 κ = 0.61 r = 0.63
Persson et al., 1987[61]	≤3 years	Self-administered n = 160	List of brand names	Prescription forms	Percentage agreement: Month begun, exactly: 85 Name: 85 Dose: 88 Duration	r = 0.98
Goodman et al., 1990[62]	1–11+ years	Personal interviews n = 964	Samples of estrogens	Medical records	Percentage agreement: Ever use: 87 Duration of use First use (±3 years): 58	κ = 0.74 r = 0.54 r = 0.57
West et al., 1995[68]	2–3 years 7–11 years	Telephone interviews n = 103	Pictures of estrogens	Pharmacy database	Recall percentage: Estrogen name: 78 (95% CI: 70–86) Estrogen name and dose: 26 (95% CI: 17–34) Agreement ±6 months ±1 year ±2 years First use: 33 33 53 Last use: 29 47 69 Duration: 53 62 68	Note: For those with multiple estrogen exposures, a single estrogen was selected as the target drug for assessing name, dose and dates of use.
Strom and Schinnar, 2004[69]	Recall of current or recent HRT use	Telephone interviews n = 154	Drug name prompt, HRT photo prompt	Pharmacy claims	Sensitivity: 82% Specificity: 95% Of the 79 women who had been dispensed an HRT during the 15-month period, 14 (17.7%) did not recall use; 12 of the 14 had only a single HRT dispensing which probably indicates that the women did not, in fact, use HRT. Removing these 14 from the analysis, 61 of the remaining 65 women (94%) accurately recalled the name of the HRT used.	κ = 0.77 95% CI: 0.67, 0.87

[a] Results for comparison with physician records only; other records were incomplete.

Postmenopausal Hormone Use

In contrast to the studies of OCs, which evaluated age, duration, and brands used, the studies of postmenopausal estrogen use focused primarily on ever/never use (Table 45.2). There have been three methodologic studies to evaluate the recall accuracy for postmenopausal estrogen use, all of which used pharmacy dispensings for comparison and some type of recall aid. The most recent study used pharmacy claims from a health maintenance organization (HMO) that served a predominantly African American population. Strom and Schinnar[69] identified two cohorts of women, 106 women with one or more hormonal replacement therapy (HRT) dispensings and 107 women who had not been dispensed HRT; 154 women (72.3%) participated in the study. Comparing the questionnaire information to pharmacy dispensings (gold standard), the sensitivity was 82% for ever use of an HRT and 95% for specificity; the concordance on estrogen name was 93.8% between the questionnaire and the pharmacy database. This study found that recall and reporting of HRT use was facilitated primarily by indication-specific questions and a drug photo prompt, but a listing of drug names was not as effective for enhancing recall.

Similar findings for HRT use were reported by West et al.,[68] with a sensitivity of 78% for accurately reporting estrogen name, but lower sensitivity for dates and duration of use, with similar results for recall periods of 2–3 years and 7–11 years. The specificity for nonsteroidal anti-inflammatory drug or estrogen exposure was 95%. As previously noted, although sensitivity was lower than specificity, the relative importance of these two measures depends on the true prevalence of exposure in the population.

Persson et al.[61] reported similar results to those of West et al. for the accuracy of reporting drug name, but much better results for reporting the exact month the estrogen was begun. The difference between the two studies may be due to study design, the questionnaire used to obtain the drug exposure information, or the recency of estrogen use.

The verification studies comparing self-reported estrogen use to medical record documentation reported percentage agreements ranging from 75% to 87% and kappas ranging from 0.51 to 0.74, indicating moderate to substantial agreement.[62,65] In particular, the Goodman et al. study verified both use as well as nonuse of estrogen exposure as part of an etiologic study of breast cancer.[62] They found that 14% of "users" and 12% of "never users" according to self-report would have been misclassified using the information from medical records for comparison. This interpretation assumes that the medical record is correct and the women's recall is inaccurate. A more likely explanation for the 14% of women whose reported estrogen use could not be confirmed is that their medical record was incomplete, i.e., it failed to document their prescriptions. In fact, this 14% error rate noted by Goodman et al. agrees very well with the results from the studies evaluating the completeness of the medical record for documenting prescriptions.[45–47]

Use of Nonhormonal Medications

There are several studies assessing the current use of different types of medications, but only a few studies have evaluated how well respondents report past use of medications other than OCs or postmenopausal estrogens (Table 45.3). Of the 14 studies in Table 45.3, only three are methodologic studies[67,68,70] whose primary goal was to evaluate the accuracy of recall of nonhormone medications. The study by West et al.[68] indicated that respondents have great difficulty accurately recalling specific information about past use of nonsteroidal anti-inflammatory drugs (NSAIDs). Despite using pictorial memory aids and a structured questionnaire, many respondents were unable to recall the name of the NSAIDs they had used in the past and had even more difficulty with the dose, duration, and dates of use.[68]

In the second methodologic study, Van den Brandt et al. compared self-report to pharmacy records of dispensed prescriptions, noting that the number of drug dispensings recalled was highest for cardiovascular medications (66%) and poorest for alimentary tract medications (48%).[67] Recall was influenced by the number of chronically used medications: 71% for one drug, 64% for two drugs, and 59% for three or more drugs, although duration of use was not related to recall. This study could evaluate only recall of current and very recent (within the past two years) medication use. Questionnaire design may have influenced the results of this study. Insufficient space in the questionnaire was allocated for the recording of all medications used in the time period under study. If the respondents were unable to record all medications due to space limitations, it would appear that they were unable to recall all medications when this self-reported information is compared to the medications dispensed according to the database.

The most recent methodologic study to evaluate recall accuracy was done by Klungel et al.[70] using the PHARMO database (see Chapter 20). The primary aim of the study was to determine whether question structure influences the recall of currently used medications. This study focused on the 372 subjects with hypertension only who had at least 90 days of dispensings in the PHARMO database. The questionnaire had indication-specific questions first, e.g., medications used for hypertension, diabetes, etc., followed by an open-ended question that asked if the subjects used any other medications not already mentioned. For hypertension,

Table 45.3. Studies of self-reported drug use other than oral contraceptives and estrogens by period of recall and type of questionnaire administration

Author	Recall period	Questionnaire and sample size	Memory aids	Comparison data source	Drugs	Findings
Hulka et al., 1975[71]	Current use	Personal interview n=357	Drug bottles	Medical records and pharmacy records	Antihistamines Antibiotics Cardiac/congestive heart failure (CHF) CNS Antidiabetics (DM) GI Vitamins	Results were not available by drug. Overall agreement and type of error (in percentages) stratified by underlying chronic condition: DM CHF Agreement 40 27 Patient omits drug(s) 21 22 MD not know of drug(s) 18 22 Patient or MD omissions 21 29 Reporting errors were less than average for cardiac and antidiabetic drugs whereas CNS, antibiotics, GI had more than the average error rate.
Adam et al., 1981[56]	Unknown	Self-administered n=676	None	Medical records	Phenothiazine	1% exposed by questionnaire 20% exposed by medical record
Paganini-Hill and Ross, 1982[64]	Unknown	Personal interview n=334	None	Medical and pharmacy records	Reserpine Other anti-hypertensives Barbiturates Thyroid medications	Percentage agreement for ever use:[a] 86, κ=0.44 87, κ=0.60 69, κ=0.38 83, κ=0.62
Landry et al., 1988[72]	Current use	Self-administered and telephone interviews n=38	None	In-home assessment	High blood pressure Arthritis/pain Tranquilizers Heart pills Seizures Diabetes pills Insulin Antibiotics Ulcer drugs Blood thinners Thyroid pills Hormones	Percentage agreement between home visit and two types of questionnaires: Self-administered (SA) Telephone 90 71 75 48 67 42 89 50 100 50 80 100 100 75 50 0 50 25 100 100 100 100 100 50 Only 16% of the total medications were missing from the SA questionnaire using the home visit as the reference and 9% of the total medications were missing from the home visit data but present on the SA questionnaire.

Table 45.3. (Continued)

Author	Recall period	Questionnaire and sample size	Memory aids	Comparison data source	Drugs	Findings		
							Sensitivity	Specificity	PPV[b]
Johnson and Vollmer 1991[73]	Current use	Self-administered $n=83$	None	Computerized pharmacy records and in-home assessment	Cardiac agents	0.85	1.00	1.00
					Diuretics	0.77	0.93	0.89
					Analgesics	0.33	1.00	1.00
					Psychotropics	0.60	0.98	0.92
					Cardiovasculars	0.75	0.98	0.94
					Anti-inflammatories	0.67	0.94	0.67
					Anti-asthmatics	0.92	0.98	0.92
					Sedatives/hypnotics	0.60	0.97	0.75
					Anti-Parkinson's	1.00	1.00	1.00
					Thyroid agents	0.83	1.00	1.00
					Hormones	1.00	0.99	0.86
Van den Brandt et al., 1991[67]	Up to 2 years	Self-administered $n=207$	None	Computerized pharmacy records		Percentage recall:		
					Alimentary	48		
					Cardiovasculars	66		
					CNS	54		
					Other	61		
Kehoe et al., 1994[74]	Current use	Personal interview $n=942$	None	Medical records		Sensitivity	Specificity	
					Insulin	0.84	0.99	
					Oral hypoglycemics	0.78	0.98	
					Aspirin	0.73	0.70	
					Oral steroids	0.66	0.96	
					Gout medications	0.68	0.98	
					Antihypertensives	0.88	0.89	
Sandvik and Hunskaar 1995[75]	Unknown	Personal interview $n=82$	None	Medical records		κ (95% CI)		
					Estrogens	0.58 (0.39–0.77)		
					Anticholinergics	0.33 (0.07–0.59)		
					Sympathomemetics	0.32 (−0.07–0.71)		
West et al., 1995[68]	2–3 years 7–11 years	Telephone interviews $n=319$	Pictures of NSAIDs	Pharmacy database	Nonsteroidal anti-inflammatory drugs (NSAIDs) For those with repeated NSAID use, a single NSAID was selected as the target drug for assessing name, dose, and dates of use.	Recall percentage for any NSAID use: 57 (95% CI: 50–64) Single NSAID dispensed in 12 year period: 41 (95% CI: 32–50) Repeated NSAID use: 85 (95% CI: 76–94) NSAID name: 30 (95% CI: 24–36) NSAID name and dose: 15 (95% CI: 10–20)		
						Agreement	±6 months	±1 year	±2 years
						First use	20	28	51
						Last use	17	24	42
						Duration	67	71	80

Study	Exposure	Method	Drug list provided	Comparison source	Drugs/Outcomes	Results
Law et al. 1996[76]	Recent use	Personal interview n=123	Name only	Computerized pharmacy records and medical records	AZT ddI ddC Acyclovir Fluconazole Ketoconazole	κ 0.83 0.80 0.95 0.74 0.76 0.64
Cotterchio et al., 1999[77]	Ever use of antidepressants (AD)	Self-administered n=147 cases with AD 119 controls with AD 57 cases with no AD 57 controls with no AD	List of 11 most common drugs	Medical records	AD use by class and by individual type AD as a class Amitriptyline Fluoxetine Imipramine Desipramine Maptroline Sertraine Doxepin Paroxetine Duration of AD use Date AD first taken	κ (95% CI) 0.60 (0.47–0.74) 0.64 (0.40–0.88) 0.69 (0.45–0.94) 0.28 (−0.24–0.79) 0.83 (0.54–1.0) 0.84 (0.54–1.0) 0.64 (0.19–1.0) 0.79 (0.38–1.0) 1.0 (1.0–1.0) 0.56 (0.32–0.79) 0.48 (0.23–0.72)
Smith et al., 1999[78]	Current use	Personal interview and medication inventory n=55 users 55 nonusers	None	Serum levels	Aspirin Propranolol Hydrochlorothiazide Digoxin	κ (95% CI) 0.16 (0.0–0.32) 0.43 (0.27–0.59) 0.62 (0.53–0.91) 0.94 (0.74–1.0)
Klungel et al., 2000[70]	Current use	Self-administered n=372 hypertensives chosen for analysis	None	Pharmacy database	Medications for thromboembolic disease, hypertension, hypercholesterolemia, diabetes, contraception	71% of all medications in current use according to the pharmacy database were mentioned on the questionnaire. 94% of all drugs mentioned on the questionnaire had been dispensed over a period of 3 to 63 months. Of those reporting no medication use on the questionnaire, 86% had no drug dispensings in the PHARMO database.
Clegg et al., 2001[79]	~6 months	Self-administered n=3196	None	Medical records	Hormone shots Hormone pills	κ2 Sens Spec PPV[b] NPV[b] 0.78 0.84 0.94 0.77 0.95 0.57 0.69 0.92 0.54 0.94 Calculated κ three ways, depending on coding of unknown in medical record or self-report. κ2 was calculated by considering unknown use in medical record as no use.

[a] Results for comparison with physician records only; other records were incomplete.

[b] Sens = sensitivity; Spec = specificity; PPV = positive predictive value; NPV = negative predictive value.

the sensitivity was 91% for indication-specific questions and 16.7% for open-ended questions. About 20% of subjects listed medications on the questionnaire that were not in the database and a similar proportion failed to list medications on the questionnaire that were in use according to the pharmacy database. Based on the results on sensitivity of recall, it appears that indication-specific questions invoke better recall accuracy. However, to adequately address the issue of question structure, the questionnaire might have been designed to query medications using an open-ended question before asking indication-specific questions. This would allow a comparison of the number of medications recalled by each question structure.

Four etiologic studies verified the accuracy of self-reported exposure to drugs other than hormones several years in the past, using medical records for comparison.[56,64,75,77] The study by Adam et al., which compared data collected by self-administered questionnaire to information from the patient history portion of the medical record, indicated that women greatly underreport use of anti-psychotic agents,[56] whereas Cotterchio et al. found substantial agreement for antidepressant use, even by drug name.[77] Paganini-Hill and Ross showed different agreement rates between self-reported information and medical record documentation depending on the medication.[64] Of course, discrepancies between the questionnaire data and medical record data can be partially attributed to the incompleteness of the medical records used for comparison.

There are several studies that evaluate the recall accuracy for current or recently used medications. The first methodologic study conducted by Hulka et al. in 1975 looked at how well drugs were reported overall and, for any errors noted, whether subjects failed to report drug use or if the omissions were due to the physicians being unaware of drugs their patients currently use.[71] The results differed by therapeutic class, but even for the cardiac and diabetic medications, there were many discrepancies between the two sources of drug data. Similar discrepant results were noted in methodologic studies,[72,73,78] and three etiologic studies[74,76,79] assessing the accuracy of self-reported current or recent drug use, comparing questionnaire data to medical records, in-home assessments, or pharmacy databases.

Medication Use in Pregnancy

Assessing the frequency and timing of pregnancy-associated exposures is important for determining the potential for teratogenic effects. Nine studies addressed how well women recall medication exposures that occurred during the three different trimesters of pregnancy. Recall accuracy for pregnancy-related exposures was evaluated by two different methods. Four studies used a pre- and post-delivery questionnaire approach, evaluating the accuracy of reporting exposures that occurred during pregnancy to that recalled at different times post-delivery.[53,80–82] Two studies used information from the obstetric or hospital records as the gold standard and evaluated self-report using questionnaires,[83,84] and four others used the interview as the standard and evaluated the completeness of obstetric, hospital, and/or pharmacy records.[53,85–87] Note that Klemetti and Saxen[53] used two techniques to assess the recall accuracy of exposures that occurred during pregnancy.

The studies that used the pre- and post-delivery approach evaluated the completeness of exposure reporting using the pre-delivery questionnaire as the criterion. All four studies found that, when questioned after delivery, women forget at least some medications that were used during gestation,[53,80–82] and there is a small tendency to overreport exposures that did not occur during the pregnancy (range: 0.4–20%). For example, 34.1% of women failed to report an antibiotic or antibacterial exposure, whereas 0.7% overreported this exposure.[80] The recall interval for these four studies spanned from weeks,[80] to months,[53,81] to eight years.[82] Feldman et al.[81] and Mackenzie and Lippman[80] reported that recall differed by type of medication. Chronically used medications were recalled more often than acute exposures, and salient exposures (those that prompted study initiation) were also more accurately recalled (81%) than were common and less disconcerting exposures (33%).[81] Similarly, Mackenzie and Lippman reported fewer deletions for prescription drugs such as antibiotics, compared with over-the-counter medications such as vitamins, analgesics, and cold preparations.

Whereas Feldman et al. found that factors such as maternal age, marital and employment status, and pregnancy outcome did not influence the reporting of pregnancy medication exposures, de Jong et al.[82] reported better recall in mothers with higher educational attainment and poorer pregnancy outcome (low birth weight, gestational age, or Apgar score). The two other papers[53,80] did not find recall differences based on pregnancy outcome.

Two studies used the obstetric record as the gold standard to assess the accuracy of self-reported medication histories.[83,84] These two studies had widely differing times between exposure and self-report. In the Tilley et al. study, women were questioned anywhere from 10 to 30 years after their pregnancy to elicit information on diethylstilbestrol use.[83] Of the women who had been exposed according to their records, 37% either did not recall or denied diethylstilbestrol exposure. Women in the Werler et al. study were interviewed during their postpartum hospital stay. Compared with the obstetric record, there was both under- and overreporting of exposures that differed by the type of exposure and by pregnancy outcome. For example, compared to women with favorable pregnancy outcomes, those with an adverse pregnancy outcome more accurately reported using birth control after conception and experiencing urinary tract infections. The Werler *et al.* study supports the potential for recall bias when using non-malformed infants as the control group for studying teratogenic exposures.

Finally, there are five studies that verified the mother's self-reported drug exposure using medical records and/or pharmacy records.[53,85–88] Klemetti and Saxen found that only 6% of the mothers' reports were incorrect when compared with medical records.[53] McCredie *et al.* used medical records to confirm Bendectin® exposure in a random sample of 30 mothers who reported use during pregnancy; 57% of the exposures were documented in the charts.[86] Of the remaining unconfirmed reports, 20% of the mothers' physicians indicated that they often prescribe the drug without recording it on the medical record and 27% of the records were unavailable. Bryant *et al.* reported moderate agreement between self-reported information and medical records for use of any prescription drugs during pregnancy ($\kappa = 0.48$), but, as expected, very poor agreement for over-the-counter medications ($\kappa = 0.02$) and vitamin supplements ($\kappa = 0.07$).[87] De Jong *et al.* reported a 50% confirmation of self-reported medication exposure using pharmacy, general practitioner, and hospital records, with the best verification noted for general practitioner and hospital records combined (69%).[85]

Of particular concern is that most studies that use medical or pharmacy records to verify exposure are only unidirectional. They confirm drug exposure if reported but typically do not evaluate whether a respondent omits reporting an exposure that actually occurred, i.e., the validation efforts typically assess sensitivity but not specificity. The most recent evaluation of the accuracy of mothers' reports of pregnancy-associated drug exposures comes from the Hungarian Case–Control Surveillance of Congenital Abnormalities study that was begun in 1980.[88] This validation study was complex and evaluated differences between control mothers who did and who did not respond to the original case–control questionnaire (no differences), as well as differences in recall between the mothers of congenital limb defect cases and their matched control mothers (slight differences). Two sources of data were compared: (i) mothers' self-report via personal interview using a structured questionnaire typically completed 12 and 24 months post-delivery for cases and controls, respectively; and (ii) the mothers' antenatal logbook containing specific

information on diagnosed pregnancy complications and medications that was completed by her clinician during the prenatal visits. They reported that women use an average of 5.26 medications during pregnancy (range 2–11). Evaluating recall, the antenatal logbooks were missing about 25% of the drugs mothers recorded on their questionnaires (50% of which were over-the-counter preparations). Conversely, mothers failed to report 23% of medications that were recorded in the logbooks. Some of the latter medications were prescribed but not used due to the mothers' concern about teratogenicity.

Influences on Accuracy

The accuracy of medication exposure reported via questionnaire is affected by several factors. Research indicates that the type of question influences how well respondents answer medication questions. Klungel *et al.* reported that most medications in current use were identified by medication-specific or indication-specific questions and that a general medication question "Have you taken any other medications?" failed to identify approximately 19% of medications the respondents were currently taking.[70] Similarly, Mitchell *et al.* reported that open-ended questions such as "Have you ever used any medications?" yielded 13–45% of the affirmative responses for use of three different medications.[16] The addition of indication-specific questions added an incremental 35–58% affirmative responses concerning exposures. Finally, 20–35% reported drug exposure only when asked medication (name)-specific questions.[16] These studies support the work by Cottler and Robins,[89] suggesting that questionnaire design influences the completeness of self-reported psychoactive medication use. Asking medication-specific questions in addition to indication-specific questions increased reported drug use by 26–36%. In particular, the medication-specific questions substantially increased reporting for certain subgroups, including 25–44-year-olds, males, African Americans, and those with eight or more years of education.

Studies have also shown that memory aids such as photographs of medications or calendars improve recall. Recently, Kimmel and colleagues found that medication pictures and listings of medications improved respondents' recall of non-aspirin nonsteroidal anti-inflammatory drugs by only 6% after previously being asked indication-specific questions.[90] The recall period for the study was relatively short, between 20 and 122 days for cases of myocardial infarction and approximately 7 days for their matched controls. Kimmel *et al.* reported that memory aids enhanced recall only if the recall period was ≤ 90 days. Using two different types of memory aids, Coulter *et al.* (see Table 45.1), noted that recall of total duration of use and date of last use were greatly improved when respondents were provided with pictures of OCs and a calendar compared with just a list of OC brands.[66] Similarly, Beresford and Coker found that only 29% of women were able to recall the name and dose of the estrogen without pictures, increasing to 71% for those who used pictures to enhance recall.[91]

Recall period, the time between when the exposure occurred and when it is reported, influences accuracy of recall. Stolley *et al.* reported that agreement on OC starting date between self-report and medical records was 55% if the OC was used within one month of hospitalization and 45% if the OC was used within the most recent two years.[60] Goodman *et al.* reported correlations of 0.7 and 0.4 for agreement on duration of estrogen use for recall periods of 0–11 and 11+ years, respectively, and similar differences in agreement for age at first use for these two recall periods ($r = 0.7$ and $r = 0.5$, respectively).[62] In the only methodologic study to evaluate recall period, West *et al.*[68] reported that the names of drugs stopped 2–3 years prior to interview were recalled more frequently than those stopped 7–11 years prior to interview (odds of recall = 3.0, 95% CI: 1.6–5.7 and 2.4, 95% CI: 0.9–6.7 for nonsteroidal anti-inflammatory drugs and estrogens, respectively). All three studies indicated greater inaccuracies as more time elapsed between occurrence of exposure and its subsequent reporting.

The extent of use as measured by number of dispensings or duration of use appears to enhance recall. Klungel *et al.* reported that currently used medications that were used for longer periods of time (92.3% for >6 months use) were better recalled than those used for <3 months (62.5%, $p < 0.01$).[70] Further analysis of the West *et al.* methodologic study indicated that individuals were better able to recall the name of the nonsteroidal anti-inflammatory drug in question (target NSAID) as the number of its dispensings increased: for every four dispensings of the target NSAID, the odds of recalling its name increased by 1.7 (95% CI: 1.3–2.2).[92] Similarly, as the number of different types of NSAIDs used increased, there was better recall: for every three different NSAIDs used, there was a 3.6-fold (95% CI: 1.3–9.9) increased odds of recalling the target NSAID name. However, this same study did not report similar findings for recalling estrogen use, which indicates that recall accuracy for past drug use and its predictors differs by therapeutic class.

The possibility of recall bias was the motivation for many validation studies of past medication use. Whereas many of the studies that addressed this issue evaluated recall accuracy for mothers of normal and abnormal infants,[53,80,81,84,86,93,94] others have assessed differences between cases and controls in case–control studies of non-pregnancy related conditions.[58–60,62,64,65,77] Overall, the literature does not strongly support a general or uniform indication of recall bias in either circumstance,[53,58,62,64,65,77,80,81,86,93] although there are some exceptions.[59,60,84,94] Rockenbauer *et al.*, using the Hungarian Case–Control Surveillance System of Congenital Abnormalities data, noted that the odds ratios were higher using medication exposures ascertained by self-report rather than from the women's antenatal logbooks.[94] This was especially evident for medications used on a short-term basis such as antimicrobial drugs. Rockenbauer and colleagues considered self-report to be the gold standard for their analysis because it captured "all" drug intake in comparison with the antenatal logbooks, which only listed drugs prescribed by obstetricians. However, the authors may have chosen self-reports as the gold standard because the antenatal logbooks included much more medication use for controls than for cases. Werler *et al.* reported differences in recall by both exposure and birth outcome (normal and malformed infants)[84] and Stolley *et al.* found that cases showed better percentage agreement between self-reports and medical records than did controls for starting date of the most recently used OC (61% versus 48%, respectively) and for duration of use (47% versus 31%, respectively).[60] Rosenberg *et al.* found similar percentage agreements for recalling the duration of past OC use between cases and controls: 94% versus 87%, respectively.[59] It seems the issue of recall bias is unresolved to this point and hinges on the accuracy and completeness of women's recall of medication use during pregnancy. Ongoing studies at two Centers for Education and Research on Therapeutics (CERTs) are evaluating whether record-linked databases can be used for studying the teratogenicity of medications to circumvent the issue of recall bias.

To date, few studies have evaluated whether demographic and behavioral characteristics influence the recall of past medication use. Cotterchio *et al.* evaluated age, household income, and education as predictors of recall accuracy for reporting ever having used an antidepressant, with inconsistent results.[77] Calculating percentage agreement using the medical record to confirm self-reported data, Goodman *et al.* noted small variations in recall accuracy for any past estrogen use by ethnicity (96% for Japanese ancestry, 91% for non-Japanese ancestry) and education, with more educated women having less accurate recall (90%) than those with without a college education (96%).[62] West *et al.* noted a similar finding for education; sensitivity was 26% for women with some college education and 47% for those without any college education recalling the NSAID name (odds of recall = 0.4, 95% CI: 0.1–1.3).[92]

Recall accuracy was affected by age in three of five studies evaluated. Clegg *et al.* found that men over age 80 had poorer recall of hormone shots and pills than did men less than age 80 (adjusted agreement for men over age 80 was 82% and 63% for hormone shots and pills, respectively, compared to 90% and >80% for men less than age 80).[79] West *et al.* reported that persons aged 50–65 years recalled the NSAID name more accurately than those aged 66–80, odds of recall = 1.8 (95% CI: 1.0–3.4).[51,68] Van den Brandt *et al.* found better recall accuracy for younger age groups as well, with sensitivities of 65%, 60%, and 58% for those aged 55–59, 60–64, and 65–69, respectively.[67] Goodman *et al.* did not report age differences in recall accuracy for past estrogen use[62] and Stolley *et al.*[60] did not find age differences in the agreement between the user and the prescriber for the name of the OC used most recently. Study design may explain the different results noted; the two studies that reported an age effect were methodologic studies evaluating recall accuracy[67,68] whereas the two that reported no age effects[60,62] were etiologic studies that reported verification of drug use as a measure of exposure misclassification for the association under study.

Few other demographic factors were evaluated consistently across studies. No differences in recall accuracy were noted by gender.[67,68] Stolley *et al.* reported racial and socioeconomic differences in reporting, with whites having better percentage agreement than nonwhites (92% versus 83.1%, respectively), and private paying users having better agreement than those receiving public health care funds (91.3% versus 77.1%, X2 = 6.6, $p < 0.04$).[60]

Behavioral characteristics such as smoking and alcohol use have been investigated as predictors of recall accuracy.[62,92] Non-smokers had better recall of ever/never use of estrogens (89.8%, $\kappa = 0.79$) than did smokers (82.2%, $\kappa = 0.64$) in the Goodman *et al.* study. This was not supported in the work of West *et al.*, which found no relationship between recall accuracy for past NSAID or estrogen use and cigarette smoking. Similarly, West *et al.* reported that current alcohol use was unrelated to recall accuracy for NSAIDs or estrogens.

With regard to predictors of recall accuracy, factors such as questionnaire design, use of memory aids, recall period, extent of past drug use, age, and education sometimes influence how well respondents remember past drug use, the effect often seeming to vary by therapeutic class. Behavioral characteristics such as smoking and alcohol use were rarely evaluated as predictors of accuracy and inconsistent findings were noted in the two studies that reported the results of their evaluation. Due to the paucity of information on predictors of recall, further research in this area is warranted.

Conclusions

It is apparent from this review, as well as an earlier review by Harlow and Linet[95], that most of the work on recall accuracy for past medication use has focused on OCs and replacement estrogens. The results of the OCs and replacement estrogens studies indicate that these medications are recalled accurately, especially if researchers allow a range of one year for agreement on age and duration of use. However, women do have difficulty recalling the brands of OC and replacement estrogens used, even if provided photos or lists of brand names. Recall of nonhormonal drugs appears potentially more problematic. Although we are beginning to see more evaluations of nonhormonal medications, there are still few studies and there are substantial differences among them. For example, recall periods ranged from one month to several years, or the exact number of years was not specified. The drugs studied were as diverse as the recall periods. As more researchers combine verification with their data collection efforts, more information will hopefully become available on the recall accuracy of other types of medications.

The methodologic literature on recall accuracy discussed above indicates that study participants have difficulty remembering drug use from the distant past, which contributes to misclassification of exposure in *ad hoc* case–control studies. A cursory review of the recent literature shows that the more recent *ad hoc* case–control studies have focused on medication use just prior to disease onset, a design feature that will improve the validity of medication exposure data. There is also a trend toward using medication-specific and indication-specific questions, along with recall enhancements, which has been shown to produce better data. Calendars and photos of drugs augment recall to a greater degree than listing only the brand names of the drugs in question. These techniques—namely photos, calendars, and the two different types of drug questions—have become the state-of-the-art for collecting self-reported drug data by personal or telephone interview.

The literature to date suggests that recall accuracy of self-reported medication exposures is sometimes, but by no means always, influenced by the type of medication, drug use patterns, the design of the data collection materials, and respondent characteristics. Differential misclassification of exposure by disease status or recall bias, as a major concern in case–control studies of medication use, appears to be a misapprehension. Given the current state of the literature, epidemiologists who plan to use questionnaire data to investigate drug–disease associations will need to consider which factors may influence recall accuracy in the design of their research protocols. Many researchers are turning to administrative databases to decrease potential exposure misclassification due to inaccurate self-report.

SELF-REPORTED DIAGNOSIS AND HOSPITALIZATION DATA FROM *AD HOC* STUDIES

Accuracy

Much of the methodologic research on the ability to remember past medical conditions and the factors that influenced this recall has been sponsored by the US National Center for Health Statistics, to determine how accurately chronic conditions were being reported in the US National Health Survey. These were large studies comparing interview data with administrative forms used by the HMOs participating in the study.[96,97] Other investigations have verified self-reported medical conditions using medical records as part of case–control or cohort studies.[98–104] The Baltimore Study[105] and Heliovaara *et al.*[106] differed from the other studies. Persons who had responded to questions regarding chronic illness were then clinically evaluated for presence or absence of the conditions under study.

Just as recall accuracy of past medication use varies by the type of drug, the ability to remember disease conditions varies by disease. The best reporting was shown for conditions that are specific and familiar, such as diabetes mellitus,[74,101,102,105–109] hypertension,[74,98,102,106,107] asthma,[101,105,106] and cancers such as breast, lung, large bowel, and prostate.[98,107,110,111] It is difficult to assess the reporting accuracy for common, symptom-based conditions such as sinusitis, arthritis, low back pain, and migraine headaches, which many people may have, or believe they have, without having been told so by a clinician.

In studies comparing self-reports to clinical evaluation, depending upon the type of condition, there is both under- and overreporting.[105,106] Studies using medical records to assess recall accuracy for common ailments typically found poor agreement, where underreporting was often the major cause of the disagreement in some studies[74,101,107,109] but overreporting occurred as well, especially for conditions where the diagnostic criteria are less explicit.[112] Similarly, comparing self-reported symptom and quality of life information at two different time periods also shows both over- and underestimation. Three separate studies found that individuals recalled having more pain than they reported previously: 3 months after total knee arthroplasty,[113] 1.5 to 3.8 years after hip replacement,[114] and 5–10 years after back pain.[115] Mancuso and Charlson

also reported that the subjects recalled better walking and function than they actually had prior to the hip replacement.[114] Thus, recollection of symptoms and function are not accurate and the direction of the error can lead to both over- and underestimation (Table 45.4).

Likewise, depending on the data source used for comparison, cardiovascular conditions may be over- or underreported as well.[74,98,99,102,106,107,109,111,117,118] Poor agreement in most studies was due to overreporting of disease[98,99,117] but some studies by design could only detect overreporting.[99] In Phase I of a cohort study to ascertain cardiovascular disease occurrence by self-report, only 61 (81%) of 75 myocardial infarctions (MIs), 20 (65%) of 31 strokes, and 29 (66%) of 44 reports of diabetes could be verified by medical record review.[99] Others noted both under- and overreporting, depending upon the cardiovascular disease being studied.[102,109,111,112] Heliovaara *et al.*[106] and Spitz *et al.*[107] noted accurate recall of cardiovascular conditions and Kehoe *et al.*[74] suggested that their results were due to underreporting of disease. In most instances of recall error, many who had incorrectly reported MIs and stroke had other conditions which they may have mistakenly understood as coronary heart disease, MI, or stroke, based upon communication with their physician during their diagnostic visits.[99,111,117,118]

Only two studies assessed the recall accuracy for mental illnesses, both comparing interview to clinical evaluation.[105,106] The results indicated poor agreement between the two data sources, with underreporting as the primary reason for poor agreement. It is unclear from these studies whether the reason for underreporting is unwillingness on the part of the respondent to admit to mental illness or whether the conditions were actually underdiagnosed.

There have been only three studies that evaluated reporting of cataracts, two assessing presence of cataract by clinical exam[105,116] and the third using medical record review for comparison.[102] Agreement was best in the Bush *et al.* study,[102] whereas the studies that used clinical assessments typically reported poor agreement. Similar to the evaluation of mental illnesses, the question remains, could the underreporting be due to underdiagnosis?

Finally, fractures were evaluated in four studies, all of which used medical records for comparison. The overall results from the studies indicated good agreement, although the one methodologic study of fracture incidence indicated a slight tendency for overreporting of hand, finger, rib, or facial fractures.[103]

Although menarche and menopause are not medical conditions per se, the age at which they occur is often of interest in pharmacoepidemiology studies. Using data from the Menstrual and Reproductive Health Study, which had recall periods ranging from 17 to 53 years (mean 33.9 years),

Table 45.4. Studies of self-reported conditions

Author	Questionnaire and sample size	Comparison data source	Conditions	Findings	
Commission on Chronic Illness, 1957[105]	Personal interview where one person reported on all those in the household $n=809$	Clinical evaluation	Selected conditions:[a]	Percentage agreement on presence of disorder comparing interview and clinical evaluation:	
			Malignant neoplasms	59	
			Asthma	99	
			Thyroid disease	10	
			Diabetes mellitus	95	
			Psychoses/neuroses	17	
			Other mental disorders	11	
			Heart disease	52	
			Chronic sinusitis	72	
			Rheumatoid arthritis	100	
			Osteoarthritis	72	
Paganini-Hill and Ross, 1982[64]	Personal interview $n=334$	Medical and pharmacy records	Ever had:	Percentage agreement	κ
			Gallbladder disease	95	0.82
			Hypertension	90	0.78
			Diabetes	96	0.70
			Benign breast disease	87	0.63
			Hysterectomy	98	0.96
			Oophorectomy	93	0.78
Tretli et al., 1982[99]	Self-administered $n=12694$	Medical records	Ever had or recently had:	Percentage agreement on ever having had disorder between self-report and medical records:	
			MI	81	
			Stroke	65	
			Diabetes	66	
				Percentage agreement between new events occurring during follow-up and self-report via questionnaire:	
			MI	74	
			Stroke	33	
Wilcox and Horney, 1984[104]	Self-administered $n=362$	Menstrual and Reproductive Health Study	Spontaneous abortion	Percentage agreement: 75 Predictors of recall (percentage of abortions recalled) Length of pregnancy when abortion occurred: ≤6 weeks: 54 >13 weeks: 93 Recall period: <10 yrs: 82 ≥20 yrs: 73	
Colditz et al., 1986[98]	Self-administered Sample size varied by disease being validated $n=121\,700$	Medical records	New report of disease between follow-ups, Nurses Health Study	Percentage agreement:	
			Breast	99	
			Large bowel	93	
			Thyroid	93	
			Ovary	87	
			Corpus uteri	74	
			Lung	67	
			MI	68	
			Stroke	66	
			Fractures	100	
			Hypertension	100 (only 60% had medical records available to confirm the diagnosis)	

Table 45.4. (Continued)

Author	Questionnaire and sample size	Comparison data source	Conditions	Findings		
Spitz *et al.*, 1988[107]	Self-administered *n*=72	Medical records	Past medical conditions Hypertension Duodenal ulcer Coronary artery disease Diabetes mellitus Gout Rheumatoid arthritis Emphysema	Percentage agreement: 82 78 100 80 60 0 100		
			Previous cancers diagnosed two or more years ago: Colorectal Genital tract Breast Melanoma Hematopoietic Lung Liver Bone Skin	100 93 100 83 100 60 0 0 0		
			Operations: Appendectomy Hysterectomy Cholecystectomy	95 96 88		
Bush *et al.*, 1989[102]	Self-administered questionnaire *n*=107	Medical records	Ever had any of the following: Angina Cancer Cataracts Diabetes Fracture Hypertension MI Stroke	Percentage agreement 85 89 76 98 91 86 94 98	κ 0.57 0.72 0.53 0.93 0.71 0.71 0.70 0.85	
Linet *et al.*, 1989[101]	Personal interview with some surrogate interviews *n*=338	Medical records	Ever had any of the following selected conditions:[a] Tuberculosis Chronic sinusitis Diverticulitis Hepatitis Rheumatoid arthritis Asthma	Percentage agreement 95 80 96 97 95 98	κ 0.49 0.24 0.53 0.59 0.00 0.39	
Linton *et al.*, 1991[116]	Self-administered *n*=3588	Ocular examination	Ever been told of having the following: Cataract Macular degeneration	Self-reported disease at the ocular exam compared to results of exam Percentage agreement 84 92	Sensitivity 0.46 0.18	Specificity 0.96 0.99

Midthjell et al., 1992[108]	Self-administered n = 507	Medical records	Presence or absence of diabetes	96.4% of diabetes cases and 99.7% of non-cases were verified. Approximately 50% of diabetics recalled the year their diabetes was diagnosed.
Nevitt et al., 1992[103]	Self-administered n = 9704	Medical records	Prospective study of non-spine fractures	78% of non-spine fractures were confirmed. False-positive report rate was 12% for all non-spine fractures. Of those with no reported fractures by self-report, medical records confirmed that no fractures occurred. Overreporting was lowest for shoulder, wrist/forearm, elbow, ankle, and hip. Overreporting was greatest for hand, finger, rib, or face.

Heliovaara et al., 1993[106]	Personal interview n = 7217	Health examination	Presence of selected chronic conditions:[a]				
				Sensitivity	Specificity	PPV	Kappa
			Arterial hypertension	0.73	0.99	0.90	0.78
			Coronary disease	0.55	0.97	0.55	0.52
			Cerebral stroke	0.58	1.00	0.65	0.61
			Any cardiovascular disease	0.80	0.94	0.80	0.74
			Bronchial asthma	0.72	0.99	0.59	0.64
			Pulmonary emphysema	0.23	0.99	0.37	0.28
			Osteoarthritis	0.34	0.97	0.53	0.37
			Low back disorder	0.56	0.92	0.44	0.43
			Any mental illness	0.20	1.00	0.93	0.30
			Diabetes	0.81	99	0.77	0.78

Paganini-Hill and Chao, 1993[111]	Self-administered	Medical records	Development of the following diseases during 2-year follow-up	Percentage agreement: 2 Questionnaires	
				1983	1985
	Sample size varied by disease being validated		Hip fracture	85	70
			Heart attack	44	36
			Cancer	80	56
			Colon	70	70
			Rectum	13	25
	Follow-up 1 n = 9734		Lung	87	57
			Breast	90	35
			Uterine	74	44
	Follow-up 2 n = 8884		Prostate	57	34
			Bladder	78	47
			Lymphoma/leukemia	65	29

Kehoe et al., 1994[74]	Personal interview n = 942	Medical records	Ever diagnosed with:	Sensitivity	Specificity
			Arthritis	0.75	0.66
			Coronary heart disease	0.64	0.96
			Hypertension	0.91	0.88
			Diabetes	0.84	0.97
			Other CVD	0.57	0.82
			Cancer	0.71	0.89

Rosamond et al., 1995[117]	Personal interview n = 1053	Medical records	Previous occurrence of an acute MI or heart attack	60% of previous acute MIs were confirmed; unconfirmed reports were confused with unstable angina, coronary heart failure, and other conditions.

Table 45.4. (Continued)

Author	Questionnaire and sample size	Comparison data source	Conditions	Findings
Kriegsman et al., 1996[109]	Personal interviews n = 2380	Medical records (physicians were sent a questionnaire to complete)	Presence or absence of: Nonspecific lung disease Cardiac disease Peripheral atherosclerosis Cerebrovascular disease Diabetes mellitus Malignant neoplasms (excluding non-melanoma skin cancer) Rheumatoid arthritis and/or osteoarthritis	κ (95% CI): 0.59 (0.53–0.65) 0.65 (0.65–0.73) 0.38 (0.30–0.46) 0.56 (0.48–0.64) 0.85 (0.81–0.89) 0.66 (0.60–0.72) 0.31 (0.27–0.35)

| Law et al., 1996[76] | Personal interview n = 123 | Medical records | Previous HIV illnesses
Hairy leukoplakia
Oral candidiasis
Herpes zoster
Pneumocystis carinii
Kaposi's sarcoma
Esophageal candidiasis | κ:
0.14
0.39
0.62
0.82
0.78
0.64 |

Author	Questionnaire and sample size	Comparison data source	Conditions	Findings	
Bergmann et al., 1998[110]	Self-administered n = 65 582	Cancer registry	MD ever diagnosed:	Sensitivity	PPV
			All cancer sites	0.79	0.75
			Colon	0.85	0.54
			Rectum	0.16	0.71
			Lung	0.90	0.72
			Melanoma	0.53	0.34
			Breast	0.91	0.85
			Uterus	0.71	0.79
			Prostate	0.90	0.80
			Bladder	0.67	0.72
			Leukemia	0.61	0.41
			Lymphoma	0.6	40.69

Author	Questionnaire and sample size	Comparison data source	Conditions	Findings		
Walker et al., 1998[118]	Self-administered n = 5787 for heart attack	Medical record	Diagnosis of heart attack or stroke during 12 year follow-up			
				κ	False-positive rate	False-negative rate
			Heart attack	0.74	33%	6%
	n = 5907 for stroke		Stroke	0.54	25%	11%

Author	Questionnaire and sample size	Comparison data source	Conditions	Findings			
Zhu et al., 1999[112]	Self-administered	Medical record	Diagnoses for selected variables by case–control status and age	Kappas			
				Age 40–64		Age 65–69	
	Prostate cancer cases, n = 181 Controls n = 297			Controls	Cases	Controls	Cases
			Vasectomy	0.53	0.61	0.52	0.71
			Benign prostatic hyperplasia	0.22	0.26	0.46	0.12
			Prostatitis	0.35	0.25	0.37	0.25
			Epididymitis/orchitis	0.31	0.33	0.44	0.22
			UTI	0.43	0.21	0.29	0.45
			Inguinal hernia	0.85	0.69	0.75	0.77
			Kidney stones	0.82	0.78	0.61	0.39

				κ	Sens	Spec	PPV[b]	NPV[b]
Clegg et al., 2001[79]	Self-administered n=3196	Medical records	Prostatectomy	0.89	0.89	0.98	0.99	0.90
			Orchiectomy	0.82	0.74	0.98	0.93	0.97

Calculated κ 3 ways, depending on coding of unknown in medical record or self-report. κ2 reported was calculated by considering unknown use in medical record as no use.

Naleway et al., 2003[119]	Telephone interview n=100	Medical records		Children or adults with atopic dermatitis or eczema, percentage recall of condition:		

	Parent guardian for child	Adult for him/herself	Adult contact for other adult
Atopic dermatitis diagnosis			
Eczema diagnosis	20%	28%	12%
Itchy, recurrent rash (≥ 6 months)	60%	50%	46%
Atopic dermatitis or eczema	37%	38%	26%
	64%	54%	50%

[a] Results for comparison with physician records only; other records were incomplete.
[b] Sens = sensitivity; Spec = specificity; PPV = Positive predictive value; NPV = negative predictive value.

Bean et al. found that the exact age of menarche was recalled by 59%, and age within one year was recalled by 90%.[54] Similarly for menopause, 45% of women were able to report their exact age at natural menopause and 75.5% reported age within one year. The percentage agreements for surgical menopause were 55.6% and 83.4%, respectively, for exact age and age within one year. The recall lengths were 7.6 years and 10.6 years for natural and surgical menopause, respectively. The lower percentage agreement for age at which natural menopause occurred compared to that for surgical menopause may be attributed to the gradual occurrence of natural menopause compared to the definitive nature of hysterectomy.[120]

Influences on Accuracy

The reporting of a medical condition during an interview is influenced by several factors, including the type of condition as well as the subject's understanding of the problem. Reporting is also dependent upon the respondent's willingness to divulge the information. Conditions such as venereal disease and mental disorders may not be reported because the respondent is embarrassed to discuss them with the interviewer or worries about the confidentiality of self-administered questionnaires.[105,121] As a result, conditions considered sensitive are likely to be underreported when ascertained by self-report.

Conditions with substantial impact on a person's life are better reported than those with little or no impact on lifestyle. Of those with current restrictions on food or beverage due to medical problems, 64.2% reported chronic conditions that were confirmed in medical records, compared with 58.2% for those without these restrictions.[96] Similarly, 71.2% of those who had restrictions on work or housework reported chronic conditions, versus 45.9% for those who did not have these restrictions.[96] The major determinant of recall for spontaneous abortions was the length of the pregnancy at the time the event occurred: 54% recalled a spontaneous abortion occurring within the first 6 weeks of pregnancy, whereas 93% remembered those occurring more than 13 weeks into the pregnancy.

Other factors that influence reporting accuracy of past diagnoses and hospitalizations include the number of physician services for that condition and the recency of services.[96,97,104,119,122,123] For peptic ulcer hospitalizations, 90% of those hospitalized 2–6 months prior to interview remembered the date of admission, compared with 80% for those hospitalized 7–18 months prior to interview, and 60% for those hospitalized 5 or more years prior to interview.[123] For reporting of diagnoses, the longer the interval between the date of the last medical visit for the condition and the date of interview, the poorer the recall was for that condition.[96,97,119] Despite the requirement that subjects have at least two diagnoses for eczematous skin conditions separated by a minimum of 60 days, Naleway and colleagues[119] found that recall of this diagnosis eroded quickly: from 90% in the first year after diagnosis to 50% approximately 15 years later. Ninety-one percent of the conditions requiring a visit within the week before interview were recalled, compared to 76% for conditions with visits 2–4 weeks prior. The numbers were 54% and 41% for conditions with visits 6 months prior and one year prior, respectively.[96]

One of the limitations of the National Center for Health Statistics study[96] is that it only assessed recall of conditions occurring in the past year. An unanswered question is the ability of respondents to recall conditions that were diagnosed and resolved more than one year previously. Using data from the Menstrual and Reproductive Health Study begun in 1935, where women reported their monthly menses and any disruption of their menses, Wilcox and Horney found that 82% of women were able to recall a spontaneous abortion that had occurred in the past 10 years, but only 73% recalled those that occurred 20 or more years previously.[104] While not large, can these differences in recall be explained by age, recall interval, a cohort effect, or some intertwining of all three? What may have been considered "sensitive" by one generation may not be considered as such by the subsequent generation. Further, terminology changes over time, with prior generations using the nomenclature "miscarriages" whereas more recent generations use "spontaneous abortions." Despite differences in recall accuracy by recall interval, Wilcox and Horney's results indicate that spontaneous abortions appear to be recalled fairly accurately, probably as a result of their emotional impact.

Perhaps as a result of the emotional stress, lifestyle changes, and potential financial strain, hospitalizations tend to be reported accurately.[122] There was only a 9% underreporting of hospitalizations where surgery was performed, compared to 16% of those without a surgical procedure. The underreporting in those with only a one-day hospital stay was 28% compared with 11% for 2–4 day stays, and approximately 6% for stays lasting 5 or more days.

There is also consensus that the type of surgery is remembered accurately.[55,79,100,123] Coulter et al. reported that 90% of the surgeries reported during interview were confirmed by general practitioner records. For the remaining 10%, there was a suggestion that the medical record lacked the information.[55] Recall of the surgery date (±1 year) was correct for 87.5%. Recall accuracy was very good for hysterectomy and appendectomy,[64,101,107] most likely because these surgeries are both salient and familiar to respondents. Cholecystectomy[107] and oophorectomy[64] were not as well recalled and were subject to some overreporting. The overreporting noted in the Paganini-Hill and Ross study[64] may have been due to the potential incompleteness of the medical records used for comparison. For induced abortions, there was only marginal agreement for the occurrence of surgical abortions as noted by records from a managed care organization, with 19% of women underreporting their abortion history, 35% overreporting abortions, and 46% reporting accurately according to their medical record.[124]

There has been a thorough evaluation of the influence of demographic characteristics on reporting of chronic illnesses, although the results are conflicting. The most consistent finding is that recall accuracy decreases with age,[74,79,109,110,116] although this may be confounded by recall interval, or cohort (generational) effects. Whether gender influences recall accuracy is uncertain. Linet et al. found men to report better than women, independent of age,[101] whereas the Baltimore Study found that women reported better than men,[105] especially in older age groups.[96] There was also a suggestion that the gender and age differences depended upon the disease under investigation,[105] with women overreporting malignancies and men overreporting stroke.[109] Unlike chronic illnesses, no difference was found for reporting of hospitalizations by age or gender.[122]

There was a consistent finding that reporting of both illnesses and hospitalizations was better for whites than for non-whites,[79,96,101,105,122] but the number of non-whites in each of the studies was relatively small. Udry et al. also reported racial differences in reporting accuracy, with non-whites underreporting surgical abortions more frequently than whites.[124]

Reporting by educational level was equivocal, with one study showing no difference,[97] another study indicating better recall for those with less education,[96] and four studies suggesting more accurate responses for those with a college education.[103,109,110,124] With the exception of the study by Nevitt et al.,[103] many studies found that reporting was more complete for self-respondents compared to proxy respondents,[97,101,105,116] including reporting for hospitalizations, where the underreporting was estimated at 7% for self-respondents and 14% for proxies.[122] For self-respondents, those with a poor or fair current health status reported conditions more completely than those with good to excellent health status.[96]

As with the validity of medication data, the validity of disease and hospitalization data obtained by self-report is also influenced by questionnaire design. Providing respondents with a checklist of reasons for visiting the doctor improves recall of all medical visits.[125] This research has also indicated that simpler questions yield better responses than more complex questions, presumably because complex questions require the respondent to first comprehend what is being asked and then provide an answer. Cannell and colleagues reported that increasing the length of the question improves recall because of the longer question's inherent redundancy and because respondents are provided with more time to develop an answer to the question.[126] However, longer questions could increase the cost of the research and could needlessly tire the respondents.

In summary, whether a person reports an illness during an interview appears to be related to age and the type of illness, when it occurred, and its saliency, but is less likely to be mediated by demographic characteristics such as gender, race, and education. Illnesses that are embarrassing and that do not substantially alter the person's lifestyle are not reported completely. Likewise, reporting accuracy is dependent upon the consistency of the terminology—from the questionnaire, to the medical records, and finally, what has been communicated to the individual. Although difficult to measure, respondent motivation appears to influence the completeness of reporting as well.[96,105,122]

VALIDITY OF PHARMACOEPIDEMIOLOGIC DRUG AND DIAGNOSIS DATA FROM COMPUTERIZED DATABASES CONTAINING ADMINISTRATIVE OR MEDICAL RECORD DATA

In addition to conducting *ad hoc* studies to evaluate drug–disease associations, a variety of computerized, administrative databases are available for pharmacoepidemiologic research, the structure, strengths, and limitations of which were reviewed in Chapters 13–22. One major advantage of using such databases for pharmacoepidemiologic research is the comparative validity of the drug data in lieu of questionnaire data, where recall bias is always a concern, as previously described.

In general, the databases differ widely on many factors, such as size (e.g., from several hundred thousand to several million covered lives), number of plans included, the type of health services provided and therefore available for analysis (e.g., prescriptions, mental health benefits, etc.),

whether out-of-plan claims are included in the main database or resident in other databases, and the timeliness of the data (e.g., the lag for prescriptions is typically in weeks whereas that for outpatient visits may be 6 or more months) (see also Chapter 24). The databases also differ on the number of demographic variables that are available, with all having age and sex, but few having race, occupation, or a measure of health status.[127] Because the plans were developed primarily for reimbursement, they all have relatively complete data on health service use and charges.

The drawbacks and limitations of the data systems discussed below are important to keep in mind. Their most critical limitation for pharmacoepidemiologic research is the manner in which health insurance is covered in the United States, typically through the place of employment. If the employer changes plans, which is often done on an annual basis, or the employee changes jobs, the plan no longer covers that employee or his or her family. Thus, the opportunity for longitudinal analyses is hindered by the continual enrollment and disenrollment of plan members.

Along these lines, the most critical elements in the selection of a database for research are the completeness and validity of the data. Completeness is defined as the proportion of all exposures and/or events that occurred in the population covered by the database that appear in the computerized data. Missing subjects, exposures, or events could introduce bias in the study results.[128] For example, completeness of the drug data might vary by income level if persons with higher incomes and drug copayments choose to obtain their medications at pharmacies not participating in a prescription plan, which is how pharmacy data are collected. Similarly, a bias may be introduced in the association between a drug and a serious adverse drug reaction if hospitalizations for that adverse reaction are missing from the database.

For the data in an administrative database to be considered valid, those who appear in the computerized files as having a drug exposure or disease should truly have that attribute and those without the exposure or disease should truly not have the attribute. Validity and completeness would be determined by comparing the database information with other data sources, such as medical records, administrative or billing records, pharmacy dispensings, procedure logs, etc. In a recent review, Rawson *et al.*[129] described the different validation analyses that could be conducted to evaluate the usefulness of administrative databases for conducting observational studies, using the Saskatchewan Health databases for illustration. These analyses include reviewing the sources noted above, i.e., medical records, billing records, etc., along with the recommendation that pharmacoepidemiologists assess three other factors as well: the consistency between data files within the same system, surrogate markers of disease such as insulin for diabetes, and time-sequenced relationships, i.e., a diagnostic procedure preceding a surgery.

The availability of validation analyses and consistency checks will be discussed briefly for each database, separately for drug and diagnosis data. For all of the pharmacy dispensation databases that will be described, it is important to realize that none of them can address adherence and drug ingestion, and that over-the-counter medications are not included typically.

An adherence issue that was first raised in the late 1980s but has received more attention recently is that of unclaimed prescriptions, estimated to occur for approximately 2% of all prescriptions.[130] In 1991, Craghead and Wartski reported that 16.5 of every 1000 new prescriptions were unclaimed, with 17.5%, 13%, and 9.2% of the unclaimed prescriptions for anti-inflammatory drugs, prenatal care medications, and antibiotics, respectively.[131] Other studies found that anti-infectives tend to be the therapeutic class most often unclaimed.[132–134] Two-thirds of the unclaimed prescriptions were for new prescriptions,[132] and a similar proportion tended to be non-essential medications.[135] Many of the unclaimed prescriptions were telephoned in,[130,132] and the most frequently cited reasons for not picking up the prescription was that they did not need the medication or they forgot to pick it up,[130,133] although cost and having a similar medication at home were often cited as well.[130,133,135]

One might ask how unclaimed prescriptions might affect the validity and completeness of the pharmacy data. Many individuals have some type of pharmacy benefits plan where reimbursement for medication costs goes through a third party payer. Entry into the reimbursement software is predicated on dispensing of the drug. However, a drug that is dispensed but is not claimed should be returned to stock and the appropriate adjustment made to the patient's pharmacy benefits plan—it is insurance fraud if this were not to happen. Unfortunately, we do not know whether this insurance adjustment has been made so there may be a substantial number of prescriptions that we, as researchers, believe were dispensed (and used) but had not been used at all. If there are dispensings in the database that were not picked up, then there is no chance that the individual had the drug exposure and our study would suffer from exposure misclassification. This is an active area of research for reasons of patient adherence and loss of revenue for pharmacies.

Drug Data in Administrative or Medical Record Databases

Group Health Cooperative of Puget Sound

The Group Health Cooperative of Puget Sound (GHC) record-linked database was developed as a medical and administrative information system. Hence its drug data have been considered to be of very high quality for pharmacoepidemiologic research (see Chapter 14).

According to a survey of GHC enrollees, more than 90% of prescription medications used for pain management, such as opioids, sedatives/muscle relaxants, and anti-inflammatory drugs, were always filled at GHC pharmacies (see Chapter 14). A later study of 936 postmenopausal women included in a case–control study found that 96% of women indicated they filled all their prescriptions through GHC pharmacies.[136] In a study comparing the recording of NSAIDs in medical records to NSAID pharmacy dispensings, West et al. reported that 89% of all NSAIDs dispensed were documented in the patient's medical record within 30 days of the dispensing.[46] The 11% that were not documented may have been due to incompleteness of the medical record or because the NSAID was prescribed more than 30 days prior to its dispensing.[46] Among 762 study subjects treated with antidepressant medications in 1996–7, only 1.5% reported obtaining antidepressants from a non-GHC pharmacy in the prior 3 months (see Chapter 14). Over time, staff model HMOs have been contracting with providers outside the system to care for GHC members in outlying areas, which results in a claim. These claims are being incorporated into GHC databases so that the pharmacy data completeness can be maintained.

Copayments were introduced for some GHC plans in 1985, and by 1993 nearly all plans required modest copayments for visits and drugs. Prior to drug copayments, 99% of all prescriptions were filled at GHC pharmacies. In contrast, as of 1986, only 89% of prescriptions for those with copayments were filled at GHC pharmacies, compared to 93% for those without drug copayments.[137] Data from a subsample of GHC enrollees with and without drug copayments indicated that the copayments did not affect out-of-plan drug dispensating but did have an effect on drug use, especially for discretionary drugs.[138] Despite the copayments, even in the Medicare population where approximately 50% of enrollees did not have pharmacy benefits, 97.5% of those over 65 filled their medications at GHC pharmacies prior to 1994, dropping slightly to 96.1% after January 1, 1994 (see Chapter 14).

Kaiser Permanente

As discussed in Chapter 15, 90% of members have prescription drug coverage and members with chronic diseases such as diabetes obtain most of their prescriptions (96.7%) from Kaiser pharmacies. Whether members who do not have chronic diseases fill all of their prescriptions at Kaiser pharmacies is unclear but for KP Northern California, as many as 15–20% of adult members filled at least some of their prescriptions at non-Kaiser pharmacies.

Harvard Pilgrim Health Care

Approximately 90% of Harvard Pilgrim Health Care members have prescription drug benefits that provide a month's supply of drug for a nominal copayment (see Chapter 16). Drug data may be missing for the 10% of members without drug benefits, for drugs which cost less than the copayment, or for those who do not submit their drug claim for reimbursement (see discussion on Group Health Cooperative, above, for the effects of copayments). However, drug exposure can be defined on the basis of either dispensing from affiliated pharmacies or prescribing, as indicated in the encounter records. This is a major advantage, and may permit the identification of drug exposures that otherwise would be missing. No formal evaluations of the completeness of these data have been performed.

UnitedHealth Group

UnitedHealth members are derived from commercial, Medicaid, and Medicare populations (see Chapter 17). The percentage of commercial and Medicaid members who have drug benefits has dropped from 93% in 2000 to 90% currently. Because Medicare pharmacy benefits vary by plan, the completeness of drug exposure data on the elderly is somewhat compromised. Like other health plans with pharmacy copayments, medications that are less expensive than the copayment are likely to be missing from the computerized claims database.

Medicaid

As discussed in Chapter 18, Medicaid databases have been used extensively for pharmacoepidemiologic research, mainly due to the validity and completeness of the drug data. Given that Medicaid covers an indigent population, it is less likely that drugs will be purchased outside of the insurance plan when the copayment may range from $0.50 to $5.00.

An FDA-funded validation study of one of the Medicaid databases was completed 20 years ago, comparing claims data from Michigan and Minnesota to its primary sources, i.e., data from hospitals, physicians, pharmacies, etc.[125] The results of this study indicated that the demographic and drug data appear to be of extremely high quality. Within pre-established limits, year of birth agreed in 94% of sampled subjects, and could not be determined from the medical records in another 2.5%; sex agreed in 95% of subjects, and could not be determined from the medical records in another 4%; and the date of a pharmacy's dispensing of each drug agreed in 97% of sampled prescriptions. A more recent study compared Oregon Medicaid dispensing data for nursing home residents with that from nursing home charts.[139] Overall percentage agreement by the therapeutic class was about 95%, with kappas of 0.79, 0.89, and 0.98 for anxiolytics, antipsychotics, and antidepressants, respectively. An important caveat is that the intended duration of the prescription, i.e., days supply, may not be accurate and must be interpreted with care.

Another indicator that pharmacy claims accurately reflect prescribing relates to the drug utilization review programs required of Medicaid programs (see Chapter 29), in which thousands of patient-specific alerts are sent each month to the physicians and pharmacists who are providing the patients' medical care. These alerts request that the practitioner verify the accuracy of the billing data, and, if they agree with the basis of the alert, modify their patients' drug therapy regimen to minimize the risks for a possible drug-induced illness. Many of the alerts are responded to by the practitioners involved in writing, and few of their responses indicate that the drug data upon which the alert was generated were erroneous.

Finally, as noted earlier in this chapter, Strom et al. found that, for 128 cases of Stevens–Johnson syndrome, the Medicaid patient's inpatient medical record had only 50% of the 234 prescriptions for drugs suspected of causing the syndrome known to be dispensed according to the computerized Medicaid pharmacy claims files.[50] However, these data probably reflect the incompleteness of the medical chart rather than poor quality of the claims data on drugs.

Of course, as with the other databases, there is no way to evaluate adherence with drugs dispensed, other than examining patterns of refills for chronically used medications, nor does Medicaid pharmacy claims data capture over-the-counter medications.

Saskatchewan Health Plan

The Saskatchewan Health Plan has been used extensively for pharmacoepidemiologic research, as was discussed in

Chapter 19. There are separate plans within the system, i.e., the Prescription Drug Plan, the Saskatchewan Hospital Services Data, etc., and each plan is responsible for verifying and validating its data. There are a series of checks on each information field on the claim submitted to the drug plan before the claim is approved for payment. These checks include verification that the person was eligible for benefits under the program and that the drug dispensed was eligible for coverage.

The Prescription Drug Plan is remarkably complete: all residents except the 9% who have their prescription drug costs paid by another agency are covered by the plan and individuals without coverage can be excluded from studies. Some drugs are listed with restricted status, i.e., they are not on the Formulary, and are covered only when certain criteria are met. Pharmacy data are included for all drugs on the Formulary that are dispensed to eligible residents regardless of the level of benefit the individual has. In 2002–2003, approximately 68% of individuals eligible to receive pharmacy benefits actually did so.

Dutch System

In the Netherlands, there is almost universal computerization of pharmacy records, enabling the compilation of drug histories as almost all patients are reimbursed for prescription medications (see Chapter 20). Despite policies that encourage competition between pharmacies for reducing drug costs, patients typically remain with one pharmacy. This enhances the longitudinal nature of the medication data. The data are believed to be of high quality for three reasons. First, the computerized dispensing records are subject to financial audit, as they are the basis of reimbursement. Second, individuals have traditionally used only one pharmacy. Third, even though there are economic incentives for identifying cost-effective pharmacy care, these incentives are not so great as to promote pharmacy switching.

There have been at least two studies that validated the Dutch pharmacy data. First, computerized pharmacy data compared favorably with information on general practitioner records.[140] Second, comparing currently used prescription drugs as ascertained by home visits to 157 elderly people with those identified by the Dutch pharmacy database, Lau *et al.* reported that 85% of all drugs in the database and 89% of oral drugs were validated, i.e., they were actually used by the study participants.[141]

Tayside Medicines Monitoring Unit (MEMO)

As explained in Chapter 21, all community prescribing is done by the general practitioners in Scotland. By devising a system for capturing and computerizing general practitioner prescriptions dispensed through community pharmacies, MEMO has developed a prescription drug database. The system is not automated, i.e., the dispensing claims for this pharmacy database are entered manually. There are several checks on the accuracy of the data entry, at the time of assigning the Community Health Index number and after entry of system drug codes, i.e., a proportion of prescriptions are dually entered for quality control. The result of this quality control exercise has not been documented.

The UK General Practice Research Database

The information for this database is amassed from general practitioners who have agreed to provide data for research (Chapter 22). The computerized drug file for this data source is based on physician prescribing, not pharmacy dispensings. Thus, a person may receive a prescription for a medication but choose not to have it filled—the database would have this person as exposed unless algorithms to deal with adherence are developed. Because this system relies on the prescribing done by general practitioners, specialist-prescribed medications would not be available in the database until the person needed to have their prescription refilled, a responsibility of the person's general practitioner. There are two potential drawbacks for using this pharmacy database for pharmacoepidemiology: (i) adherence, as drug prescribing does not equate with drug use, and (ii) specialist-prescribed medications are not available in the database unless the specialist provides a consultant letter to the person's general practitioner and the general practitioner enters the information from the letter into the database. However, adherence does not appear to be a major impediment to using the GPRD for research. As noted in Chapter 22, there is 90% concordance between the prescriptions from the GPRD pharmacy database and the UK Prescription Prescribing Authority, indicating that individuals do fill most of the prescriptions written by their general practitioners.

Diagnoses and Hospitalizations in Administrative Databases

Unlike the drug data in administrative databases, where most researchers are comfortable with data accuracy and completeness, there is considerable concern regarding the inpatient and outpatient diagnoses in these databases. The accuracy of the outpatient diagnoses is more uncertain than the inpatient diagnoses for several reasons. Hospitals employ experienced persons to code diagnoses for reimbursement, which may not occur in individual physicians' offices where outpatient diagnoses are determined. Also, inpatient diagnoses are scrutinized for errors by hospital personnel,[142] monitoring that would not occur typically in the outpatient setting.

Systematic errors as a result of diagnostic coding may influence the validity of both inpatient and outpatient diagnostic data. For example, diseases listed in record-linked databases are often coded using the International Classification of Disease (ICD) coding system. Poorly defined diseases are difficult to code using the ICD system and there is no way to indicate that an ICD code is coded for "rule-out" purposes. It is not clear how health care plans deal with "rule-out" diagnoses, i.e., are they included or excluded from the diagnoses in the physician claims files? In a study of transdermal scopolamine and seizure occurrence, Strom and colleagues found that many patients with ICD codes indicating seizures had this diagnosis as a "rule-out" code when medical records were reviewed to confirm the diagnosis, indicating that "rule-out" codes do become part of administrative claims data.[143] In addition, the selection of ICD codes for billing purposes may be influenced by reimbursement standards and patient insurance coverage limitations.[144] The potential for abuse of diagnostic codes, especially outpatient codes, may occur when physicians apply to either an insurance carrier or the government for reimbursement and would be less likely to occur in staff/group model HMOs such as Group Health Cooperative or Kaiser Permanente. Lastly, ICD version changes may produce systematic errors, the effects of which were discussed in Chapter 22.

Group Health Cooperative of Puget Sound

The Group Health Cooperative (GHC) outpatient diagnosis information was discussed in detail in Chapter 13. The inpatient diagnostic database has records for all discharges from GHC-owned hospitals (Chapter 13).

Another file contains outside billing information for all admissions to hospitals not affiliated with GHC, especially emergency admissions. The data from this outside claims file are not incorporated into the inpatient database but are available as an annual utilization data set since June 1989. Table 45.5 provides information from some studies done using the GHC database that validated diagnoses.

Kaiser Permanente

As discussed in Chapter 14, the Kaiser Permanente Medical Care Program (KP) is divided into eight administrative regions, with Northern California KP and the Center for Health Research (KP Northwest) having the oldest research

programs. The plan's clinical and administrative databases are typically used to identify health outcomes for the inpatient and outpatient setting. Researchers using these databases confirm the diagnoses using medical record validation, although the results of the validation may not be published. Table 45.5 lists some of the studies that validated outcomes as part of their research design. Other studies used the medical record to confirm the computerized diagnosis but did not provide the sensitivity or positive predictive value of the ICD codes used for case identification.[145–152]

Harvard Pilgrim Health Care

Harvard Pilgrim Health Care is nearly unique in that epidemiologic analyses use the same automated records that are used by health care providers to deliver care. Therefore, these records are likely to be more complete than information from databases derived from billing diagnoses only. However, they will also suffer from the problems described above regarding the potential incompleteness of medical records. As Table 45.5 indicates, researchers at Harvard Pilgrim do compare the information available from the automated medical record with that available as the full-text medical record as part of their quality control during project initiation.

UnitedHealth Group

To date, there has only been one published study that has formally evaluated the usefulness of UnitedHealth Group data for pharmacoepidemiologic research. Quam *et al.* noted that a combination of medical and pharmacy claims was most productive for identifying hypertensive patients (96%), than medical claims (74%) or pharmacy claims (67%) alone as compared with medical record abstraction.[153] Combining a diagnosis with a marker drug has become a very common technique in pharmacoepidemiologic research to assess the correspondence between a database diagnosis as indicated by an ICD code and actual occurrence of disease.

UnitedHealth Group-affiliated health plans are typically independent practice associations but have also offered gatekeeper or capitated models in addition to their open access or discounted fee-for-service models. The different financial incentives for the varying model structures may affect the completeness of the diagnosis data available in the databases. For example, when billing for reimbursement in capitated plans, the individual's diagnosis may not be provided and, as a result, is not available in the research databases. Alternatively, in a discounted fee-for-service plan, there may be a financial incentive to code diagnoses according to the most profitable reimbursement schedules. In using this data source for research, it would be optimal to restrict the study design to members of one model so that differential incentives and policies do not provide an additional source of potential error when using these databases for conducting observational studies.

Medicaid

As noted previously, an FDA-funded validation study compared claims data from Michigan and Minnesota to its primary sources, i.e., data from hospitals, physicians, pharmacies, etc.[125] For medical services, diagnostic agreement to at least three digits of the ICD code occurred in only 41% of claims, agreement within a broad diagnostic category in another 16% (i.e., same body system and/or type of illness), no diagnosis was present on the provider record in 12%, a single diagnosis in 3%, and there was no agreement in 28%. Clearly, this study raised important doubts about the validity of the diagnosis data in Medicaid files. As the authors defined agreement simply on the basis of ICD coding, they considered a diagnosis of myocardial infarction or chest pain in one of the data sources and a diagnosis of angina pectoris in the other as "disagreement." This is discussed in more detail in Chapter 18.

As a way to manage the escalating costs of the Medicaid program, capitated programs have been put in place to pay for services to Medicaid beneficiaries. As discussed in Chapter 18, because providers are paid per person treated rather than paying for each encounter with the provider, some of the encounters, e.g., outpatient visits and hospitalizations, may be missing and which are missing may vary by the plan under study. This occurs despite the requirement from the Centers for Medicare and Medicaid Services that all encounters be recorded even for those in capitated plans.

Considerable effort has been expended on exploring the accuracy of the diagnoses in these Medicaid claims files. Some of the results are presented in Chapter 18. Typically, there is 95% agreement for hospital diagnoses between Medicaid claims and discharge diagnoses. The validity of the discharge diagnoses recorded on outpatient medical charts is much more uncertain. The validity of laboratory-driven diagnoses (e.g., neutropenia) is high. However, for diagnoses which are difficult to make correctly or are defined poorly in the ICD system, the validity is much poorer. For this, as well as other reasons, obtaining medical records for Medicaid studies is felt to be mandatory (see Chapter 18).

Obtaining medical or hospital records to validate diagnoses has become much more difficult as a result of the Privacy Rule of the Health Insurance Portability and Accountability Act (HIPAA) of 1996, which went into effect April 2003. Although researchers can obtain these records legally, they must have the appropriate documentation, which includes a data use agreement from the organization supplying the claims data, a waiver of informed consent from the researcher's institutional review board, and for health information acquired since April 2003, a waiver of HIPAA authorization from the researcher's IRB. This will be discussed in more detail in the section on "The future."

Saskatchewan Health Plan

Validation substudies were built into the design of several analyses using this database (see Chapter 19). Overall, there appears to be a very high correlation between the information on the charts and that coded in the hospital services system (Table 45.5). However, this is not true for all conditions, and validity should be ascertained with each new condition evaluated.

Dutch System

Through collaboration between the Department of Medical Informatics and the Pharmacoepidemiology Unit of the Erasmus University Medical School, the Integrated Primary Care Information (IPCI) system was established for research. This system consists of computerized patient records from approximately 150 GPs covering 500 000 patients. There are two validation studies that compared inpatient diagnoses from the electronic file to diagnoses in the hospital charts (Table 45.5). Straus *et al.* used computerized medical data from the IPCI practitioners to identify sudden cardiac death and validated the diagnoses by manual review of medical records but they did not provide the sensitivity and positive predictive value in their publication.[154]

The Tayside Medicines Monitoring Unit (MEMO)

The Scottish Morbidity Record (SMR) contains information on all acute inpatient admissions based on the discharge diagnoses, which are abstracted by trained coding clerks. To maintain high quality and accuracy, the SMR databases are audited frequently by the Information and Statistics Division of the NHS National Services Scotland. Researchers have conducted validation studies of this data, comparing the coded diagnoses with the actual medical chart data (Table 45.5 and Chapter 21). Depending on the diagnosis under study, the validation studies have shown the computerized data to be fairly accurate.

Table 45.5. Validation of conditions in database studies

Author	Comparison data source	Conditions	Findings
Group Health Cooperative of Puget Sound			
Psaty, et al., 1994[136]	Medical records	Probable or definite MI Cardiac diagnoses other than MI	There were 60 MI and 40 other cardiac diagnoses Number (%) meeting standard criteria for MI 58 (96.7%) 3 (7.5%) Using clinical history, cardiac enzyme levels, and electrocardiograms
Newton et al., 1999[160]	Medical records		Based on mentioned or confirmed diagnosis in the medical record within 60 days before or after the date first noted in the automated record. 97.7% of 471 records were available for validation.

	Sensitivity (%)	Specificity (%)	PPV (%)
Myocardial infarction	86.5	85.4	54.2
Any ischemic heart disease	83.3	96.0	50.3
Essential hypertension	60.7	50.0	23.5
Foot/lower extremity ulcer	64.2	82.8	60.8
Osteomyelitis	53.6	96.3	58.3
Amputation	85.7	97.3	87.8
Peripheral vascular disease	57.3	81.0	47.4
End stage renal disease	40.0	85.1	14.1
Cerebrovascular disease	85.5	85.0	51.3
Transient ischemic attack	57.1	95.7	45.5
Other cerebrovascular disease	33.3	94.3	22.6
Background retinopathy	52.4	78.8	26.2
Macular edema	36.5	87.4	28.8
Proliferative retinopathy	42.1	87.9	25.4
Retinal detachment, vitreous hemorrhage, or vitrectomy	71.2	84.2	37.4
All eye diseases combined	63.4	79.4	46.4

Author	Comparison data source	Conditions	Findings
Leveille et al., 2000[161]	Medical records	Antibiotic-treated infections identified via pharmacy records using a decision rule excluding continuous or prophylactic use, long-term prevention or suppression of recurrent infection, tuberculosis infections, etc.	Of 150 women (120 with antibiotic dispensing and 30 without an antibiotic dispensing), 54% had no infections according to the medical record. Of the 69 women with at least 1 infection based on medical records, all had at least 1 infection according to pharmacy records (sensitivity = 100%). Of the 81 women with no infections according to medical records, 61 had no infections according to the pharmacy database (specificity = 75.3%).

Table 45.5. (Continued)

Author	Comparison data source	Conditions	Findings
Kaiser Permanente			
Friedman *et al.*, 1976[162]	Medical records	Diarrhea subsequent to clindamycin use	300 clindamycin users, 3.3% cases of diarrhea based on medical records. 0.67% based on computerized diagnoses. Difference attributed to the omission of diarrhea on the clinic form.
Levin, *et al.*, 1997[163]	Medical records	Acid-related disorders: Peptic ulcer Gastroesophageal reflux Gastritis/dyspepsia	Percentage verified (1511 patients): 90 88 71 5.2% with a diagnosis of acid-related disorders could not be confirmed by medical records.
Sidney *et al.*, 1997[164]	Medical records and in-patient interview	Myocardial infarction (MI) as identified through hospital admission logs, emergency room visits, and hospital discharge codes for overnight stays.	Of the 735 potential MIs identified, 685 (93.2%) were confirmed as definite or probable based on medical record review.
Go *et al.*, 1999[165]	Medical records	Ambulatory nonvalvular atrial fibrillattion based on: • an ICD-9-CM code 427.31 from the outpatient database and an electrocardiogram showing atrial fibrillation from the electrocardiographic database or • more than one outpatient diagnosis of atrial fibrillation	A random sample of 50 charts from patients who had several outpatient diagnoses of atrial fibrillation but who did not have documentation of an electrocardiogram in the database were reviewed. At least 80% had at least one 12-lead electrocardiogram demonstrating atrial fibrillation and most of these tests predated the electrocardiographic database.
Go, *et al.*, 2001[166]	Medical records	Nontransient atrial fibrillation as identified by: • at least 1 outpatient diagnosis of atrial fibrillation • at least 1 electrocardiogram in the electrocardiographic database	The records of 50 patients from each mode of identification were reviewed. 78% 56%
Harvard Pilgrim Health Care			
Donahue *et al.*, 1995[167]	Outpatient medical record transcripts and hospital and emergency department records	Herpes zoster	A random sample of 130 persons with a herpes zoster code were selected, whether the diagnosis was made by an outpatient, urgent care, or emergency department visit, hospitalization, or a telephone encounter. Medical record review showed that 87% of the cases were confirmed, 9% were possible. The age-specific positive predictive values are: ≤14 years: 100% 15–24 years: 86%

Donahue et al., 1997[168]	Paper copies of patient records	Asthma	25–34 years: 92% 35–54 years: 100% 55–64 years: 95% ≥65 years: 100% Of 100 persons with both an asthma diagnosis and at least one asthma medication dispensing, 86 (86%) were confirmed to have asthma, 4 had chronic obstructive pulmonary disease, 2 had bronchitis, and 2 had allergic rhinitis. The diagnosis for the remaining 6 patients was unclear.

HMO Research Network or studies using multiple large HMOs

Andrade et al., 2002[169]	Full-text medical records from eight HMOs	Peptic ulcers and bleeding based on hospitalizations, three-level review: 1. Trained medical reviewers to confirm cases via surgery, endoscopy, X-ray or autopsy. 2. Generalist to identify peptic ulcer and upper GI bleeding. 3. Gastroenterologist to confirm uncertain cases.	Medical records abstracted for 884 (77%) of 1152 hospitalizations: 1. n = 239 (27%) had no discharge diagnosis of peptic ulcer and bleeding. 2. n = 438 (49.5%) peptic ulcer and bleeding not confirmed. 3. n = 207 (23%) patients with confirmed peptic ulcer and bleeding.
Donahue et al., 2002[170]	Medical record review	Hospitalizations for upper gastrointestinal perforation, ulcer, or bleeding	Records were reviewed for 1041 (76%) of the 1376 hospitalizations from the three study cohorts (exposed, unexposed, and fracture cohorts); the remaining records were unavailable for review. 167 (28%) of the upper GI perforation, ulcer, or bleeding cases from the exposed and unexposed cohorts were confirmed.
Bohlke et al., 2003[171]	Chart review	Anaphylaxis subsequent to vaccination	664 cases were identified and medical charts were reviewed for 657 cases. Chart review indicated that 6 of the 657 cases were probable or possible anaphylaxis; more detailed evaluation indicated that 2 cases had anaphylaxis that was not vaccine-related and 2 cases were probably not anaphylaxis based on presenting symptoms.
Chan et al., 2003[172]	Full-text medical records from five HMOs	Incident liver disease due to hypoglycemic agents as assessed by a three-level review: 1. Trained medical reviewers to eliminate those without liver disease (coding error, normal biopsy, nonhepatic cause of jaundice. 2. Generalist to identify those without liver disease and chronic liver disease.	1287 records available for review (92%) 1. n = 106 (8.2%) had no liver disease; n = 245 (19.0%) had evidence that liver disease predated April 1, 1997 2. n = 824 (64.0%) due to another chronic condition

Table 45.5. (Continued)

Author	Comparison data source	Conditions	Findings
		3. Hepatologists identify serious acute liver failure.	3. Of 91 patients, 26 patients had acute liver failure and 9 had acute liver injury
UnitedHealth Group Quam et al., 1993[153]	Survey response and medical record review	Essential hypertension as indicated by both ICD-9-CM codes 401, 401.0, 401.1, or 401.9 and at least one pharmacy claim for an antihypertensive medication	Of the 818 persons who were randomly selected for the mail survey, 95.7% confirmed a hypertension diagnosis. Of the 84 randomly selected for medical record review, hypertension was confirmed for 96.4%.
Medicaid Griffin et al., 1991[173]	Medical records	Peptic ulcer disease as ICD-9-CM codes: 531: Gastric ulcer 532: Duodenal ulcer 533: Peptic ulcer, site unspecified 534: Gastrojejunal ulcer 536: Disorders of function of stomach 537: Other disorders of stomach and duodenum 578: Gastrointestinal hemorrhage	Of the 4195 cases, the largest number of exclusions were due to hospitalization in prior 30 days (n=662, 15.8%), ulcer either developed in the hospital or found incidentally (n=206, 4.9%), missing records (n=192, 4.5%), and 105 (2.5%) due to other reasons. 53% of the remaining 3030 patients were excluded because they did not meet diagnostic criteria; 1415 patients were analyzed for peptic ulcer disease.
Strom et al. 1991[174]	Medical records	Hospital discharge diagnosis of erythema multiforme (ICD-9-CM code 695.1), which includes erythema iris, herpes iris, Lyell's syndrome, staphylococcal scalded skin syndrome (SSSS), Stevens–Johnson syndrome (SJS), and/or toxic epidermal necrolysis.	Medical records were sought for 249 cases, of which 128 were obtained (51.4%). The following table compares the hospital discharge diagnosis with a dermatologist's assessment.
Strom et al., 1991[50]	Medical records	Erythema multiforme major, SJS, or staphylococcus scalded skin syndrome identified by ICD-9-CM code 695.1.	There were 367 potential cases, of which records were requested from 249 cases; 128 (51.4%) records were obtained. 75% of the missing records were due to hospital refusal, transcription error, and inability to identify patients. Of the 128 possible cases, only 19 (14.8%) were found to have SJS or erythema multiforme.

	Hospital discharge	Clinical assessment
Erythema multiforme or SJS	20 (15.6%)	19 (14.8%)
Erythema multiforme minor	0 (0%)	35 (27.3%)
Erythema multiforme NOS	62 (48.4%)	2 (1.6%)
Toxic epidermal necrosis	9 (7.0%)	2 (1.6%)
SSSS	17 (13.3%)	20 (15.6%)
Other 695.1 skin diagnosis	2 (1.6%)	0 (0%)
Other skin diagnosis	12 (9.4%)	43 (33.6%)
Truly misclassified	6 (4.7%)	7 (5.5%)

Study	Data source	Definition	Comments
Strom et al., 1991[143]	Medical records	Seizures	Study focused on the risk of seizures due to transdermal scopolamine exposure. Of the 15 persons with seizures after exposure, records were available for 9 of the 12 seizure cases from Michigan but no records were available from Florida (n=3). Further evaluation of the medical records indicated that none of the potential cases was actually seizure related.
Strom et al., 1992[175]	Medical records	Hospital discharge of agranulocystosis, including neutropenia (ICD-9-CM code 288.0).	198 (55.3%) of the 358 records were obtained. Of those not obtained, for 44.4% the hospitals refused access and the hospital was unable to identify the patient for 46.9%. There were numerous reasons for the inability to obtain the remaining records including lost records, dating problems, etc. 192 (97.0%) of the 198 had neutropenia, of which 26 (13.5%) had recurrent disease, 19 (9.9%) had chronic disease, 31 (16.1%) were not valid, leaving 116/147 (78.9%) as valid incident cases.
Staffa et al., 1995[176]	Death certificates and medical record review	Cardiac events including paroxysmal ventricular tachycardia, ventricular fibrillation and flutter, cardiac death, sudden death of unknown cause, or unattended death of unknown cause.	Two cohorts were identified, those with sedating antihistamines and a second with astemizole. 18 cases were identified from Medicaid claims in these cohorts and medical records were obtained for 11 (61%) cases. The 8 cases with a validated diagnosis consisted of 7 cases of cardiac arrest or sudden death and 1 case of ventricular arrhythmia.
Brown et al., 1996[177]	Medical records	Angioedema, ICD-9-CM code 995.1.	Records were retrieved for 91 (84%) of the 108 patients with an angioedema code. Of these, 82 cases met the study definition of angioedema providing an average positive predictive value of 90% (PPV = 98% in African American patients and 78% in white patients).
Steinwachs et al., 1998[178]	Medical records	Diagnoses based on ambulatory Maryland Medicaid claims for adults and children.	A total of 2407 persons were sampled. The eligibility requirements for the study were such that there was a high probability that the person was covered by Medicaid during the time period under study and that the person's usual care provider could be identified for medical record review. Interrater reliability for medical record abstraction was >90%.

	Percentage of billed visits in record on the same date	Percentage of billed visits with same diagnosis in record on same date
Asthma	90.9	82.8
Diabetes	87.4	78.3
Otitis media	91.3	81.6
Hypertension	91.4	84.4
Pregnancy	87.2	80.8
Well child	92.1	85.4

Study	Data source	Definition	Comments
Griffin et al., 2000[179]	Hospital records	Acute renal failure as identified by ICD-9-CM codes 250.4, 274.1, 403, 404, 580–589, 590.0, 590.8, 593.9, 753.1 in persons ≥65 years old • Admission creatinine level ≥180 μmo/liter and a change of ≥20% (increase from baseline or decrease during hospitalization). • End-stage renal disease patients were excluded, as were those with hospital-acquired acute renal failure.	Of the 7145 patients with acute renal failure ICD-9-CM codes on discharge, only 2314 (32%) met the definition of community-acquired disease for this study. Most (48%) were eliminated based on creatinine levels (lack of, baseline level <180 μ mol/liter, or no change), there was missing data on 11% of patients, and 9% did not meet the definition for other reasons. As 515 patients had disease that was unlikely to be a result of prostaglandin inhibition (obstruction, interstitial nephritis, glomerulonephritis, etc.), data from 1799 patients remained for analysis.

Table 45.5. (Continued)

Author	Comparison data source	Conditions	Findings
Ray et al., 2001[180]	All medical care encounters, including hospitalizations, emergency department visits, medical examiner reports	Probable sudden cardiac death: sudden pulse-less condition (arrest) fatal within 48 hours consistent with ventricular tachyarrhythmia without a known noncardiac condition as proximal cause Possible sudden cardiac death: Not witnessed Found to be unconscious or dead Alive in preceding 24 hours	Of the 4404 deaths, 614 (14%) were excluded because they did not involve medical intervention, as were 822 (19%) because records could not be obtained. Of the 2968 deaths where records were reviewed, 505 (22%) were due to other causes, 802 (27%) lacked information on time or circumstances of death, and 174 (5.8%) of deaths occurred in other institutions; 1487 deaths were used for analysis. Of these, 701 were probable and 786 were possible sudden cardiac deaths.
Wang et al., 2001[181]	Reliability comparing Medicaid and Medicare data with cancer registry data	Incident breast cancer was identified in the Medicaid and Medicare files using ICD-9-CM diagnostic codes for breast neoplasm. ICD-9-CM and Current Procedural Terminology (CPT) codes were used for breast cancer screening, surgical procedures, radiation therapy, chemotherapy, and nuclear medicine procedures; disease-related group codes for breast cancer hospitalizations, and National Drug Codes for therapies used to treat breast cancer. For the cancer registry, codes indicating incident breast cancer were used.	Cases identified from Medicaid or Medicare: 8265 Cancer registry: 8872 Either source: 11 109 Both sources: 6028 κ: 0.70
Ngo et al., 2003[182]	Medicaid Behavioral Risk Factor Survey (MBRFS)	Diabetes using ICD-9-CM codes 250, 357.2, 362, 366.41.	Medicaid claims data for 2154 patients were linked to the MBRFS using Medicaid identification numbers. Percentage agreement between the two data sources was 96.6%, κ = 0.81 (95% CI: 0.77, 0.85) using 24 months of claims data.
Rogers et al., 2004[183]	Hospital medical records	Histologically-confirmed adenocarcinoma of the colon or rectum.	Of the 2114 potential hospitalizations for incident colorectal cancer, 249 (11.8%) records were missing. Of the 1865 records that were reviewed, 145 (7.8%) had prevalent disease, 141 (7.6%) were not histologically confirmed, 421 (22%) were for hospitalizations other than incident colon cancer; 1164 incident colon cancers were used for analysis.
Health Databases in Saskatchewan			
Guess et al., 1988[51]	Hospital records and autopsy reports	Fatal upper gastrointestinal hemorrhage specified as such on the discharge summary; hematemesis or melena as documented by gastroscopy, surgery, or autopsy; perforation of the duodenum or stomach confirmed at surgery or autopsy.	95 cases based on defined criteria, 46 of which had autopsies, 73 (76.8%) of which met the case definition.

Rawson et al., 1995[184]	Hospital charts	Acute myocardial infarction and chronic obstructive pulmonary disease.	4968 with ischemic heart disease, 224 randomly selected for medical record abstraction. 4569 with COPD, 227 randomly selected for medical record abstraction. 217 (96.9%) showed exact agreement for acute myocardial infarction. 212 (94.2%) showed exact agreement for COPD.
Edouard and Rawson, 1996[185]	Hospital charts	Hysterectomy	A random sample of 227 of 1905 charts from tertiary and referral hospitals was randomly selected for review. The type of hysterectomy was concordant for 220 of 226 cases (97.3%). Primary discharge diagnosis from the Hospital Services file matched a chart diagnosis for 71.2% of cases at the 4-digit level and 84.5% at the 3-digit level.
Rawson et al., 1997[186]	Hospital records 200 records for each diagnosis	Hospitalized with a diagnosis of schizophrenia or nonspecific depressive disorder.	There were 646 and 828 patients discharged in 1986 with a diagnosis of schizophrenia and depressive disorder, respectively. Abstraction focused on patients discharged from regional hospitals to minimize cost. Access to medical records was limited in several hospitals, resulting in 131 and 156 charts being abstracted for schizophrenia and depressive disorder, respectively.

Schizophrenia

ICD	Agreement	κ
4-digit	101 (77.1%)	NA
3-digit	123 (93.9%)	0.76

Depression

	Agreement	κ
4-digit	91 (58.3%)	NA
"Depression"	146 (93.6%)	NA

Rawson et al., 1998[129]	Hospital records	Hospitalizations for aplastic anemia or agranulocytosis:

	Aplastic anemia	Agranulocytosis
Discharge code from Hospital Services file	257	140
Other blood dyscrasias, cancer, etc.	166	72
Not confirmed by laboratory results	44	30
Cases meeting hematologic criteria	38	28

Walker et al., 1999[187]	Hospital or outpatient records	Serious cardiac arrhythmias, including ventricular fibrillation, sustained ventricular tachycardia, torsade de pointes, cardiac arrest, and death.	199 cases, 27 confirmed cases of serious cardiac arrhythmias.
West et al., 2000[188]	Outpatient medical records	Depression as indicated by ICD-9-CM codes and antidepressant use. Depression was defined in two ways, by ICD-9-CM codes 296, 309, or 311 or by these codes in addition to anxiety (300).	Of the 293 physicians contacted to validate the depression diagnosis, 170 (58%) consented, 101 (34.5%) refused because their records were unavailable or they were uninterested, 22 (7.5%) did not respond. Using only the three depression ICD-9-CM codes, agreement was 77% (κ=0.54, 95% CI: 0.48, 0.61). Adding ICD-9-CM code 311, agreement was 75.5% (κ=0.50, 95% CI: 0.43, 0.57). We conducted dual review on the records of 60 patients with 93.3% agreement for a depression diagnosis (κ=0.86).

Table 45.5. (Continued)

Author	Comparison data source	Conditions	Findings
Automated Pharmacy Record Linkage in the Netherlands			
Van der Klauw et al., 1993[189]	Hospital medical records	Anaphylaxis as identified by ICD-9-CM codes: Anaphylactic shock: 995.0 Shock due to anesthesia: 995.4 Anaphylactic shock due to sera: 999.4 Anaphylactic shock due to venom: 989.5 A random sample of those with: Dermatitis due to drugs: 693.0 Toxic erythema: 695.0 Allergic urticaria: 708.0 Angioneurotic edema: 995.1 Unspecified adverse effect of drug: 995.2 Allergy, unspecified: 995.3	Of the 934 admissions consistent with anaphylaxis, discharge summaries were received for 811 (87%), with 727 (77.8%) having sufficient details for classifying anaphylaxis. Probable anaphylaxis: 153/727 (21.0%) Possible anaphylaxis: 238/727 (32.7%) Anaphylaxis unlikely: 309/727(42.5%) Unclassifiable: 27/727 (3.8%)
Heerdink et al., 1998[190]	Hospital medical records	Congestive heart failure (CHF) as the primary or secondary discharge diagnosis where CHF was identified using ICD-9-CM code 428.	A random sample of 138 cases were selected for medical record review. The authors used two different sets of criteria for assessing validity—81.2 % of cases were valid according to the Boston criteria and 79.7% according to the Framingham criteria.
Van der Klauw et al., 1999[191]	Hospital charts for index admission and records from physicians involved in patient's care	Agranulocytosis, probable, possible, unlikely, or unclassifiable.	From January 1, 1987 until December 31, 1999, 923 admissions for four ICD-9 codes: 288.0, 288.1, 288.2 and 288.9. Information was received from the hospital or the physician for 753 admissions (81.6%), although additional follow-up was required to retrieve data for 678 (90%) of admissions. Exclusion of subsequent admissions for agranulocytosis, insufficient data, and age (<2 years) resulted in 478 patients available for analysis.
Movig et al., 2003[192]	Clinical laboratory data	Hyponatremia, ICD-9-CM code 276.1, as identified in hospital administrative files.	Only 48 patients were identified with hyponatremia based on discharge diagnoses. Sodium level ≤135 mmol/L is considered the cutoff for hyponatremia. In reviewing the records of the 48 patients identified through the hospital files, 44 were true cases (positive predictive value 92%). PPV decreases as sodium level decreases.
Tayside Medicines Monitoring Unit (MEMO)			
Dornan et al., 1995[193]	Hospital records	Upper gastrointestinal hemorrhage and perforation.	Diagnoses were identified from the Scottish Morbidity Record, a hospital database, and verified using the original hospital records. Of the 3447 GI events, agreement was found for 1608 (46.6%) events.
Evans et al., 1995[194]	Hospital medical records	Upper gastrointestinal bleeding and perforation using codes for acute, chronic, or unspecified gastric ulcer, duodenal ulcer, or gastrojejunal ulcer with hemorrhage, with hemorrhage and perforation, or with perforation. Codes also included hematemesis and melena.	There were 1103 patients admitted for upper gastrointestinal bleeding. The validation study found a sensitivity of 68% for the 542 acute bleeding events confirmed and 79% for the 75 perforations confirmed. The specificity was 98%.

Study	Validation source	Case definition	Results
Evans et al., 1997[195]	Histological confirmation from hospital medical records	Acute appendicitis identified as an emergency admission for an appendectomy with an ICD-9-CM code for acute appendicitis, including 540.0, 540.1, 540.9, and 541.9.	161 (72.2%) of 223 patient records were validated, of which 138 (85.7%) had histologically confirmed appendicitis.
Evans et al., 1997[196]	Hospital medical records	Colitis due to inflammatory bowel disease identified using ICD-9-CM codes: Crohn's of the large intestine: 555.1; Crohn's, small and large intestine: 555.2; Crohn's unspecified: 555.9; Ulcerative colitis: 556.0 and 556.9; Other non-infective colitis: 558.9; Allergy, unspecified: 995.3.	Of 587 potential cases, 200 (34.1%) were colitis due to inflammatory bowel disease. Of the remaining 387 cases, approximately 80% had an ICD-9-CM of 558 indicative of other colitis, and inflammatory bowel disease could not be confirmed in the other 20%.
Morris et al., 1997[197]	Registers of diabetes patients from primary care providers	Diabetes	Primary aim was to determine whether electronic record linkage of multiple sources could identify diabetes cases.
McMahon et al., 2001[198]	Hospital medical records	Hypersensitivity reactions identified by ICD-9-CM codes: Anaphylactic shock: 995.0; Angioneurotic edema: 995.1; Unspecified adverse effect of drug: 995.2; Allergy, unspecified: 995.3.	Of 47 patients who had been dispensed naproxen, 12 had a hypersensitivity reaction in close proximity to the dispensing. Similarly, 10 of 66 patients dispensed ibuprofen had a hypersensitivity reaction. However, records were only available for 9 of the 12 naproxen patients and 7 of the 10 ibuprofen patients. Only 3 naproxen and 2 ibuprofen cases were validated but none of the 5 were felt to be induced by these NSAIDs.
Struthers et al., 2002[199]	Hospital medical records	Chronic heart failure (CHF) defined as those with at least one hospitalization for myocardial infarction and having been dispensed a loop diuretic.	Of an unknown number of CHF charts validated, 95% were confirmed with the diagnosis.
Steinke et al., 2002[200]	Hospital medical records	A primary or secondary hospital discharge code of liver disease from the Scottish Morbidity Record, including hepatitis A, B, or C; autoimmune hepatitis; abnormal liver function or fatty liver; fulminate liver failure; hepatocellular carcinoma; alcoholic liver disease; primary sclerosing cholangitis; primary biliary cirrhosis; and liver disease complications. Patients with these diagnoses were entered into the Tayside Epidemiology of Liver Disease database (ELDIT).	Of 110 patients with liver disease who were randomly selected from the ELDIT database, 90 (81.8%) were confirmed and 18 (16.4%) could not be confirmed.

Detail for Morris et al., 1997[197]:

	Sensitivity	Specificity
Prescriptions	0.69	0.97
Hospital clinics	0.63	0.99
Mobile eye units	0.72	0.99
Biochemistry data	0.67	0.98
Clinic and eye units	0.91	0.98
Clinic and biochemistry	0.82	0.98
Prescriptions and biochemistry	0.96	0.96
Prescriptions, clinic, biochemistry	0.96	0.96
All data sources	0.96	0.95

Table 45.5. (Continued)

Author	Comparison data source	Conditions	Findings
General Practice Research Database			
Van Staa et al., 1994[159]	Copies of discharge letters in GP medical records and completion of a questionnaire	Hospitalizations for hypoglycemia or possible hypoglycemia and a random sample of subjects with hospitalizations for other conditions.	Of the 553 discharge letters received, a hospitalization was noted in the computerized records for 539 (97.5%). Of the 43 discharge letters for hypoglycemic subjects, 24 questionnaires listed hypoglycemia (55.8%) and 19 of these 24 listed the diagnosis in the computerized records (79.2%). Of the 510 persons with diagnoses other than hypoglycemia, the principal diagnosis was matched for 459 (90%), was not recorded for 7.3%, and no hospitalization was listed for 2.3%. Below, sensitivity refers to the percentage of time the discharge summary was adequately listed in the database for each condition and the positive predictive value (PPV) refers to the accuracy of the codes in the database.

Conditions	Sensitivity (%)	PPV (%)
Hypoglycemia	90.7	88.6
Diabetes	90.6	98.6
Cerebrovascular disorders	96.0	92.7
Respiratory tract infection	95.7	97.2
Myocardial infarction	89.3	85.3
Congestive heart failure	100	100
Chronic ischemic heart disease	93.1	100
Chronic obstructive airway disease	100	100
Urinary tract infection	83.3	100
Fracture	100	100
Malignant neoplasm	69.2	100
Dysrrhythmias	90.9	100
Dementia	77.8	100
Depression	100	100

Author	Comparison data source	Conditions	Findings
Meier et al., 1998[201]	Medical record information captured via questionnaire	Systemic lupus erythematosus or discoid lupus	Clinical records were received[a] for 151 lupus cases. For 76 patients, there was insufficient information to confirm the diagnosis (n = 36), record indicated prevalent disease (n = 32), lupus was drug-induced (n = 3), or woman was premenopausal (n = 5).
Derby and Maier, 2000[202]	Medical record information captured via questionnaire	Cataract	Clinical records were received[a] for 225 cases of cataract that were randomly selected for validation, of which 97% were confirmed.
Lawrenson et al., 2000[203]	Medical record information captured via questionnaire	Venous thromboembolism (VTE)	277 nonfatal cases of VTE, of which 186 were still registered with a general practitioner in the GPRD; information was received on 169 patients. The questionnaire confirmed a hospital admission for 99% of the patients whereas the computerized record indicated that only 81% of the patients had been hospitalized. The 8 fatalities were confirmed by death certificate review and, for some cases, by postmortem.

Reference	Method	Condition	Description
García-Rodríguez and Huerta-Alvarez, 2001[204]	Medical record information captured via questionnaire	Colorectal cancer	Medical records were requested from a random sample of 70 cases with colorectal cancer, information was received for 68 patients. 65 patients were confirmed with colorectal cancer (96%), 2 had colorectal polyps and one had hemorrhoids.
Seshadri et al., 2001[205]	Request for medical record information	Alzheimer's disease (AD), senile dementia, or presenile dementia	Manual records were reviewed for 128 women with a new diagnosis of dementia or possible AD. 49 were classified as probable and 13 were possible according to National Institutes of Health criteria; 66 did not have AD or dementia. Of those with an AD diagnosis according to GPRD data, 43 of 51 (84.3%) cases had probable or possible AD according to the NIH criteria.
Soriano et al., 2001[206]	Medical record information captured via questionnaire	Chronic obstructive pulmonary disease	Questionnaires were sent to the GPs of 300 patients to confirm whether they had ever had COPD, emphysema, chronic bronchitis, or asthma. The response rate was 85.7%. Concordance between the GPRD algorithm and medical records was $\kappa = 0.46$. Of the 57 patients whose COPD diagnosis was not confirmed, the GP had diagnosed asthma in 28 (49.1%); the remaining patients did not have respiratory disease.
Huerta et al., 2002[207]	Medical record information captured via questionnaire	Acute liver injury in type 2 diabetic patients compared with general population controls without diabetes	165 patients identified as having an episode of acute liver disease according to electronic files: 94 patients with diabetes and 71 from the general population. 157 (95%) questionnaires were returned, of which 76.4% had sufficient information to differentiate those with normal liver function ($n=44$) or diagnoses meeting exclusion criteria ($n=49$) from those eligible for further study ($n=27$).
Lewis et al., 2002[208]	Medical record information captured via questionnaire	Inflammatory bowel disease (IBD), including Crohn's disease (CD), ulcerative colitis (UC), or IBD not otherwise specified. Highly probable or probable IBD Highly probable or probable CD Highly probable or probable UC	Questionnaires were sent to the GPs of 85 prevalent cases and 85 presumed incident cases asking about the type of disorder and when it was first diagnosed. 167 (98%) of the questionnaires were returned and of those, 157 (94%) had usable data. 144/157 = 92% 44/49 = 94% 82/88 = 93% 20% of the nonspecific IBD could not be confirmed by medical records, compared with 3% and 6% of the UC and CD diagnoses, respectively.
Margolis et al., 2002[209]	Medical record information captured via questionnaire	Patients with and without pressure ulcer	Questionnaires were sent to the GPs of a random sample of 65 persons with and 65 persons without pressure ulcers. Analyzable data were returned for 47 pressure ulcer patients and 54 patients without a pressure ulcer. Sensitivity: 91% (95% CI: 83%, 99%) Specificity: 100% (95% CI: 93%, 100%) PPV[b]: 100% (95% CI: 92%, 99%) NPV[b]: 95% (95% CI: 85%, 99%)

Table 45.5. (Continued)

Author	Comparison data source	Conditions	Findings
Ruigómez et al., 2002[210]	Medical record information captured via questionnaire	Chronic atrial fibrillation, either chronic or paroxysmal	Questionnaires were requested from the GPs of 1714 and completed responses received from 1606 (94%). 1035 (64.4%) were incident chronic atrial fibrillation, 388 were paroxysmal (24.1%), 117 (7.3%) were prevalent atrial fibrillation, and 66 (4.1%) did not have atrial fibrillation.
Van Staa et al., 2002[211]	Medical record information captured via questionnaire	Paget's disease of the bone	Questionnaires were sent to the GPs of 150 with a GPRD diagnosis of Paget's disease, to differentiate between Paget's disease of the breast, intraepidermal epithelioma, or bone. Responses were received from 140 (93%) GPs, but questionnaire responses were provided for 133 patients. Paget's disease of bone was confirmed in 120 patients (90.2%), 5 patients had breast carcinoma, and 2 patients had suspected but unconfirmed Paget's disease.
Watson et al., 2002[212]	Medical record information captured via questionnaire	Rheumatoid arthritis (RA) and thromboembolic cardiovascular events (TCE)	Questionnaires were sent to the GPs of all persons with an RA diagnosis who had naproxen use ($n = 100$), and approximately 70 GPs of RA patients who had not used naproxen, and 230 GPs of patients selected to be controls for the RA cases. Although there is no information on the return rate for the questionnaires, the diagnosis was confirmed in 80% of the exposed RA patients, 74% of unexposed RA patients, and 77% of controls. The TCE diagnosis was confirmed in 80% of the exposed cases and 78% of the unexposed cases.
Gelfand et al., 2003[213]	Diagnosis of psoriasis compared with treatments for psoriasis	Psoriasis	Using a 10% random sample of persons 65 years and older ($n = 107\,921$), there were 2718 patients with psoriasis. This represents a psoriasis prevalence of 2.52%, which is similar to prevalence estimates from population-based studies. In addition, 92% of the psoriasis patients were treated with psoriasis medications.

Huerta et al., 2003[214]	Medical record information captured via questionnaire	Irritable bowel syndrome (IBS)	620 patients with a diagnosis of IBS according to the database. Information was received from 96% of clinicians and confirmed IBS in 78% of patients with a computerized IBS diagnosis.
Ruigómez et al., 2003[215]	Medical record information captured via questionnaire	IBS	GPs provided information for 98% of the 877 questionnaires sent to validate an incident IBS diagnosis, of which 660 (75.3%) diagnoses were confirmed. 136 (15.5%) were prevalent cases, 12 (1.4%) were not IBS, and there was no available information for 49 (5.6%) patients.
Yang et al., 2003[216]	Information from medical records	Newly diagnosed depression	458 patients with newly diagnosed depression. Medical record information was requested for a random sample of 30 patients, 83.3% had newly diagnosed depression.
Ronquist et al., 2004[217]	Information from medical records	Prostate cancer	1015 patients with prostate cancer. 100 patients were randomly selected for review, of which information was returned for 90 patients. Prostate cancer was confirmed in 88 of the 90 cases.
Peng and Jick, 2004[218]	Information from medical records	Anaphylaxis	898 with a diagnosis of anaphylaxis or a mention of anaphylaxis in the comment field. A random sample of 70 records that had an anaphylaxis diagnostic code on the database was selected for validation; an additional 50 patients were selected because anaphylaxis was mentioned in the comments section of the record. Usable information was provided in 90% of the medical records. Of the 120 records reviewed, 86 were deemed to have anaphylaxis and the remainder either had a history of anaphylaxis or did not have anaphylaxis at all.

[a] Unclear how many clinic records were requested for validation effort.
[b] PPV = Positive predictive value; NPV = negative predictive value.

The UK General Practice Research Database

As a database derived from the general practitioner's primary medical record, one expects very complete documentation of diagnostic information based on visits to these clinicians. However, before this data could be used for research, there needed to be an assessment of its quality. The first determination of quality was done when the database was initiated, at which time the "up to standard" qualification was designated (see Chapter 22). Quality evaluations included a detailed review of the recorded data[155] to ensure that both diagnostic and pharmacy data were being consistently recorded in the electronic medical records. Currently, for a practice to be considered up to standard, it must record a minimum of 95% of the prescribing and patient encounters that occur in the practice. Although quality evaluations began in 1987, most practices did not receive the up to standard designation until 1990 to 1991.

Many studies have formally evaluated the usefulness of the GPRD for conducting pharmacoepidemiologic research (see Table 45.5 and Chapter 21). A particular concern is the completeness of the database with regard to diagnoses made by consultants. Jick and colleagues[156,157] conducted a validation study to assess whether the consultant diagnoses as documented in letters to the patient's general practitioner actually appeared in the GPRD. The earlier of the two very similar studies indicated that 87% of these diagnoses appeared in the database; the smaller 1992 study showed that 96% of the consultant diagnoses appeared in the database. These two studies left unknown what proportion of the individuals might have seen a consultant who did not provide a consultant letter to the person's general practitioner.

Besides the studies validating specific diagnoses that are listed in Table 45.5, a publication is under development that will provide a systematic review of all the GPRD studies that have validated outcomes.[158]

Conclusions

Validating the case definition developed for observational studies using administrative databases with original documents such as inpatient or outpatient medical records is a necessary step for enhancing the quality and credibility of the research. Since the previous edition of *Pharmacoepidemiology* in 2000, many studies have included the review of original documents to validate the diagnoses under study, which is especially true for the GPRD, as indicated in Table 45.5.

Evaluating the completeness of the databases is much more difficult as it requires an external data source that is known to be complete. When completeness is assessed, it is typically for a particular component of a study, such as the effect of drug copayments on pharmacy claims[137,138] or the availability of discharge letters in GPRD.[159] These three studies are more than 10 years old and there has been little research on the completeness of administrative databases since then, with the exception of periodic evaluations of the completeness of the GHC pharmacy database. A study published 20 years ago[125] indicated that pharmacy data from administrative databases was of high quality, and because claims are used for reimbursing pharmacy dispensings, this should continue to be so today. We realize that adherence is an issue (see Chapter 46), that not every dispensing indicates exposure, but we do not know the extent of unclaimed prescriptions and whether this might affect our research. Although administrative databases have greatly expanded our ability to do pharmacoepidemiologic research, we need to ensure that our tools, the databases, are complete and of the highest quality.

THE FUTURE

The methodologies for conducting pharmacoepidemiology studies have shifted over the past 25 to 30 years from total reliance on studies requiring data collection from individuals to the extensive use of electronic data from either administrative health claims or electronic medical records. Yet, there is still a need to collect data from individuals, especially for herbals and over-the-counter medications and for inexpensive generic medications that may be purchased outside drug plans. This chapter describes the methodologic work that continues to be published on the most valid approaches for collecting medication data via questionnaires, focusing on question design and recall period, i.e., the time between drug exposure and query by questionnaire. Current evidence suggests that recall accuracy for medications diminishes with time so that researchers should focus on recent medication use to reduce the potential for measurement error. We have also discussed techniques such as sensitivity analysis that can inform the potential magnitude of measurement error when data are collected de novo. The availability of these analytic tools will allow investigators to provide quantitative estimates of measurement error when describing the limitations of their research rather than a qualitative comment reflecting the potential for measurement bias.

In contrast with de novo data collection for pharmacoepidemiologic research, the availability, use, and richness of electronic data sources has increased exponentially. It was about 20 years ago that we realized how useful administrative claims could be for conducting pharmacoepidemiology studies,[219,220] yet there were critics.[222] With time, we found that careful and systematic evaluation of data accruing for administrative purposes could be used to study drug–disease relationships without having to take the time or spend the money to collect data de novo. We learned how to develop algorithms containing ICD-9 diagnosis, procedure, and external causes of injury codes that were used as billing codes in the administrative claims to identify individuals with certain diseases, notably acute myocardial infarction.[222,223] Just the occurrence of the procedure code, without the results of the procedure, provided useful knowledge on whether or not the individual had the disease under study.

Capitalizing on the potential that administrative claims afforded us came with pitfalls and a steep learning curve. Funded by the Food and Drug Administration, Lessler and colleagues conducted a concordance study to evaluate the accuracy of drug and diagnosis codes in Medicaid claims data.[125] The results of this landmark study are described in other chapters of this text but the primary message is that the drug claims were reliable, i.e. there was concordance between the drugs prescribed and dispensed, but the concordance for diagnosis claims was not very good. This study undermined our confidence in the validity of using record-linked databases for pharmacoepidemiologic research and dampened our initial enthusiasm. Ultimately, researchers realized that any study using electronic data would require some type of medical record verification to ensure the validity of the case definition. However, even this extra burden of abstracting medical records that increased both the timeline and budget for our record-linked database studies was nowhere comparable to the increased time and budget required for full data collection. Besides, record-linked databases with their automated pharmacy files could minimize measurement error for exposures because drug data would be identified by dispensing records and not by self-reports, with the potential for recall bias and exposure underascertainment.

The improved computer technology that resulted in faster processor speeds and increased storage capacity not only led to the efficient merging of data from multiple health plans but also to the storage of health care data in an electronic format, i.e., electronic medical records. The availability of these data for research has improved our ability to conduct studies that require knowledge not only about whether a procedure or laboratory test was done, but the results of these clinical events. The obvious advantage of access to electronic clinical data is less reliance on the need to confirm diagnoses using paper medical records, especially when there is little or no paper copy backup to review! Although clinical practice in the US is slowly moving toward electronic medical records, the paper version of the medical record will continue to be used for some time to come. Yet, as described below, the new data privacy regulations are having a negative impact on research endeavors involving personal health information derived from medical records and/or health care databases.

With the increasing use of individual health data from databases or medical records for pharmacoepidemiologic and health services research came the concern over data privacy issues. Prior to the passing of the Health Insurance Portability and Accountability Act (HIPAA) of 1996, confidentiality was an issue primarily left within the discretion and control of the researcher's organization. The public relied on the Common Rule[224] as overseen by institutional review boards (IRBs) to provide oversight of the confidential nature of the data and to protect the privacy of research subjects. However, confidentiality and privacy protection were only a small part of the IRB review process.

The HIPAA Privacy Rule protects the use and disclosure of information about the health of individuals that is derived by health care providers during the course of treatment, i.e., individualized medical information from which the identity of persons can be determined (see Chapter 38). These HIPAA standards, enforceable since April 14, 2003, have had a significantly negative effect on clinical research, as described in Chapter 18 with regard to obtaining medical records for diagnosis validation. The Association of American Medical Colleges has been documenting the effects of HIPAA on biomedical and scientific research and has noted that research activities involving data access and patient recruitment have been adversely influenced by HIPAA implementation (Washington Fax, May 6, 2004). In a statement prepared by the American College of Epidemiology for a November 20, 2003 public hearing of the Privacy and Confidentiality Subcommittee of the National Committee on Vital Statistics on the impact of HIPAA on research, Dr Martha Linet noted problems with access to electronic databases such as Medicare and Medicaid, difficulties in obtaining access to medical records by health providers, and increased difficulties with obtaining patient informed consent.[225]

We are seeing the ramifications of HIPAA implementation in all of our research activities. Chapter 38 provides a detailed description of the Privacy Rule and describes the processes that researchers need to follow to be able to access data useful for pharmacoepidemiologic research. It is clear that the process for acquiring research data has become much more onerous and time-consuming for researchers and IRBs as well. Currently, we are in a transitional phase where many covered entities, i.e. health care providers and those who house the medical records that researchers need to review or those who maintain large data sets for research, are uncertain about HIPAA requirements. In early 2004, denying researchers access to clinical data was the safest option, given the high financial penalty for breach of confidentiality that is levied solely on the covered entity. More than a year after HIPAA implementation, we can look back and see that research is getting done, albeit at a slower pace, as covered entities and investigators undergo a steep learning curve to identify the most efficient ways to meet the HIPAA privacy standards with the least impact on research process and progress.[226]

For the future, the major hurdle we face with regard to data validity for pharmacoepidemiologic research is our ability to obtain medical records to validate health outcomes that are derived from administrative claims. Until experience accrues with how to conduct HIPAA-compliant research and health care consumers and providers become better informed about the Privacy Rule through education and dissemination programs, the validation of health outcomes may be extremely difficult to accomplish or may become so expensive and time consuming that research costs will escalate tremendously.

REFERENCES

1. Gordis L. Assuring the quality of questionnaire data in epidemiologic research. *Am J Epidemiol* 1979; **109**: 21–4.
2. Keeble W, Cobbe SM. Patient recall of medication details in the outpatient clinic. Audit and assessment of the value of printed instructions requesting patients to bring medications to clinic. *Postgrad Med J* 2002; **78**: 479–82.
3. Brody DS. An analysis of patient recall of their therapeutic regimens. *J Chronic Dis* 1980; **33**: 57–63.
4. Warnecke RB, Sudman S, Johnson TP, O'Rourke D, Davis AM, Jobe JB. Cognitive aspects of recalling and reporting health-related events: Papanicolaou smears, clinical breast examinations, and mammograms. *Am J Epidemiol* 1997; **146**: 982–92.
5. Tourangeau R. Cognitive sciences and survey methods. In: Janine TB, Straf ML, Tanur JM, Tourangeau R, eds, *Cognitive Aspects of Survey Methodology: Building a Bridge between Disciplines*. Washington, DC: National Academy Press, 1984; pp. 73–100.
6. Willis GB, Royston P, Bercini D. The use of verbal report methods in the development and testing of survey questionnaires. *Appl Cognit Psychol* 1991; **5**: 251–67.
7. Tourangeau R, Rips LJ, Rasinski K. *The Psychology of Survey Response*. Cambridge, MA: Cambridge University Press, 2000.
8. Wheeler MA, Stuss DT, Tulving E. Toward a theory of episodic memory: the frontal lobes and autonoetic consciousness. *Psychol Bull* 1997; **121**: 331–54.
9. Belli RF. The structure of autobiographical memory and the event history calendar: potential improvements in the quality of retrospective reports in surveys. *Memory* 1998; **6**: 383–406.
10. Conway MA. Sensory–perceptual episodic memory and its context: autobiographical memory. *Philos Trans R Soc Lond B Biol Sci* 2001; **356**: 1375–84.
11. Tulving E. Episodic memory: from mind to brain. *Annu Rev Psychol* 2002; **53**: 1–25.
12. Allen PA, Sliwinski M, Bowie T. Differential age effects in semantic and episodic memory, Part II: Slope and intercept analyses. *Exp Aging Res* 2002; **28**: 111–42.
13. Allen PA, Sliwinski M, Bowie T, Madden DJ. Differential age effects in semantic and episodic memory. *J Gerontol B Psychol Sci Soc Sci* 2002; **57**: 173–86.
14. Kelsey JL, Thompson WD, Evans AS. Methods in observational epidemiology. In: *Monographs in Epidemiology and Biostatistics*, vol. 10. New York: Oxford University Press, 1986.
15. Sackett DL. Bias in analytic research. *J Chronic Dis* 1979; **32**: 51–63.
16. Mitchell AA, Cottler LB, Shapiro S. Effect of questionnaire design on recall of drug exposure in pregnancy. *Am J Epidemiol* 1986; **123**: 670–6.
17. Chavance M, Dellatolas G, Lellouch J. Correlated nondifferential misclassifications of disease and exposure: application to a cross-sectional study of the relation between handedness and immune disorders. *Int J Epidemiol* 1992; **21**: 537–46.
18. Kristensen P. Bias from nondifferential but dependent misclassification of exposure and outcome. *Epidemiology* 1992; **3**: 210–15.
19. Dosemeci M, Wacholder S, Lubin JH. Does nondifferential misclassification of exposure always bias a true effect toward the null value? *Am J Epidemiol* 1990; **132**: 746–8.
20. Rothman KJ, Greenland S. Precision and validity in epidemiologic studies. In: *Modern Epidemiology*, 2nd edn. Philadelphia, PA: Lippincott, Williams & Wilkins, 1998; pp. 129–30.
21. Poole C. Exceptions to the rule about nondifferential misclassification. *Am J Epidemiol* 1985; **122**: 508.
22. Rodgers A, MacMahon S. Systematic underestimation of treatment effects as a result of diagnostic test inaccuracy: implications for the interpretation and design of thromboprophylaxis trials. *Thromb Haemost* 1995; **73**: 167–71.
23. Thomas DC. Re: "When will nondifferential misclassification of an exposure preserve the direction of a trend?". *Am J Epidemiol* 1995; **142**: 782–4.
24. Weinberg CR, Umbach DM, Greenland S. Weinberg *et al.* Reply—Re: "When will nondifferential misclassification of an exposure preserve the direction of a trend?". *Am J Epidemiol* 1995; **142**: 784.
25. Wacholder S, Armstrong B, Hartge P. Validation studies using an alloyed gold standard. *Am J Epidemiol* 1993; **137**: 1251–8.
26. Rothman KJ, Greenland S. Basic methods for sensitivity analysis and external adjustment. In: *Modern Epidemiology*, 2nd edn. Philadelphia, PA: Lippincott, Williams & Wilkins, 1998; pp. 343–57.
27. Maclure M, Willett WC. Misinterpretation and misuse of the κ statistic. *Am J Epidemiol* 1987; **126**: 161–9.

28. Bland JM, Altman DG. Statistical methods for assessing agreement between two methods of clinical measurement. *Lancet* 1986; **1**: 307–10.

29. Landis JR, Koch GG. The measurement of observer agreement for categorical data. *Biometrics* 1977; **33**: 159–74.

30. Copeland KT, Checkoway H, McMichael AJ, Holbrook RH. Bias due to misclassification in the estimation of relative risk. *Am J Epidemiol* 1977; **105**: 488–95.

31. Greenland S, Kleinbaum DG. Correcting for misclassification in two-way tables and matched-pair studies. *Int J Epidemiol* 1983; **12**: 93–7.

32. Willett W. An overview of issues related to the correction of non-differential exposure measurement error in epidemiologic studies. *Stat Med* 1989; **8**: 1031–40.

33. Raphael K. Recall bias: a proposal for assessment and control. *Int J Epidemiol* 1987; **16**: 167–70.

34. Greenland S. Basic methods for sensitivity analysis of biases. *Int J Epidemiol* 1996; **25**: 1107–16.

35. Lash TL, Fink AK. Semi-automated sensitivity analysis to assess systematic errors in observational data. *Epidemiology* 2003; **14**: 451–8.

36. Horwitz RI, Feinstein AR. Alternative analytic methods for case–control studies of estrogens and endometrial cancer. *N Engl J Med* 1978; **299**: 1089–94.

37. Hutchison GB, Rothman KJ. Correcting a bias? *N Engl J Med* 1978; **299**: 1129–30.

38. Greenland S. A mathematic analysis of the "epidemiologic necropsy." *Ann Epidemiol* 1991; **1**: 551–8.

39. Greenland S. Sensitivity analysis, Monte Carlo risk analysis, and Bayesian uncertainty assessment. *Risk Anal* 2001; **21**: 579–83.

40. Phillips CV. Quantifying and reporting uncertainty from systematic errors. *Epidemiology* 2003; **14**: 459–66.

41. Phillips CV, LaPole LM. Quantifying errors without random sampling. *BMC Med Res Methodol* 2003; **3**: 9.

42. Greenland S. The impact of prior distributions for uncontrolled confounding and response bias: a case study of the relation of wire codes and magnetic fields to childhood leukemia. *J Am Stat Assoc* 2003; **98**: 47–54.

43. Steenland K, Greenland S. Monte Carlo sensitivity analysis and Bayesian analysis of smoking as an unmeasured confounder in a study of silica and lung cancer. *Am J Epidemiol* 2004; **160**: 384–92.

44. Kirking DM, Ammann MA, Harrington CA. Comparison of medical records and prescription claims files in documenting prescription medication therapy. *J Pharmacoepidemiol* 1996; **5**: 3–15.

45. Monson RA, Bond CA. The accuracy of the medical record as an index of outpatient drug therapy. *JAMA* 1978; **240**: 2182–4.

46. West SL, Strom BL, Freundlich B, Normand E, Koch G, Savitz DA. Completeness of prescription recording in outpatient medical records from a health maintenance organization. *J Clin Epidemiol* 1994; **47**: 165–71.

47. Christensen DB, Williams B, Goldberg HI, Martin DP, Engelberg R, LoGerfo JP. Comparison of prescription and medical records in reflecting patient antihypertensive drug therapy. *Ann Pharmacother* 1994; **28**: 99–104.

48. Buchsbaum DG, Boling P, Groh M. Residents' underdocumentation in elderly patients' records of prescriptions for benzodiazepine. *J Med Educ* 1987; **62**: 438–40.

49. Lau HS, Florax C, Porsius AJ, De Boer A. The completeness of medication histories in hospital medical records of patients admitted to general internal medicine wards. *Br J Clin Pharmacol* 2000; **49**: 597–603.

50. Strom BL, Carson JL, Halpern AC, Schinnar R, Snyder ES, Stolley PD *et al.* Using a claims database to investigate drug-induced Stevens–Johnson syndrome. *Stat Med* 1991; **10**: 565–76.

51. Guess HA, West R, Strand LM, Helston D, Lydick EG, Bergman U *et al.* Fatal upper gastrointestinal hemorrhage or perforation among users and nonusers of nonsteroidal anti-inflammatory drugs in Saskatchewan, Canada 1983. *J Clin Epidemiol* 1988; **41**: 35–45.

52. Lloyd SS, Rissing JP. Physician and coding errors in patient records. *JAMA* 1985; **254**: 1330–6.

53. Klemetti A, Saxen L. Prospective versus retrospective approach in the search for environmental causes of malformations. *Am J Public Health Nations Health* 1967; **57**: 2071–5.

54. Bean JA, Leeper JD, Wallace RB, Sherman BM, Jagger H. Variations in the reporting of menstrual histories. *Am J Epidemiol* 1979; **109**: 181–5.

55. Coulter A, McPherson K, Elliott S, Whiting B. Accuracy of recall of surgical histories: a comparison of postal survey data and general practice records. *Community Med* 1985; **7**: 186–9.

56. Adam SA, Sheaves JK, Wright NH, Mosser G, Harris RW, Vessey MP. A case–control study of the possible association between oral contraceptives and malignant melanoma. *Br J Cancer* 1981; **44**: 45–50.

57. Glass R, Johnson B, Vessey M. Accuracy of recall of histories of oral contraceptive use. *Br J Prev Soc Med* 1974; **28**: 273–5.

58. Nischan P, Ebeling K, Thomas DB, Hirsch U. Comparison of recalled and validated oral contraceptive histories. *Am J Epidemiol* 1993; **138**: 697–703.

59. Rosenberg MJ, Layde PM, Ory HW, Strauss LT, Rooks JB, Rubin GL. Agreement between women's histories of oral contraceptive use and physician records. *Int J Epidemiol* 1983; **12**: 84–7.

60. Stolley PD, Tonascia JA, Sartwell PE, Tockman MS, Tonascia S, Rutledge A *et al.* Agreement rates between oral contraceptive users and prescribers in relation to drug use histories. *Am J Epidemiol* 1978; **107**: 226–35.

61. Persson I, Bergkvist L, Adami HO. Reliability of women's histories of climacteric oestrogen treatment assessed by prescription forms. *Int J Epidemiol* 1987; **16**: 222–8.

62. Goodman MT, Nomura AM, Wilkens LR, Kolonel LN. Agreement between interview information and physician records on history of menopausal estrogen use. *Am J Epidemiol* 1990; **131**: 815–25.

63. Horwitz RI, Feinstein AR, Stremlau JR. Alternative data sources and discrepant results in case–control studies of estrogens and endometrial cancer. *Am J Epidemiol* 1980; **111**: 389–94.

64. Paganini-Hill A, Ross RK. Reliability of recall of drug usage and other health-related information. *Am J Epidemiol* 1982; **116**: 114–22.

65. Spengler RF, Clarke EA, Woolever CA, Newman AM, Osborn RW. Exogenous estrogens and endometrial cancer: a case–control study and assessment of potential biases. *Am J Epidemiol* 1981; **114**: 497–506.

66. Coulter A, Vessey M, McPherson K, Crossley B. The ability of women to recall their oral contraceptive histories. *Contraception* 1986; **33**: 127–37.

67. Van den Brandt PA, Petri H, Dorant E, Goldbohm RA, Van de Crommert S. Comparison of questionnaire information and pharmacy data on drug use. *Pharm Weekbl Sci* 1991; **13**: 91–6.

68. West SL, Savitz DA, Koch G, Strom BL, Guess HA, Hartzema A. Recall accuracy for prescription medications: self-report compared with database information. *Am J Epidemiol* 1995; **142**: 1103–12.

69. Strom BL, Schinnar R. An interview strategy was critical for obtaining valid information on the use of hormone replacement therapy. *J Clin Epidemiol*. 2004; **57**: 1210–13.

70. Klungel OH, de Boer A, Paes AH, Herings RM, Seidell JC, Bakker A. Influence of question structure on the recall of self-reported drug use. *J Clin Epidemiol* 2000; **53**: 273–7.

71. Hulka BS, Kupper LL, Cassel JC, Efird RL. Medication use and misuse: physician–patient discrepancies. *J Chronic Dis* 1975; **28**: 7–21.

72. Landry JA, Smyer MA, Tubman JG, Lago DJ, Roberts J, Simonson W. Validation of two methods of data collection of self-reported medicine use among the elderly. *Gerontologist* 1988; **28**: 672–6.

73. Johnson RE, Vollmer WM. Comparing sources of drug data about the elderly. *J Am Geriatr Soc* 1991; **39**: 1079–84.

74. Kehoe R, Wu SY, Leske MC, Chylack LT. Comparing self-reported and physician-reported medical history. *Am J Epidemiol* 1994; **139**: 813–18.

75. Sandvik H, Hunskaar S. General practitioners' management of female urinary incontinence. Medical records do not reflect patients' recall. *Scand J Prim Health Care* 1995; **13**: 168–74.

76. Law MG, Hurley SF, Carlin JB, Chondros P, Gardiner S, Kaldor JM. A comparison of patient interview data with pharmacy and medical records for patients with acquired immunodeficiency syndrome or human immunodeficiency virus infection. *J Clin Epidemiol* 1996; **49**: 997–1002.

77. Cotterchio M, Kreiger N, Darlington G, Steingart A. Comparison of self-reported and physician-reported antidepressant medication use. *Ann Epidemiol* 1999; **9**: 283–9.

78. Smith NL, Psaty BM, Heckbert SR, Tracy RP, Cornell ES. The reliability of medication inventory methods compared to serum levels of cardiovascular drugs in the elderly. *J Clin Epidemiol* 1999; **52**: 143–6.

79. Clegg LX, Potosky AL, Harlan LC, Hankey BF, Hoffman RM, Stanford JL *et al*. Comparison of self-reported initial treatment with medical records: results from the prostate cancer outcomes study. *Am J Epidemiol* 2001; **154**: 582–87.

80. Mackenzie SG, Lippman A. An investigation of report bias in a case–control study of pregnancy outcome. *Am J Epidemiol* 1989; **129**: 65–75.

81. Feldman Y, Koren G, Mattice K, Shear H, Pellegrini E, MacLeod SM. Determinants of recall and recall bias in studying drug and chemical exposure in pregnancy. *Teratology* 1989; **40**: 37–45.

82. de Jong PCMP, Berns MPH, van Duynhoven YTHP, Nijdam WS, Eskes TKAB, Zielhuis GA. Recall of medication during pregnancy: validity and accuracy of an adjusted questionnaire. *Pharmacoepidemiol Drug Saf* 1995; **4**: 23–30.

83. Tilley BC, Barnes AB, Bergstralh E, Labarthe D, Noller KL, Colton T *et al*. A comparison of pregnancy history recall and medical records. Implications for retrospective studies. *Am J Epidemiol* 1985; **121**: 269–81.

84. Werler MM, Pober BR, Nelson K, Holmes LB. Reporting accuracy among mothers of malformed and nonmalformed infants. *Am J Epidemiol* 1989; **129**: 415–21.

85. de Jong PCM, Prevoo MLL, Zielhuis GA, Roeleveld N, Gabreels F. Accessibility and validity of data on medical drug use during pregnancy collect from various sources. *J Pharmacoepidemiol* 1991; **2**: 45–57.

86. McCredie J, Kricker A, Elliott J, Forrest J. The innocent bystander. Doxylamine/dicyclomine/pyridoxine and congenital limb defects. *Med J Aust* 1984; **140**: 525–7.

87. Bryant HE, Visser N, Love EJ. Records, recall loss, and recall bias in pregnancy: a comparison of interview and medical records data of pregnant and postnatal women. *Am J Public Health* 1989; **79**: 78–80.

88. Czeizel AE, Petik D, Vargha P. Validation studies of drug exposures in pregnant women. *Pharmacoepidemiol Drug Saf* 2003; **12**: 409–16.

89. Cottler LB, Robins LN. The effect of questionnaire design on reported prevalence of psychoactive medication. *NIDA Res Monogr* 1984; **55**: 231–7.

90. Kimmel SE, Lewis JD, Jaskowiak J, Kishel L, Hennessy S. Enhancement of medication recall using medication pictures and lists in telephone interviews. *Pharmacoepidemiol Drug Saf* 2003; **12**: 1–8.

91. Beresford SA, Coker AL. Pictorially assisted recall of past hormone use in case–control studies. *Am J Epidemiol* 1989; **130**: 202–5.

92. West SL, Savitz DA, Koch G, Sheff KL, Strom BL, Guess HA *et al*. Demographics, health behaviors, and past drug use as predictors of recall accuracy for previous prescription medication use. *J Clin Epidemiol* 1997; **50**: 975–80.

93. Zierler S, Rothman KJ. Congenital heart disease in relation to maternal use of Bendectin and other drugs in early pregnancy. *N Engl J Med* 1985; **313**: 347–52.

94. Rockenbauer M, Olsen J, Czeizel AE, Pedersen L, Sorensen HT. Recall bias in a case–control surveillance system on the use of medicine during pregnancy. *Epidemiology* 2001; **12**: 461–6.

95. Harlow SD, Linet MS. Agreement between questionnaire data and medical records. The evidence for accuracy of recall. *Am J Epidemiol* 1989; **129**: 233–48.

96. Madow WG. Interview data on chronic conditions compared with information derived from medical records. *Vital Health Stat 1* 1967; **2**: 1–84.

97. Watson DL. Health interview responses compared with medical records. *Vital Health Stat 1* 1965; **46**: 1–74.

98. Colditz GA, Martin P, Stampfer MJ, Willett WC, Sampson L, Rosner B *et al*. Validation of questionnaire information on risk factors and disease outcomes in a prospective cohort study of women. *Am J Epidemiol* 1986; **123**: 894–900.

99. Tretli S, Lund-Larsen PG, Foss OP. Reliability of questionnaire information on cardiovascular disease and diabetes: cardiovascular disease study in Finnmark county. *J Epidemiol Community Health* 1982; **36**: 269–73.

100. Wingo PA, Ory HW, Layde PM, Lee NC. The evaluation of the data collection process for a multicenter, population-based, case–control design. *Am J Epidemiol* 1988; **128**: 206–17.

101. Linet MS, Harlow SD, McLaughlin JK, McCaffrey LD. A comparison of interview data and medical records for previous medical conditions and surgery. *J Clin Epidemiol* 1989; **42**: 1207–13.

102. Bush TL, Miller SR, Golden AL, Hale WE. Self-report and medical record report agreement of selected medical conditions in the elderly. *Am J Public Health* 1989; **79**: 1554–6.

103. Nevitt MC, Cummings SR, Browner WS, Seeley DG, Cauley JA, Vogt TM *et al*. The accuracy of self-report of fractures in elderly women: evidence from a prospective study. *Am J Epidemiol* 1992; **135**: 490–9.

104. Wilcox AJ, Horney LF. Accuracy of spontaneous abortion recall. *Am J Epidemiol* 1984; **120**: 727–33.

105. Commision on Chronic Illness. *Chronic Illness in the United States*, Vol. IV. *Chronic Illness in a Large City: The Baltimore Study*. Cambridge, MA: Harvard University Press, 1957; pp. 297–328.

106. Heliovaara M, Aromaa A, Klaukka T, Knekt P, Joukamaa M, Impivaara O. Reliability and validity of interview data on chronic diseases. The Mini-Finland Health Survey. *J Clin Epidemiol* 1993; **46**: 181–91.

107. Spitz MR, Fueger JJ, Newell GR. The development of a comprehensive, institution-based patient risk evaluation program: II. Validity and reliability of questionnaire data. *Am J Prev Med* 1988; **4**: 188–93.

108. Midthjell K, Holmen J, Bjorndal A, Lund-Larsen G. Is questionnaire information valid in the study of a chronic disease such as diabetes? The Nord-Trondelag diabetes study. *J Epidemiol Community Health* 1992; **46**: 537–42.

109. Kriegsman DM, Penninx BW, van Eijk JT, Boeke AJ, Deeg DJ. Self-reports and general practitioner information on the presence of chronic diseases in community dwelling elderly. A study on the accuracy of patients' self-reports and on determinants of inaccuracy. *J Clin Epidemiol* 1996; **49**: 1407–17.

110. Bergmann MM, Calle EE, Mervis CA, Miracle-McMahill HL, Thun MJ, Heath CW. Validity of self-reported cancers in a prospective cohort study in comparison with data from state cancer registries. *Am J Epidemiol* 1998; **147**: 556–62.

111. Paganini-Hill A, Chao A. Accuracy of recall of hip fracture, heart attack, and cancer: a comparison of postal survey data and medical records. *Am J Epidemiol* 1993; **138**: 101–6.

112. Zhu K, McKnight B, Stergachis A, Daling JR, Levine RS. Comparison of self-report data and medical records data: results from a case–control study on prostate cancer. *Int J Epidemiol* 1999; **28**: 409–17.

113. Lingard EA, Wright EA, Sledge CB. Pitfalls of using patient recall to derive preoperative status in outcome studies of total knee arthroplasty. *J Bone Joint Surg Am* 2001; **83-A**: 1149–56.

114. Mancuso CA, Charlson ME. Does recollection error threaten the validity of cross-sectional studies of effectiveness? *Med Care* 1995; **33** (suppl 4): AS77–88.

115. Dawson EG, Kanim LE, Sra P, Dorey FJ, Goldstein TB, Delamarter RB *et al*. Low back pain recollection versus concurrent accounts: outcomes analysis. *Spine* 2002; **27**: 984–93.

116. Linton KL, Klein BE, Klein R. The validity of self-reported and surrogate-reported cataract and age-related macular degeneration in the Beaver Dam Eye Study. *Am J Epidemiol* 1991; **134**: 1438–46.

117. Rosamond WD, Sprafka JM, McGovern PG, Nelson M, Luepker RV. Validation of self-reported history of acute myocardial infarction: experience of the Minnesota Heart Survey Registry. *Epidemiology* 1995; **6**: 67–9.

118. Walker MK, Whincup PH, Shaper AG, Lennon LT, Thomson AG. Validation of patient recall of doctor-diagnosed heart attack and stroke: a postal questionnaire and record review comparison. *Am J Epidemiol* 1998; **148**: 355–61.

119. Naleway AL, Belongia EA, Greenlee RT, Kieke BA, Jr, Chen RT, Shay DK. Eczematous skin disease and recall of past diagnoses: implications for smallpox vaccination. *Ann Intern Med* 2003; **139**: 1–7.

120. Colditz GA, Stampfer MJ, Willett WC, Stason WB, Rosner B, Hennekens CH *et al*. Reproducibility and validity of self-reported menopausal status in a prospective cohort study. *Am J Epidemiol* 1987; **126**: 319–25.

121. Jabine TB. Reporting chronic conditions in the National Health Interview Survey. A review of findings from evaluation studies and methodological test. *Vital Health Stat 2* 1987; **105**: 1–45.

122. Biering-Sorensen U. Reporting of hospitalization in the Health Interview Survey. *Vital Health Stat 1* 1965; **61**: 1–71.

123. Corwin RG, Krober M, Roth HP. Patients' accuracy in reporting their past medical history, a study of 90 patients with peptic ulcer. *J Chronic Dis* 1971; **23**: 875–9.

124. Udry JR, Gaughan M, Schwingl PJ, van den Berg BJ. A medical record linkage analysis of abortion underreporting. *Fam Plann Perspect* 1996; **28**: 228–31.

125. Lessler JT, Harris BSH. *Medicaid Data as a Source for Postmarketing Surveillance Information*. Research Triangle Park, NC: Research Triangle Institute, 1984.

126. Cannell CF, Marquis KH, Laurent A. A summary of studies of interviewing methodology. *Vital Health Stat 1* 1977; series 2, i–viii; 1–78.

127. Bonito AJ, Farrelly MC, Han J, Lohr KN, Lubalin JS, Lux L. Assessment of the feasibility of creating a managed care encounter-level databas, RTI Project Report 6703-003, prepared for the Center for Organization and Delivery Studies, Agency for Health Care Policy and Research, Rockville, MD, 1997.

128. Stergachis AS. Record linkage studies for postmarketing drug surveillance: data quality and validity considerations. *Drug Intell Clin Pharm* 1988; **22**: 157–61.

129. Rawson NS, Harding SR, Malcolm E, Lueck L. Hospitalizations for aplastic anemia and agranulocytosis in Saskatchewan: incidence and associations with antecedent prescription drug use. *J Clin Epidemiol* 1998; **51**: 1343–55.

130. Schering Laboratories. *The Phantom Patient and Community Pharmacy Practice, Schering Report XVII*. Kenilworth, NJ, 1996.

131. Craghead RM, Wartski DM. An evaluative study of unclaimed prescriptions. *Hosp Pharm* 1991; **26**: 616–17, 632.

132. Farmer KC, Gumbhir AK. Unclaimed prescriptions: an overlooked opportunity. *Am Pharm* 1992; **NS32**: 55–9.

133. Hamilton WR, Hopkins UK. Survey on unclaimed prescriptions in a community pharmacy. *J Am Pharm Assoc (Wash)* 1997; **NS37**: 341–5.

134. Kirking MH, Kirking DM. Evaluation of unclaimed prescriptions in an ambulatory care pharmacy. *Hosp Pharm* 1993; **28**: 90–91, 94, 102.

135. Kinnaird D, Cox T, Wilson JP. Unclaimed prescriptions in a clinic with computerized prescriber order entry. *Am J Health Syst Pharm* 2003; **60**: 1468–70.

136. Psaty BM, Heckbert SR, Atkins D, Lemaitre R, Koepsell TD, Wahl PW *et al*. The risk of myocardial infarction associated with the combined use of estrogens and progestins in postmenopausal women. *Arch Intern Med* 1994; **154**: 1333–9.

137. Stergachis AS. Evaluating the quality of linked automated databases for use in pharmacoepidemiology. In: Hartzema AG, Porta MS, Tilson HH, eds, *Pharmacoepidemiology: An Introduction*, 2nd edn. Cincinnati, OH: Harvey Whitney, 1991; pp. 222–34.

138. Harris BL, Stergachis A, Ried LD. The effect of drug co-payments on utilization and cost of pharmaceuticals in a health maintenance organization. *Med Care* 1990; **28**: 907–17.

139. McKenzie DA, Semradek J, McFarland BH, Mullooly JP, McCamant LE. The validity of medicaid pharmacy claims for estimating drug use among elderly nursing home residents: the Oregon experience. *J Clin Epidemiol* 2000; **53**: 1248–57.

140. Hoes AW, Grobbee DE, Lubsen J, Man in 't Veld AJ, van der Does E, Hofman A. Diuretics, beta-blockers, and the risk for sudden cardiac death in hypertensive patients. *Ann Intern Med* 1995; **123**: 481–7.

141. Lau HS, de Boer A, Beuning KS, Porsius A. Validation of pharmacy records in drug exposure assessment. *J Clin Epidemiol* 1997; **50**: 619–25.

142. Bright RA, Avorn J, Everitt DE. Medicaid data as a resource for epidemiologic studies: strengths and limitations. *J Clin Epidemiol* 1989; **42**: 937–45.

143. Strom BL, Carson JL, Schinnar R, Snyder ES, Shaw M, Waiter SL. No causal relationship between transdermal scopolamine and seizures: methodologic lessons for pharmacoepidemiology. *Clin Pharmacol Ther* 1991; **50**: 107–13.

144. Wynia MK, Cummins DS, VanGeest JB, Wilson IB. Physician manipulation of reimbursement rules for patients: between a rock and a hard place. *JAMA* 2000; **283**: 1858–65.

145. Go AS, Hylek EM, Chang Y, Phillips KA, Henault LE, Capra AM *et al*. Anticoagulation therapy for stroke prevention in atrial fibrillation: how well do randomized trials translate into clinical practice? *JAMA* 2003; **290**: 2685–92.

146. Ferrara A, Quesenberry CP, Karter AJ, Njoroge CW, Jacobson AS, Selby JV. Current use of unopposed estrogen and estrogen plus progestin and the risk of acute myocardial infarction among women with diabetes: the Northern California Kaiser Permanente Diabetes Registry, 1995–1998. *Circulation* 2003; **107**: 43–8.

147. Friedman GD, Habel LA. Barbiturates and lung cancer: a re-evaluation. *Int J Epidemiol* 1999; **28**: 375–9.

148. Goodwin FK, Fireman B, Simon GE, Hunkeler EM, Lee J, Revicki D. Suicide risk in bipolar disorder during treatment with lithium and divalproex. *JAMA* 2003; **290**: 1467–73.

149. Sidney S, Petitti DB, Soff GA, Cundiff DL, Tolan KK, Quesenberry CP, Jr. Venous thromboembolic disease in users of low-estrogen combined estrogen–progestin oral contraceptives. *Contraception* 2004; **70**: 3–10.

150. Petitti DB, Sidney S, Bernstein A, Wolf S, Quesenberry C, Ziel HK. Stroke in users of low-dose oral contraceptives. *N Engl J Med* 1996; **335**: 8–15.

151. Sidney S, Petitti DB, Quesenberry CP, Jr, Klatsky AL, Ziel HK, Wolf S. Myocardial infarction in users of low-dose oral contraceptives. *Obstet Gynecol* 1996; **88**: 939–44.

152. Keith DS, Nichols GA, Gullion CM, Brown JB, Smith DH. Longitudinal follow-up and outcomes among a population with chronic kidney disease in a large managed care organization. *Arch Intern Med* 2004; **164**: 659–63.

153. Quam L, Ellis LB, Venus P, Clouse J, Taylor CG, Leatherman S. Using claims data for epidemiologic research. The concordance of claims-based criteria with the medical record and patient survey for identifying a hypertensive population. *Med Care* 1993; **31**: 498–507.

154. Straus SM, Bleumink GS, Dieleman JP, van der Lei J, t Jong GW, Kingma JH *et al*. Antipsychotics and the risk of sudden cardiac death. *Arch Intern Med* 2004; **164**: 1293–7.

155. Jick SS, Kaye JA, Vasilakis-Scaramozza C, Garcia Rodriguez LA, Ruigomez A, Meier CR *et al*. Validity of the general practice research database. *Pharmacotherapy* 2003; **23**: 686–9.

156. Jick H, Terris BZ, Derby LE, Jick SS. Further validation of information recorded on a general practitioner based computerized data resource in the United Kingdom. *Pharmacoepidemiol Drug Saf* 1992; **1**: 347–9.

157. Jick H, Jick SS, Derby LE. Validation of information recorded on general practitioner based computerised data resource in the United Kingdom. *BMJ* 1991; **302**: 766–8.

158. Schoonen WM, Hall AJ. Validity of the General Practice Research Database: a systematic review. Presented at the 20th International Conference on Pharmacoepidemiology and Theraupeutic Risk Management Annual Meeting, Bordeaux, France, August 22–25, 2004.

159. van Staa TP, Abenhaim L. The quality of information recorded on a UK database of primary care records: a study of hospitalizations due to hypoglycemia and other conditions. *Pharmacoepidemiol Drug Saf* 1994; **3**: 15–21.

160. Newton KM, Wagner EH, Ramsey SD, McCulloch D, Evans R, Sandhu N *et al.* The use of automated data to identify complications and comorbidities of diabetes: a validation study. *J Clin Epidemiol* 1999; **52**: 199–207.

161. Leveille SG, Gray S, Black DJ, LaCroix AZ, Ferrucci L, Volpato S *et al.* A new method for identifying antibiotic-treated infections using automated pharmacy records. *J Clin Epidemiol* 2000; **53**: 1069–75.

162. Friedman GD, Gerard MJ, Ury HK. Clindamycin and diarrhea. *JAMA* 1976; **236**: 2498–2500.

163. Levin TR, Schmittdiel JA, Kunz K, Henning JM, Henke CJ, Colby CJ *et al.* Costs of acid-related disorders to a health maintenance organization. *Am J Med* 1997; **103**: 520–8.

164. Sidney S, Petitti DB, Quesenberry CP, Jr. Myocardial infarction and the use of estrogen and estrogen–progestogen in postmenopausal women. *Ann Intern Med* 1997; **127**: 501–8.

165. Go AS, Hylek EM, Borowsky LH, Phillips KA, Selby JV, Singer DE. Warfarin use among ambulatory patients with nonvalvular atrial fibrillation: the anticoagulation and risk factors in atrial fibrillation (ATRIA) study. *Ann Intern Med* 1999; **131**: 927–34.

166. Go AS, Hylek EM, Phillips KA, Chang Y, Henault LE, Selby JV *et al.* Prevalence of diagnosed atrial fibrillation in adults: national implications for rhythm management and stroke prevention: the Anticoagulation and Risk Factors in Atrial Fibrillation (ATRIA) study. *JAMA* 2001; **285**: 2370–5.

167. Donahue JG, Choo PW, Manson JE, Platt R. The incidence of herpes zoster. *Arch Intern Med* 1995; **155**: 1605–9.

168. Donahue JG, Weiss ST, Goetsch MA, Livingston JM, Greineder DK, Platt R. Assessment of asthma using automated and full-text medical records. *J Asthma* 1997; **34**: 273–81.

169. Andrade SE, Gurwitz JH, Chan KA, Donahue JG, Beck A, Boles M *et al.* Validation of diagnoses of peptic ulcers and bleeding from administrative databases: a multi-health maintenance organization study. *J Clin Epidemiol* 2002; **55**: 310–13.

170. Donahue JG, Chan KA, Andrade SE, Beck A, Boles M, Buist DS *et al.* Gastric and duodenal safety of daily alendronate. *Arch Intern Med* 2002; **162**: 936–42.

171. Bohlke K, Davis RL, Marcy SM, Braun MM, DeStefano F, Black SB *et al.* Risk of anaphylaxis after vaccination of children and adolescents. *Pediatrics* 2003; **112**: 815–20.

172. Chan KA, Truman A, Gurwitz JH, Hurley JS, Martinson B, Platt R *et al.* A cohort study of the incidence of serious acute liver injury in diabetic patients treated with hypoglycemic agents. *Arch Intern Med* 2003; **163**: 728–34.

173. Griffin MR, Piper JM, Daugherty JR, Snowden M, Ray WA. Nonsteroidal anti-inflammatory drug use and increased risk for peptic ulcer disease in elderly persons. *Ann Intern Med* 1991; **114**: 257–63.

174. Strom BL, Carson JL, Halpern AC, Schinnar R, Snyder ES, Shaw M *et al.* A population-based study of Stevens–Johnson syndrome. Incidence and antecedent drug exposures. *Arch Dermatol* 1991; **127**: 831–8.

175. Strom BL, Carson JL, Schinnar R, Snyder ES, Shaw M. Descriptive epidemiology of agranulocytosis. *Arch Intern Med* 1992; **152**: 1475–80.

176. Staffa JA, Jones JK, Gable CB, Verspeelt JP, Amery WK. Risk of selected serious cardiac events among new users of antihistamines. *Clin Ther* 1995; **17**: 1062–77.

177. Brown NJ, Ray WA, Snowden M, Griffin MR. Black Americans have an increased rate of angiotensin converting enzyme inhibitor-associated angioedema. *Clin Pharmacol Ther* 1996; **60**: 8–13.

178. Steinwachs DM, Stuart ME, Scholle S, Starfield B, Fox MH, Weiner JP. A comparison of ambulatory Medicaid claims to medical records: a reliability assessment. *Am J Med Qual* 1998; **13**: 63–9.

179. Griffin MR, Yared A, Ray WA. Nonsteroidal antiinflammatory drugs and acute renal failure in elderly persons. *Am J Epidemiol* 2000; **151**: 488–96.

180. Ray WA, Meredith S, Thapa PB, Meador KG, Hall K, Murray KT. Antipsychotics and the risk of sudden cardiac death. *Arch Gen Psychiatry* 2001; **58**: 1161–7.

181. Wang PS, Walker AM, Tsuang MT, Orav EJ, Levin R, Avorn J. Finding incident breast cancer cases through US claims data and a state cancer registry. *Cancer Causes Control* 2001; **12**: 257–65.

182. Ngo DL, Marshall LM, Howard RN, Woodward JA, Southwick K, Hedberg K. Agreement between self-reported information and medical claims data on diagnosed diabetes in Oregon's Medicaid population. *J Public Health Manag Pract* 2003; **9**: 542–4.

183. Rogers SO, Ray WA, Smalley WE. A population-based study of survival among elderly persons diagnosed with colorectal cancer: does race matter if all are insured? (United States). *Cancer Causes Control* 2004; **15**: 193–9.

184. Rawson NS, Malcolm E. Validity of the recording of ischaemic heart disease and chronic obstructive pulmonary disease in the Saskatchewan health care datafiles. *Stat Med* 1995; **14**: 2627–43.

185. Edouard L, Rawson NS. Reliability of the recording of hysterectomy in the Saskatchewan health care system. *Br J Obstet Gynaecol* 1996; **103**: 891–7.

186. Rawson NS, Malcolm E, D'Arcy C. Reliability of the recording of schizophrenia and depressive disorder in the Saskatchewan health care datafiles. *Soc Psychiatry Psychiatr Epidemiol* 1997; **32**: 191–9.

187. Walker AM, Szneke P, Weatherby LB, Dicker LW, Lanza LL, Loughlin JE *et al.* The risk of serious cardiac arrhythmias among cisapride users in the United Kingdom and Canada. *Am J Med* 1999; **107**: 356–62.

188. West SL, Richter A, Melfi CA, McNutt M, Nennstiel ME, Mauskopf JA. Assessing the Saskatchewan database for outcomes research studies of depression and its treatment. *J Clin Epidemiol* 2000; **53**: 823–31.

189. van der Klauw MM, Stricker BH, Herings RM, Cost WS, Valkenburg HA, Wilson JH. A population based case–cohort study of drug-induced anaphylaxis. *Br J Clin Pharmacol* 1993; **35**: 400–8.

190. Heerdink ER, Leufkens HG, Herings RM, Ottervanger JP, Stricker BH, Bakker A. NSAIDs associated with increased risk of congestive heart failure in elderly patients taking diuretics. *Arch Intern Med* 1998; **158**: 1108–12.

191. van der Klauw MM, Goudsmit R, Halie MR, van't Veer MB, Herings RM, Wilson JH *et al*. A population-based case–cohort study of drug-associated agranulocytosis. *Arch Intern Med* 1999; **159**: 369–74.

192. Movig KL, Leufkens HG, Lenderink AW, Egberts AC. Validity of hospital discharge International Classification of Diseases (ICD) codes for identifying patients with hyponatremia. *J Clin Epidemiol* 2003; **56**: 530–5.

193. Dornan S, Murray FE, White G, McGilchrist MM, Evans JM, McDevitt DG *et al*. An audit of the accuracy of upper gastrointestinal diagnoses in Scottish Morbidity Record 1 data in Tayside. *Health Bull (Edinb)* 1995; **53**: 274–9.

194. Evans JM, McMahon AD, McGilchrist MM, White G, Murray FE, McDevitt DG *et al*. Topical non-steroidal anti-inflammatory drugs and admission to hospital for upper gastrointestinal bleeding and perforation: a record linkage case–control study. *BMJ* 1995; **311**: 22–6.

195. Evans JM, Macgregor AM, Murray FE, Vaidya K, Morris AD, MacDonald TM. No association between non-steroidal anti-inflammatory drugs and acute appendicitis in a case–control study. *Br J Surg* 1997; **84**: 372–4.

196. Evans JM, McMahon AD, Murray FE, McDevitt DG, MacDonald TM. Non-steroidal anti-inflammatory drugs are associated with emergency admission to hospital for colitis due to inflammatory bowel disease. *Gut* 1997; **40**: 619–22.

197. Morris AD, Boyle DI, MacAlpine R, Emslie-Smith A, Jung RT, Newton RW *et al*. The diabetes audit and research in Tayside Scotland (DARTS) study: electronic record linkage to create a diabetes register. DARTS/MEMO Collaboration. *BMJ* 1997; **315**: 524–8.

198. McMahon AD, Evans JM, MacDonald TM. Hypersensitivity reactions associated with exposure to naproxen and ibuprofen: a cohort study. *J Clin Epidemiol* 2001; **54**: 1271–4.

199. Struthers AD, Donnan PT, Lindsay P, McNaughton D, Broomhall J, MacDonald TM. Effect of allopurinol on mortality and hospitalisations in chronic heart failure: a retrospective cohort study. *Heart* 2002; **87**: 229–34.

200. Steinke DT, Weston TL, Morris AD, MacDonald TM, Dillon JF. The epidemiology of liver disease in Tayside database: a population-based record-linkage study. *J Biomed Inform* 2002; **35**: 186–93.

201. Meier CR, Sturkenboom MC, Cohen AS, Jick H. Postmenopausal estrogen replacement therapy and the risk of developing systemic lupus erythematosus or discoid lupus. *J Rheumatol* 1998; **25**: 1515–19.

202. Derby L, Maier WC. Risk of cataract among users of intranasal corticosteroids. *J Allergy Clin Immunol* 2000; **105**: 912–16.

203. Lawrenson R, Todd JC, Leydon GM, Williams TJ, Farmer RD. Validation of the diagnosis of venous thromboembolism in general practice database studies. *Br J Clin Pharmacol* 2000; **49**: 591–6.

204. García-Rodríguez LA, Huerta-Alvarez C. Reduced risk of colorectal cancer among long-term users of aspirin and non-aspirin nonsteroidal antiinflammatory drugs. *Epidemiology* 2001; **12**: 88–93.

205. Seshadri S, Zornberg GL, Derby LE, Myers MW, Jick H, Drachman DA. Postmenopausal estrogen replacement therapy and the risk of Alzheimer disease. *Arch Neurol* 2001; **58**: 435–40.

206. Soriano JB, Maier WC, Visick G, Pride NB. Validation of general practitioner-diagnosed COPD in the UK General Practice Research Database. *Eur J Epidemiol* 2001; **17**: 1075–80.

207. Huerta C, Zhao SZ, Garcia Rodriguez LA. Risk of acute liver injury in patients with diabetes. *Pharmacotherapy* 2002; **22**: 1091–6.

208. Lewis JD, Brensinger C, Bilker WB, Strom BL. Validity and completeness of the General Practice Research Database for studies of inflammatory bowel disease. *Pharmacoepidemiol Drug Saf* 2002; **11**: 211–18.

209. Margolis DJ, Bilker W, Knauss J, Baumgarten M, Strom BL. The incidence and prevalence of pressure ulcers among elderly patients in general medical practice. *Ann Epidemiol* 2002; **12**: 321–5.

210. Ruigómez A, Johansson S, Wallander MA, Rodriguez LA. Incidence of chronic atrial fibrillation in general practice and its treatment pattern. *J Clin Epidemiol* 2002; **55**: 358–63.

211. van Staa TP, Selby P, Leufkens HG, Lyles K, Sprafka JM, Cooper C. Incidence and natural history of Paget's disease of bone in England and Wales. *J Bone Miner Res* 2002; **17**: 465–71.

212. Watson DJ, Rhodes T, Cai B, Guess HA. Lower risk of thromboembolic cardiovascular events with naproxen among patients with rheumatoid arthritis. *Arch Intern Med* 2002; **162**: 1105–10.

213. Gelfand JM, Berlin J, Van Voorhees A, Margolis DJ. Lymphoma rates are low but increased in patients with psoriasis: results from a population-based cohort study in the United Kingdom. *Arch Dermatol* 2003; **139**: 1425–9.

214. Huerta C, Garcia Rodriguez LA, Wallander MA, Johansson S. Users of oral steroids are at a reduced risk of developing irritable bowel syndrome. *Pharmacoepidemiol Drug Saf* 2003; **12**: 583–8.

215. Ruigómez A, Garcia Rodriguez LA, Johansson S, Wallander MA. Is hormone replacement therapy associated with an increased

risk of irritable bowel syndrome? *Maturitas* 2003; **44**: 133–40.

216. Yang CC, Jick SS, Jick H. Lipid-lowering drugs and the risk of depression and suicidal behavior. *Arch Intern Med* 2003; **163**: 1926–32.

217. Ronquist G, Rodriguez LA, Ruigomez A, Johansson S, Wallander MA, Frithz G *et al.* Association between captopril, other antihypertensive drugs and risk of prostate cancer. *Prostate* 2004; **58**: 50–6.

218. Peng MM, Jick H. A population-based study of the incidence, cause, and severity of anaphylaxis in the United Kingdom. *Arch Intern Med* 2004; **164**: 317–19.

219. Strom BL, Carson JL, Morse ML, LeRoy AA. The computerized on-line Medicaid pharmaceutical analysis and surveillance system: a new resource for postmarketing drug surveillance. *Clin Pharmacol Ther* 1985; **38**: 359–64.

220. Ray WA, Griffin MR. Use of Medicaid data for pharmacoepidemiology. *Am J Epidemiol* 1989; **129**: 837–49.

221. Shapiro S. The role of automated record linkage in the post-marketing surveillance of drug safety: a critique. *Clin Pharmacol Ther* 1989; **46**: 371–86.

222. Iezzoni LI, Burnside S, Sickles L, Moskowitz MA, Sawitz E, Levine PA. Coding of acute myocardial infarction. Clinical and policy implications. *Ann Intern Med* 1988; **109**: 745–51.

223. Pladevall M, Goff DC, Nichaman MZ, Chan F, Ramsey D, Ortiz C *et al.* An assessment of the validity of ICD Code 410 to identify hospital admissions for myocardial infarction: The Corpus Christi Heart Project. *Int J Epidemiol* 1996; **25**: 948–52.

224. Department of Health and Human Services. *Protection of Human Subjects*, Title 45 Part 46: Revised. Code of Federal Regulations, 1991.

225. Linet MS. Testimony on impact of HIPAA on research, American College of Epidemiology, 2003.

226. Lydon-Rochelle M, Holt VL. HIPAA transition: challenges of a multisite medical records validation study of maternally linked birth records. *Matern Child Health J* 2004; **8**: 35–8.

46

Variable Compliance and Persistence with Prescribed Drug Dosing Regimens: Implications for Benefits, Risks, and Economics of Pharmacotherapy

JOHN URQUHART

Maastricht University, Maastricht, The Netherlands, Biopharmaceutical Sciences, UCSF, San Francisco, USA, and AARDEX Ltd, Zug, Switzerland.

INTRODUCTION

Hippocrates recognized that some of his patients failed to take the drugs he prescribed, some of whom blamed him later for a poor outcome. He assumed, of course, that the prescribed drugs were effective if taken according to his dosing instructions. Given the state of therapeutics until the mid-20th century, that assumption was probably more often wrong than right, making more or less irrelevant the question of whether or not the patient actually took the prescribed drug. As we now know from reliable measurements, and as Hippocrates and his successors had to guess about, the vast majority of deviations from prescribed dosing regimens are omissions or delays of scheduled doses, with only a relatively small minority of errors involving the taking of extra doses.[1] That generalization naturally does not apply to drugs of abuse, which are a special case not considered here.

Here, we are concerned with the diverse ways in which patients use or misuse pharmaceuticals that are prescribed in ambulatory care, including those in clinical trials. There are two main topics: (i) how well or poorly patients execute prescribed drug regimens in trials and practice, and (ii) how long they persist in taking prescribed medicines in practice (short persistence in trials usually being far less common than in everyday practice). They have gained in importance in direct relation to the growing therapeutic power of available drugs. These two topics are subsumed in a new discipline: pharmionics, which is the study of how patients use or misuse prescription drugs in ambulatory care. A second factor that is propelling pharmionics into therapeutic prominence is the availability of reliable methods for compiling

Pharmacoepidemiology, Fourth Edition   Edited by B.L. Strom
© 2005 John Wiley & Sons, Ltd

drug dosing histories in ambulatory patients, because the field would be stymied without reliable methods, which have only been available since the latter 1980s.

The dosing history is the logical starting point for assessing the quality of a patient's execution of the prescribed regimen. The dosing history also shows both when dosing starts and either stops or declines to a sufficient degree of underdosing as to be considered as having, for practical purposes, stopped.

SOME METHODOLOGICAL MATTERS

Until about 1980, estimates of patients' dosing histories were based, directly or indirectly, on what patients disclosed, which meant what their recall allowed them to disclose, and what they chose to disclose. For more or less obvious reasons, interviews, histories, and diaries have been repeatedly shown to provide overestimates of ambulatory patients' intake of prescribed drugs.[1-5] Returned tablet counts, which continue to be widely used as a measure of drug intake in drug trials, were resoundingly discredited in 1989 by results of an extensive three-trial study using low-dose phenobarbital as a chemical marker of drug intake as, in the authors' words, "grossly overestimating patient compliance" in drug trials.[6] The reason for the failure of returned tablet counts is that a substantial proportion of patients discard or hoard untaken drug—easily done in a few seconds—and return an empty or nearly empty container.

The use of a low-dose, slow-turnover chemical marker substance has provided unequivocal, objective evidence for pervasive underdosing,[3,7,8] but the marker method cannot reveal when doses were taken—it can only reveal the aggregate intake of drug during a certain time window prior to blood sampling. Pharmacokinetic theory teaches that the width of that time window is 3–4 times the plasma half-life of the drug (see Chapter 4); practical experience teaches that about 7 in 8 drugs in active use have plasma half-lives of less than 12 hours,[9] which means that most drugs have a time window of 36–48 hours or less. The chemical marker method developed by Pullar and Feely relies upon phenobarbital added in subpharmacological doses (2 mg) to dosage forms. It has good absorption properties and a low-variance plasma half-life of about 100 hours, giving a time window that is not only generously wide but also one that can indicate drug intake well prior to the onset of the phenomenon of "white-coat compliance",[10] which is the strong tendency for patients who ordinarily omit many scheduled doses to start dosing per prescription in the day or two prior to a scheduled medical visit. White-coat compliance effectively nullifies the value of

using scheduled, single-point measurements of the concentrations of most drugs in plasma ("therapeutic drug monitoring") as indicators of how well patients are executing prescribed drug regimens. Obviously, if the measured concentration is low or zero, it signifies that one or more doses were omitted during the drug's pharmacokinetic time window, but the much more likely error is a normal or even high level of drug in a patient who usually omits many doses at other times.

White-coat compliance only came to light[11,12] after the advent of electronic monitoring,[13-15] a method which has become the de facto gold standard for compiling dosing histories.[1,3,5,16-18] Electronic monitoring is achieved by incorporating a time-stamping microcircuit into the pharmaceutical package so that performance of the maneuvers necessary to remove a dose of drug from the package is detected by microswitches, which signal the microcircuit to record time and date. The upshot is that, of the two objective methods, a chemical marker provides unambiguous evidence of aggregate drug intake during the time window, but cannot indicate when doses were taken, and so provides no information on time of day or day of week when errors are made, nor on intervals between doses. As experience has grown with statistical analyses of electronically compiled dosing history data,[19-22] it has become evident that the aspect of dosing history data which has the greatest amount of explanatory power for clinical events is the intervals between doses, with overly long intervals accounting for much or most of the untoward clinical events evoked by what many refer to as "poor adherence" to prescribed drug dosing regimens.

There are two principal objectives of this chapter. The first is to understand the ways in which ambulatory patients' drug dosing histories differ from prescribed or protocol-specified dosing regimens. The second objective is to understand the clinical and economic consequences of these differences, how they should be factored into the estimation and communication of the safety and efficacy of the drug in question, and the roles they may play as triggers of adverse reactions.

The orientation of this chapter is almost exclusively pharmacometric, i.e., identifying the pharmacological and clinical effects of patients' common deviations from prescribed dosing regimens, gaining quantitative understanding of the pharmacokinetics and pharmacodynamics of those deviations, and learning what can be done to prevent or minimize clinically/economically important deviations from recommended dosing regimens. The first of these considerations is: what are the temporal patterns of dosing and what are their evident clinical consequences? The remaining considerations have to do with hazardous effects of the frequently recurring "holiday" pattern of three or more days of sequentially omitted doses in the midst of a prescribed course of ongoing dosing.

Note that efforts to drive a patient's drug dosing into close correspondence with the prescribed dosing regimen can proceed on an empirical basis, guided by measurements that show whether a given intervention is or is not effective, and for how long close correspondence continues before it is necessary to repeat the intervention or try something different. In so doing, one needs also to know how close the correspondence must be to achieve full benefits of the prescribed drug dosing regimen. Many hold the false belief, arising from repetition, not evidence, that taking more than 80% of prescribed doses is "good enough". However, there is no general answer to this question,[23–25] but rather answers that are not only drug-specific, but sometimes product-specific, because of the influence that the use of special drug formulations can have on a product-by-product basis.[26] For example, based on what we know about the consequences of delaying or omitting doses of the widely used, low-dose, combined estrogen–progestin oral contraceptives (as discussed below), women who omit 10–20% of their daily pills can expect imminent conception because the time gaps between doses are too long for the steroidal blockade of ovulation to be maintained.

Yet another focus—for another chapter and another time—has to do with reasons why patients frequently delay or omit doses from their prescribed dosing regimens, and why they commonly discontinue their taking of medicines that have been prescribed for indefinitely long use. At some happy time in the future, behavioral theories may enrich or improve the efficiency of efforts to drive into correspondence with the recommended regimen ambulatory patients' execution of, and persistence with, prescribed dosing regimens. For the present, behavioral theories, of which a generous sample can be found,[27] are for the most part overly complex and ill informed by reliable data on patients' dosing histories, bringing little of practical utility to measurement, analysis, or measurement-guided intervention. Furthermore, those with a primarily behavioral perspective have complicated the search for satisfactory taxonomy by strong advocacy of the fuzzily defined term "adherence," which has been enveloped in a cloak of political correctness. The literature is cluttered with statements such as "adherence in this trial was 87%," which is inherently uninterpretable: does it mean that 13% of patients never started taking the protocol-specified treatment, or that on average among those who did start (however many of those there might have been) 87% of patients took the drug against some criterion of how much drug intake is "enough" for a satisfactory outcome, or that patients who did start treatment omitted, on average, 13% of prescribed doses? Or did it mean that 13% of patients who started treatment quit after a period of treatment deemed "too short" by some criterion? When "adherence" is explicitly defined, it is usually equated with a percentage of prescribed doses taken, which, as discussed later, often falls far short of providing the full clinical explanatory power contained in dosing history data.

NEED FOR SOUND TERMINOLOGY THAT SUPPORTS MEASUREMENT AND QUANTITATIVE ANALYSIS

Given the pharmacometric focus of this chapter, it is essential to employ coherent terminology that supports quantitative analysis of both the dosing patterns and their clinical/economic correlates. To that end, the frequently used term "adherence" is probably best defined as the percentage of prescribed doses taken by those patients who are still persisting with execution of the prescribed dosing regimen. This definition at least gives the term a quantitative basis, lifting it out of the usual murky definition as "conforming to medical advice," or words to that effect. Yet, as such, it does not distinguish the three dynamically distinct, key attributes of patients' dosing histories: (i) acceptance of the principle of treatment and the start of dosing, (ii) ongoing execution of the prescribed dosing regimen, and (iii) discontinuation of dosing.

"Acceptance" and "discontinuation" are essentially dichotomous events; with the exception that some patients tend to wobble temporarily in indecision, both occur at more or less distinct moments in time. In contrast, "execution of the prescribed dosing regimen" is an ongoing process that, over time within a single patient, can sometimes correspond closely to the prescribed dosing regimen, and at other times deviate widely. Thus, it is possible for a patient to accept and start the dosing regimen, but execute more or less poorly, even though continuing for years with the dosing regimen. In contrast, a patient can accept and start the dosing regimen, execute consistently well, but discontinue after too short a period of time for clinical benefit to occur. Another patient may never accept and thus not ever start the treatment. These different results preclude the use of a single, blanket term, e.g., "adherence," for the simple reason that poor adherence is consistent with: (i) non-acceptance (with nothing known about either execution or persistence because they never occurred); (ii) acceptance but poor execution, though long persistence; (iii) acceptance and good execution, but short persistence; or (iv) acceptance but poor execution and short persistence. The effective and economical targeting of interventions to achieve a close correspondence between the patient's dosing history and the recommended dosing regimen requires that the targets be crisply defined.

To that end, this chapter uses several measurement-supporting definitions. The first is "acceptance," which signifies whether or not the patient ever starts the dosing regimen. The second is "compliance," defined as the extent to which the patient's drug dosing history conforms to the prescribed dosing regimen. One of the basic reasons for preserving the use of the term "compliance" is that it is the indexing term used by the Index Medicus, regardless of the terms used by authors of indexed papers. Moreover, the American Heart Association has routinely used the term as the descriptor of the field having to do with how well or poorly patients take prescribed drugs. This definition indicates the comparison of two time series, the prescribed dosing regimen and the dosing history, the outcome of which specifies compliance, as defined. The third definition is "persistence," defined in principle as the time between the first dose and the last dose. In practice, however, it is difficult to ascertain when a last dose occurs, and so the operational definition is that the end of "execution" occurs when compliance (as defined) falls below a certain de minimus level. These points have previously been discussed in,[19] and at the National Cancer Institute Conference on Causal Inference at Snowbird, Utah in 2001 by Vrijens and me.

If the term "adherence" is used, it can only be in the qualitative sense that "poor" adherence signifies something wrong with acceptance, execution, and/or persistence, and that "good" adherence signifies that all three were satisfactory. Those who would talk in terms of "percent adherence" risk being smitten by thunderbolts from the gods who defend terminological purity. The term "adherence rate," as used by the World Health Organization (WHO),[27] is ill considered and essentially meaningless.

PHARMACOLOGICAL BASICS

Two pharmacological basics underlie this discussion. They are the dose dependency and the time dependency of drug actions. Clinical pharmacologists emphasize the dose–response relation, and generate such data usually by varying the dose and keeping constant the time interval between doses (see Chapter 4). In contrast, the dosing patterns of ambulatory patients show that patients usually hold the dose constant, but vary the time intervals between doses.[1] These two means of varying a patient's exposure to the drug in

question are often not equivalent pharmacodynamically, even though the two types of variation can produce equal aggregate quantities of drug ingested within a given time. This inequivalence is consistent with the fact that dose timing data generally have more clinical explanatory power than aggregate dosing data.[19–22] Notwithstanding long past practice, the natural priority in clinical pharmacological research should be reassigned to learning the clinical correlates of what patients predominantly do with their prescription drugs, i.e., holding the dose constant and varying the interval between doses. So here we have, as it were, a "pharmacoepidemiological imperative" for clinical pharmacologists.

A key concept in pursuing these objectives is that of "drug exposure," which has two natural foci: external and internal. The external focus considers the time history of dosing: dose(s) taken and intervals between doses, both of which may vary. Most pharmaceuticals in current use are based on drugs that have relatively rapid turnover within the body, e.g., as noted above, 87% of frequently prescribed drugs have a plasma half-life of 12 hours or less,[9] and are formulated in dosage forms that release drug within several hours. Patients create two principal deviations from the medical intentions that motivate prescriptions and protocols: (i) delayed or omitted doses during the patient's ongoing execution of the dosing regimen,[1–5] and (ii) early discontinuation of dosing.[28–31] These two principal deviations—the former called "variable compliance with the prescribed dosing regimen," the latter called "variable persistence with the prescribed dosing regimen"—have quite different dynamics, clinical consequences, and economic consequences.[32,33] During patients' ongoing execution of prescribed dosing regimens, the average shortfall in drug intake is about 22%,[32] relative to the intake that would occur with strictly punctual execution of the prescribed dosing regimen. In addition to the product-specific clinical and public health impact of this shortfall, it creates a corresponding 22% average shortfall in revenues for the manufacturer, and, of course, a percentage decline in profits that is much higher than 22%, because of the many fixed overheads in the research-based pharmaceutical business. Prevailing patterns of short persistence, i.e., early discontinuation of treatment, show that one-half to three-quarters of patients who start treatment with antihypertensive or lipid-lowering drugs stop treatment within two years of the start of their treatment.[28–31] Thus, underlying the year-by-year growth in a chronic-use product's revenues is a large, ongoing turnover of patients and high marketing costs. If the published data on persistence with simvastatin are applicable to the entire population of treated patients, then an effective intervention to prolong persistence could treble such a chronic-use product's revenues.[34] Obviously there is an urgent need for verification of such a huge effect, and of the reliability and associated costs of the mechanisms required to achieve it.

CLINICAL PROBLEMS TO BE ADDRESSED BY PHARMACOEPIDEMIOLOGIC RESEARCH

SOME BACKGROUND

The epidemiologically informed reader will recognize from the foregoing that patients, in their varied deviations from prescribed dosing regimens, create recurring natural experiments in varied time intervals between usually constant doses. The taxonomically informed reader will recognize that these considerations define the need for a new biopharmaceutical subdiscipline, which has been called "pharmionics"—the quantitative study of patients' self-administration of prescription drugs, to learn the magnitudes and frequencies of deviations from prescribed dosing regimens.[35] One of the first pharmionic findings, though not referred to in those terms at the time of its discovery, is white-coat compliance—the improvement in compliance that occurs during the day or two prior to, and a day or two after, a scheduled visit to the doctor or investigator. This finding was first described in 1986,[11] confirmed in 1990,[12] and given the name of "white-coat compliance" by the late Alvan Feinstein.[10]

IMPACT OF WHITE-COAT COMPLIANCE ON THERAPEUTIC DRUG MONITORING

The discovery of white-coat compliance and its incidence effectively demolished much of the presumed utility of measuring the concentration of prescribed drug in plasma (therapeutic drug monitoring). Blood samples for this method are conventionally drawn at a scheduled visit, and interpreted without reliable knowledge of the patient's dosing history in the several preceding days. Those several days comprise the time period, equivalent to 3–4 plasma half-lives of the drug in question, during which the patient's intake of any of the vast majority of drugs that have plasma half-lives less than 12 hours determines the concentration of drug in blood at a particular moment (see also Chapter 4). Drug intake could have been zero during preceding weeks, but if the intake of drug is correct in the 1–2 days prior to a blood sample, the measured concentration can be in the therapeutic range. Of course, if white-coat compliance is

exuberant, and the patient opts to take extra doses to "make up" for previously omitted doses, the measured concentration may be higher than the therapeutic concentration range. In either case, measured concentration data can mislead the prescriber about the usually prevailing situation. Yet the hypnotic power of a numerical value is such that many do not recognize the lack of utility of therapeutic drug monitoring data unadjusted by reliable data on the patient's dosing history during the drug's prior 3–4 plasma half-lives. Thus, one clinical problem to be addressed by pharmacoepidemiologic research is rationalization of the uses of therapeutic drug monitoring in dosing optimization.

GETTING THE RECOMMENDED DOSE RIGHT

A broader clinical and economic problem is the identification of each new pharmaceutical product's optimal label-recommended drug dosing regimen. Recent work showed that, since 1980, one in about 4.5 newly introduced drugs has, after market introduction, undergone a 50% or greater reduction in recommended dosing regimen.[36,37] Furthermore, the frequency of such reductions has been rising steadily since 1990,[37] indicating that methods of premarketing drug development have not satisfactorily solved the problem of identifying optimal dosing regimens during premarketing drug development.

These errors in setting recommended doses not only have the obvious result that excessive drug is administered to patients prior to the discovery that a lower dose will suffice, but they also create major economic problems for the drug developer. Most pharmaceuticals are priced on the basis of drug content. Thus, a 50% reduction in prescribed dose results in more or less a 50% fall in revenues. Then, because of the many fixed overheads in pharmaceutical firms, the fall in profits is proportionately larger. In principle, the firm could compensate for a fall in recommended dose by seeking a compensating rise in the per-milligram price of the product, but this maneuver is usually unsuccessful in countries where pricing is negotiated and set at the time of product registration.

TURNING THE NATURAL EXPERIMENT IN VARIABLE DOSE TIMING TO ADVANTAGE IN EARLY DRUG DEVELOPMENT

One promising but still neglected approach to identifying the optimal dosing regimen early in drug development is to compile trial patients' drug dosing histories routinely, with a careful analysis of the magnitude and time course of the associated drug actions. In effect, this maneuver amounts to "tuning in" on the natural experiment in variable dose timing. If, for example, patients who are only taking half the prescribed dose are still experiencing the full therapeutic benefits of the drug, then one must regard such a finding as a strong indication that the prescribed dose has been set higher than necessary. The natural experiment in variable dose timing also serves to reveal the actual variability in trials that have been designed as fixed-dose studies, but in fact are revealed by pharmionic data to have widely variable intervals between doses.

THE DRUG HOLIDAY AND ITS POTENTIAL FOR MISCHIEF

A temporal pattern brought to light from the earliest studies with electronic monitoring is the drug holiday—defined as 3 or more consecutive days of omitted doses in the course of a much longer running regimen of drug administration.[1,38] The holiday has three key facets: (i) sudden discontinuation of drug intake, (ii) a period in which drug concentrations in plasma and drug actions fade away—not necessarily synchronously—and then remain absent until, (iii) a sudden resumption of dosing, sometimes accompanied by one or more extra doses.

The holiday pattern of interrupted dosing thus has the potential to trigger hazardous rebound effects in the wake of abrupt discontinuation, or hazardous recurrent first-dose effects in the wake of abrupt resumption of dosing. Naturally, only some drugs are prone to rebound effects, and perhaps only those with recognized first-dose effects are subject to recurrent first-dose effects. But all drugs' actions will fade, sooner or later, during a holiday that lasts long enough. Naturally, therapeutic benefits of treatment come to a halt, with clinical and economic consequences that are specific to the product in question, and to the therapeutic field in which it is being used. The hazardous potential of drug holidays is, in effect, toxicity from underdosing.

Among the anti-infective drugs, drug holidays appear to be a major stimulus to the emergence of drug-resistant microorganisms, given that (i) holidays recur, and (ii) each holiday twice takes the patient through a zone of antimicrobial drug concentration that is at once low enough to allow microbial replication, but still high enough to exert selection pressure for emergence of drug-resistant microorganisms.[22] Understanding the dynamics of emergent antimicrobial drug resistance in infective microorganisms is a leading worldwide medical problem.

The incidence of drug holidays in medically unselected patients is about 2.4 holidays per patient per year, concentrated in the roughly one-third of such patients who are "holiday prone," and hyper-concentrated in about half of that one-third.[1,35] The meaning of "medically unselected" is that the patients in question were not previously in major, prior treatment programs, emerging either as treatment failures or successes. Among failures, dose omissions are likely to recur frequently, some of which break into frank holidays; among those whose treatment has been successful, dose omissions and holidays are likely to be relatively infrequent. It is not surprising that the outcome of a prior course of ambulatory pharmacotherapy would be a source of selection bias toward either exceptionally high (in the case of successful treatment) or exceptionally low (in the case of failed treatment) compliance. These attributes can be expected usually to carry over into a next course of ambulatory drug treatment. A practical consequence of this behavior is the need for both caution and reliable compilation of drug dosing histories in trials designed to assess a new medicine in patients who have failed to respond to an existing treatment. Obviously, if treatment failure had its origins in poor compliance with the dosing regimen for a prior treatment, it is likely that compliance will be poor with the dosing regimen for the new treatment.

The foregoing principles arise from the fact that compliance, as defined, can now be seen, based on reliable dosing history data, to be almost entirely a patient attribute, not a drug or disease attribute, although of course the patient behavior could be encouraged by the effects of their disease or drug.[1] For several decades, pharmaceutical promotion and expert sayings (unperturbed by reliable data) have maintained that compliance problems would be solved by the advent of convenient, side-effect-free pharmaceuticals. We now have numerous such products in a variety of therapeutic fields, but compliance problems appear to continue.

Finding the temporal sequence of drug holiday leading to adverse reaction is necessary though not sufficient for proof of the holiday's causal role in the adverse reaction. These precepts have been neglected in the consideration of adverse drug reactions, and warrant focused future research. It seems reasonable to expect that some otherwise valuable drugs are rejected on safety grounds because of adverse events in the small minority of holiday-prone patients, who, if identified *a priori*, could be either managed satisfactorily, or, if not, the drug in question could (should?) be deemed contraindicated in holiday-prone patients.

The best documented example of holiday-triggered adverse effects, aside from emergent antimicrobial drug resistance, is provided by the class of β-adrenergic receptor antagonists that lack intrinsic sympathomimetic activity (ISA). This class of agents—usually referred to as the non-ISA β-blockers—includes the most widely used β-blockers, propranolol, metoprolol, atenolol, and others. Each of these drugs carries an emphasized warning (by means of its being placed in its own box, separate from the main text of the labeling) in its US labeling, cautioning against sudden discontinuation of the drug. Two key mechanisms underlie this hazard. First, during prolonged use of non-ISA β-blockers there occurs a gradual upregulation of β-adrenergic receptors, which has no perceptible effect as long as the receptor blockade is maintained by ongoing dosing. Second, when the intake of the β-blocking agent suddenly stops, the drug concentrations decay with a plasma half-life of a few hours, so that within a day or less there is no β-blocker detectable in plasma, thus unblocking the upregulated receptors, so that they become hyperresponsive to surges of epinephrine or norepinephrine release, as occur physiologically during exercise or in response to various stimuli, classically epitomized as "fight, flight, or fear." With the β-adrenergic receptor blockade ended, the upregulated adrenergic receptors start to return to their normal level, but they do so with a half-life of about 1 week. Thus, there is a period of several weeks after abrupt cessation of β-receptor blocker intake during which unblocked, still upregulated receptors generate excessive adrenergic activity, which includes increased aggregation of platelets and vascular spasm—both recognized triggers of worsened coronary heart disease, onset of angina pectoris, and/or myocardial infarction. The magnitude of risk created by drug holidays in patients prescribed non-ISA β-adrenergic receptors has yet to be quantified, because it offsets the very considerable benefit that these drugs have in the management of coronary heart disease, trials of which have been run without attempting to identify holiday-prone patients.

The only quantitative risk assessment of this phenomenon comes from Psaty et al., who found a relative risk of 4–6 of incident coronary heart disease in partially compliant hypertensive patients prescribed non-ISA β-blockers.[39] In that study, compliance was estimated from pharmacy data on intervals between refills of β-blocker prescriptions—a relatively error-prone measure of aggregate drug intake, not capable of identifying which patients were prone to have multi-day drug holidays, as opposed to patients who occasionally missed a single dose. Thus, the holiday-linked risk in the subset of patients who were holiday-prone was probably underestimated in this study.

THE IMPORTANCE OF OFFSET TIMES: HOW LONG DRUG ACTION CONTINUES AFTER A LAST-TAKEN DOSE

The foregoing considerations have revealed how little is known about how long it takes for drug actions to fade, after

a multi-week period of dosing stops, to therapeutically de minimus levels. We certainly have extensive information on how drug concentrations decline and fade away, but only the naïve believe that such information suffices as a comprehensive description of how drug actions decline after dosing halts. Certainly there are a few drugs, e.g., theophylline, whose actions wax and wane synchronously with the waxing or waning of concentrations of the drug in plasma, but many drugs' actions lag well behind changes in their concentrations in plasma.[40]

Basic and clinical pharmacologists usually provide detailed descriptions of the time course of onset of drug action, but, aside from descriptions of the effects of a single dose, relatively little attention has been paid, until recently, to the time course of offset of drug actions, after a period of relatively long running dosing is halted. The clinical response to a single dose of drug does not provide an adequate description of the offset times that prevail after weeks or months of drug use, during which various physiological counterregulatory adaptations to the drug's primary actions develop and modulate, to a greater or lesser extent, its pharmacodynamics.[40] An illustrative example is provided by the widely used β-adrenergic antagonists, e.g., timolol maleate and levobunolol, which have single-dose ocular hypotensive effects that last for 12–24 hours, but, after some weeks of use, the post-dose ocular hypotensive effect lengthens to several days or longer.[41]

A group of widely used drugs with surprising differences in post-dose duration of effect are the three leading serotonin-reuptake inhibitor antidepressant drugs, paroxetine, sertraline, and fluoxetine. Each of these drugs requires several weeks of dosing for antidepressant actions to develop fully, but paroxetine loses its antidepressant effects essentially completely within 48 hours after a last-taken once-daily dose.[42] Sertraline's actions have substantially waned by 4–5 days after the last-taken dose, but fluoxetine's actions were still fully expressed at the end of the 7-day period of the "placebo-substitution-for- active" trial that provided these data.[42]

No one would or could have guessed that such a short offset time might be possible, given the uniformly very slow onset of action of antidepressant drugs. It required experimental demonstration, the clinical consequences of which are presently the subject of headlines.[43] Such marked dynamic asymmetries between onset and offset times are a hallmark of nonlinear pharmacodynamics,[40] making it impossible to predict offset times from onset times with any confidence—in stark contrast to the generally linear characteristics of pharmacokinetics, where the accuracy of such extrapolations is the rule rather than the exception (see Chapter 4). The current controversy over suicide hazards of antidepressant treatment of adolescents has not been adequately informed about these marked differences in offset times, especially when seen in the context of the much more erratic drug regimen compliance that prevails in adolescents versus adults.[44] It would seem that paroxetine's use in adolescents is potentially explosive, on the basis of available evidence on adolescent compliance patterns and the stunningly rapid loss of antidepressant drug actions after brief cessation of paroxetine dosing. It is reassuring to know that fluoxetine's use in adolescents is both effective and free of severe adverse reactions, including suicide,[45] but, in light of the markedly longer offset time of fluoxetine's actions, relative to other leading SSRI antidepressant drugs, one cannot conclude that what is true for fluoxetine is also true for other drugs in the class.

DESIGNING DRUG REGIMENS FOR OPTIMAL FORGIVENESS

Drug regimen design has a long and justified reputation for being difficult, and, as noted above, may be getting more so. The rising incidence of postmarketing dose reductions since 1990 has two major alternative explanations. First, it may be the consequence primarily of more mistakes being made during drug development. Or, it may be that increasingly great scrutiny is applied to recommended regimens, in hopes of finding a justification for cutting the recommended dose, and thereby cutting costs, as pharmaceutical prices spiral upward. Underlying reasons for both explanations are discussed elsewhere.[37] Of course, these potential reasons are not necessarily mutually exclusive.

An underlying but largely neglected issue is that of how much forgiveness to design into a drug regimen. "Forgiveness" is defined as the drug's post-dose duration of effective therapeutic action minus the recommended dosing interval.[1] As one can infer from points already discussed, forgiveness values vary widely. For example, the data of Rosenbaum *et al.*[42] indicate that the forgiveness for paroxetine is <24 hours, whereas that for fluoxetine is >7 days. The forgiveness for the widely prescribed β-adrenergic receptor blocker atenolol is about 6 hours, whereas that for the little-used drug of the same class betaxolol is >24 hours.[46] The forgiveness for the low-dose estrogen–progestin oral contraceptive pill is 12–24 hours.[47] One of the probably counterproductive consequences of the prevailing strong desires, especially in the hypertension field, to formulate for once-daily dosing has been to put into the market, as we see with atenolol, quite unforgiving products, which, of course, do not provide continuity of action when subjected to common, relatively small variations in intervals between doses. Thus, we have the paradox that the quest for once-daily dosing is done in the name of "better compliance," but seems to have resulted in many relatively unforgiving once-daily products that cannot provide continuity of action in any but the most punctual of patients who use such products. Only one patient in about 6 is categorically punctual, in remedicating at virtually constant intervals of 24 hours;[1] others manifest different degrees of variation in interdose intervals and thus risk interruptions in the actions of less forgiving products.

Tomorrow's drug regimen designer must work against, and resolve, a set of conflicting quantitative considerations. On the one hand, a product with a large degree of forgiveness can be expected to nullify the negative effects of all but the most egregious errors in compliance—a recipe, all other things being equal, for exceptional effectiveness, in contrast to relatively unforgiving products that can be expected to provide full effectiveness only in the most punctual of patients, who can be as few as 15% of a trial or treatment population. On the other hand, a product with a large degree of forgiveness is a natural target for dose-cutters who want to minimize pharmaceutical costs. Naturally, cutting doses also cuts forgiveness. Thus, a key task of the regimen designer is to find the right middle ground, where forgiveness is large enough to ensure full effectiveness in a substantial majority of patients, which means that full effectiveness prevails in not only the strictly punctual, but also in those whose interdose intervals sometimes wobble, and will sometimes involve single omitted doses.

The crucial information for taking a proactive approach to designing regimens with optimized forgiveness is the drug's post-dose duration of effective therapeutic action. Estimating this parameter can be difficult and error prone. Note that post-dose duration of action can, with some drugs, be predominantly a pharmacodynamic parameter, not a pharmacokinetic one. Those who believe that a drug's plasma half-life provides sufficient information for setting its interdose interval are doomed to overestimate the dosing requirements for many drugs. It is a matter of conjecture how much this "kinetocentric" view has misled regimen definitions, being perhaps a leading reason for the progressive rise in postmarketing dose-reductions since 1990.[37]

METHODOLOGIC PROBLEMS TO BE ADDRESSED BY PHARMACOEPIDEMIOLOGIC RESEARCH

Good and multiply repeated results from small studies confirm the prevalence of errors in each of the three phases of ambulatory pharmacotherapy. Many patients for whom one or another type of long-term pharmacotherapy is indicated and prescribed fail to begin treatment: a failure of acceptance. Many other patients commence treatment, but execute the prescribed (and presumably optimal) regimen poorly: a failure of compliance, and of all patients who commence treatment, a majority (it would seem from published data) discontinue treatment early, often too soon to derive benefit from the treatment: a failure of persistence.

Electronic monitoring provides a reliable basis for compiling drug dosing histories, which, in turn, provide the evidential basis for judging each of these three types of therapy-compromising errors. Usually these errors escape clinical detection.

When a patient walks out of the physician's office/ surgery with a written prescription in hand into a community with multiple pharmacies, there is no way, unless special arrangements are made, for the physician to know that the prescription was taken to a pharmacy, dispensed, and collected by the patient. Some medical groups rely on faxed prescriptions, which alert a chosen pharmacy that the patient should soon appear to collect dispensed medicine. In principle, if the prescription is not collected by the patient, the pharmacy can notify the prescriber, but how often such a link actually operates, and its effectiveness, are pharmacoepidemiologic research topics. It is not just a matter of counting dispensed but uncollected medicines, because many prescriptions are for medicines of modest efficacy for minor indications, where it is a medically trivial issue whether the patient takes the prescribed medicine or not. There are, however, other situations in which the medicines are medically crucial: antihypertensives, cardiac antiarrhythmics, oral hypoglycemics, antidepressants, antipsychotics, lipid lowering agents, bone-conserving agents, and the like. There is a clear need not only for expanded pharmacoepidemiology studies to demonstrate the extent and magnitude of the problems at this point in the pharmacotherapeutic chain, but also to devise permanent methods that can identify therapeutic lapses and direct a suitable alert to a responsible professional in the chain.

The prevalence of errors in drug regimen execution is another area of disconnect between clinical awareness and the many studies documenting the prevalence of delayed and omitted doses in many fields of pharmacotherapy, emphasizing much more the cross-field commonality of the error patterns than field-specific error patterns.[1] This body of work supports the view that the patterns of dose omission are similar across various therapeutic fields in the range of aggregate omissions and frequency of multi-day holidays. Field-specific error patterns do not appear to be a prominent

feature, though further studies may modify this view somewhat. Here again, however, prescribers have no reliable way to detect such errors. They can inquire of the patient, but in doing so they encounter the twin problems of patients' recall and willingness to disclose dosing lapses. Perhaps electronic monitoring should be routinely used with new prescriptions for medicines above a certain degree of therapeutic importance, so that both prescriber and pharmacist can identify compliance problems early, and move to minimize their occurrence. Here, too, there is a need for expanded pharmacoepidemiologic and pharmacoeconomic studies to demonstrate the extent and magnitude of the problems at this further point in the pharmacotherapeutic chain, and to transcend the study mode, by devising methods suitable for use in routine practice, to identify regimen-execution problems early on, and move, by the most cost-efficient ways, to minimize their occurrence.

Finally, there is the problem of short persistence. In this arena, there is a need for much more basic pharmacoepidemiologic research to understand the big differences in persistence between the large clinical trials and everyday practice. Taking the major trials of drugs in the statin class as examples, these trials have routinely reported that over 90% of enrolled patients complete the protocol's treatment plan—usually a 5-year treatment period. In contrast, the published studies on everyday practice have been designed to exclude the economic considerations arising from the patient's need to pay. The upshot of this design feature has been that the enrolled patients are essentially on some kind of social assistance program, which provides full payment for prescription drugs. That selection feature brings in its wake patients who tend to come from the lowermost socioeconomic stratum, where many more things go wrong, and with greater consequence, than at higher socioeconomic levels. The results of these studies speak for themselves: more than half the patients started on antihypertensive[28,29] or statin[30,31] treatment have discontinued the treatment before the second anniversary of their commencement of treatment. Pharmacoepidemiologic studies on drug regimen persistence are needed at all socioeconomic levels, designed with recognition that the economic factors are an integral part of the story and so need to be studied and understood, not treated as extraneous. A final point in respect to the seemingly long persistence in the big trials: the vast majority of patients do indeed complete the series of scheduled visits called for by the protocol, but whether or not they are actually continuing to take the trial medications will continue to be an open question as long as trialists naively continue to rely on returned tablet counts to estimate compliance. It is quite possible for patients to go through the motions of continuing with the trial while taking little or none of the protocol-specified medicines, but returning empty medicine bottles at each visit.

CURRENTLY AVAILABLE SOLUTIONS

AVAILABLE METHODS

With the exception of electronic monitoring, none of the available methods for estimating ambulatory patients' dosing histories can provide information on dose timing and interdose intervals. Instead, they provide a variably reliable estimate of aggregate drug intake during a defined period of observation. These methods are described earlier, in the second section of the introduction.

APPLICATIONS OF AVAILABLE METHODS

To have an overview of currently available solutions, it is useful to recognize that "solutions" imply a three-step process. The first is defining a problem, in this case reliable evidence that patients' faulty execution of prescribed drug regimens creates clinical and economic problems in ambulatory drug trials and routine medical care. The second is bringing together adequate methods of measurement and interventional procedures that can identify where such problems exist and what steps can be taken to improve them. The third is communicating those findings and translating them into medical practice.

Defining the Impact of Poor Compliance

The Example of Oral Steroidal Contraceptives
Oral steroidal contraception is the sole major therapeutic field in which all three steps have been taken. The history of this accomplishment is exemplary for other fields, both in terms of experimental design to produce sound evidence on which to base labeling instructions, and how the instructions have been written. It is also noteworthy because oral steroidal contraception is the mode of pharmaceutical intervention with which we have more use-experience, in both length of exposure and numbers of patients exposed, than any other pharmaceutical field.

By 1970, after about 8 years of marketing of oral contraceptives, it had become evident that users of the combined estrogen–progestin oral contraceptives, as then formulated, were at elevated risk of sometimes catastrophic thromboembolic phenomena: sudden death, pulmonary emboli, acute myocardial infarctions, and stroke. It was also evident that oral steroidal contraception enjoyed great popularity, as it provided essentially complete protection against unwanted conception, except in women who missed many doses from the once-daily dosing regimen. Return to fertility, for women seeking to conceive, was prompt and uncomplicated. A consensus formed among contraceptive researchers and regulators that the underlying blood clotting disorder could be normalized by considerably reducing the estrogen content of the daily pill. That change was made in 1970–71. It reduced the risk of catastrophic thromboembolic events to, or very near to, levels in untreated women— obviously a major pharmacoepidemiologic success story in its own right, but beyond the scope of this discussion.

Not long thereafter, contraceptive researchers began observing that minor lapses in dosing were leading to unprecedented numbers of conceptions, whereas such errors with the previous high-dose pills had not.[47] Those observations led to a series of controlled studies, starting in 1979 and continuing through the 1980s, in which placebo pills were substituted for active pills. Volunteers in these studies underwent serial sampling of plasma to detect how soon after cessation of active drug intake one would see the surge in luteinizing hormone concentration in plasma, which is the recognized hormonal trigger for ovulation. The timing of the surge in luteinizing hormone levels thus indicated the end of the pill-induced, steroidal blockade of ovulation, allowing "breakthrough" ovulation and the possibility of conception. Most of the placebo-substitution-for-active-drug studies were done in volunteers who had previously had a tubal ligation, thus precluding an unwanted conception. Five such studies were done during the 1980s, and are referenced in the summary paper by Guillebaud,[48] which also gives the consensus interpretation of the five placebo-substitution-for-active-drug studies: the risk of breakthrough ovulation begins to rise at about the 36th hour after a last-taken active pill, i.e., 12 hours after a missed daily pill. A fundamental assumption in the interpretation of these studies is that the blinded substitution of one or a series of placebo pills for active pills has effects bioequivalent to those that occur when a patient, in routine clinical use of a low-dose oral contraceptive, spontaneously omits one or more once-daily doses. That assumption has never been challenged— an important point, as the placebo-substitution-for-active-drug design has subsequently been carried over into a number of other therapeutic fields, as discussed below.

These results prompted a revision of the UK labeling of the low-dose, combined oral contraceptive products to include the following instructions to patients, varying with when the patient discovers that the daily dose has been delayed, or omitted. In summary,[48] they inform patients to start a 7-day course of back-up barrier contraception (foam and/or diaphragm) when they are more than 12 hours late in taking their regular daily pill; if yesterday's dose was omitted, the patient should take both yesterday's and today's pills and institute a 7-day course of back-up barrier contraception; if two days of pills have been omitted, the patient is to take two pills today and two pills tomorrow, and institute a 7-day course of back-up barrier contraception; if more than two pills have been omitted, the patient is instructed to discard the pill-pack, institute back-up barrier contraception, continue it until the next menstrual period occurs, and then start on a new pill-pack.

In the US, the motivation for including such information in oral contraceptive labeling came from several nonprofit foundations, which worked with FDA staff to write acceptable labeling that was then mandated for all products in the class. The oral contraceptive manufacturers remained aloof from this process. The specific wording can be found in the "instructions for patients" section of the labeling of any of the combined estrogen-progestin oral contraceptive products. One difference between the US and UK labeling is that the former does not call for any special steps to be taken until the 48th hour after a last-taken pill.

In retrospect, it would appear that the forgiveness of the old, high-dose oral contraceptives was on the order of several days, whereas the low-dose products provide only about 12 hours of forgiveness. The US labeling blurs that point by its implication of 24 hours of forgiveness. The difference arises from variance in the original placebo-substitution-for-active-drug studies, which might usefully be repeated with today's methods, which now include direct visualization of ovulation by ultrasonic scan.

Against the background of the foregoing discussion, Table 46.1 shows the estimated conception rates with the low-dose oral steroidal contraceptives, together with the conception rates measured in the premarketing trials of the 5-year norgestrel implant, which is the ultimately forgiving product, because of its automatic provision of continuous exposure to the contraceptive progestin, d-norgestrel.

Unless the patient opts for early discontinuation, human involvement with the implant is limited to the decision to replace or not the implant at the 5-year point. The 0.05% (1 in 2000 per year) conception rate is the lowest conception rate of any of the steroidal contraceptive products.[49] The implant has, however, many problems, which are summarized in Urquhart,[26] so it is not very widely used, after a brief initial surge in popularity. The daily, low-dose estrogen–progestin pill remains by far the leading pharmaceutical contraceptive.

For reference, the conception rate in pregnancy-seeking women of reproductive age is about 80% per year.

If the British interpretation of the placebo-substitution-for-active-drug studies is correct, it means that patients can take 100% of prescribed doses of the low-dose, combined oral contraceptive but still have unwanted conceptions due simply to erratic timing of doses, leading to intervals between doses that sometimes exceed 36 hours. Moreover, one can have 363 days of absolutely punctual dosing, then miss 2 days' doses and conceive. It is a cautionary lesson for researchers who believe that taking at least 80% of prescribed doses is an across-the-board satisfactory level of compliance with prescribed dosing regimens. With the low-dose oral contraceptives, missing 20% of the scheduled doses could be expected to permit many episodes of breakthrough ovulation and conception usually occurring within a few months of such misuse.

A natural question, of course, concerns the effectiveness of the labeling information, in giving women a series of steps to follow to minimize the risk of unwanted conception when they have delayed or omitted scheduled doses. The information provided in the labeling is the evidence-based foundation for sound intervention, but clearly not a complete program for helping patients maintain fully effective contraception. Limited studies with electronically monitored pill packs demonstrate the potential utility of having exact dose timing information for both patients and their caregivers,[50,51] but more needs to be done to learn how best to integrate a patient's dosing history with the evidence-based instructions for avoiding breakthrough ovulation.

The provision of evidence-based information on "what to do if you miss a dose" in oral contraceptive labeling establishes an important precedent for other chronic-use pharmaceuticals for ambulatory care. The same question invariably applies for any chronic-use medicine prescribed in ambulatory care. A proposal has been made to FDA to include evidence-based information on "what to do if you miss a dose" in conjunction with their plans to revise the format of labeling of drugs primarily used in ambulatory care.[52]

Other Studies Defining the Clinical Impact of Poor Compliance

Table 46.2 lists drugs for which there is reasonable evidence that deviations from prescribed dosing regimens result in

Table 46.1. Annualized conception rate[49]

Mode	Perfect use	Typical use
Daily pill	0.1%	5.0%
5-year implant	0.05%	0.05%

Table 46.2. Drugs whose actions are or appear to be compliance-dependent

---

Placebo-substitution-for-active-drug (PSA) study results
Combined estrogen–progestin oral contraceptive steroids[47–49]
Atenolol[46]
Betaxolol[46]
Trandolapril[53]
Enalapril[53,54]
Amlodipine[53–55]
Diltiazem[56]
Bendroflumethazide[55]
Nifedipine[55]
Paroxetine[42,57]
Sertraline[42]
Fluoxetine[42]

Comparison with assured exposure
Penicillin[58]
Sulfadiazine[58]
Norgestrel[59]
Anti-tuberculosis drugs[60,61]

Successful measurement-guided intervention in failed therapy
Triple-drug therapy for arterial hypertension[62]

Drug regimen intensification studies
Insulin[63]
Risedronate[64–66]

Compliance-stratified outcomes of randomized, placebo-controlled drug trials
Cholestyramine[67]
Gemfibrozil[68]

Observed clinical correlates of variable compliance
Warfarin[69]
Estradiol[70]
Phenytoin[13]
Carbamazepine[13]
Pilocarpine[71,72]
Cyclosporin A[73–75]
Azathiaprine[76]
Allopurinol[77]
Inhaled corticosteroids for asthma[78,79]
Anti-retroviral drugs[80–83]

---

substantive clinical problems. Its listings are discussed in the following sections.

Methodologic Lessons

Demonstrating that partial, poor, or variable compliance influences the magnitude and timing of drug actions, and therefore clinical outcomes, has been a methodological challenge. One of the strongest methods, where ethical considerations allow it to be used, is the placebo-substitution-for-active-drug protocol. We have already seen its application in the oral contraceptive field, and the central role it

played in establishing evidence-based labeling for patients, informing them of the steps needed to minimize the risk of conception when they have delayed or omitted oral contraceptive doses. Naturally, there are ethical constraints on placebo-substitution-for-active-drug applications, but it has been successfully carried over from the contraceptive field into the evaluation of antihypertensive and antidepressant drugs, with some notable surprises. One, already mentioned, is the stunningly rapid offset of action of paroxetine, within 48 hours after dosing stops.[41] Another is the strikingly long post-dose duration of the antihypertensive effect of bendrofluthiazide[55]—6 days of continuing antihypertensive action after placebo substitution, yet the drug in question has a plasma half-life of about 3 hours.[9] It is a striking example of a drug whose pharmacodynamics completely dominate in determining its post-dose duration of therapeutic action.

It is remarkable, however, that none of the placebo-substitution-for-active-drug studies to date have included the study of what happens when, after a period of placebo substitution, active drug is reinstituted. This sequence, after all, is the one followed by most patients when they enter into a drug holiday. It is not a minor point, as we can see with the remarkable story of paroxetine, and the striking rapidity of its loss of antidepressant action after dosing is interrupted.[42] Suppose, having incurred that sudden loss of antidepressant action, a patient resumes punctual dosing: how long will it take for full antidepressant action to be restored? Will it be the 10–20 days that are required when dosing first starts, or will it be some shorter period? There is no way to judge the answer, which can only be provided by experiment. If it were to turn out that a short lapse of 2–3 days in paroxetine dosing leads to a fortnight of loss of full antidepressant drug action, one would have to conclude that paroxetine is a poor choice of drug in patients who are less than fully punctual in dosing.

Another strong method, though limited to special circumstances, is a randomized, controlled trial that includes one arm in which the drug in question is unequivocally provided in strict continuity. The comparative statistics between "perfect" and "typical" use with the low-dose oral contraceptives[49] approximate that design, as do the data from the 5-year norgestrel implant, as discussed above. A direct comparison, within a single trial, was reported many years ago by the late Alvan Feinstein and colleagues, who followed 453 patients for 5 years, randomized between (i) monthly depot injections of penicillin, professionally administered, or patient-administered regimens of either (ii) daily oral penicillin or (iii) daily oral sulfadiazine, for the prevention of recurrent streptococcal infections and recurrent acute rheumatic fever.[58] Assured continuity of drug exposure establishes what is called "method effectiveness," which, in the case of penicillin and d-norgestrel, is essentially complete, though that desirable outcome may not be realized with other agents.

Feinstein's work additionally showed major differences in clinical outcome between good and poor compliers with the oral regimens as evidence of dose-dependent drug action, where the recipients of the oral regimens were found to be divided roughly equally between good and poor compliance. The randomization of patients among the three groups assured that any hidden variable, e.g., a "noncompliant lifestyle" or other "mystery factor," associated with poor compliance was equally distributed in all three groups. The hypothesis that any such factor might interfere with penicillin's beneficial actions is refuted by the essentially complete prevention of both streptococcal infections and recurrent acute rheumatic fever when exposure was assured, notwithstanding that about half of the recipients of the depot injections would have been poor compliers with an oral dosing regimen.

Refutation of the "hidden variable" concern is an important point, because the naturally occurring variations in drug exposure, created by patients' dosing patterns, can be a rich source of information on dose- and time-dependent actions of the drug in question. Yet this view is only tenable if we can be assured that there is no hidden variable, associated with both outcome and poor or partial compliance, which can serve as a confounder or effect modifier, modifying the ordinary dose- and time-response relations of the drug in question. This possibility is a natural consequence of the fact that a patient's dosing history is an observational phenomenon, not an experimentally controlled variable. In seeking to infer pharmacometric causality, i.e., that observed drug responses can be interpreted as dose- and time-dependent consequences of those dosing histories, one has to be cautious and look for discrepancies between the drug's known pharmacokinetic and pharmacodynamic attributes and the observed exposure–response relations. Substantive discrepancies would point to the operation of some kind of "mystery factor," rather than drug exposure itself.

It is also noteworthy that the once-daily oral form of progestin-only oral contraceptives has the poorest contraceptive efficacy of any of the steroidal contraceptive products.[49,59] These of course are not side-by-side comparisons, but their joint interpretation is facilitated by the fact that product-specific, contraceptive efficacy data are generally stable over time. The logical interpretation is that assured exposure to norgestrel provides reliable contraception, and that the vagaries of mistimed or omitted doses, as inevitably occur with oral dosing regimens, result in unreliable contraception. The conclusion is strengthened by the fact that oral norgestrel is the least forgiving of all pharmaceutical products for which forgiveness values are known; its forgiveness averages a miniscule 3 hours.[59] Finally, the conception rates measured in patients receiving the 3-monthly injectable progestin, DepoProvera, are only slightly higher than the rate found in recipients of the 5-year implant.[49] Thus, believers in a "mystery factor" must explain how it is that the factor appears when oral regimens are prescribed, but disappears when depot or implant formulations are prescribed. The plausible explanation is that drug exposure, not an undefined hidden variable, is the crucial factor—a long-recognized pharmacological imperative, not a fantasy of pharmacometrically challenged trial analysts. The logical time for invoking hidden variables that modify drug response will arrive when pharmacometric projections of the time course based on reliable pharmionic data cannot satisfactorily account for observed drug responses.

When ethical considerations preclude the placebo-substitution-for-active-drug method, and depot or implant methods of drug administration are not available, one is left to rely on other approaches to estimating the effects of variable drug exposure on clinical outcomes and their surrogates.

Probably the most powerful approach is to bring to bear measurement-guided efforts to improve compliance and persistence, looking to see the clinical and economic changes that follow in the wake of substantial improvements therein. For research purposes, it is important to compile pre-intervention baseline data, so that the effect of a subsequent intervention is clear. Alternatively, a parallel design is possible, with one group receiving treatment as usual, while another group receives the compliance-persistence enhancing intervention. There are pros and cons to both approaches. Burnier et al. used the serial approach.[62] While he and his colleagues never established a pre-intervention baseline of compliance data in their "drug refractory" patients, they reasonably inferred from the consistent lack of response to the sequence of prior escalations of antihypertensive treatment that poor compliance had been responsible for prior non-response in those patients whose hypertension was suddenly corrected when they achieved full compliance.

Capturing the consequences of spontaneously occurring drug holidays is facilitated by the unidirectional flow of causality, so that demonstration of the sequence of holiday followed by effects, plus pharmacological plausibility, provide strong support for causal inference. The fact that holidays recur frequently in some holiday-prone patients[1] provides the opportunity for repetition. Cramer *et al.* reported that their observation of the sequence of drug holiday leading to epileptic seizure accounted, in their view, for 12 of 16 epileptic seizures that occurred during their periods of electronic monitoring in a group of epileptics.[13] Of course, it is not an easy task to have the requisite measurement capabilities in place to capture clinical events that occur before, during, and after a drug holiday whose occurrence must, for ethical reasons, be spontaneous. Patient diaries are an obvious choice for capturing such data, but one must recognize that their use is fraught with inaccuracies, captured in a recent study using electronically monitored diaries that time-stamped each entry, showing that only 11% of entries were close enough in time to the actual events recorded to be plausible.[84] Also, a devastating error for the inference of causality is to misrecord the time of a clinical event, so that the recorded sequence is effects followed by holiday. On a hopeful note, the increasing number of automatic or semi-automatic monitoring devices may facilitate the reliable capture of holiday-triggered events.

Developing Methods to Improve Compliance

The advent and successive reductions in the cost of electronic monitoring methods for compiling ambulatory patients' dosing histories represent one cornerstone of effective attack on the problems created by patients' variable execution and persistence with prescribed regimens, especially so when those errors are clinically unrecognized. The question of interventional procedures to improve compliance and persistence appears to be much simpler and more straightforward than behaviorists have long been predicting, as noted earlier. The study by Cramer and Rosenheck of an especially difficult group of patients—alcoholic psychotics—shows that about 75% of such patients, who had been selected for taking half or less of their prescribed medicines, could be brought up to nearly full compliance by a simple scheme of showing each patient how to link his/her dosing to routines in his/her daily life.[85] This simple maneuver cannot be expected to work in all patients, as there are clearly some who have few or no daily routines, but the ability to bring three-quarters or more of formerly poor compliers up to a level of drug exposure sufficient for them to realize full or nearly full benefits of prescribed medicines projects a major advance in the quality of ambulatory medicine.

As for short persistence, the IMPACT study,[64–66] the results of which have been subsequently confirmed by the THAMES study,[86] show that simple forms of motivational reinforcement can succeed in achieving extended persistence.

The key to both the Cramer–Rosenheck work and the IMPACT and THAMES studies is reliable compilation of patients' dosing histories, so that intervention is targeted to real, not imaginary, errors. Also, feedback of the dosing history data to patients as well as to caregivers is a basic element in the interventional process; its objectivity and precision preclude hyperbole about the dosing history.

A great deal of practical learning remains to be done, aimed at converging on what measurement-guided methods work best. It is very much a work in progress that is presently gaining impetus from growing recognition of the economic costs involved, especially of short persistence, and the interactions between poor compliance and short persistence.

Applying Approaches to Improve Compliance

Forcing Continuity of Exposure through Directly Observed Therapy

Tuberculosis provides a different source of evidence for the importance of maintaining continuity of drug exposure for good outcomes of treatment, and an example of a successful intervention. Observational data around 1980 indicated a looming public health crisis in major cities in the US, from increasing prevalence of multi-drug resistant tubercle bacilli. The problem worsened with the advent of AIDS in the late 1970s. These problems led the New York City Public Health Department to launch an empirical counterattack on TB, in the form of "directly observed therapy" (DOT), which simplified the drug dosing regimens from their original several times daily versions to four much larger doses per week, given at the TB clinic under direct observation of the staff. The markedly improved results, both in terms of cure rate and emergence of multi-drug resistance,[60] led to essentially worldwide adoption of the DOT scheme, which has subsequently been simplified further into the so-called short-course DOT, known as DOTs.[61]

Note that condensing a once to thrice per day dosing regimen into a several times a week dosing regimen involves a large increase in each dose taken. Fortunately, the anti-TB drugs have wide enough therapeutic indices to permit this revision to be safely made, but there are many anti-infective drugs in current use that would pose unacceptable toxicity if the same maneuver were applied to them. Thus, the DOT approach has remained largely a one-off solution for TB, not generalizable to other major infectious diseases. The key element in the DOT story, however, is the dramatic improvement in treatment results when the dosing regimen was shifted from unobserved, patient-administered, once- to thrice-daily dosing, to professionally observed, four times weekly administration. There is no evident basis for assuming that compliance-linked lifestyle or other mystery factors change when DOT is instituted, so the logical conclusion is that, here too, assured continuity of drug action is the crucial factor in the improved outcomes of DOT versus conventional dosing regimens.

Successful Measurement-Guided Intervention in Failed Therapy

As another example of a successful intervention, Burnier and his colleagues at the University Hospital in Lausanne, Switzerland, showed the prominent role played by clinically unrecognized noncompliance with prescribed antihypertensive drug dosing regimens.[62] They studied a series of 53 patients who had sequentially been referred to their hypertension clinic for evaluation of their "drug-resistant hypertension." The admitting diagnosis was made on the basis of each patient's failure to respond to a series of antihypertensive drug regimens, escalated in steps to so-called "triple therapy," in which three drugs of proven efficacy were eventually prescribed to each nonresponding patient. Burnier et al. interposed 60 days of electronic monitoring to compile dosing histories of each patient, prior to launching the usual diagnostic workup, looking for rare causes of drug-resistant hypertension: renal artery stenosis, elevated intracranial pressure, or a catecholamine-secreting adrenal medullary tumor. They made it clear to patients from the outset that the electronically monitored drug packages were meant to inform both them and the hypertension specialist of how well the patient was executing the prescribed drug regimens. About a third of the patients took that information as the basis for deciding that the time had come to start taking the medicines; several had episodes of hypotension, as the three-drug regimen was, when actually executed, clearly too powerful. Some patients returned with empty bottles but a sparse dosing record, which became the basis for pointed instructions on how/why to take the drugs. The upshot was that slightly over half the patients, initially diagnosed as being drug refractory hypertensives, were instead identified as clinically unrecognized noncompliers, who ended up achieving satisfactory blood pressure control.[62] The remaining patients, who complied satisfactorily but continued to have hypertension, went on to the usual diagnostic workup.

The economics of this approach are favorable, since it avoids the cost of the usual workup for drug refractory hypertension in about half the patients presenting with that presumptive diagnosis. The direct cost of electronic monitoring of each of the three drugs is about $300. The direct cost of the diagnostic workup is about $1600, according to Burnier. Thus, in a group of 100 "drug refractory" hypertensives, about half of whom would be identified by electronic monitoring as clinically unrecognized noncompliers, the aggregate direct cost of electronic monitoring is $30 000, but the avoidance of the diagnostic workup in these 50 patients saves $80 000 in direct costs. If single-drug electronic monitoring proves sufficient, as Cramer et al. found in a multiple-drug epilepsy study,[87] the electronic monitoring cost drops to $10 000, giving a nominal 8:1 cost advantage of interposed electronic monitoring.

Several conclusions are suggested by the foregoing. One is the dubious wisdom of relying on stepped-care dosing regimens when they are uninformed by reliably compiled dosing histories. The odds that inadequate compliance with the step-1 drug regimen is responsible for a patient's failure to respond are already higher than 1 in 3–4.[35] Proceeding up the steps of a stepped-care regimen, the odds increase that inadequate compliance is the basis for nonresponse, to reach 1 in about 2, if Burnier's experience[62] is generalizable. As for interpretation of dosing history data, it is straightforward when the patient is discovered to have taken very little or no drug. The interpretation of intermediate levels of compliance with prescribed dosing regimen(s) will require product-specific information on the impact of dose delays and omissions on the magnitude and timing of drug response—a pharmacometric challenge.

Regimen Intensification Studies

In a sense, the work of Burnier et al. is a form of "regimen intensification," in that a whole subgroup of patients has undergone a process that intensifies their exposure to the drug in question. The work of Reichard et al.,[63] based on this approach, is one of the cornerstones of modern treatment of type I diabetes. In the IMPACT study, the intensification of the risedronate regimen, through a simple motivational program, achieved not only improved compliance and persistence,[64–66] but also significantly reduced incidence of fracture in the intensification group, relative to the control group.[88] Obviously, it is a point of basic importance to show that an intervention that improves compliance and persistence also has a favorable clinical effect.

PHARMACOMETRIC CHALLENGES

An important use of reliable dosing history data arises from the eventuality that such data will be the basis of predicting the time course of drug action from the dosing history, with, of course, the help of the drug's pharmacokinetic and pharmacodynamic models. An early pharmacometric view of this challenge is the Harter–Peck model of the sources of variance in drug response.[89] The model recognizes that patients' variable execution of prescribed drug regimens is one of the two leading sources of variation in drug response—the other being variations in pharmacokinetics, which integrates drug absorption, distribution, metabolism, and excretion. The first of two steps in implementing the Harter–Peck model is to use the patient's dosing history as input to a suitable pharmacokinetic model for the drug in question, to predict the time course of drug concentration in plasma. The second problem is to use the time course of drug concentration in plasma as input to a suitable pharmacodynamic model for the drug in question, to predict the time course of drug action(s), and then to explore the impact of varying model parameters and compliance.[40,89]

Great progress has been made in solving the first of the two problems. A decade ago, Weintraub and colleagues used electronic monitoring-compiled dosing history data as input to a pharmacokinetic model for the calcium antagonist diltiazem, and showed that the resulting projections of the time course of diltiazem concentration in plasma corresponded well to intermittent point-measurements of diltiazem concentrations in the plasma of the trial participants.[90] This achievement was neglected, and only within the past two years has Vrijens used the method with several of the protease inhibitors used to treat HIV infections. His work,[19–22] based on year-long, electronic monitoring dosing history data, generated year-long projections of protease inhibitor concentrations in plasma that were confirmed in approximately 95% of trial volunteers by periodic point-measurements of protease inhibitor concentration in plasma. The few deviations represent either unstable pharmacokinetic model parameters or artifactual dosing history data arising from some form of misusage of electronic monitoring.

One of the benefits of this work is that it makes explicit the periods of time in which protease inhibitor concentration falls below a minimum effective level, which has good explanatory power for predicting rises in viral load.[19–22] Another benefit is that it exposes the frequency with which the concentration of protease inhibitor in patients' plasma passes through a critical zone, within which the concentrations of protease inhibitor are low enough to permit resumption of viral replication, with its associated increase in viral mutations, but with still high enough protease inhibitor concentrations to

exert selection pressure for drug resistant mutants. A lapse in dosing will, with short half-life drugs, result in a prompt fall in protease inhibitor concentration and passage through the critical concentration zone, with a second pass through the critical concentration zone when dosing resumes. An important additional finding is that, as patients' aggregate intake of drug rises, the lengths of gaps in dosing decrease, but the frequency of their occurrence increases, leading to an increasing frequency of passages through the critical concentration zone, and thus greater likelihood of emergent resistance.[22,91,92] As the percentage of prescribed doses taken rises into the mid-90s, and above, there is an abrupt fall in the incidence of lapses long enough to allow the protease inhibitor concentration to reach the critical concentration zone, and so there is a sharp fall in the emergence of drug-resistant mutants.[22]

These findings force reinterpretation of the saying that "poor compliance with prescribed antimicrobial drug regimens is the main cause of emergent drug resistance." The statement is qualitatively correct, but if compliance is expressed in terms of the percentage of prescribed doses taken, as is often done, then the statement is wrong, for there is an inverse relation between the percentage of prescribed doses taken and emergent drug resistance.[91,92] The evident basis of this paradox signifies the importance of having reliable data not only on dose taking, but also dose timing, and that sayings based only on dose taking data can mislead.

Another practical expression of the importance of having dose timing information lies in answering the often-asked question: is a once-daily dosing regimen superior to a twice-daily regimen? If one defines the question in terms of which regimen has the higher percentage of prescribed doses taken, then the answer is that the once-daily regimen is superior, for it almost invariably, in side-to-side comparisons, shows a small numerical superiority over the twice-daily regimen. The practical therapeutic question, however, is: which regimen is more likely to maintain drug concentrations within a purported therapeutic range? Then the answer clearly is that the twice-daily regimen is superior. The reason lies in the fact that the impact on drug concentrations of missing a single once-daily dose is much greater than the impact of missing a single twice-daily dose. Instead, it takes the missing of two sequential twice-daily doses to produce essentially the same impact on drug concentrations as missing a single once-daily dose. The probability of missing two sequential twice-daily doses is much lower than the probability of missing a single once-daily dose.[93] Thus, one can expect better maintained concentrations of drug in plasma with a twice-daily regimen than with a once-daily regimen.

Some Pertinent History on the Use of Measured Drug Exposure Data in Randomized Controlled Trials

A noteworthy result in the Wood and colleagues trial of depot penicillin versus oral penicillin versus oral sulfadiazine[58] was the finding that poor compliers with oral sulfadiazine, even though they had high rates of streptococcal infections, nevertheless had very low rates of recurrent acute rheumatic fever, in sharp contrast to the poor compliers with oral penicillin, who had high rates of both streptococcal infection and recurrent acute rheumatic fever. This surprising result, which has never been explained, is probably the first demonstration of a forgiving drug, in that one could delay or omit many doses in an oral sulfadiazine regimen without losing protection against acute rheumatic fever. It has also resulted in oral sulfadiazine's being still considered a realistic treatment alternative to penicillin in the prevention of recurrent acute rheumatic fever[94]—an example of a valuable finding arising from careful use of compliance data in a randomized, controlled trial.

Several other early trials—the Lipid Research Clinics Coronary Primary Prevention Trial (LRC-CPPT) of cholestyramine[67] and the Helsinki Heart study trial of gemfibrozil for lipid disorders[68]—included careful attempts to estimate intake of the test drugs and placebos, and to stratify trial results by estimated drug intake. The careful analysis of LRC-CPPT[67] is exemplary of how one can probe beyond an intent-to-treat analysis to learn more about the underlying pharmionic and pharmacometric aspects of a major study. One of the results of this analysis, coming out of the compliance-stratification of the cholesterol and coronary risk reduction data, supported the communicational theme that "each 1% reduction in total cholesterol levels results in a 2% reduction in coronary risk." This message has subsequently been modified, in light of cholesterol fractionation into LDL, HDL, and other components, each with its own estimated impact on coronary risk, but in 1984, when the cholesterol hypothesis was still controversial (cf. Meier[95]), it was a useful way to begin communication of the value of reducing total cholesterol levels. The many subsequent pharmaceutical developments during the past 20 years in the lipids modification field have confirmed and reconfirmed the essential findings from LRC-CPPT.

The association of poor compliance with topical pilocarpine to deteriorating glaucoma[71,72] is biologically plausible, but, on its own, open to debate regarding the primary causal role of drug exposure. Similar debate surrounds the association between low exposure to inhaled corticosteroids and complications of asthma,[78,79] though it, too, has biological plausibility. Of course, if we see increasing numbers of such associations in a variety of drug-managed diseases, it will lend increasing credence to the primary role of drug exposure in determining good versus bad outcomes of patient care.

After the publication in 1980 of a re-analysis of the Coronary Drug Project results,[96] trialists abandoned the attempt to use measured drug exposure as an explanatory variable. The reasons for this change, and the faulty thinking involved, are a complex topic in trials design that is beyond the scope of this chapter. The reader is referred to Urquhart[97] for an in-depth discussion of the matter. It was not until the landmark publication of Efron and Feldman,[98] who received the 1990 JASA Applications Award from the American Statistical Association, that variations in drug exposure, which have long been recognized as a (or the) leading source of variance in drug response,[38,89,99–101] began to be reconsidered as an explanatory variable in trials analysis. Reflections of this change have been the points made in discussion of the Efron–Feldman paper,[87,98,102] the landmark paper of the late Lewis Sheiner on learning versus confirming in clinical drug development,[103] and the growth in biostatistical research on causal inference.[104–106] The basic principles were reflected many years ago in the landmark paper by Bradford Hill on causality, which is conveniently reproduced on Professor Edward Tufte's website.[107]

Meanwhile, the cholestyramine and gemfibrozil trials were already under way by 1980.[67,68] Both showed strong compliance dependence of drug-induced lipid changes and, in the case of the cholestyramine trial, strong compliance dependence of coronary risk, without evidence in either trial of compliance-related differences in lipid levels or coronary risk within the corresponding placebo groups. The impact of the lipid changes on coronary risk in the gemfibrozil trial can be inferred from models that link lipid levels to coronary risk, but that linkage was not published at the time. There are many complexities in these two big trials, which have been reviewed in detail, along with the re-analysis of the Coronary Drug Project Trial.[96]

The compliance-stratified results of the cholestyramine trial were included in the relabeling of the product after the trial's publication in 1984. That labeling change was hailed by Peter Barton Hutt and the late Louis Lasagna as a landmark evolution in full-disclosure labeling, for it informed patients who comply fully with the recommended regimen that they could expect a 39% coronary risk reduction instead of the all-patient (intention-to-treat) average risk reduction of 19%.[108] In such a long-term prophylaxis program, the patient who complies fully knows what his/her level of compliance is, pays the full-compliance cost of the medicine, and experiences the full-compliance side effects, of which dose-dependent colonic gas production is the main one. Yet patients have no way to experience the benefit of the treatment, which is an actuarial phenomenon called "coronary risk reduction." For that, they must rely on labeling information, which the original, compliance-stratified labeling provided. In the early 1990s, the FDA was convinced by sponsors of other modes of lipid modification to omit the compliance-stratified effectiveness data from the cholestyramine label in the interests of "comparability," which it may have brought, but at the cost of a step backwards in the sometimes tortuous path toward full-disclosure labeling. Much more useful would have been to press for compliance-stratified effectiveness data, carefully analyzed for hidden biases, in the labeling of statins and other modes of lipids modification, together with information on what patients should do when they realize that they have missed one or more scheduled doses.

The pharmacoeconomic correlates of variable compliance in the cholestyramine and gemfibrozil trials are analyzed in Urquhart.[109] One striking result of this analysis arises from the unusual linearity of the exposure–response characteristics of cholestyramine: the drug acquisition cost to prevent a coronary event (sudden death, acute myocardial infarction, onset of angina) appears to be independent of compliance with the cholestyramine dosing regimen. In effect, patients in the lowest quartile of compliance take on average about one-fourth of the prescribed daily dose, but the linearity of the exposure–risk relation means that it takes four times as many people taking one-fourth the recommended dose to prevent a coronary event, compared with full compliers. Thus, the drug acquisition cost to prevent a coronary event is essentially the same in partial compliers as in full compliers. Of course, poor compliers deprive themselves of most of the possible reduction in coronary risk that the drug can provide at full dose.

Not All Prescribed Drug Regimens Are Optimal

A wild card in the search for clinical explanatory power of dosing history data is the fact that many recommended drug regimens are suboptimal, erring mostly on the side of higher than necessary (or more frequent than necessary) dosing.[36,37] One likely reflection of this aspect of the story is given by the title of the following study: "Measured versus self-reported compliance with doxycycline therapy for chlamydia-associated syndromes: high therapeutic success rates despite poor compliance."[110] On the face of

it, this study's findings suggest that the recommended dose of doxycycline has been set considerably higher than necessary for the treatment of chlamydial infections. One would want to look carefully at the associations, patient by patient, between interdose intervals and evidence for treatment failure, as reviewed by Vrijens and Urquhart.[22] As such, it could be the first in a series of steps to revise the recommended dosing regimen. This work also serves as a warning that one cannot simply assume that all recommended dosing regimens are optimal, as there is now good evidence that 1 product in about 4.5, launched since 1980, has undergone at least a 50% reduction in recommended dose.[36,37]

Pharmaceutical scientists concerned with defining optimal dosing regimens for new pharmaceuticals appear still to be excessively focused on pharmacokinetic properties as the basis for defining dosing regimens. Instructive examples that this approach can sometimes mislead are omeprazole, which has a plasma half-life of less than one hour, and a 2–3 day duration of therapeutic action,[111] and bendrofluthiazide, which has about a 3-hour plasma half-life[9] and a post-dose duration of antihypertensive action of 6 days.[55] These are further striking examples of how some drugs' pharmacodynamic properties dominate in determining how long drug action continues at therapeutically effective levels after a last-taken dose, thus providing important constraints on the definition of an optimal dosing regimen.

Serious Prognosis Does Not Enforce Good Compliance

The findings that poor compliance with immunosuppressant regimens is a major source of post-transplant rejection reactions[73–76] were a major surprise, near the end of the era in which the field we would now call pharmionics was dominated by armchair speculation. Similar surprise was elicited by the first demonstration of drug holidays in HIV-infected patients prescribed protease inhibitors.[80] Earlier, Waterhouse et al. had found similar results in breast cancer patients prescribed tamoxifen.[112]

Ruling In or Out Poor Compliance as a Reason for Failed Proof of Efficacy

Olivieri et al. used electronic monitoring to demonstrate that the failure to reject the null hypothesis in a placebo-controlled, randomized trial could not be explained by prevalent poor compliance among the trial subjects.[113] In the absence of reliable data on trial subjects' actual dosing histories, it is always a question whether a failed trial has resulted from the test agent's intrinsic lack of pharmacological effectiveness or from underdosing due to poor/partial compliance with the protocol-specified dosing regimen. A relatively unforgiving drug, e.g., atenolol, with its approximately 30-hour post-dose duration of antihypertensive action and its once-daily dosing regimen,[46] would be likely to come off badly in a comparison with a much more forgiving, like-acting agent, simply because relatively short lapses in dosing can be expected to undermine the effectiveness of the less forgiving agent to a much greater extent than the more forgiving agent. Given that short lapses in dosing are much more common than longer ones,[1] the beneficial actions of a less forgiving agent are likely to be more frequently interrupted than those of a more forgiving agent. Such considerations are basic ones that should be incorporated into modeling and simulation of later-stage clinical trials.[40]

Is it Always Bad News that Compliance Is Poor?

A common approach taken by many researchers and editorialists is to assume that all drug regimens and all prescribers' choices of what to prescribe are optimal, and that poor compliance with prescribed drug regimens *ipso facto* results in poorer outcomes than would have occurred with correctly executed, recommended dosing regimens. This theme is a main interpretative feature of the recent monograph of the WHO.[27] Unfortunately, it is only a qualitative approach to a problem that is inherently and fundamentally quantitative in nature. Whence the need for *pharmionics*, to give quantitative expression to the kinds of deviations patients have made from prescribed regimens, and for *pharmacometrics*, which is the quantitative study of exposure–effect relations.

Prescribing Quality

I have said nothing of the quality of prescribing, which is a topic beyond the scope of this chapter. One can imagine that some instances of nonacceptance or noncompliance or very short persistence are beneficial compensations for unsatisfactory prescribing. Many years ago Michael Weintraub wrote of this under the title "intelligent non-compliance."[114] Relying on patients' errors to offset physicians' errors is not, however, a satisfactory solution to the problem of unsatisfactory prescribing. See Chapters 28, 29, and 34 for more on evaluating and changing the quality of prescribing.

THE FUTURE

In ambulatory pharmacotherapy, prevalent underdosing, in various temporal patterns, creates a challenging and diverse series of problems. Perforce, it is a major aspect of ambulatory therapeutics and drug trials, notwithstanding its having been long neglected, and still ignored by many. The general progression in pharmaceutical innovation has been, and inevitably will continue to be, toward steadily more powerful agents, thus heightening the importance of having sound pharmionic information and acting upon it in labeling, dosage form and drug regimen design, and clinical practice.

The reader may regard Table 46.2 as being a long list of drugs that presently have some form of evidential basis for concluding compliance-dependent drug actions or outcomes of prescribed ambulatory drug treatment. From another perspective, it is a remarkably short list, considering the size of the pharmacopoeia and the basic pharmacological fact that all drugs have dose- and time-dependent actions: in effect, essentially all drugs will sooner or later find places in Table 46.2. There are approximately 1000 drugs in today's pharmacopoeia, perhaps about half of which are in fairly active use. Many of the medicines based on these drugs are used for minor indications, as "comfort medicines," in which case variable compliance is probably clinically unimportant, but compliance and persistence with many other medicines are medically important, and sometimes crucial. Sound therapeutic analysis can separate the medically important drugs, and sound pharmionic and pharmacometric analyses can sort out which drugs pose substantive hazards when underdosed in certain patterns.

Recognition of the magnitude and diversity of patients' misuse of prescription drugs has thus led to new methods, new concepts, new terminology, and a new path to the ever-present goals of rational pharmacotherapy and full-disclosure labeling of pharmaceuticals used in ambulatory care. Its application will hopefully continue to expand in the future.

REFERENCES

1. Urquhart J. The electronic medication event monitor—lessons for pharmacotherapy. *Clin Pharmacokinet* 1997; **32**: 345–56.
2. Norell SE. Methods in assessing drug compliance. *Acta Med Scand* 1984; (suppl 683): 35–40.
3. Pullar T, Feely M. Problems of compliance with drug treatment: new solutions? *Pharm J* 1990; **245**: 213–15.
4. Cramer JA. Microelectronic systems for monitoring and enhancing patient compliance with medication regimens. *Drugs* 1995; **49**: 321–7.
5. Kastrissios H, Blaschke TF. Medication compliance as a feature in drug development. *Ann Rev Pharmacol Toxicol* 1997; **37**: 451–75.
6. Pullar T, Kumar S, Tindall H, Feely M. Time to stop counting the tablets? *Clin Pharmacol Ther* 1989; **46**: 163–8.

7. Feely M, Cooke J, Price D, Singleton S, Mehta A, Bradford L *et al.* Low-dose phenobarbitone as an indicator of compliance with drug therapy. *Br J Clin Pharmacol* 1987; **24**: 77–83.

8. Pullar T, Kumar S, Chrystyn H, Rice P, Peaker S, Feely M. The prediction of steady-state plasma phenobarbitone concentrations (following low-dose phenobarbitone) to refine its use as an indicator of compliance. *Br J Clin Pharmacol* 1991; **32**: 329–33.

9. Benet LZ, Øie S, Schwartz J. Design and optimization of dosage regimens; harmacokinetic data. In: Hardman JG, Limbird LE, Molinoff PB, Ruddon RW, Gilman AG, eds, *Goodman and Gilman's The Pharmacological Basis of Therapeutics*, 9th edn. New York: McGraw-Hill, 1996; pp. 1707–92.

10. Feinstein AR. On white-coat effects and the electronic monitoring of compliance. *Arch Intern Med* 1990; **150**: 1377–8.

11. Kass MA, Gordon M, Meltzer DW. Can ophthalmologists correctly identify patients defaulting from pilocarpine therapy? *Am J Ophthalmol* 1986; **101**: 524–30.

12. Cramer JA, Scheyer RD, Mattson RH. Compliance declines between clinic visits. *Arch Int Med* 1990; **150**: 1509–10.

13. Cramer JA, Mattson RH, Prevey ML, Scheyer RD, Ouellette VL. How often is medication taken as prescribed? A novel assessment technique. *JAMA* 1989; **261**: 3273–7.

14. Kruse W, Weber E. Dynamics of drug regimen compliance— its assessment by microprocessor-based monitoring. *Eur J Clin Pharmacol* 1990; **38**: 561–5.

15. Averbuch M, Weintraub M, Pollack DJ. Compliance assessment in clinical trials: the MEMS device. *J Clin Res Pharmacoepidemiol* 1990; **4**: 199–204.

16. Liu H, Golin CE, Miller LG, Hays RD, Beck CK, Sanandaij S *et al.* A comparison study of multiple measures of adherence to HIV protease inhibitors. *Ann Intern Med* 2001; **134**: 968–77.

17. Arnsten J, Demas P, Farzadegan H, Grant R, Gourevitch M, Chang C *et al.* Antiretroviral therapy adherence and viral suppression in HIV-infected drug users: comparison of self-report and electronic monitoring. *Clin Infect Dis* 2001; **33**: 1417–23.

18. Wagner GJ. Predictors of antiretroviral adherence as measured by self-report, electronic monitoring, and medication diaries. *AIDS Patient Care STDS* 2002; **16**: 599–608.

19. Vrijens B. Analyzing time-varying patterns of human exposure to xenobiotics and their biomedical impact, PhD thesis, University of Gent, Belgium, 2002.

20. Vrijens B, Tousset E, Rode R, Bertz R, Mayer S, Urquhart J. Successful projection of the time-course of drug concentration in plasma during a one-year period from electronically compiled dosing-time data used as input to individually parameterized pharmacokinetic models. *J Clin Pharmacol* 2005; **45**: 461–7.

21. Vrijens B, Tousset E, Rode R, Bertz R, Mayer SL. Within-patient variance reduced in an ARV PK study by switching from patient-reported to electronically-compiled dosing times. In: Proceedings of the 2nd IAS Conference on HIV Pathogenesis and Treatment, Paris, France, July 13–16, 2003.

22. Vrijens B, Urquhart J. Patient adherence to prescribed antimicrobial drug dosing regimens. *J Antimicrobial Chemotherapy* 2005; **55**: 616–27.

23. Urquhart J. Ascertaining how much compliance is enough with outpatient antibiotic regimens. *Postgrad Med J* 1993; **68** (suppl 3): 49–59.

24. Urquhart J. Pharmacodynamics of variable patient compliance: implications for pharmaceutical value. *Adv Drug Deliv Rev* 1998; **33**: 207–19.

25. Urquhart J. Defining the margins for errors in patient compliance with prescribed drug regimens. *Pharmacoeepidemiol Drug Saf* 2000; **9**: 565–8.

26. Urquhart J. Controlled drug delivery: pharmacologic and therapeutic aspects. *J Intern Med* 2000; **248**: 357–76.

27. World Health Organization. *Adherence to Long-term Therapies.* Geneva: World Health Organization, 2004.

28. Jones JK, Gorkin L, Lian JF, Staffa JA, Fletcher AP. Discontinuation of and changes in treatment after start of new courses of antihypertensive drugs: a study of a United Kingdom population. *BMJ* 1995; **311**: 293–5.

29. Caro JJ, Salas M, Speckman JL, Raggio G, Jackson JD. Persistence with treatment for hypertension in actual practice. *Can Med Assoc J* 1999; **160**: 31–7.

30. Catalan VS, LeLorier J. Predictors of long-term persistence on statins in a subsidized clinical population. *Value Health* 2000; **3**: 417–26.

31. Benner JS, Glynn RJ, Mogun H, Neumann PJ, Weinstein MC. Long-term persistence in use of statin therapy in elderly patients. *JAMA* 2002; **288**: 455–61.

32. Urquhart J. Some economic consequences of noncompliance. *Curr Hypertens Rep* 2001; **3**: 473–80.

33. Vrijens B, Tousset E, Koncz T, Métry JM, Urquhart J. Differential economic impact of variable compliance and variable persistence with prescribed, long-term drug regimens. Abstract. *Value Health* 2003; **6**: 200–1.

34. Arlington S, Barnett S, Hughes S, Palo J. *Pharma 2010: The Threshold of Innovation.* London: IBM Pharmaceutical Consulting Services, 2003.

35. Urquhart J. The odds of the three nons when an aptly prescribed medicine isn't working: noncompliance, nonabsorption, nonresponse. *Br J Clin Pharmacol* 2002; **54**: 212–20.

36. Cross J, Lee H, Westelinck A, Nelson J, Grudzinskas C, Peck C. Postmarketing drug dosage changes of 499 FDA-approved new molecular entities, 1980–1999. *Pharmacoepidemiol Drug Saf* 2002; **11**: 439–46.

37. Heerdink ER, Urquhart J, Leufkens HG. Changes in prescribed drug dose after market introduction. *Pharmacoepidemiol Drug Saf* 2002; **11**: 447–53.

38. Urquhart J, Chevalley C. Impact of unrecognized dosing errors on the cost and effectiveness of pharmaceuticals. *Drug Inf J* 1988; **22**: 363–78.

39. Psaty BM, Koepsell TD, Wagner EH, LoGerfo JP, Inui TS. The relative risk of incident coronary heart disease associated with recently stopping the use of beta blockers. *JAMA* 1990; **263**: 1653–7.

40. Urquhart J. History-informed perspectives on the modeling and simulation of therapeutic drug actions. In: Kimko HC,

Duffull S, eds, *Simulation for Designing Clinical Trials*. New York: Marcel Dekker, 2002; pp. 245–69.

41. Wandel T, Charap AD, Lewis RA, Partamian L, Cobb S, Lue J *et al*. Glaucoma treatment with once-daily levobunolol. *Am J Ophthalmol* 1986; **101**: 298–304.

42. Rosenbaum JF, Fava M, Hoog SL, Ascroft RC, Krebs WB. Selective serotonin reuptake inhibitor discontinuation syndrome: a randomized clinical trial. *Biol Psychiatry* 1998; **44**: 77–87.

43. Is GSK guilty of fraud? Editorial. *Lancet* 2004; **363**: 1919.

44. Cromer B. Behavioral strategies to increase compliance in adolescents. In: Cramer JA, Spilker B, eds, *Patient Compliance in Medical Practice and Clinical Trials*. New York: Raven Press, 1991; pp. 99–106.

45. March J. Treatment for adolescents with depression study, in process. *New York Times*, science section, June 2, 2004.

46. Johnson BF, Whelton A. A study design for comparing the effects of missing daily doses of antihypertensive drugs. *Am J Ther* 1994; **1**: 260–7.

47. Potter LS. Oral contraceptive compliance and its role in the effectiveness of the method. In: Cramer JA, Spilker B, eds, *Compliance in Medical Practice and Clinical Trials*. New York: Raven Press, 1991; pp. 195–207.

48. Guillebaud J. Any questions. *Br Med J* 1993; **307**: 617.

49. Anonymous. Ten great public health achievements—US, 1900–99: Family planning. *Morb Mortal Wkly Rep* 1999; **48**: 1073–80.

50. Potter L, Oakley D, de Leon-Wong E, Canamar R. Measuring compliance among oral contraceptive users. *Fam Plann Perspect* 1996; **28**: 154–8.

51. Wong E, Moeng S, Johnson A. *Do Self-Reports of Oral Contraceptive Compliance Agree with Electronic Reports?* Tables and statistical report. Report of the Biostatistics and Information Technology Office, Family Health International, Research Triangle Park, NC, October 1995.

52. Peck CC, Urquhart J. Importance of inclusion of information concerning non-compliance with the label-recommended drug regimen. FDA Docket No. 00N-1269, RIN 0910-AA94. Comments on Proposed Rule "Requirements on Content and Format of Labeling for Human Prescription Drugs and Biologics; Requirements for Prescription Drug Product Labels," 2001.

53. Vaur L, Dutrey-Dupagne C, Boussac J, Genes N, Bouvier d'Yvoire M, Elkik F, Meredith PA. Differential effects of a missed dose of trandolapril and enalapril on blood pressure control in hypertensive patients. *J Cardiovasc Pharmacol* 1995; **26**: 127–31.

54. Hernandez-Hernandez R, Armas de Hernandez MJ, Armas-Padilla MC, Carvajal AR, Guerrero-Pajuelo J. The effects of missing a dose of enalapril versus amlodipine on ambulatory blood pressure. *Blood Press Monit* 1996; **1**: 1121–6.

55. Girvin BG, Johnston GD. Comparison of the effects of a 7-day period of noncompliance on blood pressure control using three different antihypertensive agents. *J Hypertens* 2004; **22**: 1409–14.

56. Leenen FHH, Fourney A, Notman G, Tanner J. Persistence of anti-hypertensive effect after "missed doses" of calcium antagonist with long (amlodipine) vs short (diltiazem) elimination half-life. *Br J Clin Pharmacol* 1996; **41**: 83–8.

57. Meijer WEE, Bouvy ML, Heerdink ER, Urquhart J, Leufkens HGM. Spontaneous lapses in dosing during chronic treatment with selective serotonin reuptake inhibitors. *Br J Psychiatry* 2001; **179**: 519–22.

58. Wood HF, Feinstein AR, Taranta A, Epstein JA, Simpson R. Rheumatic fever in children and adolescents: a long-term epidemiologic study of subsequent prophylaxis, streptococcal infections, and clinical sequelae. III. Comparative effectiveness of three prophylaxis regimens in preventing streptococcal infections and rheumatic recurrences. *Ann Int Med* 1964; **60** (suppl 5): 31–46.

59. McCann MF, Potter LS. Progestin-only oral contraception: a comprehensive review. *Contraception* 1994; **50** (suppl 1): 9–195.

60. Weis SE, Slocum PC, Blais FX, King B, Nunn M, Matney GB, Gomez E, Foresman BH. The effect of directly observed therapy on the rates of drug resistance and relapse in tuberculosis. *N Engl J Med* 1994; **330**: 1179–84.

61. What is DOTs? Available at: http://www.who.int/gtb/publications/whatisdots. Accessed: August 18, 2004.

62. Burnier M, Schneider MP, Chiolero A, Fallab Stubi CL, Brunner HR. Electronic compliance monitoring in resistant hypertension: the basis for rational therapeutic decisions. *J Hypertens* 2001; **19**: 335–41.

63. Reichard P, Nilsson B-Y, Rosenqvist U. The effect of long-term intensified insulin treatment on the development of microvascular complications of diabetes mellitus. *N Engl J Med* 1993; **329**: 304–9.

64. Delmas PD, Vrijens B, van de Langerijt L, Roux C, Eastell R, Ringe JD *et al*. Effect of reinforcement with bone turnover marker results on persistence with risedronate treatment in postmenopausal women with osteoporosis: improving the measurements of persistence on actonel treatment: the Impact study. Presented at the European Calcified Tissues Society Meeting, Rome, May 8–12, 2003.

65. Eastell R, Garnero P, Vrijens B, van de Langerijt L, Pols HAP, Ringe JD *et al*. Influence of patient compliance with risedronate therapy on bone turnover marker and bone mineral density response: the Impact study. Presented at the European Calcified Tissues Society Meeting, Rome, May 8–12, 2003.

66. Vrijens B, Ringe JD, Watts NB, Pols HAP, Roux C, Eastell R *et al*. Electronic monitoring of adherence to therapy in postmenopausal osteoporosis: the Impact study. Presented at the European Calcified Tissues Society Meeting, Rome, May 8–12, 2003.

67. The Lipid Research Clinics Coronary Primary Prevention Trial results: (I) Reduction in incidence of coronary heart disease; (II) The relationship of reduction in incidence of coronary heart disease to cholesterol lowering. *JAMA* 1984; **251**: 351–74.

68. Manninen V, Elo MO, Frick H, Haapa K, Feinonen OP, Heinsalmi P *et al*. Lipid alterations and decline in the incidence

of coronary heart disease in the Helsinki Heart Study. *JAMA* 1988; **260**: 641–51.

69. Kumar S, Haigh JRM, Rhodes LE, Peaker S, Davies JA, Roberts BE, Feely MP. Poor compliance is a major factor in unstable outpatient control of anticoagulant therapy. *Thromb Haemost* 1989; **62**: 729–32.

70. Kruse W, Eggert-Kruse W, Rampmaier J, Runnebaum B, Weber E. Compliance with short-term high-dose oestradiol in young patients with primary infertility—new insights from the use of electronic devices. *Agents Actions* 1990; (suppl 29): 105–15.

71. Granstrom P-A. Progression of visual field defects in glaucoma: relation to compliance with pilocarpine therapy. *Arch Ophthalmol* 1985; **103**: 529–31.

72. Priddy JT, Kass MA, Gordon MO, Meltzer DW, Morley RE. Factors related to compliance with topical pilocarpine treatment. *Invest Ophthalmol Vis Sci* 1987; **28**: 377.

73. Didlake RH, Dreyfus K, Kerman RH, Van Buren CT, Kahan BD. Patient noncompliance: a major cause of late graft failure in cyclosporine-treated renal transplants. *Transplant Proc* 1988; **20** (suppl 3): 63–9.

74. Rovelli M, Palmeri D, Vossler E, Bartus S, Hull D, Schweizer R. Noncompliance in organ transplant recipients. *Transplant Proc* 1989; **21**: 833–4.

75. De Geest S, Abraham I, Moons P, Vandeputte M, Van Cleemput J, Evers G, Daenen W, Vanhaecke J. Late acute rejection and subclinical noncompliance with cyclosporine therapy in heart transplant recipients. *J Heart Lung Transplant* 1998; **17**: 854–63.

76. Nevins E, Kruse L, Skeans MA, Thomas W. The natural history of azathioprine compliance after renal transplantation. *Kidney Int* 2001; **60**: 1565–70.

77. Richardson JL, Shelton DR, Krailo M, Levine AM. The effect of compliance with treatment on survival among patients with hematologic malignancies. *J Clin Oncol* 1990; **8**: 356–64.

78. Milgrom H, Bender B, Ackerson L, Bowry P, Smith B, Rand C. Non-compliance and treatment failure in children with asthma. *J Allergy Clin Immunol* 1996; **98**: 1051–7.

79. Suissa S, Ernst P, Kezouh A. Regular use of inhaled corticosteroids and the long term prevention of hospitalisation for asthma. *Thorax* 2002; **57**: 880–4.

80. Vanhove GF, Schapiro JM, Winters MA, Merigan TC, Blaschke TF. Patient compliance and drug failure in protease inhibitor monotherapy. *JAMA* 1996; **276**: 1955–6.

81. Paterson DL, Swindells S, Mohr J, Brester M, Vergis EN, Squier C, Wagener MM, Singh N. Adherence to protease inhibitor therapy and outcomes in patients with HIV infection. *Ann Int Med* 2000; **133**: 21–30.

82. Gross R, Bilker QB, Friedman HM, Strom BL. Effect of adherence to newly initiated antiretroviral therapy on plasma viral load. *AIDS* 2001; **15**: 2109–17.

83. Arnsten R, Demas J, Farzadegan P, Grant H, Gourevitch R, Chang M *et al*. Antiretroviral therapy adherence and viral suppression in HIV-infected drug users: comparison of self-report and electronic monitoring. *Clin Infect Dis* 2001; **33**: 1417–23.

84. Stone AA, Shiffman S, Schwartz JF, Broderick JF, Hufford MR. Patient noncompliance with paper diaries. *BMJ* 2002; **324**: 1193–4.

85. Cramer JA, Rosenheck R. Enhancing medication compliance for people with serious mental disease. *J Nerv Ment Dis* 1999; **187**: 53–4.

86. De Klerk E, Lesaffre E, Van den Enden M. Improved compliance and persistence with atorvastatine through a pharmacy-based intervention. *Value Health* 2003; **6**: 635–809.

87. Zeger SL, Liang K-Y. Comment: dose–response estimands. *J Am Stat Assoc* 1991; **86**: 18–19.

88. Delmas PD, Vrijens B, Roux C, Le-Moigne-Amrani A, Eastell R, Grauer A *et al*. Osteoporosis treatment using reinforcement with bone turnover marker data reduces fracture risk: the IMPACT study. Abstracts of the 2004 Annual Meeting of the American Society of Bone Metabolism Research, Miami Beach, FL, November 2004.

89. Harter JG, Peck CC. Chronobiology: suggestions for integrating it into drug development. *Ann N Y Acad Sci* 1991: **618**: 563–71.

90. Rubio A, Cox C, Weintraub M. Prediction of diltiazem plasma concentration curves from limited measurements using compliance data. *Clin Pharmacokinet* 1992; **22**: 238–46.

91. Bangsberg DR, Deeks SG. Is average adherence to HIV antiretroviral therapy enough? *J Gen Intern Med* 2002; **17**: 812–13.

92. Harrigan PR, Dong WY, Alexander C *et al*. The association between drug resistance and adherence determined by two independent methods in a large cohort of drug naïve individuals starting triple therapy. Abstract of the 2nd IAS Conference on HIV Treatment, Paris, France, July 2003.

93. Comté L, Reners C, Tousset E, Vrijens B. Once-daily versus twice-daily regimens: which is best for HIV infected patients? Abstracts of the Belgian Statistical Society annual meeting, Vielsalm, Belgium, Oct 8–9, 2004.

94. *British National Formulary 44*. British Medical Association: London, 2002; p. 261.

95. Meier P. Discussion. *J Am Stat Assoc* 1991; **86**: 19–22.

96. Coronary Drug Project Research Group. Influence of adherence to treatment and response of cholesterol on mortality in the coronary drug project. *N Engl J Med* 1980; **303**: 1038–41.

97. Urquhart J. Patient compliance as an explanatory variable in four selected cardiovascular studies. In: Cramer JA, Spilker B, eds, *Compliance in Medical Practice and Clinical Trials*. New York: Raven Press, 1991; pp. 301–22.

98. Efron B, Feldman D. Compliance as an explanatory variable in clinical trials. *J Am Stat Assoc* 199; **86**: 7–17.

99. Joyce CRB. Patient co-operation and the sensitivity of clinical trials. *J Chron Dis* 1962; **15**: 1025–36.

100. Lasagna L, ed. *Patient Compliance*. Mount Kisco, NY: Futura, 1976.

101. Haynes RB, Taylor DW, Sackett DL, eds. *Compliance in Health Care*. Baltimore, MD: Johns Hopkins University Press, 1979.

102. Rubin D. Comment: dose–response estimands. *J Am Stat Assoc* 1991; **86**: 22–4.

103. Sheiner LB. Learning versus confirming in clinical drug development. *Clin Pharmacol Ther* 1997; **61**: 275–91.

104. Mark SD, Robins JM. A method for the analysis of randomized trials with compliance information—an application to the multiple risk factor intervention trial. *Control Clin Trials* 1993; **14**: 79–97.

105. Goetghebeur E, Loeys T. Beyond intention to treat. *Epidemiol Rev* 2002; **24**: 85–90.

106. Loeys T, Goetghebeur E. Causal proportional hazards estimator for the effect of treatment actually received in a randomized trial with all-or-nothing compliance. *Biometrics* 2003; **59**: 100–5.

107. Hill AB. (The environment and disease: association or causation? *Proc R Soc Med* 1965; **58**: 295–300. Available at: http://www.edwardtufte.com/tufte/hill/. Accessed: September 4, 2004.

108. Lasagna L, Hutt PB. Health care, research, and regulatory impact of noncompliance. In: Cramer JA, Spilker B, eds, *Compliance in Medical Practice and Clinical Trials*. New York: Raven Press, 1991; pp. 393–403.

109. Urquhart J. Pharmacoeconomic consequences of variable patient compliance with prescribed drug regimens. *Pharmacoeconomics* 1999; **15**: 217–28.

110. Bachmann LHY, Stephens J, Richey CM, Hook EW. Measured versus self-reported compliance with doxycycline therapy for chlamydia-associated syndromes: high therapeutic success rates despite poor compliance. *Sex Transm Dis* 1999; **26**: 272–8.

111. PRILOSEC® (omeprazole) delayed- release capsules. *Physicians' Desk Reference*, 58th edn. Montvale, NJ: Thomson PDR, 2004; pp. 633–8.

112. Waterhouse DM, Calzone KA, Mele C, Brenner DE. Adherence to oral tamoxifen: a comparison of patient self-report, pill counts, and microelectronic monitoring. *J Clin Oncol* 1993; **11**: 1189–97.

113. Olivieri NF, Brittenham GM, Matsui D, Berkovitch M, Blendis LM, Cameron R, *et al.* Iron-chelation therapy with oral deferiprone in patients with thalassemia major. *N Engl J Med* 1995; **332**: 918–22.

114. Weintraub M. Intelligent noncompliance and capricious compliance. In: Lasagna L, ed., *Patient Compliance*. Mount Kisco, NY: Futura, 1976; pp. 39–47.

47

Bias and Confounding in Pharmacoepidemiology

ILONA CSIZMADI[1], JEAN-PAUL COLLET[2] and JEAN-FRANÇOIS BOIVIN[2]

[1] Population Health and Information, Alberta Cancer Board, Calgary, Canada; [2] Department of Epidemiology and Biostatistics, McGill University, Montréal, Canada, and Centre for Clinical Epidemiology and Community Studies, SMBD Jewish General Hospital.

INTRODUCTION

A major objective of pharmacoepidemiology is to estimate the effects of drugs when they are prescribed after marketing. This is difficult because drug exposure is not a stable phenomenon and may be associated with factors that may also be related to the outcome of interest, such as indication for prescribing. Other examples of factors that must be taken into account include compliance, publicity, and the natural course of the disease. The great challenge of pharmacoepidemiology is thus to obtain an accurate estimate, i.e., "without error," of the relationship between drug exposure and health status. There are two types of error: *random error* relates to the concepts of precision and reliability, while *systematic error* is related to the concepts of validity and bias. *Accuracy* itself is absence of both random and systematic error. The question of measurement has always represented a key point in epidemiology; Rothman wrote that "an epidemiologic study is properly viewed as an exercise in measurement, with accuracy as the goal."[1]

CLINICAL PROBLEMS TO BE ADDRESSED BY PHARMACOEPIDEMIOLOGIC RESEARCH

In 1981, Alderslade and Miller presented the results of the National Childhood Encephalopathy Study (NCES), a nationwide case–control study conducted in the United Kingdom initiated to answer the question of a possible association between diphtheria–tetanus–pertussis (DTP) vaccine and the subsequent development of neurologic disorders.[2] This report received tremendous publicity because of the importance of the question, but it also raised a large international controversy because several potential biases affected the credibility of the results.

In the NCES, physicians of England, Scotland, and Wales reported on 1182 cases of severe acute neurologic illnesses in infants and children aged 2 to 35 months; two controls were selected for each case, matched on age, gender, and residential area. The NCES found that the risk of severe acute neurologic event was significantly increased within the seven days following DTP vaccine (relative risk (RR)

Pharmacoepidemiology, Fourth Edition   Edited by B.L. Strom
© 2005 John Wiley & Sons, Ltd

2.3; 95% confidence interval (CI), 1.4–3.2), and that, one year after the vaccine, 7 of the 241 cases (2.9%) who had died or had a developmental deficit had begun their disease within the seven days following a DTP vaccine compared to only 3 of 478 controls (0.6%), yielding a relative risk of 4.7 (95% CI, 1.1–28.0). The results have been used in many court trials by parents of disabled children who were seeking compensation.

It was, however, the beginning of an important controversy. First, the NCES's results were not confirmed in several other, but smaller, studies.[3–6] In addition, several biases were considered possible explanations, partial or total, for what was observed. The following problems, in particular, were discussed:

- The fact that the participating physicians knew the objectives of the study may have increased the reporting of cases that occurred shortly after vaccination. This referral bias would have increased the apparent relative risk.
- Information bias was also considered possible. The exact date of onset of the neurological problem was occasionally difficult to ascertain precisely. Also, the interviewers and data collectors were not blinded to the study's objectives, nor to the participants' clinical status. It is thus possible that the date of onset was sometimes shifted toward a shorter post-vaccine time window. The fact that the immediate high-risk post-vaccine period was followed by a subsequent low-risk period has been considered as evidence that this bias actually occurred.
- The main concern was selection bias. Children who had previous neurologic disorders (e.g., seizures) were more likely to go unvaccinated and were also more likely to develop permanent brain damage. This selection bias would have favored the inclusion of non-vaccinated individuals in the case group, reducing the apparent relative risk. It is also possible that the previous neurologic disorder was present and occasionally the case "event" was the first expression of the disease. In that situation, these children should have been excluded from the study because the disease in fact preceded the exposure (see "Protopathic bias," below). Of course, in this situation the subclinical neurologic disease could not have biased the choice of whether or not to vaccinate.
- Several other issues were also of concern in the interpretation of the NCES results. These include, for example, the lack of precision of the disease definitions as well as the inclusion of cases which were not thought to be plausibly related to DTP vaccine (such as Reye's syndrome, hypsarrhythmia, or acute viral encephalopathies), with a

possible dilution of any vaccine-specific association. The fact that the odds ratio for the risk of permanent brain damage was based on only seven cases and three controls was of particular concern, because among the seven cases there was one case of Reye's syndrome and two cases of well-identified viral encephalitis.

The NCES represents an example of how pharmacoepidemiology studies may contribute to data needed by clinicians, public health administrators, and lawyers. The controversy surrounding it, however, shows that a well thought out and designed pharmacoepidemiology study can raise many questions and lose an important part of its credibility because of the possibility of biases. Once a study is completed, some biases can only be discussed in terms of likelihood and importance, and cannot be estimated precisely, nor controlled at the analysis stage. The possibility of biases in a study raises doubts about its results, and provides an opportunity for subsequent debate based upon convictions rather than evidence.

Generally speaking, questions raised about the quality of studies, as exemplified above, have important implications for clinicians, regulators, public health administrators, and health economists. For example, when a case–control study shows that the risk of a severe adverse event is different in patients treated, respectively, with drugs A and B, the following questions should be raised:

- Was the clinical indication that led to the prescription of drug A or B considered in the analysis? Different drugs are likely to be prescribed to different types of patients, with different diseases or different degrees of severity or clinical expression of the same disease; such differences in baseline characteristics may lead to the patients being at different risks of developing an adverse outcome, independently of the prescription of drug A or B.
- Were all eligible cases included? Was the exclusion of some patients related to drug exposure?
- How precisely was exposure measured? Exposure is often reduced to a dichotomous classification, which is not very precise.
- Could previous knowledge of the problem have influenced the reporting of cases or the recall of previous exposure?
- Was the exposure time window defined in relation to the onset of outcome or in relation to the onset of drug exposure?
- Was temporal information about drug exposure included in the analysis? This information is very

important because the risk is probably very different in new users, in long-term chronic users of the same drug, and in those who have shifted from one drug to another.

- Was the strength of the association constant in all categories of patients (i.e., independent of age, comorbidity, coprescription, different forms of the disease, etc.)?

The study of the sources of bias and the different approaches to preventing bias is thus a fundamental aspect of pharmacoepidemiology. The question of bias in epidemiology has been covered in several good classical epidemiology textbooks,[1,7–11] and discussed in some important articles.[12–16] Pharmacoepidemiology studies, however, may be affected more often by some particular biases than other epidemiologic studies. Moreover, the dynamic of bias occurrence over time seems to represent a particularly important phenomenon in pharmacoepidemiology. In this chapter, we will first describe the most important biases that may affect pharmacoepidemiology studies. We will then focus on confounding and show that it is sometimes not very easy to separate this category from other types of bias (especially selection bias). We will also discuss the

dynamics of bias in pharmacoepidemiology and we will show how to deal with the problem of bias and confounding at the design and the analysis stage.

METHODOLOGIC PROBLEMS TO BE ADDRESSED BY PHARMACOEPIDEMIOLOGIC RESEARCH

BIASES IN PHARMACOEPIDEMIOLOGY

Several potential biases are likely to affect pharmacoepidemiology studies, for example referral bias, recall bias, nondifferential or differential follow-up bias, protopathic bias, and prevalence study bias. For the purpose of our discussion, however, we will classify these biases into three groups: selection bias, information bias, and confounding. Figure 47.1 shows that selection bias is related to the recruitment of study subjects or losses to follow-up. Information bias is related to the accuracy of the information that is collected on exposure, health status, and also covariates such as confounding variables or effect modifiers. Confounding is related to the pathophysiological mechanisms

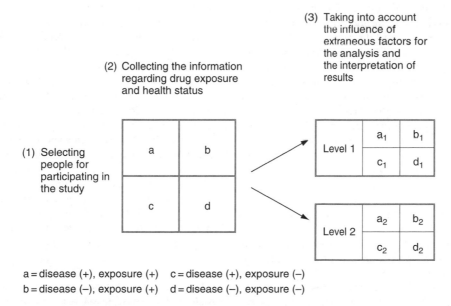

a = disease (+), exposure (+)   c = disease (+), exposure (−)
b = disease (−), exposure (+)   d = disease (−), exposure (−)

Figure 47.1. Biases in pharmacoepidemiology. (1) *Selection bias* is related to the way people are recruited for the study or are retained during the course of the study; (2) *information bias* is related to the way the information about study variables is measured during the study; (3) *confounding* is related to the influence of other variables that are related to both drug use and the outcome, and may be responsible for part or all of the observed effect, the lack of observed effect, or a reversal of the effect.

of disease development, which may be affected by several factors acting together; what is observed is not due to the exposure of interest, but to other factors.

Selection Bias

Selection bias is a distortion of the measurement of an estimate of effect, which is due to the selection into the study of groups of subjects who have an unusual and unequal relationship between drug exposure and outcome. Hence, the estimate of the association in the study group differs from the estimate in the target population (this bias is also called *sample distortion bias*). In pharmacoepidemiology, four types of selection bias seem particularly important: referral bias, self-selection, and prevalence study bias, with the special case of "protopathic bias."

Referral Bias

Referral bias can occur if the reasons for referring a patient, to the hospital for instance, may be related to the drug exposure status, e.g., when the use of the drug contributes to the diagnostic process. This is a particular problem when an illness presents in a manner such that an accurate diagnosis is not always obtained. For instance, a patient taking nonsteroidal anti-inflammatory drugs and presenting with abdominal pain may be more likely to be suspected as having a gastric ulcer. This patient is therefore more likely to be sent to the hospital for tests for this diagnosis than other patients with similar pain who are not using nonsteroidal anti-inflammatory drugs. A study using patients in the hospital may thus show a strong, but biased, association between mild nonbleeding gastric ulcers and the use of nonsteroidal anti-inflammatory drugs. On the other hand, if one were studying serious gastrointestinal bleeding, this might not be a problem.

The same problem may occur with diagnoses of deep venous thrombosis in women using oral contraceptives who present with leg pain. Knowledge of a well-established association between the disease and the drug makes the use of an oral contraceptive a key element in the diagnosis, such that these women may be more likely to be subjected to diagnostic tests for venous thrombosis.

This referral bias problem may even be more generalized. It is possible, for instance, that in older people taking many drugs, the occurrence of "any change in health status" or "any suspicious side effect" may lead to hospitalization just because of exposure to a large number of drugs. In these circumstances, there will be a positive association between drug use in general and any health condition.

Appreciating the potential for referral bias helps in interpreting the results of successive epidemiologic studies conducted at different points in time. We can imagine a situation in which only the first study was unbiased because the association was not yet known. When the first publication shows a positive association between drug and disease, the referral bias phenomenon begins and is likely to increase after each new report of a positive association. In this context, we may observe an increase in the strength of the association over time, even if the true association remains constant and even if it is actually null.

This phenomenon of referring "exposed cases" may occasionally have a very large impact in pharmacoepidemiology. It has been shown, for example, that the publication of a letter in a medical journal may affect a physician's ability to find new cases of the condition and increase the probability of his or her reporting them. This type of alert is also likely to increase the referral of these "interesting" patients to the hospital; hospitalized patients will then represent a biased group with a strong positive association between drug exposure and health event. Reports on side effects of triazolam, for example, are likely to have been affected by referral bias: after the first publication,[17] several authors reported other single case experiences,[18,19] and then Sunter *et al.* reported a series of cases in 1988.[20] While these were all spontaneous reports of adverse reactions, not formal epidemiologic studies, one could speculate that subsequent formal studies could have been affected by referral bias.

One mechanism to prevent this type of *publicity bias* would consist of keeping confidential the reports of single cases of possible adverse events until a good epidemiologic study has confirmed them. From this perspective, confidentiality related to the publication of a single case report should not be viewed as a protection of the manufacturer but as a protection of the scientific truth. This is because once the first case report has been "mediatized," the situation is intrinsically biased and, in some situations, the question cannot be answered any more, or only with a great deal of difficulty. Of course, whether such a confidential treatment of case reports would be appropriate from a public health perspective can be debated. A general solution to the question of referral bias is to restrict the study to more serious cases of the disease. It can be expected that for most diseases, all serious cases will eventually be diagnosed correctly.

Self-Selection

When patients decide themselves to participate or to leave a study, a type of selection bias may occur, because this decision may be related both to drug exposure and to change in health status. Hence, the association observed in the study sample may not be representative of the real association in the source population. This problem is particularly important in interview-based historical case–control studies, because both outcome and exposure are already manifest when study subjects are recruited. It could be the case where, for instance, birth defects are studied; we can easily imagine that mothers of affected children who also have "something to report" (i.e., use of medications) may be more (or less) likely to participate. Such a situation is not unusual in pharmacoepidemiology. The problem must be controlled at the design level by systematically identifying and including all the cases suffering from the condition. Having a registry is an excellent way to cope with this problem of selection. A similar problem may occur in historical cohort studies relying on volunteers or in clinical trials that rely on volunteers. Losses to follow-up may also bias the results similarly in cohort studies, if those who drop out belong to a special disease–exposure category.

Prevalence Bias

Another type of selection bias may occur in case–control studies when prevalent cases rather than new cases of a condition are selected for a study. An association with prevalence may be related to the duration of the disease rather than to its incidence, because prevalence is proportional to both incidence and duration of the disease. An association between drug use and prevalent cases could thus reflect an association with a prognostic factor rather than with incidence. It is possible that a positive association with "good prognosis prevalent cases" might not be confirmed in the whole group of patients defined by incidence. The situation could even be worst if only one group of patients defined by their disease duration gets the medication. It would be the case, for example, if only survivors get the medication; there will obviously be a positive association between drug use and outcome.

Another similar bias may occur when patients are recruited through a screening procedure. The population selected by screening may be different from the one identified by clinically manifest symptoms. There may be different relationships between drug exposure and adverse effects in these two subpopulations.

Generally speaking, criteria for inclusion, even those which are not clearly stated, must be considered with the highest attention when interpreting the results from nonexperimental studies; preventing selection bias or dealing with it is an essential stage in the development of a protocol in pharmacoepidemiology.

"Protopathic Bias"

The term *protopathic bias* was first used by Feinstein.[8] It may occur "if a particular maneuver was started, stopped, or otherwise changed because of the baseline manifestation caused by a disease or other outcome event." Confusion between cause and effect may then arise. For instance, people could stop taking aspirin because of the presence of blood in their stools. If the presence of blood were the first expression of colon cancer, we would find a negative association between current aspirin use and colon cancer. This type of bias is a consequence of selecting only clinically manifest cases, and of the difficulty of precisely ascertaining exposure that occurred in the past. This situation may occur in pharmacoepidemiology because diseases are often identified late after their first clinical expression and exposure to drugs may change from day to day. Such possibilities demonstrate the paramount importance of as full an understanding as possible of the pathophysiologic mechanism of disease development in designing pharmacoepidemiology studies.

Information and Misclassification Bias

Each time participants in a study are classified with regard to their exposure and disease status, there is a possibility of error, i.e., unexposed people may be considered exposed, and sick people may be considered normal (and the reverse). This type of error may lead to a *misclassification bias*. It may equally affect case–control and cohort studies. When the error occurs randomly (i.e., independently of the exposure–outcome relationship), it leads to what is referred to as *nondifferential misclassification*. When the degree of error in measuring disease or exposure is influenced by knowledge of the exposure or the outcome status, the misclassification that results is said to be *differential misclassification*, which means systematically biased. For example, this may occur in cohort studies during the process of data collection, when knowledge of the exposure influences systematically the quality of the information collected about disease outcome. Alternatively, this may occur in case–control studies when knowledge of the disease status influences the quality of the information collected about exposure. This differential misclassification is also called *information bias*. We will describe these two types of misclassification bias in more detail.

Nondifferential Misclassification

When the degree of misclassification is similar for all patients and independent of both exposure and health status conditions (because the instrument is not very reliable, for instance), it is called nondifferential or random misclassification. It may lead to a decrease in the strength of the association between drug and outcome (bias toward the null value). In extreme circumstances, it may even reverse the measure of effect. This tendency is very important to consider when the conclusion of the study is that there is "no statistically significant association." This may merely be due to important random misclassification. In pharmacoepidemiology, the assessment of drug exposure is likely to be affected by an important rate of nondifferential misclassification because it is related to many factors that are difficult to control. Figure 47.2 shows the different possibilities for misclassifying drug exposure. This is also discussed in more detail in Chapter 45.

Another important misclassification may occur when dichotomizing a patient's exposure as "exposed/not exposed" without taking into account the timing of the exposure. The International Agranulocytosis and Aplastic Anemia Study (IAAAS)[21] was criticized because the authors defined their time window only in relation to the occurrence of outcome and not in relation to the onset of drug exposure, ignoring patients' history of previous exposure.[22] The fact that previous, especially long-term, exposure to the drug was likely to be associated with a lower risk of severe events could have distorted the results. This lack of accuracy in defining exposure may result in an important information bias which may lead to a nonsignificant association overall while, in fact, within a specific time window, there is a very strong association between the drug and the outcome.

Figure 47.3 shows different hazard functions related to drug exposure. Anaphylactic reactions occur rapidly after drug exposure, the risk being very high during a short period of time and null after this period. For other outcomes, the risk is likely to decrease with time. For instance, chronic long-term users of a given anti-inflammatory drug are likely to be at a lower risk of gastrointestinal bleeding than new users. It is also possible that in some circumstances the risk steadily increases with time, due for instance to the cumulative effect of drug exposure (e.g., risk of myocardial toxicity after the use of doxorubicin). In the examples shown in Figure 47.3, the instantaneous risk is completely different in each situation but the average risk for the full period is similar. The average risk for the total period of follow-up does not represent the real risk faced by the patients. This mis-measurement is likely to decrease the strength of the association between drug exposure and adverse event.

Differential Misclassification

When misclassification is related to the exposure–outcome association, we refer to it as differential or systematic misclassification. This possibility occurs each time the knowledge about the outcome status in a case–control study, or the exposure status in a cohort study, influences the validity of the information collected. In pharmacoepidemiology, two

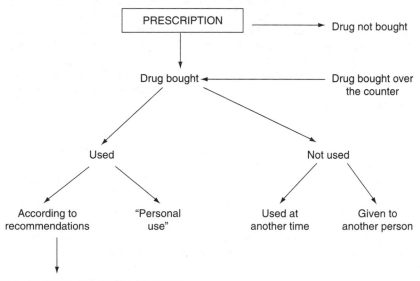

Figure 47.2. Factors influencing drug exposure.

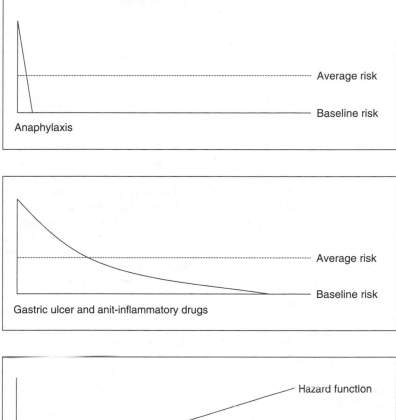

Figure 47.3. Hazard functions related to drug exposure.

situations are commonly responsible for this type of bias: "differential recall" and "differential detection."

• *Recall bias* is an important concern in retrospective studies, e.g., in case–control studies, cases and controls may have a different memory of their past exposures. In studies of birth defects, for example, mothers with an impaired child may give a more valid and complete report of their exposure to drugs during pregnancy. This has nothing to do with deliberate lies or a desire to mislead, but to memory being better when there is good reason for it. This problem

must be controlled at the design level by choosing, for instance, a control group which is likely to have the same memory of the past, if possible, (e.g., alternative birth defects) (see also Chapter 32).

• *Detection bias* can affect either cohort or case–control studies. It occurs in case–control studies when the procedures for exposure assessment are not similar in cases and controls (e.g., more attention is given to assessing exposure in the cases). In cohort studies, it occurs when the follow-up procedures for detecting adverse events differ according to the exposure status of the participants. For instance, women taking postmenopausal hormonal supplements are likely to see their doctors more often than other women. These women are therefore more likely to be examined for breast or endometrial cancer, or for the risk of cardiovascular disease. This differential follow-up may lead to an excess number of diagnosed diseases in the treated group and a falsely elevated risk, or to more complete preventive care, leading to a decreased risk. Differential follow-up may sometimes be very subtle. For instance, if a drug is responsible for the development of side effects that require specific care (e.g., abdominal pain requiring radiologic examination or medical visits), the differential follow-up induced by this condition may be responsible for an excess of diagnoses of several other already prevalent conditions that would not have been identified otherwise (e.g., cholelithiasis).

CONFOUNDING

Confounding occurs when the estimate of a measure of association between drug exposure and health status is distorted by the effect of one or several other variables that are also risk factors for the outcome of interest. Confounding occurs when the distribution of these risk factors is unbalanced across the different levels of the drug exposure. In this case, the occurrence of the outcome is changing from one level of the drug exposure to the other in relation (partly or totally) to the cofactors. Without good information on the other risk factors, i.e., valid and precise measurement of their magnitude, it is not possible to separate the respective effect of each component. The estimate measured in this condition is said to be "confounded" by the other cofactors.

In the next section of the chapter, we will present some numerical examples aimed at showing the mechanism of confounding and the statistical principles for correcting its effect. We will also describe some important confounders in pharmacoepidemiology and we will show that it is sometimes difficult to distinguish confounding and selection bias.

Mechanism of Confounding

For a variable to be a confounder, it must be associated with both the drug exposure and the outcome of interest, without being in the causal pathway between the drug exposure and the outcome. In other words, it must represent an independent risk factor. Figure 47.4 shows the classical relationship between the three variables. For example, when studying the relationship between the use of nonsteroidal antiinflammatory drugs and the occurrence of a gastric ulcer,

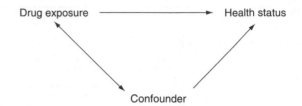

Figure 47.4. Mechanism of confounding.

personal history of gastric problems can be a confounder, because: (i) personal history of gastric problems is a risk factor for gastric ulcers, and (ii) a history of gastric problems will modify the probability of physicians' prescribing nonsteroidal anti-inflammatory drugs.

In such a situation, the measure of association between nonsteroidal anti-inflammatory drugs and gastric ulcers can be affected by the confounder. In the extreme situation, physicians could decide never to use nonsteroidal antiinflammatory drugs in patients with a history of gastric problems. These drugs could then appear as protective for peptic ulcer. The result in this case would obviously be biased. A confounder may be responsible for a part or all of the effect observed. It may exaggerate, mitigate, or reverse a true effect. The existence of confounding is generally established by comparing the crude estimate of the association with the estimate obtained after controlling for the potential confounder.

Table 47.1 presents a fictitious example of confounding. A cohort study of deaths associated with the use of drug A was conducted. The comparison group consisted of patients treated with drug B. When data for all patients were considered together, the following results were observed: the risk of death was 202/1100 = 18% among patients using drug A, and it was 8/110 = 7% among drug B users. The relative risk was therefore 18%/7% = 2.5, indicating a harmful effect of drug A. The study population was then subdivided into two

Table 47.1. A cohort study of drug use and risk of death (hypothetical)

Stratum	Treatment	Death		Total	Relative risk
		Yes	No		
All	A	202	898	1100	18%/7% = 2.5
	B	8	102	110	
Severe disease	A	200	800	1000	20%/40% = 0.5
	B	4	6	10	
Benign disease	A	2	98	100	2%/4% = 0.5
	B	4	96	100	

strata: subjects with a severe form of the disease being treated, and those with a more benign form of the disease. When the analysis was conducted within each of these two strata, the direction of the effect was reversed. Among subjects with severe disease, the risks of death were 20% and 40%, respectively, for drugs A and B, for a relative risk of 0.5. The risks of death were lower for subjects with a benign form of the disease, but the relative risk was also 0.5.

These data represent an extreme example of confounding. Obviously, if the estimate of the measure of effect, i.e., the relative risk, is 0.5 among subjects with severe disease and also 0.5 among those with benign disease, the overall estimate of effect, when the data for all subjects are pooled, should also be 0.5. The estimate of 2.5 is not valid, because of confounding by the severity of the disease. An inspection of Table 47.1 shows that subjects with severe disease experience a death rate that is much higher than the rate among those with benign disease. In addition, however, the distribution of study subjects by drug category is not balanced. One thousand subjects with severe disease received drug A. The numbers of subjects in the other subsets of the study population are much smaller. Because of this, the crude estimate of relative risk obtained when the data from the two strata are pooled is heavily influenced by the mortality experience among the 1000 subjects, and this results in the distorted estimate of 2.5.

Table 47.2 gives another example of confounding. In this cohort study, the association between the use of a drug and the risk of allergy was determined. Subjects with and subjects without drug treatment were compared. These data show confounding due to age. Older subjects experienced a high risk of allergy, and a very large group of old subjects without drug treatment was included in the study. Because of this, the overall relative risk was less than the relative risk among young subjects, and also less than the relative risk among old subjects. The confounding was, however, weaker than in the previous example. In the present

example, the direction of the association was the same for the overall study population and for the two strata. In the previous example, there was a reversal of effect.

Table 47.2 shows another phenomenon. The estimate of relative risk is not the same for young and for old subjects (4 and 2, respectively). This represents *effect modification* or *interaction*: the magnitude of the drug effect on the risk of allergy varies between strata. Statistical tests of heterogeneity (e.g. Breslow–Day or Woolf) are usually used to assess whether such variation between strata can be attributed to random fluctuations, or whether it represents a true effect.

Important Confounders in Pharmacoepidemiology

Confounding by the Reason for Prescription

The indication for a prescription is probably the most important confounding factor in pharmacoepidemiology since, theoretically, there is always a reason for prescription and because the reason is often associated with the outcome of interest. The situation has been the object of important considerations in the discussion of study results[23–26] (see also Chapter 40). It has also received several different names such as "indication bias," "channeling," or "confounding by severity." All these labels, as well as others like "contraindication bias," just represent the fact that there is a reason for prescribing a drug.

The problem of confounding by indication can be considered in the same perspective as selection bias, because the decision to prescribe can be viewed as one way to select a group of patients. If this selection process is also related to the outcome (which is often the case, especially when considering drug efficacy; see Chapter 40), there is a bias. This perspective shows that, for a given drug, the possibility of bias is not universal, but is directly related to the outcome studied and may also change over time, or from one country to another. It also shows the extreme difficulty of adjusting for this type of confounding. Miettinen[24] has discussed this problem in the context of a study of intended effects: "Thus, perceived high risk or poor prognosis tends to constitute an indication for intervention .... Where such an indication does guide the use of intervention, it constitutes a confounder: it is, by definition, a correlate of the determinant at issue, the intervention, and it is a predictor of the null outcome in so far as it indeed does imply the presumed high risk or poor prognosis."

The term "confounding by indication" implies that we could control for the reason for the prescription at the analysis stage. Although this is theoretically possible, it

Table 47.2. A cohort study of drug use and allergy risk (hypothetical)

Stratum	Treatment	Allergy		Total	Relative risk
		Yes	No		
All	Drug	28	172	200	14%/9% = 1.6
	No drug	102	998	1100	
Young	Drug	8	92	100	8%/2% = 4
	No drug	2	98	100	
Old	Drug	20	80	100	20%/10% = 2
	No drug	100	900	1000	

is in practice often impossible to obtain a sufficiently accurate estimate of the effect of this confounder, even when the reason for prescribing seems very straightforward. That is because "indication" is a very complex and multifactorial phenomenon involving the physician's knowledge and many factors, sometimes not rational, which act in different directions. Miettinen provided an example that the preventive use of warfarin can be associated with a 27-fold increase in the risk of thrombotic events, a condition that should actually be prevented by anticoagulation.[24] This paradoxical result was explained by a strong negative confounding effect, i.e., only highly susceptible patients, or those already presenting the first symptoms of thrombosis (see "protopathic bias") were receiving the therapy. Miettinen showed further in that example that controlling for the information available related to the reasons for the prescription, e.g., previous history of blood clotting, reduced the bias but could not change the direction of the association: after adjustment, the risk in treated patients was still four times higher than in nontreated patients.

The example illustrates that it can be very difficult to measure accurately the reasons for prescribing. This rather pessimistic conclusion has two consequences. The first one is related to the scope of research in pharmacoepidemiology, in which the study of the determinants of prescribing is a domain requiring much attention. The second is related to the desirability of randomized clinical trials, rather than nonexperimental studies, whenever the results from nonexperimental studies are likely to be biased and "inconclusive" because of confounding by the indication. A more positive view of this situation would, on the other hand, consider that, even when confounding by indication is present, the resulting information can be useful for other purposes. For example, it has been postulated that the reported association between β-agonists and asthma mortality was confounded by disease severity.[25] Even in the presence of such a bias, however, the fact that β-agonists were positively correlated with asthma deaths can be very useful information for physicians, as the amount of drug use becomes a good indicator of prognosis. This issue is discussed in much more detail in Chapter 40.

Confounding by Comedication and Other Cofactors

Patients often take more than one drug at a time and it is sometimes difficult to isolate the effect of a specific drug. This question was discussed in the analysis of the Coronary Drug Project,[27] which showed that in the placebo group, the risks of death in the 5 years following randomization were 15% and 28.2%, respectively, among compliant patients and noncompliant patients. Beyond a possible selection bias that would relate the better survival to some hypothetical and undetermined factors, the main reason postulated as an explanation for this difference was the fact that patients who were compliant with one drug were also very likely to be compliant with other interventions (e.g., other very effective drugs, diet, physical exercise, etc.). As in the problem of confounding by indication, it is possible to control in part the effect of all other cofactors, but the feasibility of doing so is limited (it is for instance very difficult to quantify compliance precisely), and residual bias is likely to remain.

Confounding and Effect Modification

Confounding and effect modification (or interaction) are both "multivariable phenomena" (i.e., there is a third variable, or group of variables, which plays a role in the observed effect between the drug exposure and the outcome of interest). It is, however, very important to distinguish between the two phenomena, as they have different consequences and require different strategies to be controlled for. As we have seen, Tables 47.1 and 47.2 present two hypothetical examples, one with confounding (Table 47.1) and the other one with interaction (Table 47.2). We can see that, as already defined, a third variable (or covariate) is a confounder when it is responsible for part or all of the observed effect. Table 47.1 shows that the "harmful effect of drug A" was in fact due to the selective exposure of patients with the most severe cases of the disease to drug A, while patients with benign disease were more likely to be exposed to drug B. In this situation, the crude estimate of the drug effect represents a combination of two effects: (drug A + severe disease) versus (drug B + benign disease). Table 47.1 also shows that the relative risks for drugs A and B remained constant across the different strata of the confounder. The relative effects of drug A and B were not modified by the severity of the disease. In this situation, severity is said to be a confounder, but not an effect modifier. It is possible to adjust for the difference in distribution of disease severity among the two groups of drug users, and obtain an overall relative risk, which in this case will be 0.5, instead of 2.5, the unadjusted crude relative risk.

Table 47.2 shows another example of confounding, but it also shows that the drug effect (measured by the relative risk) varies across the different strata of age. In this situation, age is said to be both a confounder and an effect modifier. It would be possible, like in the previous example, to combine the stratum-specific effects into an overall measure of effect, adjusted for the difference in age distribution. This overall adjusted result, however, is meaningless and may be misleading, as the average result represents a combination of a positive effect for certain patients and negative effects for others. When there is effect modification, the stratum-specific effect provides more information, and is also more interpretable than the single summary figure.

Effect modification corresponds to the statistical concept of interaction. An important point related to interaction is that it is model-dependent: interaction may exist with one parameter measuring the effect, the risk ratio for instance, but not with another parameter, like the risk difference. Moreover, interaction is often a finding at the time of the analysis, as there is generally not enough information for suspecting and quantifying *a priori* its presence. Effect modification, thus, is often useful for generating new hypotheses and is generally presented as a finding that may be worth being further studied.

Through these considerations it appears that confounding is a nuisance and a threat in pharmacoepidemiology because it may affect the validity of the results. On the other hand, effect modification indicates a variation in the drug effect, according to different levels of a third variable. If it is confirmed, this change of effect may be the source of important findings regarding the use of the drug and its mechanism of action. Effect modification is thus an important piece of information that deserves high consideration, adequate study, and careful interpretation.

Effect Modification by Dose or Drug Potency
Different dosage and potency are likely to have different effects that should be presented in the analysis. Reducing the information related to exposure into a dichotomous expression (i.e., exposed versus not exposed) increases the rate of misclassification and it biases the results toward the null. Spitzer *et al.*, for instance, concluded that use of both fenoterol and albuterol were associated with an excess risk of death in asthmatic patients, probably in relation to the severity of the patient's condition.[25] Table 47.3 shows that the dichotomous classification of drug exposure was associated with a three-fold excess risk of death with fenoterol compared to albuterol. However, taking into account (i) the number of inhalers used, and also (ii) the concentration of drug per inhalation (100 μg for albuterol and 200 μg for fenoterol) completely modified the results, such that the

Table 47.3. Risk of death in asthmatic patients treated by fenoterol and albuterol: change in study results with change in measurement of drug exposure

		Odds ratio	95% Confidence interval
Crude association exposed versus not exposed			
Fenoterol		9.1	3.0–28.1
Albuterol		2.8	1.0–7.6
Results per number of inhalers dispensed			
Fenoterol	0	1.0	Reference group
	1–12	4.7	1.1–20.6
	13–24	40.5	5.1–319
	≥25	113.2	17.0–754
Albuterol	0	1.0	Reference group
	1–12	3.4	0.9–13.3
	13–24	10.0	2.1–46.5
	≥25	29.4	5.1–171
Model of continuous exposure			
Fenoterol 100 μg		2.3	1.6–3.4
Albuterol 100 μg		2.4	1.5–3.8

Source: Original data from Spitzer *et al.*[25]

risk of death appears similar with the two drugs. This demonstrates the importance in pharmacoepidemiologic research of considering the possibility of differences in drug dose and drug potency in studying drug effects (see also Chapter 4).

CURRENTLY AVAILABLE SOLUTIONS

HOW CAN ONE DEAL WITH SELECTION BIAS?

Selection bias must be prevented at the design stage, because it cannot be corrected at the analysis stage. The objective is to prevent over- or underrepresentation of the people who have a particular drug exposure–outcome relationship. This can be achieved in several ways, which all result in selecting a study population that accurately represents the target population concerning the drug exposure–outcome relationship.

• Random sampling of the cases and controls (or exposed and non-exposed patients) to be included in the study from the source population.
• Systematically recruiting a series of consecutive patients (to prevent self-selection).
• Adopting a well-codified accrual procedure (to be adapted according to the nature and severity of the disease). Having

a geographic definition of the incident cases goes a long way toward reducing referral bias.

- Minimizing the number of subjects lost to follow-up in cohort studies.
- Implementing a tracking procedure for those who drop out of the study, in order to know the reason and, if possible, to measure their health status.
- Selecting only incident cases of the condition.
- Random allocation of drug exposure, which prevents both self-selection and referral bias.

This "perfect" situation, however, is very difficult to implement, and is generally limited to a small number of people who are followed for a short period of time. Besides ethical, cost, and logistic problems, the experimental design often also creates situations far from real life (see also Chapter 2).

HOW CAN ONE DEAL WITH INFORMATION BIAS?

As with selection bias, the problem of information bias must be resolved at the design stage, since its presence irremediably affects the study validity. Several techniques facilitate an unbiased collection of information:

- *Blinding* (or *masking*) is the most important strategy, as it is easier to be neutral when it is not known who is exposed, who is sick, and what are the objectives of the study. In a cohort study, the data collector should be blind as to the patient's exposure status and the patient should be unaware of the study objectives. In a case–control study, the data collector should be blind to the disease status and, if possible, the information related to the past exposure should be collected without knowing the specific objectives of the study. Blinded assessment of the information is often difficult, however, in nonexperimental designs.
- *Standardization of the measurement process* for both cases and controls, or exposed and unexposed people, is an essential step when implementing a pharmacoepidemiology study. It includes, for instance, the use of standard structured questionnaires, specific training of interviewers, the participation of different observers for different measurements, etc.
- The choices of the criteria for defining drug exposure and disease outcomes are important. Priority should be given to objective, previously defined, standardized criteria.

HOW CAN ONE DEAL WITH CONFOUNDING?

In contrast with information bias and selection bias, it is possible to control the effect of confounding at both the design and the analysis levels. We will present an overview of the different strategies that may be used; we will also describe several approaches that were developed to deal with confounding when working with large although incomplete (no information on confounding) databases, a frequent condition in pharmacoepidemiology.

Dealing with Confounding at the Design Level

There are several ways of controlling for confounding when preparing the design of pharmacoepidemiology studies: randomization, matching, and restriction will successively be described.

Randomization
Random allocation of exposure should equalize the distribution of all potential confounders, even unknown ones, across the different levels of drug exposure. *Randomization* is thus aimed at making the two groups perfectly similar apart from the independent intervention variable under assessment as exposure. This shows that the problem of confounding is in this way similar to selection bias. The distinction between the two situations may be subtle and, as Rothman wrote, a practical distinction between confounding and other biases is to consider bias as confounding if it can be controlled in the data analysis.[1]

Matching
Matching is another way to control for confounding at the design stage. The objective of matching for both cohort and case–control studies is to make the two compared groups similar with regard to the distribution of selected known extraneous factors. A matched design requires a matched analysis if the matching variable was truly a confounder. In practice, matching may be difficult, especially when there are several factors to match for; it may then become costly and time consuming. In case–control studies matching may also lead to a new distorting phenomenon called "overmatching": similarity with regard to exposure may also be related to disease status. In this case, there is artifactually no apparent difference between the exposure level of cases and controls (with regard to the exposure of interest) because of the matching.

Restriction
Restriction of the design to only one level of the confounding factor is the simplest, but also the most reductive, way of dealing with confounding. For instance, studying the effect of a drug in only one category of age will protect against the occurrence of confounding by age. The generalizability of the study, however, may be confined to this age group.

Dealing with Confounding at the Analysis Level

Standardization

Standardization represents a classical method of controlling for confounding; it is often used for comparing vital statistics from populations that have different age or sex distributions, especially in occupational epidemiology. A standardized (or summary) rate is thus a weighted average of stratum-specific rates.

Standardized rate = $\Sigma_i W_i I_i / \Sigma_i W_i$ where W_i and I_i represent, respectively, the stratum-specific weight and the stratum-specific incidence rate. The ratio of standardized rates gives one an estimate of the effect of the exposure, where the ratio of standardized rates = $\Sigma_i W_i (a_i/N_{1i}) / \Sigma_i W_i (b_i/N_{0i})$ and N_{1i} and N_{0i} represent, respectively, the stratum-specific size of the populations which are exposed (N_{1i}) and not exposed (N_{0i}) to the drug, and a_i and b_i represent the number of cases in each stratum which are, respectively, exposed (a_i) and not exposed (b_i) to the drug.

There are two methods of standardization: direct and indirect. Table 47.4 shows the principle of each method and the requirements for their computation. The number of factors that can be managed by standardization is limited (i.e., two or three). Pharmacoepidemiologic research usually requires the manipulation of more than three factors and often, therefore, requires the use of other techniques like mathematical modeling.

Stratification

Stratification is another way of obtaining a summary rate ratio that adjusts for confounding. It is performed in two stages: the first stage requires the computation of a stratum-specific rate ratio for each level of the stratifying (confounding) variable. The second stage involves pooling the results into a single estimate that represents the "overall" effect of the drug, adjusted for the effect of the confounding factor. Standardization and stratification both pursue the same objective of obtaining a pooled estimate of the drug effect.

There are several ways of pooling the stratum-specific measures of effect into an overall estimate.[1,7–10] A classic approach consists of defining the weights as proportional to the inverse of each stratum's variance, (i.e., weighting the contribution of each stratum by its statistical stability). The most popular approach to this has been proposed by Mantel and Haenszel for the odds ratio in case–control studies,[28] and provides a formula which is easy to compute:

$$\text{Adjusted rate ratio} = [\Sigma_i W_i (a_i/N_{1i})(b_i/N_{0i})]/\Sigma_i W_i$$

$$\text{Mantel–Haenszel odds ratio} = \Sigma_i a_i (N_{0i}/T_i)/\Sigma_i b_i (N_{1i}/T_i)$$

where T_i, N_{0i} and N_{1i} represent, respectively, the stratum sample size, the number of unexposed controls, and the number of exposed controls; a_i and b_i represent the number of cases in, respectively, the exposed and the unexposed groups.

Stratification is performed in order to have very little or no variation of the confounder within each stratum of the confounding variable. When this is the case, no or very little confounding remains in each stratum. Stratification, therefore (like "adjustment," described below), requires an accurate measurement of the confounding variable to fulfill its objective. Nondifferential misclassification of a confounder may lead to the persistence of some confounding.[15]

Table 47.4. Standardizing because of difference in age distribution

Methods of standardization	Requirements	Principles
Direct	Age-specific rates in each age stratum A standard population with its age distribution	The age-specific rates for the two compared groups are applied to the standard population. For each age stratum of the standard population an expected number of events is obtained for each observed group; it is the one that would have been observed if the standard population had the age-specific rates of the observed groups. The sum of these expected cases in each group is then divided by the size of the standard population. This provides one age-adjusted mortality rate for each group, which may then be compared.
Indirect	Distribution by age in each of the two compared groups Age-specific rates of a standard population	The population of each stratum of the two compared groups is multiplied by the age-specific rate of a standard population. The computation gives an expected number of events in each group, which is the number that would have occurred if these groups had the age-specific rates of the standard population. In each studied population the expected number is then divided by the observed number of events. The values are called standardized mortality (or incidence) ratios.

The limitation of stratified analysis is that, each time a new factor is added, stratum-specific cell sizes become smaller, and the probability of having people not exposed or not sick in each stratum becomes larger. The stratum-specific estimate of the measure of association cannot then be computed, and the stratum does not provide any statistical information. In this situation, it is better to use a multivariate approach, modeling the relationship between exposure to all factors of interest and the outcome.

Multivariate Analysis and Modeling

Determining the relationship between risk factors and outcomes using a mathematical model allows the assessment of many factors at the same time. According to the prespecified model of relationship (this choice is a crucial one), a parameter of effect will be estimated for each risk factor. This estimate represents the individual contribution of the factor for the risk of the outcome, adjusted for all other factors in the model. However, in order to maintain reasonably stable estimates of parameters there are general rules of thumb for ensuring an optimal sample size: approximately 10 observations are required per factor in a multiple regression model where the outcome is continuous and approximately 10 events per factor for logistic regression models where the outcome is binary. Hence, while multivariate analysis provides a more efficient means of controlling for several factors simultaneously, the adequacy of the data in meeting these requirements must be examined. Most of the important models are derived from *general linear* equations and are very powerful tools that require sophisticated skills in biostatistics and epidemiology, which are beyond the scope of this chapter but are well dealt with in books on multivariate statistical methods.

Dealing with Confounding when Working with Large Drug Databases

Standardization, stratification, and modeling all require an accurate measurement of the confounding variable. Recently, a large number of pharmacoepidemiology studies have been performed using large databases of previously collected data (see Chapters 13–22). One of the major limitations of these studies is the impossibility of adjusting for potential confounders not included in the database. An example would be a study of the relationship between low-dose oral contraceptives (OC) and the risk of myocardial infarction. Databases are likely to provide accurate information for OC prescription and the occurrence of myocardial infarction, for example, but are very unlikely to provide any information on smoking habits, a strong risk factor for myocardial infarction which is also related

to OC use. Not being able to control for such an important confounder prevents studying this association, because the results will obviously be biased: OC users are also heavy smokers. When information on the confounder is available for the cases only,[29] Ray and Griffin showed how to use this information to assess the presence of confounding. If it can be assumed there is no effect modification then, if there is no association between the confounder and exposure among the cases, there is no confounding, and a valid analysis can be carried out. This suggestion is interesting because pharmacoepidemiologists often have more information for the cases (because of hospitalization records) than for the controls (see also Chapter 45).

When information on confounders is not available, it is possible to simulate the effect that the confounder could have by incorporating into a model the information related to the strength of the association of the confounding variable with both the outcome and the exposure of interest, as well as the proportion of people exposed to the confounder. Fine and Chen,[30] for instance, reconsidered the relationship between the risk of pertussis vaccine and the occurrence of sudden infant death syndrome (SIDS). Most studies have shown a significant protective effect of the vaccine, with relative risks as low as 0.15 and a 95% confidence interval of 0.05 to 0.45.[31] Despite the strength of this association, almost no causal inference has been drawn from these results; it is generally assumed that other external factors might be responsible for either avoidance or delay of vaccination, and further development of SIDS. Fine and Chen identified a list of seven potential confounders that had been shown to be related to "failure or delay in receiving vaccines," and also were risk factors for SIDS. They further focused on what they identified as "contraindications to vaccine" and built a model for correcting the crude relative risk. They could study the variation of the adjusted relative risk for different values of: (i) the percentage of children with vaccination; (ii) the relative risk of SIDS associated with vaccination, and (iii) the percentages of vaccination among children with and without contraindications. These models are certainly interesting for assessing the magnitude of the problem; they are, however, limited for providing an accurate adjusted estimate.

In 1982, White[32] and Walker[33] suggested sampling a fraction of the study population to gather information about confounding variables, and using this information in the analysis to obtain covariable-adjusted estimates of the parameters of interest. This approach, referred to as "two-stage sampling,"[34,35] was further developed by Cain and Breslow[36] for multivariate analysis. Efficiency is the essence of this approach, motivated by the desire to use resources optimally. In this approach, stage 1 represents the study population, for example the cases and controls in a case–control study. Individuals for stage 2 are selected according to their disease–exposure characteristics. The balanced design is often more efficient than random and disease- or exposure-based sampling; it consists in having an equal number of individuals in each cell of the second stage 2×2 table. This strategy decreases the occurrence of small cells (responsible for large variance) by forcing an overrepresentation of individuals who belong to small groups in the exposure–disease cross-classification. The sampling fractions that lead to the second stage sample are typically different for each exposure–disease category, creating a selection bias which must be corrected in the analysis. The two-stage design permits the detection of, and adjustment for, confounding. Interaction can also be evaluated. Schaubel *et al.* proposed software for sample size estimation for two-stage sampling.[37]

Propensity Scores for Efficient Adjustment

The propensity score, proposed and developed by Rosenbaum and Rubin,[38] is an innovative statistical approach that can be used to increase the comparability of treatment groups in the absence of randomized treatment assignment. Defined as the conditional probability of being treated, given an individual's covariates, the objective of propensity score analysis is to simulate randomized controlled trial treatment groups in order to estimate a causal treatment effect. One should caution, however, that this objective is achievable only to the extent that all covariates related to treatment assignment have been well measured.[39] Unmeasured relevant covariates will remain potential sources of bias in the estimation of effect. Recently, propensity scores have been used in clinical,[40–46] health services,[47] and pharmacoepidemiologic[48–50] research.

The propensity score is estimated using logistic regression where the exposure or treatment of interest is the dependent variable and covariates related to treatment assignment are the independent variables. The probability or propensity of receiving a treatment, given the observed covariates, is then determined for each subject. Individuals with similar propensity scores are comparable since they are similar in their propensity to receive the treatment under study. The effect of treatment can be estimated using this propensity score (i) as a matching variable prior to analysis, (ii) during analysis to define quintiles for stratification, or (iii) as a covariate in regression analysis. By using the propensity score in the analysis, the effects of all of the prognostic covariates used in estimating it are removed from the estimation of the treatment effect, thus

reducing bias. For any given value of the propensity score the unbiased average treatment effect is estimated for that propensity score if the treatment is "strongly ignorable", given the covariates. Rosenbaum and Rubin[51] define strongly ignorable as the condition where all variables related to both treatment assignment and outcomes have been accounted for by the covariates used to estimate the propensity score. In other words, the probability of being assigned a treatment is dependent only on the propensity score covariates and otherwise treatment assignment is random.

A number of studies have used propensity score matching as a means of controlling for confounding.[45,50] Stamou *et al.*[45] and Gum *et al.*[50] were successful in matching 72% and 58% of eligible treated subjects, respectively, on propensity scores. However, in these studies other multivariate analyses were also performed using all of the subjects, and estimates of treatment effect were similar to those obtained with propensity score matching.

In the above studies the advantages of using matched samples may be debatable. A clear advantage of propensity score matching is described by D'Agastino,[52] in an example where data are available on a small number of treated subjects, a larger number of controls, and an extensive but incomplete array of covariates. In this case, and in similar such cases, estimating and matching on propensity score, and then collecting additional covariate information from only matched pairs would reduce the cost and increase the statistical efficiency of the study.

Using Monte Carlo simulations to simulate observational studies with a variation in the number of covariates, number of events, and sample size, Cepeda *et al.*[53] compared the statistical performance of conventional logistic regression with results from analyses where propensity scores were used. Results from propensity score analysis were less biased, more precise, and less sensitive to a misspecification of the regression model compared with logistic regression analysis, only when there were seven or fewer events per confounder.[53] When there were at least eight events per covariate, logistic regression performed better, with estimates less biased than those obtained with propensity score methods.

Propensity score analysis is not intended to replace well-designed randomized controlled trials (RCTs). Rather, it is a viable and appropriate tool that should be considered in clinical and pharmacoepidemiologic research when RCTs are not feasible due to ethical or cost concerns or when outcomes are extremely rare. It is also an analysis that can be conducted to generate hypotheses for future clinical trials or to provide sufficient evidence to establish clinical equipoise in order to justify an RCT.

Sensitivity Analysis

In this chapter we have discussed the various sources of bias and confounding that can affect pharmacoepidemiology studies. While threats to validity need to be minimized at the design stage of a study, potential biases that have not been accounted for need to be addressed in the presentation of results and discussion. Theoretical models have been proposed to facilitate the identification of unaccounted for biases.[54–56]

Traditionally, the "uncertainty" about study findings has only been addressed in "Discussion" sections of research reports and publications. The limited scope and impact of this practice has recently been highlighted in epidemiology literature.[57] Sensitivity analysis, defined as a quantitative analysis of the potential for systematic error, is a more formal approach used to communicate this uncertainty with respect to the validity of findings. There are several advantages to using this quantitative approach compared with limiting the discussion to a qualitative assessment when presenting results. Sensitivity analysis not only brings to the forefront the important issues related to the validity of results but it also provides a means for presenting objective evidence that may be used by readers to evaluate the magnitude of the threat to validity. In addition, the results of a sensitivity analysis can provide direction for, or suggest, areas of future research.

Not infrequently, sensitivity analysis is carried out to test how robust specific assumptions are in a study; for example, whether or not point estimates vary with the choice of statistical tests (parametric versus nonparametric), definitions of prescription adherence, or definitions of time windows. However, sensitivity analyses, performed with the objective of assessing the potential role of bias in producing an observed effect, is not routinely practiced. Explanations that have been proposed for this under-utilization of sensitivity analyses include the lack of demand from the scientific community, specifically as outlined in the Uniform Requirements for Manuscripts Submitted to Biomedical Journals, the increased need for journal space, and the lack of availability of statistical programs that automate the process.[58]

In a discussion of basic methods that can be used in sensitivity analysis, Greenland, an advocate of its use, illustrates with simple calculations, analyses that can be carried out to assess the potential impact of uncontrollable confounding, misclassification of exposures, diseases and covariates, and selection bias in observational studies.[59] In order to gain an understanding of the potential impact of an unmeasured confounder on estimates of exposure–disease associations, his approach involves the recalculation of adjusted exposure–disease associations at various hypothetical or known levels of prevalence of the confounder in exposure groups, while also varying the strength of association for exposure–specific confounder–disease odds ratios. Using his methods, Hennessy *et al.*[60] conducted a sensitivity analysis to assess the degree of confounding that would have had to be present in studies to account for an observed increase in risk of venous thromboembolism (VTE) with desogestrel and gestodene OC use compared with levonorgestrel. After carrying out a meta-analysis that included data from twelve studies, the summary odds ratio (OR) of 1.7 (1.4–2.0) was adjusted by varying the assumptions about the prevalence of an unmeasured confounder and the OR for the association between the unmeasured confounder and the occurrence of VTE. In a tabular form the authors provided estimates of ORs that accounted for an unmeasured potential confounder present in 5–40% of women taking levonorgestrel and 1.5, 2, or 3 times more common in women receiving desogestrel or gestodene and in which the unmeasured confounder increased the risk of VTE by a factor of 2, 3, 5, or 10. Quantifying bias in such a way clearly has the advantage of allowing readers to judge for themselves the plausibility that an unmeasured confounder may explain the results. In this example and in other recent publications[58,61–63] it is clear that sensitivity analysis facilitates the pursuit of more in-depth discussion than would otherwise arise if unmeasured confounding were addressed merely in the Discussion section of the meta-analysis.

As articulated by Greenland,[59] "it [sensitivity analysis] can be viewed as an attempt to bridge the gap between conventional statistics, which are based on implausible randomization and random-error assumptions, and the more informed but informal inferences that recognize the importance of biases, but do not attempt to estimate their magnitude."

THE FUTURE

One great challenge facing the future in pharmacoepidemiology is the ability to control adequately for "indication for prescribing" at the analysis stage. This requires obtaining a valid and complete ascertainment of the reasons for prescribing drugs. This could be accomplished by adopting very strict, standardized, and measurable criteria for prescribing drugs. Whenever it is not possible to clearly differentiate the respective effects of the drug and the underlying medical conditions, implementing randomized clinical trials in the postmarketing phase should be considered (see Chapter 39).

It is also interesting to consider bias and confounding in pharmacoepidemiology under a dynamic perspective. We have already described the change in referral patterns after the publication of a single case report. Confounding is susceptible to change with time as well, as the decision to prescribe depends directly on the physician. We could even conceptualize the ultimate objective of research in medicine and pharmacoepidemiology as to bias the prescribing of physicians, as only patients who may benefit from the drug should receive it. With this perspective, identification of a change in efficacy or variability in drug effect according to a patient's characteristics or other factors (i.e., the presence of effect modification) should subsequently induce a change in physicians' prescribing to take into account this information. A recent example of this is the change in hormone replacement therapy prescribing since the release of the Women's Health Initiative results in July 2001.[64] This change is normal and expected, as obtaining a more accurate definition of the treatment target population is an objective of pharmacoepidemiologic research.[65] Any further studies of the effect of the drug can then be biased by this new reason for prescribing. We may therefore view confounding by indication as a natural and positive consequence of integrating the results of research into medicine, rather than simply a nuisance while estimating the real effect of a drug.

Another important issue facing pharmacoepidemiology is the ability to measure drug exposure accurately (see also Chapter 45). This should be accomplished by more accurately defining exposure time windows, by better considering dosage and potency, and by accurately measuring drug use; the study of compliance represents thus a highly promising domain of research with regard to the study of drug effects (see Chapter 46). The development of population pharmacokinetics and pharmacodynamics (see Chapter 4), as well as pharmacogenetics (see Chapter 37), should also provide useful information for interpreting pharmacoepidemiologic results with regard to drug exposure. Finally, propensity scores opened a new way for efficient adjustment. This approach could in the future allow adjusting for reasons of prescribing drugs, but only to the degree that indication can be measured. In the end, since it is usually not possible in any study to be certain that confounding has been completely controlled for, sensitivity analyses should be routinely incorporated into the discussion section of study of results.

REFERENCES

1. Rothman KJ. *Modern Epidemiology*. Boston, MA: Little, Brown, 1986.
2. Committee on Safety of Medicines and the Joint Committee on Vaccination and Immunization. *Woophing Cough*. London: Her Majesty's Stationery Office, 1981.
3. Pollock TM, Morris J. A 7-year survey of disorders attributed to vaccination in North West Thames region. *Lancet* 1983; 1: 753–7.
4. Shields WD, Nielsen C, Buch D, Jacobsen V, Christenson P, Zachau-Christenson B *et al*. Relationship of pertussis immunization to the onset of neurological disorders. A retrospective epidemiologic study. *J Pediatr* 1988; **113**: 801–5.
5. Walker AM, Jick H, Petra DR, Knauss TA, Thompson RS. Neurologic events following diphtheria–tetanus–pertussis immunication. *Pediatrics* 1988; **81**: 345–9.
6. Griffin MR, Ray WA, Morimer EA, Fenchel GM, Schafner W. Risk of seizures and encephalopathy after immunization with the diphtheria–tetanus–pertussis vaccine. *JAMA* 1990; **263**: 1641–5.
7. Kleinbaum DG, Kupper LL, Morgenstern H. *Epidemiologic Research*. New York: Van Nostrand Reinhold, 1982.
8. Feinstein AR. *Clinical Epidemiology: The Architecture of Clinical Research*. Philadelphia, PA: WB Saunders, 1985.
9. Kramer MS. *Clinical Epidemiology and Biostatistics*. Heidelberg: Springer-Verlag, 1988.
10. Checkoway H, Pearce NE, Crawford-Brown DJ. *Research Methods in Occupational Epidemiology*. New York: Oxford University Press, 1989.
11. Walker AM. Observation and inference. In: *An Introduction to the Methods of Epidemiology*. Chestnut Hill, MA: Epidemiology Resources, 1991.
12. Miettinen OS. Confounding and effect modification. *Am J Epidemiol* 1972; **100**: 350–3.
13. Copeland KT, Checkoway H, McMichael AJ, Holbrook RH. Bias due to misclassification in the estimation of relative risk. *Am J Epidemiol* 1977; **105**: 488–95.
14. Miettinen OS, Cook F. Confounding: essence and detection. *Am J Epidemiol* 1981; **114**: 593–603.
15. Greenland S. The effect of misclassification in the presence of covariates. *Am J Epidemiol* 1980; **112**: 564–9.
16. Greenland S, Robins JM. Confounding and misclassification of covariates. *Am J Epidemiol* 1985; **122**: 495–506.
17. Van der Kroef C. Reactions to triazolam. *Lancet* 1979; **2**: 526.
18. Schoght B. Paranoid symptoms associated with triazolam. *Can J Psychiatry* 1985; **30**: 462–3.
19. Weiburg JB, Sachs F, Falk WE. Triazolam-induced brief episodes of secondary mania in a depressed patient. *J Clin Psychiatry* 1987; **48**: 492–3.
20. Sunter JP, Bal TS, Cowan WK. Three cases of triazolam poisoning. *BMJ* 1988; **297**: 719.
21. The International Agranulocytosis and Aplastic Anemia Study. Risks of agranulocytosis and aplastic anemia: a first report of

their relation to drug use with special reference to analgesics. *JAMA* 1986; **256**: 1749–57.

22. Guess HA. Behavior of the exposure odds ratio in a case–control study when the hazard function is not constant over time. *J Clin Epidemiol* 1989; **42**: 1179–84.

23. Strom BL, Carson JL, Morse ML, West SL, Soper KA The effect of indication on hypersensitvity reactions associated with zomepirac sodium and other nonsteroidal antiinflammatory drugs. *Arthritis Rheum* 1987; **30**: 1142–9.

24. Miettinen OS. The need for randomization in the study of intended effects. *Stat Med* 1983; **2**: 267–71.

25. Spitzer WO, Suissa S, Ernst P, Horwitz RI, Habbick B, Cockcroft D, *et al*. The use of beta-agonists and the risk of death and near death from asthma. *N Engl J Med* 1992; **326**: 501–6.

26. Petri H, Urquhart J, Herings R, Bakker A. Characteristics of patients prescribed three different inhalational beta-2 agonists: an example of the channeling phenomenon. *Post-Mark Surveil* 1991; **5**: 57–66.

27. Coronary Drug Project Research Group. Influence of adherence to treatment and response of cholesterol on mortality in the coronary drug project. *N Engl J Med* 1980; **303**: 1038–41.

28. Mantel N, Haenszel W. Statistical aspects of the analysis of data from retrospective studies of disease. *J Natl Cancer Inst* 1959; **22**: 719–48.

29. Ray W, Griffin MR. Use of Medicaid data for pharmacology. *Am J Epidemiol* 1989; **129**: 837–49.

30. Fine PEM, Chen RT. Confounding in studies of adverse reactions to vaccines. *Am J Epidemiol* 1992; **136**: 121–35.

31. Walker AM, Jick H, Perera DR, Thompson RS, Knauss TA. Diphtheria–tetanus–pertussis immunization and sudden infant death syndrome. *Am J Public Health* 1987; **77**: 945–51.

32. White JE. A two-stage design for the study of the relationship between a rare exposure and a rare disease. *Am J Epidemiol* 1982; **115**: 119–28.

33. Walker AM. Anamorphic analysis: sampling and estimation for covariate effects of both exposure and disease are known. *Biometrics* 1982; **38**: 1025–32.

34. Zhao LP, Lipsitz S. Design and analysis of two-stage studies. *Stat Med* 1992; **11**: 769–82.

35. Wacholder S, Carroll RJ, Pee D, Gail MH. The partial questionnaire design for case–control studies. *Stat Med* 1994; **13**: 623–4.

36. Cain KC, Breslow NE. Logistic regression analysis and efficient design for two-stage studies. *Am J Epidemiol* 1988; **28**: 1198–1206.

37. Schaubel D, Hanley J, Collet JP, Sharpe C, Boivin JF. Controlling confounding when studying large pharmacoepidemiologic databases: the two-stage sampling design *Am J Epidemiol* 1997; **146**: 450–8.

38. Rosenbaum PR, Rubin DB. The central role of the propensity score in observational studies for causal effects. *Biometrika* 1983; **70**: 41–55.

39. Joffe MM, Rosenbaum PR. Invited commentary: propensity scores. *Am J Epidemiol* 1999; **150**: 327–33.

40. Winkelmayer WC, Glynn RJ, Mittleman MA, Levin R, Pliskin JS, Avorn J. Comparing mortality of elderly patients on hemodialysis versus peritoneal dialysis: a propensity score approach. *J Am Soc Nephrol* 2002; **13**: 2353–62.

41. Grunkemeier GL, Payne N, Jin R, Handy JR, Jr. Propensity score analysis of stroke after off-pump coronary artery bypass grafting. *Ann Thorac Surg* 2002; **74**: 301–5.

42. Teufelsbauer H, Prusa AM, Wolff K, Polterauer P, Nanobashvili J, Prager M *et al*. Endovascular stent grafting versus open surgical operation in patients with infrarenal aortic aneurysms: a propensity score-adjusted analysis. *Circulation* 2002; **106**: 782–7.

43. Karthik S, Musleh G, Grayson AD, Keenan DJ, Hasan R, Pullan DM *et al*. Effect of avoiding cardiopulmonary bypass in non-elective coronary artery bypass surgery: a propensity score analysis. *Eur J Cardiothorac Surg* 2003; **24**: 66–71.

44. Schwarz RE, Smith DD, Keny H, Ikle DN, Shibata SI, Chu DZ *et al*. Impact of intraoperative radiation on postoperative and disease-specific outcome after pancreatoduodenectomy for adenocarcinoma: a propensity score analysis. *Am J Clin Oncol* 2003; **26**: 16–21.

45. Stamou SC, Jablonski KA, Pfister AJ, Hill PC, Dullum MK, Bafi AS *et al*. Stroke after conventional versus minimally invasive coronary artery bypass. *Ann Thorac Surg* 2002; **74**: 394–9.

46. Normand ST, Landrum MB, Guadagnoli E, Ayanian JZ, Ryan TJ, Cleary PD *et al*. Validating recommendations for coronary angiography following acute myocardial infarction in the elderly: a matched analysis using propensity scores. *J Clin Epidemiol* 2001; **54**: 387–98.

47. Coyte PC, Young W, Croxford R. Costs and outcomes associated with alternative discharge strategies following joint replacement surgery: analysis of an observational study using a propensity score. *J Health Econ* 2000; **19**: 907–29.

48. Jasmer RM, Saukkonen JJ, Blumberg HM, Daley CL, Bernardo J, Vittinghoff E *et al*. Short-course rifampin and pyrazinamide compared with isoniazid for latent tuberculosis infection: a multicenter clinical trial. *Ann Intern Med* 2002; **137**: 640–7.

49. Perkins SM, Tu W, Underhill MG, Zhou X-H, Murray MD. The use of propensity scores in pharmacoepidemiology research. *Pharmacoepidemiol Drug Saf* 2000; **9**: 93–101.

50. Gum PA, Thamilarasan M, Watanabe J, Blackstone EH, Lauer MS. Aspirin use and all-cause mortality among patients being evaluated for known or suspected coronary artery disease: a propensity analysis. *JAMA* 2001; **286**: 1187–94.

51. Rosenbaum PR, Rubin DB. Reducing bias in observational studies using subclassification on the propensity score. *J Am Stat Assoc* 1984; **79**: 516–24.

52. D'Agostino RB, Jr. Propensity score methods for bias reduction in the comparison of a treatment to a non-randomized control group. *Stat Med* 1998; **17**: 2265–81.

53. Cepeda MS, Boston R, Farrar JT, Strom BL. Comparison of logistic regression versus propensity score when the number

of events is low and there are multiple confounders. *Am J Epidemiol* 2003; **158**: 280–7.

54. Greenland S, Pearl J, Robins JM. Causal diagrams for epidemiologic research. *Epidemiology* 1999; **10**: 37–48.

55. Phillips CV. Quantifying and reporting uncertainty from systematic errors. *Epidemiology* 2003; **14**: 459–66.

56. Maclure M, Schneeweiss S. Causation of bias: the episcope. *Epidemiology* 2001; **12**: 114–22.

57. Phillips CV, LaPole LM. Quantifying errors without random sampling. *BMC Med Res Methodol* 2003; **3**: 9.

58. Lash TL, Fink AK. Semi-automated sensitivity analysis to assess systematic errors in observational data. *Epidemiology* 2003; **14**: 451–8.

59. Greenland S. Basic methods for sensitivity analysis and external adjustment. In: *Modern Epidemiology*, 2nd edn. Philadelphia, PA: Lippincott-Raven, 1998; pp. 343–57.

60. Hennessy S, Berlin JA, Kinman JL, Margolis DJ, Marcus SM, Strom BL. Risk of venous thromboembolism from oral contraceptives containing gestodene and desogestrel versus levonorgestrel: a meta-analysis and formal sensitivity analysis. *Contraception* 2001; **64**: 125–33.

61. Wright CC, Sim J. Intention-to-treat approach to data from randomized controlled trials: a sensitivity analysis. *J Clin Epidemiol* 2003; **56**: 833–42.

62. Lash TL, Silliman RA. A sensitivity analysis to separate bias due to confounding from bias due to predicting misclassification by a variable that does both. *Epidemiology* 2000; **11**: 544–9.

63. Psaty BM, Koepsell TD, Lin D, Weiss NS, Siscovick DS, Rosendaal FR *et al*. Assessment and control for confounding by indication in observational studies. *J Am Geriatr Soc* 1999; **47**: 749–54.

64. Hersh AL, Stefanick ML, Stafford RS. National use of postmenopausal hormone therapy: annual trends and response to recent evidence. *JAMA* 2004; **291**: 47–53.

65. Collet JP, Boissel JP. Populations: evaluation and treatment. The need for a better definition. *Eur J Clin Pharmacol* 1991; **41**: 267–71.

48

Novel Approaches to Pharmacoepidemiology Study Design and Statistical Analysis

SAMY SUISSA

Department of Epidemiology and Biostatistics, Department of Medicine, and McGill Pharmacoepidemiology
Research Unit, McGill University, Montreal, Canada.

INTRODUCTION

The past two decades have witnessed an explosion of methodological advances in the design and analysis of epidemiological studies. Several of these contributions have been fundamental to the field of epidemiology in general, thus transcending content area, such as cancer, cardiovascular, occupational, or infectious disease epidemiology, to name a few. Further methodological advances have, on the other hand, arisen specifically from questions posed by pharmacoepidemiology applications or simply found a niche in pharmacoepidemiology because of the distinct nature of the available (and unavailable) data in this field, as well as its specific needs. Several of these advances have already played an important role in the conduct of research on drug effects, and will certainly take a greater place in future applications. In this chapter, we introduce some of these approaches.

First, we present various strategies of sampling within a large cohort, as an alternative to analyzing the full cohort.

These sampling schemes are crucial in pharmacoepidemiology, where cohorts are necessarily large and the related expense and time of data collection and analysis for every single member of the cohort can be prohibitive. Even if all the data were available, the fact that exposure, namely drug use, varies over time and often involves multiple uses, implies very complex measures of exposure and formidable technical challenges in data analysis. Consequently, it becomes indispensable to use strategies based on the collection and analysis of data for a sample of the cohort. The nested case–control and case–cohort techniques are discussed for both internal and external comparisons of adverse event rates. We also discuss the role of time in sampling within the cohort.

Second, we describe techniques of design and analysis for situations where only partial data are available on confounders. The first, an approach developed around specific problems in pharmacoepidemiology, is a practical method that permits the investigator to assess whether a factor is a confounder, and to adjust for this confounder, when data on this factor are only available in the cases and not in the controls of a case–control study. This situation is commonly encountered in pharmacoepidemiology, particularly when using computerized databases where data, in both quantity and quality, are more readily available for the cases than non-cases. We also briefly introduce the two-stage sampling technique, which deals with confounder data available on a sample of the cases and controls of the study population.

Third, we describe new designs that use within-subject comparisons to estimate risk, namely the case-crossover and case–time–control designs. These designs, dealing with the study of transient drug effects on the risk of acute adverse events, are useful when there is uncertainty about the proper selection of controls under the traditional case–control approach or when unmeasured confounders are deemed to be important. We also briefly describe methods based solely on prescription drug databases, namely prescription sequence analysis and prescription sequence symmetry analysis, to assess the risk of a drug as well as the phenomenon of channeling of drugs.

Fourth, we describe a problem in the analysis of data from cohort studies of drug effectiveness, namely that of immortal time bias. Several recent studies have attempted to use observational data for cohorts in an attempt to emulate the randomized controlled trial design. In doing so, the approach to data analysis used an intent-to-treat approach that was found to be subject to an important bias because of the time-varying nature of the drug exposure.

CLINICAL PROBLEMS TO BE ADDRESSED BY PHARMACOEPIDEMIOLOGIC RESEARCH

Pharmacoepidemiology deals with several facets of drug research, including the utilization, benefits, and risks of drugs. The primary focus of pharmacoepidemiology, however, and the one that receives the greatest attention and interest, is that of assessing the risk of uncommon, at times latent, and often unexpected adverse conditions resulting from the use of medications. Whereas the more common conditions are usually studied prior to drug marketing using experimental research designs such as randomized clinical trials, for the study of uncommon adverse conditions, the mainstay of pharmacoepidemiology, we must rely on methods based on nonexperimental designs. The greatest challenge of this field is then to quantify the risk of a drug accurately, relative to one or a variety of alternatives. Four features of nonexperimental

research methods, affecting the degree of uncertainty in this risk assessment process, have recently been the object of methodological development and are the subject of this chapter.

First, because of the rarity of the adverse conditions under study, source populations and study cohorts must be extremely large to permit the control of statistical uncertainty arising from random error. It is not unusual to require population or cohort sizes in the tens or even hundreds of thousands of subjects to identify a sufficiently large number of subjects with the adverse condition under study to yield stable results. For example, the Cancer Prevention Study II cohort used 1.2 million persons to assess the effect of aspirin use on the risk of colon cancer,[1] while the Nurses' Health Study cohort used 121 700 subjects to study the effect of oral contraceptives on the risk of cardiovascular diseases.[2] As described in Part III of this book, hurdles in forming these massive cohorts have been reduced by the use of computerized databases. Such databases have in fact revolutionized risk assessment research in pharmacoepidemiology, where conclusive information about a drug's potential risks cannot be delayed by the lengthy process of classical epidemiologic methods. Nevertheless, even if much of these data are already computerized, they sometimes remain expensive and time-consuming to collect in such mega-sized cohorts. Moreover, drug exposure often varies over time and involves multiple agents, which complicates the analysis of cohort data. Further, sometimes supplemental data are needed on confounders or other variables, which are not practical to obtain on such large numbers. Accordingly, efficient designs to sample a manageable number of study subjects within such cohorts have been devised and can be used effectively in pharmacoepidemiology, providing accurate results more rapidly and at less expense. The first part of this chapter deals with these more efficient designs.

The second source of uncertainty is related to the presence of confounding factors, which may possibly bias risk estimates and distort corresponding conclusions. For example, most epidemiologists accept unconditionally the finding that cervical clear-cell carcinoma in young women is caused by the use of diethylstilbestrol (DES) by their mothers during pregnancy.[3] A few, however, still suggest that this is an unresolved issue, as the association may be confounded by the mother's history of spontaneous abortions and of bleeding during pregnancy.[4] Analysis of such crucial studies requires a thorough knowledge and accurate measurements of the potential clinical confounders. Since data on confounders may be difficult to obtain on all subjects, a novel approach based on confounder data measured only on cases has been proposed and a formula to estimate the corresponding adjusted rate ratios has been devised. We describe this technique here, since it is particularly suited to pharmacoepidemiology, where this situation is most often met. In addition, the two-stage sampling technique, which measures confounders on a sample of the case–control study population, will also be introduced as an alternative tool to address this challenge.

Third, pharmacoepidemiology is frequently faced with the assessment of the risk of rare acute adverse events resulting from transient drug effects. For example, we may wish to study the risk of ventricular tachycardia in association with the use of inhaled β-agonists in asthma. This possible effect has been hypothesized on the basis of clinical study observations of hypokalemia and prolonged Q–T intervals in patients after β-agonist exposure.[5] These unusual cardiac deviations were observed only in the 4-hour period following drug absorption. Although the case–control approach can be used to address this question, the acuteness of the adverse event and the length of the drug's effect, as well as difficulties in determining the timing of drug exposure, induce uncertainty about the proper selection of controls. Moreover, confounding by indication may often be a problematic issue in such a design. We will review a recently proposed approach that addresses these difficulties, the case-crossover design. We also review the case–time–control design, which was devised to counter the time-trend biases inherent in the case-crossover design. The concept of comparing exposures within subjects used by these approaches also led to the development of several techniques applied to prescription drugs database studies.

Fourth, assessing drug effectiveness using observation study designs is particularly challenging, even beyond the issue of confounding by indication discussed in Chapter 40. A recent such cohort study included over 22 000 elderly patients hospitalized for COPD in Ontario, Canada, of whom around 8000 either died or were readmitted for COPD.[6] The question was whether the use of inhaled corticosteroids after discharge could prevent readmission and all-cause mortality. It was found that around 11 000 of the subjects were dispensed inhaled corticosteroids within the 90-day period after discharge. The study found, using an intention-to-treat analysis, that the subjects who received these drugs had a 29% reduction in the rate of all-cause mortality. We will show the impact of immortal time bias in this study and address

the ways this time-varying exposure can be taken into account in the data analysis.

METHODOLOGIC PROBLEMS TO BE ADDRESSED BY PHARMACOEPIDEMIOLOGIC RESEARCH

SAMPLING WITHIN A COHORT

Cohort studies are essential to pharmacoepidemiology, as they form the basis for the quantification of drug risk assessment. By following users of the drug under investigation who are originally free of the adverse condition of concern until the occurrence of the adverse condition, a cohort enables the estimation of the rate of occurrence of this adverse event. Because of the usual rarity of the adverse events under study, the cohort must be composed of very large numbers of subjects (see also Chapter 3). For example, to quantify the risk of an adverse event occurring at the rate of 2 per 10 000 per year with a precision of ± 1 per 10 000 with 95% probability, necessitates a cohort of close to 80 000 subjects followed for 1 year (or 160 000 subjects followed for 6 months). This type of requirement explains the infrequent use of the cohort design in pharmacoepidemiology. Examples of authentic cohorts are scant. The Cancer Prevention Study II cohort of 1.2 million persons enrolled in 1982 was used to assess the effect of aspirin use on the risk of colon cancer.[1] The Nurses' Health Study cohort of 121 700 female nurses established in 1976 evaluated several associations, notably the effect of oral contraceptives on the risk of cardiovascular diseases.[2] The McGill Hodgkin's Disease cohort of 10 472 patients was formed to assess the effects of chemotherapy on the risk of second cancers[7] and of coronary artery disease.[8] The Oxford Family Planning Association cohort of 17 032 women assessed mortality associated with oral contraceptive use.[9] Other examples exist, but the list is short.

Complementing such authentic cohorts formed from actually following a group of "live" subjects over time, the "computerized" cohort has become a popular alternative. Most of Part III of this book is devoted to the description of national and regional computerized health databases, frequently used to form cohorts for drug risk assessment, from which we derive the distinguishing designation "computerized" cohort. In fact, because of the urgent nature of several drug risk assessment situations, the "live" cohort approach, with its prospective nature, cannot address the problem sufficiently rapidly in a majority of instances, unless of course if it happens to have been already formed and followed up for another purpose. Accordingly, the "computerized" cohort has become an indispensable instrument in the armamentarium of many investigators in pharmacoepidemiology.

In any cohort study, the cost, time, and resources necessary to collect data on all cohort members can be prohibitive. Moreover, even with computerized cohorts, most studies will need to supplement and validate data obtained from the computer databases with data from hospital records, medical records, and physician or patient interview questionnaires. When, as in the majority of instances, the cohort size is considerable, such additional data gathering can become a formidable task, if not next to impossible. More importantly, however, is when the exposure varies over time and includes several drugs. The analysis of such a cohort with time-dependent exposure measures can be infeasible, if not impossible. To counter these obvious cost, time, and feasibility constraints, designs based on sampling subjects within a cohort have been proposed and recently applied successfully in pharmacoepidemiology. These designs are based on the selection of all cases with an adverse event in the cohort, but differ in the selection of a small subset of non-cases. Generally, they permit the precise estimation of relative risk measures with negligible losses in precision. Below, we discuss structural aspects of cohorts and present two sampling designs within a cohort, the nested case–control and case–cohort designs.

PARTIAL CONFOUNDER DATA

The most important limitation of the nonexperimental research methods frequently used in pharmacoepidemiology is the concern about error in the final risk estimate. Invariably, questions are posed as to whether an important confounding factor that was not considered in the study design is biasing the reported results. A factor is considered a *confounder* if it is associated with the adverse event irrespective of exposure to the drug under study, and with exposure to the drug itself (see Chapter 47).

Essentially, two classical solutions exist to address the problem of confounding variables in nonexperimental studies, once all such potential confounders have been identified *a priori*. We will use the case–control design to illustrate the problem, although the principles discussed in this section apply equally well to a cohort design. The first solution is to design the study to account for the confounder, e.g., selecting controls that are matched to the cases with respect to all these confounding factors and then using the appropriate corresponding techniques

of analysis for matched data. The second solution is to select controls unmatched with respect to these confounding factors, but to measure these confounders in the course of the study for all subjects and use statistical techniques, either based on stratification or regression, permitting one to remove their effect on the risk from the effect of the drug under study. The advantage of the first approach over the second is that, for strong confounders, fewer subjects will be needed to attain a desired level of power and simpler techniques of data analysis will be necessary. The second approach will permit one to assess the relative contribution of the confounders to the risk, which is impossible with the first approach. Irrespective, both standard approaches require the measurement of each confounding factor for each subject in the study, case and control, whether at the design stage for the first or at the analysis phase for the second solution.

However, it is at times impossible to obtain data on certain important confounding variables. This limitation could be fatal to a study that is already based on fragile nonexperimental methodology. A frequent situation encountered in pharmacoepidemiologic research is the availability of a wealth of data for the cases but a shortage of data for the controls. This is particularly true for "computerized" studies based on administrative databases, where cases have likely been hospitalized, and thus have an extensive medical chart, or died and have lengthy coroner or autopsy reports. For these cases, the investigator will have access to abundant information on potential confounding variables. However, if the controls are population based, as is usually the practice with "computerized" studies, it is unlikely they were hospitalized and, even if they were, probably not as extensively as the cases. The controls will therefore not be able to provide comparable data on confounders on the basis of medical charts only. Since, in such studies, we rarely contact subjects directly but rather rely exclusively on charts and records to supplement the computerized information, confounder data will typically only be available in the cases, and not in the controls. This chapter will describe a strategy of analysis to assess whether a factor is a confounder based on data available uniquely for the cases and the formula to estimate the rate ratio adjusted for this partially available confounder. Another closely related situation is when the confounders can be measured on both cases and controls, but resources only allow this measure for a sample of subjects. The two-stage sampling approach has been advanced as a strategy to efficiently select this sample and obtain adjusted estimates of the rate ratio. This approach will also be briefly described.

WITHIN-SUBJECT DESIGNS

When conducting a conventional case–control study (as distinct from the one nested within a cohort), the selection of controls is usually the most challenging task. The fundamental principle used in this process is that selected controls should be representative of the source population which gave rise to the cases,[10] a principle which derives from the case-base paradigm, i.e., that controls should provide valid exposure information on the source population.[11] Although elementary in theory, the principle is often extremely complex to implement in practice, irrespective of whether one decides to select population or hospital controls.

For population controls, specific hurdles make it difficult to apply the principle. First, we can often expect significant non-response or non-participation rates in the control group, particularly if the data collection instrument is burdensome, as it frequently is. This is rarely acceptable since the reasons for acceptance of participation as a control are not easily known and could be associated with exposure to the drug of interest, while the corresponding case selection is usually comprehensive with essentially complete response and acceptance rates. Consequently, the source population could have been well identified on theoretical grounds, but the practical results of the sampling exercise could result in a control population unrepresentative of this source population.

Second, when dealing with acute adverse events, the timing of the interview or data collection is crucial. For our example of the risk of ventricular tachycardia in association with the use of inhaled β-agonists in asthma, which was conjectured after observations of hypokalemia and prolonged Q–T intervals in patients within the 4-hour period following β-agonist absorption,[5] a case–control study may be attempted. Indeed, one would first select cases with this adverse event and easily probe whether they took the drug during the 4-hour span preceding the event. For controls, on the other hand, the investigator must define a time point of reference for which to ask the question about use of this drug in the "past 4 hours." If, as a simple example, the drug is more likely to be required during the day, but controls can only be reached in the evening, the questioning process may become invalid since it will produce differential response patterns for cases and controls.

For hospital controls, similar obstacles could invalidate the study. Choosing an array of diagnoses suitable for control subjects is not simple. Acute conditions could be associated with an elevated prevalence of use of the drug under study. Alternatively, hospitalizations for chronic diseases could be planned with specific contraindications against use of the drug. In addition, problems related to timing as discussed above can be as or more complicated in this context. Consequently, when dealing with the study of transient drug effects on the risk of acute adverse events, the case-crossover design will be presented as a solution to these obstacles, along with the case–time–control design, which adjusts for exposure time trends. Moreover, other within-subject techniques based solely on prescription drug databases will also be discussed.

IMMORTAL TIME BIAS

The analysis of cohort studies of drug effectiveness is a challenge if the drug exposure of interest changes over time. Such time-varying exposure is not simple to incorporate in the analysis. Several recent studies employed instead a time-fixed definition of exposure, by invoking the principle of intention-to-treat analysis borrowed from randomized clinical trials. This principle is based on the premise that subjects are exposed to the drug under study immediately at the start of follow-up, which is not the case in observational database studies. One must look forward after cohort entry for the first prescription of the drug under study. For instance, in the context of COPD, a prescription for inhaled corticosteroids during the period of 90 days after cohort entry was used to define exposure.[6] In this way, a subject who was dispensed a prescription within 90 days was considered exposed and a subject who was not was considered unexposed. This approach, however, leads to immortal time bias, a major source of distortion in the rate ratio estimate.[12]

This bias arises from the introduction of immortal time in defining exposure. Immortal time refers to follow-up time during which, by definition or design, outcome events cannot occur. For example, in the above-mentioned study of inhaled corticosteroids in COPD, an exposed subject who was dispensed their first prescription for an inhaled corticosteroid 80 days after cohort entry necessarily had to be alive on day 80, which generates an 80-day immortal time period. On the other hand, unexposed subjects do not have any immortal time. In particular, the subjects who die soon after cohort entry will have too little time to receive the drug under study. Therefore, the exposed subjects will have a major survival advantage over their unexposed counterparts because they are guaranteed to survive at least until their drug was dispensed. This presence of immortal time in exposed subjects, but not in the unexposed subjects, causes both underestimation of the rate of the outcome among the exposed subjects and overestimation of the rate among the unexposed subjects, making a drug appear effective.

CURRENTLY AVAILABLE SOLUTIONS

SAMPLING WITHIN A COHORT

A cohort is defined by subjects meeting a set of eligibility criteria and by entry and exit time points. Consider, for example, the 13-year cohort study, spanned by the period 1978–1990, of the risks of human insulin in diabetes.[13] For illustrative purposes, consider the subcohort of newly diagnosed diabetics only. The eligibility criteria may be one or more of disease status (insulin-dependent diabetes mellitus), age (diabetics less than 40 years of age), drug use (regular users of insulin), geographical location (urban/rural residence), etc. Entry into the cohort may be defined by calendar time (spanned by the study, e.g., any time after January 1, 1978), by age (any age before 40th birthday), by events (the first use of a certain form of insulin), or by disease status (the date of diagnosis of diabetes). Exit from the cohort may be defined by the first occurrence of specific calendar time (e.g., December 31, 1990), age (exit at 40th birthday), events (death; exit from the study; the first use of an oral hypoglycemic agent), or disease status (onset of nephropathy).

Types and Structures of Cohorts

This cohort of newly diagnosed diabetics may be illustrated graphically as in Figure 48.1. This figure, based on 21 subjects, is plotted in terms of calendar time, with subjects ranked according to their date of entry into the cohort, which corresponds to disease diagnosis. Cohorts with this form of illustration, where the time axis of interest is calendar time (zero-time is January 1, 1978), depicting the chronological nature of the cohort, may be called *variable-entry cohorts*. An alternative depiction could be based on

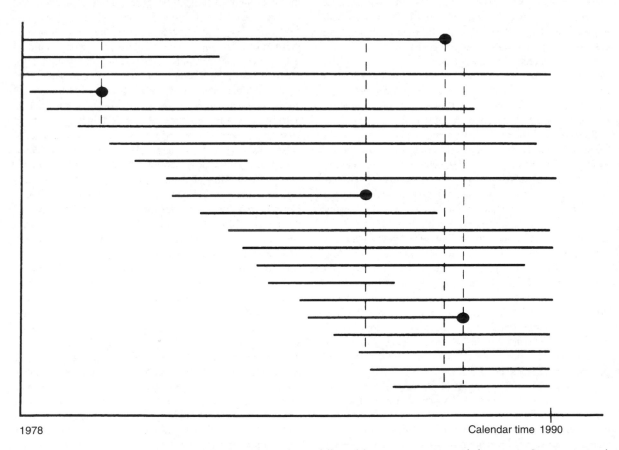

1978   Calendar time 1990

Figure 48.1. Illustration of a variable-entry cohort of 21 subjects followed from 1978 to 1990 with four cases (●) occurring and related risk sets (---).

duration of disease (i.e., time since diagnosis or first exposure to insulin), which may be more relevant to the risk factor under study. In this instance, the illustration given in Figure 48.2 for the same cohort, using duration of disease as the new time axis, is significantly different from the previous one. Here, the subjects are ranked according to the length of follow-up time in the study and zero-time is the time of diagnosis. Such cohorts may be called *fixed-entry cohorts*. Alternatively, if a specific drug is of interest, zero-time can be redefined as the start of exposure to that drug, irrespective of when this occurs with respect to the time of disease diagnosis.

The question of which of the two forms one should use for the purposes of data analysis rests on one's judgment of the more relevant of the two time axes, called the primary time axis, with respect to risk and drug exposure. This decision is important, since it affects the demarcation of "risk sets," which are fundamental to the analysis of data

from cohorts and consequently the sampling designs within cohorts. A risk set is formed by the members of the cohort who are at-risk of the adverse event at a given point in time, that is they are free of the adverse event and are members of the cohort at that point in time. The only relevant risk sets for data analysis are those defined by the time of occurrence of each case. It is clear that Figures 48.1 and 48.2 produce distinct risk sets for the same cases in the same cohort, as illustrated by the different sets of subjects crossed by the vertical broken line for the same case under the two forms of the cohort. In Figure 48.1, for example, case 1 has in its risk set only the first 6 subjects to enter the cohort, while in Figure 48.2, all 21 cohort members belong to its risk set. In classical epidemiology, the second form (fixed-entry) based on disease duration is used almost exclusively in these situations, primarily because this time axis is the more important determinant of risk and exposure is assumed to be stable in time. In pharmacoepidemiology, on the other hand,

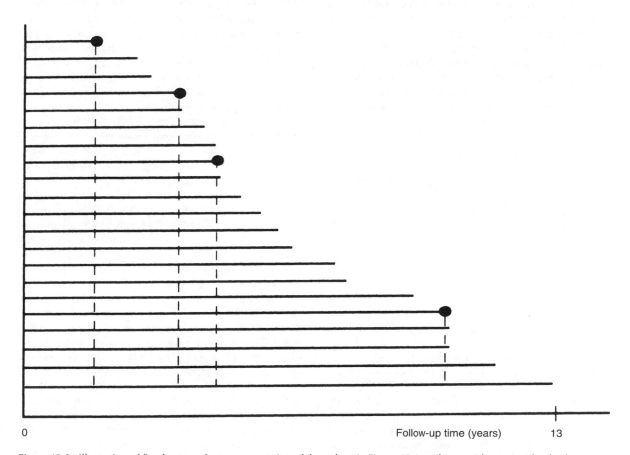

0   Follow-up time (years)   13

Figure 48.2. Illustration of fixed-entry cohort representation of the cohort in Figure 48.1, with new risk sets (---) for the four cases.

drug exposure can vary substantially over calendar time, thus adding a "cohort effect." Consequently, the first form (variable-entry) may be as relevant for the formation of risk sets and data analysis as the second form. Regardless, an advantage of having data on the full cohort is that we can change the primary time axis according to the question being posed, using calendar time for one analysis, duration of disease or drug exposure for another.

This "cohort effect," important as a result of potentially significant drug exposure variation over calendar time, can be sufficiently accounted for by simply partitioning the cohort into several subcohorts, each having its own zero-time defined by entry date, analyzing duration within each subcohort. We could, for example, partition the cohort displayed in Figures 48.1 and 48.2 into four subcohorts, according roughly to 3-year intervals, to combine the two alternative forms of variable-entry and fixed-entry cohorts illustrated in Figures 48.1 and 48.2. The risk sets from such a partition will necessarily depend on both disease duration and calendar time. Arguments for variable-entry cohorts can then be made by repeating the fixed-entry argument, conditional on each subcohort, and combining the results by stratification or regression methods. This would correspond to analyses controlling for calendar year. Because of the possibility of analyzing a variable-entry cohort as several fixed-entry subcohorts, we will focus the remaining presentation on a single fixed-entry cohort.

The Nested Case–Control Design

The idea of a nested case–control design within a cohort was first introduced by Mantel,[14] who proposed an unmatched selection of controls and called it a synthetic retrospective study. It was developed further and formalized by Liddell et al.[15] in the context of a cohort study of asbestos exposure and the risks of lung cancer and mortality. The nested case-control design involves four steps:

1. defining the cohort's time axis;
2. selecting all cases in the cohort, i.e., all subjects with an adverse event;
3. forming all risk sets corresponding to the cases;
4. randomly selecting one or more controls from each risk set.

Figure 48.3 illustrates the selection of a nested case–control sample from a cohort, with one control per case (1 : 1 matching). It is clear from the definition of risk sets that a future case is eligible to be a control for a prior case, as illustrated in the figure for the fourth case, and that a subject may be selected as a control more than once. If, instead, controls are forced to be selected only from the non-cases and subjects are not permitted to be used more than once in the nested case–control sample, a bias is introduced in the estimation of the relative risk, because the control exposure prevalence will be slanted to that of longer term subjects who do not become cases during the study follow-up.[16] The magnitude of the bias depends on the frequency of the adverse event in the cohort; the more frequent the event the larger the potential for bias.

This property leading to subjects possibly being selected more than once in the sample may be problematic when the exposure and covariate factors are time-dependent, particularly when the data are obtained by questionnaire where the respondent would have to answer questions regarding multiple time points in their history. We faced this problem in a study of the risks of severe adverse events in asthma associated with the use of inhaled β-agonists.[17] A cohort of 12 301 asthmatics spanning the period 1978–87 was identified from the Saskatchewan Health computerized databases, of whom 129 were cases (death or near-death from asthma). To permit the feasible collection of additional data from hospital charts and questionnaires sent to all physicians who saw these patients, it was necessary to sample from the cohort. These additional data were specifically focusing on the two-year period prior to the risk set date. A standard nested case–control sample of six controls per case, as described above, would have produced some case and control subjects who contributed multiple times as controls in the sample. This would have been problematic vis-à-vis the questioned physicians, for example, who would have had to respond to questions about the same patient's asthma severity in different two-year periods, a clearly confusing and potentially unreliable data collection scheme. To circumvent this difficulty, we stratified the cohort according to various potential confounding factors, namely age, area of residence, social assistance, prior asthma hospitalization, and, of course, calendar date of entry into the cohort. This extremely fine stratification resulted in 129 subcohorts, one for each case. We thus selected between 2 and 8 controls per case (some risk sets contained only 2 eligible controls, mostly because of the matching by prior hospitalization). Since each subcohort contained a single risk set (only one case) and the subcohorts were mutually exclusive, a selected subject was guaranteed to appear only once in the nested case–control sample. This stratified nested case–control design strategy is commonly needed in pharmacoepidemiology since calendar time matching for cohort entry is often essential to account for disease duration and drug exposure time trends.

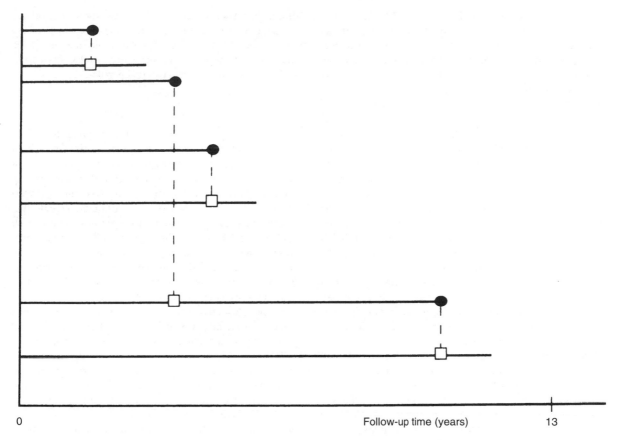

Figure 48.3. Nested case–control sample of one control (□) per case (●) from the cohort in Figure 48.2.

The analysis of data from a nested case–control study must conserve the matched nature of the selection of cases and controls, particularly if the risk of the adverse event changes with disease duration and drug exposure varies in calendar time. This also applies to the stratified nested case–control design, which is based on other matching criteria as well. The method of analysis is identical to that of a conventional matched case–control study, not nested within a cohort. The conditional logistic regression method for this design is appropriate, as it uses the risk set as the fundamental unit of analysis, in agreement with the proportional hazards model of the full cohort.[18] Simple formulae exist to estimate the relative risk for 1 : 1 matching.[10] When more than one control is matched to each case, however, sophisticated computer packages such as EGRET[19] SAS or STATA are required to fit the necessary conditional logistic regression model. This technique was used in our nested case–control study of β-agonist risks in asthma,[17] where the number of controls per case varied between 2 and 8.

The question of the required number of controls per case is important (see also Chapter 3). Although selecting one control per case will greatly simplify the data analysis, a large number of cases will be required to attain an acceptable level of power. Since the number of cases in the cohort is fixed and cannot be increased to satisfy this requirement, the only remaining alternative is to increase the control-to-case ratio. Tables for determining the power for given numbers of controls are given in Breslow and Day.[20] It can be readily seen from these sample size tables that the gain in power is significant for every additional control up to four controls per case, but becomes negligible beyond this ratio. For example, if we consider an exposure prevalence in the controls to be 30% and we target detecting a relative risk of 2 with 5% significance and 80% power, the required numbers of cases are 122, 90, 74, 65, and 62, respectively, for $1:1$, $2:1$, $4:1$, $10:1$, and $20:1$ control-to-case ratios. These translate to total study sizes (cases and controls combined) of 244, 270, 370, 715, and 1302, with clear cost implications and related optimality decisions. Of course, the number of cases in a cohort is frequently fixed *a priori* by the study constraints, thus eliminating this option to increase the number of cases. However, although this general rule of an optimal $4:1$ control-to-case ratio is appropriate in the majority of instances, one should be prudent when exposure to the drug under study is infrequent, when the hypothesized relative risk moves further from unity, or when several factors or other drugs are being assessed simultaneously. In these situations, the ratio could easily be required to increase to 10 or more controls per case. This was the case in two recent studies. In our study of the risks of fatal or near-fatal asthma associated with the use of inhaled β-agonists,[17] the low rate of use of fenoterol, believed to be around 5%, dictated the selection of up to 8 controls per case. In a proposed study of the cardiovascular risks of oral contraceptives,[21] the relative infrequency of newer oral contraceptives with lower estrogen dose and new progestins, coupled with the strong confounding effect of age, led to a requirement of 10 controls per case.

Like the cohort, the nested case–control design is used primarily to conduct internal comparisons (within the cohort) between exposures to different drugs. At times, however, it is of interest to contrast exposure to a drug to no exposure, or to some average exposure. This is not possible using methods for internal comparisons when all subjects in the cohort are exposed to the drug under study. Instead, external comparisons are performed, comparing the rate of adverse experience in the cohort to that of an external population, with appropriate adjustment for only a few available key factors, such as age, sex, and calendar time. The result is usually called the standardized mortality rate (SMR) when the adverse event is death, or the standardized incidence rate (SIR) when it is not. Techniques to estimate these measures using the full cohort are described in most textbooks of epidemiology.[10,11] The nested case–control design, however, is not a simple random sample from the cohort and thus cannot use the same techniques to estimate these measures. Indeed, it is evident from Figure 48.3 that those cohort members with the longest follow-up have a greater chance of being selected in the nested case–control sample, since they belong to all the risk sets. If their drug exposure pattern is different from that of other cohort members, the members of the nested case–control sample will not be representative of the cohort, which may substantially bias the resulting analyses. The appropriate method to perform external comparisons using data from a nested case–control

design has been described.[22] It uses knowledge about the sampling structure to yield an unbiased estimate of the adverse event rate in the full cohort, thus permitting the estimation of the necessary standardized relative measure with respect to the selected external population.

The Case–Cohort Design

The first recognized application of a sampling design we currently call *case–cohort* was made by Hutchison,[23] in performing external comparisons of leukemia rates in patients treated by radiation for cervical cancer. It was ultimately developed and formalized by Prentice,[24] who coined the name "case–cohort." Although recent, this design has already been used effectively in some drug risk studies.[25–28] The case–cohort design involves two steps: (i) selecting all cases in the cohort, i.e., all subjects with an adverse event; and (ii) randomly selecting a sample of predetermined size of subjects from the cohort. Figure 48.4 depicts the selection of a case–cohort sample of six subjects from the illustrative cohort. Note that it is possible that some cases selected in step 1 are also selected in the step 2 sample, as illustrated in the figure for the third case.

The case–cohort design resembles a reduced version of the cohort, with all cases added. It can also be perceived as an unmatched version of the nested case–control design. Although these aspects suggest a possible resemblance of the data analysis approach with either the established cohort or case–control methods, the techniques are in fact distinct, each requiring specific software. This is because the method of analysis for a case–cohort sample is extremely complex, as it must take into account the overlap of cohort members between successive risk sets induced by this sampling strategy. This handicap has severely limited the use of the case–cohort design. However, a statistical software package called EPICURE[29] has been released, which includes a module for the analysis of case–cohort data. As well, statisticians of the US National Cancer Institute are developing a user-friendly program called EPITOME, which performs this analysis. These advances will facilitate and undoubtedly encourage the future use of the case–cohort design, which offers some interesting advantages over the nested case–control design.[30]

The first advantage of the case–cohort design is its capacity to use the same sample to study several different types of events. Indeed, the cases can be split into several subcategories and each can be analyzed with the same "control" subcohort. In contrast, the nested case–control design requires different control groups for each type of event because the selection depends on event times. For

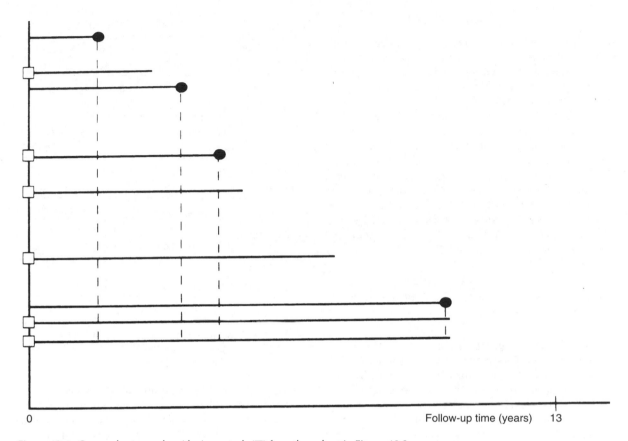

Figure 48.4. Case–cohort sample with six controls (□) from the cohort in Figure 48.2.

example, the β-agonist risks nested case–control study had two distinct control groups, one of size 233 for the 44 asthma deaths, the other of size 422 for the 85 asthma near-deaths.[17] Another useful advantage is that the case–cohort design permits one to change the primary time axis of analysis from calendar to disease time and vice versa, depending on either the assumed model or the targeted outcome. This is not possible with the nested case–control study, where the primary time axis must be set *a priori* to permit the risk set construction. This is less of a problem in pharmacoepidemiology, however, where the cohort can be divided into subcohorts of successive calendar time, as was discussed earlier. Yet another example is its simplicity in sampling, which has advantages in both comprehensibility and computer programming. Finally, external comparisons are simple to perform with the case–cohort approach.[31]

The nested case–control design does have some advantages. The first is the simplicity of power calculation, or equivalently sample size determination. The nested case–control design is independent of the size of the cohort, while for the case–cohort design knowledge about overlap in risk sets is essential, thus greatly complicating these calculations. Second, data on time-dependent exposure and covariates need only be collected up to the time of the risk set for the nested case–control study, while the collection must be exhaustive for the case–cohort. Finally, despite the accessibility of software for data analysis of case–cohort data, these can quickly become surpassed and even infeasible with larger sample sizes and time-dependent exposures. In this situation, the nested case–control design, with its single risk set per case, is not only advantageous but also the only solution. A study of benzodiazepine use and motor vehicle crashes, initially designed as a case–cohort study, had to be analyzed as a nested case–control study because of technical limitations of the case–cohort analysis software and hardware.[32]

PARTIAL CONFOUNDER DATA

A strategy of analysis exists, on the basis of data available solely for the cases of a case–control or a cohort study, to assess whether a factor is a confounder or not. The rationale is that, if the factor is not found to be a confounder in the cases by this method, the final analysis will not need to adjust for its effect when estimating the risk of the drug under study. The approach is described by Ray and Griffin[33] and was used in the context of a study of nonsteroidal anti-inflammatory drugs and the risk of fatal peptic ulcer disease.[34] The strategy is based on the definition[18] of a confounder C (C+ and C– denote presence and absence) in the assessment of the association between a drug exposure E (E+ and E– denote exposure or not to the drug) and an adverse condition D (D+ and D– denote presence and absence). Confounding is present if both of the following conditions are satisfied:

1. C and E are associated in the control group (in D–);
2. C and D are associated in E+ and in E–.

Because confounding assumes a common E : D odds ratio in C+ and in C–, condition 1 becomes equivalent to: C and E are associated in the case group (in D+). Thus, if in the cases we find no association between the potential confounder and drug exposure, confounding by this factor can be excluded outright, without having to verify the second condition. In this instance, the analysis involving drug exposure in cases and controls can be performed directly without any concern for the confounding variable. If, on the other hand, an association is found between C and E in the cases, confounding is not necessarily confirmed (since condition 2 must also be satisfied), but is very likely since a potential confounder is usually selected for its property of being a known risk factor for D.

As an example of this approach, we use data from a case–control study of estrogen use and the risk of endometrial cancer.[35] These data, restricted to the effect of former estrogen exposure, were used previously to illustrate confounding[36] by simulating hypothetical stratifications by a third factor. They are displayed in Figure 48.5. The crude odds ratio between estrogen use and endometrial cancer is 3.3 in this study of 17 cases and 60 controls. When the study population is partitioned according to the hypothetical potential confounding factor parity, the odds ratios are 1.1 in the low parity group and 1.0 in the high parity group, indicating a strong confounding effect of parity. This is a result of the strong association, using the odds ratio as the measure of association, between

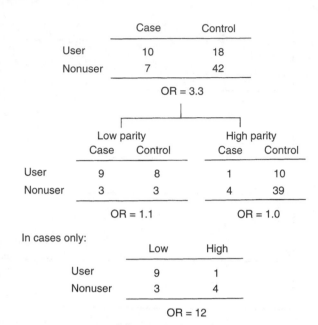

Figure 48.5. Data from case–control study of former estrogen use and endometrial cancer with hypothetical stratification by parity (confounding present).[33]

parity and estrogen exposure in the control group (OR = $8 \times 39/(3 \times 10)$ = 10.4) and the strong association between parity and endometrial cancer in subjects exposed to estrogen (OR = 11.3) and subjects not exposed (OR = 9.8). The bottom section of the figure displays the data *for the cases only*, where the odds ratio between estrogen exposure and parity is 12, demonstrating analogously the strong confounding role of parity. If the parity data were only available in the cases, this finding would invalidate the crude odds ratio of 3.3. Conversely, the same example could be used with smoking as another hypothetical confounder, as displayed in Figure 48.6. It is clear that the crude odds ratio of 3.3 is not affected by stratification by smoking, which is therefore not a confounder. This is confirmed by the lack of association between estrogen exposure and smoking *in the cases only*, with an odds ratio of 1.1.

This strategy to assess confounding is extremely valuable for several case–control studies in pharmacoepidemiology since, if confounding is excluded by this technique, crude methods of analysis can be used to obtain a valid estimate of the odds ratio. However, if confounding is found to be present, the crude estimate is biased. A new method was recently developed to obtain an adjusted estimate of the rate ratio in the absence of

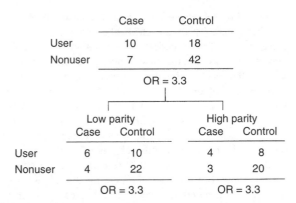

In cases only:

	Low	High
User	6	4
Nonuser	4	3

OR = 1.1

Figure 48.6. Data from case–control study of former estrogen use and endometrial cancer with another hypothetical stratification by parity (no confounding).[33]

confounder data among the controls.[37] The adjusted odds ratio is given by:

$$OR_{adj} = P_0(w - y) / [(1 - P_0) y]$$

where $y = \{v - [v^2 - 4(r-1) rwx]^{1/2}\} / [2(r-1)]$, $v = 1 + (r-1)(w+x)$ when $r \neq 1$ (and $y = wx$ when $r = 1$), r is the odds ratio between exposure and confounder among the cases, x is the probability of exposure among the controls, and w is the prevalence of the confounder among the controls. The latter (w) is the only unknown and must be estimated from external sources. An estimate of the variance of OR_{adj} exists.[37] As an example, we use data from a case–control study conducted using the Saskatchewan computerized databases to assess whether theophylline, a drug used to treat asthma, increases the risk of acute cardiac death.[38] In this study, the 30 cases provided data on theophylline use, as well as on smoking, possibly an important confounder. On the other hand, the 4080 controls only had data available on theophylline use and not on smoking. Table 48.1 displays the data from this study. The crude odds ratio between theophylline use and cardiac death is 4.3 [(17/13)/(956/3124)]. Because of the missing data on smoking, it is only possible to partition the cases, but not the controls, according to smoking. The odds ratio between theophylline use and smoking among the cases is estimable and found to be 7.5 [(14/5)/(3/8)], thus

Table 48.1. Data from a case–control study of theophylline use and cardiac death in asthma, with the smoking confounder data missing for controls[36]

	Cases		Controls	
	Use	Non-use	Use	Non-use
All subjects	17	13	956	3124
Stratified by smoking:				
Smokers	14	5	a	a
Non-smokers	3	8	a	a

[a] These frequencies are missing for controls.

indicating that smoking is indeed a strong confounder. An external estimate of smoking prevalence among asthmatics, obtained from a Canadian general population health survey, is 24%. Using this estimate and the formula given above, the adjusted odds ratio is 2.4, much lower than the crude estimate of 4.3, with 95% confidence limits 1.0–5.8.

An alternative approach is available when the confounders can be measured on both cases and controls, albeit only for a sample of subjects. This technique, developed more than a decade ago but not widely used, is the two-stage sampling approach, in which stage 1 is the collection of information on drug exposure and outcomes, and stage 2 is the collection of confounder data on a subset of the stage 1 sample. This situation is common with database studies, where the database provides data on exposure and outcome for all subjects, but confounders are missing and need to be obtained directly on a subset of subjects. The balanced design, wherein equal numbers of individuals are selected from each exposure–outcome category, is usually the most efficient strategy by which to select the stage 2 sample. This method has recently been used in pharmacoepidemiology.[39] An analogous method has been devised in the context of verifying the validity of the case status in studies where both outcome and exposure are rare. In this instance, validating the case status of all cases would be inefficient when most cases are unexposed. Validating all exposed cases and a sample of the unexposed cases turns out to be an efficient means of estimating the rate ratio.[40]

WITHIN-SUBJECT DESIGNS

When dealing with the study of transient drug effects on the risk of acute adverse events, Maclure[41] submits that the best representatives of the source population that produced the cases would be the cases themselves: this is the premise of the case-crossover design. This is a design where comparison between exposures are made within subjects. Other within-subject methods such as the case–time–control design and prescription symmetry analysis have been proposed and are also briefly presented here.

The Case-Crossover Design

To carry out a case-crossover study, three critical points must be considered. First, the study must necessarily be dealing with an acute adverse event that is alleged to be the result of a transient drug effect. Thus, drugs with regular patterns of use which vary only minimally between and within individuals are not easily amenable to this design. Nor are latent adverse events, which only occur long after exposure. Second, since a transient effect is under study, the effect period (or time window of effect) must be precisely determined. For example, in our hypothetical study of the possible acute cardiotoxicity of inhaled β-agonists in asthmatics (see above), we identified this effect period to be 4 hours after having taken the usual dose of 2 inhalations of 100 μg of the product. An incorrect specification of this time window can have important repercussions on the risk estimate, as we will show in the example below. Third, one must be able to obtain reliable data on the usual pattern of drug exposure for each case, over a sufficiently long period of time. For our example, we could seek the frequency of use of β-agonists during the year preceding the adverse event.

The case-crossover study is simply a crossover study *in the cases only*. The subjects alternate at varying frequencies between exposure and non-exposure to the drug of interest, until the adverse event occurs, which happens for all subjects in the study, since all are cases by definition. With respect to the timing of the adverse event, each case is investigated to determine whether exposure was present within the predetermined effect period, namely within the previous 4 hours in our example. This occurrence is then classified as having arisen either under drug exposure or non-exposure on the basis of the effect period. Thus, for each case, we have either an exposed or unexposed status, which represents for data analysis the first column of a 2×2 table, one for each case. Since each case will be matched to itself for comparison, the analysis is matched and thus we must create separate 2×2 tables for each case.

With respect to control information, the data on the average drug use pattern are necessary to determine the typical probability of exposure to the time window of effect. This is done by obtaining data for a sufficiently stable period of time. In our example, we may find out the average

number of times a day each case has been using β-agonists (2 inhalations of 100 μg each) in the past year. Note that there are six 4-hour periods (the duration of the effect period) in a day. Such data will determine the proportion of time that each asthmatic is usually spending time in the effect period and thus potentially "at risk" of ventricular tachycardia. This proportion is then used to obtain the number of cases expected on the basis of time spent in these "at risk" periods, for comparison with the number of cases observed during such periods. This is done by forming a 2×2 table for each case, with the corresponding control data as defined above, and combining the tables using the Mantel–Haenszel technique as described in detail by Maclure.[41]

We generated data for a hypothetical case-crossover study of 10 asthmatics who experienced ventricular tachycardia. These were all queried regarding their use of two puffs of inhaled β-agonist in the last 4 hours and on average over the past year. The data are displayed in Table 48.2. The fact of drug use within the effect period for the event classification is straightforward. The usual frequency of drug use per year is converted to a ratio of the number of "at risk" periods to the number of "no risk" periods, the total number of 4-hour periods being 2190 in one year. Thus, for example, the content of the 2×2 table for the first case, who is not found to have been exposed in the prior 4-hour period, is (0,1,365,1825), while for the second case, who is exposed, it is (1,0,6,2184). Using the Mantel–Haenszel technique to combine the 10 2×2 tables, the estimate of relative risk is 3.0 (95% CI = 1.2–7.6).

This method is sensitive to the specification of the time window of effect. For example, if this effect period is in fact

Table 48.2. Hypothetical data for a case-crossover study of β-agonist exposure in last 4 hours and the risk of ventricular tachycardia in asthma

Case no.	β-agonist use[a] in last 4 hours (a_i)	Usual β-agonist use in last year	Periods of risk (N_{1i})	Periods of no-risk (N_{0i})
1	0	1/day	365	1825
2	1	6/year	6	2184
3	0	2/day	730	1460
4	1	1/month	12	2178
5	0	4/week	208	1982
6	0	1/week	52	2138
7	0	1/month	12	2178
8	1	2/month	24	2166
9	0	2/day	730	1460
10	0	2/week	104	2086

[a] Inhalations of 200 μg: 1 = yes, 0 = no. RR $= \Sigma a_i N_{0i} / \Sigma (1 - a_i) N_{1i}$.

only 2 hours, then the data of Table 48.2 would be affected in two ways: some cases may not be considered exposed anymore, and the exposure probabilities will change. By considering as unexposed cases 2 and 4, for instance, who may have been exposed 3 hours before ventricular tachycardia, and recalculating the appropriate exposure probabilities, the relative risk becomes 2.0 (95% CI=0.3–12.0). On the other hand, if this effect period is in fact 6 hours long, then the data of Table 48.2 would be affected in two ways: some new cases may now be considered exposed, and the exposure probabilities will change. By considering as exposed cases 3 and 5, for instance, who may have been exposed 5 hours before ventricular tachycardia, and recalculating the appropriate exposure probabilities, the relative risk becomes 5.0 (95% CI=2.0–12.2). The difference in the magnitude of the risk and the corresponding statistical significance between the various scenarios is indicative of the importance of the need for an accurate specification of the length of the effect period.

This method is extremely valuable when studying an acute adverse event that is alleged to be the result of a transient drug effect. Consequently, it excludes drugs with regular patterns of use that vary minimally between and within individuals or adverse events which can only result from long extended exposure. Moreover, the case-crossover design requires precise knowledge about the effect period (or time window of effect), although the latter can be varied to investigate the optimum window to use. The design is also very useful when the selection of controls in the usual sense is uncertain. A significant advantage of this design is that it eliminates the problem of confounding by factors that do not change over time. It cannot, however, easily address the problem of confounding by factors that do change over time. In this instance, time dependent data will be required for such confounders, a possibly difficult task. The case-crossover design is automatically free of selection bias, which occurs when controls are not representative of the base population from which the cases arose. However, although such control selection bias (in the usual control sense) is eliminated, case selection bias could be present if case selection is related to the exposure under study, such as the exposure being associated with the detection of the outcome (exposure, detection procedure, and outcome identification all by the same physician). Finally, information bias resulting from the differential quality of recent and past drug exposure data can be problematic if the exposure collection system is not robust. This source of bias can, however, be dismissed if one uses, for example, drug exposure data from computerized databases. Greenland[42] presented examples where the odds ratio estimates from this approach can be biased. Nevertheless, this approach is being used successfully in several studies.[43–46] It has also been adapted for application to the risk assessment of vaccines.[47]

The Case–Time–Control Design

One of the limitations of the case-crossover design is the assumption of the absence of a time trend in the exposure prevalence. An approach that adjusts for such time trends is the case–time–control method. By using cases and controls of a conventional case–control study as their own referents, the *case–time–control design* eliminates the biasing effect of unmeasured confounding factors, such as drug indication, while addressing the time trend assumption.[48] In fact, the method is an extension of the case-crossover analysis that uses, in addition to the case series, a series of controls to adjust for exposure time trends.

The approach is illustrated with data from the Saskatchewan Asthma Epidemiologic Project,[17] a study conducted to investigate the risks associated with the use of inhaled β-agonists in the treatment of asthma. Using a cohort of 12 301 asthmatics followed during 1980–87, 129 cases of fatal or near-fatal asthma and 655 controls were identified. The amount of β-agonist used in the year prior to the index date was used for exposure. Table 48.3 displays the data comparing low (12 or less canisters per year) with high (more than 12) use of β-agonists. The crude odds ratio for high β-agonist use is 4.4 (95% CI: 2.9–6.7). Adjustment for all available markers of severity, such as oral corticosteroids and prior asthma hospitalizations as confounding factors, lowers the odds ratio to 3.1 (95% CI: 1.8–5.4), the "best" estimate one can derive from these case–control data using conventional tools.

Table 48.3. Illustration of a case–time–control analysis of data from case–control study of fatal or near-fatal asthma and β-agonist use

	Cases		Controls		Adjusted		
	High	Low	High	Low	OR	OR	95% CI
Current β-agonist use	93	36	241	414	4.4	3.1	1.8–5.4
Discordant[a] use (case–crossover)	29	9				3.2	1.5–6.8
Discordant[a] use (control–crossover)			65	25	2.6		1.6–4.1
Case–time–control	29	9	65	25	1.2		0.5–3.0

[a] Discordant from exposure level during reference time period.

To apply the case–time–control design, exposure to β-agonists was obtained for the one-year current period and the one-year reference period prior to the current period. First, a case-crossover analysis is performed using the discordant subjects among the 129 cases, namely the 29 who were current high users of β-agonists and low users in the reference period and the 9 cases who were current low users of β-agonist and high users previously. This analysis is repeated for the 655 controls, of which there were 90 discordant in exposure; that is, 65 were current high users of β-agonists and low users in the reference period and 25 were current low users of β-agonists and high users previously. The case–time–control odds ratio, using these discordant pairs frequencies for a paired-matched analysis, is given by $(29/9)/(65/25) = 1.2$ (95% CI: 0.5–3.0). This estimate, which excludes the effect of unmeasured confounding by disease severity, indicates a minimal risk for these drugs.

The case–time–control approach provides an unbiased estimate of the odds ratio in the presence of confounding by indication, despite the fact that the indication for drug use (in our example, disease severity) is not measured, because of the within-subject analysis. It also controls for time trends in drug use. Nevertheless, its validity is subject to several assumptions, including the absence of time-dependent confounders, so that caution is recommended in its use.[42,49]

Drug Database Designs

One of the distinguishing features of pharmacoepidemiology is the use of computerized administrative health databases to answer research questions reliably with sufficient rapidity (see Part III). The usual urgency of concerns related to drug safety makes these databases essential to perform such risk assessment studies. In contrast to the databases described in Part III, some databases contain only information on prescriptions dispensed to patients, and no outcome information on disease diagnoses, hospitalizations, or vital status. These standalone prescription drug databases are more numerous and usually more easily accessible than the fully linked databases. They have been the object of recent methodological developments.

A technique that was developed specifically for the drug databases is prescription sequence analysis.[50] Prescription sequence analysis is based on the situation when a certain drug A is suspected to cause an adverse event that itself is treated by a drug B. To apply this technique, the computerized drug database is searched for all patients with a drug history who used drug A. For these subjects, all patients prescribed drug B in the course of using drug A are

identified and counted. Under the null hypothesis that drug A does not cause the adverse event treated by drug B, the number of subjects should be proportional to the duration of use of drug A relative to the total period of observation. This extremely rapid method of assessing the association between drug A and drug B is assessed for its random error with a Monte Carlo simulation analysis. This technique was applied to assess whether using the anti-vertigo or anti-migraine drug flunarizine (drug A) causes mental depression, as measured by the use of antidepressant drugs (drug B). The authors found that the number of patients starting on antidepressant drugs during flunarizine use was in fact lower than expected.[50] They thus concluded, using this rapid approach based solely on drug prescription data, that this drug probably does not cause mental depression. An extension of prescription sequence analysis, called prescription sequence symmetry analysis, was recently proposed.[51] Using a population of new users of either drug A or B, this approach compares the number of subjects who used drug A before drug B to those who used B before A. Under the null hypothesis, this distribution should be symmetrical and the numbers should be equal. It has recently been applied to the question of screening for drug-related dyspepsia.[52]

Another function of these databases is to use the prescriptions as covariate information to explain possible confounding patterns. The concept of *channeling* of drugs was put forward as an explanation of unusual risk findings.[53] For example, a case–control study conducted in New Zealand found that fenoterol, a β-agonist bronchodilator used to treat asthma attacks, was associated with an increased risk of death from asthma.[54] Using a prescription drug database, Petri and Urquhart found that severe asthmatics, as deemed from their use of other asthma medications prescribed for severe forms of the disease, were in fact channeled to fenoterol, probably because fenoterol was felt by prescribers to be a more potent bronchodilator than other β-agonists.[55] Conceptually the same as a selection bias due to uncontrolled confounding by indication (see Chapter 40), this phenomenon of channeling can be assessed rapidly in such databases, provided medications can be used as proxies for disease severity. This approach can be subject to bias, however, as it has been used with cross-sectional designs that cannot differentiate the directionality of the association.

An application of channeling using a longitudinal design was recently presented.[56] It indicated that channeling can vary according to the timing of exposure, namely that disease severity was not associated with first-time use of a drug, but subsequently severe patients were more likely to be switched to that drug. This type of research into patterns of drug prescribing and drug use can be very useful in understanding the results of case–control studies with limited data on drug exposures and subject to confounding by indication. The presence of the phenomenon of channeling implies that at the design stage of a study the entire history of drug exposures must be obtained for each subject and the analysis must account for changes in medication use and confounders (if available) as of the beginning of therapy.

IMMORTAL TIME BIAS

The analysis of cohort studies of drug effectiveness, where drug exposure is time varying, must necessarily be based on time-dependent methods. In the example of the COPD cohort, the "exposed" subjects who received their first prescription for an inhaled corticosteroid 80 days after cohort entry had to be alive on day 80. Thus, the subject was in fact unexposed for the first 80 days, which must be classified accordingly. Indeed, the rate of death among the exposed computed from an intention-to-treat perspective should in fact be divided into two rates. The first is the true rate, based on the person-time cumulated after the date of drug dispensing that defines exposure, while the second is that based on the person-time cumulated from cohort entry until the date of drug dispensing that defines exposure. The second rate will by definition be based on zero events. The zero component of the rate will necessarily bias downward the exposed rate. This zero component of the exposed rate is thus misclassified and should in fact be classified in the unexposed group since subjects should be considered unexposed to the drug until the date of drug dispensing. Thus, the combination of misclassification of unexposed person-time as exposed and the fact that this misclassified person-time is immortal will produce rate ratios lower than 1, thus creating an appearance of effectiveness for the drug.

Immortal time bias is thus the result of improper exposure definitions and analyses that cause serious misclassification of exposure and outcome events. This results from the attempt to emulate the randomized controlled trial to simplify the analysis of complex time-varying drug exposure data. However, observational studies rarely permit such simple paradigms. Instead, time-dependent methods for analyzing risks, such as the Cox proportional hazard models with time-dependent exposures or nested case–control designs (see above), must be used to account for complex changes in drug exposure and confounders over time.[12,57] Alternatively, one should be certain that one is dealing with a true inception cohort, i.e., follow-up time begins with initiation of therapy.

THE FUTURE

The growing importance and awareness of pharmacoepidemiology in the medical, regulatory, and industry settings have led to a greater need and emphasis on solid methodology. As well, specific situations have induced the development of significant advances in the design and analysis of epidemiological studies of drug effects. We have described four recently developed methodologic approaches that facilitate the conduct of research in pharmacoepidemiology. First, we presented three strategies of sampling within a large cohort, as alternatives to analyzing the full cohort, namely the nested case–control and case–cohort techniques, as well as the stratified nested case–control approach, which has been proposed specifically to circumvent a restriction inherent in the nested case–control strategy. Future developments in this area will provide user-friendly tools to facilitate the estimation of risk difference or excess risk measures, in addition to the standard risk ratio measures routinely produced by these sampling schemes. As well, we can anticipate statistical models of analysis that take into account two or more time axes simultaneously, for example calendar time and disease duration, so that we do not have to resort to schemes based on cohort stratification. Finally, techniques to provide the optimal number of controls for each case have been proposed but have yet to be implemented.[58]

We also described methods useful in dealing with confounders when data on these factors are only available in the cases of a case–control study or in a sample of subjects. Development in this area is crucial in view of the limitations of databases. It should be directed to the situation of multiple confounders and should address the issue of effect modification, which eludes current techniques.

We described the case-crossover and case–time–control designs, alternatives to the classical case–control design, which are valuable when dealing with the study of transient drug effects on the risk of acute adverse events. Extensions and refinements of these designs should address their assumptions, as well as modifications for chronic effects and latent events. We also introduced novel techniques devised for standalone prescription drugs databases. Such innovative methods should be given priority in view of the importance of these databases in pharmacoepidemiology.

Lastly, we showed that the study of drug effectiveness from observational data can lead to immortal time bias if the analysis does not account for the time-varying nature of drug exposure. We must thus remain vigilant with respect to the possible introduction of subtle yet important biases in the conduct of such research, as it appears to become more prevalent.[59–62]

When used judiciously, these approaches can expand the limits inherent in the more traditional methods of epidemiology and generally optimize the conduct of research in pharmacoepidemiology. In the future, we can expect further enhancements of these methods and yet more effective tools in pharmacoepidemiology's unique search for the balance between high quality research and rapid results. This balance is fundamental to sound decision making around the management of drugs by clinicians, patients, industry, and regulators.

ACKNOWLEDGMENT

Samy Suissa is the recipient of a Distinguished Scientist award from the Canadian Institutes of Health Research (CIHR).

REFERENCES

1. Thun MJ, Namboodiri MM, Heath CW. Aspirin use and reduced risk of fatal colon cancer. *N Engl J Med* 1991; **325**: 1593–6.
2. Stampfer MJ, Willett WC, Colditz GA, Speizer FE, Hennekens CH. A prospective study of past use of oral contraceptive agens and risk of cardiovascular diseases. *N Engl J Med* 1988; **319**: 1313–17.
3. Herbst AL, Ulfelder H, Poskanzer DC. Adenocarcinoma of the vagina. Association of maternal stilbestrol therapy with tumor appearance in young women. *N Engl J Med* 1971; **284**: 878–81.
4. McFarlane MJ, Feinstein AR, Horwitz RI. Diethylstilbestrol and clear cell vaginal carcinoma. Reappraisal of the epidemiologic evidence. *Am J Med* 1986; **81**: 855–63.
5. Aelony Y, Laks MM, Beall G. An electrocardiographic pattern of acute myocardial infarction associated with excessive use of aerosolized isoproterenol. *Chest* 1975; **68**: 107–10.
6. Sin DD, Tu JV. Inhaled corticosteroids and the risk of mortality and readmission in elderly patients with chronic obstructive pulmonary disease. *Am J Respir Crit Care Med* 2001; **164**: 580–4.
7. Boivin JF, Hutchison GB, Lyden M, Godbold J, Chorosh J, Schottenfeld D. Second primary cancers following treatment of Hodgkin's disease. *J Natl Cancer Inst* 1984; **72**: 233–41.
8. Boivin JF, Hutchison GB, Lubin JH, Mauch P. Coronary artery disease mortality in patients treated for Hodgkin's disease. *Cancer* 1992; **69**: 1241–7.
9. Vessey MP, Villard-Mackintosh L, McPherson K, Yeates D. Mortality among oral contraceptive users: 20 year follow-up of women in a cohort study. *Br Med J* 1989; **299**: 1487–91.
10. Rothman KJ, Greenland S. *Modern Epidemiology*, 2nd edn. Hagerstown, MD: Lippincott-Raven, 1998.
11. Miettinen OS. *Theoretical Epidemiology: Principles of Occurrence Research in Medicine*. New York: John Wiley & Sons, 1985.
12. Suissa S. Effectiveness of inhaled corticosteroids in chronic obstructive pulmonary disease: immortal time bias in observational studies. *Am J Respir Crit Care Med* 2003; **168**: 49–53.
13. Suissa S, Spitzer WO, Abenhaim L, Downey W, Gardiner RJ, Fitzgerald, D. *Risk of Death from Human Insulin*. New York: John Wiley & Sons, 1992; pp. 169–75.
14. Mantel N. Synthetic retrospective studies and related topics. *Biometrics* 1973; **29**: 479–86.
15. Liddell FDK, McDonald JC, Thomas DC. Methods of cohort analysis appraisal by application to asbestos mining. *J R Stat Soc A* 1977; **140**: 469–91.
16. Lubin JH, Gail MH. Biased selection of controls for case–control analyses for cohort studies. *Biometrics* 1984; **40**: 63–75.
17. Spitzer WO, Suissa S, Ernst P, Horwitz RI, Habbick B, Cockcroft D *et al.* The use of beta-agonists and the risk of death and near death from asthma. *N Engl J Med* 1992; **326**: 501–6.
18. Breslow N, Day NE. *Statistical methods in cancer research*, vol. 1: *The Analysis of Case–Control Studies*, 2nd edn. Lyon: International Agency for Research on Cancer, 1980.
19. EGRET. Statistical and Epidemiology Research Corporation, Seattle, Washington, 1990.
20. Breslow N, Day NE. *Statistical Methods in Cancer Research*, vol. 2: *The Design and Analysis of Cohort Studies*, 2nd edn. Lyon: International Agency for Research on Cancer, 1987.
21. Suissa S, Hemmelgarn B, Spitzer WO, Brophy J, Collet JP, Côte R *et al.* The Saskatchewan oral contraceptive cohort study of oral contraceptive use and cardiovascular risks. *Pharmacoepidemiol Drug Saf* 1993; **2**: 33–49.
22. Suissa S, Edwardes MD, Boivin JF. External comparisons from nested case–control designs. *Epidemiology* 1998; **9**: 72–8.
23. Hutchinson GB. Leukemia in patients with cancer of the cervix uteri treated with radiation. *J Natl Cancer Inst* 1968; **40**: 951–82.
24. Prentice RL. A case–cohort design for epidemiologic cohort studies and disease prevention trials. *Biometrika* 1986; **73**: 1–11.
25. Bergkvist L, Adami HO, Persson I, Hoover R, Schairer C. The risk of breast cancer after estrogen and estrogen–progestin replacement. *N Engl J Med* 1989; **321**: 293–7.
26. van der Klauw MM, Stricker BH, Herings RM, Cost WS, Valkenburg HA, Wilson JH. A population based case–cohort study of drug-induced anaphylaxis. *Br J Clin Pharmacol* 1993; **35**: 400–8.
27. Moulton LH, Wolff MC, Brenneman G, Santosham M. Case-cohort analysis of case-coverage studies of vaccine effectiveness. *Am J Epidemiol* 1995; **142**: 1000–6.
28. Strom BL, Schinnar R, Bilker WB, Feldman H, Farrar JT, Carson JL. Gastrointestinal tract bleeding associated with naproxen sodium vs ibuprofen. *Arch Intern Med* 1997; **157**: 2626–31.
29. EPICURE. Risk regression and data analysis software. Seattle, WA: Hirosort International Corporation, 1991.
30. Wacholder S. Practical considerations in choosing between the case–cohort and nested case–control designs. *Epidemiology* 1991; **2**: 155–8.

31. Wacholder S, Boivin JF. External comparisons with the case-cohort design. *Am J Epidemiol* 1987; **126**: 1198–209.

32. Hemmelgarn B, Suissa S, Huang A, Boivin JF, Pinard G. Benzodiazepine use and the risk of motor vehicle crash in the elderly. *JAMA* 1997; **278**: 27–31.

33. Ray WA, Griffin MR. Use of Medicaid data for pharmaco-epidemiology. *Am J Epidemiol* 1989; **129**: 837–49.

34. Griffin MR, Ray WA, Schaffner W. Nonsteroidal anti-inflammatory drug use and death from peptic ulcer in elderly persons. *Ann Intern Med* 1988; **109**: 359–63.

35. Jick H, Watkins RN, Hunter JR, Dinan BJ, Madsen S, Rothman KJ *et al*. Replacement estrogens and endometrial cancer. *N Engl J Med* 1979; **300**: 218–22.

36. Suissa S. Statistical methods in pharmacoepidemiology. Principles in managing error. *Drug Saf* 1991; **6**: 381–9.

37. Suissa S, Edwardes M. Adjusted odds ratios for case–control studies with missing confounder data in controls. *Epidemiology* 1997; **8**: 275–80.

38. Suissa S, Hemmelgarn B, Blais L, Ernst P. Bronchodilators and acute cardiac death. *Am J Respir Crit Care Med* 1996; **154**: 1598–602.

39. Collet JP, Schaubel D, Hanley J, Sharpe C, Boivin JF. Controlling confounding when studying large pharmacoepidemiologic databases: a case study of the two-stage sampling design. *Epidemiology* 1998; **9**: 309–15.

40. Bilker WB, Berlin JA, Gail MH, Strom BL. An efficient design for verifying disease outcome status in large cohorts with rare exposures and low disease rates. *Stat Med* 1999; **18**: 3021–36.

41. Maclure M. The case-crossover design: a method for studying transient effects on the risk of acute events. *Am J Epidemiol* 1991; **133**: 144–53.

42. Greenland S. Confounding and exposure trends in case-crossover and case–time–control design. *Epidemiology* 1996; **7**: 231–9.

43. Ray WA, Fought RL, Decker MD. Psychoactive drugs and the risk of injurious motor vehicle crashes in elderly drivers. *Am J Epidemiol* 1992; **136**: 873–83.

44. Sturkenboom MC, Middelbeek A, de Jong van den Berg LT, van den Berg PB, Stricker BH, Wesseling H. Vulvo-vaginal candidiasis associated with acitretin. *J Clin Epidemiol* 1995; **48**: 991–7.

45. Meier CR, Jick SS, Derby LE, Vasilakis C, Jick H. Acute respiratory-tract infections and risk of first-time acute myocardial infarction. *Lancet* 1998; **351**: 1467–71.

46. Barbone F, McMahon AD, Davey PG, Morris AD, Reid IC, McDevitt DG *et al*. Association of road-traffic accidents with benzodiazepine use. *Lancet* 1998; **352**: 1331–6.

47. Farrington CP, Nash J, Miller E. Case series analysis of adverse reactions to vaccines: a comparative evaluation. *Am J Epidemiol* 1996; **143**: 1165–73.

48. Suissa S. The case–time–control design. *Epidemiology* 1995; **6**: 248–53.

49. Suissa S. The case–time–control design: further assumptions and conditions. *Epidemiology* 1998; **9**: 441–5.

50. Petri H, De Vet HCW, Naus J, Urquhart J. Prescription sequence analysis: a new and fast method for assessing certain adverse reactions of prescription drugs in large populations. *Stat Med* 1988; **7**: 1171–5.

51. Hallas J. Evidence of depression provoked by cardiovascular medication: a prescription sequence symmetry analysis. *Epidemiol* 1996; **7**: 478–84.

52. Hallas J, Bytzer P. Screening for drug related dyspepsia: an analysis of prescription symmetry. *Eur J Gastroenterol Hepatol* 1998; **10**: 27–32.

53. Urquhart J. ADR crisis management. *Scrip* 1989; **1388**: 19–21.

54. Crane J, Pearce N, Flatt A, Jackson R, Ball M, Burgess C *et al*. Prescribed fenoterol and death from asthma in New Zealand 1981–1983: case–control study. *Lancet* 1989; **1**: 917–22.

55. Petri H, Urquhart J. Channeling bias in the interpretation of drug effects. *Stat Med* 1991; **10**: 577–81.

56. Blais L, Ernst P, Suissa S. Confounding by indication and channeling over time: the risks of beta-agonists. *Am J Epidemiol* 1996; **144**: 1161–9.

57. Samet JM. Measuring the effectiveness of inhaled corticosteroids for COPD is not easy! *Am J Respir Crit Care Med* 2003; **168**: 1–2.

58. Miettinen OS. Principles of epidemiologic research I: study design. Course notes, McGill University, Montreal, Canada, 1993.

59. Soriano JB, Vestbo J, Pride NB, Kiri V, Maden C, Maier WC. Survival in COPD patients after regular use of fluticasone propionate and salmeterol in general practice. *Eur Respir J* 2002; **20**: 819–25.

60. Soriano JB, Kiri VA, Pride NB, Vestbo J. Inhaled corticosteroids with/without long-acting ß-agonists reduce the risk of rehospitalization and death in COPD patients. *Am J Respir Med* 2003; **2**: 67–74.

61. Suissa S. Inhaled steroids and mortality in COPD: bias from unaccounted immortal time. *Eur Respir J* 2004; **23**: 391–5.

62. Burney P, Suissa S, Soriano JB, Vollmer WM, Viegi G, Sullivan SD *et al*. The pharmacoepidemiology of COPD: recent advances and methodological discussion. *Eur Respir J* 2003; **43** (suppl): 1–44.

Part VI

CONCLUSION

49

The Future of Pharmacoepidemiology

BRIAN L. STROM and SEAN HENNESSY

University of Pennsylvania School of Medicine, Philadelphia, Pennsylvania, USA.

> We should all be concerned about the future because we will have to spend the rest of our lives there.
>
> Charles Franklin Kettering, 1949

Speculating about the future is at least risky and possibly foolish. Nevertheless, the future of pharmacoepidemiology seems apparent in many ways, judging from past trends and recent events. Interest in the field by the pharmaceutical industry, government agencies, new trainees, and the public is truly exploding, as is realization of what pharmacoepidemiology can contribute. Indeed, as this book goes to press, international attention on drug safety has been higher than at any time in recent memory, as the safety of one analgesic after another is thrown into doubt, and with it the effectiveness of our entire system of drug approval and drug safety monitoring.

As the functions of academia, industry, and government become increasingly global, so does the field of pharmacoepidemiology. The number of individuals attending the annual International Conference on Pharmacoepidemiology has increased from approximately 50 in the early 1980s to nearly 900 in 2004. The International Society for Pharmacoepidemiology (ISPE), only two decades old, has grown to over 800 members from 37 countries. It has developed a set of guidelines for Good Epidemiologic Practices for Drug, Device, and Vaccine Research in the United States in 1996,[1] and updated these guidelines in 2004. Many national pharmacoepidemiology societies have been formed as well. The journal *Clinical Pharmacology and Therapeutics*, the major US academic clinical pharmacology journal, actively solicits pharmacoepidemiology manuscripts, as does the *Journal of Clinical Epidemiology*. The major journal of the field, *Pharmacoepidemiology and Drug Safety*, ISPE's official journal, is now indexed on Medline. The number of individuals seeking to enter the field is rapidly increasing, as is their level of training. The number of programs of study in pharmacoepidemiology is increasing in schools of medicine, public health, and pharmacy. While two decades ago the single summer short course in pharmacoepidemiology at the University of Minnesota was sometimes cancelled because of insufficient interest, more recently the University of Michigan School of Public Health summer course in pharmacoepidemiology attracted 10% of all students in the entire summer program, and now McGill University, Erasmus University Rotterdam, and the Johns Hopkins Bloomberg School of Public Health all conduct summer short courses in pharmacoepidemiology. Several other short courses are given as well, including by ISPE

Pharmacoepidemiology, Fourth Edition   Edited by B.L. Strom
© 2005 John Wiley & Sons, Ltd

itself. Regulatory bodies around the world have expanded their internal pharmacoepidemiology programs. The number of pharmaceutical companies forming their own pharmacoepidemiology units has also increased, along with their support for academic units and their funding of external pharmacoepidemiology studies. Requirements that a drug be shown to be cost effective (see Chapter 41) have been added to many national health care systems, provincial health care systems, and managed care organizations, either to justify reimbursement or even to justify drug availability. Drug utilization review is being widely applied (see Chapter 29), and many hospitals are becoming mini-pharmacoepidemiology practice and research laboratories (see Chapter 35).

Thus, from the perspective of those in the field, the future of pharmacoepidemiology looks remarkably bright, although many important challenges remain. In this chapter, we will briefly give our own views on the future of pharmacoepidemiology. Following the format of Part II of the book, we explore this future from the perspectives of academia, the pharmaceutical industry, regulatory agencies, and then the law.

THE VIEW FROM ACADEMIA

SCIENTIFIC DEVELOPMENTS

Methodologic Advances

Methodologically, the array of approaches available for performing pharmacoepidemiology studies will continue to grow. Each of the methodologic issues discussed in Part V can be expected to be the subject of more development. The future is likely to see ever more advanced ways of performing and analyzing epidemiologic studies across all content areas, as the field of epidemiology continues to expand and develop. Some of these new techniques will, of course, be particularly useful to investigators in pharmacoepidemiology (see Chapters 47 and 48). The next few years will likely see expanded use of neural networks, propensity scores, sensitivity analysis, and novel methods to analyze time-varying exposures and confounders. In addition, we believe that we will see increasing application of pharmacoepidemiologic insight in the conduct of clinical trials, as well as increased use of the randomized trial design to examine questions traditionally addressed by observational pharmacoepidemiology (see Chapter 39), especially given the recent controversies resulting from apparent inconsistencies between nonexperimental studies versus experimental studies, in some cases seeing inconsistencies where they would not

really exist, if one took into account the selection bias identified by the authors of the nonexperimental studies.

The field of pharmacoepidemiology has enthusiastically embraced the concept of therapeutic risk management (see Chapter 33). Yet, this field is very much in its infancy, with an enormous amount of work needed to develop new methods to measure, communicate, and manage the risks and benefits associated with medication use. Studies (i.e., program evaluations) evaluating the effectiveness of risk management programs are also badly needed. Development of this area will require considerable effort from pharmacoepidemiologists as well as those from other academic fields.

We will probably see developments in the processes used to assess causality from individual case reports (see Chapters 9, 10, and 36). We are also likely to see new guidelines emerge for the publication of spontaneous reports. "Data mining" approaches will be used increasingly in spontaneous reporting databases to search for early signals of adverse reactions. Hopefully, we will see data evaluating the utility of such approaches. The need for newer methods to screen for potential adverse drug effects, such as those using health care claims or medical record data, is also clear.

We are likely to see increasing input from pharmacoepidemiologists into policy questions about drug approval (see Chapter 25). We anticipate that emphasis will shift from studies evaluating whether a given drug is associated with an increased risk of a given event to those that examine patient- and regimen-specific factors that affect risk.[2] Such studies are crucial because, if risk factors for adverse reactions can be better understood before a safety crisis occurs, or early in the course of a crisis, then the clinical use of the drug may be able to be repositioned, avoiding the loss of useful drugs.

With recent developments in molecular biology and bioinformatics, and their application to the study of pharmacogenetics, exciting developments have occurred in the ability of researchers to identify genetic factors that predispose patients to adverse drug reactions[3] (see Chapter 37). However, few of these discoveries have yet been shown useful in improving patient care. Pharmacogenetics has evolved from studies of measures of slow drug metabolism as a contributor to adverse reactions[4] to more recent molecular genetic markers.[5] This has been aided by the development of new, noninvasive methods to collect DNA, such as buccal swabs, making population-based genetic studies feasible. We believe that clinical measurement of genetic factors will ultimately complement existing approaches to tailoring therapeutic approaches for individual patients. However, it is unlikely that genotype will be the only, or even the major, factor that determines the optimal drug or dose for a given patient. Future years are likely to see much more of this cross-fertilization between pharmacoepidemiology and molecular biology. From a research perspective, we can easily envision pharmacogenetic studies added to the process of following up on spontaneous reports of adverse reactions. We also anticipate the availability of genotypic information for members of large patient cohorts for whom drug exposures and clinical outcomes are recorded electronically, and even for selected patients from automated databases, such as those described in Part IIIb of this book.

Advances can also be expected in the measurement of drug exposures in human tissue. Blood and urine have long been available for this purpose, but their collection in large ambulatory populations is difficult, and detection is largely limited to the interval shortly following exposure. For case–control studies in particular, where the exposure is measured some time after it actually occurred, such sampling is of little or no use. In recent years, however, researchers have explored the usefulness of measuring drug levels in samples of other tissues, such as hair, in which drugs or their metabolites may persist and accumulate.

New Content Areas of Interest

In addition, there are a number of new content areas that are likely to be explored more and developed more. Studies of drug utilization will continue to grow and become more innovative (see Chapter 27). Particularly as the health care industry becomes more sensitive to the possibility of over-utilization, underutilization, and inappropriate utilization of drugs, and the risks associated with each, one would expect to see an increased frequency of and sophistication in drug utilization review programs, which seek to improve care (see Chapter 29). This is especially likely to be the case for studies of antibiotic misuse, as society becomes ever more concerned about the development of organisms resistant to our currently available drugs.

The US Joint Commission on Accreditation of Healthcare Organizations revolutionized US hospital pharmacoepidemiology through its standards requiring adverse reaction monitoring and drug use evaluation programs in every hospital[6,7] (see Chapter 35). Hospitals are also now experimenting with different methods of organizing their drug delivery systems to improve their use of drugs, e.g., use of computerized physician order entry and the addition of pharmacists to ward teams[8] (see Chapter 34).

Interest in the field of "pharmacoeconomics," i.e., the application of the principles of health economics to the study of drug effects, is continuing to explode (see Chapter 41). Society is realizing that the acquisition cost of drugs is often a very minor part of their economic impact, and that their beneficial and harmful effects can be vastly more important. Further, more governments and insurance programs are requiring economic justification before permitting reimbursement for a drug. As a result, the number of studies exploring this is increasing dramatically. As the methods of pharmacoeconomics become increasingly sophisticated, and its applications clear, this could be expected to continue to be a popular field of inquiry.

More nonexperimental studies of beneficial drug effects, particularly of drug effectiveness, can be expected, as the field becomes more aware that such studies are possible (see Chapter 40). This is being encouraged by the rapid increase in the use of propensity scores to adjust for confounding by indication, although investigators using this method often place more confidence in that technique than is warranted, not recognizing that its ability to control for confounding by indication remains dependent on one's ability to *measure* the true determinants of exposure (see Chapter 40).

We will also see more use of pharmacoepidemiology approaches prior to drug approval, e.g., to understand the baseline rate of adverse events that one can expect to see in patients who will eventually be treated with a new drug (see Chapters 7 and 26).

Recent years have seen an explosion in the worldwide use of herbal and other complementary and alternative medications. These are essentially pharmaceuticals sold without conventional standardization, and with no premarketing testing of safety or efficacy. In a sense, for these products, this is a return to a preregulatory era. Therefore, it is quite likely that the next few years will see an analogous set of safety disasters associated with their use, and society will turn to pharmacoepidemiologists to help evaluate the use and effects of these products.

Research interest in the entire topic of patient noncompliance (nonadherence) with prescribed drug regimens goes back to about 1960, but little fruitful research could be done until about just a decade ago because the methods for ascertaining drug exposure in individual ambulatory patients were grossly unsatisfactory. The methodologic impasse was broken by two quite different developments. The initial one was to use very low doses of a very long half-life agent, phenobarbital, as a chemical marker, since a single measurement of phenobarbital in plasma is indicative of aggregate drug intake during the prior two weeks.[9] The other, more recent, advance has been to incorporate time-stamping microcircuitry into pharmaceutical containers, which records the date and time each time that the container is opened.[10] Perhaps as a consequence of its inherent simplicity and economy, electronic monitoring is increasingly emerging as the *de facto* gold standard for compiling dosing histories of ambulatory patients, from which one can judge the extent of compliance with the prescribed drug regimen. Future years are likely to see a dramatic increase in the use of this technique (see Chapter 46) in research, and perhaps in clinical practice.

The next few years are also likely to see the increasing ability to target drug therapy to the proper patients. This will involve both increasing use of statistical methods, and increasing use of techniques from laboratory sciences, as described above. Statistical approaches will allow us to use predictive modeling to study, from a population perspective, who is statistically most likely to derive benefit from a drug, and who is at greatest risk of an adverse outcome. Laboratory science will enable us to determine individuals' genotypes, to predict responses to drug therapy (i.e., molecular susceptibility). From the perspective of pre-approval testing, these developments will allow researchers to target specific patient types for enrollment into their studies, those subjects most likely to succeed with a drug. From a clinical perspective, it will enable health care providers to incorporate genetic factors in the individualization of choice of regimens.

The past few years have seen the increased use of intermediate markers, presumed to represent increased risk of rarer serious adverse effects when drugs are used in broader numbers of patients. These range from mild liver function test abnormalities, used as predictors of serious liver toxicity, to QTc prolongation on the electrocardiogram, as a marker of risk of suffering the arrhythmia torsade de pointes, which can lead to death. Indeed, some drugs have been removed from the market, or from development, because of the presence of these intermediate markers. Yet, the utility of these markers as predictors of serious clinical outcomes is poorly studied. The next few years are likely to see data emerge addressing some of these.

In addition, with the growth of concerns about patient safety (see Chapter 34), there has been increasing attention to simultaneous use of two drugs which have been shown in pharmacokinetic studies (see Chapter 4) to cause increased or decreased drug levels. Yet, there are few data indicating which, if any, of these potential interactions are of clinical importance. The next few years are likely to see the emergence of data beginning to answer this question.

Finally, in the past few years, society has increasingly turned to pharmacoepidemiology for input into major policy decisions. For example, pharmacoepidemiology played a major role in the evaluations by the Institute of Medicine of the US National Academy of Sciences of the anthrax vaccine[11] and the smallpox vaccine program.[12] This is likely to occur even more often in the future.

Logistical Advances

Logistically, with the increased computerization of data in society in general and within health care in particular, and the increased emphasis on using computerized databases for pharmacoepidemiology[13] (see Part IIIb), some data resources will disappear (e.g., the Rhode Island Drug Use Reporting System and the inpatient databases discussed in prior editions of this book have disappeared), and a number of new computerized databases will undoubtedly emerge as major resources for pharmacoepidemiologic research, e.g., the databases from Denmark and Ontario. The importance of these databases to pharmacoepidemiology is now clear: they enable researchers to address, quickly and relatively inexpensively, questions about drug effects that require large sample sizes, with excellent quality data on drug exposures, although the data on outcomes is less certain.

Nevertheless, even as the field increases its use of databases, it is important to keep in mind the importance of studies that collect their data *de novo*. Each approach to pharmacoepidemiology has its advantages and its disadvantages, as described in Part III. No approach is ideal, and often a number of complementary approaches are needed to answer any given research question. To address some of the problems inherent in any database, we must maintain the ability to perform *ad hoc* studies as well. Preferably other, perhaps better, less expensive, and complementary approaches to *ad hoc* data collection in pharmacoepidemiology will be developed. For example, a potential approach that has not been widely used is the network of regional and national poison control centers. In particular, poison control centers would be expected to be a useful source of information about dose-dependent adverse drug effects. Others will probably be developed as well.

It is likely that new types of research opportunities will emerge. For example, as the US finally implements a drug benefit as part of Medicare, its health program for the elderly, government drug expenditures will suddenly be incremented by over \$40 billion annually. The Medicare drug benefit is already generating a huge new interest in pharmacoepidemiology and, if structured correctly, should generate an enormous new data resource that potentially could be useful for pharmacoepidemiologic research. Outside the US, as well, many different opportunities to form databases are being developed. There is also an increased interest in the importance of pharmacoepidemiology in the developing world. Many developing world countries spend a disproportionate amount of their health care resources on drugs,[14] yet these drugs are often used inappropriately.[15] There have been a number of initiatives in response to this, including the World Health Organization's development of its list of "Essential Drugs"[16,17] (see also Chapter 25).

FUNDING

For a number of years, academic pharmacoepidemiology suffered from limited research funding opportunities. With the increasing interest in the field, this situation appears to be changing, at least in the US. Much more industry funding is available, as perceived need for the field within industry grows (see below). This is likely to increase, especially as the FDA expands its own pharmacoepidemiology program, and more often requires industry to perform postmarketing studies. This will be particularly true, if these new postmarketing studies are used to permit earlier drug marketing, as has been proposed for drugs used to treat life threatening illnesses, and has been implemented in selected situations, most notably zidovudine.[18]

There is, of course, a risk associated with academic groups becoming too dependent on industry funding, both in terms of choice of study questions and credibility. Fortunately, in the US the Agency for Healthcare Research and Quality (AHRQ) has begun to fund pharmacoepidemiologic research as well, as part of an initiative in pharmaceutical outcomes research. In particular, the AHRQ Centers for Education and Research on Therapeutics (CERTs) program appears particularly promising, to begin to provide Federal support for ongoing pharmacoepidemiology activities (see also Chapter 6). While still small relative to industry expenditures on research, it is large relative to the US Federal funding previously available for pharmacoepidemiology, and is likely to expand in the next few years.

Even the National Institutes of Health (NIH) has begun to fund pharmacoepidemiology projects more often. NIH is the logical major US source for such support, as it is the major funding source for most US biomedical research. Its funds are also accessible to investigators outside the US, via the same application procedures. However, NIH's current organizational structure represents an obstacle to pharmacoepidemiology support. In general, the institutes within NIH are organized by organ system. Earlier in the development of pharmacoepidemiology, the National Institute of General Medical Sciences provided most of the US government support for our field. It remains perhaps the most appropriate source of such support, since it is the institute that is intended to fund projects that are not specific to an organ system, and

it is the institute that funds clinical pharmacology research. However, over the past few years it has not funded epidemiologic research, as it has focused much of its funding on molecular biology. This remains a problem for the field of pharmacoepidemiology that badly needs to be addressed. In the meantime, NIH funding is now available if one tailors a project to fit an organ system or in some other way fit the priorities of one of the individual institutes.

As the US government begins to pay for drugs as part of Medicare, and therefore becomes concerned about the use, effects, and costs of drugs, it is likely that there will be substantial new funding for pharmacoepidemiology available.

Finally, but of critical importance, there is increasing concern about confidentiality in many countries. The regulatory framework for human research is actively changing, in the process. As discussed in Chapter 38, this is already beginning to make pharmacoepidemiologic research more difficult, whether it is access to medical records in database studies, or access to a list of possible cases with a disease to enroll in *ad hoc* case–control studies. This will be an area of great interest and rapid activity over the next few years, and one in which the field of pharmacoepidemiology will need to remain very active, or risk considerable interference with its activities.

PERSONNEL

With the major increase in interest in the field of pharmacoepidemiology, accompanied by an increased number of funding opportunities, a major remaining problem, aggravated by the other trends, is one of inadequate personnel resources. There is a desperate need for more well-trained people in the field, with employment opportunities available in academia, industry, and government agencies. Some early attempts have been made to address this. The Burroughs Wellcome Foundation developed the Burroughs Wellcome Scholar Award in Pharmacoepidemiology, a faculty development award designed to bring new people into the field. This program, now discontinued, did not provide an opportunity for fellowship training of entry-level individuals, but was designed for more experienced investigators. Unfortunately, it is no longer an active program.

Outside of government, training opportunities are limited. In the US, the NIH is the major source of support for scientific training but, as noted above, the National Institute of General Medical Sciences, which funds training programs in clinical pharmacology, has not recently supported pharmacoepidemiology. This results in the dependence of pharmacoepidemiology training on non-Federal sources of funds. There are a few institutions now capable of carrying out such training, for example universities with faculty members interested in pharmacoepidemiology, including those with clinical research training programs supported by, for example, an NIH Clinical Research Curriculum Award and organ system-specific training grants. Young scientists interested in undergoing training in pharmacoepidemiology, however, can only do so if they happen to qualify for support from such programs. No ongoing support is normally available from these programs for training in pharmacoepidemiology *per se*. This is being addressed, primarily through the leadership and generosity of some pharmaceutical companies. Modest funding is also available through the CERTs program. Much more is needed, however.

THE VIEW FROM INDUSTRY

It appears that the role of pharmacoepidemiology in industry is and will continue to be expanding rapidly. All that was said above about the future of pharmacoepidemiology scientifically, as it relates to academia, obviously relates to industry as well. The necessity of pharmacoepidemiology for industry has become apparent to many of those in industry (see Chapters 5 and 7). In addition to being useful for exploring the effects of their drugs, manufacturers are beginning to realize that the field can contribute not only to identifying problems, but also to documenting drug safety and developing and evaluating risk management programs. An increasing number of manufacturers are mounting pharmacoepidemiology studies "prophylactically," to have data available in advance of when crises may occur. Proper practice would argue for postmarketing studies for all newly marketed drugs used for chronic diseases, and all drugs expected to be either pharmacologically novel or sales blockbusters, because of the unique risks that these situations present. Pharmacoepidemiology also can be used for measuring beneficial drug effects (see Chapter 40) and even for marketing purposes, in the form of descriptive market research and analyses of the effects of marketing efforts. Perhaps most importantly for the industry's financial bottom line, pharmacoepidemiology studies can be used to protect the major investment made in developing a new drug against false allegations of adverse effects, protecting good drugs for a public that needs them. Further, even if a drug is found to have a safety problem, the legal liability of the company may be diminished if the company has, from the outset, been forthright in its efforts to learn about that drug's risks.

In light of these advantages, most major pharmaceutical firms have formed their own pharmacoepidemiology units. Of course, this then means that industry confronts and, in fact, aggravates the problem of an insufficient number of well-trained personnel described above. Many pharmaceutical companies are also increasing their investment in external pharmacoepidemiologic data resources, so that they will be available for research when crises arise. All of this is likely to continue. A risk of the growth in the number of pharmacoepidemiology studies for industry is the generation of an increased number of false signals about harmful drug effects. This is best addressed by having adequately trained individuals in the field, and by having personnel and data resources available to address these questions quickly, responsibly, and effectively, when they are raised.

THE VIEW FROM REGULATORY AGENCIES

It appears that the role of pharmacoepidemiology in regulatory agencies is also expanding (see Chapter 8). Again, all of what was said above about the future of pharmacoepidemiology scientifically, as it relates to academia, obviously relates to regulatory agencies as well. In addition, there have been a large number of major drug crises, described throughout this book. Many of these crises resulted in the removal of the drugs from the market. The need for and importance of pharmacoepidemiology studies have become clear. Again, this can be expected to continue in the future. It has even been suggested that postmarketing pharmacoepidemiology studies might replace some premarketing Phase III studies in selected situations, as was done with zidovudine.[18] We are also seeing increasing governmental activity and interest in pharmacoepidemiology, outside the traditional realm of regulatory bodies. For example, in the US, pharmacoepidemiology now plays an important role within the AHRQ, the Centers for Disease Control and Prevention, and the NIH, and there is increasing debate about the wisdom of developing an independent new Center for Drug Surveillance.

As noted above, the use of therapeutic risk management approaches (see Chapter 33) has been aggressively embraced by regulatory bodies around the world. This will continue to change regulation as more experience with it is gained.

Finally, as this book goes to press, there is an enormous increase in attention to drug safety, driven by drug safety issues identified with COX-2 inhibitors and even traditional NSAIDs. The net result is likely to be major regulatory changes, and possibly even new legislation, either now or in response to a new Institute of Medicine study that is just being commissioned as this book goes to press.

THE VIEW FROM THE LAW

Finally, the importance of pharmacoepidemiology to the law has also been increasing. The number of lawsuits related to adverse drug effects is very large. There are an increasing number of drugs on the market, an increasing sensitivity to the adverse effects they can have, and an increasing awareness of the legal system's ability to obtain substantial remuneration for those who suffered from those adverse effects. Litigation has shifted from, say, pelvic inflammatory disease caused by intrauterine devices to the cardiac valvular effects of diet drugs and estrogen-induced breast cancers and vascular disease. The financial payments have been enormous, and indeed put entire companies at risk. The recent attention to the analgesics will create yet a new wave of litigation. It is clear that the interest in the field and the need for more true experts in the field will, therefore, increase accordingly.

CONCLUSION

There are no really "safe" biologically active drugs. There are only "safe" physicians.

Harold A. Kaminetzsky, 1963

All drugs have adverse effects. Pharmacoepidemiology will never succeed in preventing them. It can only detect them, hopefully early, and thereby educate health care providers and the public, which will lead to better medication use. The net results of increased activity in pharmacoepidemiology will be better for industry and academia but, most importantly, for the public's health. The next "thalidomide disaster" cannot be prevented by pharmacoepidemiology. However, pharmacoepidemiology can minimize its adverse public health impact by detecting it early. At the same time, it can improve the use of drugs that have a genuine role, protecting against the loss of useful drugs. The past few decades have demonstrated the utility of this new field. They also have pointed out some of its problems. With luck, the next few years will see the utility accentuated and the problems ameliorated.

REFERENCES

1. Andrews EB, Avorn J, Bortnichak EA, Chen R, Dai WS, Dieck GS *et al*. Guidelines for Good Epidemiology Practices for Drug, Device, and Vaccine Research in the United States. *Pharmacoepidemiol Drug Saf* 1996; **5**: 333–8.
2. Strom BL, West SL, Sim E, Carson JL. The epidemiology of the acute flank pain syndrome from suprofen. *Clin Pharmacol Ther* 1989; **46**: 693–9.
3. Spielberg SP. Idiosyncratic drug reactions: interaction of development and genetics. *Semin Perinatol* 1992; **16**: 58–62.
4. Woosley RL, Drayer DE, Reidenberg MM, Nies AS, Carr K, Oates JA. Effect of acetylator phenotype on the rate at which procainamide induces antinuclear antibodies and the lupus syndrome. *N Engl J Med* 1978; **298**: 1157–9.
5. Leeder JS, Riley RJ, Cook VA, Spielberg SP. Human anti-cytochrome P450 antibodies in aromatic anticonvulsant-induced hypersensitivity reactions. *J Pharmacol Exp Ther* 1992; **263**: 360–7.
6. Strom BL, Gibson GA. A systematic integrated approach to improving drug prescribing in an acute care hospital: a potential model for applied hospital pharmacoepidemiology. *Clin Pharmacol Ther* 1993; **54**: 126–33.
7. Classen DC, Pestotnik SL, Evans RS, Burke JP. Computerized surveillance of adverse drug events in hospital patients. *JAMA* 1991; **266**: 2847–51.
8. Bates DW, Leape LL, Cullen DJ, Laird N, Petersen LA, Teich JM, Burdick E, Hickey M, Kleefield S, Shea B, Vander Vliet M, Seger DL. Effect of computerized physician order entry and a team intervention on prevention of serious medication errors. *JAMA* 1998; **280**: 1311–16.
9. Pullar T, Feely M. Problems of compliance with drug treatment: new solutions? *Pharm J* 1990; **245**: 213–15.
10. Urquhart J. The electronic medication event monitor—lessons for pharmacotherapy. *Clin Pharmacokinet* 1997; **32**: 345–56.
11. Joellenbeck LM, Zwanziger LL, Durch JS, Strom BL, eds. *The Anthrax Vaccine: Is it Safe? Does it Work?* Washington, DC: National Academies Press, 2002.
12. Institute of Medicine. *The Smallpox Vaccination Program: Public Health in an Age of Terrorism.* Washington, DC: National Academies Press, 2005.
13. Strom BL, Carson JL. Use of automated databases for pharmacoepidemiology research. *Epidemiol Rev* 1990; **12**: 87–107.
14. Yudkin JS. The economics of pharmaceutical supply in Tanzania. *Int J Health Serv* 1980; **10**: 455–77.
15. Yudkin JS. Use and misuse of drugs in the Third World. *Dan Med Bull* 1984; **31** (suppl 1): 11–17.
16. Lunde PKM. WHO's programme on essential drugs. Background, implementation, present state and prospectives. *Dan Med Bull* 1984; **31** (suppl 1): 23–7.
17. Howard NJ, Laing RO. Changes in the World Health Organization essential drug list. *Lancet* 1991; **338**: 743–5.
18. Young FE. The role of the FDA in the effort against AIDS. *Public Health Rep* 1988; **103**: 242–5.

Appendix A

Sample Size Tables

Table A1. Sample sizes for cohort studies[a]

Incidence in control group	Relative risk to be detected															
	0.2	0.3	0.5	0.75	1.25	1.5	2.0	2.5	3.0	3.5	4.0	5.0	7.5	10.0	20.0	50.0
0.00001	1 970 717	2 788 497	6 306 290	29 429 320	37 837 603	10 510 431	3 153 120	1 634 946	1 051 034	756 742	583 904	394 133	211 445	142 727	61 134	22 318
0.00005	394 133	557 684	1 261 219	5 885 657	7 567 179	2 101 980	630 585	326 965	210 189	151 334	116 768	78 816	42 280	28 538	12 220	4 458
0.0001	197 060	278 832	630 585	2 942 699	3 783 376	1 050 923	315 268	163 467	105 083	75 657	58 376	39 401	21 135	14 264	6 106	2 225
0.0005	39 401	55 751	126 078	588 332	755 333	210 078	63 015	32 669	20 999	15 117	11 662	7 870	4 219	2 845	1 215	439
0.001	19 694	27 865	63 015	294 037	377 953	104 973	31 483	16 320	10 488	7 549	5 823	3 928	2 104	1 418	603	216
0.005	3 928	5 557	12 564	58 600	75 249	20 888	6 257	3 240	2 080	1 495	1 152	775	412	276	114	37
0.01	1 957	2 769	6 257	29 170	37 411	10 378	3 104	1 605	1 028	738	568	381	201	133	53	15
0.05	381	538	1 212	5 627	7 140	1 969	582	297	188	133	101	65	32	19	4	—
0.10	184	259	582	2 684	3 357	918	266	133	82	57	42	26	10	4	—	—
0.15	118	166	372	1 703	2 095	568	161	79	47	32	23	13	—	—	—	—
0.20	85	120	266	1 212	1 465	393	109	52	30	19	13	6	—	—	—	—
0.25	65	92	203	918	1 086	287	77	35	19	12	7	—	—	—	—	—
0.30	52	73	161	722	834	217	56	24	12	6	—	—	—	—	—	—
0.35	43	60	131	582	654	167	41	16	7	—	—	—	—	—	—	—
0.40	36	50	109	477	519	130	30	11	—	—	—	—	—	—	—	—
0.45	30	42	91	395	414	101	21	6	—	—	—	—	—	—	—	—
0.50	26	36	77	329	329	77	14	—	—	—	—	—	—	—	—	—
0.55	22	31	66	276	261	58	8	—	—	—	—	—	—	—	—	—
0.60	19	27	56	231	203	42	2	—	—	—	—	—	—	—	—	—
0.65	17	23	48	194	155	29	—	—	—	—	—	—	—	—	—	—
0.70	15	20	41	161	113	17	—	—	—	—	—	—	—	—	—	—
0.75	13	17	35	133	77	7	—	—	—	—	—	—	—	—	—	—
0.80	11	15	30	109	46	—	—	—	—	—	—	—	—	—	—	—
0.85	10	13	25	87	18	—	—	—	—	—	—	—	—	—	—	—
0.90	8	11	21	68	—	—	—	—	—	—	—	—	—	—	—	—
0.95	7	9	17	51	—	—	—	—	—	—	—	—	—	—	—	—

[a] $\alpha = 0.05$ (two-tailed), $\beta = 0.10$ (power = 90%), control : exposed ratio = 1 : 1. The sample size listed is the number of subjects needed in the exposed group. An equivalent number would be included in the control group.

Table A2. Sample size for cohort studies[a]

Incidence in control group	Relative risk to be detected															
	0.2	0.3	0.5	0.75	1.25	1.5	2.0	2.5	3.0	3.5	4.0	5.0	7.5	10.0	20.0	50.0
0.00001	1 529 057	2 153 636	4 825 616	22 279 822	28 149 090	7 764 537	2 302 889	1 183 563	755 529	540 883	415 381	278 329	147 626	99 000	41 938	15 197
0.0001	152 896	215 349	482 527	2 227 804	2 814 625	776 367	230 258	118 337	75 539	54 077	41 528	27 825	14 756	9 895	8 384	3 036
0.0005	30 570	43 057	96 475	445 402	562 673	155 196	46 024	23 651	15 095	10 805	8 297	5 558	2 946	1 974	4 189	1 516
0.001	15 280	21 521	48 218	222 602	281 179	77 550	22 994	11 815	7 540	5 396	4 143	2 774	1 469	984	834	300
0.005	3 047	4 292	9 613	44 362	55 984	15 433	4 571	2 346	1 496	1 069	820	548	288	192	414	148
0.01	1 518	2 138	4 787	22 082	27 834	7 668	2 268	1 163	740	528	404	269	141	93	79	26
0.05	295	415	927	4 258	5 315	1 456	426	216	136	95	72	47	23	14	37	11
0.10	142	200	444	2 030	2 500	680	196	97	60	41	31	19	8	3	3	—
0.15	91	128	283	1 287	1 561	421	119	58	35	23	17	9	—	—	—	—
0.20	66	92	203	916	1 092	291	80	38	22	14	10	4	—	—	—	—
0.25	50	70	155	693	811	214	57	26	14	9	5	—	—	—	—	—
0.30	40	56	123	545	623	162	42	18	9	4	—	—	—	—	—	—
0.35	33	46	100	439	489	125	31	12	5	—	—	—	—	—	—	—
0.40	27	38	82	359	388	97	22	8	—	—	—	—	—	—	—	—
0.45	23	32	69	297	310	76	16	—	—	—	—	—	—	—	—	—
0.50	20	27	58	248	248	58	11	—	—	—	—	—	—	—	—	—
0.55	17	23	49	207	196	44	5	—	—	—	—	—	—	—	—	—
0.60	15	20	42	173	154	32	—	—	—	—	—	—	—	—	—	—
0.65	13	17	36	145	117	22	—	—	—	—	—	—	—	—	—	—
0.70	11	15	31	120	86	13	—	—	—	—	—	—	—	—	—	—
0.75	9	13	26	99	59	—	—	—	—	—	—	—	—	—	—	—
0.80	8	11	22	80	35	—	—	—	—	—	—	—	—	—	—	—
0.85	7	10	18	64	—	—	—	—	—	—	—	—	—	—	—	—
0.90	6	8	15	49	—	—	—	—	—	—	—	—	—	—	—	—
0.95	5	7	12	36	—	—	—	—	—	—	—	—	—	—	—	—

[a] $\alpha = 0.05$ (two-tailed), $\beta = 0.10$ (power = 90%), control : exposed ratio = 2 : 1. The sample size listed is the number of subjects needed in the exposed group. Double this number would be included in the control group.

Table A3. Sample sizes for cohort studies[a]

Incidence in control group	Relative risk to be detected															
	0.2	0.3	0.5	0.75	1.25	1.5	2.0	2.5	3.0	3.5	4.0	5.0	7.5	10.0	20.0	50.0
0.00001	1 369 471	1 930 847	4 322 614	19 888 657	24 913 372	6 843 626	2 014 756	1 029 014	653 418	465 696	356 275	237 254	124 571	83 030	34 793	12 510
0.00005	273 886	386 158	864 495	3 977 589	4 962 452	1 368 657	402 927	205 788	130 673	93 131	71 248	47 445	24 910	16 602	6 955	2 499
0.0001	136 938	193 072	432 230	1 988 706	2 491 087	684 286	201 449	102 885	65 330	46 560	35 619	23 719	12 452	8 299	3 476	1 248
0.0005	27 380	38 603	86 418	397 599	497 995	136 790	40 266	20 563	13 055	9 303	7 117	4 738	2 486	1 656	692	247
0.001	13 685	19 294	43 192	198 711	248 859	68 352	20 118	10 272	6 521	4 646	3 554	2 365	1 240	825	344	122
0.005	2 729	3 847	8 611	39 600	49 549	13 603	4 030	2 040	1 294	921	703	467	244	161	66	21
0.01	1 359	1 916	4 288	19 711	24 636	6 759	1 985	1 011	640	455	347	230	119	78	31	9
0.05	264	372	830	3 800	4 705	1 284	373	188	117	82	62	40	19	12	2	—
0.10	127	179	398	1 811	2 213	600	171	85	52	36	26	16	7	3	—	—
0.15	81	114	254	1 148	1 383	372	104	50	30	20	14	8	—	—	—	—
0.20	58	82	181	817	968	257	71	33	19	12	8	4	—	—	—	—
0.25	45	63	138	618	719	189	50	23	13	7	4	—	—	—	—	—
0.30	36	50	109	485	552	143	37	16	8	4	—	—	—	—	—	—
0.35	29	41	89	391	434	111	27	11	4	—	—	—	—	—	—	—
0.40	24	34	73	319	345	86	20	7	—	—	—	—	—	—	—	—
0.45	20	28	61	264	275	67	14	—	—	—	—	—	—	—	—	—
0.50	17	24	52	220	220	52	9	—	—	—	—	—	—	—	—	—
0.55	15	21	44	184	175	39	—	—	—	—	—	—	—	—	—	—
0.60	13	18	37	154	137	29	—	—	—	—	—	—	—	—	—	—
0.65	11	15	32	128	105	19	—	—	—	—	—	—	—	—	—	—
0.70	10	13	27	106	77	10	—	—	—	—	—	—	—	—	—	—
0.75	8	11	23	87	53	—	—	—	—	—	—	—	—	—	—	—
0.80	7	10	19	71	31	—	—	—	—	—	—	—	—	—	—	—
0.85	6	8	16	56	—	—	—	—	—	—	—	—	—	—	—	—
0.90	5	7	13	43	—	—	—	—	—	—	—	—	—	—	—	—
0.95	4	6	11	31	—	—	—	—	—	—	—	—	—	—	—	—

[a] $\alpha = 0.05$ (two-tailed), $\beta = 0.10$ (power = 90%), control : exposed ratio = 3 : 1. The sample size listed is the number of subjects needed in the exposed group. Triple this number would be included in the control group.

Table A4. Sample sizes for cohort studies[a]

Incidence in control group	Relative risk to be detected															
	0.2	0.3	0.5	0.75	1.25	1.5	2.0	2.5	3.0	3.5	4.0	5.0	7.5	10.0	20.0	50.0
0.00001	1 285 566	1 815 876	4 068 209	18 690 665	23 293 643	6 381 472	1 869 238	950 463	601 217	427 061	325 766	215 895	112 429	74 554	30 945	11 048
0.00005	257 106	363 164	813 616	3 737 999	4 658 521	1 276 231	373 825	190 079	120 234	85 404	65 147	43 174	22 482	14 907	6 186	2 207
0.0001	128 548	181 575	406 791	1 868 916	2 329 131	638 076	186 899	95 031	60 111	42 697	32 569	21 583	11 238	7 451	3 091	1 102
0.0005	25 702	36 304	81 332	373 649	465 619	127 552	37 358	18 993	12 013	8 532	6 507	4 311	2 244	1 487	615	218
0.001	12 846	18 145	40 650	186 741	232 680	63 737	18 665	9 488	6 000	4 261	3 249	2 152	1 119	741	306	107
0.005	2 562	3 618	8 104	37 214	46 329	12 684	3 711	1 884	1 190	844	643	425	220	145	58	19
0.01	1 276	1 802	4 035	18 523	23 035	6 303	1 842	934	589	417	318	209	107	70	27	8
0.05	248	349	781	3 571	4 399	1 198	346	174	108	76	57	36	17	10	2	—
0.10	119	168	374	1 702	2 070	560	159	78	48	33	24	15	6	2	—	—
0.15	76	107	238	1 079	1 294	347	97	47	28	19	13	7	—	—	—	—
0.20	55	77	171	767	905	240	66	31	18	11	8	3	—	—	—	—
0.25	42	59	130	580	672	177	47	21	12	7	4	—	—	—	—	—
0.30	33	47	103	456	517	134	34	15	7	—	—	—	—	—	—	—
0.35	27	38	83	366	406	103	25	10	3	—	—	—	—	—	—	—
0.40	23	32	69	300	323	81	18	6	—	—	—	—	—	—	—	—
0.45	19	27	58	248	258	63	13	—	—	—	—	—	—	—	—	—
0.50	16	23	48	206	206	48	8	—	—	—	—	—	—	—	—	—
0.55	14	19	41	172	164	37	—	—	—	—	—	—	—	—	—	—
0.60	12	16	35	144	128	27	—	—	—	—	—	—	—	—	—	—
0.65	10	14	30	120	98	18	—	—	—	—	—	—	—	—	—	—
0.70	9	12	25	99	72	7	—	—	—	—	—	—	—	—	—	—
0.75	8	10	21	81	50	—	—	—	—	—	—	—	—	—	—	—
0.80	6	9	18	66	29	—	—	—	—	—	—	—	—	—	—	—
0.85	6	8	15	52	—	—	—	—	—	—	—	—	—	—	—	—
0.90	5	6	12	39	—	—	—	—	—	—	—	—	—	—	—	—
0.95	4	5	10	28	—	—	—	—	—	—	—	—	—	—	—	—

[a] $\alpha = 0.05$ (two-tailed), $\beta = 0.10$ (power = 90%), control : exposed ratio = 4 : 1. The sample size listed is the number of subjects needed in the exposed group. Quadruple this number would be included in the control group.

Table A5. Sample sizes for cohort studies[a]

Incidence in control group	Relative risk to be detected															
	0.2	0.3	0.5	0.75	1.25	1.5	2.0	2.5	3.0	3.5	4.0	5.0	7.5	10.0	20.0	50.0
0.00001	1 472 091	2 082 958	4 710 686	21 983 178	28 264 016	7 851 105	2 355 325	1 221 276	785 104	565 273	436 166	294 411	157 946	106 615	45 666	16 672
0.00005	294 411	416 580	942 108	4 396 481	5 652 548	1 570 142	471 036	244 238	157 008	113 044	87 224	58 875	31 583	21 318	9 129	3 330
0.0001	147 201	208 283	471 036	2 198 144	2 826 115	785 022	235 500	122 108	78 496	56 515	43 606	29 433	15 788	10 656	4 562	1 663
0.0005	29 433	41 645	94 178	439 474	564 968	156 925	47 071	24 404	15 686	11 292	8 712	5 879	3 152	2 126	908	329
0.001	14 711	20 816	47 071	219 641	282 325	78 413	23 518	12 191	7 835	5 639	4 350	2 935	1 572	1 060	451	162
0.005	2 935	4 152	9 385	43 774	56 210	15 604	4 675	2 421	1 554	1 117	861	579	309	207	86	28
0.01	1 463	2 069	4 675	21 790	27 946	7 752	2 319	1 199	769	552	425	285	151	100	40	12
0.05	285	402	906	4 204	5 334	1 471	435	222	141	100	76	49	24	15	3	—
0.10	138	194	435	2 005	2 508	686	200	100	62	43	32	20	8	4	—	—
0.15	89	125	278	1 273	1 566	425	121	59	36	24	17	10	—	—	—	—
0.20	64	90	200	906	1 095	294	82	39	23	15	10	5	—	—	—	—
0.25	49	69	152	686	812	215	58	27	15	9	6	—	—	—	—	—
0.30	40	55	121	540	623	163	42	19	10	—	—	—	—	—	—	—
0.35	33	45	99	435	489	125	31	13	—	—	—	—	—	—	—	—
0.40	27	38	82	357	388	97	23	8	—	—	—	—	—	—	—	—
0.45	23	32	69	295	309	76	16	—	—	—	—	—	—	—	—	—
0.50	20	27	58	247	247	58	11	—	—	—	—	—	—	—	—	—
0.55	17	24	50	207	195	44	—	—	—	—	—	—	—	—	—	—
0.60	15	20	42	173	152	32	—	—	—	—	—	—	—	—	—	—
0.65	13	18	36	145	116	22	—	—	—	—	—	—	—	—	—	—
0.70	11	15	31	121	85	—	—	—	—	—	—	—	—	—	—	—
0.75	10	13	27	100	58	—	—	—	—	—	—	—	—	—	—	—
0.80	9	12	23	82	35	—	—	—	—	—	—	—	—	—	—	—
0.85	8	10	19	66	14	—	—	—	—	—	—	—	—	—	—	—
0.90	7	9	16	51	—	—	—	—	—	—	—	—	—	—	—	—
0.95	6	8	14	38	—	—	—	—	—	—	—	—	—	—	—	—

[a] $\alpha = 0.05$ (two-tailed), $\beta = 0.20$ (power = 80%), control : exposed ratio = 1 : 1. The sample size listed is the number of subjects needed in the control group. An equivalent number would be included in the exposed group.

Table A6. Sample sizes for cohort studies

Incidence in control group	Relative risk to be detected															
	0.2	0.3	0.5	0.75	1.25	1.5	2.0	2.5	3.0	3.5	4.0	5.0	7.5	10.0	20.0	50.0
0.00001	1 190 356	1 663 432	3 680 447	16 792 779	20 878 641	5 726 194	1 683 582	859 799	546 209	389 547	298 242	198 909	104 767	69 986	29 458	10 630
0.00005	238 065	332 677	736 066	3 358 436	4 175 543	1 145 183	336 697	171 948	109 233	77 903	59 643	39 777	20 950	13 994	5 889	2 124
0.0001	119 028	166 332	368 018	1 679 143	2 087 655	572 556	168 336	85 967	54 611	38 947	29 818	19 886	10 473	6 995	2 943	1 061
0.0005	23 799	33 257	73 580	335 708	417 346	114 455	33 648	17 182	10 914	7 783	5 958	3 973	2 091	1 396	586	210
0.001	11 895	16 622	36 775	167 779	208 557	57 193	16 812	8 584	5 452	3 887	2 975	1 983	1 043	696	292	104
0.005	2 372	3 315	7 332	33 436	41 526	11 382	3 343	1 705	1 082	771	589	392	205	136	56	19
0.01	1 182	1 651	3 651	16 643	20 647	5 656	1 659	845	536	381	291	193	100	66	26	8
0.05	230	321	707	3 208	3 944	1 075	312	157	99	69	52	34	17	10	2	—
0.10	111	154	339	1 529	1 856	503	144	71	44	30	23	14	6	3	—	—
0.15	71	99	216	969	1 160	312	88	43	26	17	13	7	—	—	—	—
0.20	51	71	155	689	812	216	60	28	17	11	8	4	—	—	—	—
0.25	39	54	118	522	603	159	43	20	11	7	4	—	—	—	—	—
0.30	31	43	93	410	464	121	32	14	7	4	—	—	—	—	—	—
0.35	26	35	76	330	365	93	23	10	4	—	—	—	—	—	—	—
0.40	21	29	63	270	290	73	17	6	—	—	—	—	—	—	—	—
0.45	18	25	52	223	232	57	13	—	—	—	—	—	—	—	—	—
0.50	15	21	44	186	186	44	9	—	—	—	—	—	—	—	—	—
0.55	13	18	38	155	148	34	5	—	—	—	—	—	—	—	—	—
0.60	11	16	32	130	116	25	—	—	—	—	—	—	—	—	—	—
0.65	10	13	27	108	89	18	—	—	—	—	—	—	—	—	—	—
0.70	9	12	23	90	66	11	—	—	—	—	—	—	—	—	—	—
0.75	8	10	20	74	46	—	—	—	—	—	—	—	—	—	—	—
0.80	7	9	17	60	28	—	—	—	—	—	—	—	—	—	—	—
0.85	6	7	14	47	—	—	—	—	—	—	—	—	—	—	—	—
0.90	5	6	12	36	—	—	—	—	—	—	—	—	—	—	—	—
0.95	4	5	9	26	—	—	—	—	—	—	—	—	—	—	—	—

[a] $\alpha = 0.05$ (two-tailed), $\beta = 0.20$ (power = 80%), control : exposed ratio = 2 : 1. The sample size listed is the number of subjects needed in the exposed group. Double this number would be included in the control group.

Table A7. Sample sizes for cohort studies[a]

Incidence in control group	Relative risk to be detected															
	0.2	0.3	0.5	0.75	1.25	1.5	2.0	2.5	3.0	3.5	4.0	5.0	7.5	10.0	20.0	50.0
0.00001	1 088 323	1 516 254	3 330 831	15 057 392	18 412 768	5 014 203	1 456 566	736 622	464 207	328 848	250 342	165 451	85 870	56 861	23 565	8 410
0.00005	217 658	303 242	666 145	3 011 370	3 682 391	1 002 792	291 297	147 315	92 835	65 764	50 064	33 087	17 171	11 370	4 711	1 681
0.0001	108 825	151 615	333 059	1 505 617	1 841 094	501 366	145 638	73 651	46 413	32 879	25 029	16 541	8 584	5 684	2 355	839
0.0005	21 759	30 314	66 590	301 015	368 057	100 225	29 111	14 721	9 276	6 570	5 001	3 305	1 714	1 134	469	166
0.001	10 875	15 151	33 281	150 439	183 927	50 082	14 545	7 354	4 634	3 282	2 498	1 650	855	566	233	82
0.005	2 169	3 021	6 635	29 979	36 623	9 968	2 892	1 461	920	651	495	326	168	111	45	15
0.01	1 080	1 505	3 304	14 922	18 210	4 954	1 436	725	456	322	245	161	83	54	21	6
0.05	210	292	639	2 876	3 480	942	271	135	84	59	44	29	14	8	2	—
0.10	101	140	306	1 370	1 638	441	125	62	38	26	19	12	5	2	—	—
0.15	65	90	195	868	1 025	274	76	37	22	15	11	6	—	—	—	—
0.20	46	64	139	617	718	190	52	25	14	9	6	3	—	—	—	—
0.25	36	49	106	466	534	140	37	17	10	6	4	—	—	—	—	—
0.30	28	39	84	366	411	107	28	12	6	3	—	—	—	—	—	—
0.35	23	32	68	294	323	83	21	9	4	—	—	—	—	—	—	—
0.40	19	26	56	240	257	65	15	6	—	—	—	—	—	—	—	—
0.45	16	22	47	199	206	51	11	—	—	—	—	—	—	—	—	—
0.50	14	19	39	165	165	39	8	—	—	—	—	—	—	—	—	—
0.55	12	16	33	138	132	30	—	—	—	—	—	—	—	—	—	—
0.60	10	14	28	115	104	23	—	—	—	—	—	—	—	—	—	—
0.65	9	12	24	96	80	16	—	—	—	—	—	—	—	—	—	—
0.70	8	10	20	79	60	9	—	—	—	—	—	—	—	—	—	—
0.75	7	9	17	65	42	—	—	—	—	—	—	—	—	—	—	—
0.80	6	7	14	52	26	—	—	—	—	—	—	—	—	—	—	—
0.85	5	6	12	41	—	—	—	—	—	—	—	—	—	—	—	—
0.90	4	5	10	31	—	—	—	—	—	—	—	—	—	—	—	—
0.95	3	4	8	22	—	—	—	—	—	—	—	—	—	—	—	—

[a] $\alpha = 0.05$ (two-tailed), $\beta = 0.20$ (power = 80%), control : exposed ratio = 3 : 1. The sample size listed is the number of subjects needed in the exposed group. Triple this number would be included in the control group.

Table A8. Sample sizes for cohort studies[a]

Incidence in control group	Relative risk to be detected															
	0.2	0.3	0.5	0.75	1.25	1.5	2.0	2.5	3.0	3.5	4.0	5.0	7.5	10.0	20.0	50.0
0.00001	1 034 606	1 440 316	3 154 116	14 188 116	17 178 604	4 657 092	1 342 104	674 194	422 454	297 814	225 764	148 182	76 019	49 975	20 438	7 223
0.00005	206 915	288 054	630 802	2 837 520	3 435 570	931 374	268 406	134 830	84 485	59 558	45 149	29 633	15 201	9 993	4 086	1 443
0.0001	103 454	144 022	315 388	1 418 696	1 717 691	465 659	134 194	67 410	42 238	29 776	22 572	14 815	7 599	4 995	2 042	721
0.0005	20 685	28 795	63 057	283 636	343 387	93 087	26 824	13 473	8 442	5 950	4 510	2 960	1 518	997	407	143
0.001	10 338	14 392	31 515	141 754	171 599	46 516	13 402	6 731	4 217	2 972	2 253	1 478	757	497	203	71
0.005	2 061	2 870	6 282	28 248	34 169	9 259	2 665	1 338	837	590	446	292	149	98	39	13
0.01	1 027	1 429	3 128	14 059	16 990	4 601	1 323	663	415	292	221	144	73	48	19	6
0.05	199	277	605	2 709	3 247	876	250	124	77	53	40	26	12	8	2	—
0.10	96	133	289	1 290	1 529	410	115	57	35	24	17	11	5	2	—	—
0.15	61	85	184	817	957	255	71	34	20	14	10	6	—	—	—	—
0.20	44	61	132	581	670	177	48	23	13	9	6	3	—	—	—	—
0.25	34	47	100	439	499	130	35	16	9	5	3	—	—	—	—	—
0.30	27	37	79	344	384	99	26	11	6	—	—	—	—	—	—	—
0.35	22	30	64	277	302	77	19	8	3	—	—	—	—	—	—	—
0.40	18	25	53	226	241	60	14	5	—	—	—	—	—	—	—	—
0.45	15	21	44	186	193	47	10	—	—	—	—	—	—	—	—	—
0.50	13	18	37	155	155	37	7	—	—	—	—	—	—	—	—	—
0.55	11	15	31	129	124	28	—	—	—	—	—	—	—	—	—	—
0.60	9	13	26	108	97	21	—	—	—	—	—	—	—	—	—	—
0.65	8	11	22	89	75	15	—	—	—	—	—	—	—	—	—	—
0.70	7	9	19	74	56	7	—	—	—	—	—	—	—	—	—	—
0.75	6	8	16	60	39	—	—	—	—	—	—	—	—	—	—	—
0.80	5	7	13	48	24	—	—	—	—	—	—	—	—	—	—	—
0.85	4	6	11	38	—	—	—	—	—	—	—	—	—	—	—	—
0.90	4	5	9	28	—	—	—	—	—	—	—	—	—	—	—	—
0.95	3	4	7	20	—	—	—	—	—	—	—	—	—	—	—	—

[a] $\alpha = 0.05$ (two-tailed), $\beta = 0.20$ (power = 80%), control : exposed ratio = 4 : 1. The sample size listed is the number of subjects needed in the exposed group. Quadruple this number would be included in the control group.

Table A9. Sample sizes for case–control studies[a]

Prevalence in control group	Odds ratio to be detected															
	0.2	0.3	0.5	0.75	1.25	1.5	2.0	2.5	3.0	3.5	4.0	5.0	7.5	10.0	20.0	50.0
0.00001	1 970 728	2 788 519	6 306 363	29 429 793	37 838 497	10 510 715	3 153 225	1 635 011	1 051 081	756 780	583 937	394 159	211 464	142 743	61 147	22 330
0.00005	394 143	557 705	1 261 292	5 886 130	7 568 072	2 102 264	630 690	327 029	210 236	151 372	116 801	78 842	42 300	28 555	12 234	4 469
0.0001	197 070	278 853	630 659	2 943 172	3 784 269	1 051 207	315 373	163 532	105 130	75 696	58 409	39 427	21 155	14 281	6 120	2 237
0.0005	39 412	55 772	126 151	588 806	757 227	210 362	63 120	32 734	21 046	15 155	11 695	7 896	4 238	2 862	1 228	451
0.001	19 704	27 887	63 088	294 510	378 847	105 257	31 588	16 384	10 535	7 587	5 856	3 954	2 124	1 435	617	228
0.005	3 939	5 579	12 638	59 074	76 145	21 173	6 363	3 304	2 127	1 533	1 184	801	432	293	128	49
0.01	1 968	2 790	6 331	29 646	38 309	10 663	3 210	1 669	1 076	777	601	407	221	150	67	27
0.05	391	560	1 288	6 111	8 059	2 261	690	363	237	172	135	93	52	37	18	9
0.10	195	281	659	3 181	4 302	1 219	379	202	133	98	77	54	32	23	13	8
0.15	129	189	451	2 215	3 072	879	278	150	100	75	60	43	26	19	11	8
0.20	97	143	348	1 741	2 476	716	230	126	85	64	52	37	23	18	11	8
0.25	77	116	287	1 465	2 137	624	203	113	77	59	48	35	23	18	12	9
0.30	64	98	248	1 289	1 930	569	188	106	73	56	46	34	23	18	13	10
0.35	56	86	222	1 174	1 802	536	180	103	72	56	46	35	24	19	14	11
0.40	49	77	203	1 097	1 727	519	177	102	72	56	47	36	25	20	15	12
0.45	44	70	191	1 048	1 694	513	178	104	74	58	49	38	27	22	17	14
0.50	40	66	182	1 023	1 696	519	182	108	77	61	52	40	29	24	19	16
0.55	38	62	178	1 019	1 732	535	191	114	82	66	56	44	32	27	21	18
0.60	36	61	177	1 035	1 806	562	203	123	89	72	61	49	36	31	25	21
0.65	35	60	180	1 077	1 927	605	222	135	99	80	69	56	42	36	29	25
0.70	34	61	188	1 149	2 110	669	248	153	113	92	79	64	49	43	35	31
0.75	35	64	203	1 268	2 390	764	287	178	133	109	94	77	59	52	43	38
0.80	37	70	230	1 465	2 831	913	348	218	164	135	117	97	75	66	55	49
0.85	43	82	278	1 811	3 591	1 168	451	285	216	179	156	129	101	90	75	68
0.90	54	108	379	2 527	5 143	1 687	659	420	320	266	233	195	154	137	116	105
0.95	93	190	690	4 717	9 851	3 257	1 288	828	635	531	466	391	313	280	238	217

[a] $\alpha = 0.05$ (two-tailed), $\beta = 0.10$ (power = 90%), control : case ratio = 1 : 1. The sample size listed is the number of subjects needed in the case group. An equivalent number would be included in the control group.

Table A10. Sample sizes for case–control studies[a]

Prevalence in control group	Odds ratio to be detected															
	0.2	0.3	0.5	0.75	1.25	1.5	2.0	2.5	3.0	3.5	4.0	5.0	7.5	10.0	20.0	50.0
0.00001	1 529 065	2 153 652	4 825 672	22 280 178	28 149 758	7 764 749	2 302 966	1 183 610	755 564	540 911	415 405	278 348	147 639	99 012	41 948	15 205
0.00005	305 811	430 731	965 148	4 456 162	5 630 233	1 553 041	460 628	236 743	151 128	108 194	83 091	55 678	29 534	19 807	8 393	3 044
0.0001	152 904	215 366	482 583	2 228 160	2 815 293	776 578	230 335	118 385	75 573	54 105	41 552	27 844	14 770	9 906	4 199	1 524
0.0005	30 578	43 073	96 531	445 759	563 340	155 407	46 101	23 698	15 130	10 833	8 321	5 577	2 960	1 986	843	307
0.001	15 288	21 537	48 274	222 959	281 846	77 761	23 072	11 862	7 574	5 424	4 167	2 793	1 483	996	424	155
0.005	3 055	4 308	9 669	44 719	56 653	15 644	4 649	2 393	1 530	1 097	844	567	302	204	88	34
0.01	1 526	2 154	4 843	22 440	28 505	7 880	2 346	1 210	775	556	428	289	155	105	46	19
0.05	303	431	984	4 623	6 001	1 674	506	264	171	124	97	66	37	26	13	7
0.10	150	216	503	2 405	3 207	904	279	148	97	71	56	39	23	17	9	6
0.15	100	145	343	1 673	2 292	653	205	111	74	55	44	31	19	14	8	6
0.20	74	110	265	1 313	1 849	533	170	93	63	47	38	28	17	13	8	6
0.25	59	89	218	1 104	1 597	465	151	84	57	44	35	26	17	13	9	6
0.30	49	75	188	971	1 443	425	140	79	55	42	34	26	17	14	9	7
0.35	42	65	168	883	1 349	401	135	77	54	42	34	26	18	14	10	8
0.40	37	58	154	825	1 294	388	133	77	54	42	35	27	19	15	11	9
0.45	33	53	144	788	1 270	385	133	78	56	44	37	28	20	17	13	10
0.50	31	50	137	768	1 272	389	137	81	58	46	39	31	22	19	14	12
0.55	28	47	133	764	1 301	402	144	86	62	50	42	33	24	21	16	14
0.60	27	45	133	775	1 357	423	154	93	68	55	47	37	28	24	19	16
0.65	26	45	135	805	1 449	456	168	103	76	61	52	42	32	28	22	19
0.70	26	45	140	859	1 588	505	188	116	86	70	61	49	38	33	27	23
0.75	26	47	151	947	1 799	577	218	136	102	84	72	59	46	40	33	29
0.80	28	51	170	1 092	2 133	690	265	166	125	104	90	74	58	51	42	38
0.85	31	60	205	1 349	2 708	884	343	218	165	137	120	100	78	70	58	53
0.90	39	78	279	1 880	3 881	1 278	503	322	246	205	180	150	119	107	90	82
0.95	66	137	506	3 505	7 438	2 472	984	635	489	410	360	303	243	218	186	169

[a] $\alpha = 0.05$ (two-tailed), $\beta = 0.10$ (power = 90%), control : case ratio = 2 : 1. The sample size listed is the number of subjects needed in the case group. Double this number would be included in the control group.

Table A11. Sample size for case–control studies[a]

Prevalence in control group	Odds ratio to be detected															
	0.2	0.3	0.5	0.75	1.25	1.5	2.0	2.5	3.0	3.5	4.0	5.0	7.5	10.0	20.0	50.0
0.00001	1 369 478	1 930 861	4 322 663	19 888 975	24 913 964	6 843 813	2 014 824	1 029 056	653 448	465 720	356 295	237 271	124 583	83 040	34 800	12 517
0.00005	273 893	386 172	864 545	3 977 907	4 933 044	1 368 844	402 996	205 830	130 703	93 155	71 268	47 461	24 922	16 612	6 963	2 506
0.0001	136 945	193 086	432 280	1 989 023	2 491 679	684 473	201 517	102 927	65 360	46 584	35 640	23 735	12 464	8 309	3 483	1 254
0.0005	27 387	38 617	86 468	397 917	498 587	136 977	40 334	20 604	13 086	9 328	7 137	4 754	2 498	1 666	700	253
0.001	13 692	19 309	43 242	199 028	249 451	68 540	20 186	10 314	6 551	4 671	3 574	2 382	1 252	836	352	128
0.005	2 736	3 862	8 661	39 918	50 143	13 790	4 068	2 082	1 324	945	724	484	256	171	73	28
0.01	1 367	1 931	4 338	20 030	25 231	6 947	2 054	1 053	671	480	368	246	131	88	39	16
0.05	271	387	881	4 125	5 313	1 477	444	231	149	108	84	57	32	22	11	6
0.10	134	194	450	2 145	2 841	799	245	129	85	62	49	34	20	14	8	5
0.15	89	130	307	1 491	2 031	577	180	97	64	48	38	27	16	12	7	5
0.20	66	98	236	1 171	1 639	471	150	82	55	41	33	24	15	12	7	5
0.25	53	79	195	984	1 417	412	133	74	50	38	31	23	15	12	8	6
0.30	44	67	168	865	1 281	376	124	70	48	37	30	23	15	12	8	6
0.35	38	58	150	786	1 197	355	119	68	47	37	30	23	16	13	9	7
0.40	33	52	137	734	1 149	345	118	68	48	37	31	24	16	14	10	8
0.45	30	47	128	700	1 128	342	119	69	49	39	32	25	18	15	11	9
0.50	27	44	122	682	1 131	346	122	72	52	41	35	27	19	16	12	10
0.55	25	42	119	679	1 156	357	128	76	55	44	38	30	22	18	14	12
0.60	24	40	118	689	1 207	377	137	83	60	49	41	33	25	21	17	14
0.65	23	40	119	715	1 289	406	150	91	67	55	47	38	28	24	20	17
0.70	23	40	124	762	1 414	450	168	104	77	63	54	44	33	29	24	21
0.75	23	42	133	839	1 602	515	195	121	91	75	65	53	41	36	29	26
0.80	24	45	150	968	1 900	616	236	149	112	93	80	66	52	45	38	34
0.85	27	52	180	1 194	2 413	789	307	195	148	123	107	89	70	62	52	46
0.90	34	68	245	1 664	3 459	1 142	450	288	220	184	161	134	107	95	80	72
0.95	57	119	444	3 100	6 632	2 208	881	569	438	367	323	271	217	194	165	150

[a] $\alpha = 0.05$ (two-tailed), $\beta = 0.10$ (power = 90%), control : case ratio = 3 : 1. The sample size listed is the number of subjects needed in the control group. Triple this number would be the number of subjects needed in the case group.

Table A12. Sample sizes for case–control studies[a]

Prevalence in control group	Odds ratio to be detected															
	0.2	0.3	0.5	0.75	1.25	1.5	2.0	2.5	3.0	3.5	4.0	5.0	7.5	10.0	20.0	50.0
0.00001	1 285 573	1 815 890	4 068 256	18 690 963	23 294 197	6 381 647	1 869 301	950 501	601 245	427 084	325 786	215 910	112 440	74 563	30 952	11 054
0.00005	257 112	363 178	813 662	3 738 297	4 659 075	1 276 406	373 889	190 118	120 262	85 427	65 166	43 189	22 493	14 916	6 193	2 213
0.0001	128 555	181 589	406 838	1 869 214	2 329 685	638 251	186 963	95 070	60 139	42 720	32 588	21 599	11 249	7 461	3 098	1 108
0.0005	25 709	36 318	81 379	373 947	466 173	127 727	37 422	19 032	12 041	8 554	6 526	4 326	2 255	1 496	622	224
0.001	12 853	18 159	40 697	187 039	233 234	63 912	18 729	9 527	6 028	4 284	3 269	2 167	1 130	750	313	113
0.005	2 568	3 632	8 151	37 513	46 884	12 860	3 775	1 923	1 219	867	662	440	231	154	65	25
0.01	1 283	1 816	4 082	18 823	23 592	6 479	1 906	973	618	440	337	224	118	79	34	14
0.05	255	363	829	3 876	4 969	1 378	412	214	137	99	77	52	29	20	10	5
0.10	126	182	423	2 015	2 658	746	228	120	78	57	45	31	18	13	7	4
0.15	83	122	289	1 401	1 901	539	168	90	60	44	35	25	15	11	7	4
0.20	62	92	222	1 099	1 534	440	140	76	51	38	31	22	14	11	7	5
0.25	50	74	183	923	1 326	385	125	69	47	36	29	21	14	11	7	5
0.30	41	63	158	812	1 200	352	116	65	45	34	28	21	14	11	7	6
0.35	35	55	140	738	1 122	333	111	63	44	34	28	21	14	12	8	6
0.40	31	49	128	688	1 077	323	110	63	45	35	29	22	15	13	9	7
0.45	28	44	120	657	1 058	320	111	65	46	36	30	23	17	14	10	8
0.50	25	41	114	640	1 060	324	114	67	48	38	32	25	18	15	11	10
0.55	23	39	111	636	1 084	335	120	72	52	41	35	28	20	17	13	11
0.60	22	38	110	645	1 132	354	128	78	57	46	39	31	23	20	15	13
0.65	21	37	111	669	1 209	381	140	86	63	51	44	35	26	23	18	16
0.70	21	37	116	713	1 326	422	158	97	72	59	51	41	31	27	22	19
0.75	21	39	125	786	1 504	483	183	114	85	70	61	50	38	33	27	24
0.80	22	42	140	905	1 784	579	222	140	105	87	75	62	48	42	35	31
0.85	25	48	168	1 117	2 266	742	289	183	139	115	101	83	65	58	48	43
0.90	31	63	228	1 556	3 248	1 073	423	271	207	173	151	126	100	89	75	67
0.95	52	110	412	2 897	6 229	2 076	829	536	412	345	303	255	203	182	154	139

[a] α = 0.05 (two-tailed), β = 0.10 (power = 90%), control : case ratio = 4 : 1. The sample size listed is the number of subjects needed in the case group. Quadruple this number would be included in the control group.

Table A13. Sample sizes for case–control studies[a]

Prevalence in control group	Odds ratio to be detected															
	0.2	0.3	0.5	0.75	1.25	1.5	2.0	2.5	3.0	3.5	4.0	5.0	7.5	10.0	20.0	50.0
0.00001	1 472 099	2 082 974	4 710 741	21 983 531	28 264 683	7 851 317	2 355 404	1 221 324	785 139	565 302	436 191	294 430	157 960	106 627	45 676	16 681
0.00005	294 418	416 596	942 163	4 396 835	5 653 216	1 570 354	471 115	244 286	157 043	113 073	87 248	58 894	31 598	21 330	9 139	3 339
0.0001	147 208	208 299	471 091	2 198 497	2 826 782	785 234	235 579	122 156	78 531	56 544	43 631	29 452	15 803	10 668	4 572	1 671
0.0005	29 440	41 661	94 233	439 828	565 636	157 137	47 150	24 452	15 721	11 321	8 736	5 899	3 166	2 138	918	337
0.001	14 719	20 831	47 126	219 994	282 992	78 625	23 596	12 239	7 870	5 668	4 375	2 954	1 587	1 072	461	171
0.005	2 943	4 168	9 441	44 128	56 879	15 816	4 753	2 469	1 589	1 146	885	599	323	219	96	37
0.01	1 470	2 085	4 730	22 145	28 617	7 966	2 398	1 248	804	581	449	305	165	113	50	20
0.05	293	419	962	4 566	6 020	1 690	516	272	177	129	101	70	39	28	14	7
0.10	146	211	493	2 377	3 214	911	283	151	100	74	58	41	24	18	10	6
0.15	97	142	337	1 655	2 295	657	208	113	75	56	45	32	20	15	9	6
0.20	73	107	260	1 301	1 850	535	172	95	64	48	39	28	18	14	9	6
0.25	58	87	215	1 095	1 597	466	152	85	58	44	36	27	17	14	9	7
0.30	49	74	186	964	1 442	425	141	80	55	42	35	26	18	14	10	8
0.35	42	65	166	877	1 346	401	135	77	54	42	35	26	18	15	11	9
0.40	37	58	152	820	1 291	388	133	77	54	42	35	27	19	16	12	10
0.45	33	53	143	784	1 266	384	133	78	56	44	37	29	20	17	13	11
0.50	31	50	137	765	1 267	388	137	81	58	46	39	31	22	19	15	12
0.55	29	47	133	761	1 294	400	143	85	62	50	42	33	25	21	16	14
0.60	27	46	133	774	1 350	421	152	92	67	54	46	37	28	24	19	16
0.65	26	45	135	805	1 440	453	166	101	75	61	52	42	32	27	22	19
0.70	26	46	141	859	1 577	500	186	115	85	69	60	49	37	32	26	23
0.75	27	48	152	948	1 785	571	215	134	100	82	71	58	45	39	33	29
0.80	28	53	172	1 095	2 115	682	260	163	123	101	88	73	57	50	42	37
0.85	32	62	208	1 353	2 683	873	337	213	162	134	117	97	76	68	57	51
0.90	41	81	283	1 888	3 842	1 260	493	314	240	200	175	146	116	103	87	79
0.95	70	142	516	3 524	7 359	2 433	962	619	475	397	349	293	234	210	179	162

[a] $\alpha = 0.05$ (two-tailed), $\beta = 0.20$ (power = 80%), control : case ratio = 1 : 1. The sample size listed is the number of subjects needed in the case group. An equivalent number would be included in the control group.

Table A14. Sample sizes for case–control studies[a]

Prevalence in control group	Odds ratio to be detected															
	0.2	0.3	0.5	0.75	1.25	1.5	2.0	2.5	3.0	3.5	4.0	5.0	7.5	10.0	20.0	50.0
0.00001	1 190 363	1 663 444	3 680 489	16 793 046	20 879 138	5 726 351	1 683 639	859 834	546 235	389 568	298 260	198 923	104 777	69 995	29 465	10 635
0.00005	238 071	332 689	736 108	3 358 703	4 176 039	1 145 339	336 754	171 983	109 259	77 923	59 660	39 791	20 960	14 003	5 896	2 129
0.0001	119 034	166 344	368 060	1 679 410	2 088 152	572 713	168 393	86 001	54 637	38 967	29 835	19 899	10 483	7 004	2 950	1 066
0.0005	23 805	33 269	73 622	335 976	417 842	114 612	33 705	17 216	10 939	7 803	5 975	3 986	2 101	1 405	593	216
0.001	11 901	16 635	36 817	168 047	209 054	57 349	16 869	8 618	5 477	3 907	2 993	1 997	1 053	705	298	109
0.005	2 378	3 327	7 374	33 704	42 024	11 540	3 400	1 740	1 107	791	607	406	215	145	63	24
0.01	1 188	1 664	3 693	16 911	21 146	5 814	1 717	880	561	402	308	207	211	75	33	14
0.05	236	333	750	3 482	4 455	1 237	371	193	125	91	70	48	27	19	10	5
0.10	117	167	383	1 810	2 383	669	205	109	71	53	41	29	17	13	7	5
0.15	77	112	261	1 258	1 704	484	152	82	54	41	32	23	14	11	7	5
0.20	58	84	201	987	1 376	396	126	69	47	35	28	21	13	10	7	5
0.25	46	68	166	829	1 190	346	112	62	43	33	27	20	13	10	7	5
0.30	38	57	143	729	1 076	316	105	59	41	32	26	20	13	11	7	6
0.35	33	50	127	662	1 006	299	101	58	40	31	26	20	14	11	8	7
0.40	29	45	116	618	966	290	99	58	41	32	27	21	15	12	9	7
0.45	26	41	108	590	949	288	100	59	42	33	28	22	16	13	10	8
0.50	24	38	103	574	951	292	103	61	44	35	30	24	17	15	11	10
0.55	22	36	100	571	973	301	108	65	47	38	32	26	19	16	13	11
0.60	21	34	99	579	1 016	318	116	70	52	42	36	29	22	19	15	13
0.65	20	34	101	601	1 085	343	127	78	58	47	40	33	25	22	18	16
0.70	20	34	105	640	1 190	380	143	89	66	54	47	38	29	26	21	19
0.75	20	35	112	705	1 350	435	166	104	78	64	56	46	36	32	26	23
0.80	21	38	126	812	1 601	520	201	127	96	80	70	58	45	40	34	30
0.85	23	44	152	1 002	2 034	667	261	167	127	106	93	77	61	55	46	42
0.90	29	58	205	1 395	2 916	965	383	246	189	158	139	117	94	84	71	65
0.95	48	100	371	2 598	5 592	1 868	750	487	376	316	279	236	190	171	147	134

[a] $\alpha = 0.05$ (two-tailed), $\beta = 0.20$ (power = 80%), control : case ratio = 2 : 1. The sample size listed is the number of subjects needed in the case group. Double this number would be included in the control group.

Table A15. Sample sizes for case–control studies[a]

Prevalence in control group	Odds ratio to be detected															
	0.2	0.3	0.5	0.75	1.25	1.5	2.0	2.5	3.0	3.5	4.0	5.0	7.5	10.0	20.0	50.0
0.00001	1 088 329	1 516 265	3 330 869	15 057 631	18 413 208	5 014 341	1 456 616	736 652	464 229	328 865	250 357	165 463	85 879	56 868	23 570	8 415
0.00005	217 664	303 253	666 182	3 011 608	3 682 831	1 002 930	291 347	147 345	92 856	65 782	50 079	33 098	17 180	11 377	4 717	1 685
0.0001	108 831	151 626	333 096	1 505 856	1 841 534	501 504	145 688	73 681	46 435	32 896	25 044	16 553	8 592	5 691	2 360	844
0.0005	21 764	30 325	66 628	301 253	368 496	100 363	29 161	14 751	9 298	6 588	5 016	3 316	1 723	1 141	474	171
0.001	10 881	15 162	33 319	150 678	134 367	50 220	14 595	7 384	4 655	3 299	2 513	1 662	864	573	239	87
0.005	2 174	3 032	6 672	30 218	37 064	10 107	2 943	1 491	942	668	510	338	177	118	50	19
0.01	1 086	1 516	3 342	15 161	18 652	5 093	1 486	755	478	340	259	173	91	61	27	11
0.05	215	303	678	3 120	3 932	1 085	323	167	107	77	60	41	23	16	8	4
0.10	107	152	345	1 620	2 105	588	179	94	62	45	35	25	15	11	6	4
0.15	70	101	235	1 125	1 507	426	132	71	47	35	28	20	12	9	6	4
0.20	52	76	181	882	1 218	349	111	60	41	31	25	18	11	9	6	4
0.25	42	62	149	741	1 053	305	99	55	37	29	23	17	11	9	6	5
0.30	35	52	128	650	954	280	92	52	36	28	23	17	12	9	7	5
0.35	30	45	114	590	892	265	89	51	36	28	23	18	12	10	7	6
0.40	26	40	104	550	857	257	88	51	36	28	24	18	13	11	8	7
0.45	23	36	97	525	843	256	89	52	37	30	25	19	14	12	9	7
0.50	21	34	92	511	846	259	92	55	39	32	27	21	15	13	10	9
0.55	19	32	89	507	866	268	97	58	42	34	29	23	17	15	12	10
0.60	18	30	88	514	905	283	104	63	46	38	32	26	19	17	13	12
0.65	18	30	89	533	967	306	114	70	52	42	36	30	23	20	16	14
0.70	17	30	92	567	1 061	339	128	80	60	49	42	35	27	23	19	17
0.75	18	31	99	624	1 204	389	149	93	70	58	51	42	32	29	24	21
0.80	18	33	111	718	1 429	466	181	115	87	72	63	52	41	37	31	28
0.85	20	38	132	884	1 817	598	235	151	115	96	84	70	56	50	42	38
0.90	25	50	179	1 230	2 607	867	345	223	172	144	127	107	85	77	65	59
0.95	41	85	323	2 288	5 002	1 678	678	442	342	288	255	215	174	157	134	123

[a] $\alpha = 0.05$ (two-tailed), $\beta = 0.20$ (power = 80%), control : case ratio = 3 : 1. The sample size listed is the number of subjects needed in the case group. Triple this number would be included in the control group.

Table A16. Sample sizes for case–control studies[a]

Prevalence in control group	Odds ratio to be detected															
	0.2	0.3	0.5	0.75	1.25	1.5	2.0	2.5	3.0	3.5	4.0	5.0	7.5	10.0	20.0	50.0
0.00001	1 034 611	1 440 327	3 154 151	14 188 340	17 179 015	4 657 221	1 342 151	674 222	422 474	297 830	225 778	148 193	76 026	49 982	20 443	7 227
0.00005	206 920	288 065	630 838	2 837 745	3 435 981	931 503	268 452	134 858	84 505	59 574	45 162	29 644	15 209	9 999	4 091	1 447
0.0001	103 459	144 032	315 424	1 418 920	1 718 102	465 788	134 240	67 438	42 259	29 792	22 585	14 825	7 607	5 002	2 047	725
0.0005	20 690	28 806	63 092	283 861	343 799	93 216	26 870	13 501	8 462	5 966	4 524	2 970	1 525	1 003	412	147
0.001	10 344	14 403	31 551	141 978	172 011	46 645	13 449	6 759	4 237	2 988	2 266	1 489	765	504	207	75
0.005	2 067	2 880	6 318	28 473	34 581	9 388	2 712	1 366	858	606	460	303	157	104	44	17
0.01	1 032	1 440	3 164	14 285	17 404	4 731	1 370	691	435	308	234	155	81	54	23	10
0.05	205	288	641	2 938	3 670	1 009	298	153	98	70	54	37	20	14	7	4
0.10	101	144	327	1 525	1 966	547	166	87	57	41	32	23	13	10	5	3
0.15	67	96	222	1 059	1 408	397	123	66	43	32	26	18	11	8	5	4
0.20	50	72	171	830	1 138	325	103	56	38	28	23	17	10	8	6	4
0.25	39	58	140	696	985	285	92	51	35	26	21	16	10	8	6	5
0.30	33	49	121	611	892	261	86	48	33	26	21	16	11	9	6	5
0.35	28	42	107	554	836	248	83	47	33	26	21	16	11	9	7	5
0.40	24	38	97	517	803	241	82	48	34	26	21	17	12	10	7	6
0.45	22	34	91	492	790	240	83	49	35	28	23	18	13	11	8	7
0.50	20	32	86	479	793	243	86	51	37	30	25	20	14	12	9	8
0.55	18	30	83	475	812	252	91	55	40	32	27	22	16	14	11	9
0.60	17	28	82	481	849	266	97	59	44	35	30	24	18	16	13	11
0.65	16	28	83	498	908	288	107	66	49	40	34	28	21	18	15	13
0.70	16	28	86	530	997	319	121	75	56	46	40	33	25	22	18	16
0.75	16	29	92	583	1 131	366	140	88	67	55	48	39	31	27	22	20
0.80	17	31	103	670	1 343	439	171	108	82	68	60	50	39	35	29	26
0.85	18	35	123	826	1 708	564	222	143	109	91	80	67	53	47	40	36
0.90	23	45	166	1 148	2 452	817	327	211	163	137	120	101	81	73	62	56
0.95	37	78	298	2 133	4 707	1 583	641	419	325	273	242	205	165	149	127	116

[a] $\alpha = 0.05$ (two-tailed), $\beta = 0.20$ (power = 80%), control : case ratio = 4 : 1. The sample size listed is the number of subjects needed in the case group. Quadruple this number would be included in the control group.

Table A17. Tabular values of 95% confidence limit factors for estimates of a Poisson-distributed variable

Observed number on which estimate is based (n)	Lower limit factor (L)	Upper limit factor (U)	Observed number on which estimate is based (n)	Lower limit factor (L)	Upper limit factor (U)	Observed number on which estimate is based (n)	Lower limit factor (L)	Upper limit factor (U)
1	0.0253	5.57	21	0.619	1.53	120	0.833	1.200
2	0.121	3.61	22	0.627	1.51	140	0.844	1.184
3	0.206	2.92	23	0.634	1.50	160	0.854	1.171
4	0.272	2.56	24	0.641	1.49	180	0.862	1.160
5	0.324	2.33	25	0.647	1.48	200	0.868	1.151
6	0.367	2.18	26	0.653	1.47	250	0.882	1.134
7	0.401	2.06	27	0.659	1.46	300	0.892	1.121
8	0.431	1.97	28	0.665	1.45	350	0.899	1.112
9	0.458	1.90	29	0.670	1.44	400	0.906	1.104
10	0.480	1.84	30	0.675	1.43	450	0.911	1.098
11	0.499	1.79	35	0.697	1.39	500	0.915	1.093
12	0.517	1.75	40	0.714	1.36	600	0.922	1.084
13	0.532	1.71	45	0.729	1.34	700	0.928	1.078
14	0.546	1.68	50	0.742	1.32	800	0.932	1.072
15	0.560	1.65	60	0.770	1.30	900	0.936	1.068
16	0.572	1.62	70	0.785	1.27	1000	0.939	1.064
17	0.583	1.60	80	0.798	1.25			
18	0.593	1.58	90	0.809	1.24			
19	0.602	1.56	100	0.818	1.22			
20	0.611	1.54						

Appendix B

Glossary

The *accuracy* of a measurement is the degree to which the measurement approximates the truth.

Ad hoc studies are studies that require primary data collection.

An *adverse drug event* or *adverse drug experience* is an untoward outcome that occurs during or following clinical use of a drug, whether preventable or not.

An *adverse drug reaction* is an adverse drug event that is judged to be caused by the drug.

Studies of *adverse effects* examine case reports of adverse drug reactions, attempting to judge subjectively whether the adverse events were indeed caused by the antecedent drug exposure.

Studies of *adverse events* explore any medical events experienced by patients and use epidemiologic methods to investigate whether any given event occurs more often in those who receive a drug than in those who do not receive the drug.

An *adverse experience* is any adverse event associated with the use of a drug or biological product in humans, whether or not considered product related.

Agreement is the degree to which different methods or sources of information give the same answers. Agreement between two sources or methods does not imply that either is valid or reliable.

Analyses of secular trends examine trends in disease events over time and/or across different geographic locations, and correlate them with trends in putative exposures, such as rates of drug utilization. The unit of observation is usually a subgroup of a population, rather than individuals. Also called ecological studies.

Analytic studies are studies with control groups, typically case–control studies, cohort studies, and randomized clinical trials.

Anticipated beneficial effects of drugs are desirable effects that are presumed to be caused by the drug. They represent the reason for prescribing or ingesting the drug.

Anticipated harmful effects of drugs are unwanted effects that could have been predicted on the basis of existing knowledge.

An *association* is when two events occur together more often than one would expect by chance.

Autocorrelation is where any individual observation is to some extent a function of the previous observation.

Bias is a systematic manner in which the two study groups have been treated differently. The presence of a bias causes a study to yield incorrect results.

Biological inference is the process of generalizing from a statement about an association seen in a population to a causal statement about biological theory.

Case–cohort studies are studies that compare cases with a disease to a sample of predetermined size of subjects randomly selected from the parent cohort, analyzing the study as a cohort study.

Pharmacoepidemiology, Fourth Edition   Edited by B.L. Strom
© 2005 John Wiley & Sons, Ltd

Case–control studies are studies that compare cases with a disease to controls without the disease, looking for differences in antecedent exposures.

Case-crossover studies are studies that compare cases with a disease to a different time period in the same individuals, looking for differences in antecedent exposures.

Case reports are reports of the experience of single patients. As used in pharmacoepidemiology, a case report describes a single patient who was exposed to a drug and experiences a particular outcome, usually an adverse event.

Case series are reports of collections of patients, all of whom have a common exposure, examining what their clinical outcomes were. Alternatively, case series can be reports of patients who have a common disease, examining what their antecedent exposures were. No control group is present.

An exposure *causes* a health event when it truly increases the probability of that event.

Changeability is the ability of an instrument to measure a difference in score in patients who have improved or deteriorated.

Channeling bias is a type of selection bias, which occurs when a drug is claimed to be safe and therefore is used in high-risk patients who did not tolerate other drugs for that indication.

Drug *clearance* is the proportion of the "apparent" volume of distribution that is cleared of drug over a specified time. The total body clearance is the sum of clearances by different routes, e.g., renal, hepatic, pulmonary, etc.

Clinical pharmacology is the study of the effects of drugs in humans.

Cohort studies are studies that identify defined populations and follow them forward in time, examining their rates of disease. Cohort studies generally identify and compare exposed patients to unexposed patients or to patients who receive a different exposure.

Confidence interval is a range of values within which the true population value probably lies.

Confidentiality is the right of patients to limit the transfer and disclosure of private information.

A *confounding variable*, or *confounder*, is a variable other than the risk factor and outcome variable under study that is related independently both to the risk factor and to the outcome. A confounder can create the appearance of an association between the risk factor and the outcome or mask a real one.

Confounding by indication can occur when the underlying diagnosis or other clinical features that trigger use of a certain drug also are related to patient outcome.

Construct validity refers to the extent to which results from a given instrument are consistent with those from other measures in a manner consistent with theoretical hypotheses.

A *cost* is the consumption of a resource that could otherwise be used for another purpose.

Cost–benefit analysis of medical care compares the cost of a medical intervention to its benefit. Both costs and benefits must be measured in the same monetary units (e.g., dollars).

Cost-effectiveness analysis of medical care compares the cost of a medical intervention to its effectiveness. Costs are determined in monetary units, while effectiveness is determined independently and may be measured in terms of any clinically meaningful unit. Cost-effectiveness analyses usually examine the additional cost per unit of additional effectiveness between two or more interventions.

Cost-identification analysis enumerates the costs involved in medical care, ignoring the outcomes that result from that care.

Criterion validity refers to the ability of an instrument to measure what it is supposed to measure, as judged by agreement with a gold standard.

Cross-sectional studies examine exposures and outcomes in populations at one point in time; they have no time sense.

Descriptive studies are studies that do not have control groups, namely case reports, case series, and analyses of secular trends. They contrast with analytic studies.

Detection bias is an error in the results of a study due to a systematic difference between the study groups in the procedures used for ascertainment, diagnosis, or verification of disease.

Differential misclassification occurs when the misclassification of one variable (e.g., drug usage) varies according to the level of another variable (e.g., disease status).

The *direct medical costs* of medical care are the costs that are incurred in providing the care.

Direct nonmedical costs are nonmedical care costs incurred because of an illness or the need to seek medical care. They can include the cost of transportation to the hospital or physician's office, the cost of special clothing needed because of the illness, and the cost of hotel stays and special housing (e.g., modification of the home to accommodate the ill individual).

Discriminative instruments are those that measure differences among people at a single point in time.

A *drug* is any exogenously administered substance that exerts a physiologic effect.

Drug utilization, as defined by the World Health Organization (WHO), is the "marketing, distribution, prescription and use of drugs in a society, with special emphasis on the resulting medical, social, and economic consequences."

Drug utilization evaluation (DUE) programs are ongoing structured systems designed to improve drug use by intervening when inappropriate drug use is detected. See also *drug utilization review programs*.

Drug utilization evaluation studies are *ad hoc* investigations that assess the appropriateness of drug use. They are designed to detect and quantify the frequency of drug use problems.

Drug utilization review programs are ongoing structured systems designed to improve drug use by intervening when inappropriate drug use is detected.

Drug utilization review studies are *ad hoc* investigations that assess the appropriateness of drug use. They are designed to detect and quantify any drug use problems. See also *drug utilization evaluation programs*.

Drug utilization studies are descriptive studies that quantify the use of a drug. Their objective is to quantify the present state, the developmental trends, and the time course of drug usage at various levels of the health care system, whether national, regional, local, or institutional.

Ecological studies examine trends in disease events over time or across different geographic locations and correlate them with trends in putative exposures, such as rates of drug utilization. The unit of observation is a subgroup of a population, rather than individuals. See also *analyses of secular trends*.

Effect modification occurs when the magnitude of effect of a drug in causing an outcome differs according to the levels of a variable other than the drug or the outcome (e.g., sex, age group). See *interaction*.

A study of drug *effectiveness* is a study of whether, in the usual clinical setting, a drug in fact achieves the effect intended when prescribing it.

A study of drug *efficacy* is a study of whether, *under ideal conditions*, a drug has the ability to bring about the effect intended when prescribing it.

A study of drug *efficiency* is a study of whether a drug can bring about its desired effect at an acceptable cost.

Epidemiology is the study of the distribution and determinants of diseases in populations.

Evaluative instruments are those designed to measure changes within individuals over time.

Experimental studies are studies in which the investigator controls the therapy that is to be received by each participant, generally using that control to randomly allocate patients among the study groups.

Face validity is a judgment about the validity of an instrument, based on an intuitive assessment of the extent to which an instrument meets a number of criteria, including applicability, clarity and simplicity, likelihood of bias, comprehensiveness, and whether redundant items have been included.

Fixed costs are costs that are incurred regardless of the volume of activity.

Generic quality of life instruments aim to cover the complete spectrum of function, disability, and distress of the patient, and are applicable to a variety of populations.

Half-life ($T_{1/2}$) is the time taken for the drug concentration to decline by half. $T_{1/2}$ is a function of both the volume of distribution and clearance of the drug.

Health profiles are single instruments that measure multiple different aspects of quality of life.

Health-related quality of life is a multifactorial concept which, from the patient's perspective, represents the end result of all the physiological, psychological, and social influences of the disease and the therapeutic process. Health-related quality of life may be considered on different levels: overall assessment of well-being; several broad domains—physiological, functional, psychological, social, and economic status; and subcomponents of each domain—for example, pain, sleep, activities of daily living, and sexual function within physical and functional domains.

A *human research subject*, as defined in US regulation, is "a living individual, about whom an investigator (whether professional or student) conducting research obtains either: 1) data through intervention or interaction with the individual, or 2) identifiable private information." [Title 45 US Code of Federal Regulations Part 46.102 (f)].

Hypothesis-generating studies are studies that give rise to new questions about drug effects to be explored further in subsequent analytical studies.

Hypothesis-strengthening studies are studies that reinforce, although do not provide definitive evidence for, existing hypotheses.

Hypothesis-testing studies are studies that evaluate in detail hypotheses raised elsewhere.

Incidence/prevalence bias, a type of selection bias, may occur in studies when prevalent cases rather than new cases of a condition are selected for a study. A strong association with prevalence may be related to the duration of the disease rather than to its incidence, because prevalence is proportional to both incidence and duration of the disease.

The *incidence rate* of a disease is a measure of how frequently the disease occurs. Specifically, it is the number of new cases of the disease which develop over a defined time period in a defined population at risk, divided by the number of people in that population at risk.

Indirect costs are costs that do not stem directly from transactions for goods or services, but represent the loss of opportunities to use a valuable resource in alternative ways. They include the cost of morbidity (e.g., time lost from work) or mortality (e.g., premature death leading to removal from the work force).

Information bias is an error in the results of a study due to a systematic difference between the study groups in the accuracy of the measurements being made of their exposure or outcome.

Intangible costs are those of pain, suffering, and grief.

Interaction, see *effect modification*.

Interrupted time-series designs include multiple observations (often 10 or more) of study populations before and after an intervention.

Medication errors are defined as any mistake in the medication use process, including prescribing, transcribing, dispensing, administering, and monitoring

Meta-analysis is the formal statistical analysis of a collection of analytic results for the purpose of integrating the findings. Meta-analysis is used to identify sources of variation among study findings and, when appropriate, to provide an overall measure of effect as a summary of those findings.

Misclassification bias is the error resulting from classifying study subjects as exposed when they truly are unexposed, or vice versa. Alternatively, misclassification bias can result

from classifying study subjects as diseased when they truly are not diseased, or vice versa.

Molecular pharmacoepidemiology is the study of the manner in which molecular biomarkers alter the clinical effects of medications.

An *N-of-1 RCT* is a randomized controlled trial within an individual patient, using repeated assignments to the experimental or control arms.

Near misses are medication errors that have high potential for causing harm but did not, either because they were intercepted prior to reaching a patient or because the error reached the patient who fortuitously did not have any observable untoward sequelae.

Nondifferential misclassification occurs when the misclassification of one variable does not vary by the level of another variable. Nondifferential misclassification usually results in bias toward the null.

Nonexperimental studies are studies in which the investigator does not control the therapy, but observes and evaluates the results of ongoing medical care. These are the study designs that do not involve random allocation, namely case reports, case series, analyses of secular trends, case–control studies, and cohort studies.

Observational studies are studies in which the investigator does not control the therapy, but observes and evaluates the results of ongoing medical care. These are the study designs that do not involve randomization, namely case reports, case series, analyses of secular trends, case–control studies, and cohort studies.

The *odds ratio* is the odds of exposure in the diseased group divided by the odds of exposure in the nondiseased group. It provides an estimate of the relative risk when the disease under study is relatively rare.

One-group, post-only study design consists of making only one observation on a single group which has already been exposed to a treatment.

An *opportunity cost* is the value of a resource's next best use, a use that is no longer possible once the resource has been used.

A *p-value* is the probability that a difference as large as or larger than the one observed in the study could have occurred purely by chance.

Pharmacodynamics is the study of the relationship between drug level and drug effect. It involves the study of the response of the target tissues in the body to a given concentration of drug.

Pharmacogenetic epidemiology is the study of the effects of genetic determinants of drug response on outcomes in large numbers of people.

Pharmacoepidemiology is the study of the use of and the effects of drugs in large numbers of people.

Pharmacogenetics is the study of genetic determinants of responses to drugs. Although it is sometimes used synonymously with pharmacogenomics, it often refers to a candidate-gene approach as opposed to a genome-wide approach.

Pharmacogenomics is the study of genetic determinants of responses to drugs. Although it is sometimes used synonymously with pharmacogenetics, it often refers to a genome-wide approach as opposed to a candidate-gene approach.

A *pharmacokinetic compartment* is a theoretical space into which drug molecules are said to distribute, and is represented by a given linear component of the log-concentration versus time curve. It is not an actual anatomic or physiologic space, but is sometimes thought of as a tissue or group of tissues that have similar blood flow and drug affinity.

Pharmacokinetics is the study of the relationship between the dose of a drug administered and the serum or blood level achieved. It includes the study of the processes of drug absorption, distribution, metabolism, and excretion.

Pharmacology is the study of the effects of drugs in a living system.

Pharmacotherapeutics is the application of the principles of clinical pharmacology to rational prescribing, the conduct of clinical trials, and the assessment of outcomes during real-life clinical practice.

Pharmionics is the study of how patients use or misuse prescription drugs in ambulatory care.

Postmarketing surveillance is the study of drug use and drug effects after release onto the market. This term is sometimes used synonymously with "pharmacoepidemiology," but the latter can be relevant to premarketing studies, as well. Conversely, the term "postmarketing surveillance" is sometimes felt to apply to only those studies conducted after drug marketing that systematically screen for adverse drug effects. However, this is a more restricted use of the term than that used in this book.

Potency refers to the amount of drug that is required to elicit a given response.

Potential adverse drug events are medication errors that have high potential for causing harm but did not, either because they were intercepted prior to reaching a patient or because the error reached the patient who fortuitously did not have any observable untoward sequelae.

The *power* of a study is the probability of detecting a difference in the study if a difference really exists (either between study groups or between treatment periods).

Precision is the degree of absence of random error. Precise estimates have narrow confidence intervals.

Pre–post with comparison group design includes a single observation both before and after treatment in a nonrandomly selected group exposed to a treatment (e.g., physicians receiving feedback on specific prescribing practices), as well as simultaneous before and after observations of a similar (comparison) group not receiving treatment.

Prescribing errors refer to issues related to underuse, overuse, and misuse of prescribed drugs, all of which contribute to the suboptimal utilization of pharmaceutical therapies.

The *prevalence* of a disease is a measurement of how common the disease is. Specifically, it is the number of existing cases of the disease in a defined population at a given point in time or over a defined time period, divided by the number of people in that population.

Prevalence study bias, a type of selection bias that may occur in studies when prevalent cases rather than new cases of a condition are selected for a study. A strong association with prevalence may be related to the duration of the disease rather than to its incidence, because prevalence is proportional to both incidence and duration of the disease.

Privacy, in the setting of research, refers to each individual's right to be free from unwanted inspection of, or access to, personal information by unauthorized persons.

Propensity scores are an approach to controlling for confounding that uses mathematical modeling to predict *exposure*, rather than the traditional approach of predicting *outcome*.

Prospective drug utilization review is designed to detect drug–therapy problems before an individual patient receives the drug.

Prospective studies are studies performed simultaneously with the events under study; namely, patient outcomes have not yet occurred as of the outset of the study.

Protopathic bias is interpreting a factor to be a result of an exposure when it is in fact a determinant of the exposure.

Publication bias occurs when publication of a study's results is related to the study's findings.

Qualitative drug utilization studies are studies that assess the *appropriateness* of drug use.

Quality of life is the description of aspects (domains) of physical, social, and emotional health that are relevant and important to the patient.

Quantitative drug utilization studies are descriptive studies of *frequency* of drug use.

Random allocation is the assignment of subjects who are enrolled in a study into study groups in a manner determined by chance.

Random error is error due to chance.

Random selection is the selection of subjects into a study from among those eligible in a manner determined by chance.

Randomized clinical trials are studies in which the investigator randomly assigns patients to different therapies, one of which may be a control therapy.

Recall bias is an error in the results of a study due to a systematic difference between the study groups in the accuracy or completeness of their memory of their past exposures or health events.

Referral bias is error in the results of a study that occurs when the reasons for referring a patient for medical care are related to the exposure status, e.g., when the use of the drug contributes to the diagnostic process.

Regression to the mean is the tendency for observations on populations selected on the basis of an abnormality to approach normality on subsequent observations.

The *relative risk* is the ratio of the incidence rate of an outcome in the exposed group to the incidence rate of the outcome in the unexposed group.

Reliability is the degree to which the results obtained by a measurement procedure can be replicated. The measurement of reliability does not require a gold standard, since it assesses only the concordance between two or more measures.

A *reporting rate* in a spontaneous reporting system is the number of reported cases of an adverse event of interest divided by some measure of the suspect drug's utilization, usually the number of dispensed prescriptions. This is perhaps better referred to as a *rate of reported cases*.

Reproducibility is the ability of an instrument to obtain more or less the same scores upon repeated measurements of patients who have not changed.

Research, as defined in US regulation, is any activity designed to "develop or contribute to generalizable knowledge" [Title 45 US Code of Federal Regulations Part 46.102 (d)].

Responsiveness is an instrument's ability to detect change.

Retrospective drug utilization review compares past drug use against predetermined criteria to identify aberrant prescribing patterns or patient-specific deviations from explicit criteria.

Retrospective studies are studies conducted after the events under study have occurred. Both exposure and outcome have already occurred as of the outset of the study.

Risk is the probability that something will happen.

A judgment about *safety* is a personal and/or social judgment about the degree to which a given risk is acceptable.

Sample distortion bias is another name for selection bias.

Scientific inference is the process of generalizing from a statement about a population, which is an association, to a causal statement about scientific theory.

Selection bias is error in a study that is due to systematic differences in characteristics between those who are selected for the study and those who are not.

Sensibility is a judgment about the validity of an instrument, based on an intuitive assessment of the extent to which an instrument meets a number of criteria, including applicability, clarity and simplicity, likelihood of bias, comprehensiveness, and whether redundant items have been included.

Sensitivity is the proportion of persons who truly have a characteristic, who are correctly classified by a diagnostic test as having it.

Sensitivity analysis is a set of procedures in which the results of a study are recalculated using alternate values for some of the study's variables, in order to test the sensitivity of the conclusions to altered specifications.

A *serious adverse experience* is any adverse experience occurring at any dose that results in any of the following outcomes: death, a life-threatening adverse experience, inpatient hospitalization or prolongation of existing hospitalization, a persistent or significant disability/incapacity, or congenital anomaly/birth defect.

Specific quality of life instruments are focused on disease or treatment issues specifically relevant to the question at hand.

Specificity is the proportion of persons who truly do *not* have a characteristic, who are correctly classified by a diagnostic test as not having it.

Spontaneous reporting systems are maintained by regulatory bodies throughout the world and collect unsolicited clinical observations that originate outside of a formal study.

Statistical inference is the process of generalizing from a sample of study subjects to the entire population from which those subjects are theoretically drawn.

Statistical interaction, see *effect modification*.

A *statistically significant difference* is a difference between two study groups that is unlikely to have occurred purely by chance.

Steady state, within pharmacokinetics, is the situation when the amount of drug being administered equals the amount of drug being eliminated from the body.

Systematic error is error introduced into a study by its design, rather than due to random variation.

The *therapeutic ratio* is the ratio of the drug concentration that produces toxicity to the concentration that produces the desired therapeutic effect.

Therapeutics is the application of the principles of clinical pharmacology to rational prescribing, the conduct of clinical trials, and the assessment of outcomes during real-life clinical practice.

Type A adverse reactions are those that are the result of an exaggerated but otherwise predictable pharmacological effect of the drug. They tend to be common, dose-related, and less serious than Type B reactions.

Type B adverse reactions are those that are aberrant effects of the drug. They tend to be uncommon, not dose-related, and unpredictable.

A *type I error* is concluding there is an association when in fact one does not exist, i.e., erroneously rejecting the null hypothesis.

A *type II error* is concluding there is no association when in fact one does exist, i.e., erroneously accepting the null hypothesis.

Unanticipated beneficial effects of drugs are desirable effects that could not have been predicted on the basis of existing knowledge.

Unanticipated harmful effects of drugs are unwanted effects that could not have been predicted on the basis of existing knowledge.

Uncontrolled studies refer to studies without a comparison group.

An *unexpected adverse experience* means any adverse experience that is not listed in the current labeling for the product. This includes an event that may be symptomatically and pathophysiologically related to an event listed in the labeling, but differs from the event because of greater severity or specificity.

Utility measures of quality of life are measured holistically as a single number along a continuum, e.g., from death (0.0) to full health (1.0). The key element of a utility instrument is that it is preference-based.

Validity is the degree to which an assessment (e.g., questionnaire or other instrument) measures what it purports to measure.

Variable costs are costs that increase with increasing volume of activity.

Apparent *volume of distribution* (V_D) is the "apparent" volume that a drug is distributed in after complete absorption. It is usually calculated from the theoretical plasma concentration at a time when all of the drug was assumed to be present in the body and uniformly distributed. This is calculated from back extrapolation to time zero of the plasma concentration time curve after intravenous administration.

Voluntariness is the concept in research ethics, that investigators must tell subjects that participation in the research study is voluntary, and that subjects have the right to discontinue participation at any time.

Index